EVERYTHING YOU NEED TO KNOW BEFORE YOU CALL THE DOCTOR

A Straightforward and Sensible Home Medical Reference for Men, Women, Children and Seniors

By 60 Doctors from All Fields of Medicine
and Verena Corazza, Renata Daimler,
Andrea Ernst, Krista Federspiel, Ph.D.,
Vera Herbst, Kurt Langbein,
Hans-Peter Martin, J.D. and Han Weis, Ph.D.

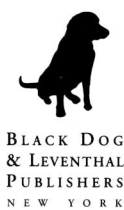

BLACK DOG
& LEVENTHAL
PUBLISHERS
NEW YORK

Published by
Black Dog & Leventhal Publishers, Inc.
151 West 19th Street
New York, NY 10011

Distributed by
Workman Publishing Company
708 Broadway
New York, NY 10003

ISBN: 1-57912-082-2
Manufactured in Spain

h g f e d c b a

Designed by Tony Meisel

Library of Congress Cataloging-in-Publication Data

    [Kursbuch Gesundheit. English]
Everything you need to know before you call the doctor / [edited by]
Hans-Peter Martin ... [et al.].
        p. cm.
Originally published as: Kursbuch Gesundheit / hrsg. Verena Corazza.
Kèoln : Kiepenheuer & Witsch, 1992.
Includes index.
    ISBN 1-57912-082-2
    1. Medicine, Popular. I. Martin, Hans-Peter, M.D. II. Corazza, Verena.
RC81.K9713 2000
610—dc21
                        00-022018

Professional Consultation, First Edition

Dr. Michael Adam, Gynecologist, Vienna

Dr. Rieke Alten, Rheumatologist, Schloßpark-Klinik, Berlin

Dr. Klaus Baum, Biology, Physiology, Physiologisches Institut der Sporthochschule, Cologne

Professor Dr. Heinz Carl Bettelheim, Ophthalmologist, Universitätsklinik, Vienna

Assistant Professor Dr. Wolfgang Bigenzahn, Ear, Nose & Throat, Universitätsklinik, Vienna

Dr. Hans Peter Bilek, Cancer Psychotherapist, Vienna

Assistant Professor Dr. Christian Dittrich, Internist, Universitätsklinik, Vienna

Dr. Ulrike Fenesz, Gynecologist, Vienna

Dr. Bernhard Frischhut, Orthopedist, Universitätsklinik, Innsbruck

Dr. Gerd Glaeske, Pharmacist, Division Head of Medical Research Fundamental Questions, Barmer Ersatzkasse, Wuppertal

Dr. Karl-Johann Hartig, Chemist, Vienna

Helmut Hirsch, Physicist, Group Ecologist, Vienna

Dr. Judith Hutterer, Dermatologist, Vienna

Assistant Professor Dr. Jochen Jordan, Psychosomatics, Universitätsklinik, Frankfurt/M.

Assistant Professor Dr. Gert Judmeier, Gastroenterologist, Universitätsklinik, Innsbruck

Dr. Wolfgang Kirchhoff, Dentist, Marburg

Frank Kuebarth, Chemist, Cologne

Dr. Ingeborg Lackinger Karger, Gynecologist, Psychotherapist, Düsseldorf

Professor Dr. Claus Leitzmann, Nutrition Researcher, Universitätsklinik, Gießen

Professor Dr. Heinz Ludwig, Internist, Wilhelminenspital, Vienna

Dr. Klaus Malek, Attorney, Freiburg i. Br.

Dr. Thomas Meisl, Nephrologist, Wilhelminenspital, Vienna

Dr. Ingrid Mühlhauser, Internist, Diabetologist, Universitätsklinik, Düsseldorf

Professor Dr. J. R. Möse, Hygienics, Universität Graz

Dr. Christine Remien, Physician, Munich

Professor Dr. Jörg Remien, Pharmacologist, Universitätsklinik, Munich

Dr. Georg Röggla, Internist, Krankenhaus Neunkirchen

Dr. Wolfgang Scheibelhofer, Internist, Cardiologist, Vienna

Marietta Schirpf, Masseuse, Advisor, Vienna

Assistant Dr. Paul Schramek, Urologist, Allgemeine Poliklinik, Vienna

Dr. Ilse Sokal, Psychotherapist, Vienna

Dr. Susanna Stadler, General Practitioner, Vienna

Dr. Kirsten Stollhoff, Pediatrician, Hamburg

Dr. Ines Stuchly, Specialist for Physical Therapy, Vienna

Professor Dr. Reinhard Ziegler, Endocrinologist, Universitätsklinik, Heidelberg

Contributors, First Edition

Katja Austerlitz, Vienna

Erica Fischer, Berlin

Martin Margulies, Vienna

Additional Professional Consultation, Revised Edition

Dr. Petra Ball, Nutrition Researcher, Frankfurt

Professor Dr. Michael Berger, Internist, Universitätsklinik, Düsseldorf

Bettina Flörchinger, Gynecologist, Düsseldorf

Professor Dr. Stefan Görres, Nursing Researcher and Gerontologist, Univeristät, Bremen

Professor Dr. Peter Kroling, Specialist for Physical Medicine, Ludwig Maximilians Universität, Munich

Dr. Bernd Laufs, Psychiatrist and Psychotherapist, Städtische Krankenanstalten Idar-Oberstein

Christa Merfert-Diete, Social Worker, Deutsche Hauptstelle gegen die Suchtgefahren, Hamm

Dr. Godske Nielsen, Hygenics, Virologist, Hamburg

Dr. Klaus Rhomberg, Environmental Medicine, Universität Innsbruck

Dr. Beatrix Tappeser, Öko-Institut, Freiburg

Dr. Karin Weigang-Köhler, Internist, Oncologist, Universitätsklinik, Nuremberg

Additional Contributors, Revised Edition

Dr. Peter Felch, Vienna

Heiner Friesacher, Bremen

Sabine Keller, Cologne

Elfriede Rometsch, Vienna

Friedhelm Scheffel, Bremen

Rosa Scheuringer, Vienna

Charlotte Uzarewicz, Bremen

Sina Vogt, Cologne

Joachim Voß, Bremen

Editorial Staff

Erika Stemann, Cologne

Nikolaus Wolter, Cologne

HOW TO USE THIS BOOK

Identifying Your Symptoms

Let's say you are experiencing pains in the abdomen. In the blue section, "Signs and Symptoms," find the listing for "Abdominal Pain." The blue section lists, in alphabetical order, the most commonly reported medical complaints.

Locate your symptoms in the left-hand column; keep looking until you locate the description that most closely matches what you are experiencing. In the middle column, you'll find the disorder(s) your complaints may indicate.

The right-hand column will tell you what actions to take: Can you take care of this condition yourself, and if so, how? Should you see a doctor, and if so, how urgently? This section will also direct you to in-depth information on this disorder elsewhere in the book.

Becoming an Informed Patient

Based on your symptoms, let's say you have reason to believe you're suffering from gastritis. Look up gastritis, either under the "Digestive System" heading in the table of contents beginning on page *viii*, or in the index beginning on page 797.

In the red section, "Complaints," you'll find the possible causes of gastritis, and read about ways of preventing it if possible. You'll also find information on home treatment, and what to do when home treatment isn't enough and professional attention is required.

Next, the treatments usually prescribed for this illness are described, together with their advantages and disadvantages.

Asking the Right Questions

Your doctor has prescribed an endoscopy to determine whether there are any obvious organic causes for your abdominal symptoms.

Look up endoscopy, either under the "Diagnostic Tests/Procedures" heading in the table of contents beginning on p. *viii*, or in the index beginning on p. 797.

In the yellow "Examination and Treatment" section you'll discover what sorts of ailments endoscopy is routinely prescribed for, and what risks may be involved.

In addition, you'll find useful information about frequently prescribed complementary therapies such as homeopathy, acupuncture, psychotherapy and physiotherapy.

Practicing Prevention

You decide to improve your lifestyle to prevent future illness as much as possible. This may involve losing weight, quitting smoking, or ridding your living space of known toxins.

Look up nutrition, smoking, or hazardous substances under the headings "Body Weight," "Mood-Altering Substances and Recreational Drugs," or "Healthy Living" in the table of contents beginning on p. *viii*, or look up specific terms such as "weight," "nicotine" or "formaldehyde" in the index beginning on p. 797.

In the green "Self-Help" section you'll find in-depth, useful information on how lifestyle and behavior affect health, together with suggestions and recommendations on changes you can make in order to avoid risks to your health and well-being wherever possible.

Signs and Symptoms

Complaints and Symptoms
The left-hand column of this section lists various symptoms. Some may be listed as "possible" (or similarly qualified) symptoms of a particular condition; the corresponding potential causes and treatment recommendations only apply if all the symptoms listed occur simultaneously.

Possible Causes
The middle column lists the conditions or illnesses that can cause symptoms like those you are experiencing. Unless stated otherwise, only one of the listed causes should be at fault.

What To Do
The right-hand column lists recommendations for self-help.

If the only action suggested is further reading elsewhere in the book, professional help is not necessary at this time, and you'll find useful information on home treatment in the designated sections.

If you read "Call your doctor" or "Call your doctor immediately" or "Call emergency medical services immediately," your symptoms require medical attention, with varying degrees of urgency.

Complaints

Complaints
Typical symptoms are given for each disease listed.

Causes
The most frequent and principal causes of the disease are given.

Who's at Risk
This section will help you determine your risk of having the disease. It includes information (if available) on the frequency of the disease and known risk factors such as lifestyle, behavior, environmental hazards, or existing medical conditions.

Prevention
Preventive measures you can take yourself, if any, are listed here.

Possible After-effects and Complications
Possible complications of the disorder are described, including those that may arise if it is untreated or treated too late.

When to Seek Medical Advice
This section lists alarm signals to watch for, alerting you that medical attention is necessary.

Self-Help
The most appropriate home treatment methods (if any) are given.

Treatment
Commonly prescribed therapies and treatment modalities are briefly described and evaluated. When possible, recommendations are made as to advisable or inadvisable methods, taking into consideration the expected results and possible risks.

Examination and Treatment

In the "Examination and Treatment" section, commonly used diagnostic and treatment methods are described.

Assessments and recommendations are given based on expected results and possible risks, according to recognized medical opinion.

Self-Help

The information on home treatment and self-help in this section has been selected to offer a range of appropriate methods of prevention and treatment for as large a population as possible.

Assessments and recommendations are given based on expected results and possible risks, according to recognized medical opinion.

CONTENTS

SIGNS AND SYMPTOMS

COMPLAINTS

Signs and Symptoms

ABDOMINAL DISORDERS

ABDOMINAL PAIN

The abdomen is also called the "belly." We cannot always pinpoint the pain, so we usually say we have a "stomach ache," meaning pain in that area. A subsection called "Stomach Ache" follows this section. Abdominal pain is usually not serious, and does not require any special treatment. In some cases, however, it is a sign of illness.

COMPLAINTS AND SYMPTOMS	POSSIBLE CAUSES	WHAT TO DO
Abdominal pain soon after overeating rich foods	Overloaded stomach • Indigestion	Loosen tight clothes and lie down for a short time. A gentle belly massage might help.
Abdominal pain and nervous tension caused by stressful activities, such as school exams or having to make important decisions • **Diarrhea**	Anxiety • Emotional stress • Nervousness	Try to avoid stressful situations; learn some relaxation techniques. If you suffer from frequent abdominal pain, **call your doctor.** → Health and Well-being, p. 182 → Irritable Bowel Syndrome, p. 403 → Nervous Stomach, p. 386 → Relaxation, p. 693
Menstrual cramps	Menstruation	If you have frequent severe pains during menstruation, **call your doctor.** → Menstrual Disorders, p. 103, 508
Abdominal pain and unexplained weight loss • **Worms in stool**	Worms	**Call your doctor.** → Worms (Parasites), p. 415
Abdominal cramps • **Anxiety** • **Belching** • **Feeling of fullness** • **Gas, bloating** • **Heartburn** • **Overburdened**	Emotional problems • Gastritis	If symptoms recur even after repeated attempts at relaxation, **call your doctor.** → Acute Gastritis, p. 387 → Health and Well-being, p. 182 → Nervous Stomach, p. 386 → Relaxation, p. 693
Abdominal pain with diarrhea	Gastrointestinal infection • Malfunction of the digestive process	Drink plenty of liquids; eat only crackers or nothing at all. If symptoms persist longer than two days, **call your doctor.** → Acute gastritis, p. 387 → Gastroenteritis, p. 599

COMPLAINTS AND SYMPTOMS	POSSIBLE CAUSES	WHAT TO DO
Abdominal pain with a hard, bloated belly • **Alternating diarrhea and constipation** • **Feeling of fullness** • **Frequent bowel movements** • **Gas, bloating**	Irritable bowel syndrome	If symptoms keep recurring, **call your doctor,** → Irritable Bowel Syndrome, p. 403

Abdominal pain after taking medicine
• **Intestinal cramps**
• **Stomach cramps**
	Side effect of medicines, especially
	• cholesterol-lowering medicines containing
	   cholestyramine
	   clofibrate
	   sitosterol
	• laxatives containing
	   alder buckthorn bark
	   bisacodyl
	   castor oil
	   phenolphthalein, rhubarb
	   senna
	   sodium picosulfate
	• potassium compounds
		Check the medicine label or insert for these substances. If your medicine is over-the-counter, *stop taking it*. If your medicine is by prescription, **call your doctor.**
		→ Medication Summary, p. 657

Abdominal cramps after taking medicines • **Blood in the urine**	Kidney stones, as a side effect of • ulcer medicines or antacids containing calcium • vitamin C overdose	Check the medicine label or insert for vitamin C and calcium. If you have this symptom, **call your doctor.** → Medication Summary, p. 657
Abdominal pain • **Alternating constipation and diarrhea** • **Blood in stool**	Diverticulitis • Intestinal cancer	**Call your doctor.** → Colon and Rectal Cancers, p. 414 → Diverticulitis, p. 409
Acute, recurring abdominal pains • **Bloody, mucous diarrhea** • **Fever** • **Weight loss**	Inflammatory bowel disease	**Call your doctor.** → Crohn's Disease, p. 412 → Ulcerative Colitis, p. 411
In women, pain in the lower abdomen • **Vaginal discharge with unpleasant odor**	Fever • Endometriosis • Inflamed fallopian tubes • Inflamed ovaries • Inflamed uterus	**Call your doctor.** → Endometriosis, p. 522 → Salpingitis, p. 525 → Uterine Inflammation, p. 520

COMPLAINTS AND SYMPTOMS	POSSIBLE CAUSES	WHAT TO DO
Abdominal pain spreading from the back to the groin • **Fever** • **Frequent urination** • **Pain while urinating**	Urinary tract infection	**Call your doctor.** ➡ Acute Pyelonephritis (Kidney Infection), p. 421 ➡ Cystitis (Bladder Infection), p. 418
Pain on the right side of the abdomen under the rib cage • **Diarrhea** • **Fever** • **Gas, bloating** • **Itching** • **Jaundice**	Hepatitis (liver infection)	**Call your doctor.** ➡ Hepatitis, p. 395
Pain in the upper abdomen, becoming stronger after eating, drinking alcohol, or lying down • **Greasy stools in large quantities**	Chronic pancreas infection	**Call your doctor.** ➡ Pancreatitis (Pancreas Inflammation), p. 400
Pain mainly in the right lower abdomen, made worse by walking, coughing, or sneezing • **Fever** • **Hard, tight abdomen** • **Nausea** • **Vomiting**	Appendicitis	If pain is severe, **call your doctor immediately.**
Sharp, piercing pain in the upper right abdomen • **Bitter-tasting vomit** • **Fever** • **Light-colored stool** • **Yellowed eyes**	Gallstones • Inflamed gallbladder	**Call your doctor immediately.** ➡ Gallstones, p. 398 ➡ Cholecystitis (Gallbladder Inflammation), p. 400
Cramps in the upper abdomen • **Extremely depressed, feeling of hopeless** • **Pain spreading throughout the abdomen and back** • **Rapid pulse** • **Vomiting of bitter stomach juices**	Acute pancreas infection	**Call emergency medical services immediately.** ➡ Pancreatitis (Pancreas Inflammation), p. 400
Severe abdominal pain with hard, tight abdomen • **Cold forehead and hands** • **Difficult breathing** • **Rapid pulse** • **Vomiting**	Peritonitis	**Call emergency medical services immediately.** ➡ Peritonitis (Inflammation of the Peritoneum), p. 409

COMPLAINTS AND SYMPTOMS	POSSIBLE CAUSES	WHAT TO DO
Abdominal pain with feelings of anxiety • **Pressure in the chest**	Heart attack (Myocardial Infarction)	**Call emergency medical services immediately.** → Heart Attack, p. 335
Sudden, strong abdominal cramping • **Abdominal swelling** • **Bitter vomiting, or vomiting of intestinal contents** • **Constipation**	Intestinal obstruction	**Call emergency medical services immediately.** → Intestinal Obstruction, Ileus, p. 407
Abdominal pain and bleeding between menstrual periods	Ectopic pregnancy • Miscarriage	**Call emergency medical services immediately.** → Ectopic Pregnancy, p. 526 → Miscarriage, p. 574

STOMACH ACHE

Pain in the stomach is nearly always caused by medicines, food, ulcers, or being forced to endure a disagreeable situation. In about half of all cases, no systemic cause for stomach ache can be found.

COMPLAINTS AND SYMPTOMS	POSSIBLE CAUSES	WHAT TO DO
Stomach pains after eating too quickly, eating overly rich foods, or drinking too much alcohol • **Vomiting**	Normal reaction of the stomach to stress • Inappropriate diet	Go without or take very little food for one day (clear soup, crackers). → Nutrition, p. 722
Stomach ache after excessive smoking or alcohol consumption	Irritation of the stomach lining	Stop smoking. Limit your alcohol intake. If symptoms persist after one week, **call your doctor.** → Acute Gastritis, p. 387 → Mood-altering Substances, Recreational Drugs, p. 754
Stomach pain • **Belching** • **Bloating** • **Coated tongue and bad breath** • **Feeling of fullness** • **Heartburn** • **Loss of appetite** • **Nausea and vomiting** • **Nervous stomach**	Gastritis • Emotional problems	When symptoms appear, try immediately to relax . This usually helps. If you often suffer from stomach aches, **call your doctor.** → Acute Gastritis, p. 387 → Health and Well-being, p. 182 → Nervous Stomach, p. 386 → Relaxation, p. 693

COMPLAINTS AND SYMPTOMS	POSSIBLE CAUSES	WHAT TO DO
Stomach pain **• Diarrhea** **• Fever** **• General weak feeling** **• Nausea or vomiting**	Stomach irritation, food poisoning from alcohol abuse poisonous mushrooms radiation sickness spoiled food viral infection	If you have eaten mushrooms, **call your doctor immediately.** If you have not eaten mushrooms, and if symptoms persist longer than two days, **call your doctor.** → Cancer, p. 470 → Poisoning, p. 708 → Stomach Irritation, p. 385
Stomach pains after exposure to hazardous materials	Toxic substances in the environment	If you often suffer from stomach aches, **call your doctor.** → Health in the Workplace, p. 789
Stomach pain after taking medicines **• Constipation** **• Diarrhea** **• Nausea** **• Vomiting**	Side effect of many medicines, especially analgesics antibiotics anti-inflammatory drugs (steroids) cardiovascular medicines cough and asthma medicines gastrointestinal medicines rheumatism medicines urinary tract disorders medicines	If your medicine is over-the-counter, and stomach ache was not mentioned as a temporary and harmless side effect, *stop taking it.* If your medicine is by prescription and you were not made aware of the possible side effects, **call your doctor**. → Medication Summary, p. 657
Stomach pain with pressure and feeling of fullness	Chronic gastritis	**Call your doctor.** → Chronic Gastritis, p. 389
Burning, cramp-like stomach pains with feeling of fullness immediately after eating **• Coated tongue and bad breath** **• Heartburn** **• Nausea or vomiting** **• Weight loss**	Gastritis • Stomach ulcer	**Call your doctor.** → Acute Gastritis, p. 387 → Stomach and Duodenal Ulcer, p. 389
Stomach pain with heartburn, made worse by lying down after eating	Excessive body weight • Hiatal hernia • Inflamed esophagus	**Call your doctor.** → Body weight, p. 727 → Esophagitis (Esophageal inflammation), p. 383 → Hernia, p. 439
Stomach pain localized between the navel and middle right ribs within two hours of eating **• Coated tongue** **• Heartburn** **• Loss of appetite** **• Vomiting and nausea** **• Weight loss**	Peptic (duodenal) ulcer	**Call your doctor.** → Stomach and Peptic Ulcer, p. 389

COMPLAINTS AND SYMPTOMS	POSSIBLE CAUSES	WHAT TO DO
Stomach pain • **Loss of appetite** • **Weight loss**	Stomach cancer	**Call your doctor.** → Stomach Cancer, p. 391

Stomach pain after taking medicines
• **Black stool**
• **Vomiting**
	Gastrointestinal hemorrhages or ulcers as side effects of many medicines, including
	  acetylsalicylic acid (ASA)
	  anti-inflammatory medicines
	    (steroids) after prolonged use
	  carbocysteine or diflunisal
	  potassium supplements
	  rheumatism medicines
	  ron supplements
		Check the medicine label or insert for these substances. When taking iron preparations, blackish stools are a normal symptom. In all other cases, **call your doctor** *immediately*.
		→ Medication Summary, p. 657

Stomach pain • **Foul-smelling, tarry stool** • **Vomiting of blood or a substance like coffee grounds**	Stomach hemorrhage	**Call emergency medical services immediately.** → Stomach and Peptic Ulcer, p. 389
Stomach pain with very hard abdomen and racing pulse • **Sweating**	Perforation of the stomach	**Call emergency medical services immediately.** → Stomach & Duodenal Ulcer, p. 389
Stomach pain with strong pressure in the chest	Heart attack (Mycardial Infarction)	**Call emergency medical services immediately.** → Heart Attack (Mycardial Infarction), p. 335

ABDOMINAL PAIN IN CHILDREN

What small children call a "tummy ache" may refer to pain in the chest or stomach, the upper or lower abdomen. Most often, they cannot differentiate where the pain really is. Careful questioning and gentle probing of the affected areas may reveal the actual source of the pain.

COMPLAINTS AND SYMPTOMS	POSSIBLE CAUSES	WHAT TO DO
Abdominal pain in a child • **Eating foods that are not easily digested** • **Overeating**	Normal reaction of the overloaded stomach	Give fennel tea, perhaps with small quantities of crackers or soup. Symptoms will pass without further treatment. → Nutrition, p. 722
Abdominal pain in a child after eating gas-producing foods (cabbage-family vegetables, fresh bread, etc.) • **Distended abdomen**	Gas, bloating	Give fennel tea and avoid gas-producing foods. → Irritable Bowel Syndrome, p. 403

COMPLAINTS AND SYMPTOMS	POSSIBLE CAUSES	WHAT TO DO
Unexplained abdominal pain with no other symptoms • **In certain situations**	Emotional issues	Make the child comfortable with a hot water bottle or compress on the belly, and try to find out whether something is bothering him or her. If abdominal pain persists over three hours, **call your doctor.** → Compresses, p. 692 → Irritable bowel syndrome, p. 403 → Health and well-being, p. 182
Abdominal pain with diarrhea • **Vomiting**	Gastrointestinal infection • Food poisoning • Reaction to medicine or household chemicals	If vomiting persists longer than one day, **call your doctor.** → Gastrointestinal infections, p. 599 → Acute gastritis, p. 387 **If you suspect poisoning, call your doctor immediately, or call your local poison center.**
Abdominal pain in a child with a cold	Symptom of the cold	If symptoms persist longer than one day, **call your doctor.** → Colds, p. 298 → Flu, p. 297
Abdominal pain and pain during urination • **Fever** • **Frequent urination**	Bladder or urinary tract infection	**Call your doctor.** → Cystitis (Bladder Infection), p. 418
Abdominal pain extending into the back or kidney area • **Fever** • **Pain when urinating**	Kidney infection	**Call your doctor.** → Acute pyelonephritis (Kidney Infection), p. 421
Abdominal pain accompanied by a painful bulge in the groin area or scrotum	Hernia • Hydrocele	**Call your doctor.** → Hernia, p. 439 → Hydrocele, Hematocele, Variocele p. 532
Abdominal cramping in a child, with folding-up of the legs • **Fever** • **Severe pain in right lower abdomen** • **Vomiting**	Appendicitis	**Call your doctor** *immediately*. → Appendicitis, p. 408

COMPLAINTS AND SYMPTOMS	POSSIBLE CAUSES	WHAT TO DO
Severe abdominal pain with hard, tight abdomen • **Stronger pain in the right lower abdomen** • **Rapid pulse** • **Cold sweat** • **Vomiting**	Ruptured appendix	**Call emergency medical services immediately.** → Appendicitis, p. 408

LOWER ABDOMINAL PAIN IN WOMEN

Lower abdominal pain can be a warning sign of either physical or psychological problems.

COMPLAINTS AND SYMPTOMS	POSSIBLE CAUSES	WHAT TO DO
A slight pulling pain in the lower abdomen in the area around the ovaries, before ovulation or before or during the menstrual period	Normal reaction	A slight pulling sensation is no reason for concern; in some women this is the regular signal for ovulation or menstruation. → Contraception, p. 551 → Menstruation, p. 506
Lower abdominal pain and no desire to sleep with partner • **Vaginal cramps** • **Pain on penetration**	The body's reaction to your psychological refusal to address your unsolved problems	Try to understand the reasons why you are avoiding your problems. If symptoms persist, **call your doctor.** → Counseling/Psychotherapy, p. 697 → Health and Well-being, p. 182 → Women's Issues, p. 537
Abdominal pain • **Frequent urination** • **Pain when urinating**	Bladder or urinary tract infection • Sexually transmitted diseases	**Call your doctor.** → Cystitis (Bladder Infection), p. 418 → Sexually Transmitted Diseases, p. 545
Pain near ovaries and fallopian tubes • **Fever** • **Pain during intercourse** • **Unusual discharge**	Inflammation of the uterine tube (salpingitis) • Endometriosis • Inflammation of the uterus • Sexually transmitted diseases	**Call your doctor.** → Endometriosis, p. 522 → Salpingitis, p. 525 → Sexually Transmitted Diseases, p. 545 → Uterine Inflammations, p. 520
Severe abdominal pain and bleeding during pregnancy	Miscarriage	**Call emergency medical services immediately.** → Miscarriage, p. 574
Severe abdominal pain on one side, and bleeding one or more weeks after menstrual period due • **Racing pulse** • **Sweating**	Ectopic pregnancy	**Call emergency medical services immediately.** → Ectopic Pregnancy, p. 526

ABDOMINAL GAS AND BLOATING

Gas and bloating are usually harmless and caused by eating habits. However, if you often experience abdominal bloating, ask yourself what is "upsetting" you. In rare cases, bloating can be a sign of illness.

COMPLAINTS AND SYMPTOMS	POSSIBLE CAUSES	WHAT TO DO
Bloating soon after eating	Gas-producing foods, especially beans cabbage fresh bread garlic lentils onions	Avoid these foods. → Nutrition, p. 722
Gas or bloating following a change in diet, or eating unfamiliar food	Normal transitional period	No cause for concern; the digestive system needs time to adjust. → Nutritional Habits, p. 722
Bloated abdomen and feeling of fullness after eating large portions • **Snacking often between meals**	Overloaded stomach	Eat only three meals a day, and chew each bite as long as possible. You will feel full sooner, and the stomach will be able to rest between meals.
Bloated abdomen and constipation	Insufficient roughage in diet	If symptoms persist longer than one week, **call your doctor.** → Constipation, p. 406 → Irritable Bowel Syndrome, p. 403
Gas and abdominal bloating along with intense emotional pressure	Emotional issues	Try to get to the root of your problems. If bloating persists after doing relaxation exercises, **call your doctor.** → Health and Well-being, p. 182 → Irritable Bowel Syndrome, p. 403 → Relaxation, p. 693
Bloated abdomen in women before or during menstruation • **Stomach ache**	Menstruation	No cause for concern. If symptoms do not disappear after menstruation, **call your doctor.** → Menstruation, p. 506
Gas or bloating after taking medicine	Side effect of diabetes medicine containing acarbose diet medicine containing methylcellulose disorders with the active ingredient probucol laxatives with lactulose medicine used for fat-metabolism	Check the medicine label or insert for these substances. If your medicine is over-the-counter, *stop taking it.* If your medicine is by prescription, **call your doctor.** → Medication Summary, p. 657

COMPLAINTS AND SYMPTOMS	POSSIBLE CAUSES	WHAT TO DO
Intestinal bloating • **Diarrhea** • **Fever** • **Intestinal cramps** • **Loss of appetite**	Intestinal inflammation or infection	**Call your doctor.** → Crohn's Disease, p. 412 → Gastroenteritis, p. 599 → Ulcerative Colitis, p. 411
Abdominal bloating • **Frequent night urination** • **Shortness of breath** • **Swelling in feet or legs**	Heart disease	**Call your doctor.** → Congestive Heart Failure, p. 337
Abdominal bloating • **Exhaustion** • **Fever** • **High blood pressure** • **Infrequent urination** • **Swelling in feet or legs** • **Swollen eyelids**	Kidney disease	**Call your doctor.**
Abdominal bloating with heavy stools • **Loss of appetite** • **Upper abdominal pain**	Inflammation of the pancreas (pancreatitis), pancreatic insufficiency	**Call your doctor.** → Pancreatic Insufficiency, p. 401 → Pancreatitis (Pancreas Infection), p. 400
Abdominal bloating with yellowish skin • **Yellowish whites of the eyes**	Liver disease	**Call your doctor.** → Fatty Liver, p. 394 → Jaundice, p. 393
Long-term abdominal bloating, distaste for meat • **Loss of appetite** • **Weight loss**	Stomach cancer	**Call your doctor.** → Stomach Cancer, p. 391
Abdominal bloating with no bowel movements for over 3 days (if this is unusual) • **Abdominal pain** • **Vomiting of intestinal contents**	Intestinal obstruction	**Call emergency medical services immediately.** → Intestinal Obstruction, p. 407

BELCHING

Belching was considered a sign of good health in the Middle Ages, and is most often a normal derivative of our digestion. It could also be an indicator of displeasure, faulty nutrition, or even illness.

COMPLAINTS AND SYMPTOMS	POSSIBLE CAUSES	WHAT TO DO
Belching after a meal	Foods that cause bloating • Eating overly rich foods • Eating too hastily • Unconsciously gulping air with the food	If you always belch after a meal, even though you are not overeating, you are probably an "air gulper." Chew slowly and swallow only small bites. Don't suppress belching – it relieves pressure.
Belching after drinking carbonated beverages	Stomach bloating	Try to avoid carbonated beverages; this may include mineral water.
Belching after taking medicines	Improper ingestion of medicines	Always take medicines with half a glass of water, or help them down with a few bites of banana. ↪ Medication Summary, p. 657
Belching up half-digested food or stomach acids (heartburn) **• Burning and pressure behind the breastbone**	Excessively acid stomach • Hiatal hernia • Overweight • Pregnancy • Weakness of the muscle that closes the esophagus	If heartburn persists after repeated belching, **call your doctor.** ↪ Acid Reflux (Heartburn), p. 383 ↪ Complaints During Pregnancy, p. 570 ↪ Hernia, p. 439
Belching with stomach pain **• Feeling of fullness** **• Gas** **• Loss of appetite** **• Nausea and vomiting**	Nervous stomach • Gastritis	Try relaxing. If symptoms persist for several weeks in spite of relaxation exercises, **call your doctor.** ↪ Acute Gastritis. p. 387 ↪ Health and Well-being, p. 182 ↪ Nervous Stomach, p. 386 ↪ Relaxation, p. 693
Belching with alternating diarrhea and constipation **• Feeling of fullness** **• Gas**	Irritable bowel syndrome	If symptoms persist, **call your doctor.** ↪ Health and Well-being, p. 182 ↪ Irritable Bowel Syndrome, p. 403
Belching of half-digested food and stomach acids **• Burning and pressure (heartburn) that may extend into the throat** **• Trouble swallowing**	Inflammation of the esophagus	If symptoms recur, **call your doctor.** ↪ Esophagitis (Esophageal Inflammation), p. 383

COMPLAINTS AND SYMPTOMS	POSSIBLE CAUSES	WHAT TO DO
Belching with pain in the upper stomach, resembling colic, from eating rich foods • **Nausea and vomiting** • **Pain extending into the right shoulder**	Gallstones	**Call your doctor.** → Gallstones, p. 398
Belching with pain in the right upper stomach • **Fatty, voluminous stools**	Inflammation of the pancreas (pancreatitis) or pancreatic insufficiency	**Call your doctor.** → Pancreatic Insufficiency, p. 401 → Pancreatitis (Pancreas Inflammation), p. 400

NAUSEA

Nausea can have various causes. It is the natural reaction of the body to anything that isn't good for it – hunger, smoking or drinking too much, or low blood pressure. Only in rare cases is nausea a symptom of serious illness.

COMPLAINTS AND SYMPTOMS	POSSIBLE CAUSES	WHAT TO DO
Nausea and stomach ache		→ Stomach, p. 385
Nausea after long periods of time not eating and/or sleeping or spent in hot, stuffy rooms	Hunger • Lack of sleep • Low blood pressure • Stale air	Your body is trying to make you aware of a deficiency. Once you eat again, or catch up on your sleep, the nausea will pass. → Health and well-being, p. 182 → Healthy living, p. 772 → Hypotension (Low Blood Pressure), p. 325
Nausea after eating or at the sight of food • **Stomach ache** • **Vomiting**	Overly rich or greasy food • Severe eating disorder • Spoiled food	If you have overeaten, fast for a day. If the sight of food makes you sick, or you repeatedly make yourself vomit, **call your doctor.** → Acute Gastritis, p. 387 → Eating Disorders, p. 202
Nausea and burning, cramp-like pain in upper stomach • **Heartburn and belching** • **Over-full feeling** • **Vomiting**	Nervous stomach • Infection of the stomach lining	If the symptoms recur, **call your doctor.** → Acute Gastritis, p. 387 → Health and Well-being, p. 182 → Nervous Stomach, p. 386
Nausea with fear, stress, or other emotional strain	Mental or emotional problems	If nausea persists for an extended period of time, **call your doctor.** → Counseling and Psychotherapy, p. 697 → Health and Well-being, p. 182

COMPLAINTS AND SYMPTOMS	POSSIBLE CAUSES	WHAT TO DO
Nausea after using alcohol, cigarettes, or drugs	Side effect of alcohol • Symptom of alcohol withdrawal • Symptom of cigarette or drug abuse	Stop smoking. If you often drink to excess or take drugs, and need help making changes, **call your doctor.** ⟶ Mood-altering Substances, Recreational Drugs, p. 754 ⟶ Addictions & Dependencies, p. 204
Nausea after breathing toxic fumes (including from unexpected sources in your home, such as a gas stove) • **Headaches**	Poisoning	If nausea persists longer than three days, or you are continuously exposed to toxic fumes at work, **call your doctor.** ⟶ First Aid, p. 704 ⟶ Common Pollutants, p. 773
In women: nausea on getting up in the morning, possibly with vomiting	Pregnancy	Nausea in the first trimester is normal. If nausea is severe, **call your doctor.** ⟶ Complaints During Pregnancy, p. 570

Nausea after taking medicines	Side effect of many medicines, including
	  antibiotics for urinary tract infections
	  antifungals
	  cough medicines
	  local anesthetics
	  medicines for cardiovascular disease
	  oral contraceptives and other hormonal medicines (for example, for menopause)
	  sedatives classified as opiates
		If your medicine is over-the-counter and nausea is not mentioned as a possible harmless, temporary side effect, *stop taking it.* If your medicine is by prescription and you were not made aware of the possible side effects, **call your doctor.**
		⟶ Medication Summary, p. 657

Nausea in conjunction with all illnesses	Often a symptom of the illness	If you are not already under medical supervision, and the nausea lasts longer than three days, **call your doctor.**
Nausea with cold sweat and racing pulse	Various life-threatening illnesses	**Call emergency medical services immediately.**

ANAL DISORDERS

Aching or itching of the anus is usually caused by irritation, fissures, hemorrhoids, worms, or, in rare cases, fistulas or abscesses. Emotional stress can also lead to anal problems.

COMPLAINTS AND SYMPTOMS	POSSIBLE CAUSES	WHAT TO DO
Anal itching when wearing tight or very warm clothing	Clothing constantly rubbing against the anus • The irritating heat that results from this friction	Wear loose clothing that isn't too warm, and switch to natural-fiber underwear. If symptoms persist, **call your doctor.**
Anal itching • **Area seldom washed** • **Area washed excessively** • **Use of hygienic wipes**	Poor hygiene • Irritation from toilet paper or hygienic wipes • Too much soap or friction used in cleaning the area	Clean the anus after bowel movements with a moist cotton cloth or under running water. If symptoms persist, **call your doctor,**

Anal itching	Chronic ailments, especially
	   diabetes
	   intestinal illnesses
	   liver disorders
	• Emotional problems
	• Irritation of the anus caused by allergic reactions to certain foods, especially
	   beer
	   citrus fruit
	   cola
	   seasonings
	   vitamin C tablets
		Keep a record of what you are eating, and try to find out which foods seem to cause the itching. Avoid strong soaps and hygienic wipes. If symptoms persist, **call your doctor.**
		→ Allergies, p. 360
		→ Health and Well-being, p. 182

Painful, bleeding cracks and splits in the anus	Hard stools • Unsafe sexual practices	Make sure you eat a fiber-rich diet (salads, vegetables, fruit, whole-grain products), and drink lots of fluids to soften bowel movements. If you have anal intercourse, use a lubricant. If anal fissures persist longer than one week, **call your doctor.** → Anal Fissures, p. 416 → Nutrition, p. 722
Irritated skin or anal itching after applying medicines	Side effect of hemorrhoid medicines, antibiotics, or topical anesthetics	If you are using an over-the-counter medicine, stop using it. If the medicine is by prescription, **call your doctor.** → Medication Summary, p. 657

COMPLAINTS AND SYMPTOMS	POSSIBLE CAUSES	WHAT TO DO
Painful anal itching • **Bumps or blisters** • **Wart-like growths**	Irritated mucous membrane • Genital warts • Herpes	If symptoms persist for more than one week, or herpes blisters and genital warts recur, **call your doctor.** ↪ Genital Herpes, p. 547 ↪ Genital Warts, p. 547
Anal itching • **White, thread-like worms in stool**	Pinworms	**Call your doctor.** ↪ Worms (Parasites), p. 415
Painful anus • **Bright red blood in stool** • **Knot-like swelling**	Hemorrhoids • Cancer	**Call your doctor.** ↪ Hemorrhoids, p. 417 ↪ Colon and Rectal Cancers, p. 414
Inflamed, tight anus • **Swelling**	Abscess	**Call your doctor.**
Pains during bowel movements because of a small, festering sore next to the anus	Fistula between the anus and the rectum	**Call your doctor.** ↪ Crohn's Disease, p. 412
Pus or mucus from anus • **Bloody, mucous diarrhea** • **Pain during bowel movements**	Inflammation of the pelvic (sigmoid) colon (proctitis)	**Call your doctor.** ↪ Ulcerative Colitis, p. 411

Signs and Symptoms • 17

APPETITE DISORDERS

EXCESSIVE APPETITE AND BULIMIA

Being very hungry and eating a lot may simply indicate your body's natural need for more food. However, extended periods of bulimia often indicate a disorder. If you consistently overeat, ask yourself what eating is compensating for in your life, or what your weight is protecting you from. Bulimia and weight gain: Eating Disorders, p. 202

COMPLAINTS AND SYMPTOMS	POSSIBLE CAUSES	WHAT TO DO
Bulimia, or excessive appetite accompanying psychological problems • **Boredom** • **Lack of motivation** • **Worries**	Compensation	Look for other ways to "nourish" yourself. If you habitually overeat, **call your doctor.** → Eating Disorders, p. 202 → Health and Well-being, p. 182
Bulimia during pregnancy • **Food cravings**	Symptom of pregnancy	Although cravings or being hungrier than usual are normal during pregnancy, you should not feel compelled to "eat for two." If weight gain is excessive, **call your doctor.** → High Blood Pressure During Pregnancy (Preeclampsia), p. 574 → Nutrition During Pregnancy, p. 568
Bulimia • **Frequent urination** • **Unusual thirst** • **Weight loss**	Diabetes	**Call your doctor.** → Diabetes, p. 483
Bulimia • **Protruding eyeballs** • **Trembling** • **Weight loss**	Hyperthyroidism	**Call your doctor.** → Hyperthyroidism (Overactive Thyroid), p. 496
Bulimia and excessive appetite • **Purging**	Bulimia	**Call your doctor.** → Eating Disorders, p. 202

LOSS OF APPETITE

When food is no longer enjoyable, and each bite seems to stick in your throat, you may have a disease or you may be suffering from emotional stress.

COMPLAINTS AND SYMPTOMS	POSSIBLE CAUSES	WHAT TO DO
Loss of appetite • **Foods taste bad or have been carelessly prepared**	Your diet lacks nutritional variety • Emotional issues • Lack of enjoyment from food • Vitamin deficiency • You are under stress • You feel lonely because you always eat alone	Eat healthy, well-balanced meals. A nutritionally unbalanced diet can lead to vitamin deficiencies. Try to alter the habits that spoil your appetite. If loss of appetite lasts longer than three weeks, **call your doctor.** ↪ Health and well-being, p. 182 ↪ Nutrition, p. 722
Loss of appetite • **Drug use** • **Excessive alcohol consumption** • **Heavy smoking** • **Side effect of alcohol and/or nicotine abuse**	Side effect of drug use	Stop smoking. If you often drink to excess or take drugs, **call your doctor.** ↪ Addictions and Dependencies, p. 204 ↪ Mood-altering Substance, Recreational Drugs, p. 754
Loss of appetite accompanying emotional problems or unhappiness • **Extreme weight loss** • **Induced vomiting (bulimia)**	Emotional problems • Anorexia	Work on resolving the situation causing your unhappiness. If loss of appetite or vomiting persist, **call your doctor.** ↪ Eating Disorders, p. 202 ↪ Emotional Problems, p. 60 ↪ Health and Well-being, p. 182 ↪ Mental Health Disorders, p. 195
Loss of appetite • **Feeling of pressure or fullness** • **Nausea** • **Stomach ache**	Emotional problems • Gastritis • Nervous stomach • Stomach or duodenal ulcer • Stomach cancer	If loss of appetite lasts longer than two weeks, **call your doctor.** ↪ Acute Gastritis, p. 387 ↪ Health and Well-being, p. 182 ↪ Nervous Stomach, p. 386 ↪ Stomach & Duodenal Ulcer, p. 389 ↪ Stomach Cancer, p. 391
Loss of appetite with chronic constipation	Effect of constipation	Eat nutritious, well-balanced meals that include plenty of bulk. Drink lots of liquids. If constipation lasts longer than five days, **call your doctor.** ↪ Constipation, p. 406 ↪ Intestinal Obstruction, p. 407 ↪ Nutrition, p. 722

COMPLAINTS AND SYMPTOMS	POSSIBLE CAUSES	WHAT TO DO

Reduced appetite after taking medicine	Side effect of
	  an overdose of vitamin A or D
	  antibiotics containing
	    metronidazole
	  cholesterol medicine containing
	    sitosterol at high doses
	  epilepsy medicine containing
	    barbexaclone
	  heart medicine to treat ventricular
	    arrhythmias containing
	    propafenone
	  phenobarbital
	  primidone
	  tuberculosis medicine containing
	    pyrazinamide
		Check the medicine label or insert for these substances. If your medicine is over-the-counter, *stop taking it*. If your medicine is by prescription, **call your doctor.**
		→ Medication summary, p. 657

Loss of appetite and mouth or throat pain	Minor wounds • Denture pressure • Inflammation of the mucous membrane • Various mouth or throat ailments	Gargle with chamomile or sage tea. If symptoms persist longer than one day, **call your doctor.** → Gingivitis (gum inflammation), p. 370 → Glossitis (tongue inflammation), p. 381 → Oral mucous membrane inflammation, p. 379 → Periodontal diseases, p. 371
Loss of appetite • **Skin has a yellow tint** • **Whites of the eyes are yellowish**	Jaundice	**Call your doctor.** → Jaundice, p. 393
Loss of appetite • **Bloating** • **Excessive stools** • **Pain in the upper abdomen**	Disorders of the pancreas • Disorders of the gallbladder	**Call your doctor.** → Cholecystitis (gall-bladder inflammation), p. 400 → Pancreatic insufficiency, p. 401 → Pancreatitis (Pancreatic Infection), p. 400

ARM PAIN AND HAND PAIN

Pain in the arms or hands can result from overexertion and pulled muscles, tendons, or ligaments; in some cases it may also signal a serious illness or disorder.

COMPLAINTS AND SYMPTOMS	POSSIBLE CAUSES	WHAT TO DO
Painful arms after unaccustomed stress, for example, from sports	Muscle soreness/stiffness	Take it easy. A charley horse will heal itself. Heat and massage often help. ➼ Massages, p. 686 ➼ Muscle Soreness/Stiffness, p. 435 ➼ Stretching, p. 765
Painful wrists after unaccustomed or repetitive actions, such as typing	Tendinitis	Rest wrist and thumb joints, and apply cold to the painful area. If symptoms persist or recur repeatedly, **call your doctor.** ➼ Cold Treatments, p. 685 ➼ Tendinitis, tenosynovitis, p. 442
Arm and shoulder pain, especially on your dominant side	Muscle spasm • Degeneration • Tennis elbow	If you frequently have such pain, **call your doctor.** ➼ Arthritis, p. 452 ➼ Fibromyalgia Syndromes (Soft Tissue Pain and Stiffness), p. 462
Red, swollen, painful elbow with possible limited mobility	Bursitis	Rest and immobilize elbow, applying cold (ice) to the painful area. If symptoms persist or recur repeatedly, **call your doctor.** ➼ Bursitis, p. 443 ➼ Cold Treatments, p. 685
Painful, whitened fingers, possibly after exposure to cold	Reaction to cold • Frostbite • Vasoconstriction • Various systemic disorders	If your fingers frequently turn white or you have had lengthy cold exposure, **call your doctor.** ➼ First aid, p. 704 ➼ Cold Injuries, frostbite, p. 264. 708 ➼ Raynaud's Disease, p. 332 ➼ Scleroderma, p. 461
Painful finger joints • **Fever** • **Red, swollen joints** • **Stiffness and pain after getting up in the morning**	Joint inflammation	**Call your doctor.** ➼ Arthritis, p. 452
Painful fingertip joints	Degeneration	**Call your doctor.** ➼ Arthritis, p. 452

COMPLAINTS AND SYMPTOMS	POSSIBLE CAUSES	WHAT TO DO
Arm pain radiating from the neck • **An ache in the back of the head** • **Confused sensations in the arms**	Ruptured disc	**Call your doctor.** → Lumbago, Sciatica, Herniated or Ruptured Disk Damage, p. 466
Arm pain extending into the hand, especially at night • **Tingling or loss of sensation in the fingers**	Carpal tunnel syndrome (pressure on a nerve in the wrist)	**Call your doctor.** → Fibromyalagia Syndromes (Soft Tissue Pain and Stiffness), p. 462
Arm pain accompanied by painful stiffness and scoliosis (curvature of the spine) • **Pain in the heels of the palms**	Chronic inflammation of the spine	**Call your doctor.** → Ankylosing Spondylitis, p. 459
Pain and swelling of the arms • **After a breast operation** • **After armpit radiation therapy** • **After chest radiation therapy**	Lymphedema	**Call your doctor.** → Breast Cancer, p. 515
Pain while stretching or bending wrists, after unaccustomed stress	Tearing of tendons and ligaments	Elevate the affected areas, apply cold (ice). **Call your doctor.** → Pulled Tendon, Torn Ligament, p. 441
Arm pain following an accident or injury • **Swelling** • **Unusual position or movement of the arm**	Fracture	**Call your doctor.** → Fractures, p. 429
Painful arm or wrist after a fall, accident or extreme movement • **Ecchymosis (bruise)** • **Near or total immobilization** • **Swelling** • **Unusual position or movement, of the arm or hand**	Sprained or twisted joint • Fracture • Pulled or torn ligament • Pulled or torn tendon	*Act immediately.* Immobilize the arm or hand. **Call your doctor** *immediately.* → Dislocations, p. 448 → Fractures, p. 429 → Pulled Ligament, Torn Ligament, p. 441 → Pulled Tendon, Torn Tendon, p. 441 → Sprain, p. 441
Pain, particularly in the left arm and radiating from the chest, with a constricting sensation as if an iron band circled the chest • **Difficulty breathing** • **Heart palpitations**	Lack of oxygen to the heart due to constriction of the coronary arteries • Emotional problems	**Call your doctor.** → Angina Pectoris, p. 333 → Tachycardia, p. 340

COMPLAINTS AND SYMPTOMS	POSSIBLE CAUSES	WHAT TO DO
Pain, particularly in the left arm, with severe chest pains • **Anxiety** • **Cold sweat** • **Feelings of oppression** • **Nausea and vomiting** • **Shortness of breath**	Heart attack (myocardial infarction)	**Call emergency medical services immediately.** ↪ Heart Attack (Myocardial Infarction), p. 335
Arm pain, shortness of breath • **Chest pains** • **Cough** • **Heart palpitations** • **Hemoptysis (coughed-up blood)** • **Preceded by cramping in the calves a few days earlier**	Lung infarction	**Call emergency medical services immediately.** ↪ Pulmonary Infarction, p. 312

BACK PAIN

Back pain can be caused by bearing heavy burdens – physical and emotional. However, wear and tear, overweight, a pinched nerve, and various general ailments can also be sources of back pain.

COMPLAINTS AND SYMPTOMS	POSSIBLE CAUSES	WHAT TO DO
Back pain after sustained sitting, standing, heavy lifting, or unaccustomed sports activity	Tension of back muscles from bad posture • Overextended or torn back muscles	Warmth, massage, and relaxation exercises usually help. If pain persists, **call your doctor.** → Back and Lower Back Pain, p. 465 → Massage, p. 686 → Physical Activity and Sports, p. 762 → Relaxation, p. 693
Back pain with stress and/or mental or emotional burdens	Strain on spinal column from tense body posture (for example, unconscious hunching of shoulders)	Be more aware of body position; psychological stress almost always shows up in your posture. If pain persists for more than a week, **call your doctor.** → Back and Lower Back Pain, p. 465 → Fibromyalgia Syndromes, p. 462 → Health and Well-being, p. 182
Back pain with overweight	Constant strain on spinal column from excessive body weight	Try to lose weight. If you are not successful on your own, **call your doctor.** → Body Weight, p. 727 → Physical Activity and Sports, p. 762
Back pain **• After menopause, with possible loss of bladder control** **• After several births** **• Before or during menstrual period** **• During pregnancy**	Strain on spinal column from increased weight • Normal symptom of menstruation • Prolapsed uterus	If pain persists, **call your doctor.** Complaints During Pregnancy → Massage, p. 686 → Menstrual disorders, p. 508 → Prolapsed Uterus, p. 523 → Relaxation, p. 693
Back pain with colds	Symptom of colds	If symptoms persist over three days, **call your doctor.** → Colds, p. 298 → Flu, p. 297
Back pain after taking medicines	Side effect of medicines containing allylestranol, dydrogesterone (to prevent premature birth) hydroxyprogesterone medrogestone, progestin (for menstrual disorders)	Check the medicine label or insert for these substances. If you were not made aware of possible side effects, **call your doctor.** → Medication Summary, p. 657

COMPLAINTS AND SYMPTOMS	POSSIBLE CAUSES	WHAT TO DO
Back pain after long-term use of medicines	Bone softening as side effect of steroids, usually prescribed for rheumatism, asthma, and allergies	When symptoms appear, **call your doctor.** → Glucocorticoids (Steroids), p. 665 → Medication Summary, p. 657
Pain in middle and lower spine after an awkward movement or heavy lifting	Tearing or tension of back musculature • Disk damage • Lumbago	Warmth, massage, and relaxation exercises usually help. If pain persists after one day or recurs, **call your doctor.** → Lumbago, Sciatica, Herniated or Ruptured Disk, p. 466
Pain in lower back spreading over buttocks into leg, possibly to foot	Tense back • Irritated sciatic nerve • Herniated disk • Spondylolisthesis	**Call your doctor.** → Lumbago, Sciatica, Herniated or Ruptured Disk, p. 466
Back pain with crooked posture (elevated shoulder or hip) and possibly a hump	Scoliosis	**Call your doctor.** → Scoliosis, p. 468
Recurring pain in entire spinal column • **Arm pain** • **Heel pain**	Chronically inflamed and stiff spine	**Call your doctor.** → Ankylosing Spondylolisthesis, p. 459
In youths, back pain after mild exertion, possibly with slightly rounded back	Changes in spinal vertebrae	**Call your doctor.** → Scheuermann's Disease, p. 467
Pain especially in lower back • **Fever** • **Painful urination**	Kidney infection	**Call your doctor.** → Acute Pyelonephritis (Kidney Infection), p. 421
Pain in back and lower abdomen • **Fever** • **Vaginal discharge**	Uterine inflammation • Inflamed fallopian tubes	**Call your doctor.** → Salpingitis, p. 525 → Uterine Inflammation, p. 520
Back pain after age 50, especially in women • **Decrease in body size** • **Frequent bone fractures**	Osteoporosis	**Call your doctor.** → Osteoporosis, p. 430
Back pain over time with an existing cancer	Metastasis to spinal column	**Call your doctor.** → Cancer, p. 470

COMPLAINTS AND SYMPTOMS	POSSIBLE CAUSES	WHAT TO DO
Severe back pain with paralysis in the legs and sensory disorders	Herniated disk	**Call your doctor.** → Lumbago, Sciatica, Herniated or ruptured disk, p. 466
Sudden back pain after a fall or back injury • **Loss of sensation** • **Paralysis of legs**	Spinal cord injury	**Call your doctor.** Remain lying flat on your back. *Do not move.* Any movement can cause serious damage. → First Aid, p. 704

BAD BREATH

Bad breath can stem from poor dental hygiene. It can also be a warning signal of serious stomach disease, lung disease, or emotional problems and stress.

COMPLAINTS AND SYMPTOMS	POSSIBLE CAUSES	WHAT TO DO
Bad breath after garlic, onions, alcohol, etc.	Normal reaction	Bad breath disappears after a day.
Bad breath after notbrushing teeth	Poor dental hygiene	Food particles between teeth. Brush teeth after each meal, or at least before bed and after breakfast. ↪ Proper Tooth Care, p. 364
Bad breath with psychological stresses	Emotional problems	Bad breath will disappear when stress is reduced. ↪ Health and Well-being, p. 182
Bad breath accompanying an illness • **Fever**	Common symptom of fevers and illness	If bad breath does not disappear by the end of the illness, **call your doctor.**
Bad breath with bleeding, painful gums	Inflammation of the gums	**Call your doctor.** ↪ Gingivitis (Gum Inflammation), p. 370
Bad breath with yellow coating on teeth • **Toothache**	• Cavities • Plaque	**Call your doctor.** ↪ Cavities, p. 366 ↪ Tooth Care, p. 364
Bad breath while wearing braces or a bridge	Food particles stuck in dental device, or between device and teeth or mouth	**Call your doctor.** ↪ Dentures, p. 376
Bad breath with sore throat • **Difficulty in swallowing** • **Fever**	Inflammation of the tonsils (tonsillitis)	**Call your doctor.** ↪ Tonsillitis, p. 302
Bad breath with pain and blisters or white coating inside mouth • **Difficulty in swallowing** • **Fever**	Infection of the oral mucous membrane	**Call your doctor.** ↪ Stomatitis (Oral Mucous-membrane Infection), p. 379
Bad breath with stomach pain	Nervous stomach • Gastritis • Peptic (duodenal) ulcer	**Call your doctor.** ↪ Acute gastritis, p. 387 ↪ Nervous Stomach, p. 386 ↪ Stomach and Duodenal Ulcer, p. 389

COMPLAINTS AND SYMPTOMS	POSSIBLE CAUSES	WHAT TO DO
Bad breath with stubborn cough • **Sputum containing pus**	Inflammation of the bronchial tubes • Pneumonia	**Call your doctor.** → Acute Bronchitis, p. 305 → Pneumonia, p. 310
Bad breath over a long period of time with none of the symptoms mentioned above • **Sensation of a foreign object in the mouth**	Tumor of the mouth or pharynx	**Call your doctor.** → Oral Cancers (Cancer of the Mouth Area), p. 382
Bad breath with difficulty in swallowing • **Hoarseness** • **Nausea** • **Pain behind the breastbone**	Cancer of the esophagus	**Call your doctor.** → Esophageal Cancer, p. 385
Breath smells like ammonia	Liver damage	**Call your doctor.** → Cirrhosis of the Liver, p. 396 → Liver Failure, p. 393
Breath smells like urine	Kidney failure	**Call your doctor.** → Kidney Failure, Uremia, p. 425
Breath smells like acetone (nail polish remover)	Diabetes	**Call your doctor** *immediately*. → Diabetes, p. 483

BODY TEMPERATURE CHANGES

CHILLS

If you often feel cold or "freezing" for no apparent reason, there are many possible causes, among them constant fatigue, circulatory or hormonal disorders, and depression.

COMPLAINTS AND SYMPTOMS	POSSIBLE CAUSES	WHAT TO DO
Chills with insufficient sleep	Exhaustion	Get plenty of sleep
Chills while dieting	Hunger	Many dieting programs are unhealthy. If you are not feeling well, you should take a break from the diet. ↪ Body Weight, p. 727
Chills in underweight persons	Insufficient protection against cold	Try gaining some weight. If you are extremely thin, **call your doctor.** ↪ Body Weight, p. 727 ↪ Eating Disorders, p. 202
Chills • **Feeling lonely** • **Feeling unloved**	Emotional issues	Try to bring love and warmth into your life. If you need guidance, **call your doctor.** ↪ Health and Well-being, p. 182 ↪ Counseling and Psychotherapy, p. 697
Chills • **Fatigue on awakening** • **Headache** • **Nausea**	Low blood pressure	Incorporate more physical activities into your life. Participate in sports; walk more frequently. If that doesn't help, **call your doctor.** ↪ Hypotension (Low Blood Pressure)p. 325 ↪ Physical Activity and Sports, p. 762

Chills after taking medicines
• **Pallor**
	Circulatory disorders as side effects of medicines
	• for heart and circulatory disorders containing
	    dihydroergocornine
	    dihydroergocristine
	    dihydroergocryptine
	    dihydroergotamine
	• for high blood pressure
	    beta-blockers
	• for migraine containing
	    dihydroergotamine
	    ergotamine
	• for Parkinson's disease and other hormonal disorders containing bromocriptine
		Check the medicine label or insert for these ingredients. If any are present, **call your doctor.**
		↪ Medication Summary, p. 657

COMPLAINTS AND SYMPTOMS	POSSIBLE CAUSES	WHAT TO DO
Chills and fever • **Shivering**	Symptom of fever	If fever persists longer than three days and exceeds 103°F, **call your doctor.**
Blue-white fingers, lips, and ears • **Anemia** • **Dark urine**	Acute or chronic hypothermia	**Call your doctor.** → Anemia, p. 345
Cold fingers that suddenly turn blue or white	Blood vessel constriction	**Call your doctor.** → Raynaud's Disease and Renaud's Phenomenon, p. 332

FEVER

Fever is the body's first line of defense against germs and illness. Medicating to reduce a fever is seldom necessary; cool compresses are usually sufficient to bring the fever down. Fever or elevated temperature over a long period of time can signify a more serious illness. Fever with skin rash: Fever in children: See the following section. Skin rash with fever, p. 33.

COMPLAINTS AND SYMPTOMS	POSSIBLE CAUSES	WHAT TO DO
Fever with general exhaustion and head cold • **Cough** • **Headache** • **Hoarseness** • **Joint pain** • **Scratchy throat**	Flu	If fever exceeds 103°F or symptoms persist after a week, **call your doctor.** → Cold, p. 298 → Compresses, p. 692 → Flu, p. 297
Fever with general exhaustion and cough • **Chest pain** • **Mucous, thick, glassy, or pus-like sputum**	Acute bronchitis • Chronic bronchitis	If fever exceeds 103°F or sputum contains pus, or if symptoms recur, **call your doctor.** → Acute Bronchitis, p. 305 → Chronic Bronchitis, p. 306
Fever with sore throat • **Difficulty swallowing** • **Headache** • **Swollen glands in throat**	Tonsillitis • Pharyngitis	If fever exceeds 103°F or symptoms persist after two days, **call your doctor.** → Pharyngitis, p. 302 → Tonsillitis, p. 302
Fever with sore throat • **Difficulty swallowing** • **Pain when speaking** • **Severe hoarseness**	Laryngitis	If fever exceeds 103°F or symptoms persist after three days, **call your doctor.** → Laryngitis (Vocal Cord Inflammation), p. 303
Fever after taking medicines	Side effect of various medicines	If you get a fever while taking medicines, **call your doctor.** → Medication Summary, p. 657

COMPLAINTS AND SYMPTOMS	POSSIBLE CAUSES	WHAT TO DO
Fever with diarrhea • **Vomiting**	Infection of the gastrointestinal tract	If fever exceeds 103°F or symptoms persist after three days, **call your doctor.** ↪ Acute Gastritis, p. 387 ↪ Gastroenteritis, p. 599
Slight fever and mucous or bloody diarrhea • **Abdominal pain** • **Loss of appetite** • **Weight loss**	Inflammatory bowel disorders	**Call your doctor.** ↪ Crohn's Disease, p. 412 ↪ Ulcerative Colitis, p. 411
Fever and earaches • **Headaches** • **Pus or watery discharge from ear**	Middle-ear infection	**Call your doctor.** ↪ Acute Otitis Media (Acute Ear Infection), p. 255
Fever with pain in forehead and/ or jaw • **Pain between eyes and cheeks (in sinuses)**	Sinus infection	**Call your doctor.** ↪ Sinusitis, p. 300
Fever with pain in forehead and/ or jaw • **Pain between eyes and cheeks (in sinuses)**	Sinus infection	**Call your doctor.** ↪ Sinusitis, p. 300
Fever • **Pain while urinating** • **More frequent urination than usual**	Infection of the bladder or urinary tract	**Call your doctor.** ↪ Cystitis (Bladder Infection), p. 418
Fever with lower back pain extending to bladder • **Pain while urinating**	Kidney inflammation	**Call your doctor.** ↪ Acute Pyelonephritis (Kidney Infection), p. 421
Fever and toothache	Abscess	**Call your doctor.** ↪ Root Tip Inflammation, p. 370
Fever, with pain experienced in waves in upper right abdomen	Gallbladder inflammation	**Call your doctor.** ↪ Cholecystitis (Gallbladder Infection), p. 400
In women, fever with pain in lower abdomen	Inflamed fallopian tubes Inflamed ovaries	**Call your doctor.** ↪ Salpingitis (Inflammation of the Fallopian Tubes, Pelvic Inflammatory Disease), p. 525
In women, fever shortly after giving birth	Breast infection • Postpartum fever	**Call your doctor.** ↪ Mastitis (Breast Infection), p. 513

COMPLAINTS AND SYMPTOMS	POSSIBLE CAUSES	WHAT TO DO
Fever and swelling • **In the armpits** • **In the groin** • **On the side of the neck**	Swollen lymph glands from viral infection	**Call the doctor.** ↪ Infectious Mononucleosis, p. 355
Fever following heavy blood loss • **Suddenly festering post-operative wounds**	Traumatic fever • Wound infection	**Call your doctor.**
Fever with prolonged joint pain	Rheumatic fever • Collagen vascular disease	**Call your doctor.** ↪ Rheumatic Fever, p. 458 ↪ Systemic Lupus Erythematosus, p. 460
Fever with cough and sputum • **Chills** • **Excessive sweating** • **Shortage of breath**	Pneumonia	**Call your doctor.** ↪ Pneumonia, p. 310
Slight fever with cough over an extended period of time (longer than three weeks) • **Night sweats** • **Weight loss**	Tuberculosis • Lung cancer	**Call your doctor.** ↪ Lung cancer, p. 314 ↪ Tuberculosis, p. 670
Slight fever over an extended period of time, with none of the symptoms listed above • **Weight loss**	Anemia • AIDS • Cancer	**Call your doctor.** ↪ AIDS, p. 357 ↪ Anemia, p. 345 ↪ Cancer, p. 470
Fever after taking medicines • **Sore throat** • **Whitish coating in throat**	Blood or bone marrow disorder as side effect of medicines	**Call your doctor.** ↪ Medication Summary, p. 657
Fever during stay in—or after return from—the tropics	Tropical illnesses	**Call your doctor.** ↪ Gastroenteritis, p. 599 ↪ Travel, p. 717
High fever and soreness in the thyroid area • **Hoarseness**	Thyroid inflammation	**Call your doctor.** ↪ Thyroiditis (Inflammation of the Thyroid Gland), p. 498
Fever and pain on right side of abdomen • **Nausea and vomiting** • **Tight, hardened abdomen**	Appendicitis	If abdomen is hard and tight, **call your doctor.** ↪ Appendicitis, p. 408

COMPLAINTS AND SYMPTOMS	POSSIBLE CAUSES	WHAT TO DO
Fever with eye pain, sudden deterioration of vision • **Dizziness** • **Headaches** • **Nausea and vomiting** • **Reddened eyes**	Abnormal pressure in the eye (glaucoma)	**Call your doctor immediately.** ↳ Glaucoma, p. 244
Fever with severe headaches that get worse when tilting head forward • **Dizziness** • **Light sensitivity** • **Nausea and vomiting** • **Stiff neck**	Meningitis	**Call your doctor immediately.** ↳ Meningitis, p. 212
High fever, hot, dry skin, dizziness, and nausea after exposure to the sun • **Disorientation**	Heat stroke	**Act immediately**: move victim into shade, loosen clothes, and splash with cold water. Place ice packs on head and neck. Give sips of cool beverage if the person is conscious. **Call your doctor immediately.** ↳ Heat Disorders (and Cold Injuries) p. 707
High fever with noticeable temperature fluctuations throughout the day	Bacteremia (sepsis)	**Call your doctor immediately.**

FEVER IN CHILDREN

Fever is the body's first line of defense against germs and illness. As long as the child's temperature is not over 103°F and there are no convulsions, there is no need to give medicine. Vinegar compresses on the forehead or cool water compresses on the calves reduce fever just as effectively as medicines, and are less risky. If your baby is under three months old and has a fever, always call your doctor. Fever with skin rash: Skin rash in children, p. 33. Fever with abdominal pain: Abdominal pain in children, p. 7.

COMPLAINTS AND SYMPTOMS	POSSIBLE CAUSES	WHAT TO DO
Fever with general exhaustion and head cold • **Cough** • **Headaches** • **Loss of appetite**	Common cold	Apply vinegar compresses to the forehead or cool water compresses to the calves. Give plenty of fluids. If child is under three years old, or temperature exceeds 103°F, or symptoms persist longer than a week, **call your doctor.** ↳ Cold, p. 298 ↳ Compresses, p. 692 ↳ Flu, p. 297

COMPLAINTS AND SYMPTOMS	POSSIBLE CAUSES	WHAT TO DO
Sudden high fever of uncertain origin that disappears after three or four days • **Skin rash of diffused spots**	Viral infection	Apply vinegar compresses to the forehead or cool water compresses to the calves. Give plenty of fluids. The so-called "three-day fever" is usually harmless. If fever persists longer than three or four days, or temperature exceeds 103°F, **call your doctor.** ➡ Three-day Fever (Roseola), p. 605 ➡ Compresses, p. 692
Fever with diarrhea • **Vomiting**	Gastrointestinal infection	Apply vinegar compresses to the forehead or cool water compresses to the calves. Give the child crackers and tea or soup. If child is under three years old or temperature exceeds 103°F, **call your doctor.** ➡ Compresses, p. 692 ➡ Gastrointestinal Infections, p. 599
Fever and sore throat in children too young to speak • **Refusal to eat** • **Screaming when being fed**	Tonsillitis • Inflammation of the pharynx • Laryngitis • Vocal cord inflammation	If child is under three years old or temperature exceeds 103°F, **call your doctor.** ➡ Laryngitis, Vocal Cord Inflammation, p. 303 ➡ Pharyngitis, p. 302 ➡ Tonsillitis, p. 302
Fevers with toothache and/or gum pain	Abscess Teething	Teething children are more susceptible to illness. If fever exceeds 103°F, **call your doctor.** ➡ Baby Teeth, p. 376 ➡ Inflammations of the Root Tip: Abscess, Granuloma, Fistula, Cyst, p. 370
Fever and pain when urinating **More frequent urination than usual**	Infection of the bladder or urinary tract	**Call your doctor.** ➡ Cystitis (Bladder Infection), p. 418
Fever and lower back pain extending to the bladder • **Pain when urinating**	Kidney inflammation	**Call your doctor.** ➡ Acute Pyelonephritis (Kidney Infection), p. 421
Fever and earache in children too young to speak • **Frequently pulling at earlobe** • **Screaming and holding hands over ears**	Middle-ear inflammation	**Call your doctor.** ➡ Acute Otitis Media (Acute Ear Infection), p. 255

COMPLAINTS AND SYMPTOMS	POSSIBLE CAUSES	WHAT TO DO
Fever with pain in forehead and/or jaw • **Pain between the eyes and cheeks (in sinuses)**	Sinus infection	**Call your doctor.** ↪ Sinusitis, p. 300
Fever and swelling • **In the armpits** • **In the groin** • **On the side of the neck**	Mumps • Swollen lymph glands from viral infection	**Call your doctor.** ↪ Infectious mononucleosis, p. 355 ↪ Mumps, p. 603
Fever following heavy blood loss • **Suddenly festering post-operative wounds**	Traumatic fever • Wound infection	**Call your doctor.**
Fever with general exhaustion and cough • **Chest pain** • **Mucous, thick, glassy, or pus-like sputum**	Acute bronchitis • Bronchiolitis • Pneumonia	**Call your doctor.** ↪ Acute bronchitis, p. 305 ↪ Bronchiolitis, p. 597 ↪ Pneumonia, p. 310
Fever with prolonged coughing attacks • **Coughing up of thick phlegm** • **Deep, whooping inhalations**	Whooping cough	**Call your doctor.** ↪ Pertussis (Whooping Cough), p. 602
Fever with barking cough • **Hoarseness** • **Shortage of breath** • **Suffocating feeling at night**	Croup • Inflamed epiglottis	Keep the child calm. **Call your doctor immediately.** ↪ Croup, p. 596 ↪ Epiglottitis, p. 597
Fever with severe headaches that worsen when head is tilted forward • **Convulsions** • **Light sensitivity** • **Nausea and vomiting** • **Stiff neck**	Meningitis	**Call your doctor immediately.** ↪ Meningitis, p. 212
High fever with noticeable temperature fluctuations throughout the day	Bacteremia (sepsis)	**Call your doctor immediately.**
High fever, hot, dry skin, dizziness and nausea after exposure to the sun • **Disorientation**	Heat stroke	**Call your doctor immediately.** ↪ Heat Stroke, p. 707

COMPLAINTS AND SYMPTOMS	POSSIBLE CAUSES	WHAT TO DO
Fever and convulsions • **Disorientation**	Convulsions	Convulsions in children are not necessarily life-threatening. Try to lower fever with cold compresses to the calves. If child is under 18 months or convulsions last longer than 5 minutes, **call emergency medical services immediately.**
Fever after ingestion of poisonous substances (toothpaste, poisonous plants, detergents, etc.)	Poisoning	**Call emergency medical services immediately.** ➥ Poisoning, p. 708
Fever after an injury • **Dizziness** • **Headaches** • **Muscle cramps**	Tetanus	**Call emergency medical services immediately.** ➥ Tetanus, p. 670

BREAST PAIN AND LUMPS

Pain or lumps in the breasts are usually harmless. They may, however, indicate a developing or existing cancer.

COMPLAINTS AND SYMPTOMS	POSSIBLE CAUSES	WHAT TO DO
Painful, sensitive breasts just before your period	Symptom of menstruation	↪ Premenstrual syndrome, p. 506
Painful, sensitive breasts during pregnancy	Normal reaction to hormonal changes	The breasts enlarge as they prepare for milk production. Tightness or constriction is normal. Wear a bra for support.
Painful, swollen breasts after childbirth, until milk comes in	Preparation for lactation	Milk ducts may take a few days to fill. Letting the baby nurse at this point may expedite milk production. ↪ Nursing, p. 584
Painful nipples while nursing • **Redness**	Normal reaction • Chapped nipples	Nipples take a while to become accustomed to nursing. If symptoms increase or persist longer than two weeks, **call your doctor.** ↪ Nursing, p. 584
Painful, swollen breasts while nursing • **Fever** • **Redness**	Milk accumulation • Blocked milk duct • Breast infection	Before nursing, apply a warm, moist compress. After nursing, apply ricotta cheese to breasts. If pain persists, **call your doctor.** ↪ Mastitis (Breast Infection), p. 513 ↪ Nursing, p. 584
Painful and/or tight breasts after taking medicines	Side effects of birth control medicine menopausal estrogen-replacement therapy	Check medicine label or inserts for these substances. If you have not been alerted to these side effects, **call your doctor.** ↪ Medication Summary, p. 657
Painful, sensitive breasts • **Swelling** • **Redness** • **Fever**	Enlarged breast tissue • Breast infection	**Call your doctor.** ↪ Breast Lumps and Cysts, p. 514 ↪ Mastitis (Breast infection), p. 513
Painless lump or lumps in the breasts	Enlarged breast tissue • Breast cancer • Fibrocystic changes • Harmless cyst • Various harmless lumps	**Call your doctor.** ↪ Breast Cancer, p. 515 ↪ Breast Lumps and Cysts, p. 514

COMPLAINTS AND SYMPTOMS	POSSIBLE CAUSES	WHAT TO DO
Painful, inverted nipple • **Discharge** • **Itching**	Breast cancer	**Call your doctor.** → Breast Cancer, p. 515

BREAST GROWTH IN MEN

Breast growth in men is usually due to hormonal disorders, inner illnesses, medicines, or alcoholism.

COMPLAINTS AND SYMPTOMS	POSSIBLE CAUSES	WHAT TO DO
Breast growth in boys during puberty	Normal change in hormones	Symptoms will subside without treatment.
Breast growth resulting from bodybuilding	Muscle growth	→ Physical Activity and Sports, p. 762
Breast growth with extreme obesity	Overweight	If you need help losing weight, **call your doctor**. → Body Weight, p. 727

Breast growth after taking medicines	Side effects of medicines containing
	    male sex hormones
	    body-building aids such as
	        clostebol
	        methenolone
	        nandrolone
	        oxabolone
	        stanozolol
	    diuretics such as
	        aldosterone antagonists
		Check to see if you are taking medicines of this type. If you were not advised of possible side effects, **call your doctor.**
		→ Medication Summary, p. 657

Breast growth associated with chronic alcoholism	Side effect of alcoholism	**Call your doctor.** → Alcoholism, p. 205
Breast growth and loss of secondary sex characteristics (for example, slowing of beard growth)	Hormonal disorders • Cirrhosis of the liver	**Call your doctor.** → Cirrhosis of the Liver, p. 396
Breast growth and lumps • **On a testicle** • **Palpable lump in breast**	Testicular tumor • Breast cancer (rare, but possible in men)	**Call your doctor.** → Testicular Cancer, p. 533 → Breast Cancer, p. 515

BREATHING (RESPIRATORY) DIFFICULTIES

From a harmless stuffy nose to pneumonia (lung infection), many things can "take your breath away." **SHORTNESS OF BREATH IS ALWAYS AN EMERGENCY.**

COMPLAINTS AND SYMPTOMS	POSSIBLE CAUSES	WHAT TO DO
Difficulty breathing during strenuous activity, with no additional symptoms	Poor physical condition • Normal reaction of the body to exceptional physical exertion	If sports aren't your thing, try bringing more movement into your daily life: bicycle instead of driving, use stairs instead of elevators. ➥ Physical Activity and Sports, p. 762
Difficulty breathing with a stuffy nose • **Cough** • **Sore throat**	Common cold Nasal polyps	Colds are harmless and last only a few days. If symptoms last longer than a week and include cough and sore throat, **call your doctor.** ➥ Cold, p. 298 ➥ Flu, p. 297 ➥ Nasal Polyps, p. 301

Difficulty breathing with the sense of not getting enough air
• **Dry cough without phlegm production**
	Air passages irritated by
	  car fumes
	  cigarette smoke
	  dust
	  emotional problems
	  environmental hazards, especially
	    ozone
	  indoor pollutants, especially
	    formaldehyde in particle
	    boards and textiles
	  solvents
	  toxic substances in the work
	    environment
		Stop smoking. Try to reduce your exposure to pollutants. If symptoms persist, **call your doctor.**
		➥ Air pollution, p. 783
		➥ Health and Well-being, p. 182
		➥ Health in the Workplace, p. 789
		➥ Healthy Living, p. 772
		➥ Smoking (Nicotine), p. 754

Heavy breathing (with the feeling of still not getting enough air) cramp-like pains in the chest • **Anxiety** • **Cramped, clenched hands** • **Tingling in the fingers**	Hyperventilation, usually due to emotional factors	**Act immediately.** Calm down. Take slow, shallow breaths. Hold a bag over your mouth to increase your carbon dioxide level. If you are concerned symptoms might recur, **call your doctor.** ➥ Counseling and Psychotherapy, p. 697 ➥ Health and Well-being, p. 182

COMPLAINTS AND SYMPTOMS	POSSIBLE CAUSES	WHAT TO DO

Breathing disorders or difficulties after taking medicines	Side effect of
	  barbiturates (at high doses)
	  beta-blockers (heart medicines)
	  cough medicine containing
	    terpin hydrate
	  diet pills (over a long period)
	  epilepsy medicine containing
	  migraine medicines containing
	    methysergide (over a long
	    period)
	  strong analgesics (opiates)
	  urinary infection medicines
	    containing nitrofurantoin
	    (over a long period)
		Check medicine label or inserts for these substances. If your medicine is over-the-counter, stop taking it. If your medicine is by prescription, **call your doctor. If breathing stops, call emergency medical services immediately.**
		➥ Allergies, p. 360
		➥ Medication Summary, p. 657

Breathing problems (shortness of breath) in babies and young children after use of medicines	Side effects of
	  many nose drops and cold sprays
	  ointments and vaporizer
	    camphor
	    eucalyptus
	    medicines containing
	    menthol
		Check medicine label or inserts for these substances. If your medicine is over-the-counter, stop taking it. If your medicine is by prescription, **call your doctor.**
		➥ Medication summary, p. 657

Difficulty in breathing, cough that produces clear or yellowish-green mucus • **Fever**	• Acute airway infection • Chronic airway infection	**Call your doctor.** ➥ Acute Bronchitis, p. 305 ➥ Chronic Bronchitis, p. 306 ➥ Pneumonia, p. 310
Spasmodic breathing, especially while exhaling • **Fear of asphyxiation, anxiety** • **Severe shortage of breath, gasping**	Asthma • Allergic reaction • Emotional disorders	**Call your doctor.** ➥ Allergies, p. 360 ➥ Asthma, p. 307 ➥ Health and Well-being, p. 182
Breathing difficulty while inhaling deeply, with painful cough • **Chills** • **Rapid breathing** • **Rapidly rising fever** • **Shortness of breath** • **Subsequent spitting up of yellowish-green mucous**	Pneumonia	**Call your doctor.** ➥ Pneumonia, p. 310

COMPLAINTS AND SYMPTOMS	POSSIBLE CAUSES	WHAT TO DO
Shallow breathing, at first only during strenuous activity, but becomes increasingly frequent and chronic • **Frequent urination at night** • **Shortness of breath at night (difficulty sleeping lying down)** • **Swollen legs**	Inadequate pumping action by the heart	**Call your doctor immediately.** ↳ Congestive Heart Failure, p. 337
Breathing difficulty in children, with difficulty swallowing and sore throat • **Barking cough** • **Hoarseness** • **Muffled voice**	Inflammation of the epiglottis (at the root of the tongue) • Croup (moderate to severe)	**Call emergency medical services immediately.** ↳ Croup, p. 596 ↳ Epiglottitis, p. 597 ↳ Laryngitis (Vocal Cord Inflammation), p. 303
Sudden breathing difficulty with severe chest pain, worse when inhaling • **Coughing up blood specks** • **Preceded some days earlier by cramping in the calves**	Pulmonary embolism (blood clot in the lung)	**Call emergency medical services immediately.** ↳ Pulmonary Embolism (Pulmonary Infarction), p. 312
Sudden shortness of breath with bloody, frothy spittle	Fluid in the lungs (pulmonary edema)	**Call emergency medical services immediately.** ↳ Pulmonary Edema, p. 313
Sudden shortness of breath with severe chest pain	Collapsed lung (pneumothorax)	**Call emergency medical services immediately.** ↳ Pneumothorax (Collapsed Lung), p. 314
Sudden shortness of breath with severe pain in the heart area, spreading to neck, arms, and shoulders • **Anxiety** • **Cold sweat** • **Nausea and vomiting**	Heart attack (myocardial infarction)	**Call emergency medical services immediately.** ↳ Heart Attack (Myocardial Infarction), p. 335
Sudden inability to breathe while eating	Foreign object in the airway	**Call emergency medical services immediately.** ↳ Everyday Accidents, p. 704

CHEST PAIN AND PRESSURE

Chest pain and pressure are usually symptoms of respiratory and circulatory diseases. However, they can also indicate strained or injured muscles. Pressure in the chest with a racing heartbeat: Heart palpitations, p. 41, below.

COMPLAINTS AND SYMPTOMS	POSSIBLE CAUSES	WHAT TO DO
Chest pains that are relieved by physical exertion • **Heart palpitations or rapid heartbeat**	Stress • Abnormal heart rhythm • Emotional problems	Ask yourself what is making your heart "heavy." If symptoms persist, **call your doctor.** → Cardiac Arrythmia (Abnormal Heart Rythms), p. 339 → Counseling and Psychotherapy, p. 697 → Health and Well-being, p. 182
Pressure in the chest, especially during physical exertion on sunny summer days	Excessive ozone stress	Avoid outdoor exertion, particularly in the early afternoon.
Pressure or subtle pains in the heart area • **Fear** • **Loss of a loved one** • **Problems in a relationship** • **Unhappiness in love**	"Heartache"	If symptoms persist even after conditions change, and you cannot cope with your problems, **call your doctor.** → Counseling and Psychotherapy, p. 697 → Health and Well-being, p. 182
Pains in the side of the chest, spreading from the spinal muscles	Muscle cramps • Torn muscle	If pain persists in spite of rest and relaxation, **call your doctor.** → Back and Lower Back Pain, p. 465 → Muscle Cramps, p. 435 → Pulled, Torn Muscles, p. 437
Chest cramps with very rapid breathing and gasping for air • **Feelings of anxiety** • **Hand cramps** • **Tingling in the fingers**	Psychologically caused hyperventilation	**Act immediately.** Calm down and take slow, shallow breaths into a paper bag held over the mouth, to stabilize carbon dioxide levels. Your health is NOT in danger. If you are worried that symptoms could reappear, **call your doctor.** → Emotional Problems, p. 60 → Health and Well-being, p. 182 → Mental Health Disorders, p. 195
Chest pain after a fall or an accident	Bruised or fractured rib	**Call your doctor.** → First Aid, p. 704 → Fractures, p. 429

COMPLAINTS AND SYMPTOMS	POSSIBLE CAUSES	WHAT TO DO
Chest pain with stubborn cough and mucous phlegm • **Raised temperature** • **Shortness of breath**	Acute or chronic bronchitis	**Call your doctor.** ➟ Acute Bronchitis, p. 305 ➟ Chronic Bronchitis, p. 306

Chest or heart pains after taking medicine	Side effect of
	    many asthma medicines
	    many flu medicines
	    medicine for angina pectoris
	        containing Isosorbide,
	        at high doses
	    medicine for low blood pressure
	        containing Etilefrin or
	        Oxedrin
	    overdose of thyroid hormones
		Check medicine label or inserts for these substances. If your medicine is over-the-counter, stop taking it. If your medicine is by prescription, **call your doctor.**
		➟ Medication Summary, p. 657

Burning chest pain is made worse by leaning forward • **Severe heartburn**	Hiatal hernia	**Call your doctor.** ➟ Hernia, p. 439
Sudden chest pain radiating from spine	Irritated nerves between ribs	**Call your doctor.** ➟ Brain and Nerve Disorders, p. 210
Pains in part of the chest, with blisters on the affected areas	Shingles	**Call your doctor.** ➟ Shingles, p. 284
Chest pain and cough • **Chills** • **Rapidly rising temperature** • **Yellow or greenish-yellow mucus**	Pneumonia	**Call your doctor.** ➟ Pneumonia, p. 310
Long-term chest pain with irritating cough and unexplained weight loss	Tuberculosis • Lung cancer	**Call your doctor.** ➟ Lung Cancer, p. 314 ➟ Tuberculosis, p. 670
Chest pains and constricting, band-like pressure, particularly during periods of stress • **Rapid heartbeat and palpitations** • **Shortness of breath**	Heart asphyxiation due to constricted coronary arteries	**Call your doctor immediately.** ➟ Angina Pectoris, p. 333
Pulling or stinging chest pain with severe shortness of breath and irritated cough	Collapsed lung	**Call emergency medical services immediately.** ➟ Pneumothorax (Collapsed Lung), p. 314

COMPLAINTS AND SYMPTOMS	POSSIBLE CAUSES	WHAT TO DO
Chest constriction and severe pain extending to neck, shoulders, and left arm • **Anxiety** • **Cold sweat** • **Feeling of impending doom** • **Nausea and vomiting** • **Shortness of breath**	Heart attack	**Act immediately.** Take a nitroglycerine tablet. **Call emergency medical services immediately.** ➙ Heart Attack (Myocardial Infarction), p. 335
Sudden, severe chest pains with breathing difficulties • **Cough and spitting up of blood** • **Rapid heartbeat** • **Tightness in the calves appeared a few days before the pains**	Blood clot in the lung	**Call emergency medical services immediately.** ➙ Pulmonary Embolism, Pulmonary Infarction, p. 312

CONSTIPATION

The term "constipation" refers to very hard stools, and the inability to move the bowels over an extended period—at least three or four days. Sluggish intestines are usually caused by faulty nutrition or a lack of roughage in the diet. Sometimes constipation is a warning signal or symptom of an illness.

COMPLAINTS AND SYMPTOMS	POSSIBLE CAUSES	WHAT TO DO
Frequent constipation when the diet is low in roughage, along with a lifestyle lacking in physical activity	Sluggish intestines	Change your eating habits; drink more water; engage in more physical activity. → Constipation, p. 406 → Nutrition, p. 722 → Physical Activity and Sports, p. 762
Frequent constipation, together with the habit of postponing bowel movement to a "more convenient" time	A change of the body's natural reflexes	Get out of the habit of suppressing the urge to defecate. → Constipation, p. 406
Constipation while traveling, or accompanying changes in climate or other changes	Product of lifestyle changes	Eat light meals including lots of roughage; drink plenty of liquids. When traveling, fight the urge to snack constantly; if possible, eat regular meals. → Constipation, p. 406 → Nutrition, p. 722
Frequent constipation, along with nervousness • **Headaches** • **Sleep disorders** • **Tiredness**	Psychological issues	If constipation persists longer than four days, **call your doctor.** → Constipation, p. 406 → Health and Well-being, p. 182
Constipation during pregnancy	Common complaint during pregnancy	If unable to stimulate digestion by increasing roughage in diet, **call your doctor.** → Complaints during pregnancy, p. 570 → Constipation, p. 406

Constipation while taking medicines	Side effect of many medicines, especially
	    analgesics and antispasmodics
	    antidepressants
	    laxatives
	    medicines containing iron
	    some medicines for Parkinson's disease
	    stomach medicines containing aluminum
		If your medicine is over-the-counter and constipation was not mentioned as a possible side effect, *stop taking it.* If your medicine is by prescription and you were not made aware of the possible side effects, **call your doctor.**
		→ Medication Summary, p. 657

COMPLAINTS AND SYMPTOMS	POSSIBLE CAUSES	WHAT TO DO
Constipation in spite of increasing use of laxatives	Sluggish digestion due to laxative use	Stop taking laxatives. If this does not help, **call your doctor.** ↝ Constipation, p. 406 ↝ Nutrition, p. 722
Constipation, alternating with diarrhea **• Abdominal cramping** **• Bloating**	Irritable bowel • Diverticulitis	**Call your doctor.** ↝ Diverticulitis, p. 409 ↝ Health and Well-being, p. 182 ↝ Irritable bowel syndrome, p. 403
Constipation with painful bowel movements **• Blood in the stool**	Hemorrhoids Small fissures on anus	**Call your doctor.** ↝ Anal Fissures, p. 416 ↝ Hemorrhoids, p. 417
Constipation over a long period of time, but without any of the symptoms mentioned above **• Blood in stool** **• Bowel incontinence**	Intestinal cancer	**Call your doctor.** ↝ Colon and Rectal Cancers, p. 414
Constipation with severe abdominal pain **• Bloated stomach** **• Vomiting of intestinal contents resembling bile or stool**	Intestinal obstruction	**Call emergency medical services immediately.** ↝ Intestinal Obstruction, p. 407

COUGH

Coughing is the body's normal reaction to irritation of the air passages by foreign objects, chemicals, viruses, etc. In children, Coughing in Children, p. 48. Coughing blood: Coughing up and spitting up blood, p. 50

COMPLAINTS AND SYMPTOMS	POSSIBLE CAUSES	WHAT TO DO
Nervous coughing along with anger or aggression that may be unconscious	Repressed feelings	→ Health and Well-being, p. 182
Sudden dry cough that worsens with time	Irritation of the air passages by cigarette smoke environmental pollution toxins in the home toxins in the workplace	Stop smoking and avoid smoke-filled areas. Try to reduce the pollutants in your environment. If the cough does not improve, **call your doctor.** → Air Pollution, p. 783 → Chronic Bronchitis, p. 306 → Health in the Workplace, p. 789 → Healthy Living, p. 772 → Mood-altering Substances and Recreational drugs, p. 754
Cough appearing over a short period of time, with mucous sputum • **Fever** • **Hoarseness** • **Runny nose**	Cold • Acute bronchitis • Flu	If symptoms persist for more than a week, **call your doctor.** → Acute Bronchitis, p. 305 → Cold, p. 298 → Flu, p. 297
Dry cough appearing over a short period of time • **Fever** • **Hoarseness** • **Loss of voice**	Laryngitis	If symptoms persist for more than three days, **call your doctor.** → Laryngitis (Vocal Cord Inflammation), p. 303

COMPLAINTS AND SYMPTOMS	POSSIBLE CAUSES	WHAT TO DO

Cough or asthma attacks after the use of medicines	Side effect of
	  high blood pressure medicines
	    containing ACE inhibitors
	    captopril
	    enalapril
	  intestinal and bladder medicines
	    containing distigmine
	    mesalamine
	    neostigmine
	    pyridostigmine
	  many cough and asthma medicines
	  nonsteroidal medicines for
	    rheumatism
	  pain and flu medicines containing
	    acetylsalicylic acid (ASA)
	    mefenamic acid
	    salicylamide
		Check the medicine label or insert for these substances. If your medicine is over-the-counter, stop taking it. If your medicine is by prescription, **call your doctor.**
		↦ Medication Summary, p. 657

Recurring cough with greenish-yellow mucous sputum	Chronic bronchitis	**Call your doctor.** ↦ Chronic Bronchitis, p. 306
Coughing attacks accompanied by shortness of breath	Asthma • Chronic bronchitis	**Call your doctor.** ↦ Asthma, p. 307 ↦ Chronic Bronchitis, p. 306
Cough with mucous sputum and a sick feeling • **Chills** • **Fever** • **Shortness of breath** • **Sweating**	Acute bronchitis • Pneumonia	**Call your doctor.** ↦ Acute Bronchitis, p. 305 ↦ Pneumonia, p. 310
Coughing and fever over an extended period of time • **Night sweats** • **Weight loss**	Tuberculosis • Lung cancer	**Call your doctor.** ↦ Lung Cancer, p. 314 ↦ Tuberculosis, p. 670
Sudden severe coughing following choking	Foreign objects in air passages	Tilt head forward and try to cough up the object. If unsuccessful, **call emergency medical services immediately.** ↦ First Aid, p. 704

COUGHING IN CHILDREN

Coughing is the body's normal reaction to irritation of the air passages by foreign objects, chemicals, viruses, etc. A cough in children under six months is unusual and could signal a more serious illness. In older children it is often a symptom of a harmless cold, unless accompanied by shortness of breath.

COMPLAINTS AND SYMPTOMS	POSSIBLE CAUSES	WHAT TO DO
Nervous cough in particular situations	Attention-seeking Repressed feelings of anger or aggression	Notice in which situations the cough appears. Try to talk to the child about his or her feelings and needs. ➙ Couple and Family Therapy, p. 698 ➙ Health and Well-being, p. 182

Sudden dry cough in children who spend time in smoky or polluted environments	Irritation of the air passages from
	  cigarette smoke
	  environmental pollution
	  toxins
		Do not smoke in the presence of children. Protect your child as much as possible from all kinds of pollutants. If cough doesn't improve, **call your doctor.**
		➙ Chronic Bronchitis, p. 306
		➙ Healthy Living, p. 722

Cough in connection with a cold, especially at night	Mucus running down the pharynx (postnasal drip)	Raise child's head by adding an extra pillow. If the child has frequent colds, **call your doctor.** ➙ Colds, p. 298
Cough appearing over a short period of time, with mucous sputum • **Fever** • **Hoarseness** • **Runny nose**	Cold • Acute bronchitis	If symptoms persist longer than one week, **call your doctor.** ➙ Acute bronchitis, p. 305 ➙ Cold, p. 298 ➙ Flu, p. 297

Cough or asthma attacks after the use of medicines	Side effect of
	  intestinal and bladder medicines
	  containing
	    distigmine
	    mesalamine
	    neostigmine
	    pyridostigmine
	  many cough and asthma medicines
	  nonsteroidal antirheumatic
	    medicines
	  pain and flu medicines containing
	    acetylsalicylic acid (ASA)
	    mefenamic acid
	    salicylamide
		Check the medicine label or insert for these substances. If medicine is over-the-counter, stop giving it. If medicine is by prescription, **call your doctor.**
		➙ Medication Summary, p. 657

COMPLAINTS AND SYMPTOMS	POSSIBLE CAUSES	WHAT TO DO
Recurring cough with greenish-yellow mucous sputum	Chronic bronchitis	**Call your doctor.** ↪ Chronic Bronchitis, p. 306
Coughing attacks accompanied by shortness of breath	Asthma	**Call your doctor.** ↪ Asthma, p. 307
Barking cough and hoarseness in children	Laryngitis	**Call your doctor.** ↪ Laryngitis (Vocal Cord Inflammation), p. 303
Coughing and breathing difficulties in children • **Fever**	Bronchiolitis	**Call your doctor.** ↪ Bronchiolitis, p. 597
Attacks of coughing, short and hard, usually after an extended cold • **Whooping sounds on breathing in**	Whooping cough	**Call your doctor.** ↪ Pertussis (Whooping Cough), p. 602
Cough appearing over a short period of time, with mucous sputum and a very sick feeling • **Chills** • **Fever** • **Shortness of breath** • **Sweating**	Acute bronchitis • Pneumonia	**Call your doctor immediately.** ↪ Acute Bronchitis, p. 305 ↪ Pneumonia, p. 310
Sudden attacks of barking cough • **Hoarseness** • **Shortness of breath**	Croup	**Call your doctor immediately.** ↪ Croup, p. 596
Sudden, severe coughing after choking	Foreign object in air passages	Have child tilt head forward while trying to cough up the object. Put infants so their head is lower than their feet; and pat their back. If unsuccessful, **call emergency medical services immediately.** ↪ Choking (Children), p. 704

COUGHING UP OR SPITTING UP BLOOD

Coughing up or spitting up blood is almost always an alarm signal. Unless the blood can be attributed to a minor mouth injury, you should definitely call your doctor.

COMPLAINTS AND SYMPTOMS	POSSIBLE CAUSES	WHAT TO DO
Spitting up small amounts of blood, with pain in the mouth or tongue	Injury of the oral mucous membrane • Tongue injury	No cause for concern. If bleeding persists, **call your doctor.** → Mouth (Oral) Cavity, p. 379
Bleeding after brushing the teeth or dental work	Gum disease • Gum injury	If bleeding persists or recurs, **call your doctor.** → Gingivitis, p. 370 → Periodontal Disease, p. 371
Spitting up blood during a nosebleed	Blood draining from nose through pharynx	No cause for concern; symptoms should disappear with the nosebleed. If they persist, **call your doctor.** → Injuries, Nosebleed, p. 296
Coughing up blood • **Fever** • **Shortness of breath**	Acute bronchitis • Chronic bronchitis • Pneumonia • Tuberculosis	**Call your doctor.** → Acute Bronchitis, p. 305 → Chronic Bronchitis, p. 306 → Pneumonia, p. 310 → Tuberculosis, p. 670
Spitting up blood after an epileptic seizure	Tongue biting	**Call your doctor.** → Epilepsy, p. 216
Spitting up blood, in those who work in certain occupations • **Asbestos** • **Ceramics** • **Stone quarrying**	Hazardous dust particles in the lung	**Call your doctor.** → Healthy Living, p. 772 → Health in the Workplace, p. 789
Spitting up blood and chronic hoarseness	Cancer of the larynx	**Call your doctor.** → Vocal Chord Polyps, nodules and Laryngeal cancer, p. 304
Coughing blood with night sweats • **Chest pain** • **Weight loss**	Tuberculosis • Lung cancer	**Call your doctor.** → Lung Cancer, p. 314 → Tuberculosis, p. 670
Coughing up blood with vomiting • **Stomach pain**	Stomach or duodenal ulcer • Bleeding from varicose vein in esophagus	**Call emergency medical services immediately.** → Cirrhosis of the Liver, p. 396 → Stomach and Duodenal Ulcer, p. 389

COMPLAINTS AND SYMPTOMS	POSSIBLE CAUSES	WHAT TO DO
Coughing up blood and shortness of breath • **Chest pain** • **Swelling on side of leg**	Lung infarction	**Call emergency medical services immediately.** → Pulmonary Embolism, Pulmonary infarction, p. 312
Bloody, frothy cough and heart palpitations • **Bluish skin** • **Cold sweats** • **Rattling in lungs** • **Shortness of breath**	Pulmonary edema (fluid in the lungs)	**Call emergency medical services immediately.** → Pulmonary Edema, p. 313
Spitting blood after an accident or injury	Internal injuries	**Call emergency medical services immediately.** → First Aid, p. 704

DIARRHEA

Diarrhea is usually caused by an intestinal infection. It can also be caused by various general illnesses, medicines, nervousness, and stress.

COMPLAINTS AND SYMPTOMS	POSSIBLE CAUSES	WHAT TO DO
Diarrhea in connection with stress and fear • **Emotional problems** • **Excessive alcohol consumption**	Stress • Alcohol misuse • Emotional problems	Drink plenty of fluids (mineral water, tea). Try and get a handle on the stress in your life. If symptoms persist more than three days, **call your doctor.** ➜ Health and Well-being, p. 182 ➜ Relaxation, p. 693 ➜ Mood-altering Substances and Recreational Drugs, p. 754
Recurring diarrhea • **Feeling of fullness** • **Gas or bloating** • **Nausea**	Irritable bowel syndrome	If you repeatedly have diarrhea, **call your doctor.** ➜ Health and Well-being, p. 182 ➜ Irritable Bowel Syndrome, p. 403 ➜ Relaxation, p. 693
Diarrhea with stomach pain • **Fever** • **Headache** • **Muscle pain** • **Vomiting**	Usually a viral infection	Drink plenty of fluids (mineral water, tea) and eat only crackers, or nothing at all. If diarrhea persists after three days, **call your doctor.** ➜ Gastroenteritis, p. 599
Diarrhea that always occurs after eating certain foods • **Skin rash** • **Stomach ache**	Allergic reaction to certain foods	Identify and avoid the allergy-producing foods. If diarrhea persists, **call your doctor.** ➜ Allergies, p. 360

Diarrhea after taking certain medicines	Side effect of many medicines, especially
	  antibiotics
	  cough and asthma medicines
	  medicines containing iron
	  medicines for heart and circulatory disorders
	  medicines for stomach and intestinal disorders
	  rheumatism and gout medicines
		If your medicine is over-the-counter and does not list diarrhea as a side effect, stop taking it. If your medicine is by prescription and you were not alerted to possible side effects, **call your doctor.**
		➜ Medication Summary, p. 657

Foul-smelling diarrhea • **Pallor** • **Weight loss**	Intestine unable to process or absorb food (absorption disorder)	**Call your doctor.** ➜ Malabsorption Syndromes, p. 410 ➜ Celiac Disease, p. 411

COMPLAINTS AND SYMPTOMS	POSSIBLE CAUSES	WHAT TO DO
Diarrhea with blood and mucus in the stool • **Fever**	Inflammation of the colon	**Call your doctor.** → Crohn's Disease, p. 412 → Ulcerative Colitis, p. 411

Diarrhea when traveling in developing countries	Unfamiliar foods, living conditions, or pathogens
	    cholera
	    dysentery
	    typhoid
		Call your doctor.
		→ Gastroenteritis, p. 599
		→ Traveling, p. 717

In children, frequent diarrhea and failure to thrive	Celiac disease • Cystic fibrosis • Lactose intolerance	**Call your doctor.** → Celiac Disease, p. 411 → Cystic Fibrosis, p. 598 → Lactose Intolerance, p. 599
Diarrhea alternating with constipation over a long period of time • **Bloody stool** • **Passing stool while passing gas** • **Weight loss**	Intestinal cancer	**Call your doctor.** → Colon and Rectal Cancers, p. 414
Diarrhea with violent vomiting and stomach pain within a few hours of eating; several individuals affected simultaneously	Food poisoning, usually from spoiled foods or mushroom poisoning	Drink plenty of fluids (mineral water, tea) and eat only crackers. If diarrhea persists after three days, **call your doctor.** If mushrooms were eaten and/or symptoms intensify, **call your doctor immediately.** → Hazardous Substances in Food, p. 729

DIZZINESS

Dizziness is usually caused by a disturbance of the organs of balance and a temporary lack of oxygen supply to the brain.

COMPLAINTS AND SYMPTOMS	POSSIBLE CAUSES	WHAT TO DO

Dizziness occurring in those who are
  at high altitudes
  consuming alcohol and/or drugs
  experiencing emotional strain
  suffering from anxiety
  traveling in a car, on a bus, on a ship
  under constant stress
	Psychological factors
	• Alcohol consumption
	• Altitude sickness
	• Drug abuse
		Try to identify the causes of your dizzy spells. If unsuccessful, **call your doctor.**
		↪ Addictions and Dependencies, p. 204
		↪ Counseling and Psychotherapy, p. 697
		↪ Health and Well-being, p. 182
		↪ Travel, p. 717

Dizziness and tiredness • **Headaches** • **Pallor or redness**	High blood pressure • Anemia • Low blood pressure	If you have low blood pressure, stimulate your circulation by activity. Take a hot shower and then switch to cold water. High blood pressure often goes undiagnosed. If dizziness persists, **call your doctor.** ↪ Hypotention (Low Blood Pressure), p. 325 ↪ Hypertension (High Blood Pressure), p. 321 ↪ Anemia, p. 345

Dizziness after taking medicines
• **Headaches**
• **Lethargy**
	Indication of falling blood pressure
	• Side effect of many medicines, especially those for
	  cardiovascular disorders
	  coughs and asthma, containing
	    terpin hydrate
	    theophylline
	  many local anesthetics
	  pain and migraines, containing
	    mefenamic acid
	    methysergide
	    tilidine
	  rheumatism
		If your medicine is over-the-counter and dizziness was not mentioned as a possible temporary side effect, *stop taking it.*
		If your medicine is by prescription and you were not made aware of the possible side effects, **call your doctor.**
		↪ Medication Summary, p. 657

COMPLAINTS AND SYMPTOMS	POSSIBLE CAUSES	WHAT TO DO
Dizziness in those who are exposed to high noise levels live in a polluted environment (for example, with high carbon monoxide levels) work with harsh or toxic chemicals	Effects of pollution or noise	**Call your doctor.** → Air Pollution, p. 783 → Hearing Loss, p. 250
Dizziness with poor vision	Incorrect eyeglasses • Acute glaucoma	**Call your doctor.** → Faulty Vision, p. 229 → Glaucoma, p. 244
Dizziness with poor hearing **• Tinnitus and/or buzzing in one or both ears**	Ménière's disease	**Call your doctor.** → Ménière's Disease, p. 258
Dizziness in those over age 50 when turning head quickly or tilting head back	Wear and tear of the cervical spinal column • Circulatory disorder in brain	**Call your doctor.** → Transient Ischemic Attacks, p. 318
Dizziness or vertigo with tingling or numbness **• Brief confusion or loss of consciousness** **• Difficulty in moving part of the body, for example, a paralyzed arm** **• Slightly slurred speech**	Circulatory disorder in brain • Sign of impending stroke • Brain tumor • Multiple sclerosis	**Call your doctor immediately.** → Transient Ischemic Attacks, p. 318 → Strokes, p. 215 → Brain Tumors, p. 221 → Multiple Sclerosis, p. 220
Frequent dizziness with severe headaches **• Nausea and vomiting**	Brain tumor	**Call your doctor immediately.** → Brain Tumors, p. 221
Sudden severe dizziness **• Confusion or loss of consciousness** **• Headaches** **• Nausea and vomiting**	Intracranial hemorrhage	**Call your doctor immediately.** → Intracranial Hemorrhage, p. 214

EARACHES

Earaches can be caused by infections, inflammations, injuries, and changes in air or water pressure.

COMPLAINTS AND SYMPTOMS	POSSIBLE CAUSES	WHAT TO DO
Earaches with a clogged sensation or deafness as a result of pressure differences (in airplanes, when diving, etc.) • **Dizziness** • **Noise in the ear**	Ear cannot equalize pressure between body and environment	Swallowing hard, chewing gum or sucking on candy often helps. If complaints do not clear up within three to five hours, **call your doctor.** → Barotrauma, p. 257
Earache with clogged feeling not relieved by swallowing • **Hearing difficulties**	Blockage of ear canal by foreign object	If you cannot remove object on your own, **call your doctor.** → Cerumen (Earwax), p. 253 → Foreign Objects in the Ear, p. 253
Itching in ear after use of medicines	Symptom of allergic reaction as side effect of many ear medicines	If your medicine is over-the-counter, stop using it. If your medicine is by prescription, **call your doctor.** → Medication Summary, p. 657
Slight earache or stinging with stuffy nose • **Pressure in ear**	Cold	If condition does not clear up after three days, **call your doctor.** → Cold, p. 298 → Flu, p. 297
Strong, throbbing earache • **Eventual drainage from the ear** • **Fever** • **Hearing loss** • **Sensation of fullness or pressure in the ear**	Ear infection	**Call your doctor.** → Acute Otitis Media (Acute Ear Infection), p. 255
Earaches as result of ear infection, with pain that spreads from behind the ear • **Fever** • **Hearing loss**	Inflammation of bone behind the ear	**Call your doctor.** → Mastoiditis, p. 256
Earaches made worse by pulling on the ear lobe • **Itching in the outer ear** • **Secretion of pus**	Inflammation of the outer ear canal	**Call your doctor.** → Inflammation of the Ear Canal (Otitis Externa), p. 254
Earache with swollen cheek	Inflammation of parotid gland	**Call your doctor.** → Mumps, p. 603

COMPLAINTS AND SYMPTOMS	POSSIBLE CAUSES	WHAT TO DO
Earache with tooth or jaw pain • **Tooth inflammation** • **Uneven bite**	Temporomandibular joint disorders	**Call your doctor.** → Baby Teeth, p. 376 → Inflammation of Tooth Root Tip: Abscess, Granuloma, Fistula, Cyst p. 370 → Pulpitis, p. 368 → Temporomandibular Joint Disease (TMJ), p. 364 → Uneven Bite, p. 372
Sudden pain in the ear, with blood or discharge • **Dizziness** • **Hearing loss** • **Ringing in ear**	Perforated eardrum (punctured by cotton-tipped swab, or other accident)	**Call your doctor immediately.** → Eardrum Injury, p. 257

EARS: HEARING LOSS

Hearing loss or deterioration is not only a symptom of aging, but can also be caused by exposure to noise or chemicals. Hearing loss accompanying earaches: Earaches, p. 56.

COMPLAINTS AND SYMPTOMS	POSSIBLE CAUSES	WHAT TO DO
Hearing loss with a clogged sensation in the ear, as a result of differences in pressure (on ski lift, in airplanes, when diving, etc.) • **Noises in the ear** • **Pain in the ear** • **Tinnitus**	Ear cannot equalize pressure between body and environment	Swallowing hard or chewing gum often helps. If hearing does not improve within three to five hours, **call your doctor.** → Barotrauma, p. 257
Hearing loss with sensation of blockage in ear, not improved by swallowing • **Earache** • **Tinnitus**	Blockage of ear canal by earwax or objects	If the wax doesn't dislodge itself, or if something is lodged in the canal, **call your doctor.** → Cerumen (Earwax), p. 253 → Foreign Objectss in the Ear, p. 253
Hearing loss after a cold or respiratory illness, with pressure in ear	Eustachian tube blockage	If hearing does not improve within three days, **call your doctor.** → Eustachian Tube Disorders, p. 254

Hearing disorders after use of medicines	Side effect of
	  aminoglycosides, antibiotics used for ear and skin disorders
	  heart medicines containing
	    ethacrinic acid
	    furosemide
	  medicines for stomach and intestinal disorders containing
	    neomycin
	    paromomycin
	  muscle relaxants containing
	    quinine
		Check medicine label or insert for these substances. **Call your doctor.**
		→ Medication Summary, p. 657

Hearing loss • **Constant or intermittent pus drainage from ear**	Chronic middle-ear infection	**Call your doctor.** → Cholesteatomas, p. 258 → Chronic Otitis Media (Chronic Infection), p. 256
Hearing loss after age 60	Symptom of aging	Poor hearing can usually be improved with a proper hearing aid. **Call your doctor.** → Hearing Loss, p. 250

COMPLAINTS AND SYMPTOMS	POSSIBLE CAUSES	WHAT TO DO
Hearing loss after frequent exposure to loud noise (in workplace, listening to loud music, living near an airport, etc.)	Ear damage due to noise	**Call your doctor.** ↪ Hearing Loss, p. 250
Hearing loss and tinnitus or buzzing in one or both ears • **Dizziness** • **Nausea** • **Vomiting**	Ménière's disease • Calcification in ear	**Call your doctor.** ↪ Ménière's Disease, p. 258 ↪ Otosclerosis, p. 259
Hearing loss and tinnitus in one or both ears • **Hissing and whistling**	Acoustic trauma from loud explosion or skull injury • Circulatory disorders in inner ear • Damage from infectious illnesses (mumps, meningitis)	If you experience poor hearing following an injury, **call your doctor immediately.** ↪ Tinnitus, p. 252
Sudden hearing loss in one ear • **Pressure in the ear** • **Tinnitus**	Sudden deafness	**Call your doctor immediately**.

EMOTIONAL PROBLEMS

ANXIETY

Fear can serve a purpose: It can protect us from danger. In most cases, however, it alerts us to an overwhelming situation or intense emotional stress. Often our body language will express hidden fears we're not aware of.

COMPLAINTS AND SYMPTOMS	POSSIBLE CAUSES	WHAT TO DO
Fear in children, especially at night	Dreams • Fear of the dark • Feeling lonely and unloved • Insecurity1	Take your child's fears seriously. What may appear insignificant to an adult can be overwhelming to a child. If unreasonable fears persist, **call your doctor.** ↪ Health and Well-being, p. 182 ↪ Mental HealthDisorders, p. 195
Unreasonable, recurring fears	Emotional problems	If you are constantly depressed by fears, or they persist longer than three to four weeks, **call your doctor.** ↪ Health and Well-being, p. 182 ↪ Neurotic Behavior, p. 195
Anxiety after excessive alcohol intake or alcohol withdrawal	Alcohol abuse • Emotional problems • Side effects of withdrawal	If you frequently drink to "drown" your fears, or if your fears result from drinking, **call your doctor.** ↪ Alcohol, p. 756 ↪ Alcoholism, p. 205

Anxiety before or after mental or physical stress, caused by events such as
  birth of a child
  exams
  loss of a job
  loss of a loved one
  new and difficult challenges
  serious illness
	Normal reaction to stress	Do not suppress your fears. Discuss your feelings with others.
		If you are unable to cope with your fears, seek counseling, or **call your doctor.**
		↪ Counseling and Psychotherapy, p. 697
		↪ Health and Well-being, p. 182
		↪ Pregnancy and Birth, p. 565

Anxiety only in certain situations, such as closed-in areas, elevators, airplanes, tunnels, top floors of tall buildings, etc.	Phobias • Anxiety attack	If the fears return regularly, **call your doctor.** ↪ Neurotic Behavior, p. 195
Anxiety after a serious illness	Side effect of the illness	Serious illnesses always affect us deeply. If anxiety persists for more than three weeks, **call your doctor.** ↪ Counseling and Psychotherapy, p. 697 ↪ Health and Well-being, p. 182

COMPLAINTS AND SYMPTOMS	POSSIBLE CAUSES	WHAT TO DO

Anxiety after taking medicines	Side effect of
	  anti-psychotic (neuroleptic)
	    medicines
	  medicines promoting blood flow,
	    containing piracetam
	  tranquilizers and sedatives
	    containing benzodiazepine, if
	    taken over long periods of time
		Check medicine labels and inserts for these substances. If they are present, **call your doctor.**
		→ Medication Smmary, p. 657

Anxiety after discontinuing a long-term medicine
• **Heart palpitations**
• **Restlessness, shaking**
• **Sleep disorders**
	Withdrawal symptoms from
	  amphetamines
	  medicines containing
	    benzodiazepine
	  tranquilizers and sedatives
		Call your doctor.
		→ Medicine Dependency, p. 657

Anxiety and shaking, with extreme weight loss • **Heavy perspiration** • **Shiny, bulging eyeballs**	Overactive thyroid	**Call your doctor.** → Hyperthyroidism (Overactive Thyroid), p. 496
Anxiety with feelings of depression • **Loss of appetite** • **Sleep disorders** • **Suicidal thoughts**	Depression	**Call your doctor.** → Depression, p. 197

CONFUSION AND DISORIENTATION

If you are unable to think clearly, have sudden memory lapses, or get events, times, and places mixed up, a serious illness may be the cause. However, alcohol, drugs, and certain medicines can also lead to confusion and disorientation. Confusion and disorientation with a high fever: Fever, p. 2.

COMPLAINTS AND SYMPTOMS	POSSIBLE CAUSES	WHAT TO DO
Confusion and disorientation • **After discontinuing alcohol and drugs** • **After excessive alcohol or drug intake**	Alcohol abuse • Drug abuse • Withdrawal symptoms	If alcohol or drug intake often results in mental confusion, **call your doctor.** → Addictions and Dependencies, p. 204

COMPLAINTS AND SYMPTOMS	POSSIBLE CAUSES	WHAT TO DO

Confusion and disorientation after taking medicine	Side effect of many medicines, especially
	   psychopharmaceuticals and
	      medicines containing them
	      (for example, flu medicines)
	   some medicines for
	      circulatory disorders
	      gastrointestinal disorders
	      urinary tract disorders
		If symptoms occur, check the medicine label or insert. If the medicine is in one of the listed groups, **call your doctor.**
		→ Medication Summary, p. 657

Confusion and disorientation that occurs when not drinking enough fluids (often in older people)	Lack of fluid intake	**Call your doctor.** → Drinks, p. 736
Confusion and disorientation in older people • **Difficulty in concentrating** • **Memory lapses** • **Speech disorders**	Circulatory disorder in the brain • Alzheimer's disease	**Call your doctor.** → Alzheimer's Disease, p. 219 → Transient Ischemic Attacks, p. 214
Confusion and disorientation with chronic kidney disorders	Electrolyte imbalance	**Call your doctor.** → Kidney Failure, Uremia, p. 425
Confusion and disorientation with bad breath ("liver" odor)	Liver disorder	**Call your doctor.** → Cirrhosis of the Liver, p. 396
Confusion and disorientation in diabetics	Extremely low blood sugar	If possible, measure blood-sugar levels. **Immediate action required:** Drink some juice. If this does not help, **call your doctor immediately.** → Diabetes, p. 483
Confusion and disorientation in older people after prolonged exposure to cold, either indoors or outdoors	Hypothermia	**Call your doctor immediately.** → Hypothermia, p. 707
Confusion and memory lapses after a head injury or fall	Concussion	**Call your doctor immediately.** → Concussion, p. 211
Confusion and disorientation following a head injury (possibly days later)	Intracranial hemorrhage	**Call emergency medical services immediately.** → Intracranial Hemorrhage, p. 214

COMPLAINTS AND SYMPTOMS	POSSIBLE CAUSES	WHAT TO DO
Confusion and disorientation • **Breathing disturbances** • **Restlessness and drowsiness** • **Sweating and trembling**	Acute poisoning due to hazardous substances affecting the nerves	**Call emergency medical services immediately.** → Hazardous Substances in Food, p. 729
Confusion and disorientation with paralysis in the arms or legs • **Speech disorders** • **Dizziness** • **Visual disorders**	Stroke	**Call emergency medical services immediately.** → Stroke, p. 215

FORGETFULNESS AND DIFFICULTY CONCENTRATING

Forgetfulness is not necessarily due to age: it can be a strategy for coping with what would otherwise be too many things at once. Memory disorders can, however, be symptomatic of an illness.

COMPLAINTS AND SYMPTOMS	POSSIBLE CAUSES	WHAT TO DO
Forgetfulness and difficulty in concentrating along with a frequent lack of sleep	Exhaustion	Lack of sleep leads to difficulties in concentrating. Get plenty of rest. → Health and Well-being, p. 182
Forgetfulness and difficulty in concentrating accompanying too many responsibilities or worries	Normal reaction	Make a list of your daily responsibilities and decide what's most important. You are probably demanding too much of yourself. → Health and Well-being, p. 182
Forgetfulness of, and difficulty in concentrating on things you'd prefer to avoid	Natural defense mechanism	If you keep forgetting certain things it is likely that you want nothing to do with them. → Health and Well-being, p. 182
Forgetfulness and difficulty in concentrating accompanying strong emotions (for example, love or grief) • **Deep absorption in a certain topic or project**	Normal reaction	Intense preoccupation with emotions or issues can cause everything else to fade into the background. → Health and Well-being, p. 182
Forgetfulness that worsens with age	Age-related memory loss	Memory loss is a common sign of aging. However, the memory can be trained and stimulated. Join a discussion group, or learn something new (for example, a foreign language). → Aging, p. 606

COMPLAINTS AND SYMPTOMS	POSSIBLE CAUSES	WHAT TO DO
Forgetfulness and difficulty in concentrating after alcohol or drug use	Alcohol abuse • Drug abuse	If you often drink to excess or abuse drugs, **call your doctor.** → Addiction to Illegal Drugs, p. 208 → Alcoholism, p. 205 → Mood-altering Substances and Recreational Drugs, p. 754
Difficulty concentrating • **General exhaustion** • **Fatigue** • **Headaches**	Hazardous substances affecting the nerves	Examine your living environment, workplace and diet. **Call your doctor.** → Hazardous Substances in Food, p. 729 → Health in the Workplace, p. 789 → Healthy Living, p. 772
Memory gaps or difficulty in concentrating after serious illnesses or surgery	Normal reaction	If forgetfulness persists longer than three months, **call your doctor.**

Decrease in reactive ability and poor concentration after taking medicines	Side effect of various medicines, including
	    anti-psychotic medicines
	        (neuroleptics)
	    epilepsy medicines containing
	        carbamazepine
	        clonazepam
	    most sleep medicines and sedatives
	    muscle relaxants containing
	        memantine
	        orphenadrine
		Check medicine label or insert for these substances. If they are present, **call your doctor.**
		→ Medication Summary, p. 657

Forgetfulness and difficulty in concentrating • **Memory gaps** • **Confusion** • **Speech disorders**	Circulation disorders in the brain • Alzheimer's disease	**Call your doctor.** → Alzheimer's Disease, p. 219 → Transient Ischemic Attacks, p. 214
Forgetfulness and difficulty in concentrating, accompanied by memory gaps, after a head injury	Aftereffects of head injury	**Call your doctor.** → Cerebral Contusions, p. 212 → Concussion, p. 211
Memory loss (no desire to recollect) after a traumatic event (accident, shock, etc.)	Psychological factors	**Call your doctor.** → Counseling and Psychotherapy, p. 697

HALLUCINATIONS

If you see things, hear voices, or feel things that others don't, there is not necessarily any cause for concern. In some cases, however, hallucinations can be a symptom of physical, mental, and emotional disorders, as well as a side effect of drugs.

COMPLAINTS AND SYMPTOMS	POSSIBLE CAUSES	WHAT TO DO
Unusual perceptions shortly before falling asleep or awakening or in connection with meditation	Unknown	No cause for concern.
Hearing or seeing a recently deceased loved one	Normal grieving process	No cause for concern. If you are unwilling or unable to go through the grieving process alone, **call your doctor.** → Counseling and Psychotherapy, p. 697
Hallucinations accompanying the intake of large amounts of alcohol, drugs, or medicines	Alcohol abuse • Drug abuse • Side effect of various medicines	**Call your doctor.** → Addictions and Dependencies, p. 204 → Mood-altering Substances and Recreational Drugs, p. 754
Hallucinations accompanied by high fever	Feverish dreams	If your fever is over 104°F for more than a day, **call your doctor.**
Visual hallucinations and hearing accusing or persecuting voices	Depression • Mania • Schizophrenia	**Call your doctor.** → Depression, p. 197 → Schizophrenia, p. 201
Hallucinations • **Break into a sweat** • **Extreme restlessness** • **General confusion** • **Trembling**	Delirium tremens	**Call your doctor.** → Alcoholism, p. 205

EMOTIONAL DISORDERS

Changes in your emotional state and behavior may be the result of physiological disorders or psychological disorders.

COMPLAINTS AND SYMPTOMS	POSSIBLE CAUSES	WHAT TO DO
Perceptual disturbances and loss of orientation • **Alcohol abuse** • **Drug abuse**	Alcohol abuse • Medicine abuse • Drug abuse	If these symptoms occur frequently, **call your doctor.** → Addiction to Illegal Drugs, p. 208 → Alcoholism, p. 205 → Medication Misuse, p. 658 → Mood-altering Substances and Recreational Drugs, p. 754
Strong craving for a specific substance • **Compulsion to search it out** • **Shame following its consumption**	Dependency • Addiction	For help in overcoming addiction, **call your doctor.** → Addictions and Dependencies, p. 204
Sexual desires and imaginings you believe to be unusual	Sexual fantasies • Sexual practices • Attraction to members of the same sex	There are no prohibitions of sexual desires and fantasies as long as those involved are in agreement. If you feel drawn to members of the same sex you may be in denial of homosexual feelings. If this is an issue for you, **call your doctor.** → Counseling and Psychotherapy, p. 697 → Desire and Love, p. 537
Uncontrollable behavior • **Eye-twitching** • **Head-shaking** • **Making faces**	Tics	If you have a tic, **call your doctor.** → Neurotic Behavior, p. 195 → Tics, p. 196
Compulsive behavior in certain areas • **Cleanliness** • **Collecting** • **Compulsive tardiness** • **Finickiness** • **Greed**	Character neurosis • Compulsion	If these habits become a problem for you, **call your doctor.** → Counseling and Psychotherapy, p. 697 → Neurotic Behavior, p. 195
Anxiety associated with specific things, places, or situations • **Closed-in spaces** • **Snakes** • **Spiders** • **Wide-open spaces**	Various phobias (claustrophia, agoraphobia, etc.) • Anxiety disorders	If your fears make life difficult for you, **call your doctor.** → Counseling and Psychotherapy, p. 697 → Neurotic Behavior, p. 195

COMPLAINTS AND SYMPTOMS	POSSIBLE CAUSES	WHAT TO DO
Feelings of • **difficulty in concentrating** • **emptiness and futility** • **exhaustion** • **headaches** • **loss of appetite** • **sadness and depression** • **self-doubt and blame** • **sleeplessness** • **withdrawal into yourself**	Depression • Hazardous substances affecting the nerves	Examine your living environment, workplace, and diet. If you need help, **call your doctor.** ↪ Counseling and Psychotherapy, p. 697 ↪ Depression, p. 197 ↪ Hazardous Substances in Food, p. 729 ↪ Health and Well-being, p. 182 ↪ Health in the Workplace, p. 789 ↪ Healthy Living, p. 772 ↪ Neurotic Behavior, p. 195

Depression after taking medicine	Side effect of
	    many psychopharmaceuticals
	    medicine for Parkinson's disease
	        containing amantadine or levodopa
	    muscle relaxants containing baclofen
	    sex hormones (for example, birth-control pills)
	    various gastrointestinal medicines
	    various hypertension medicines
		Check the medicine label or insert for these substances. If they are present, **call your doctor.**
		↪ Medication Summary, p. 657

Loss of composure • **Aggressive and destructive reactions** • **Screaming** • **Trembling** • **Uncontrollable crying**	Nervous breakdown	**Call your doctor.** ↪ Counseling and Psychotherapy, p. 697 ↪ Nervous Breakdown, p. 195 ↪ Psychoses, p. 200
Perceptual disorders • **Hearing strange voices** • **Seeing things others do not** • **The sensation of being followed**	Schizophrenia	**Call your doctor.** ↪ Psychoses, p. 200 ↪ Schizophrenia, p. 201
Exaggerated moods alternating between depression and periods of unfocused, frenetic activity	Manic-depressive disorder (bipolar disorder)	**Call your doctor.** ↪ Mania, p. 199 ↪ Psychoses, p. 200

EMOTIONAL (BEHAVIORAL) DISORDERS IN CHILDREN

A child's behavior that parents call "disturbed" may actually be normal for that particular child. This may make child-rearing very difficult. Sometimes behavioral disorders can indicate that a child is reacting to unrealistic expectations on the part of parents. Take such a cry for help seriously; punishment will only make it worse.

COMPLAINTS AND SYMPTOMS	POSSIBLE CAUSES	WHAT TO DO
Extreme liveliness in a child who is always in motion • **Unable to sit still** • **Hyperactive** • **Requiring very little sleep**	Normal behavior • Nervousness • Overstimulation (for example, watching lots of TV)	"Normal behavior" varies greatly from child to child. Your child's activity level may be normal for him or her, though it may seem unusual or a nuisance to care-givers. However, if your child never seems to calm down, or often reacts excessively or impulsively, **call your doctor.** ➜ Health and Well-being, p. 182 ➜ Hyperactivity, p. 589
Petulant or rebellious behavior	Normal symptom of a certain age (for example, "terrible twos") • Autocratic, authoritarian parental behavior • Puberty	In a child under four years of age, rebellious behavior indicates the discovery of the self as a separate person. Puberty is also a time of separation and self-definition. In both cases, strictness is not appropriate. If you are accustomed to giving orders, your child's recalcitrance is a normal reaction. If you have constant problems with your child and need help, **call your doctor.** ➜ Couple and Family Therapy, p. 698
Aggressive behavior	Jealousy • Desire for attention • Insufficient or inappropriate limits • Reaction to unexpressed aggression in adults	Aggressions usually mask insecurity and reflect a desire for approval. If your child consistently exhibits aggressive behavior, **call your doctor.** ➜ Couple and Family Therapy, p. 698
Inexplicably withdrawn, unapproachable behavior	Problems the child can't or won't discuss (for example, low grades) • Drug problems • Grief • Shock (for example, from abuse)	Try to talk to your child, or find someone in whom your child can confide. If behavior persists longer than a week, **call your doctor.** ➜ Addiction to Illegal Drugs, p. 208 ➜ Counseling and Psychotherapy, p. 697 ➜ Health and Well-being, p. 182

COMPLAINTS AND SYMPTOMS	POSSIBLE CAUSES	WHAT TO DO
Frequent thumb-sucking and bed-wetting (without a bladder infection) in children older than four or five years	Desire for attention • Anxiety • Reaction to new situation • Stress	If thumb-sucking or bed-wetting persists, try to determine the cause. (Punishing or forbidding the behavior is no solution.) If you are unsuccessful, **call your doctor.** ↪ Baby Teeth, p. 376 ↪ Bed-wetting, p. 587 ↪ Couple and Family Therapy, p. 698 ↪ Health and Well-being, p. 182
Frequent sucking on or playing with hair, and nail-biting	Nervousness • Anxiety • Desire for attention • Stress (usually school-related)	If your child exhibits this behavior over a period of time, try to determine what's wrong. If you are unsuccessful and your child rarely seems happy, **call your doctor.** ↪ Couple and Family Therapy, p. 698 ↪ Health and Well-being, p. 182
Apparent unhappiness in a child who shuts himself or herself off from the environment and has little interest in playing • **Loss of appetite** • **Sleep disorders**	Depression	**Call your doctor.** ↪ Couple and Family Therapy, p. 698
Unresponsiveness and expressionlessness in a small child who acts unaware of his/her environment • **Uncommunicative (or lacks speech)**	Severe disorder (autism)	**Call your doctor.** ↪ Autism, p. 590

EYE DISORDERS

Sore eyes and deteriorating vision are caused by eye injuries, inflammations, contusions, incorrect or missing eyeglasses, medicines, pollution, illnesses, stress, and emotional issues.

COMPLAINTS AND SYMPTOMS	POSSIBLE CAUSES	WHAT TO DO
Tired eyes • **Straining to see**	Exhaustion • Emotional difficulties • Incorrect eyeglasses or contact lenses • Medicines • Stress • Unconscious squinting • Undiagnosed faulty vision	Rest your eyes, and relax with your eyes closed. If symptoms persist or reappear, **call your doctor.** ↪ Eye Strain, p. 228 ↪ Faulty Vision, p. 229

Dry eyes
• **Stinging**
• **Sensation of a foreign object**
	Overheated rooms
	• Irritation from
	    air conditioning
	    drafts
	    dust
	    perfume
	    smoke
	• Medicines (for example, birth-control pills)
		Glasses can protect the eyes from drafts. If symptoms persist or recur, **call your doctor.**
		↪ Eye Strain, p. 228

Teary eyes
• **Red eyes**
	Overexertion
	• Allergic reaction
	• Blocked tear duct
	• Mechanical irritations
	    contact lenses
	    dust
	    eyelashes
	• Pollutants, especially
	    car fumes
	    cigarette smoke
	    formaldehyde
	    ozone
		If symptoms persist more than a few days, **call your doctor.**
		↪ Blocked Tear Duct, p. 240
		↪ Eye Strain, p. 228

Itchy eyes • **Red eyes**	Incorrect eyeglass prescription • Allergic reaction • Eyelid inflammation (blepharitis) • Incompatible contact lenses • Irritation from contact-lens solution • Irritation from cosmetics • Medicines	If symptoms persist more than a few days, **call your doctor.** ↪ Allergies, p. 360 ↪ Contact Lenses, p. 236 ↪ Eyelid Inflammation, p. 239 ↪ Faulty Vision, p. 229

COMPLAINTS AND SYMPTOMS	POSSIBLE CAUSES	WHAT TO DO
Swollen eyelids	Stye • Chalazion (tarsal cyst, cyst on the eyelid) • Contusions (for example, a black eye) • Inflammations on or in the eye • Kidney disorders	If symptoms persist for more than a few days, **call your doctor.** ↪ Acute or Chronic Glomerulonephritis, p. 422, 423 ↪ Blocked Tear Duct, p. 240 ↪ Chalazion (Tarsal Cyst, Cyst on the Eyelid), p. 238 ↪ Stye, p. 238
Red eyes • **Itching** • **Mild pain** • **Worsening eyesight**	Fatigue from very detailed close-up work • Allergy • Conjunctivitis • Conjunctival hemorrhage • Faulty vision • Incorrect glasses or contact lenses • Inflamed tear ducts • Irritation of the conjunctiva (by dust, wind, light) • Keratitis, corneal inflammation	If symptoms persist more than one day or additional symptoms appear, **call your doctor.** ↪ Allergies, p. 360 ↪ Blocked Tear Duct, p. 240 ↪ Conjunctivitis, p. 240 ↪ Keratitis (Corneal Iinflammation), p. 241 ↪ Eye Strain, p. 228 ↪ Faulty Vision, p. 229
Gluey, sticky eyes • **Itching** • **Pain** • **Redness**	Eyelid inflammation (blepharitis) • Conjunctival disorders • Corneal herpes infection	Cool, moist compresses on the closed eyes will help alleviate symptoms. If they persist more than three days, **call your doctor.** ↪ Conjunctivitis, p. 240 ↪ Eyelid Inflammation (Blepharitis), p. 239 ↪ Keratitis (Corneal Inflammation), p. 241
Yellow pigmentation of the whites of the eyes	Jaundice	**Call your doctor.** ↪ Jaundice, p. 393
Protruding eyeballs	Inflammations • Bleeding after an accident • Cancer • Thyroid disorders	**Call your doctor.** ↪ Cancer, p. 470 ↪ Graves' Disease, p. 496

EYE PAIN

Painful eyes and vision are often alarm signals. These symptoms may be caused by serious eye disorders; they could also indicate less serious general ailments.

COMPLAINTS AND SYMPTOMS	POSSIBLE CAUSES	WHAT TO DO
Painful eyes • **Headache**	Changeable weather • Weather sensitivity	If symptoms recur regularly, **call your doctor.** ⤳ Health and well-being, p. 182
Painful eyes • **Itching** • **Stinging**	Insufficient tear production • Hay fever	Avoid air-conditioned rooms, car ventilation fans, wind, tobacco smoke, perfume. If symptoms recur, **call your doctor.** ⤳ Allergies, p. 360 ⤳ Eye Strain, p. 228 ⤳ Sinusitis, p. 300

Painful eyes after taking medicines	Side effect of
	  incompatible eye drops
	  many anti-inflammatory
	    medicines (steroids) for
	    rheumatism, asthma,
	    and allergies after long-term
	    use
	  migraine medicine containing
	    pizotyline
		Check the medicine label or insert for these substances. If your medicine is over-the-counter, stop taking it. If your medicine is by prescription, **call your doctor.**
		⤳ Medication Summary, p. 657

Eye pain made worse by bending the head forward, extending into forehead and cheeks • **Pressure sensitivity**	Sinus infection	**Call your doctor.** ⤳ Sinusitis, p. 300
Painful eyes • **Pain in the upper jaw**	Facial neuralgia	**Call your doctor.** ⤳ Neuralgia, p. 224
Eye pain when moving eyes	Onset of multiple sclerosis	**Call your doctor.** ⤳ Multiple Sclerosis, p. 220
Painful eyes with deterioration of eyesight	Injury or inflammation of the cornea • Acute glaucoma • Inflammation of the optic nerve • Iris inflammation	**Call your doctor.** ⤳ Glaucoma, p. 244 ⤳ Keratitis (Corneal Inflammation), p. 241

COMPLAINTS AND SYMPTOMS	POSSIBLE CAUSES	WHAT TO DO
Painful, red eyes • **Cramping eyelid** • **Deterioration of eyesight** • **Tears**	Conjunctivitis • Burns of the eyeball • Conjunctival hemorrhage • Corneal inflammation • Foreign bodies in the eye • Iris inflammation	**Call your doctor immediately.** → Conjunctivitis, p. 240 → Keratitis (Corneal Inflammation), p. 241
Painful, red eyes • **Deteriorating eyesight** • **Headache** • **Nausea to the point of vomiting**	Acute glaucoma	**Call your doctor immediately.** → Glaucoma, p. 244

EYES: VISUAL DISTURBANCES

Visual disturbances include distorted, veiled, blurred, or double vision, and often result from harmless eye fatigue. In rare cases, they can also indicate a serious eye disorder. Emotional problems also can distort your vision.

COMPLAINTS AND SYMPTOMS	POSSIBLE CAUSES	WHAT TO DO
Shining, shimmering dots in the field of vision	Normal vision • Pressure on the eyes • Onset of detached retina	These symptoms are usually harmless. If they persist longer than one day, **call your doctor.** → Retinal Detachment, p. 247
Lightning and shining zig-zag patterns in the field of vision • **Headaches**	Migraine	These symptoms pass on their own. If you suffer from frequent migraines, **call your doctor.** → Migraine, p. 225

Disturbed vision after taking medicines	Side effect of a large number of medicines, primarily
	    acne medicines
	    birth-control pills
	    cold or flu medicines
	    many anti-depressant medicines
	    many anti-inflammatory
	        medicines (steroids) after
	        long-term use
	    many muscle relaxants
	    many rheumatism medicines
	    most eye medicines
		If your medicine is over-the-counter and does not list visual disturbances as a side effect, *stop taking it.*
		If your medicine is by prescription and you were not alerted about possible side effects, **call your doctor.**
		→ Medication Summary, p. 657

Defective night vision	Myopia • Vitamin A deficiency • Sign of aging • Jaundice	Be careful driving at night. If symptoms worsen, **call your doctor.** → Night Blindness, p. 235

COMPLAINTS AND SYMPTOMS	POSSIBLE CAUSES	WHAT TO DO
Blurred vision	Faulty vision • Cataracts • Corneal disorders • Diabetes • Disorders of the optic nerve • Incorrect glasses or contact lenses • Nervous disorders • Retinal disorders	**Call your doctor.** ↪ Blood Vessel Disorders of the Retina, p. 246 ↪ Cataract, p. 243 ↪ Diabetes, p. 483 ↪ Faulty Vision, p. 229 ↪ Keratitis (Corneal Inflammation), p. 241 ↪ Macular Degeneration, p. 246 ↪ Multiple Sclerosis, p. 220 ↪ Retinal Detachment, p. 247
Seeing rainbow rings around light sources	Glaucoma	**Call your doctor.** ↪ Glaucoma, p. 244
Disturbed vision and extreme light-sensitivity • **Neck stiffness** • **Skin rash**	Measles • Meningitis	**Call your doctor immediately.** ↪ Measles, p. 601 ↪ Meningitis, p. 212
Sudden poor vision or loss of sight in one eye	Closing of the retinal artery • Acute glaucoma • Disorder or injury of the optic nerve (due to inflammation or other factors) • Inflammation of blood vessels • Retinal hemorrhage	**Call your doctor immediately.** ↪ Blood Supply Disorders of the Retina, p. 246 ↪ Glaucoma, p. 244 ↪ Polymyalgia Rheumatica, p. 461
Sudden poor vision or loss of sight in both eyes	Disorders of blood vessels or hemorrhages in the field of vision • Paralysis of lens muscle	**Call your doctor immediately.** ↪ Poor Circulation, p. 326
Blurred vision • **Pain** • **Redness** • **Tears**	Inflammation of the iris	**Call your doctor immediately.**
Double vision	Multiple sclerosis • Brain tumor • Intracranial hemorrhage • Myasthenia gravis	**Call your doctor immediately.** ↪ Brain Tumors p. 221 ↪ Intracranial Hemorrhage, p. 214 ↪ Multiple Sclerosis, p. 220 ↪ Myasthenia Gravis, p. 438

COMPLAINTS AND SYMPTOMS	POSSIBLE CAUSES	WHAT TO DO
Worsening vision with part of the visual field missing, or sudden blindness	Retinal disorders • Alcoholism • Chronic glaucoma • Diabetes • Disorders of the optic nerve • Stroke	**Call your doctor immediately.** ➵ Blood Supply Disorders of the Retina, p. 246 ➵ Diabetes, p. 483 ➵ Glaucoma, p. 244 ➵ Macular Degeneration, p. 246 ➵ Retinal Detachment, p. 247 ➵ Retinitis Pigmentosa (Hereditary Retina Disorders), p. 248 ➵ Stroke, p. 215

FAINTING, LOSS OF CONSCIOUSNESS

Fainting and loss of consciousness can be caused by fear, weakness, heat, or humid, oppressive air. In some cases, loss of consciousness can signal serious illness or a life-threatening situation. A fainting spell lasting more than one minute is always an emergency and calls for immediate, urgent intervention.

COMPLAINTS AND SYMPTOMS	POSSIBLE CAUSES	WHAT TO DO
Fainting after reclining for a while, then getting up abruptly	Cardiovascular disorder	No cause for concern. Stretch your legs before getting up and rise slowly. If fainting spells recur, **call your doctor.**
Fainting that recurs with no identifiable cause • **Lethargy** • **Pallor**	Emotional problems • Anemia	**Call your doctor.** → Anemia, p. 345 → Health and Well-being, p. 182
Fainting • **After a shocking or traumatic event** • **During fright or panic** • **In a hot, humid environment**	Cardiovascular disorder	If fainting spell lasts longer than one minute, **call your doctor immediately.**
Fainting after many gasping breaths • **Muscle cramps (hands in claw-like position)**	Hyperventilation due to psychological factors	Hold a paper bag over your mouth to increase carbon dioxide level. If fainting spell lasts longer than one minute, **call your doctor immediately.** → Counseling and Psychotherapy, p. 697 → Health and Well-being, p. 182
Fainting after prolonged exposure to heat or sun • **High fever** • **Nausea** • **Vomiting**	Heatstroke • Sunstroke	**Immediate action required.** Move victim into shade, loosen clothes, and apply cool compress to forehead. **Call your doctor immediately.** → First Aid, p. 704 → Heatstroke, p. 707 → Sunstroke, p. 707

COMPLAINTS AND SYMPTOMS	POSSIBLE CAUSES	WHAT TO DO
Loss of consciousness after excessive alcohol consumption or after ingesting or breathing poisonous substances	Symptoms of poisoning	If the victim cannot be awakened, **call emergency medical services immediately.** → Alcoholism, p. 205 → Fainting and Loss of Consciousness, p. 76 → Poisoning, p. 708

Loss of consciousness after
   accident
   electric shock
   injury
	Concussion
	• Arrhythmia
	• Brain injury
		Call emergency medical services immediately.
		→ Cerebral Contusion, p. 212
		→ Concussion, p. 211
		→ Electrical Injuries, p. 708
		→ Fainting and Loss of Consciousness, p. 76

Fainting
   after a coughing fit
   after extremely strong pain
	Circulatory disorder
	• Circulatory failure
		If fainting spell lasts longer than one minute, **call emergency medical services immediately.**
		→ Fainting and Loss of Consciousness, p. 76

Fainting with convulsions and foaming mouth	Epilepsy	**Immediate action required.** If the seizure lasts longer than three minutes, or recurs, **call emergency medical services immediately.** Protect the patient from injury. Do not hold the patient tightly or force anything between the teeth to prevent tongue biting. Much sleep is required after the seizure. → Epilepsy, p. 216
In children: fainting and muscle cramping with high fever	Febrile seizures	Febrile seizures in children are not life-threatening. Try to bring the fever down using cold compresses. If the child is under 18 months of age, or the seizure lasts longer than 5 minutes or recurs, **call emergency medical services immediately.**
Fainting with distinctive head movements (head twisting or eyes looking back and up)	Cerebrovascular accident	If fainting spell lasts longer than one minute, **call emergency medical services immediately.** → Fainting and Loss of Consciousness, p. 76

COMPLAINTS AND SYMPTOMS	POSSIBLE CAUSES	WHAT TO DO
Loss of consciousness in diabetics who inject insulin	Critically low blood–sugar level	**Immediate action required.** If possible, measure blood-sugar level. If the victim wakes, give juice. Give glucagon injection, if available. If consciousness is not restored within five minutes of glucagon injection, **call emergency medical services immediately.** → Diabetes, p. 483

Loss of consciousness after taking medicines
Skin rash
• **Fever**
• **Pallor**
• **Perspiring**
• **Shortness of breath**
	State of shock as side effect of many medicines, including
	  analgesics
	  antispasmodics
	  flu medicines containing
	    aminopyrine
	    antipyrone
	    dipyrone
	    propyphenazone
	  injected local anesthetics
	    benzocaine
	    lidocaine
	    procaine
	  migraine medicines
		Call emergency medical services immediately.
		→ First aid, p. 704
		→ Medication Summary, p. 657

Loss of consciousness preceded by markedly quicker, slower or irregular pulse	Cardiac dysrhythmia • Tachycardia	**Call emergency medical services immediately.** → Fainting and Loss of Consciousness, p. 76 → Heart block, p. 341
Loss of consciousness • **Cold swea** • **Racing pulse**	Shock due to various disorders	**Call emergency medical services immediately.** → Fainting and Loss of Consciousness, p. 76

Loss of consciousness and partial paralysis, preceded by
  confusion
  speech disorders
	Stroke	**Call emergency medical services immediately.**
		→ First Aid, p. 704
		→ Stroke, p. 215

FATIGUE

If you constantly feel fatigued or exhausted, even when you haven't done any kind of work, the lack of physical activity, poor nutrition, excessive body weight, or even the weather may be responsible. Perhaps a change in your lifestyle will restore your energy. However, this drained, worn-out feeling can also be a sign of a serious illness.

COMPLAINTS AND SYMPTOMS	POSSIBLE CAUSES	WHAT TO DO
Fatigue after overworking or missing sleep	The body's normal reaction	Get plenty of sleep. Make time for relaxation. → Health and Well-being, p. 182 → Relaxation, p. 693
Fatigue that occurs when there has been no physical exercise • **A diet high in fats or limited in variety** • **Overweight**	Lack of exercise • Poor nutrition • Excessive body weight	Work on bringing more physical activity into your life. Change your eating habits. Gain control of your weight. → Body Weight, p. 727 → Exercise and Sports, p. 762 → Healthy Nutrition, p. 722
Fatigue during changing weather • **Headaches** • **Irritability**	Weather sensitivity	Respect your body's needs and slow down. Cancel all appointments that are not absolutely necessary. → Health and Well-being, p. 182 → Relaxation, p. 693
Exhaustion or fatigue while dieting	Side effects of the diet • Over-stressed metabolism • Toxins released from metabolism of fats	Many diets are unbalanced and therefore unhealthy. Get the facts. → Body Weight, p. 727
Exhaustion and/or fatigue after drinking large quantities of alcohol heavy smoking taking drugs	Side effects of substance abuse	Reduce your alcohol consumption. Stop smoking. Take no other drugs. If you are unable to control your addictions, **call your doctor.** → Addictions and Dependencies, p. 204 → Mood-altering Dubstances and Recreational Drugs, p. 754
Fatigue in certain situations or with specific people • **A lack of incentive** • **A sense of oppression** • **Feelings of reluctance**	The body's defense reaction against mental or emotional discomfort • Excessive demands or expectations by others • Inner conflicts • Repressed conflicts	Notice what seems to trigger your fatigue. Pay attention to your own needs. If you are unable to cope with your problems, **call your doctor.** → Counseling and Psychotherapy, p. 697 → Emotional Problems, p. 60 → Health and Well-being, p. 182 → Mental Health Disorders, p. 195

COMPLAINTS AND SYMPTOMS	POSSIBLE CAUSES	WHAT TO DO

Dizziness and fatigue after taking medicines	Side effects of a large number of medicines, especially
	  antihistamines
	  benzodiazepines, including
	    many cold medicines
	    many cough medicines
	    many flu medicines
	    most allergy medicines
	    most sedatives and sleeping medicines
	    several migraine medicines
		If your medicine is over-the-counter and does not list fatigue as a side effect, *stop taking it.*
		If your medicine is by prescription and you were not alerted about possible side effects, **call your doctor.**
		→ Medication Summary, p. 657

Fatigue after taking medicines
• **Dizziness**
• **Headaches**
	May indicate a drop in blood pressure
	• A side effect of many medicines, especially
	  cough and cold medicine
	  hypertension medicine
	  sleeping medicines and sedatives
	  some motion sickness and nausea medicine
		If your medicine is over-the-counter and does not list lowered blood pressure as a side effect, *stop taking it.*
		If your medicine is by prescription and you were not alerted about possible side effects, **call your doctor.**
		→ Medication Summary, p. 657

Fatigue upon awakening • **Dizziness when standing up quickly** • **Headache**	Low blood pressure	Stimulate your circulation through regular exercise. Switch between warm and cool showers, or take a cold shower. Drink plenty of liquids. If low blood pressure persists, **call your doctor.** → Hypotension (Low Blood Pressure), p. 325
Fatigue with a general feeling of low spirits • **Raised temperature or fever**	Onset of an illness • Various inflammations	If complaints persist for more than three days, **call your doctor.**
Exhaustion or fatigue after recovery from an illness, or accompanying a chronic disease	Side effect of the ailment	Take it easy until you are feeling better. If you suffer from a chronic disease and are unusually tired, **call your doctor.**

Fatigue with weight loss, when not dieting	Emotional problems
	• Cancer
	• Various general ailments, especially
	  intestinal illness
	  tuberculosis
	  ulcer
		If the tiredness and weight loss persist longer than two weeks, **call your doctor.**
		→ Emotional Problems, p. 60
		→ Health and Well-being, p. 182
		→ Mental Health Disorders, p. 195

COMPLAINTS AND SYMPTOMS	POSSIBLE CAUSES	WHAT TO DO
Fatigue after moving into a new home or work space, or making major renovations • **Inability to concentrate**	Indoor pollutants	If your symptoms worsen and persist more than two weeks, **call your doctor.** → Health in the workplace, p. 789 → Healthy Living, p. 772
Fatigue over a long period of time • **Feelings of emptiness or meaninglessness** • **Headache or other physical complaints** • **Listlessness** • **Self-absorption, retreat from the world** • **Sleep disorders**	Depression	If you are not already receiving medical treatment for your depression, **call your doctor.** → Depression, p. 197 → Health and Well-being, p. 182 → Counseling and Psychotherapy, p. 697
Fatigue • **Feeling of impending collapse** • **Pallor** • **Weakness**	Anemia	**Call your doctor.** → Anemia, p. 345
Fatigue • **Feelings of cold** • **Weight gain**	Hypothyroidism	**Call your doctor.** → Hypothyroidism (Underactive Thyroid), p. 495

FOOT PAIN

If your feet just won't carry you any more, maybe you've been putting too many demands on them. Causes of foot pain also include injury from something you stepped on, wear and tear on joints, and various illnesses.

COMPLAINTS AND SYMPTOMS	POSSIBLE CAUSES	WHAT TO DO
Foot pain after prolonged standing or walking • **Overweight** • **Uncomfortable shoes**	Fatigue • Ill-fitting shoes • Overweight	Wear only shoes that fit correctly and give your feet plenty of room. Put your feet up. Take a foot bath. → Body Weight, p. 727 → Feet, p. 443
Foot pain from incorrect foot placement	Various incorrect placements, including broad feet flat feet	**Call your doctor.** → Feet, p. 443
Pain in the sole of the foot • **Infected area** • **Raised, horny callus** • **Small callus**	Plantar wart • Callus • Corn • Foreign object (for example, glass sliver)	If symptoms persist longer than one week or you cannot remove the foreign object, **call your doctor.** → Calluses, p. 266 → Corns, p. 266 → Warts, p. 267
Itching feet • **Between the toes** • **Cracked, reddened, peeling skin**	Fungus ("athlete's foot")	Treat the affected areas with fungus medicine for two to three weeks. If symptoms persist, **call your doctor.** → Athlete's Foot, p. 265
Pain in the toes • **Red, infected cuticle**	Cuticle infection	Take a warm foot bath with chamomile tea. If the infection does not lessen, **call your doctor.** → Paronychia, p. 294
Foot pain • **Tingling in arms and legs after taking medicine**	Nerve disorders as side effects of prolonged use of vitamin B6 rheumatism medicine containing chloroquine tuberculosis medicine containing isoniazide methaniazide	Check the medicine label or insert for these ingredients. If the symptoms are present, **call your doctor.** → Medication Summary, p. 657
Ankle pain, slight or severe, brief or prolonged • **Swelling**	Sprained ankle	Keep the foot still, and apply cold compresses. If the joint is still swollen and sore after three days, **call your doctor.** → Sprains and Strains, p. 447

COMPLAINTS AND SYMPTOMS	POSSIBLE CAUSES	WHAT TO DO
Pain when moving the ankles, increasing with advancing age • **Simultaneous pain in knees and hips**	Deterioration	**Call your doctor.** → Arthritis, p. 452
Pain, swelling, and redness in ankles • **Fever** • **Pain in other joints**	Rheumatism • Gout (usually affects the big toe)	**Call your doctor.** → Gout, p. 454 → Inflamed joints, p. 449 → Rheumatism (Disorders of Joints and Connective Tissue), p. 449 → Rheumatoid Arthritis, p. 455 → Systemic Lupus Erythematosus, p. 460
Pain in the heels and the back, especially in young men	Ankylosing spondylitis	**Call your doctor.** → Ankylosing Spondylitis, p. 459
Foot pain • **Tingling and burning in the legs**	Nerve disorders in diabetics and alcoholics	**Call your doctor.** → Alcoholism, p. 205 → Diabetes, p. 483 → Peripheral Nerve Disorders, p. 224
Pain in the foot after a fall or accident • **Inability to use the foot** • **Incorrect position of the foot** • **Swelling**	Pulled or torn tendon or ligament • Bone fracture • Twisted joint bones	**Call your doctor immediately.** → First aid, p. 704 → Fracture, p. 429 → Pulled or Torn Ligament, p. 441 → Pulled or Torn Tendon, p. 441 → Sprains and Strains, p. 447

SWOLLEN FEET

Swollen feet are not only a sign of inflammation or injury to the feet, but can also be a warning signal of other illnesses.

COMPLAINTS AND SYMPTOMS	POSSIBLE CAUSES	WHAT TO DO
Swollen feet • **After prolonged standing or walking** • **In extreme heat**	Fatigue • Swelling caused by heat	Put your feet up. Take a cool foot bath. → Water Therapy, p. 692
Swollen feet with varicose veins • **Aches or pains**	Symptom of varicose veins	If feet are frequently swollen, **call your doctor.** → Varicose Veins, p. 328

COMPLAINTS AND SYMPTOMS	POSSIBLE CAUSES	WHAT TO DO

In women, swollen feet
   before and during
      menstruation
   during pregnancy
   while taking birth-control
      medicines
	Water retention
	• Normal symptom
		If there are additional complaints, **call your doctor.**
		→ Birth-control Pills, p. 556
		→ Complaints During Pregnancy, p. 570
		→ Menstruation, p. 506

Swollen feet during pregnancy, with sudden weight gain in spite of not eating more • **Dizziness** • **Headaches**	Pregnancy-related high blood pressure	**Call your doctor.** → Pregnancy-related High Blood Pressure (Pre-eclampsia), p. 574
Swollen ankle after an injury (possibly months later)	Stretched or pulled ligaments	**Call your doctor.** → Sprains and Strains, p. 447
Unexplained swelling in both ankles (no injury or strain) • **Shortness of breath**	Weak heart	**Call your doctor.** Congestive Heart Failure, p. 337
Swollen ankles and eyelids exhaustion • **Cloudy urine** • **Fever** • **Headaches**	Kidney inflammation	**Contact your doctor.** → Acute Glomerulonephritis, p. 422

HAIR
EXCESSIVE HAIR GROWTH IN WOMEN

Excessive hair growth in women is seldom a sign of illness. However, an unusual increase in body hair could indicate a disorder.

COMPLAINTS AND SYMPTOMS	POSSIBLE CAUSES	WHAT TO DO
Thick hair growth beginning at a young age, possibly with similar cases among female relatives	Hereditary predisposition	No cause for concern, fashion need not dictate how you look. Hair can also be bleached or removed.
Hair growth after age 45, especially on upper lip and chin	Hormonal changes	No cause for concern. If unusual body hair growth bothers you, **call your doctor.** → Menopause, p. 510

Excessive hair growth after taking medicines	Side effect of
	    epilepsy medicines containing
	        mephenytoin
	        phenytoin
	    infertility medicines containing
	        danazol
	    male sex hormones, such as
	        clostebol
	        methenolone
	        mesterolone,
	        methyltestosterone
	        nandrolone
	        testosterone
	    medicines for menstrual disorders
	    containing
	        lynestrenol
	        medrogestone
	        norethindrone
		Check medicine labels and inserts for these substances. If you were not made aware of these side effects, **call your doctor.**
		→ Medication Summary, p. 657

Excessive hair growth • **Absence of menstruation** • **Lowered voice tone** • **Masculine characteristics**	Disorder of the pituitary gland • Disorder of the adrenal glands • Disorder of the ovaries	**Call your doctor.** → Acromegaly, p. 501 → Cushing's Syndrome, p. 503 → Fallopian Tubes and Ovaries, p. 525
Thick hair growth accompanying malnutrition	Malnutrition • Anorexia	**Call your doctor.** → Eating Disorders, p. 202

HAIR LOSS

Finding a few hairs in your comb is usually no cause for concern; "hair loss" refers to thinning hair or bald spots.

COMPLAINTS AND SYMPTOMS	POSSIBLE CAUSES	WHAT TO DO
Especially in men, hairline slowly receding with age, beginning at temples and crown	Heredity • Normal aging process	There is no miracle cure. → Hair Loss, Baldness, p. 290
Hair loss after harsh treatment • **Dyes and colorings** • **Hot blow dryers** • **Perms** • **Strong shampoos**	Damaged hair from mistreatment	Avoid harsh treatments and hair loss will stop. → Hair and Beard Care, p. 289
In women, hair loss after giving birth	Hormonal changes	No need for concern. Hair loss will stop within a few months.
Hair loss some time after a serious infectious illness	Symptom of the illness	No need for concern. Hair loss will stop within a few months.
Hair loss in connection with alcoholism and liver diseases	Symptom of the disease	If you are not already in medical treatment, **call your doctor.** → Alcoholism, p. 205 → Cirrhosis of the Liver, p. 396
Sudden, heavy hair loss	Hormone disorder	**Call your doctor.** → Hair Loss, Baldness, p. 290 → Menopause, p. 510
Sudden, circular hair loss	The disease called "alopecia areata"	**Call your doctor.** → Alopecia Areata, p. 291
Hair loss after use of medicine	Side effect of 　blood clotting medicines 　containing 　　acenocoumarol 　　heparin 　　phenprocoumon 　chemotherapy for cancer 　treatment 　dandruff medicine containing 　　cadmium sulfide 　　selenium sulfide 　epilepsy medicines containing 　　valproic acid 　skin medicines containing 　　etretinate 　thyroid medicines containing 　　carbimazole 　　methimazole	Check the medicine label or insert for these substances. If your medicine is over-the-counter, *stop taking it.* If your medicine is by prescription, **call your doctor.** → Medication Summary, p. 657

COMPLAINTS AND SYMPTOMS	POSSIBLE CAUSES	WHAT TO DO
Hair loss and brittle hair • **Brittle nails** • **Pallor** • **Tiredness**	Anemia	**Call your doctor.** → Anemia, p. 345
Hair loss • **Aching joints, especially fingers** • **Fever** • **Red, slightly scaly spots, especially on face, nose, and cheekbones**	Connective tissue disorders	**Call your doctor.** → Systemic Lupus Erythematosus, p. 460
Hair loss with bald spots • **Pus blisters** • **Scalp inflammations** • **Scaly scalp**	Fungal infections	**Call your doctor.**

HEART PALPITATIONS

Palpitations of the heart—when the heart races, seems to skip a beat, or the rhythm is irregular—can be symptoms of a serious disorder.

COMPLAINTS AND SYMPTOMS	POSSIBLE CAUSES	WHAT TO DO
Palpitations or racing heart after physical exertion	Normal reaction	No need for concern. Get some rest.
Palpitations or rapid heartbeat after drinking 　　**heavy drinking** 　　**heavy smoking** 　　**large quantities of coffee** 　　　　**or tea** 　　**taking drugs**	Misuse of alcohol, nicotine, caffeine and drugs	Drink less alcohol. Stop smoking. Reduce coffee, tea, or cola consumption. Stop taking other drugs. If this creates difficulties, **call your doctor.** ➙ Addictions and Dependencies, p.204 ➙ Mood-altering Substances and Recreational Drugs, p.754
Palpitations, racing heart or irregular heartbeat, accompanying stress or emotional problems • **Anxiety** • **Sensation of pressure in the chest**	Stress • Emotional problems • Heart rhythm disorders	Notice what situations bring on symptoms. Try to avoid them, or work on your problems. If unsuccessful or if irregular heartbeat recurs, **call your doctor.** ➙ Cardiac Arrhythmias (Abnormal Heart Rhythms), p. 339 ➙ Counseling and Psychotherapy, p. 697 ➙ Health and Well-being, p. 182 ➙ Tachycardia, p. 340
Rapid heartbeat with fever	Symptom of fever	If you are not already in medical treatment, **call your doctor.**
Racing heart and paleness • **Exhaustion** • **Difficulty in concentrating** • **Headaches**	Anemia	If you are not already in medical treatment, **call your doctor.** ➙ Anemia, p. 345
Palpitations after discontinuing long-term medicines • **Anxiety** • **Restlessness and trembling** • **Sleep disorders**	Symptoms of withdrawal from sleep medicines and sedative medicines containing 　　appetite suppressants 　　codeine 　　diazepam 　　oxazepam 　　phenobarbital 　　tetrazepam	**Call your doctor.** ➙ Medication Dependencies, p. 206

COMPLAINTS AND SYMPTOMS	POSSIBLE CAUSES	WHAT TO DO

Irregular pulse (irregular heart-beat, palpitations) after taking medicines	Side effect of many medicines, especially
	    appetite suppressants
	    cold medicines containing
	        ephedrine
	        phenylpropanolamine
	        phenylephrine
	        pseudoephedrine
	    flu medicines containing
	        etilefrine
	        ephedrine
	        methylephedrine
	        norfenefrine
	    many antispasmodics
	    many cough and asthma medicines
	    many heart medicines (glycosides) in excessive doses
	    most heart-rhythm disorder medicines
	    many high blood pressure and angina pectoris medicines
	    many low blood pressure medicines
	    thyroid hormones in excessive doses
		If your medicine is over-the-counter and irregular pulse (palpitations) was not mentioned as a possible side effect, *stop taking it.*
		If yourmedicine is by prescription and you were not made aware of the sideeffects, **call your doctor.**
		→ Medication Summary, p. 657

Tremors and profuse sweating in diabetics	Low blood sugar levels	**Immediate action required:** If possible, measure blood sugar level; drink a glass of juice, followed by a slice of bread or an apple (two bread units). If blood sugar levels are repeatedly low, **call your doctor.** → Diabetes, p. 483
Palpitations accompanying high blood pressure	Rising blood pressure	If you do not know how to measure your blood pressure, **call your doctor.** → Hypertension (High Blood Pressure), p. 321
Repeatedly racing heart that occurs with an unexplained weight loss but with no loss of appetite • Shiny, slightly protruding eyeballs • Trembling	Hyperthyroidism	**Call your doctor.** → Hyperthyroidism, p. 496

COMPLAINTS AND SYMPTOMS	POSSIBLE CAUSES	WHAT TO DO
Repeatedly racing heart or palpitations, made worse by physical exertion • **Shortness of breath** • **Swollen legs**	Congestive heart failure • Heart muscle inflammation • Heart valve disorder	**Call your doctor.** → Congestive Heart Failure, p. 337 → Heart Valve Disorders, p. 343 → Myocarditis, Endocarditis, Pericarditis (Heart Inflammations) p. 341
Racing heart with dizziness and near-loss of consciousness (blackness before the eyes)	Heart rhythm disorder	**Call your doctor immediately.** → Tachycardia, p. 340
Repeatedly racing heart or palpitations with shortness of breath and tight pain around the chest	Asphyxiation of the heart due to constriction of the coronary arteries	**Immediate action required:** take a nitroglycerine tablet. If the situation does not improve, **call emergency medical services immediately.** → Angina Pectoris, p. 333

HEADACHES

Headaches usually appear independently of other illnesses and are seldom of organic origin. Your headaches may be an alarm signal of physical or emotional stress. Medicines, diseases, or pollutants can also cause headaches.

COMPLAINTS AND SYMPTOMS	POSSIBLE CAUSES	WHAT TO DO
Headaches • **Nervousness** • **Sleep disorders**	Overwork • Psychological problems • Stress	Get plenty of rest. Try to solve the problems that have you "banging your head against the wall." ↪ Headaches, p. 193 ↪ Health and Well-being, p. 182 ↪ Relaxation, p. 693

Headaches with neck and shoulder pain	Body tension due to
	    emotional problems
	    incorrect posture or sitting too
	      long
		Take breaks and change position frequently. Try to identify the "burdens" weighing on your neck and shoulders.
		↪ Health and Well-being, p. 182
		↪ Relaxation, p. 693

Headaches **Heavy caffeine consumption (coffee, tea, cola)** • **Stopping caffeine consumption**	• Effects of caffeine • Effects of caffeine withdrawal	Reduce caffeine consumption. ↪ Caffeine, p. 758
Headaches • **Heavy drinking** • **Heavy smoking** • **Taking drugs**	Side effects of nicotine • Aftereffects of alcohol • Aftereffects of drugs	If this scenario recurs often, **call your doctor.** ↪ Alcoholism, p. 205 ↪ Drug Addiction, p. 204 ↪ Mood-altering Substances and Recreational Drugs, p. 754
Headaches with slight dizziness	Weather sensitivity • Low air pressure • "Santa Ana winds" • Too much sun	Get plenty of rest. In case of overexposure to sun, **move into shade immediately.** If symptoms persist after one day, **call your doctor.** ↪ Sunstroke, p. 707
Strong, pulsating headaches, usually localized in the temples or eye area • **Nausea or vomiting**	Migraines	Get rest and take some time off. If you often suffer from migraines, **call your doctor.** ↪ Health and Well-being, p. 182 ↪ Migraines, p. 225

COMPLAINTS AND SYMPTOMS	POSSIBLE CAUSES	WHAT TO DO

Sudden, sharp pain, usually on one side of face, while
     chewing
     sneezing
     speaking
     yawning
	Damaged facial nerve (trigeminal nerve)	**Call your doctor.**
		 ➙ Nerve Disorders, p. 210

Headaches with runny or stuffy nose • **Cough** • **Fever** • **Teary eyes**	A cold	If symptoms persist for more than one week, **call your doctor.** ➙ Colds, p. 298 ➙ Flu, p. 297
Headaches, usually with a flicker-ing in front of the eyes during severe eyestrain • **Detailed needlework** • **Extended periods of reading** • **Video screen work**	Eyestrain • Faulty eyesight	Take more frequent breaks; insist on your legal right to take breaks at work. If headaches recur often, or eyesight is failing, **call your doctor.** ➙ Eyestrain, p. 228 ➙ Faulty Eyesight, p. 229
Headaches, usually connected with a feeling of dull pressure or stinging pain • **Living in a polluted environment** • **Working with chemicals**	Airborne pollutants	If headaches recur often, **call your doctor.** ➙ Air Pollution, p. 783 ➙ Health in the Workplace, p. 789 ➙ Healthy Living, p. 772
Headaches and nervousness accompanying high noise levels, at home or work	Noise-related stress	If headaches recur often or hearing is impaired, **call your doctor.** ➙ Hearing Loss (Impaired Hearing), p. 250

Headaches after taking medicines	Side effect of numerous medicines, especially
	     birth-control pills
	     high-blood-pressure medicine
	     many medicines for cardiovascular disorders
	     many medicines for stomach and intestinal disorders
	     many rheumatoid medicines
	     painkillers
		If your medicine is over-the-counter and headaches were not mentioned in the insert as a possible temporary and harmless side effect, *stop taking it.* If your medicine is by prescription and you were not made aware of possible side effects, **call your doctor.**
		 ➙ Medication Summary, p. 657

COMPLAINTS AND SYMPTOMS	POSSIBLE CAUSES	WHAT TO DO
Headaches that occur with low or high blood pressure and dizziness	Low blood pressure • High blood pressure	If you have low blood pressure, get your circulation going. Exercise or walk after rising. If you have high blood pressure, **call your doctor.** ➥ Hypertension (High Blood Pressure), p. 321 ➥ Hypotension (Low Blood Pressure), p. 325 ➥ Physical Activity and Sports, p. 762
Headaches in diabetics • **Breaking into a sweat** • **Restlessness** • **Trembling**	Low blood sugar levels	**Immediate action required:** If possible, measure blood sugar level drink a glass of juice, followed by a slice of bread or an apple. If blood sugar levels are repeatedly low, **call your doctor.** ➥ Diabetes, p. 483
Headaches with pain around the eyes and cheekbones, made worse by tilting the head forward • **Elevated temperature** • **Yellowish-green nasal mucus**	Frontal sinusitis • Sinus infection	**Call your doctor.** ➥ Sinusitis, p. 300
Headaches during pregnancy • **Swollen eyelids** • **Swollen legs**	Pregnancy-related high blood pressure	**Call your doctor.** ➥ Preeclampsia, p. 574
Headaches following a head wound (usually after a fall) • **Dizziness or nausea** • **Lethargy** • **Memory lapses**	Concussion	**Call your doctor immediately.** ➥ Concussion, p. 211 ➥ First Aid, p. 704
Headaches made worse by tilting the head • **Fever** • **Sensitivity to light** • **Stiff neck**	Meningitis	**Call your doctor immediately.** ➥ Meningitis, p. 212
Severe headaches in those not suffering from migraines • **Confusion** • **Dizziness** • **Visual disturbances** • **Vomiting**	Intracranial hemorrhage • Brain tumor	**Call your doctor immediately.** ➥ Brain Tumors, p. 221 ➥ Intracranial Hemorrhage, p. 214

COMPLAINTS AND SYMPTOMS	POSSIBLE CAUSES	WHAT TO DO

Headaches after using medicines
• **Nosebleeds**
• **Visual disturbances**
	Indication of rising blood pressure as a side effect of
	    birth-control pills
	    decongestants and cold medicines
	    flu and pain medicines containing
	        caffeine
	        etilefrine
	        phenylephrine
	        pholedrine
	    low blood pressure medicines
	    medicines for menstrual or
	    menopausal symptoms containing
	        estrogen
	        estrogen compounds
		Check the medicine label or insert for these substances. If your medicine is over-the-counter, *stop taking it.* If your medicine is by prescription, **call your doctor immediately.**
		↪ Medication Summary, p. 657

INFERTILITY

A couple trying to conceive a child are considered infertile if, after a year or two of having intercourse several times a week, they are unsuccessful. The source of infertility can lie with either partner, so both should be examined. Before starting infertility treatments, consider whether any subconscious issues may be affecting your ability to conceive. Sometimes couples are able to conceive after a perceived pressure to "perform" is lifted.

COMPLAINTS AND SYMPTOMS	POSSIBLE CAUSES	WHAT TO DO
Infertility when you are unsure which days are optimal for conception, or practice sex that is counterproductive	Lack of understanding of physiology	There are only a few days in a woman's cycle when the egg can be fertilized. Intercourse at these times, using techniques to facilitate fertilization, can increase chances of becoming pregnant. → Contraception, p. 551 → Infertility, p. 559
Infertility with no organic cause • **A baby is seen as an emotional substitute for a healthy relationship** • **Only one partner wants a child, and the other is just "going along" with the idea** • **The relationship is not doing well and a baby is seen as a way of improving or cementing it**	Unconscious rejection of pregnancy	The desire for a child might be superficial. Try to establish whether it really makes sense to launch a complicated campaign to become pregnant. If you need help resolving this, **call your doctor.** → Consultation and Psychotherapy, p. 687 → Infertility, p. 559
Infertility • **Constant stress** • **Drug abuse** • **Heavy drinking of alcohol** • **Heavy smoking** • **Overburdened**	Side effect of stress • Alcohol and nicotine abuse • Drug abuse	Take time for one another. Do not use alcohol and other dependencies as your path to relaxation. If you need help with this, **call your doctor.** → Addictions and Dependencies, p. 204 → Health and Well-being, p. 182 → Infertility, p. 559 → Mood-altering Substances and Recreational Drugs, p. 754

COMPLAINTS AND SYMPTOMS	POSSIBLE CAUSES	WHAT TO DO
Infertility • **Constant dieting** • **Serious overweight condition** • **Serious underweight problem**	Hormonal disorders	If you are overweight, enter a weight-loss program under your physician's care. Avoid extreme or "fad" diets, or chronic undereating just to maintain your weight. If you need help with this, **call your doctor.** → Body Weight, p. 727 → Eating Disorders, p. 202 → Infertility, p. 559
Infertility in individuals working with hazardous substances, in industries • **Agriculture** • **Anesthesiology** • **Clinical or chemistry labs** • **Dentistry** • **Forestry** • **Grape farming** • **Horticulture** • **Textiles**	Effects of hazardous substances	**Call your doctor.** → Infertility, p. 559
Infertility if one partner suffers from a chronic or long-term disease	Effect of the illness	Chronic or severe illnesses can cause fertility disorders. Be patient. If this is difficult, **call your doctor.** → Infertility, p. 559
Infertility *in men* • **Always wearing tight pants** • **Hernia** • **High-riding testicle** • **Inflammation of the testicles, prostate, urethra, or seminal vesicles** • **Sexually transmitted disease** • **Taking various medicines** • **Varicocele**	Disorder in sperm production • Ejaculatory disorder	Avoid tight pants or those made from fabrics that don't "breathe." It takes about three months to restore production of viable sperm. If any of the other conditions listed apply to you, **call your doctor.** → Male Infertility, p. 560
Infertility *in women* • **Chronic fallopian tube inflammation** • **Ectopic pregnancy** • **Miscarriage** • **Sexually transmitted disease** • **Taking medicines**	Effects of medicine • Consequence of surgery • Illness	**Call your doctor.** → Female Infertility, p. 562

ITCHING

Itching can be caused by fabrics, chemicals, inflammations, parasites, fungi, and internal illnesses. If you frequently itch, however, recurring psychological issues could also be a source of irritation. Itching with a rash: Skin rashes, p. 136. Vaginal itching: Vaginal itching and/or burning, p. 167. Itching penis: Men's Illnesses, p. 529.

COMPLAINTS AND SYMPTOMS	POSSIBLE CAUSES	WHAT TO DO
Itching with dry and sensitive skin	Strong oil-removing cleansers • Age-related symptom • Dry air from central heating and air conditioning • Wool and other fabrics	Avoid dry air, central heating, and air conditioning. Bathe as little as possible and avoid foaming bath products. Moisturize after bathing. Test your tolerance of various fibers on skin. ➟ Powerstations and Private Home Heating, p. 786 ➟ Skin care, p. 261
Itching over entire body • **Emotional problems** • **Nervousness** • **Stress**	Reaction to a situation that's driving you "up the wall"	Work on solving your problems. If you need help, **call your doctor.** ➟ Health and Well-being, p. 182
Itchy scalp	Flaking scalp • Head lice	If itching continues or you discover lice or nits, **call your doctor.** ➟ Dandruff, p. 290 ➟ Lice, p. 268

Anal itching	Insufficient hygiene
	• Allergies (to toilet paper, for example)
	• Bacteria
	• Chronic disorders, for example
	  diabetes
	  intestinal disorders
	  liver disorders
	• Emotional problems
	• Food intolerance, for example
	  beer
	  citrus fruits
	  colas
	  seasonings
	  vitamin C
	• Fungi (yeast)
	• Genital herpes
	• Hemorrhoids
	• Pinworms
		Wash anus carefully with a mild soap. Avoid skin-care products with harsh chemicals. If itching persists for more than three days, **call your doctor.**
		➟ Allergies, p. 360
		➟ Genital Herpes, p. 547
		➟ Health and Well-being, p. 182
		➟ Hemorrhoids, p. 417
		➟ Vaginal Candidiasis, p. 545
		➟ Worms (Parasites), p. 415

COMPLAINTS AND SYMPTOMS	POSSIBLE CAUSES	WHAT TO DO
Itching in a specific area on one side of the body	Preliminary stage of shingles (before rash appears)	**Call your doctor.** → Shingles, p. 284

Itchy skin after use of medicines	Usually indicates an allergic reaction
	• Side effect of numerous internal and external medicines, especially
	    first-aid medicines containing mercury
	    many acne medicines
	    many fungus medicines
	    many skin medicines
	    most ointments for muscle and joint pain
		If your medicine is over-the-counter and itching was not listed as a possible side effect, *stop using it.*
		If your medicine is by prescription and you were not made aware of possible side effects, **call your doctor.**
		→ Medication Summary, p. 657

Itching after taking medicines
• **Discolored stool and urine**
• **Yellow-tinged skin**
	Indication of liver disorders as a side effect of numerous medicines, especially
	    antibiotics (especially tetracyclines)
	    antipsychotic medicines (neuroleptics)
	    antispasmodic medicines
	    cholesterol medicines
	    diarrhea medicines
	    estrogen compounds, especially birth-control pills
	    migraine medicines
	    pain medicines
	    rheumatoid medicines
	    vitamin A (extended use)
		Check the medicine label or insert for these substances. If they are present and symptoms occur, **call your doctor.**
		→ Medication Summary, p. 657

Itching with yellow-tinged skin and yellowish whites of the eyes	Jaundice	**Call your doctor.** → Jaundice, p. 393
Itching over entire body • **Bulimia** • **Frequent urination** • **Strong thirst** • **Weight loss**	Diabetes	**Call your doctor.** → Diabetes, p. 483
Itching over entire body, with a feeling of severe illness • **Swollen lymph nodes** • **Weight loss**	Lymph node cancer	**Call your doctor.** → Hodgkin's Lymphoma, p. 356
Itching over entire body **Discolored skin** **Frequent urination or complete lack of urination** **Nausea and loss of appetite** **Tiredness**	Kidney failure	**Call your doctor immediately.** → Kidney Failure, p. 425

KNEE PAIN AND SWELLING

Knee pain is usually due to injury, degeneration, or inflammation of the knee joint.

COMPLAINTS AND SYMPTOMS	POSSIBLE CAUSES	WHAT TO DO
Knee pain after strenuous activity such as hiking, skiing, sports	Strained knee joint	Rest the knee; apply cool compresses. If pain persists for more than one day, **call your doctor.** ↪ Cold Tratments, Ice Packs, p. 685
Pain and swelling in knee following an injury	Injured ligament • Injured meniscus • Injured tendon • Knee joint effusion • Sprain	**Call your doctor.** ↪ Meniscal Injury, p. 448 ↪ Pulled or Torn Tendon, Pulled or Torn Ligament, p. 441 ↪ Sprain, Strain, p. 441
Frequent knee pain, worsening over the years, with restricted knee movement	Gradual degeneration due to normal wear and tear	**Call your doctor.** ↪ Arthritis, p. 452
Red, swollen, very painful knee with restricted movement	Bursitis	**Call your doctor.** ↪ Bursitis, p. 443
Red, swollen, very painful knee with sensation of heat **• Additional swollen joints, such as fingers** **• Fever**	Joint inflammation	**Call your doctor.** ↪ Gout, p. 454 ↪ Rheumatoid Arthritis, p. 455
Pain and swelling in knee after a fall or accident	Pulled ligament • Fracture • Torn ligament	**Call your doctor immediately.** ↪ Fracture, p. 429 ↪ Pulled or Torn Ligament, p. 441

LEG PAIN AND SWELLING

Pain in the legs can be caused by overexertion, injury, or inflammation. Or it may be that you really need a rest and simply can't manage to "stand up for" something right now.

COMPLAINTS AND SYMPTOMS	POSSIBLE CAUSES	WHAT TO DO
Tingling pain in the leg after sitting or lying for a long period • Leg "falling asleep"	Muscle cramp from an awkward position • Restricted circulation	Normal reaction. Pain usually lessens after changing position. → Massage, p. 686 → Physical Activity and Sports, p. 762
Leg cramps after unusual exertion (for example, playing sports)	Muscle cramp or muscle soreness/ stiffness from overexertion • Pulled muscle	Heat applications, sauna treatments, or gentle massage may alleviate the pain. A pulled muscle usually heals without further treatment. → Massage, p. 686 → Muscle Cramps, p. 435 → Pulled, Torn Muscle, p. 437
Leg pain, especially after sitting or lying for a long period • Calf cramps at night • Heavy, swollen legs • Protruding veins	Varicose veins	Do leg exercises and increase your physical activity by bicycling and walking, etc. as much as possible. Wear support stockings. If varicose veins worsen, **call your doctor.** → Physical Activity and Sports, p. 762 → Varicose Veins, p. 328
Leg pain extending into the thighs and lower back	Lumbago • Sciatica	If pain persists, **call your doctor.** If signs of paralysis appear, **call your doctor immediately.** → Lumbago, Sciatica, Herniated or Rupured Disc Damage, p. 466 → Massage, p. 686
Cramps in the calf • Perspiring heavily	• Dieting • Taking diuretics	Disruption of the body's salt and water balance If cramps persist, **call your doctor.** → Muscle Cramps, p. 435
Calf cramps in alcoholics or diabetics	Nerve damage	If you are not already in medical treatment, **call your doctor.** → Alcoholism, p. 205 → Diabetes, p. 483
Leg pains in women taking hormones • Swelling and sensation of warmth in the calf	Thrombosis • Side effect or overdose of medicines, especially birth-control medicines menopausal hormone-replacement therapy	**Call your doctor.** → Medication Summary, p. 657

COMPLAINTS AND SYMPTOMS	POSSIBLE CAUSES	WHAT TO DO
Leg pain when bending or stretching • **Fall or accident** • **Overexertion**	Pulled or torn tendon • Pulled or ruptured disc	Keep leg still and apply cold to the painful area. **Call your doctor.** ↪ Tendons and ligaments, p. 441 ↪ Sprains and Strains, p. 441 ↪ Cold Treatments, p. 685
Calf pain due to incorrect foot placement	Mobile or rigid flat feet, paralytic drop-foot, broad foot	**Call your doctor.** ↪ Feet, p. 443
Leg pains while walking, alleviated by rest • **Cold feet**	Bad circulation in the legs	**Call your doctor.** ↪ Circulatory Disorders (Intermittent Claudication), p. 326
Swollen legs • **Shortness of breath during exertion**	Weak heart	**Call your doctor.** ↪ Congestive Heart Failure, p. 337
Pain in legs, radiating from hip joints	Deterioration of hip joints	**Call your doctor.** ↪ Arthritis, p. 452
Ankle pain • **Fatigue** • **Fever** • **Pain and swelling in fingers or other joints** • **Pain upon arising in the morning**	Joint inflammation	**Call your doctor.** ↪ Rheumatoid Arthritis, p. 455
Constant leg pain concentrated in one spot • **Fever**	Bone inflammation • Bone cancer	**Call your doctor.**
Leg pain with redness and swelling around a hard, inflamed vein	Phlebitis with developing blood clot	**Call your doctor.** ↪ Superficial Phlebitis, p. 329
Pain, swelling, and sensation of heat in one calf • **Pain in sole of the foot**	Venous obstruction	**Call your doctor immediately.** If pain extends to the thigh, **call emergency medical services immediately.** ↪ Deep Vein Thrombosis, p. 330
Pulling sensation in lower back and thighs, usually extending to the feet • **Difficulty walking (limping to ease the pain)** • **Numbness**	Disc pressing on a nerve • Prolapsed disc	**Call your doctor.** ↪ Lumbago, Sciatica, Herniated or Ruptured Disc Damage, p. 466

COMPLAINTS AND SYMPTOMS	POSSIBLE CAUSES	WHAT TO DO
Leg pain following a fall or accident, severe enough to prevent standing • Restricted movement or immobilization • Swelling • Unnatural position of the leg	Dislocation • Fracture • Torn tendon	Call your doctor immediately. → Dislocation, p. 448 → Fracture, p. 429 → Sprains and Strains, p. 441
Sudden, severe leg pain, with unusually pale, cold skin	Arterial embolism	Call emergency medical services immediately.

LIMPING

Limping is often a natural protective action when walking is painful. There might be other reasons for "dragging one's feet," however. If children are limping, they should see a doctor immediately.

COMPLAINTS AND SYMPTOMS	POSSIBLE CAUSES	WHAT TO DO
Limping • Faulty foot placement • Stepping on a splinter or thorn • Too-tight shoes, either currently or for a prolonged period in the past • Warts or corns	Painful shoes • Corns • Crippled feet • Flatfoot • Warts • Wounds on the sole	Wear only roomy, comfortable shoes. If feet are incorrectly placed or other symptoms cannot be solved without help, call your doctor. → Corns, p. 266 → Feet, p. 443 → Warts, p. 267
Limping in children	Developmental hip dislocation • Inflammation of the hip	Call your doctor. → Developmental Dislocation of the Hip, p. 592
Limping and leg pain after a fall or accident • Redness • Swelling	Pulled muscle • Pulled tendons or ligaments	Apply cool compresses. Call your doctor. → Cold Treatments, p. 685 → First aid, p. 704 → Pulled Tendon or Ligament, p. 441 → Pulled, Torn muscles, p. 437
Limping after a long walk Calf pain alleviated by resting the leg	Circulatory disorders	Call your doctor. → Circulatory Disorders, p. 326
Sudden limping due to weak legs • Crooked mouth • Difficulty in speaking • Tingling or numbness on one side of the body	Sign of a stroke	Call your doctor immediately. → Stroke, p. 215 → Transient Ischemic Attacks, p. 318

MENSTRUAL DISORDERS

Menstrual periods are a time of heightened sensitivity. Illnesses, medicines, and emotional problems can all affect your cycle.

COMPLAINTS AND SYMPTOMS	POSSIBLE CAUSES	WHAT TO DO
Irregular periods between the ages of 13 and 20	Hormones not yet in balance • Inflammations • Psychological factors • Physical changes through puberty	Fluctuations of up to six weeks are normal in young girls. If your periods are farther apart, **call your doctor.** ➙ Health and Well-being, p. 182 ➙ Menstrual Disorders, p. 508
Irregular menstruation **• Pain during the period**	Stress and overload • Exhaustion • Hormonal problems (possibly caused by toxins) • Location and/or climate change • Psychological factors • Side effects of illnesses	If pain does not decrease, or periods do not normalize over time, **call your doctor.** ➙ Hazardous Substances in Food, p. 729 ➙ Health and Well-being, p. 182 ➙ Menstrual Disorders, p. 508
Irregular periods between ages 45 and 55	Irregular or decreased hormone production at onset of menopause	If periods stay irregular, or start up again one year or more into menopause, **call your doctor.** ➙ Menopause, p. 510

Menstrual disorders after taking medicines	Side effect of many medicines, including
	    antipsychotics containing
	        sulpiride
	    diuretics containing
	        potassium canrenoate
	        spironolactone
	    high doses of liothyronine
	    hormone replacement therapy
	    oral contraceptives
	    thyroid medicines containing
	        levothyroxine
		Check the medicine label or insert for these substances. If they are present, **call your doctor.**
		➙ Medication Summary, p. 657

Heavy periods of long duration	Side effect of IUD • Blood coagulation disorders • Polyps and myomas • Uterine inflammations	If periods are consistently long and heavy, **call your doctor.** ➙ IUD (Intrauterine Device), p. 555 ➙ Menstrual Disorders, p. 508 ➙ Polyps, p. 521 ➙ Salpingitis (Inflammation of the Fallopian Tubes, Pelvic Inflammatory Disease), p. 525 ➙ Uterine Inflammations, p. 520

COMPLAINTS AND SYMPTOMS	POSSIBLE CAUSES	WHAT TO DO
Heavy bleeding one week or longer after the period is expected	Heavier bleeding due to delayed period • Hormonal changes • (In rare cases) early miscarriage • Psychological factors	If the flow is very heavy, **call your doctor.** → Health and Well-being, p. 182 → Menstrual Disorders, p. 508 → Miscarriage, p. 574
Bleeding or spotting between periods	Irritation from IUD • Cancer or precancerous stage • Cervicitis • Hormonal changes • Psychological factors • Side effect of oral contraceptive • Vaginal infection • Vaginitis	If pain or spotting continues or recurs, **call your doctor.** → Health and Well-being, p. 182 → IUD (Intruterine Device), p. 555 → Menstrual Disorders, p. 508 → Oral Contraceptives (Birth-control Pills, p. 556 → Salpingitis (Inflammation of the Fallopian Tubes, Pelvic Inflammatory Disease), p. 525 → Uterine Cancer, p. 525 → Uterine Inflammations, p. 520 → Vaginitis (Vaginal Inflammation), p. 518
Absence of period	Psychological factors • Discontinuing oral contraceptives • Hormonal changes • Intensive sports training or performance • Menopause • Pregnancy • Serious illness • Weight loss or fasting	**Call your doctor.** → Amenorrhea (Absence of Period), p. 509 → Body weight, p. 727 → Health and Well-being, p. 182 → Menopause, p. 510 → Menstrual disorders, p. 508 → Oral contraceptives (Birth-control Pills), p. 556 → Pregnancy and Birth, p. 565
Heavy bleeding or spotting one week or more after period is expected • **Racing pulse** • **Severe pain on one side of lower abdomen** • **Sweating**	Ectopic pregnancy	**Call emergency medical services immediately.** → Ectopic Pregnancy, p. 526

MENSTRUAL PAIN

Menstrual pain is usually caused by tumors, hormonal disorders, ovulation disturbances, diseases of the pelvic organs, and, sometimes, emotional stress.

COMPLAINTS AND SYMPTOMS	POSSIBLE CAUSES	WHAT TO DO
Cramping pains or subtle aches in the lower abdomen occurring regularly with each period • **Backache** • **Circulatory disorders** • **Headaches** • **Vomiting**	Tumors • Endometriosis • Infection • Systemic dysfunctions	Get rest. Sometimes a hot water bottle on the abdomen helps. If symptoms are severe, **call your doctor.** → Dysmenorrhea (Menstual Pain), p. 507 → Health and Well-being, p. 182
Cramping pains or subtle aches in lower abdomen, occurring suddenly and without precedent during menstruation	Polyps or myomas • Emotional problems • Endometriosis • Hormonal changes (menopause) • Miscarriage	If complaints continue or recur, **call your doctor.** → Dysmenorrhea (Menstual Pain), p. 507 → Endometriosis, p. 522 → Health and Well-being, p. 182 → Menopause, p. 182 → Miscarriage, p. 574 → Polyps, p. 521
Cramping in lower abdomen after intrauterine device (IUD) insertion	Adjustment to IUD • IUD incompatibility	If pain does not lessen after two days or bleeding is excessive (more than six sanitary pads in two hours), **call your doctor.** → Dysmenorrhea (Menstrual Pain), p. 507 → IUD (Intrauterine Device), p. 555
Painful period after discontinuing oral contraceptives	Hormonal changes • Psychological problems	"The pill" lessens menstrual pain. When you stop taking it, former sensations return. If you have difficulties with this, **call your doctor.** → Health and Well-being, p. 182 → Oral Contraceptives (Birth-control Pills), p. 556

MOUTH AND TONGUE PAIN

Pain in or around the mouth is usually caused by inflammation, and only rarely by allergies or general illness.

COMPLAINTS AND SYMPTOMS	POSSIBLE CAUSES	WHAT TO DO
Fissures at corners of mouth (possibly inflamed)	Vitamin deficiency • Iron deficiency	If fissures do not heal after one week, **call your doctor.** ↠ Anemia, p. 345 ↠ Vitamins, p. 740
Pain and red, swollen, bleeding gums, especially between teeth	Gum inflammation • Periodontal disease	Gargle with sage tea and use a soft toothbrush. If pain persists for more than two weeks, **call your doctor.** ↠ Gingivitis (Gum Inflammation), p. 370 ↠ Periodontal Disease, Trench Mouth, p. 371
Burning tongue without having eaten anything too hot	Iron deficiency • Allergies • Emotional problems • Vitamin deficiency	If the sensation persists after one week, **call your doctor.** ↠ Allergies, p. 360 ↠ Anemia, p. 345 ↠ Health and Well-being, p. 182 ↠ Vitamins, p. 740
White-coated tongue with stomach ache	Fever • Constipation • Intestinal disorders • Nervous stomach • Stomach or peptic ulcer	If coating does not clear up after one week, **call your doctor.** ↠ Constipation, p. 406 ↠ Nervous Stomach, p. 386 ↠ Stomach & Duodenal Ulcer, p. 389
Red, swollen mouth lining	Allergy • Environmental toxins • Irritation from dentures	If pain persists after one week, **call your doctor.** ↠ Air Pollution, p. 783 ↠ Allergies, p. 360 ↠ Dentures, p. 376 ↠ Partial Dentures, p. 374
Painful swelling under the tongue, which can be felt at the angle of the lower jaw	Salivary gland inflammation	Chew gum or a slice of lemon to stimulate saliva flow. If symptoms persist after three days, **call your doctor.** ↠ Parotitis, p. 381
Painful, whitish, red-rimmed spots inside mouth	Viral disease	If symptoms persist after a few days of rest, **call your doctor.** ↠ Canker Sores, p. 380

COMPLAINTS AND SYMPTOMS	POSSIBLE CAUSES	WHAT TO DO

Dry mouth after taking medicines	Side effect of many of medicines, especially
	    allergy medicines
	    antidepressants
	    antihistamines
	    antispasmodics
	    flu, cold, and cough medicines
	    medicines for stomach and
	        intestinal disorders
	    sedatives containing
	        sleep aids
		If your medicine is over-the-counter, and dry mouth was not mentioned as a possible harmless side effect, *stop taking it.*
		If your medicine is byprescription and you were not made aware of possible side effects, **call your doctor.**
		→ Medication Summary, p. 657

Mouth and tongue complaints after applying topical medicines
• **Discoloration of the mouth cavity or tongue**
• **Rash or itching in mouth area**
	Side effect of
	    many mouth and throat treatments
	    skin preparations containing
	        etretinate
		If your medicine is over-the-counter, *stop taking it.* If your medicine is by prescription and you were not made aware of the possible side effects, **call your doctor.**
		→ Medication Summary, p. 657

Inflamed mouth with white coating in some spots • **Swelling of lymph nodes in the neck**	Mycosis, fungal infections	**Call your doctor.** → Thrush, p. 380
Painful, swollen oral mucous membrane with blisters • **Bad breath** • **Coated tongue** • **Difficulty in swallowing** • **Fever**	Stomatitis	**Call your doctor.** → Stomatitis (Oral Mucus Menbrane Inflammation), p. 379
Itchy blisters in the mouth and on the tongue • **Fever** • **On the body** • **On the face** • **On the scalp**	Chickenpox	**Call your doctor.** → Chickenpox, p. 604

Blue-white spots in the mouth and on the tongue	Chronic irritation of the mouth and the tongue from
	    heavy-metal poisoning
	    metal fillings or crowns
	    sharp edges on teeth
	    tobacco
		Call your doctor.
		→ Dental Care, p. 364
		→ Glossitis (Tongue Inflammation), p. 381
		→ Health in the Workplace, p. 789
		→ Smoking, p. 754
		→ Stomatitis (Oral Mucus Menbrane Inflammation), p. 379

COMPLAINTS AND SYMPTOMS	POSSIBLE CAUSES	WHAT TO DO
Painful, smooth, dark-red tongue • Red, swollen mouth lining	Glossitis • Intestinal disorders • Liver disorders • Vitamin B-12 deficiency	**Call your doctor.** → Glossitis (Tongue Inflammation), p. 381 → Liver Failure, p. 393 → Ulcerative Colitis, p. 411 → Vitamins, p. 740
Hard spots, nodes, or small tumors on the tongue and in the mouth	Tongue cancer	**Call your doctor.** → Oral Cancers (Cancers of the Mouth Area), p. 382
Bright-red tongue • Speckled, scarlet skin rash	Scarlet fever	**Call your doctor.** → Scarlet Fever, p. 602

LIP AILMENTS

Irritation and inflammation can cause lips to become cracked and sore. Blue lips or ulcers can be symptoms of serious illness.

COMPLAINTS AND SYMPTOMS	POSSIBLE CAUSES	WHAT TO DO
Chapped lips	Climatic conditions • Dry air due to heating or air conditioning • Pollutants	Select a high-emollient lip salve or cream. → Power Stations and Private Home Heating, p. 786
Inflamed or irritated lips after application of lipstick or lip balm	Intolerance to a cosmetic ingredient	Switch brands. You probably cannot tolerate some substance in the cosmetic. → Allergies, p. 360
Red, swollen lips	Iron deficiency • Environmental toxins • Food intolerance • Insect bites • Vitamin deficiency	If symptoms persist after two weeks, **call your doctor.** → Air Pollution p. 783 → Allergies, p. 360 → Anemia, p. 345 → Vitamins, p. 740
Painful, raised areas on lips topped by multiple blisters	Fever blister (herpes)	If you suffer frequently from fever blisters, **call your doctor.** → Herpes Simplex, p. 285
Fissures at corners of mouth, inflamed	Iron deficiency Vitamin deficiency	If symptoms persist longer than two weeks, **call your doctor.** → Anemia, p. 345 → Vitamins, p. 740
Blue lips (not associated with exposure to cold)	Heart or lung disorder	**Call your doctor immediately.**

MUSCLE PAINS AND CRAMPS

Muscle pains or cramps are generally harmless and are usually caused by over-exertion of the muscles, or extended periods of time in an uncomfortable position.

COMPLAINTS AND SYMPTOMS	POSSIBLE CAUSES	WHAT TO DO
Muscle cramps after extended sitting or lying down	Cramping from an uncomfortable position	This is a normal reaction. Cramping will ease when you change position.
Muscle pain after unaccustomed strain (for example, sports)	Muscle soreness	This is a normal reaction. Warmth or gentle massage can alleviate the pain. ⇢ Massages, p. 686 ⇢ Muscle Cramps, p. 435
Muscle cramps • **Dieting** • **Heavy perspiration** **(for example, after a sauna)** • **Prolonged exposure to sun** • **Taking diuretics**	Improper electrolyte balance	Drink lots of liquids (tea or mineral water). Eat salty foods. If complaints persist for more than a day, **call your doctor.** ⇢ Muscle Cramps, p. 435 ⇢ Sunstroke, p. 707
Muscle cramps • **Alcoholics** • **Diabetics**	Nerve disorders	If you are not already under medical supervision, **call your doctor.** ⇢ Alcoholism, p. 205 ⇢ Diabetes, p. 483

Muscle cramps after taking medicines	Side effect of many medicines, including those for
	     asthma and bronchitis, containing
	         theophylline
	     migraine, containing
	         methysergide
	     mite or head lice infestation,
	         containing
	         carbaryl
	         lindane (in overdose)
	     poor circulation, containing
	         bencyclane
	     psychosis (neuroleptics)
	     urinary disorders, containing
	         norfloxacin
	         ofloxacin
	         pipemidic acid
		Check the medicine label or insert for these substances. If your medicine is over-the-counter, *stop taking it.* If your medicine is by prescription, **call your doctor.**
		 ⇢ Medication Summary, p. 657

COMPLAINTS AND SYMPTOMS	POSSIBLE CAUSES	WHAT TO DO

Muscle cramps or weakness after taking medicines	Symptoms of electrolyte imbalance as side effect of
	    diuretics
	    high blood-pressure medicines
	        containing
	        diuretics
	        reserpine
	    many laxatives
	    medicines for diarrhea containing
	        carob
	        kaolin
	        pectin
		Check the medicine label or insert for these substances. If your medicine is over-the-counter, *stop taking it.* If your medicine is by prescription, **call your doctor.**
		→ Medication Summary, p. 657

Muscle cramps in babies and small children after use of medicines	Side effect of
	    medicines for nausea, vomiting,
	        and motion sickness containing
	        chlorphenoxamine
	        cyclizine
	        dimenhydrinate
	        hydroxyzine
	        megadoses of meclozine
	    rubbing/inhalation medicines
	        containing
	        camphor
	        eucalyptus oil
	        menthol
		Check medicine label or insert for these substances. If your medicine is over-the-counter, *stop taking it.* If your medicine is by prescription, **call your doctor.**
		→ Medication Summary, p. 657

Nightly cramps with varicose veins	Varicose veins	**Call your doctor.** → Varicose Veins, p. 328
Muscle pain while walking, alleviated by rest	Circulatory disorders	**Call your doctor.** → Circulatory Disorders (Intermittent Claudication), p. 326
Muscle cramps with shaking • **Heavy perspiration** • **Goiter** • **Shiny, protruding eyeballs** • **Weight loss**	Hyperthyroidism	**Call your doctor.** → Hyperthyroidism (Overactive Thyroid), p. 496

MUSCLE SPASMS

Partial or complete loss of bodily control is always uncomfortable and can in some cases be life-threatening.

COMPLAINTS AND SYMPTOMS	POSSIBLE CAUSES	WHAT TO DO
Spasms (tetany) in the hands • **Anxiety** • **Extremely rapid breathing** • **Numbness and tingling in arms and legs**	Hyperventilation (usually due to emotional factors)	**Immediate action required.** Calm down. Take slow, shallow breaths. Hold a paper bag over your mouth to increase the carbon dioxide level. If you are concerned symptoms might recur, **call your doctor.** → Counseling and Psychotherapy, p. 697 → Health and Well-being, p. 182
Muscle spasms that initially appear only in localized areas (for example, corners of the mouth, hand, or foot), then spread to the whole area or limb	Brain tumor • Epilepsy	**Call your doctor immediately.** → Brain Tumors, p. 221 → Epilepsy, p. 216
Muscle spasms and high fever *in children* • **Momentary loss of consciousness**	Febrile seizures	Febrile seizures in children are not life-threatening. Try to lower temperature with cold compresses. If the child is younger than 18 months, or convulsions last longer than five minutes, **call emergency medical services immediately.**
A spasm of the whole body (as in seizures) • **Frothing at the mouth** • **Shortness of breath** • **Tongue biting** • **Unconsciousness** • **Uncontrolled urinating**	Epileptic seizures	**Immediate action required:** Protect the patient from injury. Do not hold tightly or force anything between the teeth to prevent tongue biting. Allow for plenty of sleep after the seizure. If the seizure lasts longer than three minutes, or recurs, **call emergency medical services immediately.** → Epilepsy, p. 216
Muscle spasms after a wound • **Back pain** • **Headaches and dizziness** • **Shivering** • **Twisted mouth (from spasms in the jaw area)**	Tetanus	**Call emergency medical services immediately.** → Tetanus, p. 670

TREMORS

Tremors—shaking, trembling, twitching, and losing muscle control—may indicate serious illness or severe anxiety.

COMPLAINTS AND SYMPTOMS	POSSIBLE CAUSES	WHAT TO DO
Shivering in cold environments or with insufficient clothing	Loss of body heat	Dress warmly; have a hot drink.
Tremors after excessive consumption of • **coffee** • **cola** • **tea**	Irritated nervous system due to caffeine	Reduce caffeine consumption. ➙ Caffeine, p. 758
Twitching of body parts while falling asleep	Involuntary muscle tension	This is normal reaction during relaxation.
Tremors accompanying strong emotions (fear, anger, excitement)	Bodily expression of inner tension	This is normal reaction during tension.
Tremors after excessive alcohol or drug use or after discontinuing alcohol and drug use	Reaction of the nervous system • Withdrawal symptom	If you frequently drink to excess or take drugs, or experience serious withdrawal symptoms, **call your doctor.** ➙ Addiction to Illegal Drugs, p. 208 ➙ Alcoholism, p. 205 ➙ Mood-altering Substances and Recreational Drugs, p. 754
Tremors soon after taking certain medicines	Side effects of numerous medicines, especially angina pectoris medicines antipsychotics (neuroleptics) asthma and bronchitis medicines barbiturates high blood pressure medicines sedatives	If your medicine is over-the-counter, *stop taking it.* If the medicine is by prescription, **call your doctor.** ➙ Medication Summary, p. 657
Tremors after long-term use of medicines • **Palpitations** • **Panic attacks** • **Sleep disorders**	Withdrawal symptoms from appetite suppressants barbiturates medicines containing benzodiazepine codeine sedatives	**Call your doctor.** ➙ Medicine Dependency, p. 658

COMPLAINTS AND SYMPTOMS	POSSIBLE CAUSES	WHAT TO DO
Uncontrollable trembling in hands, more pronounced when precise movements are attempted • **Trembling of head**	Nervous disorder • Multiple sclerosis	**Call your doctor.** ↪ Multiple Sclerosis, p. 220 ↪ Parkinson's Disease, p. 218
Muscular tremors • **Difficulty in concentrating** • **General exhaustion** • **Sleep disorders**	Constant exposure to loud noise • Stressed nervous system due to toxic substances	Examine your living and working environment, and diet, for possible causes. **Call your doctor.** ↪ Hazardous Substances in Food, p. 729 ↪ Health in the Workplace, p. 789 ↪ Healthy Living, p. 772
Trembling or twitching of a single muscle • **Chin** • **Eyelid** • **Mouth**	Fatigue • Stress • Tic	If symptoms keep recurring or last longer than two weeks, **call your doctor.** ↪ Health and Well-being, p. 182 ↪ Neurotic Behavior, p. 195
Tremors in diabetics	Low blood sugar level	**Immediate action required:** If possible, measure blood sugar level. Drink some juice. If low blood sugar levels keep recurring, **call your doctor.** ↪ Diabetes, p. 483
Tremors with profuse sweating • **Goiter** • **Shiny, slightly protruding eyeballs** • **Weight loss in spite of a good appetite**	Hyperthyroidism	**Call your doctor.** ↪ Hyperthyroidism (Overactive Thyroid), p. 496
Sudden trembling and twitching • **Cramped muscles** • **Falling to the ground** • **Foaming at the mouth** • **Unconsciousness**	Epileptic seizure	**Immediate action required:** Protect the patient from injury. Do not hold tightly or force anything between the teeth to prevent tongue biting. Allow for plenty of sleep after the seizure. If the seizure lasts longer than three minutes, or recurs, **call emergency medical services immediately.** ↪ Epilepsy, p. 216

NAIL PROBLEMS

Although nails are in fact dead tissue, they can serve as an indicator of overall health. Dry, discolored or misshapen nails can be a sign of illness.

COMPLAINTS AND SYMPTOMS	POSSIBLE CAUSES	WHAT TO DO
Matte, dull nails after wearing nail polish	Nail polish • Nail polish remover	Paint your nails less often.
Ingrown toenails • **Inflamed nail bed**	Cutting nails too short at the corners • Tight-fitting shoes	Wear better-fitting, more comfortable shoes. → Feet, p. 443 → Ingrown Toenail, p. 294
Brittle nails	Hereditary predisposition • Exposure to degreasing substances or solvents • Hypothyroidism • Vitamin or trace-element deficiencies (especially iron)	Wear gloves while working. Swab nails with sunflower or olive oil occasionally. If you suffer from broken nails over the course of several months, **call your doctor.** → Anemia, p. 345 → Hazardous Substances, p. 773 → Hypothyroidism (Underactive Thyroid), p. 495 → Mineral Substances, p. 744 → Nails, p. 293 → Trace Elements, p. 747 → Vitamins, p. 740
Misshapen or discolored nails • **Horizontal grooves** • **Spoon-like shape** • **Transparent nails** • **White spots**	Various harmless disorders	If nails keep growing back discolored or misshapen, **call your doctor.**
Thickened nails • **Discolored nails** • **Misshapened nails**	Injury to the root of nail from constant pressure (ill-fitting shoes) • Nail fungus • Symptom of aging (arteriosclerosis)	Avoid pressure on nail. If nail keeps growing back thickened, **call your doctor.** → Paronychia, p. 294
Red, swollen nail bed • **Pain** • **Pus**	Injury and consequent infection of nail bed	**Call your doctor.** → Paronychia, p. 294
Detached nail	Psoriasis • Inflammation of the nail fold (paronychia) • Injuries from excessive pressure on nail	**Call your doctor.** → Paronychia, p. 294 → Psoriasis, p. 278

NECK PAIN

Neck pains almost always have various kinds of tension as their root cause. In some cases, neck pains or a stiff neck may be symptoms of a more serious disease.

COMPLAINTS AND SYMPTOMS	POSSIBLE CAUSES	WHAT TO DO
Neck pain after long periods of sitting or lying (for example, at a work station or in bed)	Tense muscles	Massage your neck. Take small breaks at work and stretch. Check your sitting posture and improve it if possible. → Health and Well-being, p. 182 → Relaxation, p. 693
Neck pain • **Exposure to drafts** • **Illness**	Drafts • Symptom of an illness (for example, a cold)	Warmth, massage, and relaxation exercises usually help. If pain persists after three days, **call your doctor.** → Massage, p. 686 → Relaxation, p. 693
Neck pain • **Anxiety** • **Emotional pressure** • **Overload** • **Stress**	Physical or psychological overload	Try to resolve any overwhelming issues or problems. If you need help, **call your doctor.** → Counseling and Psychotherapy, p. 697 → Health and Well-being, p. 182 → Relaxation, p. 693
Sudden neck pain • **Stiff or tilted neck**	Muscle tension • Pulled, torn muscle	Lie down and apply heat treatment. If pain does not subside after a few days, **call your doctor.** → Pulled, Torn Muscles, p. 437
Neck pain more pronounced in the morning • **Headache localized at temples** • **Shoulder and pelvic pain** • **Worsening eyesight**	Connective-tissue disorder of muscle • Blood vessels	**Call your doctor immediately.** → Polymyalgia Rheumatica, p. 461
Neck pains worsening over time • **Pain, weakness, or sensitivity to touch in the arms** • **Stiff neck**	Intervertebral disk damage in cervical vertebrae	**Call your doctor immediately.** → Lumbago, Sciatica, Herniated or Ruptured Disc Damage, p. 466
Neck pain after a severe impact or fall	Pulled neck muscles or ligaments	**Call your doctor immediately.** → Pulled Muscles, p. 437

COMPLAINTS AND SYMPTOMS	POSSIBLE CAUSES	WHAT TO DO
Neck pain made worse by bending head forward • **Confusion** • **Fever** • **Nausea** • **Sensitivity to light** • **Severe headaches and exhaustion** • **Vomiting**	Meningitis	**Call your doctor immediately.** → Meningitis, p. 212
Neck pain after a severe impact or fall • **Partial or complete paralysis of the limbs**	Spinal cord injury	Lie quietly and do not move the head. Any movement could cause severe damage. **Call emergency medical services immediately.** → First Aid, p. 704

NERVOUSNESS AND IRRITABILITY

Nervousness and irritability can be signals that it's high time to make some changes in lifestyle, attitude, or workplace.

COMPLAINTS AND SYMPTOMS	POSSIBLE CAUSES	WHAT TO DO
Nervousness and irritability after little or poor sleep	Exhaustion	Sleep requirements differ for each individual; determine your own needs. → Health and Well-being, p. 182 → Sleep Disorders, p. 190
Nervousness and irritability linked to certain climatic conditions	Weather sensitivity	If possible, limit activity on these days. Do something to reduce stress. → Health and Well-being, p. 182
Nervousness after smoking too much or drinking too much coffee	Symptom of excessive use or abuse • Caffeine • Smoking (nicotine abuse)	Mild nicotine and coffee poisoning. Quit smoking; drink less coffee. → Mood-altering Substances and Recreational Drugs, p. 754
Nervousness and dissatisfaction with emotional stress	Psychological factors Inner conflicts	Try to get a handle on your problems or issues. If you need help, **call your doctor.** → Counseling and Psychotherapy, p. 697 → Health and Well-being, p. 182
Nervousness and irritability associated with constant pressure and lack of personal time	Overload • Burnout	Take stock of your situation and decide whether all your activities and obligations are strictly necessary. Make time for relaxation. If this seems impossible, determine whether you are making yourself busy in order to avoid issues like loneliness or low self-esteem. If you need help with these issues, **call your doctor.** → Counseling and Psychotherapy, p. 697 → Health and Well-being, p. 182
Nervousness and irritability when subjected to constant noise • **Industrial noise at the workplace** • **Living near an airport**	Noise-related nervous tension	Take measures to reduce the noise level in your environment. If your hearing is suffering, **call your doctor.** → Health and Well-being, p. 182 → Hearing Loss, p. 250

COMPLAINTS AND SYMPTOMS	POSSIBLE CAUSES	WHAT TO DO
Nervousness and irritability in a hazardous environment	Symptoms of poisoning	Determine the source and take measures to protect yourself. If irritability does not ease, **call your doctor.** → Hazardous Substances, p. 773
Nervousness and irritability after an illness	Not enough time to recuperate	Arrange to convalesce longer. If symptoms do not lessen and you need help, **call your doctor.** → Health and Well-being, p. 182
Nervousness and irritability associated with drug abuse or stopping use • **Drug abuse** • **Excessive drinking (alcohol)** • **Excessive smoking (tobacco)**	Symptoms of withdrawal	If you have problems with addiction, **call your doctor.** → Alcoholism, p. 205 → Drug Addiction, p. 208 → Mood-altering Substances and Recreational Drugs, p. 754
Nervousness and irritability while dieting	Symptom of dieting	If excessive nervousness is a problem, eat small low-calorie snacks between meals. If your quality of life is seriously affected and your diet was prescribed by a doctor, **call your doctor.** → Body Weight, p. 727 → Eating Disorders, p. 202

Nervousness and restlessness after taking medicines	Side effect of a large number of medicines, especially medicines used to treat
	    cardiovascular disorders
	    circulatory disorders
	    common cold (including analgesics)
	    cough and asthma
	and the following medicines
	    overweight problems ("diet pills")
	    pain (local anesthetics)
	    psychosis (neuroleptics)
		If your medicine is over-the-counter and restlessness or nervousness was not mentioned as a harmless, temporary symptom, *stop taking it.*
		If your medicine is by prescription and you were not made aware of the possible side effects, **call your doctor.**
		→ Medication Summary, p. 657

Nervousness *in older people* after taking medicines	Side effect of
	    sedatives containing benzodiazepines
	    sleep medicines
		If you are taking such medicines, **call your doctor.**
		→ Medication Summary, p. 657

COMPLAINTS AND SYMPTOMS	POSSIBLE CAUSES	WHAT TO DO
Nervousness *in children* **after taking medicines**	Side effect of medicines for various complaints, including itching nausea travel sickness weight regulation, containing chlorphenoxamine cyclizine cyproheptadine dimenhydrinate diphenhydramine, hydroxyzine meclizine at high dosages	Check the medicine label or insert for these substances. If the medicine is over-the-counter, *stop using it.* If the medicine is by prescription, **call your doctor.** ↪ Medication Summary, p. 657
Nervousness *in babies* **after use of medicines**	Side effect of decongestants	If medicine is over-the-counter, *stop using it.* If medicine is by prescription, **call your doctor.** ↪ Medication Summary, p. 657
Nervousness and weight loss with normal appetite • **Protruding eyeballs** • **Trembling**	Hyperthyroidism	**Call your doctor.** ↪ Hyperthyroidism (Overactive Thyroid), p. 496

NOSE PROBLEMS

NOSEBLEED

A nosebleed in adults or children is usually not serious. It can be a symptom of infection, high blood pressure, head injury, polyps, or allergy.

COMPLAINTS AND SYMPTOMS	POSSIBLE CAUSES	WHAT TO DO

Nosebleed	Burst blood vessel in the nasal passage lining from
	    abrasion
	    accident
	    high blood pressure
	    infection
	    medicines
		Immediate action: Lean head forward and pinch nose shut for a few minutes. If nosebleed does not stop after 20 minutes, **call your doctor.**
		➟ Nosebleed, p. 296

Nosebleed after fall or blow to the head (without a direct nasal injury)	Skull fracture	**Call emergency medical services immediately.** ➟ Skull Fracture, p. 212

RUNNY NOSE

A runny nose can be caused by colds, dust, smoke, chemical vapors, allergies, and emotional strain.

COMPLAINTS AND SYMPTOMS	POSSIBLE CAUSES	WHAT TO DO

Runny nose
• **Scratchy throat**
• **Sore throat**
	Colds
	• Adenoids
	• Allergies
	• Deviated septum
	• Irritated nasal passage from
	    chemical vapors
	    dust
	    smoke
	• Side effect of
	    aerosol inhalers (after prolonged use)
	    nose drops
	    sprays
	• Stress
		If you often have a runny nose, **ascertain the cause by calling your doctor.**
		➟ Allergies, p. 360
		➟ Colds, p. 298
		➟ Hazardous substances, p. 773
		➟ Health and Well-being, p. 182
		➟ Nasal polyps, p. 301

Runny nose and sneezing • **Itchy eyes** • **Teary eyes**	Hay fever	**Call your doctor.** ➟ Allergies, p. 360 ➟ Colds, p. 298
Runny nose • **Cough** • **Fever** • **Headache** • **Joint pain**	Cold • Flu • Sinusitis	If the cold does not improve after one week, **call your doctor.** ➟ Colds, p. 298 ➟ Flu, p. 297 ➟ Sinusitis, p. 300

NUMBNESS

Numbness (and tingling) is most frequently caused by temporary lack of circulation, usually due to sitting or standing in a particular position. However, when accompanied by other symptoms, prolonged numbness could be a sign of a more serious illness.

COMPLAINTS AND SYMPTOMS	POSSIBLE CAUSES	WHAT TO DO
Tingling or numbness upon waking, or after sitting in an uncomfortable position for a long time	Restricted blood flow • Pressure on a nerve	Symptoms will disappear on their own when you change position.

Numbness in the arms and legs
 • **Foot pain**
	Nerve damage as side effect of medicines, including those for treatment of
	    long-term use of vitamin B6
	    rheumatism (containing
	        chloroquine)
	    tuberculosis (containing
	        methaniazide)
		Check the medicine label or insert for these substances. If your medicine is over-the-counter, *stop taking it.* If your medicine is by prescription, **call your doctor.**
		 → Medication Summary, p. 657

Numbness in your hands and toes • **Bluish tinge to your hands or feet when cold**	Temporary circulatory disorders • Low blood pressure • Muscle spasm	**Call your doctor.** → Hypotention (Low Blood Pressure), p. 325 → Raynaud's Disease, p. 332
Tingling or numbness in both arms • **Pain spreading from shoulder to arm** • **Headaches**	Spinal column disorders involving cervical vertebrae	**Call your doctor.** → Back and Lower Back Pain, p. 465 → Lumbago, Sciatica, Herniated or Ruptured Disc Damage, p. 466
Tingling or numbness in the hand • **Index finger** • **Middle finger** • **Morning swelling** • **Pain (especially at night) spreading from the wrist up the arm** • **Thumb**	Damaged nerve in the hand (carpal tunnel syndrome)	**Call your doctor.** → Fibromyalgia Syndromes (Soft-tissue Pain and Stiffness), p. 462

Tingling or numbness in the arms or legs
 • **Pain**
	Diabetes
	 • Alcoholism
	 • Insecticides
	 • Nerve disorders
	    multiple sclerosis
	 • Pollutants and toxins
	    lead
	    mercury
		Call your doctor.
		 → Air Pollution, p. 783
		 → Alcoholism, p. 205
		 → Brain and Nerve Disorders, p. 210
		 → Diabetes, p. 483
		 → Multiple Sclerosis, p. 220

COMPLAINTS AND SYMPTOMS	POSSIBLE CAUSES	WHAT TO DO
Numbness and tingling in arms and legs • **Anxiety** • **Cramps in the hands (Trousseau's phenomenon)** • **Extremely rapid breathing**	Hyperventilation (usually due to mental or emotional factors)	**Immediate action required.** Calm down. Take slow, shallow breaths. Hold a paper bag over mouth to increase carbon dioxide level. If you are concerned symptoms might recur, **call your doctor.** ➙ Counseling and Psychotherapy, p. 697 ➙ Health and Well-being, p. 182
Numbness in arms or legs • **Pain in the back and lower back spreading to the legs** • **Partial paralysis**	Ruptured disc	**Call your doctor immediately.** ➙ Lumbago, Sciatica, Herniated or Ruptured Disc Damage, p. 466
Numbness on one side of the body • **Confusion, disorientation** • **Crooked mouth** • **Difficulty speaking** • **Partial paralysis of the arm or leg** • **Visual disturbances**	Stroke-like attack, temporary circulatory disorders (TIA) • Brain tumors • Stroke	**Call emergency medical services immediately.** ➙ Brain Tumors, p. 221 ➙ Stroke, p. 215 ➙ Transient Ischemic Attack, p. 318
Pain in back or spine after an accident or fall • **Difficulty in moving**	Numbness in arms and/or legs and paraplegia	**Call emergency medical services immediately.** ➙ First Aid, p. 704 ➙ Spinal Cord Injuries, p. 221

PARALYSIS

Any instance of physical paralysis calls for **immediate emergency help**.

COMPLAINTS AND SYMPTOMS	POSSIBLE CAUSES	WHAT TO DO
Paralysis with numbness in both legs (rarely in the arms) • **Pain in the back and lower back spreading to the legs**	Ruptured disc	**Call your doctor immediately.** ➙ Lumbago, Sciatica, Herniated or Ruptured Disc Damage, p. 466
Paralysis with loss of feeling in the arms or legs • **Difficulty in speaking** • **Dizziness** • **Fever** • **Headaches**	Encephalitis • Brain abscess	**Call your doctor immediately.** ➙ Brain Abscess, p. 213 ➙ Encephalitis, p. 213

COMPLAINTS AND SYMPTOMS	POSSIBLE CAUSES	WHAT TO DO
Paralysis of one side of the face • **Other facial muscles**	Nerve damage • Tick bite	**Call your doctor immediately.** → Facial Paralysis (Bell's Palsy), p. 226 → Lyme Disease, p. 223
Partial paralysis and unconsciousness after a head injury	Damage to blood vessels in brain	**Call your doctor immediately.** → Cerebral Contusion, p. 212

Paralysis following an accident	Injury to spinal cord due to
	    internal bleeding
	    severed cord
	    swelling
		Call emergency medical services immediately.
		→ Spinal Cord Injuries, p. 221

Paralysis of one arm or leg or entire side of body • **Confusion** • **Difficulty in speaking** • **Unconsciousness** • **Visual disturbances**	Temporary circulatory disorders • Intracranial hemorrhage • Stroke	**Call emergency medical services immediately.** → Intracranial Hemorrhage, p. 214 → Stroke, p. 215 → Transient Ischemic Attack, p. 214

PERSPIRATION

Breaking into a heavy sweat is often the body's reaction to stress, anxiety, or agitation. Excessive body weight, physical exertion, unsuitable clothing, hormonal changes, and various illnesses can also be the cause.

COMPLAINTS AND SYMPTOMS	POSSIBLE CAUSES	WHAT TO DO
Heavy perspiration • **Agitation** • **Fear** • **Stress**	Normal reaction of the body	Breaking into a sweat is a form of "body language." Be considerate of this. → Health and Well-being, p. 182
Regular heavy perspiration when you are overweight	Symptom of being overweight	Try to lose some weight. → Body Weight, p. 727
Heavy perspiration when wearing certain clothes	Fabric that prevents skin from breathing • Tight clothing	Choose clothing in fibers that absorb sweat. Avoid excessively tight clothing.
Heavy perspiration *in women* • **After age 45** • **During menstruation**	Symptom of menstruation	Hormonal changes during menopause → Menopause, p. 510 → Menstruation, p. 506

Heavy perspiration after taking medicines	Side effect of
	  analgesics, especially those
	    containing
	      ASA (acetylsalicylic acid)
	      diabetes medicines
	      dipyrone
	      distigmine
	  intestinal and bladder
	    medicines containing
	    neostigmine
	    pyridostigmine
	    thyroid hormones
	  liver medicines containing
	    papaverine
	    xenytropium bromide
	  medicines for circulatory disorders
	    containing
	    pirazetam
		Check the medicine label or insert for these substances. If your medicine is over-the-counter, *stop taking it.* If your medicine is by prescription, **call your doctor.**
		→ Medication Summary, p. 657

Heavy perspiration following a stomach operation • **Trembling**	Food passing through the stomach too quickly	Eat smaller portions, and eat frequently. If sweating persists, **call your doctor.**
Heavy perspiration *in infants* • **While drinking**	Metabolic disorder	**Call your doctor.** → Cystic Fibrosis, p. 598

COMPLAINTS AND SYMPTOMS	POSSIBLE CAUSES	WHAT TO DO
Heavy perspiration in diabetics	Low blood sugar	**Immediate action required:** If possible, measure blood sugar level. Drink some juice, or administer glucagon by injection if available and not improving. If low blood sugar recurs, **call your doctor.** ↪ Diabetes, p. 483
Heavy perspiration in alcoholics after cessation of drinking • **Confusion** • **Restlessness** • **Trembling**	Symptom of withdrawal	If you are not already in medical treatment, **call your doctor.** ↪ Alcoholism, p. 205
Heavy perspiration • **Nervousness** • **Protruding eyeballs** • **Trembling** • **Weight loss**	Overactive thyroid	**Call your doctor.** ↪ Hyperthyroidism (Overactive Thyroid), p. 496
Sweating, itching, and extremely sick feeling • **Weight loss**	Lymphoma	**Call your doctor.** ↪ Hodgkin's Lymphoma, p. 356
Heavy perspiration with constant coughing, especially at night • **Weight loss**	Tuberculosis • Lung cancer	**Call your doctor.** ↪ Tuberculosis, p. 670 ↪ Lung Cancer, p. 314
Profuse sweating, including cold sweats • **Hard abdomen** • **Racing pulse** • **Severe abdominal pain** • **Vomiting**	Ruptured/perforated internal organ • Appendix • Stomach	**Call emergency medical services immediately.** ↪ Appendicitis, p. 408 ↪ Stomach and Duodenal Ulcers, p. 389
Profuse sweating with severe pains spreading into the heart area • **Cold sweats** • **Nausea** • **Shortness of breath**	Heart attack	**Immediate action required:** Take a sublingual nitroglycerin tablet. **Call emergency medical services immediately.** ↪ Heart Attack (Myocardial Infarction), p. 335

SEX

PAINFUL SEX IN WOMEN

If love-making isn't enjoyable because intercourse is painful, the underlying causes may be fear, inhibitions, an inconsiderate partner, or lower abdominal illnesses.

COMPLAINTS AND SYMPTOMS	POSSIBLE CAUSES	WHAT TO DO
Painful intercourse because of insufficient vaginal lubrication	Insufficient arousal • Problems with partner • Menopause • Psychological factors	Various illnesses with drier mucous membrane as symptom. Tell your partner what you find exciting. If you cannot resolve your issues together, **call your doctor.** ↪ Health and Well-being, p. 182 ↪ Menopause, p. 510 ↪ Women's Issues, p. 537

Pain on penetration
• **Vaginal spasms**
• **Tension**
	Psychological factors
	    fear
	    insensitive partner
	    rejection
	    unresolved conflicts
		Your body is defending itself. If you don't understand why, **call your doctor.**
		↪ Health and Well-being, p. 182
		↪ Women's Issues, p. 537

Painful intercourse after childbirth	Painful episiotomy • Problems with partner • Psychological factors	If pain does not ease with time, **call your doctor.** ↪ Episiotomy, p. 581 ↪ Health and Well-being, p. 182 ↪ Postdelivery Period, p. 584 ↪ Women's Issues, p. 537
Pain on penetration	Problems with your partner • Growths in the uterus • Psychological factors • Shortened or narrowed vagina after surgery	If pain persists, **call your doctor.** ↪ Women's Issues, p. 537
Painful intercourse • **Pain when urinating** • **Unusual discharge** • **Vaginal itch or burning**	Bladder infection • Sexually transmitted disease (STD) • Vaginal infection	**Call your doctor.** ↪ Cysts, p. 527 ↪ Vaginitis (Vaginal Inflammation), p. 518 ↪ Sexually Transmitted Diseases, p. 545
Painful intercourse with simultaneous pain in abdomen	Salpingitis • Endometriosis • Uterine inflammations	**Call your doctor.** ↪ Endometriosis, p. 522 ↪ Salpingitis (Inflammation of the Fallopian Tubes, Pelvic Inflammatory Disease, p. 525 ↪ Uterine Inflammations, p. 520

PAINFUL SEX IN MEN

If physical love-making is painful, possible causes include a variety of illnesses, chemical sensitivity, and feelings of fear, guilt, or shame.

COMPLAINTS AND SYMPTOMS	POSSIBLE CAUSES	WHAT TO DO
Pain during sex due to excessive friction	Insufficient arousal • Anal intercourse • Insufficient lubrication of partner • Problems with partner	If you are inexperienced, ask your partner for guidance. If you have anal intercourse, use a lubricant. **Call your doctor.** → Health and Well-being, p. 182 → Men's Issues, p. 541 → Women's Issues, p. 537
Pain after sex from a sore glans or foreskin	Allergy to chemical contraceptive • Allergy to condom • Unusual sexual practices	Change contraceptives. Try a different brand of condom. If pain does not ease after a day, **call your doctor.** → Balanitis and Posthitis (Inflammation of Glans and Foreskin), p. 530
Pain during sex • **Red and swollen glans and foreskin** • **Whitish coating on the penis**	Inflammations of the glans or foreskin • Fungal infection	**Call your doctor.** → Balanitis and Posthitis (Inflammation of the Glans and Foreskin), p. 530 → Candidiasis, p. 545
Pain during sex with little blisters on the glans and foreskin	Herpes virus	**Call your doctor.** → Genital Herpes, p. 547
Pain during ejaculation • **Burning or pain when urinating** • **Unusual discharge from the urethra**	Infection of the urethra • Inflammation of the prostate • Sexually transmitted disease	**Call your doctor.** → Prostatitis (Inflammation of the Prostate Gland), p. 534 → Sexually Transmitted Diseases, p. 545 → Urethritis (Inflammation of the Urethra), p. 530
Pain on erection	Fibrous thickening that may extend into the erectile tissue (Peyronie's disease) • Crooked penis • Phimosis	**Call your doctor.** → Phimosis, p. 594

SEXUAL PROBLEMS IN WOMEN

Low sex drive, trouble having orgasms, or pain during intercourse are almost always caused by conflicts in the relationship, inhibitions, or negative attitudes about sex. In some cases, psychological problems or physical illnesses can also take the joy out of love-making. Painful intercourse: lack of desire, painful intercourse, p. 537.

COMPLAINTS AND SYMPTOMS	POSSIBLE CAUSES	WHAT TO DO
Low or nonexistent sex drive • Apathy	Normal reaction to exhaustion and feeling overwhelmed • Preoccupation due to major life changes	If your sex drive is low, try to relax and explore what you find stimulating. ➥ Health and Well-being, p. 182 ➥ Relaxation, p. 693
Lack of interest in sex, in a previously successful sexual relationship	Unconscious rejection of partner Negative associations with (or attitudes about) sex • Boredom with sexual relationship • Exhaustion • Problems with partner • Psychological factors • Temporary lull in sex drive	Try to discover the source. If this seriously interferes with your quality of life, seek help at a women's counseling center or from a therapist. ➥ Counseling and Psychotherapy, p. 697 ➥ Health and Well-being, p. 182 ➥ Women's Issues, p. 537
Low sex drive after a serious illness, or accompanying a chronic illness	Normal reaction of a weakened body • Symptom of chronic illness	If lack of sexual desire persists for more than two months after recovery, **call your doctor.** ➥ Women's Issues, p. 537
Low sex drive or difficulties reaching orgasm after childbirth	Normal reaction • Exhaustion and preoccupation with the child • Painful episiotomy sutures	Taking care of a newborn requires a lot of time and energy. It's natural that your role as lover take second place. Also, episiotomy sutures can be painful. If sexual desire is not rekindled after three months, **call your doctor.** ➥ Postdelivery Period, p. 584 ➥ Women's Issues, p. 537
Difficulties reaching orgasm with a new partner	Normal reaction	Stop worrying about performance. Letting yourself go takes a lot of trust both in yourself and your partner, as well as practice. Be patient and tell your partner what feels good. If you never, or only rarely, experience orgasm, and this becomes an issue, **call your doctor.** ➥ Counseling and Psychotherapy, p. 697 ➥ Women's Issues, p. 537

COMPLAINTS AND SYMPTOMS	POSSIBLE CAUSES	WHAT TO DO
Inability to climax, or infrequent orgasms	Negative associations with sex • Belief that there's only one "right" way to climax • Fear of loss of self, or loss of control • Insensitive partner • Psychological factors • Sexual feelings you can't admit to • Unconscious rejection of partner	Tell your partner what excites you, or what makes you uncomfortable. Anything that takes place between consenting adults is fine. If, in spite of a comfortable sexual life, you are still unable to achieve orgasm and this becomes an issue, **call your doctor.** → Counseling and Psychotherapy, p. 697 → Women's Issues, p. 537
Vaginal spasms and pain at penetration, or penetration is not possible	Psychological factors • Fear or rejection of partner • Insensitive partner • Negative associations with sex	To break the cycle of fear, pain, and rejection, **call your doctor.** → Counseling and Psychotherapy, p. 697 → Health and Well-being, p. 182 → Women's Issues, p. 537

Sexual problems after taking medicines	Side effect of
	  medicines for psychoses (neuroleptics)
	  sedatives and allergy medicines containing promethazine
		Check the medicine label or insert for these substances. If they are present, **call your doctor.**
		→ Medication Summary, p. 657

SEXUAL PROBLEMS IN MEN

Sexual-performance pressure and anxiety are common in males. Fear of not being able to meet expectations is often the cause of impotence or difficulty in having erections. Other factors that can have an impact are stress, psychological factors, and some illnesses. Problems with erection in conjunction with penile disorders or diseases: Penile Disorders, p. 541. Painful sexual intercourse, p. 127.

COMPLAINTS AND SYMPTOMS	POSSIBLE CAUSES	WHAT TO DO
Problems with erection • **Exhaustion** • **Fever** • **Stress**	Normal reaction	Condition will clear up on its own. → Health and Well-being, p. 182 → Men's Issues, p. 541
Problems with slow erection or premature ejaculation	Overstimulation (in young men) • Exhaustion • Normal symptom of aging • Psychological factors	Unless you're under great pressure to perform, a slower erection should not be a problem. If ejaculation is consistently too early, and this is causing problems with your partner, **call your doctor.** → Counseling and Psychotherapy, p. 697 → Health and Well-being, p. 182 → Men's Issues, p. 541

COMPLAINTS AND SYMPTOMS	POSSIBLE CAUSES	WHAT TO DO

Problems with erection when using
    alcohol
    drugs
    tobacco
	Alcohol abuse
	 • Drug abuse
	 • Nicotine abuse
		Drink less alcohol. Quit smoking. Try not to abuse any more drugs. If unsuccessful, **call your doctor.**
		 ↪ Addictions and Dependencies, p. 204
		 ↪ Health and Well-being, p. 182
		 ↪ Men's Issues, p. 541

Long-term problems with erection • **Emotional issues** • **Performance anxiety** • **Relationship conflicts** • **Stress**	Fear • Psychological factors	Try to address your problems. Talking with your partner can help. If unsuccessful, **call your doctor.** ↪ Counseling and Psychotherapy, p. 697 ↪ Men's Issues, p. 541
Sexual problems due to unacknowledged sexual preferences or practices	Social taboos, pressures, or inhibitions	If you have a partner, talk things through. Be honest. Anything that takes place between consenting adults is okay. If you have preferences you're unsure about, or that could be harmful to your partner, **call your doctor.** ↪ Counseling and Psychotherapy, p. 697
Long-term problems with erection in conjunction with illness	Symptom of the illness, for example, nerve disorders from injury or surgery circulatory disorders of the genitals	If you are not already getting medical treatment, **call your doctor.**
Problems with erection and difficulties in urinating	Prostate disorders	**Call your doctor.** ↪ Prostate Enlargement, p. 534 ↪ Prostatitis, p. 534

COMPLAINTS AND SYMPTOMS	POSSIBLE CAUSES	WHAT TO DO

Sexual and/or erection problems after taking medicines	Side effect of various medicines, including
	    beta-blockers
	    diuretics containing
	        potassium canrenoate
	        spironolactone
	        thiazides
	    male sex hormones
	    medicines for epilepsy containing
	        carbamazepine
	    medicines for gastrointestinal
	        problems containing
	        cimetidine
	        famotidine
	        metoclopramide
	        ranitidine
	    medicines for high blood pressure
	    medicines for psychosis
	        (neuroleptics)
	    sedatives and allergy medicines
	        containing
	        promethazine
		Check the medicine label or insert for these substances. If they are present, **call your doctor.**
		→ Medication Summary, p. 657

SHOULDER PAIN

Pains or aches in the shoulders are usually due to tension, but can also be a symptom of degeneration or various illnesses.

COMPLAINTS AND SYMPTOMS	POSSIBLE CAUSES	WHAT TO DO
Shoulder pain after spending the day sitting or standing in a tense position (at the office, at the conveyor belt in a factory, running a cash register, etc.)	Muscle tension	Try to take frequent five-minute relaxation breaks if possible. Make sure your seat height and distance from work station are ergonomically correct. → Fibromyalgia Syndrome (Soft-tissue Pain and Stiffness), p. 462 → Relaxation, p. 693
Shoulder pain after unaccustomed activity (sports, gardening, housework, etc.)	Using unfamiliar muscles	Take a warm bath. A massage can help. → Massage, p. 686 → Muscle Soreness/Stiffness, p. 435
Shoulder pain over a period of time, spreading into the arm or from the neck down the back, with headaches • **Anxiety** • **Emotional strain** • **Stress**	Unconsciously hunched or tense shoulders • Psychological factors	Try to reduce the load weighing you down. If you need help, **call your doctor.** → Back and Lower Back Pain, p. 465 → Fibromyalgia Syndrome (Soft-tissue Pain and Stiffness), p. 462 → Health and Well-being, p. 182 → Relaxation, p. 693
Shoulder pain when moving arm, worsening over the years • **Stiffness**	Symptom of wear	**Call your doctor.** → Arthritis, p. 452 → Fibromyalgia Syndrome (Soft-tissue Pain and Stiffness), p. 462
Shoulder pain with simultaneous aching and swelling in other joints	Rheumatism	**Call your doctor.** → Rheumatism (Disorders of Joints and Connective Tissue), p. 449
Shoulder pain after a fall or accident	Pulled or torn muscle or ligament	**Call your doctor.** → Pulled, Torn Muscles, p. 437 → Tendons and Ligaments, p. 441
Shoulder pain after a fall, accident, or extreme movement • **Barely moveable arm** • **Dislocated arm**	Sprain • Dislocation • Fracture	**Call your doctor immediately.** → Dislocations, p. 448 → Fractures, p. 429 → Sprains and Strains, p. 441
Shoulder pain, severe in the morning • **Neck and lower back pain** • **Rapidly worsening eyesight**	Disease of blood vessels in muscular connective tissue	**Call your doctor immediately.** → Polymyalgia Rheumatica, p. 461

COMPLAINTS AND SYMPTOMS	POSSIBLE CAUSES	WHAT TO DO
Severe pain in left shoulder • Sensation of constriction and pressure in chest	Heart attack	**Call emergency medical services immediately.** → Heart Attack (Myocardial Infarction), p. 335

SKIN

GENERAL SKIN PROBLEMS

Dry, oily, or flaky skin isn't always genetically determined. Many skin-protection options are available, and most problems are completely manageable.

COMPLAINTS AND SYMPTOMS	POSSIBLE CAUSES	WHAT TO DO
Dry skin • **Flaky** • **Rough spots**	Genetic predisposition • Decreased oil-gland function (for example, due to aging) • Dry air from central heating or air conditioning • Strong, drying skin cleansers	Avoid dry air (central heating and air conditioning), or invest in a humidifier. Bathe as infrequently as possible, and avoid foaming bath products. Apply moisturizing cream after washing. → Skin Care, p. 261
Oily skin, often in distinct areas • **Oily, yellowish, scaly patches**	Genetic predisposition • Seborrheic eczema	Use oil-removing skin care products. If symptoms recur, **call your doctor.** → Seborrheic Dermatitis, p. 276
Skin impurities and eruptions • **Blackheads** • **Pimples** • **Pustules**	Oily skin • Acne	Avoid oily or greasy skin-care products. If acne is severe, **call your doctor.** → Acne, p. 274
Areas of tough skin (calluses) • **Painful (corns)**	Friction or pressure, such as from too-tight shoes	Calluses can be softened with warm water and removed with a pumice stone; corn bandages usually alleviate corn pain. If symptoms persist, **call your doctor.** → Calluses, p. 266 → Corns, p. 266 → Feet, p. 443

Facial rash or acne breakout after taking medicines	Side effect of
	  hormone preparations containing
	    mesterolone
	    methyltestosterone
	    testosterone
	  medicines with iodine or bromine
	    compounds
	  psychopharmacological agents
	    containing lithium
	  some anti-epileptic medicines
	  vitamins
	    B6, B12, D2
		Check the medicine label or insert for these substances. If your medicine is by prescription, **call your doctor.**
		→ Acne, p. 274
		→ Medication Summary, p. 657

COMPLAINTS AND SYMPTOMS	POSSIBLE CAUSES	WHAT TO DO
Rough, dry skin with whitish, non-flaking scales ("lizard skin")	Transmitted severe dry skin disorder	**Call your doctor.** ↪ Ichthyosis (Dry Skin), p. 277

Spotty, reddened pores, with pimples, especially on
    cheeks
    forehead
    nose
	Rosacea	**Call your doctor.**
		↪ Rosacea, p. 281

Thick, swollen veins under the skin, usually painful	Varicose veins	**Call your doctor.** ↪ Varicose Veins, p. 328
Open sores on lower leg	Ulcers from varicose veins • Lack of circulation	**Call your doctor.** ↪ Diabetes, p. 483 ↪ Leg Ulcers, p. 287 ↪ Varicose Veins, p. 328
Red, swollen skin or open sores in bed-ridden persons	Continuous pressure on skin	**Call your doctor.** ↪ Bedsores (Decubitis Ulcers), p. 288
Thin skin showing stripes or striations • **Acne** • *In women,* **profuse hair growth and menstrual disorders**	Hormone imbalance due to adrenal gland disorder	**Call your doctor.** ↪ Cushing's Syndrome, p. 503
Tough, inflexible skin • **Dry eyes and mouth** • **Vaginal dryness** • **Difficulty in swallowing** • **Open sores on fingers**	Connective tissue disorder	**Call your doctor.** ↪ Scleroderma, p. 461
Red skin after a burn • **Blisters** • **Oozing**	Burns	**Immediately** rinse affected areas with cold water, for up to half an hour or until pain stops. **Warning:** Do not apply creams, powders, or oils. Cover serious burns with sterile bandage. If over 20 percent of skin surface is affected (5 percent in children), **call emergency medical services immediately.** ↪ Burns, p. 264 ↪ First Aid, p. 704

SKIN RASHES

The skin clearly shows your emotions. It is emotions that make you blush, turn pale, and get goosebumps. Skin rashes may be caused by infections, viruses, fungi, allergies, or emotional problems.

COMPLAINTS AND SYMPTOMS	POSSIBLE CAUSES	WHAT TO DO
Sudden rash after eating	Allergic reaction to certain foods or food additives	Notice which foods cause you to react and avoid them. If you encounter difficulties, **call your doctor.** → Allergies, p. 360
Rash with emotional problems • **Stress**	Reaction of skin to stress	Try to address your problems and lessen stress. If you need help, **call your doctor.** → Counseling and Psychotherapy, p. 697 → Emotional Problems, p. 60 → Health and Well-being, p. 182 → Mental Health Disorders, p. 195
Bright red rash, usually with itching • **Blisters** • **Skin becoming thickened, infected, dry, and scaly**	Contact dermatitis	Try to identify the cause of the rash: watch, jewelry, cosmetics, detergents? **Call your doctor.** → Contact Dermatitis, p. 271
Red or white, fleetingly itchy, raised skin	Urticarial rash	If symptoms are uncomfortable or keep recurring, **call your doctor.** → Hives (Uticaria), p. 282
Red, extremely itchy bump with red dot (puncture point) on skin, often several close together	Insect bites	If itching is severe, **call your doctor.** → Insect Bites, p. 268
Itchy, infected, reddened skin • **Backs of hands** • **Backs of knees** • **Elbows** • **Face** • **Neck** • **With small lumps**	Atopic dermatitis	**Call your doctor.** → Eczema (Atopic Dermatitis), p. 272

COMPLAINTS AND SYMPTOMS	POSSIBLE CAUSES	WHAT TO DO

Skin rash and blisters after the use of medicines	Often signs of an allergic reaction, for instance, extreme light sensitivity
	• Side effect of numerous medicines, especially
	    antibiotics and medicines containing antibiotics
	    many varicose vein medicines
	    most ointments for muscle and joint pain
	    most skin medicines
	    some analgesics
	    some cold medicines
	    some cough and asthma medicines
	    some heart and circulation medicines
	    some laxatives
	    some rheumatism and gout medicines
	    some stomach and intestinal medicines
		If you bought the medicine over the counter and skin problems were not mentioned as a side effect, *stop taking it.*
		If the medicine was prescribed and you were not made aware of the side effects, **call your doctor.**
		↪ Medication Summary, p. 657

Greasy, yellowish, scaly, slightly reddened skin, with slight itchiness, mostly on the head but also
    eyebrow area
    eyelids
    In men, **also in beard area, on chest and back**
    mouth area
    nose
	Seborrheic dermatitis	**Call your doctor.**
		↪ Seborrheic Dermatitis, p. 276

Bright red to pale pink scaly spots, usually starting on torso and spreading over body	Pityriasis rosea	**Call your doctor.** ↪ Pityriasis Rosea, p. 277
Brick-red raised spots, especially on head, elbows, and lower back, with silver-white scales, usually not itchy	Psoriasis	**Call your doctor.** ↪ Psoriasis, p. 278
Very painful red rash with groups of blisters, usually on one side of torso or face	Shingles	**Call your doctor.** ↪ Shingles, p. 284
Small blisters, usually around mouth and nose, that quickly pop open and form yellow crusts	Bacterial skin infection	**Call your doctor.** ↪ Impetigo, p. 283

COMPLAINTS AND SYMPTOMS	POSSIBLE CAUSES	WHAT TO DO

Small, red, extremely itchy lumps and pustules in linear formation, on
  ankles
  buttocks
  genital area
  wrists
	Scabies	**Call your doctor.**
		→ Scabies, p. 270

Red, cracked skin between toes • Itching • Oozing • Peeling • Unpleasant odor	Fungal infection (athlete's foot)	Treat affected areas two to three weeks with fungus medicine. If infection persists, **call your doctor.** → Athlete's Foot, p. 265
Itchy, red, inflamed skin especially behind the ears • White dots (nits) visible in hair	Head lice	**Call your doctor.** → Lice, p. 268
Bluish, itchy dots in genital area	Crab lice (pubic lice)	**Call your doctor.** → Lice, p. 268
Swollen, reddened skin over entire body after an insect bite • Fainting • Itching • Shortness of breath	Allergic reaction	**Call emergency medical services immediately.** → Allergies, p. 360

SKIN RASHES IN CHILDREN

Children's skin responds sensitively to all kinds of influences. One moment it can be red and blotchy, the next, unnaturally pale. However, rashes may also be caused by irritations from foods and various childhood diseases. If you can't find an obvious reason, try to identify psychological factors that may be causing the reaction.

COMPLAINTS AND SYMPTOMS	POSSIBLE CAUSES	WHAT TO DO
Sudden rash with red spots, subsiding after some time	The body is overheated • The child is too excited.	Remove excess clothing; move the child into the shade. Cool drinks and rest will help.
Rash associated with emotional stress or specific situations	Skin reaction to overwhelming situations	Support your child in avoiding (or at least talking about) stressful situations. If the rash persists over time, **call your doctor.** → Counseling and Psychotherapy, p. 697 → Emotional Problems, p. 60 → Health and Well-being, p. 182 → Mental Health Disorders, p. 195

COMPLAINTS AND SYMPTOMS	POSSIBLE CAUSES	WHAT TO DO
Itchy, painful, red area of skin	Insect bite	Insect bites are not dangerous unless a child is allergic to them; the pain and redness will soon subside. ↪ Insect Bite, p. 268
Blotchy, sometimes itchy, rash after eating certain foods • **Chocolate** • **Strawberries** • **Tomatoes**	Poorly tolerated foods	Notice when rash appears; avoid associated foods. If rash recurs, **call your doctor.** ↪ Allergies, p. 360
Permanent red spot on face, usually on forehead or base of nose, present since birth	Birthmark	Birthmarks are harmless. In time they will fade or disappear. If you are concerned or uncertain, **call your doctor.**
Yellowish skin in babies a few days old	Newborn jaundice	Slight jaundice is harmless and common in newborns; serious jaundice requires treatment. **Call your doctor.** ↪ Jaundice in Newborns, p. 594
In babies, rash with small, red pimples, especially in groin area and buttocks • **White coating in the mouth**	Thrush and yeast diaper rash	Sterilize pacifiers and bottles by immersing in boiling water. Leave diapers off baby as often as possible. Switching diaper brands, and changing baby more frequently, may also help. If rash persists after one week, **call your doctor.** ↪ Thrush, Yeast Candial Diaper Rash, p. 595
Red, dry, itchy, scaly skin with thickened patches	Cradle cap, eczema	Prevent child from scratching. Moist compresses, cool baths with soothing oils, and cotton clothing may alleviate itching. If rash oozes and recurs repeatedly, **call your doctor.** ↪ Cradle cap, p. 596 ↪ Eczema (Atopic Dermatitis), p. 272
Rash with scattered spots • **High fever lasting three to four days**	Harmless symptom of a viral infection	If temperature exceeds 103°F, **call your doctor.** ↪ Cold, p. 298 ↪ Flu, p. 297
Rash after use of medicines	Usually indicates an allergic reaction	**Call your doctor.** ↪ Medication summary, p. 657

COMPLAINTS AND SYMPTOMS	POSSIBLE CAUSES	WHAT TO DO
Rash with red spots • **Itching**	Allergies	**Call your doctor.** ➥ Allergies, p. 360
Inflamed, scaly, red or oily, yellow skin patches • **Face** • **Groin** • **Neck** • **Scalp**	Seborrheic eczema	**Call your doctor.** ➥ Seborrheic Dermatitis, p. 276
Itchy rash with fine, slightly raised lines, between the fingers	Scabies	**Call your doctor.** ➥ Scabies, p. 270
Small, itchy, pus-filled blisters mostly around the mouth and nose	Bacterial skin infection	**Call your doctor.** ➥ Impetigo, p. 283
Rash with red, clearly defined, pea-sized spots, beginning on face and spreading over the entire body • **Slight fever** • **Swollen lymph nodes in the throat**	German measles	**Call your doctor.** ➥ German Measles, p. 601
Itchy rash with red lumps, mostly on face and torso, that turn into raised, fluid-filled blisters, which dry out and crust over • **Fever** • **Headaches** • **Joint pain** • **Lower back pain**	Chicken pox	**Call your doctor.** ➥ Chicken Pox, p. 604
Rash with small, red, irregular spots starting on face and behind ears, spreading over entire body • **Dry cough** • **Fever** • **Headaches** • **Red eye (conjunctiva)** • **Sensitive to light**	Measles	**Call your doctor.** ➥ Measles, p. 600

COMPLAINTS AND SYMPTOMS	POSSIBLE CAUSES	WHAT TO DO
Sandpaper-like scarlet spots starting on chest and groin, spreading over the entire body • **Bright red tongue** • **Chills** • **Fever** • **Sore throat**	Scarlet fever	**Call your doctor.** ↪ Scarlet Fever, p. 602
Redness and swelling over entire body following an insect bite • **Fainting** • **Itching** • **Shortness of breath**	Allergic reaction	**Call emergency medical services immediately.** ↪ Allergies, p. 360
Itchy, painful, red skin in throat or pharynx following an insect bite or sting	Insect bite	If the child was stung in mouth or throat, give ice to suck on. **Call emergency medical services immediately.** ↪ Insect Bite, p. 268

SKIN RASHES WITH FEVER

If your skin breaks out into a rash accompanied by fever, a so-called childhood disease may be at fault. Occasionally these symptoms are also caused by other disorders.

COMPLAINTS AND SYMPTOMS	POSSIBLE CAUSES	WHAT TO DO
Rash accompanying most fevers during illness	Viral infection	If rash and/or fever persist over three days, **call your doctor.**
Rash with fever and red spots, blotches or blisters	Sign of a childhood disease • Chicken pox • German measles • Measles	**Call your doctor.** ↪ Chicken Pox, p. 604 ↪ German Measles, p. 601 ↪ Measles, p. 600
Localized, painful, red swelling with inflamed streaks spreading from it, often in the lower leg • **High fever**	Infected skin injury	**Call your doctor.** ↪ Erysipelas, p. 283
Rash with fever and swollen lymph nodes • **Armpits** • **Enlarged tonsils** • **Groin** • **Sore throat** • **Throat**	Infectious mononucleosis	**Call your doctor.** ↪ Infectious Mononucleosis, p. 355

COMPLAINTS AND SYMPTOMS	POSSIBLE CAUSES	WHAT TO DO
Sandpaper-like, scarlet spots • **Bright red tongue** • **Chills** • **Fever** • **Sore throat**	Scarlet fever	**Call your doctor.** ↣ Scarlet Fever, p. 602
Dark red dots on skin • **Confusion** • **Headaches** • **High fever** • **Light sensitivity** • **Stiff neck**	Meningitis	**Call your doctor immediately.** ↣ Meningitis, p. 212

SKIN SPOTS AND DISCOLORATIONS

If you turn pale with rage, red with anger, or blue with cold, the changes in your skin are easily explained. However, spots or discolored skin can also be symptoms of several illnesses.

COMPLAINTS AND SYMPTOMS	POSSIBLE CAUSES	WHAT TO DO
Constant pallor • **Tiredness**	Genetic predisposition • Anemia • Cardiovascular disorders • Low blood pressure	Your skin might be naturally pale. However, if your skin is unusually pale over a period of time, **call your doctor.** ↣ Anemia, p. 345 ↣ Hypotention (Low Blood Pressure), p. 325
Red spots appearing under specific conditions, subsiding after a short time	Agitation • Allergies	Notice under what circumstances the rash appears. You may be allergic to certain environmental conditions, foods, cosmetics, etc. **Call your doctor.** ↣ Allergies, p. 360 ↣ Health and Well-being, p. 182
Redness with eventual white spots in conditions of extreme cold • **Fingertips** • **Nose** • **Toes**	Frostbite	**Warning:** Do **not** massage frostbitten areas, rub with snow, or apply direct heat from sources such as electric blankets or hair dryers. Drink hot liquids (no alcohol); slowly and carefully warm affected areas. If these methods prove ineffective, **call your doctor.** ↣ Cold Injuries (Frostbite), p. 264 ↣ First Aid, p. 704

COMPLAINTS AND SYMPTOMS	POSSIBLE CAUSES	WHAT TO DO
Hot, red, painful skin after prolonged exposure to sun	Sunburn	Keep skin moistened and cover red areas with damp cloths. If additional symptoms appear, **call your doctor.** ↪ First Aid, p. 704 ↪ Sunburn, p. 263
Shiny, bluish spots under skin following an injury	Blood collecting in tissues	If blue spots persist longer than seven days, or appeared without an injury, **call your doctor.** ↪ Muscle Contusion, Bruise, Ecchymosis, p. 436
Red dots or small spots of bleeding under skin	Changes in skin blood vessels • Blood clotting disorders • Blood platelet deficiency	If spots did not follow an injury, **call your doctor.** ↪ Hemophilia, p. 348 ↪ Thrombocytopenia, p. 349
Highly visible blue veins snaking under the skin	Varicose veins	If varicose veins are painful or cause discomfort, **call your doctor.** ↪ Varicose Veins, p. 328

Reddish to purplish stripes on the skin, later becoming white	Stretch marks due to
	    abnormal hormone production
	    adrenal disorders
	    large fluctuations in weight
	    side effects of cortisone
		If uncertain as to the cause of the stretch marks, **call your doctor.**
		↪ Cushing's Syndrome, p. 503
		↪ Striae (Stretch Marks), p. 279

Yellowish-brown spots, mainly in the face	Cosmetic sensitivity to sun • Pigmentation disorders (melasma), common during pregnancy and in those taking birth control pills	Brown skin spots are usually harmless and disappear on their own. If you are concerned, or symptoms develop further, **call your doctor.** ↪ Pigmentation Disorders, p. 280
Stretch marks and skin spots after taking medicines • **Bluish spots** • **Delicately wrinkled, parchment-like skin** • **Delayed healing of wounds**	Side effect of all cortisone-containing skin medicines	Check whether your medicine contains cortisone, or ask your pharmacist. If these symptoms appear, **call your doctor.** ↪ Medication Summary, p. 657
After taking medicines, skin discolors to yellowish or reddish	Side effect of many medicines	If your medicine is by prescription, **call your doctor.** ↪ Medication Summary, p. 657
Brown spots, often present since birth • **Growing hairs**	Birthmarks • Freckles	Birthmarks are usually harmless. If they grow, bleed, or itch, **call your doctor.**

COMPLAINTS AND SYMPTOMS	POSSIBLE CAUSES	WHAT TO DO
Brown spots • **Bleeding** • **Increasing in size** • **Itching**	Melanoma	**Call your doctor.** ↪ Skin Cancer, p. 286
Distinct white spots, often darker around the edges	Cause unknown; probably an immune disorder	**Call your doctor.** ↪ Vitiligo, p. 280
Painful, dark red to blue spots after extreme cold • **Ears** • **Feet** • **Hands** • **Nose**	Frostbite	**Call your doctor.** ↪ Cold Injuries (Frostbite), p. 264 ↪ First Aid, p. 704
Yellow-tinged skin • **Yellow whites of eyes**	Jaundice	**Call your doctor.** ↪ Jaundice, p. 393
Yellowish-brown tinge to the skin, not due to sun	Chronic diseases • Various medicines	If you are not already receiving medical care, **call your doctor.** ↪ Kidney Failure (Uremia) p. 425
Spider angiomas • **Yellow whites of eyes** • **Tingling in hands and feet** • **Loss of appetite** • **Weight loss** • **Breast development in men**	Cirrhosis of the liver	**Call your doctor.** ↪ Cirrhosis of the Liver , p. 396

SKIN GROWTHS, NODULES, AND WARTS

Skin growths, nodules, and warts are harmless in most cases and often disappear without treatment. Rarely are they symptoms of a serious illness.

COMPLAINTS AND SYMPTOMS	POSSIBLE CAUSES	WHAT TO DO
Small, soft, unchanging nodules under the skin	Fatty tissue lipoma	To be certain of this diagnosis, **call your doctor.** ↪ Skin Growths, Nodules and Warts, p. 144
Small, fairly hard, painless, unchanging, movable nodules under the skin	Connective tissue lipoma	To be certain of this diagnosis, **call your doctor.** ↪ Skin Growths, Nodules and Warts, p. 144

COMPLAINTS AND SYMPTOMS	POSSIBLE CAUSES	WHAT TO DO
Nodules in the skin, often containing one hair, possibly inflamed	Superficial folliculitis	If nodules cause discomfort or pain, **call your doctor.** → Boils and Carbuncles, p. 284 → Folliculitis, Pseudofolliculitis Barbae, p. 291
Warts (uneven, cracked, calloused raised skin)	Viral disease	Warts are usually harmless, but if you are over 45, they should be checked by a skin doctor. **Call your doctor.** → Warts, p. 267
Mole-like, soft, fatty growths	Warts • Birthmarks	To be certain of this diagnosis, **call your doctor.** → Warts, p. 267

Nodules in
    armpit
    groin area
    neck
	Swollen lymph nodes	**Call your doctor.**
		→ Lymphatic System Disorders, p. 355

Brown, mole-like growths resembling birthmarks, that may bleed when scratched • **Itch**	Melanoma	**Call your doctor.** → Skin cancer, p. 286
Deep-seated, infected, pus-filled, painful lump	Boils	**Call your doctor.** → Boils and Carbuncles, p. 284
Nodes under the skin near elbows, wrists, and finger joints • **Fever** • **Pain after getting up in the morning** • **Red, painful and swollen joints** • **Tiredness**	Inflamed joints	**Call your doctor.** → Rheumatism, disorders of joints and connective tissue, p. 449 → Rheumatoid Arthritis, p. 455
Reddish-blue, sponge-like lump	Hemangioma	**Call your doctor.**
Small, pointy, wart-like, calloused skin growths in the genital area and the anus	Genital warts (condyloma accuminata)	**Call your doctor.** → Genital Warts, p. 547
Red swelling on lips or genitals, with little blisters that pop open into painful sores	Herpes simplex • Genital herpes	**Call your doctor.** → Genital Herpes, p. 547 → Herpes Simplex, p. 285

COMPLAINTS AND SYMPTOMS	POSSIBLE CAUSES	WHAT TO DO

Nodes
  anus
  labia
  penis
	Syphilis	**Call your doctor.**
		→ Syphilis, p. 548

Reddish, waxy nodules, usually on face	Skin cancer (basal cell carcinoma)	**Call your doctor.** → Skin Cancer, p. 286

SLEEP DISORDERS

If you have trouble falling asleep, or awaken frequently during the night, a variety of factors may be at fault: excessive worries, bedroom temperature or noise level, a bad mattress, medicine, or illness. People's sleep requirements differ, so the quantity of sleep is not as important as its quality; the term "sleep disorder" only really applies if you are dazed and exhausted the next day.

COMPLAINTS AND SYMPTOMS	POSSIBLE CAUSES	WHAT TO DO
You cannot fall asleep • **A heavy meal** • **Alcohol consumption** • **Caffeine consumption (coffee, tea, colas)** • **Overloaded stomach**	Too much alcohol or caffeine	Eat earlier and eat lighter meals. Consume fewer alcoholic and caffeinated beverages. ➙ Mood-altering Substances and Recreational Drugs, p. 754 ➙ Nutrition, p. 722 ➙ Sleep Disorders, p. 190
Trouble sleeping after eating little or nothing	Hunger	Eat light foods that won't strain the stomach, such as broth or crackers. ➙ Body Weight, p. 727 ➙ Sleep Disorders, p. 190
Trouble sleeping after unaccustomed physical or mental exertion	Overstimulation	Often a soothing bath or herbal tea will help. ➙ Sleep Disorders, p. 190
Trouble sleeping and restlessness • **Thoughts that keep "going round and round"**	Unresolved problems	Often a soothing bath or herbal tea will help. Try writing down your thoughts or talking them over. ➙ Sleep Disorders, p. 190
Sleep disorders with no recognizable cause over a period of time, or in a new environment	Bad mattress • Noise • Pollutants in air or diet • Uncomfortable room temperature or insufficient ventilation	Buy a firm mattress on a wood-slat frame. Try to eliminate all disturbing factors. ➙ Hazardous Substances, p. 729 ➙ Healthy Living, p. 772 ➙ Sleep Disorders, p. 190
Sleep disorders that occur when you stop drinking alcohol or taking drugs	Symptoms of withdrawal	If you encounter problems, or sleep disorders do not lessen, **call your doctor**. ➙ Addiction to Illegal Drugs, p. 208 ➙ Alcoholism, p. 205 ➙ Mood-altering Substances and Recreational Drugs, p. 754

COMPLAINTS AND SYMPTOMS	POSSIBLE CAUSES	WHAT TO DO
Trouble sleeping through the night • **Anxiety** • **Listlessness** • **Loss of appetite** • **Nervousness** • **Tiredness**	Depression	If you still have trouble sleeping even after trying various self-help measures,**call your doctor.** → Counseling and Psychotherapy, p. 697 → Depression, p. 197
Sleeping problems due to snoring	Frequent sleeping on your back • Alcohol consumption • Nasal congestion (possibly due to polyps)	If you or your partner suffer from this, **call your doctor.** → Alcoholism, p. 205 → Nasal Polyps, p. 301
In women, **sleep disorders during menopause, possibly with night sweating**	Hormonal changes	If your quality of life is seriously affected, **call your doctor.** → Menopause, p. 510

Trouble sleeping with various illnesses	Symptoms depending on the illness, such as
	    aches
	    coughing
	    frequent urination
	    pains
	    shortness of breath
		If you are not already in medical treatment and disorders persist, **call your doctor.**

Sleep disorders after taking medicines	Side effect of many medicines, especially
	    many cough and asthma medicines
	    many medicines for cardiovascular disorders
	    sleep medicines and sedatives after extended use
		If your medicine is over-the-counter and sleep disorders were not mentioned as a possible harmless side effect, stop taking it. If your medicine is by prescription and you were not made aware of the possible side effects, **call your doctor.**
		→ Medication Summary, p. 657

Sleep disorders after discontinuing long-term medicines
• **Anxiety**
• **Palpitations**
• **Restlessness and trembling**
	Withdrawal symptoms from sleep medicine and sedatives
	    diet pills containing
	        diethylpropion
	        fenfluramine
	        norpseudoephedrine
	        phentermine
	        phenylpropanolamine
	    medicines containing
	        benzodiazepine
	        codeine
		Call your doctor.
		→ Medicine Dependency, p. 658

NIGHTMARES

Nightmares can be caused by medicines and certain illnesses.

COMPLAINTS AND SYMPTOMS	POSSIBLE CAUSES	WHAT TO DO

Nightmares before or after a stressful event such as
    car accident
    exams
    loss of a job
    new and difficult challenges
    separation from a loved one
	Normal processing of life events through dreams	The dream may recur several times; No cause for concern. If nightmares continue for several months, **call your doctor.**
		→ Emotional Problems, p. 60
		→ Health and Well-being, p. 182
		→ Mental Health Disorders, p. 195

Nightmares in conjunction with an illness • **Fever**	Side effect of illness	No cause for concern. The nightmares usually disappear along with the illness. If they persist, **call your doctor.** → Health and Well-being, p. 182
Nightmares • **Drinking to excess** • **During withdrawal from alcohol, drugs, or sedatives** • **Overeating**	Full stomach • Alcohol abuse • Side effects of withdrawal from alcohol, drugs, or sedatives	If nightmares persist for more than a few weeks, **call your doctor.** → Addictions and Dependencies, p. 204 → Health and Well-being, p. 182 → Mood-altering Substances and Recreational Drugs, p. 754 → Sleep Disorders, p. 190

Nightmares after taking medicine	Side effect of
	    nose drops for young children
	    medicines for
	        dizziness
	        itching
	        motion sickness
	        nausea
	        containing
	            cyclizine
	            diphenhydramine
	            hydroxyzine
	            meclizine
		Check medicine label or inserts for these substances. If your medicine is over-the-counter, *stop taking it.* If your medicine is by prescription, **call your doctor.**
		→ Medication Summary, p. 657

SPEECH DISORDERS

Speech problems can be the result of physical or emotional disorders in children and adults alike.

COMPLAINTS AND SYMPTOMS	POSSIBLE CAUSES	WHAT TO DO
Unclear diction in children up to age three	Normal development	Some children take longer to speak correctly. If your child doesn't seem to hear well, **call your doctor.** ⇢ Hearing Loss, p. 250
Delayed speech development or unusually limited vocabulary in children	Insufficient linguistic stimulation • Hearing loss	If your child speaks very little, **call your doctor.** ⇢ Hearing Loss, p. 250
Speech impairment in children (lisp, or inability to form sounds like a hard "g," "k," or "l")	Speech impairment with physical or mental and emotional origins	If the impediment does not clear up by age four, **call your doctor**. ⇢ Counseling and Psychotherapy, p. 697 ⇢ Health and Well-being, p. 182
Excessive nasal speech (speaking through one's nose)	Imitation of friends or family members • Physical causes	If this is not due to imitating the speech of others, **call your doctor.** ⇢ Nasal Polyps, p. 301
Stuttering in children and adults	Emotional problems	If stuttering is constant, **call your doctor.** ⇢ Counseling and Psychotherapy, p. 697 ⇢ Health and Well-being, p. 182
Speech disorders accompanying cleft lip or palate	Malformation	If you are not already receiving medical treatment, **call your doctor.** ⇢ Cleft Palate, p. 620
Speech disorders after excessive drug or alcohol intake	Alcohol abuse • Drug abuse	If you frequently drink to excess or have a drug problem, **call your doctor.** ⇢ Addiction to Illegal Drugs, p. 208 ⇢ Alcoholism, p. 205 ⇢ Mood-altering Substances and Recreational Drugs, p. 754
Delayed speech development or speechlessness in children • **Lack of interest in environment** • **Limited mimicking** • **Unresponsiveness**	Autism	**Call your doctor.** ⇢ Autism, p. 590

COMPLAINTS AND SYMPTOMS	POSSIBLE CAUSES	WHAT TO DO
Speech disorder accompanied by paralysis of half of the face • **Crooked mouth** • **Inability to close eye**	Paralysis of facial nerves	**Call your doctor.** → Facial Paralysis (Bell's Palsy), p. 226
Speech disorders (slurred speech) • **Trembling** • **Weakness or numbness in arms and legs**	Multiple sclerosis	**Call your doctor.** → Multiple Sclerosis, p. 220
Speech disorders and a stiff face • **Expressionless voice** • **Trembling hands**	Parkinson's disease	**Call your doctor.** → Parkinson's Disease, p. 218
Speech disorders in older people • **Confusion** • **Difficulty in concentrating** • **Memory lapses**	Isolation and loneliness • Circulatory disorders in the brain	**Call your doctor.** → Aging, p. 606 → Alzheimer's Disease, p. 219
Speech disorders accompanied by paralysis in one arm or leg • **Confusion** • **Dizziness** • **Visual disturbances**	Temporary circulatory disorder • Brain tumor • Stroke	**Call emergency medical services immediately.** → Brain Tumors, p. 221 → Stroke, p. 215 → Transient Ischemic Attacks, p. 214

STOOL ABNORMALITIES

Bowel movements give important clues as to what is going on in the body. Different colors or strong odor aren't necessarily cause for alarm (certain foods or an unbalanced diet can be factors), although sometimes they can point to a serious illness.

COMPLAINTS AND SYMPTOMS	POSSIBLE CAUSES	WHAT TO DO
Unusually colored stool (for example, nearly black or reddish), after eating foods that discolor stool (for example, dark leafy vegetables, beets, carrots)	Normal digestion	No need for concern; the color will normalize.
Loose and foul-smelling stool	Digestive problems due to poor nutrition	Try to eat a more balanced diet. ↣ Nutrition, p. 722
Excessively loose—or hard—stool	Too much or not enough roughage in your diet • Change of diet • Symptom of various illnesses	If stool does not normalize after three days, **call your doctor.** ↣ Constipation, p. 406 ↣ Gastroenteritis, p. 599 ↣ Nutrition, p. 722
Discolored stool after taking medicine • **Itchy skin** • **Yellow skin**	Signs of liver damage as side effect of many medicines	If you have these complaints, **call your doctor.** ↣ Medication Summary, p. 657
Worms in stool	Worm (parasite) infestation	**Call your doctor.** ↣ Worms (Parasites), p. 415
Yellow, greasy stool • **Huge amount and foul-smelling**	Digestive problems due to pancreatitis	**Call your doctor.** ↣ Pancreatitis (Pancreas Infection), p. 400
Yellow stool • **Dark urine** • **Yellow-tinged skin and whites of the eyes**	Jaundice	**Call your doctor.** ↣ Hepatitis, p. 395 ↣ Jaundice, p. 393
Fresh blood in the stool • **Pain while eliminating** • **Itchy anus**	Hemorrhoids • Anal fissures	**Call your doctor.** ↣ Anal Fissures, p. 416 ↣ Hemorrhoids, p. 417
Blood and mucus in diarrhea • **Abdominal cramps** • **Fever**	Severe gastrointestinal infection (for example, dysentery) • Crohn's disease • Ulcerative colitis	**Call your doctor.** ↣ Crohn's Disease, p. 412 ↣ Gastroenteritis, p. 599 ↣ Ulcerative Colitis, p. 411

COMPLAINTS AND SYMPTOMS	POSSIBLE CAUSES	WHAT TO DO
Blood in stool • **Alternating between diarrhea and constipation** • **Nodes on anus**	Intestinal cancer	**Call your doctor.** → Colon and Rectal Cancers, p. 414
Black stool after taking some medicines	Side effect of all medicines containing iron charcoal • *In rare cases:* symptoms of stomach or intestinal bleeding as side effect of various medicines	Check the medicine label or insert to see if discoloration of stool is mentioned as a harmless, temporary side effect. If not, **call your doctor immediately.** → Medication Summary, p. 657
Black, tarry stool (not diet-related) • **Vomiting of a substance that looks like coffee grounds** • **Vomiting of blood**	Stomach ulcer • Peptic ulcer	**Call your doctor immediately.** If you are vomiting: **Call emergency medical services immediately.** → First aid, p. 704 → Stomach and Duodenal Ulcers, p. 389
Black stool or blood in stool after an accident or injury to the abdomen	Intestinal injury	**Call your doctor immediately.** → First Aid, p. 704

SWELLINGS AND NODES UNDER THE SKIN

Nodes and swelling that you can feel and see are usually due to enlarged lymph nodes fighting infections. Swellings that you are not sure of need to be checked by your doctor. Skin nodes, warts, growths: Skin nodes, warts, growths, p. 267. *In women:* Pain or lumps in breast: Breast pain or lumps in women, p. 514.

COMPLAINTS AND SYMPTOMS	POSSIBLE CAUSES	WHAT TO DO
Small, unchanging, painless lumps under skin, either soft or medium hard	Lipoma • Connective-tissue tumor	To be certain of this diagnosis, **call your doctor.** → Moles (Nevi), p. 286
Swelling between the ear and the jaw • **Fever**	Swollen parotid gland (mumps)	**Call your doctor.** → Mumps, p. 603
Soft, painful swelling in groin that subsides with pressure	Hernia	**Call your doctor.** → Inguinal Hernia, p. 439
Swelling or lump • **Armpit** • **Groin** • **Throat**	Swollen lymph nodes in connection with various infections	**Call your doctor.** → Lymphatic System Disorders, p. 355
Swelling in armpit after breast surgery or radiation	Blocked lymphatic duct	**Call your doctor.** → Breast Cancer, p. 515
Swelling on the throat, under the arm, or in the groin • **Fever** • **Loss of appetite** • **Night sweats** • **Tiredness** • **Weight loss**	Lymphatic cancer • AIDS	**Call your doctor.** → AIDS, p. 357 → Lymphoma, p. 356

TESTICLE PAIN AND SWELLING

The testicles produce semen and male sex hormones. Any testicular aching, swelling or changing shape should always be taken seriously, as they are alarm signals.

COMPLAINTS AND SYMPTOMS	POSSIBLE CAUSES	WHAT TO DO
Painful, enlarged scrotum and lump on the testicles or worm-like thickened veins	Hydrocele • Hematocele • Varicocele	**Call your doctor.** ➜ Hydrocele, Hematocele, Varicocele, p. 532
Testicle pain and swelling • **Reddened scrotum** • **Fever**	Testicular inflammation	**Call your doctor.** ➜ Orchitis, (Testicular Inflammation) p. 531
Painful swelling of one testicle with hard, reddened epididymis	Epididymitis	**Call your doctor.** ➜ Epididymitis, p. 532
Ulcer on the scrotum	Sexually transmitted disease	**Call your doctor.** ➜ Venereal Diseases, p. 545
Swollen testicle, usually not painful • **Hardening** • **Lump**	Testicular cancer	**Call your doctor.** ➜ Testicular Cancer, p. 533
Usually in children, sudden, stinging pain on side of testicle, often following a sudden movement, with quick swelling of the testicle	Testicular torsion	**Call your doctor immediately.** ➜ Accidents and Injuries of the Genital Organs, p. 529
Testicle pain after a contusion or injury • **Open wound** • **Swelling**	Injury or contusion	If pain and swelling persist longer than an hour, **call your doctor immediately.** ➜ Accidents and Injuries of the Genital Organs, p. 529

THIRST

Thirst is almost always a natural signal that your body needs more water. However, excessive thirst can signal serious illness.

COMPLAINTS AND SYMPTOMS	POSSIBLE CAUSES	WHAT TO DO
Excessive thirst **• At high temperatures (for example, in a sauna)** **• During sweating from physical exertion**	Natural regulatory mechanism	Drink mineral water or tea
Excessive thirst after very salty foods	High sodium intake	Drink mineral water or tea
Excessive thirst after alcohol consumption	Side effect of alcohol consumption	If you drink alcohol frequently and want to cut back, **call your doctor.** ↳ Alcohol, p. 756 ↳ Alcoholism, p. 205
Excessive thirst with recurring diarrhea	Natural regulatory mechanism	Drink as much mineral water or tea as possible. If you are not already receiving medical treatment, **call your doctor.** ↳ Gastroenteritis, p. 599
Excessive thirst with fever	Natural regulatory mechanism	Drink plenty of mineral water or tea. If fever persists longer than three days, **call your doctor.**
Excessive thirst **• Fatigue** **• Frequent urination** **• Weight loss**	Diabetes	**Call your doctor.** ↳ Diabetes, p. 483
Excessive thirst **• Fatigue** **• Frequent urination** **• Sharp kidney pain** **• Stomach pain**	Overactive parathyroid glands	**Call your doctor.** ↳ Parathyroid Glands, p. 500
Excessive thirst with chronic kidney disorders	Symptom of the illness	**Call your doctor.**
Excessive thirst **• Large volume of urine**	Hormone disorder (specifically, diabetes insipidus)	**Call your doctor.**

THROAT DISORDERS

SORE THROAT

Sore throats are usually the result of irritated or inflamed airways.

COMPLAINTS AND SYMPTOMS	POSSIBLE CAUSES	WHAT TO DO
Sore throat with hoarseness • **Excessive alcohol consumption** • **Excessive smoking**	Irritated mucous membranes	Quit smoking; drink less. Gargling with chamomile or sage tea will ease the pain. → Healing with Herbs, p. 688 → Mood-altering Substances and Recreational Drugs, p. 754
Sore throat and hoarseness • **Lengthy talking** • **Shouting** • **Singing**	Strained vocal chords	Rest your voice. Gargle with chamomile or sage tea. → Healing with Herbs, p. 688
Stinging, scratchy sore throat • **Constant need to clear throat** • **Dry throat** • **Trouble swallowing**	Irritated pharynx from dry, over-heated air • Chemicals • Dust	Gargle with chamomile or sage tea. If chemical stress is acute (for example, exposure to irritating gases), **call your doctor.** → Air Pollution p. 783 → Pharyngitis, p. 302
Sore throat with runny nose • **Cough** • **Fever** • **Headaches** • **Muscle aches** • **Sneezing** • **Trouble swallowing**	Cold or flu	Gargle with chamomile or sage tea. Drink plenty of tea or other liquids. If complaints persist for more than one week, **call your doctor.** → Cold, p. 298 → Flu, p. 297 → Healing with Herbs, p. 688 → Pharyngitis, p. 302
Sore throat after taking medicines • **Increased susceptibility to infections** • **Pallor, tiredness, and dizziness**	Signs of blood or bone-marrow disorders as side effects of many medicines	**Call your doctor.** → Medication summary, p. 657
Sore throat with trouble swallowing • **Red, swollen, pus-coated tonsils** Fever • **Swollen lymph glands in neck**	Inflammation of the tonsils • Infectious mononucleosis	**Call your doctor.** → Infectious Mononucleosis, p. 355 → Tonsillitis, p. 302

COMPLAINTS AND SYMPTOMS	POSSIBLE CAUSES	WHAT TO DO
Sore throat with swelling between ear and jaw • **Fever**	Mumps	**Call your doctor.** ➥ Mumps, p. 603
Sore throat and fever in children • **Papular, sandpaper-like red skin rash**	Scarlet fever	**Call your doctor.** ➥ Scarlet Fever, p. 602
Sore throat • **Gradual changes in voice** • **Pain when speaking** • **Severe hoarseness** • **Trouble swallowing**	Vocal cord inflammation • Laryngitis • Polyps or nodules on larynx or vocal cords	**Call your doctor.** ➥ Laryngitis (Vocal Cord Inflammation), p. 303 ➥ Vocal Cord Polyps, Nodules, and Laryngeal Cancer, p. 304
Sore throat in thyroid area	Thyroid inflammation	**Call your doctor.** ➥ Thyroiditis (Inflammation of the Thyroid Gland), p. 498
Severe sore throat and coughing attacks after choking	Foreign objects or particles of food in the windpipe	Bend forward and try to cough up the object. Lift and support small children so their head is lower than their feet, patting the back. If this is unsuccessful and signs of asphyxiation appear, **call emergency medical services immediately.** ➥ First Aid, p. 704
In children, **sore throat with trouble swallowing** • **Barking cough** • **Hoarseness** • **Shortness of breath** • **Thick voice**	Croup • Inflamed epiglottis	If shortage of breath is present, or the child's voice is thick, **call emergency medical services immediately.** ➥ Croup, p. 596 ➥ Epiglottitis, p. 597

SWALLOWING DIFFICULTIES

Swallowing difficulties are usually symptoms of various throat disorders.

COMPLAINTS AND SYMPTOMS	POSSIBLE CAUSES	WHAT TO DO
Difficulty swallowing with the sensation of a lump in the throat • **Belching** • **Heartburn**	Psychological factors • Nervous stomach	Try to identify what it is you "can't swallow." If unsuccessful, **call your doctor.** ➥ Counseling and Psychotherapy, p. 697 ➥ Health and Well-being, p. 182 ➥ Nervous Stomach, p. 386

COMPLAINTS AND SYMPTOMS	POSSIBLE CAUSES	WHAT TO DO
Difficulty swallowing accompanied by heartburn • **Chest pain** • **Sour belches**	Stomach juices entering esophagus	If symptoms persist, **call your doctor.** → Acid Reflux (Heartburn), p. 383 → Esophagitis (Esophageal Inflammation), p. 383
Difficulty swallowing after eating, with pressure or sense of something stuck in the esophagus • **Scratchy throat**	Food particle in esophagus	Drink copious amounts of liquid. If symptoms persist for more than an hour, or recur, **call your doctor.** → Esophagus, p. 383 → Esophageal Pouches, p. 384
Difficulty swallowing and raw, sore throat • **Coughing** • **Fever** • **Hoarseness**	Common cold • Inflamed vocal cords • Laryngitis • Pharyngitis • Tonsilitis	If symptoms persist after three days, **call your doctor.** → Colds, p. 298 → Flu, p. 297 → Pharyngitis, p. 302 → Tonsillitis, p. 302 → Laryngitis, Vocal Cord Inflammation, p. 303
Difficulty swallowing accompanied by blisters in mouth • **Bad breath** • **Fever**	Stomatitis (inflamed oral mucous membrane)	**Call your doctor.** → Stomatitis (Oral Mucus-membrane Inflammation), p. 379
Difficulty in swallowing with a goiter	Narrowed esophagus due to goiter	**Call your doctor.** → Goiter, p. 494
Difficulty in swallowing when you have anemia	Iron deficiency	**Call your doctor.** → Anemia, p. 345
Difficulty swallowing with cramped throat • **Facial palsy** • **Feeling of pressure** • **Retching**	Narrowed esophagus • Scleroderma	**Call your doctor.** → Esophageal Stenosis (Narrowing), p. 384 → Scleroderma, p. 461
Difficulty in swallowing over a period of time • **Bad breath** • **Hoarseness** • **Vomiting** • **Unexplained weight loss**	Esophageal cancer • Laryngeal cancer	**Call your doctor.** → Esophageal Cancer, p. 385 → Vocal Cors Polyps, Nodules, and Laryngeal Cancer, p. 304

COMPLAINTS AND SYMPTOMS	POSSIBLE CAUSES	WHAT TO DO
Difficulty in swallowing • **Cold sweats** • **Double vision** • **Drooping eyelids** • **Intestinal paralysis and constipation** • **Nausea**	Severe food poisoning (botulism)	**Call emergency medical services immediately.** → Acute Gastritis, p. 387
Difficulty in swallowing • **Severe cough** • **Shortness of breath**	Food particles blocking airways	Bend forward and try coughing up the foreign object. For infants: Hold them so their head is lower than the rest of their body, and perform back blows and chest thrusts. If attempts are unsuccessful and asphyxiation follows, **call emergency medical services immediately.** → First Aid, p. 704

TOOTHACHES AND TOOTH PROBLEMS

Toothaches always require attention. Even if an ache is mild or disappears, the underlying disease—in most cases, destructive cavities—will continue unabated unless treated.

COMPLAINTS AND SYMPTOMS	POSSIBLE CAUSES	WHAT TO DO
Brown-stained teeth	Smoking • Discoloration due to medicine • Tartar	Quit smoking. If stains are a source of distress, they can be removed by a dentist. → Cavities, p. 366 → Smoking (Nicotine), p. 754
Slight toothache • **Limited to certain days** • **Sensitivity to cold, sweet, or sour drinks or foods**	Hypersensitivity of the tooth pulp • Change in climate • Emerging cavities • Psychological factors • Stress	If pain does not subside or recurs frequently, **call your doctor.** → Cavities, p. 366 → Health and Well-being, p. 182
Hypersensitive, aching base of tooth after tartar removal	Normal reaction to treatment	If symptoms persist more than a few days, **call your doctor.** → Gum Disease: Periodontitis, Periodontal Disease, Trench Mouth, p. 371
Slight toothache and tooth-grinding at night • **Pain in jaw** • **Tense chewing muscles**	Psychological problems • Protruding filling • Uneven bite	If symptoms persist longer than a few days, **call your doctor.** → Cavities, p. 366 → Health and Well-being, p. 182 → Uneven Bite, p. 372
In children: **itching, red, swollen gums**	Irritation due to emerging teeth • Irritation due to eruption of cysts	Give teething babies a hard rubber ring to bite. If you notice an uneven bite, **call your doctor.** → Baby Teeth, p. 376

Gum damage after taking medicine	Side effect of
	    epilepsy medicines containing
	        cyclosporine
	        mephenytoin
	        phenytoin
	        primidone
		Check the medicine label or insert for these substances. If they are present, **call your doctor.**
		→ Medication Summary, p. 657

Sharp, piercing pain or dull ache in tooth • **Pus discharge from gums** • **Swollen cheek**	Advanced tooth decay	Inflamed pulp, root, or jawbone, **call your doctor.** If pain is extremely severe, request same-day treatment. → Cavities, p. 366 → Inflammations of Root Tip: Abscess, Granuloma, Fistula, Cyst, p. 370 → Pulpitis (Inflammation of the Tooth Pulp), p. 368

COMPLAINTS AND SYMPTOMS	POSSIBLE CAUSES	WHAT TO DO
Painful gums that bleed during hard biting or tooth brushing **• Swelling between teeth**	Gum inflammation due to allergies diabetes epilepsy medicine protruding fillings or crowns stress tartar vitamin deficiency	**Call your doctor.** → Cavities, p. 366 → Crowns, p. 373 → Gingivitis (Gum Inflammation), p. 370 → Health and Well-being, p. 182
Painful pulling sensation in jaw **• Inflamed gums** **• Loosening teeth**	Gum disease	**Call your doctor.** → Gum Disease: Periodontitis, Periodontal Disease, Trench Mouth, p. 371
Spreading pain in jaw **• Jaw cracking**	Uneven bite • Clenching or grinding of teeth • Dislocated jaw	**Call your doctor.** → Disorders of the Temporomandibular Joint, p. 372 → Uneven Bite, p. 372
Pain under dentures	Ill-fitting dentures • Cancer • Irritation due to synthetics in dentures • Poor hygiene • Shifting jaw position	**Call your doctor.** → If a Tooth is not Salvageable, p. 373 → Oral Cancers (Cancer of the Mouth Area), p. 382

URINATION PROBLEMS

An unusually frequent need to urinate, or the inability to control the bladder, do not necessarily indicate an illness; however, pain while urinating is always an alarm signal.

COMPLAINTS AND SYMPTOMS	POSSIBLE CAUSES	WHAT TO DO
Frequent urination • **Large amounts of tea, coffee, or alcohol** • **Stress or anxiety**	Diuretic effect of drinks • Psychological stress	If you need to use the toilet frequently and this causes problems for you, **call your doctor.** → Health and Well-being, p. 182
In women: **frequent urination during pregnancy**	Normal side effect of pregnancy	→ Complaints During Pregnancy, p. 570

Frequent urination after taking medicines	Intended effect of diuretics
	• Side effect of
	  heart medicines
	  low-blood-pressure medicines
	   containing midodrine
	  medicine for urinary disorders
	   containing methenamine
		Check the medicine label and insert for these substances. **Call your doctor.**
		→ Medicine Summary, p. 657

Uncontrolled urination in toilet-trained children over four years old	Psychological causes • Congenital malformation of the urinary tract • Urinary tract infection	Try to identify the cause of the bed-wetting. If you need help with this, or suspect an underlying illness, **call your doctor.** → Cystitis (Bladder Infection), p. 418 → Health and Well-being, p. 182

Uncontrolled urination during
  coughing
  lifting
  other physical strains
  pushing
  sneezing
	Weak bladder sphincter muscle
	• *In women:* prolapsed uterus
		If you frequently urinate unintentionally, **call your doctor.**
		→ Prolapsed Uterus, p. 523
		→ Urinary Incontinence, p. 419

In men: **Discomfort when urinating**	Constriction of foreskin (phimosis)	**Call your doctor.** → Phimosis, p. 594
Constant urgent need to urinate in spite of passing urine frequently • **Bloody, strong-smelling urine** • **Burning sensation when urinating**	Cystitis • Bladder infection • Prostatitis	**Call your doctor.** → Cystitis (Bladder Infection), p. 418 → Prostatitis (Inflammation of the Prostate Gland), p. 534

COMPLAINTS AND SYMPTOMS	POSSIBLE CAUSES	WHAT TO DO
Pain when urinating and frequent urination • **Backache in kidney area** • **Fever**	Kidney infection	**Call your doctor.** → Acute pyelonephritis (Kidney Infection), p. 421
In women: **pain when urinating** • **Vaginal discharge** • **Vaginal itching** • **Holding back of urine**	Vaginitis • Sexually transmitted disease	**Call your doctor.** → Vaginitis(Vagina Inflammation), p. 518 → Sexually Transmitted Diseases, p. 545
In men: **pain when urinating, accompanied by discharge**	Urethritis • Sexually transmitted disease	**Call your doctor.** → Urethritis (Infection of the Urethra), p. 530 → Sexually Transmitted Diseases, p. 545
In men: **frequent urgent need to urinate** • **Dribbling** • **Smaller and smaller amount of urine passed** • **Thin urine stream**	Prostate enlargement • Prostate cancer	**Call your doctor.** → Prostate Enlargement, p. 534 → Prostate Cancer, p. 535
Frequent urination • **Excessive thirst** • **Weight loss**	Diabetes	**Call your doctor.** → Diabetes, p. 483
Frequent urination at night • **Breathlessness associated with physical strain** • **Shortness of breath at night (worse if head is not elevated)** • **Swollen legs**	Insufficient pumping ability of heart	**Call your doctor.** → Congestive Heart Failure, p. 337
In women: **uncontrolled "urination" toward end of pregnancy, either in droplets or gushing**	Breaking water	**Call your doctor immediately.** Transport in horizontal position only. → Labor and Delivery, p. 575

ABNORMAL URINE

Discolored urine after eating certain foods or taking medicine can be harmless. In many instances, however, changes in color or odor signify illness.

COMPLAINTS AND SYMPTOMS	POSSIBLE CAUSES	WHAT TO DO
Discolored urine for a brief period after eating foods containing natural or artificial color (for example, beets and carrots)	Color of food	No need for concern. The color will normalize after a few days.
Urine reddening or discoloration after taking certain medicines	Laxatives containing senna • Analgesics containing dipyrone	Check the medicine label or insert for these substances. The urine discoloration is a temporary, harmless side effect.
Dark yellow urine • **Diarrhea** • **Fever** • **Heavy perspiration** • **Low fluid intake** • **Vomiting**	Highly concentrated urine due to lack of fluids	Drink plenty of liquids and urine will return to its normal color. If color does not normalize after heavy fluid intake, **call your doctor.**
Red or brownish urine • **Foul-smelling** • **Milky or cloudy** • **Pain when urinating**	Bladder infection • Bladder cancer • Kidney cancer • Kidney infection • Kidney injury • Kidney stones • Permanent catheter	**Call your doctor.** ➥ Acute or Chronic glomerulonephritis, p. 422 ➥ Acute Pyelonephritis (Kidney Infection), p. 421 ➥ Cystitis (Bladder Infection), p. 418 ➥ Kidney Injuries, p. 424 ➥ Kidney Stones, p. 424 ➥ Tumors of the Kidney and Bladder, p. 427
Clear, dark brown urine and light-colored stool • **Yellow cast to skin and whites of the eyes**	Jaundice	**Call your doctor.** ➥ Jaundice, p. 393

VAGINAL DISORDERS

VAGINAL DISCHARGE

A slight vaginal discharge with no unpleasant odor is quite normal, in spite of what advertisements claim. If the discharge increases, possible causes include emotional stress, fungi and bacteria, or anxiety about sexuality. An unpleasant-smelling discharge indicates infection of the reproductive organs.

COMPLAINTS AND SYMPTOMS	POSSIBLE CAUSES	WHAT TO DO
Slight discharge with no unpleasant odor	The vaginal opening normally produces a discharge	Slight discharge is normal. Wear cotton underwear and avoid strong soaps or deodorants.
Slight, watery, mucous discharge with no unpleasant odor, which appears or increases in the middle of the menstrual cycle	Ovulation	This is a normal function of the body. During ovulation, a discharge can appear or become heavier. ↪ Contraception, p. 551
Discharge with no unpleasant odor • **Emotional problems** • **Overwork** • **Stress**	Reaction of the body to excessive demands or emotional issues	The discharge will disappear once stress is removed. ↪ Health and Well-being, p. 182
Discharge with no unpleasant odor, during use of an IUD or while taking birth-control pills	Irritation from the IUD • Harmless changes in the uterus • Hormonal changes due to birth-control pills	If the discharge is bothersome, or if you simultaneously have abdominal pain, **call your doctor.** ↪ Contraception, p. 551
Discharge during pregnancy	Hormonal changes	Heavier discharge during pregnancy is normal. If you have additional problems or the discharge has an unpleasant odor, **call your doctor.** ↪ Complaints During Pregnancy, p. 570
Whitish vaginal discharge • **Itching** • **Stinging**	Red, inflamed vaginal lips • Bacterial or fungal infection of the vagina	**Call your doctor.** ↪ Vaginitis (Vaginal Inflammation), p. 518
Yellow-greenish discharge with unpleasant odor • **Itching** • **Stinging**	Bacterial infection of vagina or uterus • Forgotten tampon or diaphragm • Gonorrhea • Trichomoniasis	**Call your doctor.** ↪ Gonorrhea, p. 549 ↪ Trichomoniasis, p. 546 ↪ Uterine Inflammation, p. 520 ↪ Vaginitis (Vaginal Inflammation), p. 518

COMPLAINTS AND SYMPTOMS	POSSIBLE CAUSES	WHAT TO DO
Slight discharge • **Frequent urination** • **Pain during intercourse** • **Painful abdomen** • **Problems in urination**	Chlamydia and ureaplasma infections	**Call your doctor.** ↪ Chlamydia and Ureaplasma Infections, p. 546
Discharge with strong abdominal pain • **Fever**	Fallopian tube infection or inflamed ovary (pelvic inflammatory disease)	**Call your doctor.** ↪ Salpingitis (Inflammation of the Fallopian Tubes), p. 525
Bloody discharge	Spotting during ovulation • Benign uterine tumors • Cancer of the uterus or cervix	**Call your doctor.** ↪ Cervical Cancer, p. 524 ↪ Menstrual Disorders, p. 508 ↪ Polyps, p. 521 ↪ Uterine Cancer, p. 525 ↪ Uterine Inflammation, p. 520
Spotty bleeding and severe abdominal pain	Ectopic pregnancy	**Call your doctor immediately.** ↪ Ectopic Pregnancy, p. 526

VAGINAL ITCHING AND BURNING

Vaginal itching or burning is always a sign of irritation and can be caused by infections, chemical substances, anxiety, and a variety of general disorders.

COMPLAINTS AND SYMPTOMS	POSSIBLE CAUSES	WHAT TO DO
Vaginal itching or burning after wearing tight or synthetic clothing • **Chemical contraceptives** • **Use of feminine deodorants** • **Vaginal douches** • **Washing with soap several times daily**	Irritation of the vaginal lips from chafing • Vaginal irritation from soap or chemicals	Avoid tight-fitting or synthetic clothing. Wash with water, or use alkaline-free products. Avoid chemicals. ↪ Contraception, p. 551 ↪ Vulva and Vagina, p. 518
Vaginal itching after age 45, with no other symptoms • **Dry vagina**	Decreased hormone levels	If the condition does not improve, **call your doctor.** ↪ Menopause, p. 510
Vaginal itching or burning when urinating • **Frequent urinating** • **Pain while urinating**	Urinary tract infection	**Call your doctor.** ↪ Acute Pyelonephritis (Kidney Infection), p. 421 ↪ Kidneys and Urinary-tract Disorders, p. 418

COMPLAINTS AND SYMPTOMS	POSSIBLE CAUSES	WHAT TO DO
Vaginal itching or burning • **Unusual discharge**	Vaginal infection • Sexually transmitted diseases (STD)	**Call your doctor.** → Vaginitis (Vagina Inflammation), p. 518 → Sexually Transmitted Diseases, p. 545
Vaginal itching or burning • **Swelling** • **Warts, boils, or painful blisters on the vaginal lips**	Condyloma • Genital herpes • Inflammation of the Bartholin's glands	**Call your doctor.** → Sexually Transmitted Diseases, p. 545 → Inflammation of the Bartholin's Glands, p. 519
Vaginal itching with open, oozing patch of skin that refuses to heal • **Swelling**	Vulva and vaginal cancer	**Call your doctor.** → Vulva and Vaginal Cancer, p. 519
Vaginal itching with strong thirst • **Weight loss**	Diabetes	**Call your doctor.** → Diabetes, p. 483

VAGINAL BLEEDING

Bleeding between menstrual periods may be a reflection of external influences or harmless hormonal changes, but it could also be a symptom of various ailments.

COMPLAINTS AND SYMPTOMS	POSSIBLE CAUSES	WHAT TO DO
Bleeding after sexual intercourse	Harmless changes in the uterus • Cancer • Cervical polyps • Injury during intercourse	If symptoms persist, **call your doctor.** → Cervical Cancer, p. 524 → Polyps, p. 521 → Uterine Cancer, p. 525
Bleeding after installation of an intrauterine contraceptive device (IUD)	Initial irritation • IUD intolerance	IUDs are usually installed during menstruation. A subsequent heavier or longer-lasting flow is no cause for concern. If symptoms persist more than ten days or flow is extremely heavy, **call your doctor.** → IUD (Intrauterine Devices), p. 555
In pregnant women, passing of mucous, bloody plug on or around due date	Normal first signs of birth process	No cause for concern. If you are uncertain or worried, **call your doctor.** → Pregnancy, p. 565

COMPLAINTS AND SYMPTOMS	POSSIBLE CAUSES	WHAT TO DO
Unusual bleeding after taking certain medicines	Side effect of excessive dosages of birth-control medicines blood-clotting inhibitors ("blood thinners") estrogen-containing menopause medicines	**Call your doctor.** ↪ Medication Summary, p. 657
Bleeding along with discharge • **Foul-smelling discharge** • **Very watery discharge**	Inflammation of the uterus • Cervical cancer • Inflamed ovary	**Call your doctor.** ↪ Cervical Cancer, p. 524 ↪ Uterine Inflammation, p. 520
Bleeding during menopause, after not menstruating for several months	Another period • Hormonal disorder • In rare cases, uterine or cervical cancer • Myomas • Polyps	**Call your doctor.** ↪ Cervical Cancer, p. 525 ↪ Menopause, p. 510 ↪ Uterine Cancer, p. 525
Slight bleeding during first three months of pregnancy	Low hormone levels • First signs of miscarriage	**Call your doctor.** ↪ Miscarriage, p. 574 ↪ First Trimester, p. 565
Bleeding during first and second trimester of pregnancy	Miscarriage • Premature birth	**Call emergency medical services immediately.** ↪ Miscarriage, p. 574 ↪ Premature Delivery, p. 574
Bleeding during last trimester of pregnancy	Premature birth • Detached placenta • Displaced placenta	**Call emergency medical services immediately.** ↪ Caesarean Section, p. 581 ↪ Premature Delivery, p. 574
Bleeding and severe abdominal pain when not menstruating	Ectopic pregnancy	**Call emergency medical services immediately.** ↪ Ectopic Pregnancy, p. 526 ↪ IUD (Intrauterine Devices), p. 555

VOICE DISORDERS

When our vocal cords don't vibrate freely, hoarseness results. The cause is usually an infection of the pharynx or larynx, but talking loudly, screaming, or singing can also contribute to hoarseness by straining the vocal cords.

COMPLAINTS AND SYMPTOMS	POSSIBLE CAUSES	WHAT TO DO
Hoarseness with rough or sore throat and cough	Dry, overheated air • Heavy smoking • Irritation from pollution	Give up smoking. ➥ Air Pollution, p. 783 ➥ Health in the Workplace, p. 789 ➥ Healthy Living, p. 772 ➥ Smoking (Nicotine), p. 754

Hoarseness associated with
  anxiety
  nervousness
  repressed anger
  tension
	Psychological issues	Try to get to the bottom of your problems. If you need help, **call your doctor.**
		➥ Counseling and Psychotherapy, p. 697
		➥ Emotional Problems, p. 60
		➥ Health and Well-being, p. 182
		➥ Mental Health Disorders, p. 195

Hoarseness after prolonged speaking, singing, or screaming	Strained vocal cords	Rest your voice. Gargle with sage or chamomile tea. If symptoms persist after two weeks, **call your doctor.**
Hoarseness and sore throat • **Difficulty in swallowing** • **Cough** • **Fever**	Cold • Flu • Laryngitis	Gargle with sage or chamomile tea. Take inhaling treatments. If symptoms persist after one week, **call your doctor.** ➥ Colds, p. 298 ➥ Flu, p. 297 ➥ Healing with Herbs, p. 688 ➥ Laryngitis (Vocal Cord Inflammation), p. 303

Change in the voice after taking medicines	Side effect of
	  asthma inhalants containing cortisone
	  diuretics containing canrenoate potassium spironolactone
		Check the medicine label or insert for these substances. If they are present, **call your doctor.**
		➥ Medication Summary, p. 657

In women, **a deeper voice after taking medicines**	Side effect of male sex hormones	If you are using these medicines and the symptom appears, **call your doctor.** ➥ Medication Summary, p. 657

COMPLAINTS AND SYMPTOMS	POSSIBLE CAUSES	WHAT TO DO

Hoarseness with
    dry skin and hair
    tiredness
    unexplained weight gain
    unusual sensitivity to cold
	Hypothyroidism	**Call your doctor.**
		↣ Hypothyroidism (Underactive Thyroid), p. 495

Hoarseness with
    difficulty in swallowing
    pain when speaking
    possible gradual change in
        voice tone
    sore throat
	Inflamed vocal cords
	• Laryngitis
	• Tumor of larynx or vocal cords
		Call your doctor.
		↣ Laryngitis, Vocal Cord Inflammation, p. 303
		↣ Vocal Cord Polyps, Nodules, and Laryngeal Cancer, p. 304

Hoarseness after goiter operation	Paralysis of the vocal cords	**Call your doctor.**
***In children,* hoarseness with barking cough** • **Croup** • **Muffled voice** • **Shortness of breath**	Epiglottitis	If shortness of breath is severe, or if voice is muffled, **call emergency medical services immediately.** ↣ Croup, p. 596 ↣ Epiglottitis, p. 597

VOMITING

Vomiting is a defense mechanism of the body, geared to rid it of toxic substances. However, vomiting can also be a symptom of various illnesses.

COMPLAINTS AND SYMPTOMS	POSSIBLE CAUSES	WHAT TO DO
Vomiting after excessive food or alcohol consumption	Normal reaction	Symptoms usually disappear on their own. Drink plenty of fluids (tea, mineral water, broth) and eat little (crackers) or nothing at all. Try to address your problems through means other than food or drink. If you need guidance, **call your doctor.** → Alcoholism, p. 205 → Counseling and Psychotherapy, p. 697 → Health and Well-being, p. 182
Vomiting primarily in the morning • **Belching** • **Gas or bloating** • **Heartburn** • **Loss of appetite** • **Stomach pain**	Nervousness • Psychological problems • Ulcer	If symptoms persist after one week, **call your doctor.** → Acute Gastritis, p. 387 → Counseling and Psychotherapy, p. 697 → Health and Well-being, p. 182 → Nervous Stomach, p. 386
In women, **vomiting and nausea primarily in the morning**	Pregnancy	If symptoms persist after the first few weeks, or if you lose weight, **call your doctor.** → Complaints During Pregnancy, p. 570
Vomiting with diarrhea and stomach pain • **Fever**	Viral infection	Drink plenty of fluids (mineral water, tea, broth) and eat crackers or nothing at all. If symptoms persist longer than three days, **call your doctor.** → Gastroenteritis, p. 404
Vomiting after prolonged exposure to the sun • **Dizziness** • **Headache**	Sunstroke	Get into the shade immediately. Apply damp cloths to forehead. Drink plenty of fluids (iced tea or mineral water). Eat something salty. If symptoms persist after a few hours, **call your doctor.** → Sunstroke, p. 707

COMPLAINTS AND SYMPTOMS	POSSIBLE CAUSES	WHAT TO DO
Violent vomiting, stomach cramps, and diarrhea • **Several individuals affected simultaneously**	Food poisoning	Drink plenty of fluids (mineral water, tea, broth). Eat crackers or nothing at all. If symptoms persist longer than three days, **call your doctor.** If mushrooms were eaten and vomiting intensifies, **call your doctor immediately.** ➜ Poisoning, p. 708

Nausea or vomiting after taking medicines	Side effect of many medicines, especially
	   antibiotics
	   excessive doses of vitamins A
	      and D
	   local anesthetics
	   many cough and asthma medicines
	   many medicines for heart and
	      circulatory disorders
	   many medicines for stomach and
	      intestinal complaints
	   many medicines for urinary-tract
	      disorders
	   medicines containing potassium
	   some migraine medicines
		If your medicine is over-the-counter and does not list vomiting as a side effect, *stop taking it.*
		If the medicine is by prescription and you werenot alerted to possible side effects, **call your doctor.**
		➜ Medicines Summary, p. 657

Vomiting with severe abdominal pain • **Diarrhea** • **Fever**	Severe intestinal infection	**Call your doctor.** ➜ Gastroenteritis, p. 404
Vomiting and nausea some time after a high-fat meal • **Sudden cramps on right side of upper abdomen**	Biliary colic	**Call your doctor.** ➜ Gallstones, p. 398
Vomiting with pain in the lower back or kidney area, sometimes radiating to the bladder • **Fever**	Kidney colic	**Call your doctor.** ➜ Acute Pyelonephritis (Kidney Infection), p. 421 ➜ Kidney Stones, p. 424
Vomiting with nausea • **Fatigue** • **Fever** • **Headaches and joint pain** • **Itching throughout whole body** • **Lack of appetite** • **Yellowing of eyes and skin**	Jaundice	**Call your doctor.** ➜ Jaundice, p. 393 ➜ Hepatitis, p. 395

COMPLAINTS AND SYMPTOMS	POSSIBLE CAUSES	WHAT TO DO
Vomiting with dizziness • **Balance disorders** • **Difficulties in hearing** • **Nausea**	Infection or disorders of the inner ear	**Call your doctor.** ➙ Ménière's Disease, p. 258
Frequent and deliberate vomiting • **Weight loss**	Serious emotional and psychological disorders	**Call your doctor.** ➙ Eating Disorders, p. 202
Vomiting with eye pain and blurred vision in one eye	Extreme pressure in eye (glaucoma)	**Call your doctor immediately.** ➙ Glaucoma, p. 244
Vomiting, usually sudden and often after excessive alcohol consumption • **Fever** • **Severe abdominal pain**	Inflammation of the pancreas	**Call your doctor immediately.** ➙ Pancreatitis (Pancreas Infection), p. 400
Vomiting with headaches after a head injury	Concussion	**Call your doctor immediately.** ➙ Concussion, p. 211
Vomiting with headaches • **Dizziness** • **Drowsiness or confusion** • **Pain in the neck when tilting head forward** • **Sensitive to light**	Meningitis • Bleeding into the brain • Pressure on the brain	**Call your doctor immediately.** ➙ Brain Tumors, p. 221 ➙ Intracranial Hemorrhage, p. 214 ➙ Meningitis, p. 212
Vomiting of blood or a liquid that looks like coffee grounds	Stomach hemorrhage • Bleeding of varicose vein in esophagus (esophageal varices)	**Call emergency medical services immediately.** ➙ Cirrhosis of the Liver, p. 396 ➙ Stomach & Duodenal Ulcer, p. 389
Vomiting with hard or tight abdomen • **Cold sweat** • **Rapid pulse** • **Severe abdominal pain**	Organ rupture	**Call your doctor immediately.** ➙ Appendicitis, p. 408 ➙ Cholecystitis, p. 400 ➙ Stomach and Duodenal Ulcer, p. 389
Vomiting with severe abdominal pain • **Bloated abdomen** • **Vomiting of brownish stool**	Intestinal obstruction	**Call emergency medical services immediately.** ➙ Intestinal Obstruction, p. 407
Vomiting with severe pain in the heart area, possibly radiating to the neck or arm • **Cold sweat** • **Nausea** • **Shortness of breath**	Heart attack	**Call emergency medical services immediately.** ➙ Heart Attack (Myocardial Infarction), p. 335

VOMITING IN SMALL CHILDREN

Occasional vomiting in babies is no cause for concern. However, frequent vomiting, or vomiting with symptoms like fever or stomach ache, is always an alarm signal.

COMPLAINTS AND SYMPTOMS	POSSIBLE CAUSES	WHAT TO DO
Vomiting of small amounts of food directly after a meal	Harmless reflux of food	No need for concern.
Vomiting in babies fed infant formula	Bottle nipple hole too large • Intolerance to formula	Replace bottle nipple. Switch to a formula your baby tolerates better. If vomiting persists, **call your doctor.** ↪ Baby Foods, Infant Formulas, p. 738
Frequent vomiting directly after feeding (in infants under three months)	Constriction of the stomach opening (pyloric stenosis)	If your baby regularly vomits after meals, **call your doctor.**
Vomiting • **Coughing** • **Runny nose**	Common cold	If vomiting persists more than two days, **call your doctor.** ↪ Colds, p. 298

Nausea or vomiting after taking medicines	Side effect of many medicines, especially
	   antibiotics
	   excessive doses of vitamins A and D
	   local anesthetics
	   many cough and asthma medicines
	   many medicines for stomach and intestinal complaints
	   many medicines for urinary-tract disorders
	   medicines containing potassium
		Give your child medicines in liquid form, or give plenty of fluids after medicine. Check the medicine label or inserts for these ingredients. If your child's medicine is over-the-counter, *stop using it.* If the medicine is by prescription, **call your doctor.**
		↪ Medication Summary, p. 657

Vomiting with watery stool • **Abdominal pain** • **Fever**	Infection of the gastrointestinal tract	**Call your doctor.** ↪ Gastrointestinal Infections, p. 599
Vomiting and abdominal pain	Food poisoning • Appendicitis	**Call your doctor.** ↪ Acute Gastritis, p. 387 ↪ Appendicitis, p. 408
Vomiting and diarrhea • **Dry mouth** • **Sunken eyes** • **No urine (dry diaper)** • **Dry skin** • **Drowsiness**	Dehydration	**Call your doctor immediately.** ↪ Gastrointestinal Infections, p. 599

COMPLAINTS AND SYMPTOMS	POSSIBLE CAUSES	WHAT TO DO
Vomiting after a fall	Concussion • Head injury	**Call your doctor immediately.** ➞ Cerebral Contusion, p. 212 ➞ Concussion, p. 211
Vomiting with severe headaches • **Drowsiness or confusion** • **High fever** • **Light sensitivity**	Meningitis	**Call emergency medical services immediately.** ➞ Meningitis, p. 212

WEIGHT

WEIGHT GAIN

Although in rare cases weight gain may be caused by hormonal disorders or other ailments, it is usually caused by excessive food, too rich a diet, and alcohol consumption. If you consistently overeat, ask yourself what eating is compensating for in your life, or what your weight is protecting you from.

COMPLAINTS AND SYMPTOMS	POSSIBLE CAUSES	WHAT TO DO
Weight gain after frequent consumption of rich foods and alcohol	Normal reaction of the body	Eat less for a few days. Try to eat well-balanced meals and be more active. Curtail alcohol consumption. → Alcohol, p. 756 → Body Weight, p. 727
Weight gain in a family with overweight parents	Bad eating habits • Emotional problems • Insufficient physical activity • Predisposition	Examine your eating habits. → Body Weight, p. 727 → Health and Well-being, p. 182 → Nutritional Habits, p. 722 → Physical Activity and Sports, p. 762
Weight gain after quitting smoking	Reaction to nicotine withdrawal	Eating or snacking is probably taking the place of smoking. Try to increase physical activities. In most cases weight will stabilize after a few months. → Physical Activity and Sports, p. 762 → Smoking (Nicotine), p. 754
Weight gain after a change in lifestyle (more relaxed pace, fewer physical activities)	Reduced demand for calories	Reduce food intake, or take up a new sport. → Body Weight, p. 727 → Physical Activity and Sports, p. 762
In women, **weight gain one week before, and during, menstruation**	Hormonal fluctuations	No need for concern. The body's water retention levels fluctuate. → Menstruation, p. 506
Weight gain • **Anxiety** • **Exhaustion** • **Lack of initiative** • **Melancholy** • **Stress**	Food as compensation • Emotional problems	Check whether eating habits have changed lately. If food is a substitute for facing problems, make an effort to deal with your issues. If you need help, **call your doctor.** → Body Weight, p. 727 → Counseling and Psychotherapy, p. 697 → Health and Well-being, p. 182

COMPLAINTS AND SYMPTOMS	POSSIBLE CAUSES	WHAT TO DO

Weight gain and noticeable increase in appetite after taking certain medicines	Side effect of
	    allergy medicines containing
	        astemizole
	    epilepsy medicines containing
	        valproic acid
	    migraine medicines containing
	        methysergide
	        pizotyline
	    rheumatism medicines containing
	        cortisone or ACTH
	    sedatives and allergy medicines
	        containing promethazine
	    women's hormone-regulating
	        medicines with danazol
		Check the medicine label or insert for these substances. If your medicine is over-the-counter, *stop taking it.* If your medicine is by prescription and you were not made aware of the side effects, **call your doctor.**
		→ Medication Summary, p. 657

Weight gain • **Heart disease** • **Kidney disease** • **Liver disease**	Water retention	**Call your doctor.** → Congestive Heart Failure, p. 337 → Cirrhosis of the Liver, p. 396 → Kidney Failure, p. 425
Weight gain • **Dry skin and hair** • **Hoarseness** • **Tiredness** • **Unusual sensitivity to cold**	Hypothyroidism	**Call your doctor.** → Hypothyroidism Underactive Thyroid), p. 495
Sudden weight gain during pregnancy, with no increase in food intake • **Puffiness in the face** • **Swollen legs, feet, and hands**	High blood pressure	**Call your doctor.** → Pre-eclampsia, p. 574

WEIGHT LOSS

Weight loss is usually due to loss of appetite. If you have lost the desire to eat or your body cannot utilize food properly, various ailments may be the cause. However, something might also be upsetting you and taking your appetite away.

COMPLAINTS AND SYMPTOMS	POSSIBLE CAUSES	WHAT TO DO
Weight loss accompanying stress or mental strain • **Difficulty in concentrating** • **Feeling downcast** • **Loss of appetite** • **Sleep disorders**	Mental or emotional problems • Environmental pollutants • Nervous stomach	If your weight has not normalized after six weeks and is connected with a move or job change, **call your doctor.** → Health and Well-being, p. 182 → Health in the Workplace, p. 789 → Nervous Stomach, p. 386

COMPLAINTS AND SYMPTOMS	POSSIBLEa CAUSES	WHAT TO DO
Weight loss accompanying heavy alcohol consumption • **Loss of appetite**	Reaction to excessive alcohol intake	If you are not already in medical treatment, **call your doctor.** ↪ Alcoholism, p. 205
Weight loss after taking certain medicines	To be expected when taking diuretics • Side effect of cholesterol medicine epilepsy medicine overdoses of thyroid hormones	If you are taking medicines for these illnesses and were not made aware of the side effects, **call your doctor.** ↪ Medication Summary, p. 657
Weight loss • **Diarrhea** • **Stomach ache** • **Vomiting**	Intestinal infection	Drink plenty of liquids (mineral water, tea) and eat little (crackers, soup). If complaints persist for more than three days, **call your doctor.** ↪ Gastroenteritis, p. 599
Weight loss and induced vomiting • **Bingeing** • **Absence of menstruation**	Anorexia • Bulimia nervosa	**Call your doctor.** ↪ Eating Disorders, p. 202
Weight loss • **Diarrhea in spurts** • **Greasy, voluminous stools**	Chronic inflammation of the pancreas	**Call your doctor.** ↪ Pancreatic Insufficiency p. 401 ↪ Pancreatitis (Pancreas Infection), p. 400
Weight loss • **Diarrhea** • **Goiter** • **Heavy perspiration** • **Shiny, slightly protruding eyeballs** • **Trembling**	Hyperthyroidism	**Call your doctor.** ↪ Hyperthyroidism, p. 496
Weight loss • **Extreme thirst** • **Frequent urination** • **Itching in genital area** • **Tiredness**	Diabetes	**Call your doctor.** ↪ Diabetes, p. 483
Weight loss • **Bloody, mucous diarrhea** • **Cramping** • **Fever** • **Loss of appetite**	Infectious intestinal disorders • Serious intestinal infection	**Call your doctor.** ↪ Crohn's Disease, p. 412 ↪ Gastroenteritis, p. 599 ↪ Ulcerative Colitis, p. 411

COMPLAINTS AND SYMPTOMS	POSSIBLE CAUSES	WHAT TO DO
Weight loss with cramping or piercing stomach pain • **Bad breath** • **Heartburn** • **Nausea and vomiting**	Stomach ulcer • Duodenal ulcer • Esophageal cancer	**Call your doctor.** → Esophageal Cancer, p. 385 → Stomach and Duodenal Ulcer, p. 389
Weight loss accompanied by cough • **Blood in sputum** • **Fever** • **Night sweats**	Tuberculosis • Lung cancer	**Call your doctor.** → Lung Cancer, p. 314 → Tuberculosis, p. 670
Severe, unexplained weight loss	Indication of almost all types of cancer • In rare cases, of AIDS	**Call your doctor.** → AIDS, p. 357 → Cancer, p. 470

Complaints

HEALTH AND WELL-BEING

People who are "well" tend to be comfortable with the relationships in their lives and have satisfying jobs; they tend to be well-adjusted socially and feel reasonably in control of their circumstances and environment. However, they are not necessarily "healthy" in the absolute sense of the word. Some people have numerous ailments or disabilities requiring constant medication and doctor visits, yet live relatively healthy lives. Others are physically "healthy" but never really "well" because of an underlying dissatisfaction with life. People or events easily irritate or overwhelm them, and they seem to be forever going from one doctor to the next.

Similarly, the influence of a so-called "healthy" and "unhealthy" lifestyle is relative. We all know someone who has lived to a ripe old age despite a lifetime of smoking, drinking, eating rich foods and physical inactivity. And we all know that person's counterpart—someone who is extremely health-conscious yet always sick, in spite of a nutritious diet, lots of exercise and no cigarette or alcohol usage.

Simply avoiding health risks, therefore, does not automatically lead to well-being and a long life; our health is influenced by a wide variety of factors. Who's to say which is the "healthier" person: the one who unwinds with a glass of wine every evening, or the one who strictly denies himself all pleasures, only to indulge occasionally with a guilty conscience?

As we can see, the deceptively simple phrase, "I feel well" or "I'm healthy" actually comprise many complex interactions between conflicting desires and attitudes, environmental influences, and physical, emotional, and social factors.

HEALTH AWARENESS

Most of us are aware of our bodies' strengths and weaknesses. Some people can overeat constantly, overburdening their stomachs without apparent ill effects, but need to be very careful of a sensitive bladder. With others, the situation is exactly reversed. Usually we are more or less aware of distress signals from our bodies, and develop strategies for avoiding or minimizing illnesses. Although each individual's approach is unique, people seem to handle the body's stress signals in one of three ways:

— The first type of person is keenly attuned to the body's slightest distress signal and responds immediately, by making behavioral and/or environmental changes until physical and emotional harmony is restored.
— The second type tries to practice "preventive medicine" by living a balanced life, getting plenty of rest, making sure all necessary support systems are in place, or perhaps seeking medical advice. This approach is effective in preventing serious trouble.
— The third type of person is oblivious to the body's subtle messages, ignoring the signals indicating minor changes; this can eventually lead to dysfunction and end in the manifestation of disease. Only a serious illness will force this person to pay attention to what's going on in his or her body.

Risk Awareness

Most people today can name various substances or behaviors that are risky to their health. Just as important as these single factors, however, is the frequency and the duration of our exposure to them. For example, occasionally getting very drunk does less damage to the liver than drinking a bottle of wine every day.

When many single risk factors are combined, their effects are compounded and consequently much stronger. To counterbalance this, individuals with a strong sense of health awareness are constantly alert, deciding which risks to take and which to avoid, and accepting responsibility for their behavior.

STRESS

This fashionable word is used to explain a wide range of unpleasant situations in our lives: too much work, not enough time, high expectations, low expectations, aggressiveness, irritability. Stress can be aggravated by excessive heat or cold, street noise, having surgery, living a life of constant opposition to the body's natural rhythms (see p. 183), impending life changes, anticipation of pleasure, and even success itself.

Stress is a basic reaction in our lives; anything we experience or feel, anything we do or don't do can trigger stress. The triggers don't determine whether the body will react positively or negatively: stress is simply the body's reaction to changes, ensuring survival.

Evolutionary Programming

Our minds and bodies are programmed by evolution to survive by coping successfully with challenging situations. Four systems cooperate for this purpose:
— The limbic system, governing our feelings, moods and subconscious impressions.
— The cerebrum, which is responsible for sensory perception and conscious action.
— The hypothalamus, which activates the autonomic nervous system and switches the body to "on."
— The control centers in the spinal cord, which regulate muscle tension and fine motor skills.

Various hormones are involved in stress reactions: adrenaline and noradrenaline from the adrenal medulla, cortisol from the adrenal cortex, and various hormones from the pituitary gland. This causes bronchodilation, accelerated heartbeat, and elevated blood pressure. Everything is on alert; the organs and muscular system are primed to handle the extra surge of oxygen and energy. Such a burst of hormones also stimulates the immune system.

Stress factors

In general, stress in modern life results from demanding too much of our bodies; in extreme situations, this can lead to physical violence or emotional overload. Intensive work taxes the entire nervous system, mobilizing reserves, and exhausting energy. Note, however, that physical or mental exhaustion in itself does not contribute to stress as long as the work being done is satisfying and fulfilling.

"Overdoing it," in any number of ways, can cause harm to our systems. Many of the diseases affecting the industrialized world have been blamed on the negative side effects of stress, especially increases in the cardio-vascular disorders and high blood pressure, which seem to affect half the population, and a long list of feelings of malaise and disorders of the various organs.

Biorhythms

Every person has his or her own daily rhythm. The autonomic nervous system requires both tension (stimulation) and relaxation. Our hormones are released in accordance with the daily alternation between day and night and the seasonal alternation between light and warmth in summer, dark and cold in winter. In general, human beings are active during the day and inactive at night during the restorative period of sleep. To this end, most of the hormone cortisol is released in the morning, to ensure lots of energy during the day. Body temperature is highest in the afternoon and lowest at night, with a normal fluctuation range of approximately 1.5°F. There is also a definite rhythm to the day, with maximum productivity in the early morning hours, a low around noon, and then an increase again in the early evening hours.

It takes time for the human organism to adjust to change.

Production of melatonin, the "rhythm hormone," is keyed to the presence or absence of light. In darkness, the pineal gland in the brain releases large quantities of sleep-inducing melatonin; in light, it releases much less. This explains our tendency to be sluggish and melancholy on dreary winter days, and impulsive and energetic in the spring and summer months.

Constant switching of waking and sleeping patterns is not in the body's best interest and can induce headaches, nervousness and sleep disorders in people who work shifts or nights. The metabolic changes brought about by jet lag are the result of changing time zones rapidly, allowing insufficient time for the body to react.

Working Time

Standard work schedules contrast starkly with our biorhythms (see above), offering us artificial light at work, night and shift work, and no vacation during the darkest time of year. The job market also does not take into consideration variables such as stamina, endurance, and productivity, which are always in flux depending on an individual's situation and age. Many people feel burdened by the strict delineation between work and

Obeying Your Light-Dark Rhythm
— Schedule major projects for the lightest months of the year.
— A winter vacation at home will encourage rest and retreat; a trip to sunnier climes can help balance winter "blues."
— Get outdoors as much as possible: even on cloudy days you absorb more light outdoors than indoors.
— Move tables at which you sit for long stretches nearer to windows. Get rid of curtains or shades. Lighten up rooms.
— Reverse your daily rhythm as little as possible (i.e. avoid staying up at night and sleeping during the day).

relaxation; we actually require regular periods of relaxation at work, just as we require some stimulation or challenge during periods of relaxation.

Shift Work

In shift workers the light-dark rhythm is disturbed. Because the body does not receive proper rest, 64 percent of all shift workers suffer from nervous disorders. These problems are made worse by the lack of truly restful sleep during the day and the limited opportunity to participate in daily family life. Therefore, if shift work is necessary, it should be occasional and not on a regular basis. For every night shift, workers should ideally be granted a compensation period of at least 24 hours during which no work is done.

Production-Line Work

Working on a production line requires patience, adaptability, endurance, precision, and the ability to meet deadlines and perform repetitive movements for hours on end. The resulting monotony does not provide sufficient stimulation for the mind; high noise levels are stressful to the body; and the need for intense concentration combined with too short breaks is stressful to the psyche.

Housework

Housework is repetitive, not highly regarded, and never-ending. It is usually an isolating experience providing little or no social contact. In addition to supplying these stress factors, family work is always situation-dependent and usually provides no monetary income. It is essential that people working inside the home have effective methods for maintaining a balanced life (see Balance is Possible, p. 185).

Underemployment

People who are insufficiently challenged, either by outside stimulation or their individual goals, are underemployed and often suffer from feelings of worthlessness and superfluousness. This happens not only in the workplace, but is present as a general condition.

Frustration

Remarkable stress levels are often the cumulative result of years of driving ambition, hard work and great personal effort, undercut by persistent feelings of not having accomplished much, or of downright failure. A lack of recognition by others, or a constant fear of criticism or failure, can be intense stress factors.

Major Life Events

Every departure from our routine threatens our basic security and is potentially stressful: Moving, switching jobs, losing a job, retirement, marriage, childbirth, separation from a partner, a child moving out, the death of a loved one—not to mention being robbed or raped or experiencing other acts of violence. It usually takes at least a year—often longer—to recover.

Serious childhood events affect many people well into adult life. Constant rejection by parents, the feeling of not being loved, tensions at home, placement in a foster home, violence or sexual abuse by a trusted person—all of these can destroy self-confidence to the point of imbalance.

Poisonous (Harmful) Substances

Besides nicotine and alcohol (see p. 754, 756), environmental substances such as lead, solvents, benzene or pesticides are very taxing to the body (see Healthy Living, p. 772; Air Pollution, p. 783; Health in the Workplace, p. 789).

BALANCE

Human beings are naturally accustomed to an alternating sequence of contrasts. The pendulum continuously swings back and forth between light and dark, tension and relaxation, hunger and satiety, sleeping and waking. A constant state of imbalance, therefore, is very damaging: As the body grows accustomed to prolonged tension, the "fight or flight reaction" becomes the norm. An advantage of this condition is that the body will no longer react to the slightest irritation; by the same token, however, chronic stress on kidneys, blood vessels and connective tissue can pass unnoticed and cause disorders with few overt symptoms.

The body's reaction to a life of unrelenting, excessive tension can manifest as headaches, nervousness, sleep disorders, difficulties functioning, or psychosomatic disorders such as backaches, asthma, high blood pressure or peptic ulcers. Excess amounts of cortisol weaken the immune system and may also provide cancer cells with a favorable growth environment.

Balance is Possible

Achieving balance in life does not necessarily mean living in an easy chair in front of the television. Rather, it means incorporating the alternation of opposites into your daily activities: Sitting for a while, then moving around; eating well, then fasting till the next meal; doing mental work, then switching to manual activities. If you work alone all day, you need to get out at night and socialize; if you are with people all day, you need some time alone.

Psychological factors are our biggest resources for managing stress. We can gain great strength from the conviction that we are in control of our situation and that our actions can make a difference in our lives and in the world. Imbalance and negative stress arise when our duties outweigh our capabilities. There are few things more oppressive than feelings of helplessness.

Avoiding Overload

Over the course of life, everyone develops individual stress management mechanisms. One very helpful strategy is to plan ahead and mentally "walk through" an anticipated stressful process or situation; this allows life changes to be enriching rather than threatening. Also, if we can find meaning in what happens to us, we can react positively to challenges. For example, a job that makes sense is a lot more satisfying and less stressful than one that seems pointless.

One obvious way to see how differently people handle stress is by observing their reactions to serious illness. Research continues to show that those gathering as much information as possible cope the best; they develop strength through knowledge and have the feeling of being active and in control. A second group of people live in complete denial, go on living as if nothing were the matter, and ignore the obvious as long as possible. Those who cope the worst, however, are those who either try to accept a bad diagnosis stoically, or let themselves slide into hopelessness.

Creating Equilibrium

The body and the psyche, the nerves, hormones, immune system, muscles, and organs are all interconnected. They work together like gears; a variation in one area affects the whole system. There are different ways of intervening in this system; one is through relaxation methods, for instance yoga (p. 695), which eases stress in body and mind while simultaneously relaxing the muscles. When practiced over the long term, it not only produces immediate relaxation but also promotes general health.

A similar effect can be brought about by regular exercise, a healthy diet, avoiding alcohol and/or tobacco, ending a stressful relationship, leaving an unsatisfying job, and so on.

PSYCHOSOMATIC DISORDERS

Many health disorders occur in our emotional life without impinging on our physical awareness—e.g., anxiety, uneasiness, nervousness, irritability, listlessness, or apathy. Functional complaints which may be closely connected to these emotional conditions are diarrhea, headaches, or circulatory problems. In these connections the autonomic nervous system plays an important role.

The autonomic nervous system regulates breathing, circulation, digestion, metabolism, body temperature, hormones, and healing processes without our involvement. It affects our muscular system and glands as well, which is why emotional complaints go hand in hand with functional disorders of the organs.

All illnesses should in principle be understood as psychosomatic events, because physical conditions constantly influence our mental and emotional well-being and vice versa. This means that an endless complex of potential disorders is presented by the many situations that arise throughout life; it is up to each individual to discover the critical situations or experiences contributing to disease.

Signals of Excessive Demands

Excessive demands on your body or psyche over a long period of time can lead to total exhaustion. Feelings of not being able (or not wanting) to cope are clear signals of this condition. Lack of interest or participation and withdrawal are symptoms that force the body and mind to rest. The body sends us "healthy" signals such as fatigue, exhaustion, and concentration problems to let us know we have reached the limit of our resources and that relaxation, rest, and healing are urgently needed.

There are four kinds of psychosomatic disorders, each of which can be traced to similar causes and can be healed or eased in a similar way as well.

Feelings of Malaise

These are uncomfortable, mostly psychological sensations and feelings not connected with an actual disease. Typical of these vague feelings of ill-health are:
— General anxiety
— Uneasiness
— Feeling downcast or sad
— Nervousness or irritation
— Fatigue or exhaustion
— Confusion or lack of concentration
— Listlessness or apathy
—Withdrawal from sexual and social life
— Changes in awareness, accuracy and judgment

Functional Disorders

In this situation the functions and interactions of various organs are disturbed without ill effect to the organs themselves. The most common functional complaints are
— Eating, swallowing and digestive disorders (diarrhea, constipation, vomiting or nausea, and changes in body weight)
— Breathing complaints, long-lasting hoarseness or loss of voice
— Palpitations, racing heartbeat, feelings of stabbing pain in the heart, poor circulation or fainting
— Painful menstruation or lack of ovulation
— Vaginal cramps, lack of orgasm, impotence or premature ejaculation

Conversion Symptoms

These include blindness, deafness, loss of voice, lameness, or apparent paralysis, not caused by organic changes. Although these "illnesses" exist exclusively in the mind, they sometimes look and act exactly like actual disabilities.

Psychosomatic Disorders

These are the "classic" psychosomatic disorders, of which the gastric ulcer is best known. Also included are arterial occlusive diseases, heart attacks, essential high blood pressure (p. 316), bronchial asthma (p. 307), stomach and duodenal ulcers (p. 389), inflammatory intestinal disorders (ulcerative colitis, p. 411; Crohn's disease, p. 412), inflammatory and allergic skin diseases (atopic dermatitis, p. 272), eating disorders (p. 202), various women's illnesses and disorders relating to mobility.

You are under stress if:

— You feel irritable and overreact to the slightest event.
— You constantly feel rushed.
— You have a hard time relaxing and feel you should be doing something even in your spare time.
— You notice you no longer have fun or enjoy activities you used to enjoy.
— You are no longer able to participate in conversations and have a hard time listening to others.
— An overriding feeling of uneasiness replaces interest in social contact.
— You start to withdraw from the world.

In these illnesses, the organs and tissues are actually affected as a result of psychological factors.

Autoimmune Diseases

It is suspected but not proven that mental processes contribute to the genesis of autoimmune disorders. In these cases, the immune system attacks its host's body and secretions, which it no longer recognizes as its own; it creates antibodies against itself, thus establishing a cycle that is hard to break. These conditions can become life-threatening as the body's processes stop working together.

Illnesses caused by this self-destructive activity include rheumatoid arthritis (p. 455), Type I diabetes (p. 483), hyperthyroidism (p. 496), systemic lupus erythematosus (p. 460), and polymyalgia rheumatica (p. 461).

Causes

The causes of "system overload" include the total exhaustion of physical, mental and emotional reserves. This can result in a constant condition of hyperactivity or overexcitement which makes it impossible to relax or sleep despite exhaustion.

Poisoning

Various chemical substances can be toxic to the nervous system and cause disorders:

Nervousness and memory disorders in the central nervous system,

Visual and sensory disorders in the peripheral nervous system,

Disturbed sense of balance, exhaustion, and depression in the autonomic nervous system (p. 211).

Medications

Many medications list drowsiness and exhaustion as side effects. Consult your health-care provider or pharmacist. Discontinuing use of tranquilizers or medications for anxiety, nervousness and restlessness can often produce precisely the conditions they were prescribed to treat (see Medication Summary, p. 657).

Illness

Weariness, listlessness or apathy often occur in conjunction with an illness: these are caused by the body's natural reaction to illness, namely to withdraw while mobilizing strength and regenerating itself.

On the other hand, exhaustion, weakness, and weariness could also signal a bodily deficiency or the onset of an illness if caused by
— Deficiency of vitamins, iron, magnesium
— Lack of exercise and a deficit of oxygen
— Metabolic disorders
— Infectious disorders

Risks of Illness

Psychosomatic complaints such as feeling under the weather, vaguely sick, or just run-down are very common. About two thirds of all patients seeking medical advice suffer from this sort of general malaise; of these complaints, half are psychosomatic. Over twice as many women as men suffer from a general sense of ill-health.

The average person experiences about 600 different "health disorders" in a lifetime, most of which clear up without medical treatment or heal on their own. Only about 140 of these require medical treatment, and only 20 lead to hospitalization or intervention by specialists.

This ratio shows us that most complaints are efficiently handled by our own self-healing powers. However, the risk of illness definitely increases when serious events occur in our lives, calling for quick adaptation. This can happen with both positive and negative changes; the more intense the event, the more time and vigor are required to withstand the strain it places on our powers of adaptation, and the higher the risk of illness. Usually illness does not manifest until 6 to 18 months after the event. A common example of this is someone retiring from the workforce; often, about a year later, one can expect to see heart problems, organic disorders, even a heart attack.

Aftereffects and Complications

Feeling under the weather can serve a useful purpose by informing us that the body needs some time off. Someone who comes down with a cold like clockwork every fall, for example, is better off than the person who, so as not to "waste" time being sick, suppresses all feelings of illness and accumulates them over several years. This can lead to a total breakdown, which takes a lot more out of the body than the occasional cold. Being sick has an important function: it creates time for rest and relaxation. Furthermore, functional disorders can actually force us to confront serious issues in our lives that need resolution.

The Upside of Illness

Psychosomatic complaints or functional disorders not only force us to make time for rest and relaxation, they also affect our environments. Being ill frees us not only from professional responsibilities, but from everyday tasks, and the job of organizing them as well. It allows us to be taken care of, even spoiled; others become more attentive, and often little things make a big difference. Stomachache? Eat only what you feel like eating. Headache? Cancel that unpleasant appointment. Sore throat? Don't have that stressful conversation now—wait till you're feeling better. Poor circulation? You're entitled to have help performing daily tasks. There is meaning to be found in functional complaints: Learning to listen to and understand the body's signals.

Ignore at Your Own Risk

If this sort of psychosocial connection is consistently ignored, symptoms can eventually involve the entire organism, affecting circulation, digestion, breathin and metabolism. These complications not only lead to chronic suffering but can also cause organic damage. Medications can effectively ease pain and eliminate the body's warning signals, but do not address causes. Chronic consumption of medications is the most common aftereffect of feeling sick or run-down.

Prevention

A feeling of general malaise is an important alarm signal indicating an imbalance between mind and body. Take this warning seriously and learn to interpret it. One basic preventive strategy is learning to let go—of unrealistic expectations, performance pressure, and the

Stress affects the entire body

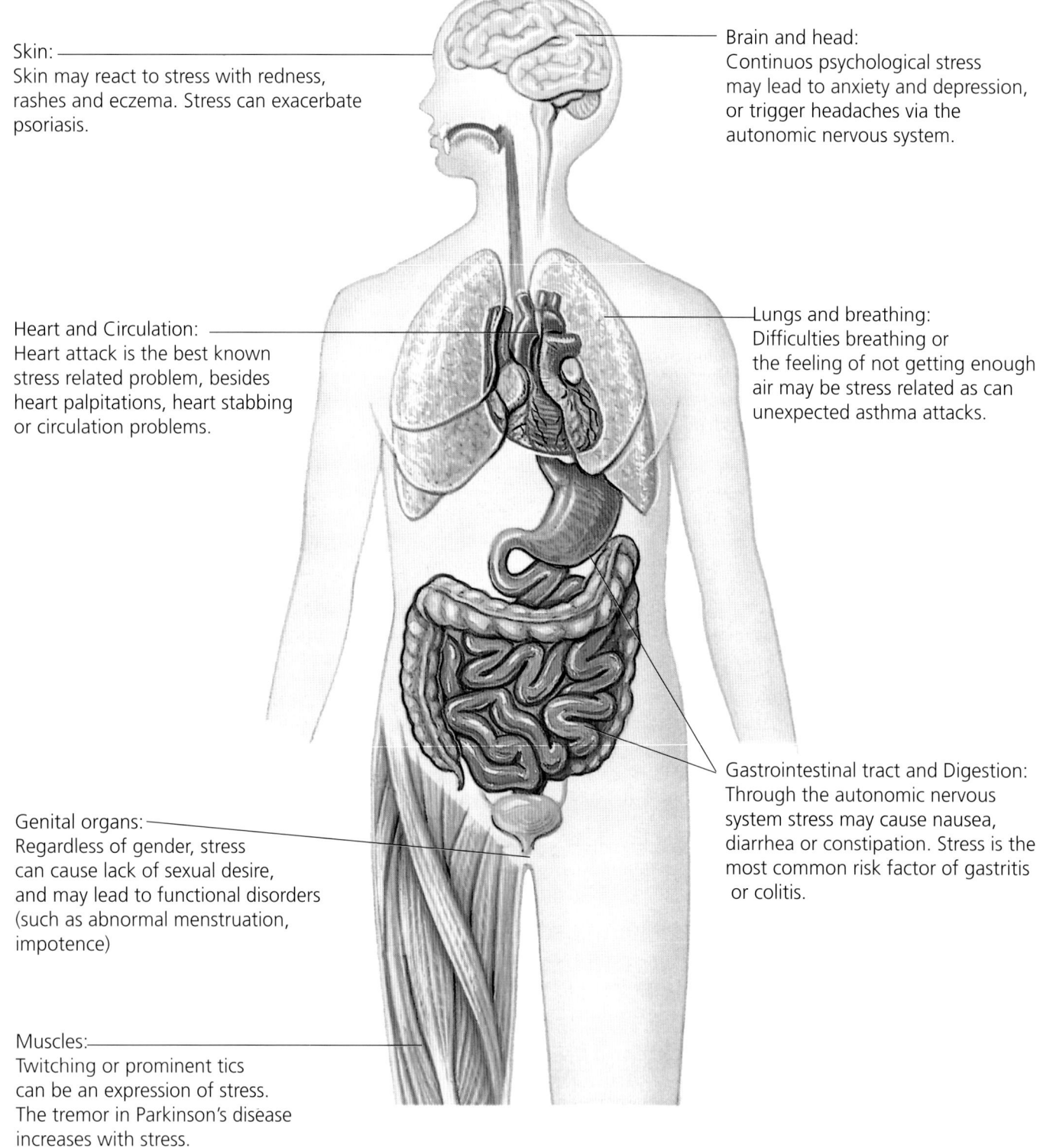

Skin:
Skin may react to stress with redness, rashes and eczema. Stress can exacerbate psoriasis.

Brain and head:
Continuos psychological stress may lead to anxiety and depression, or trigger headaches via the autonomic nervous system.

Heart and Circulation:
Heart attack is the best known stress related problem, besides heart palpitations, heart stabbing or circulation problems.

Lungs and breathing:
Difficulties breathing or the feeling of not getting enough air may be stress related as can unexpected asthma attacks.

Genital organs:
Regardless of gender, stress can cause lack of sexual desire, and may lead to functional disorders (such as abnormal menstruation, impotence)

Gastrointestinal tract and Digestion:
Through the autonomic nervous system stress may cause nausea, diarrhea or constipation. Stress is the most common risk factor of gastritis or colitis.

Muscles:
Twitching or prominent tics can be an expression of stress. The tremor in Parkinson's disease increases with stress.

need to be organized, disciplined, and in control. Constant pressure to conform to some external norm or ideal can be hazardous to your health. The more you ignore the subtler psychological symptoms, the more intense physical complaints tend to become. Often people's problems are not taken seriously until they have proof of an actual physiological disorder—which means organ damage has already occurred. Don't let it get to this point: Take immediate action if you start feeling overtaxed, overwhelmed, or unfairly dealt with. Go ahead and explode if you need to; if something is aggravating you, deal with it as soon as possible. Fight any tendency toward passivity or debilitating self-pity.

Self-help

A long and intense work week, moving into a new home, or exhaustion after childbirth are commonly stressful situations whose effects can be counterbalanced. Feeling run-down or sick at times like these can be relieved by:
— Sleep (p. 147, 190, 588)
— Relaxation (p. 693)
— Physical Activity and Sports (p. 762)
— "Natural" supplements—Teas (p. 688)

A change of scenery: A trip to the country, weekend with friends, or a short vacation

Treat yourself to a nurturing, pampering experience:
— A long, hot bath or sauna can work relaxing, rejuvenating wonders.
— Talking things over can take a big load off your mind. See friends regularly and don't be afraid to discuss personal issues or worries.
— Don't choke back your emotions. Sadness, anxiety, anger, and pain lessen when shared.
— Ask for help and support—whether you need someone just to listen, or to look after your children on a regular basis.
— Get out of the house. Make an effort to broaden your horizons. Accept social invitations, let yourself be entertained and taken care of, go dancing, take a risk, make a new friend, enjoy a new relationship.

If you've "gone without" for a long time, you may need more time off—a six-week vacation, for example—to relax thoroughly and get yourself back in sync with life.

When to Seek Medical Advice

Functional disorders of the bodily organs, no matter which ones, need to be investigated by a health-care provider as soon as possible.

Affective complaints such as restlessness, nervousness, or apathy need to be approached differently. If attempts at self-help bring no relief, seek the advice of a professional, be it a health-care provider or a counselor (p. 626). Taking medications, even over-the-counter ones, will not help resolve the underlying causes of your symptoms.

Treatment of Emotional Situation Disorders

Even though a feeling of general, pervasive illness only rarely has an organic cause, emotional complaints such as restlessness, nervousness, and exhaustion tend to be treated medically in our society and are given labels like neurodystonic complaints, neurovegetative dystonia, neurovegetative disturbed regulation, or autonomic dystonia.

Critics have called such diagnoses a thinly veiled excuse for prescribing psychopharmaceutical drugs (tranquilizers, for example) which in most cases relieve or mask pain but do nothing to heal it. The underlying causes of the anxiety, confusion or apathy almost always remain buried, and in the long run such treatment can cause more harm than good by leading to drug dependence and addiction.

Sedatives/Tranquilizers

The most commonly prescribed tranquilizers are those in the benzodiazepine group: Diazepam (e.g. Valium), Bromazepam, and Lorazepam

The effect of all these drugs is similar. They:
— Dull feelings and awareness
— Lessen anxiety and tension
— Relax muscles
— Calm aggressions

Tranquilizers can be helpful in acute psychological crises, as well as before surgery or after a heart attack. Due to the risk of dependency, however, they should be discontinued as soon as possible. Even after only 4 to 6 weeks, stopping these medications can result in aggravated symptoms such as panic attacks, severe anxiety, restlessness and sleep disorders. Although it can be tempting merely to renew the prescription, this just sets in motion the spiral of addiction. Unlike other addictive drugs whose dosages must constantly be increased to provide relief, the effect of tranquilizers does not diminish over time—but neither can the dose be reduced without a loss of effectiveness.

Treatment Alternatives

Resources for resolving long-term psychosomatic illness, general malaise, and similar disorders include:
— Psychotherapists
— Women's crisis centers
— Community health centers
— Social services
— See Counseling and Psychotherapy, p. 697.

SLEEP DISORDERS

When we fall asleep, many of our bodily functions slow down. Body temperature and blood pressure drop slightly; pulse and breathing rates grow slower. Our senses are not as attuned to the environment as they are when we are awake, and the nervous system is less responsive. Our bodily functions switch to "minimum," allowing us to relax and conserve energy.

Sleep patterns are culturally determined. In some cultures people arise early, sleep in the middle of the day, and stay up late in the evening; in others, they arise later, stay awake at midday and retire earlier. In addition, each individual has different sleep needs; age is also a factor. Determining how many hours of sleep are "normal" for everyone, therefore, is an impossible task.

Morning People–Evening People

In today's society, a standard workday is from 9 A.M. to 5 P.M., and a standard night's sleep is eight hours. These standards have evolved slowly throughout history, and today they dictate the rhythms of public life and determine our patterns of eating, resting, working, going to school, and everything else. There is little room for individual deviation; this can be inconvenient. So-called "evening people" are simply obeying their inner clocks, and may go to bed and get up two hours later than "morning people"; both types are "normal" and will sleep as long as necessary for them. Old saws such as "Early to bed and early to rise makes a man healthy, wealthy, and wise" are therefore bogus.

Sleep Duration

Sleep duration is age-dependent. Babies sleep almost

two thirds of the time; small children need between 10 and 12 hours of sleep, older children 8 to 10 hours, and adults about 8 hours. In older adults, the need for sleep diminishes to 5 to 6 hours after age 70.

Sleep Structure

A night's sleep is structured into four to six 90-minute cycles that alternate between deep—and light-sleep. During the light-sleep phase, the eyes move rapidly beneath the eyelids; this is referred to as rapid eye movement (REM) sleep and is primarily a time to process mental and emotional experiences. The deep-sleep phase serves to refresh and renew the body.

Complaints

— Trouble falling asleep (tossing and turning, sometimes for hours)
— Sporadic sleep (superficial and interrupted, with frequent waking)
— Premature waking (much too early, with inability to go back to sleep)

A Common Misperception

At night our sense of time is distorted, and periods of light sleep or wakefulness may seem much longer than they really are. How you feel in the morning is really the only yardstick for judging the quality of sleep: As long as you wake up cheerful and productive, you don't have a sleep disorder, no matter how many times you awaken at night.

Causes

Alcohol

Alcohol is a common cause of sleep disorders. A single glass of wine or beer can cause drowsiness and induce sleep, but larger quantities of alcohol can disturb sleep. Although we usually fall asleep quickly after a drink, alcohol takes its toll on the nervous system (and indeed the entire organism) as it is broken down by the body. The drinker soon wakes, and sleep is disturbed from then on as the important REM phase is suppressed and normal sleep patterns change.

Psychosocial Problems

Sleep quality is heavily influenced by mental and emotional states.

Difficult life situations, even those we can't readily

define, will eventually disturb our sleep. Lasting troubles in a relationship, smoldering family conflicts, increased pressure at work, unrewarding friendships, an unsatisfying sex life, and loneliness can all affect the quality of sleep.

A clear indicator of psychological problems is the following scenario: Going to sleep is an agonizing, even fear-inducing experience; a chaos of thoughts and images churns in your head; you get up continually. Only in the early morning do you finally doze off into a deep sleep.

Sadness or depression will affect sleep differently: Though you may have little or no trouble falling asleep, you soon wake and lie there agonizing, tossing and turning. Sleep disorders are often the sole symptom of depression (see p. 197).

Noise
Although it is commonly believed that we can get used to constant noise ("I don't even hear it any more"), the autonomic nervous system is negatively affected by chronic high noise levels, and even when the rest of us goes to sleep, our sense of hearing stays "awake." The physical effects of noise include fluctuations in blood pressure, trembling, and perspiring; psychological effects include difficulty concentrating, sleep disorders, exhaustion, distress, and heightened aggression.

In a quiet neighborhood the noise level drops to 30 to 35 decibels at night; street noise raises it to 70 to 80 decibels; construction noise, to 90 decibels (Hearing Loss, p. 58, 250). A noise level of 50 decibels already compromises deep sleep.

Environmental Factors
Excessive heat, dry air, or poor-quality air affect sleep negatively. So do beds that are too soft; they cause circulatory and back problems.

Shift Work
Shift work disturbs the natural rhythm of sleep because it drives our inner clocks out of sync with the rhythm of light and dark. Daytime sleep is usually superficial or curtailed, and cannot compensate for the loss of nighttime sleep.

Toxins
One of the first symptoms of poisoning by environmental toxins is a sleep disorder (see pp. 147, 588).

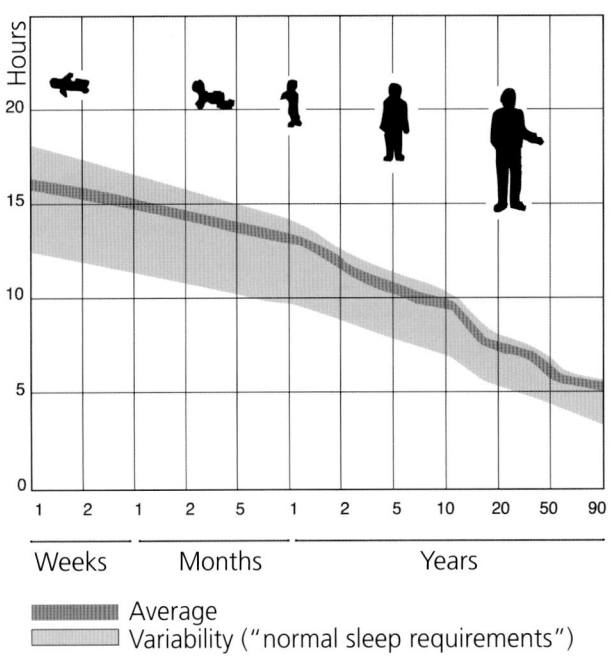

Sleep requirements

Average
Variability ("normal sleep requirements")

Medication
Analgesics and cold medications containing caffeine are stimulants and can cause sleep problems. So can preparations containing ephedrine, theophylline or related substances usually found in cold, cough, bronchitis, and asthma medications, and occasionally in medications to improve circulation. Diet pills almost always cause sleep disorders. If you suffer from sleep disorders, check whether any medications you are taking contain stimulants.

Tranquilizers can help you sleep, but often have adverse aftereffects. If you take them for some time and then stop, your complaints may recur or worsen (see Medication Summary, p. 657).

Illnesses
Worrying about your health can be just as sleep-disturbing as the symptoms of many illnesses.

Aftereffects and Complications
The direct results of sleep deprivation are well known: feeling worn out and exhausted, being unable to concentrate, and taking hours to feel halfway normal. Continuous sleep deprivation affects the entire nervous system, distorts awareness and sense perception, and feels like torture (in fact, sleep deprivation and disturbances are still common torture methods). The most frequent

result of sleep disorders is use of sleeping medications, which can lead to drug dependency and a long-term alteration in sleep patterns.

Prevention

— Keep evening meals light, with easily digested foods.
— Avoid alcohol, coffee, black or green tea, and cola in the evening.
— Spend evenings relaxing: reading, visiting, playing, bathing, or just hanging out.
— Do sports or physical activities; take an evening walk.
— Make sure your bedroom gets plenty of fresh air; if you can't open the windows, make sure air circulates freely.
— Keep bedroom temperatures on the cool side.
— The spine is supported best on a flat mattress or futon on slats. If you can't lie completely flat, the mattress supporting your upper body should be raised slightly.
— Buy mattresses and bedding of natural fibers that absorb perspiration.
— Often forgotten: Sex, tenderness, skin contact, and human warmth are relaxing and help you sleep better.

When to Seek Medical Advice

If sleep disorders persist more than 2–3 weeks in spite of your efforts to prevent them, see your health-care provider. It's useful to keep a journal of your sleep disorders and bring it along to your appointments.

If your symptoms (particularly early waking and restless sleep) coincide with problems such as loss of weight or appetite, apathy or difficulty concentrating, they may signal a serious depression: definitely see a medical professional, for medication alone will not solve the problem.

Self-Help

The following may help relieve sleep disorders:
— Relaxing evening rituals (playing a board game, having someone read to you, sipping warm milk, listening to soft music)
— Body relaxation (see p. 693)
— A warm bath with essential oils
— Massages (see p. 686)
— Physical activity and sports (see p. 762)
  Anything that soothes your body and soul will sup-

port sleep. Some people need various pillows, cushions and blankets to get comfortable. Accommodate your body's needs.

As mentioned, keeping a journal for several weeks may help you pinpoint the causes of long-term sleep disorders.

Sleep Disorders as Opportunity

If psychological problems are affecting your sleep quality, you can turn sleepless nights to your advantage by using them for major problem-solving. The night's stillness fosters uninterrupted contemplation, and unresolved conflicts, grief, problems, decisions, and crises work issues appear in a new light. Don't do this work while lying in bed, however: Go into another room, concentrate on developing some basic strategies for handling your problems, and write your thoughts down, perhaps as a "letter" to yourself. It's always helpful to share stressful situations and experiences.

Treatment

If your sleep is disturbed as a result of a physical ailment, you need to seek help for that ailment. If the disorder is caused by work-related stress or environmental toxins, enlist the help of coworkers, the human resources department, or the company doctor. When sleep disorders are due to psychosocial problems, counseling and psychotherapy are probably the answer (see p. 697).

Sleep Laboratories

People who suffer from serious sleep disorders may find

What to Track in Your Sleep Journal

When did you go to sleep? When did you awaken?
Which foods and beverages did you have after 5 p.m.?
What medications did you take throughout the day?
What did you do during the day—what kind of work, etc.?
How was your mood during the day?
Were there any especially stressful situations or experiences?
Did you take a nap?
If your sleep was affected, were you unable to fall asleep or stay asleep?
Did you awaken too early?
What were some of the thoughts churning in your head as you lay awake?
How did you feel the next day, on the whole?

relief at a sleep laboratory staffed by experts who can teach various sleep-improving techniques. In a sleep lab, the various phases of sleep and their sequence, duration, and intensity are analyzed. Electroencephalograms (EEGs) reveal electrical currents in the brain. Eye, jaw, arm, and leg movements are measured, as are heartbeat and breathing.

Medications

Many health-care providers prescribe sedatives for sleep disorders, even though medications tend to make matters worse after a short time.

If the condition fails to improve, the dosage is often increased, and a night's sleep simply becomes a narcotic stupor.

Sedatives interfere with the phases of sleep. Benzodiazepines affect deep sleep; others affect REM sleep.

Discontinuing benzodiazepines after only three weeks can cause withdrawal symptoms including serious sleep disturbances, dizziness, headaches, trembling, diarrhea, nausea, weight loss, anxiety, and panic attacks.

These symptoms can lead to resumed medication use, starting the insidious spiral of dependence and addiction.

Slow-release sedatives take longer to break down in the body, causing grogginess, confusion, and reduced productivity the following day.

Some medications accumulate in the body, retaining their effects for many hours after ingestion.

Ask your health-care provider or pharmacist about possible side effects of any medications (see Medication Summary, p. 657).

The bottom line is that sedatives should be used only to treat
— short-term stresses or changes (e.g. after flying across several time zones); usually a single dose is enough
— short-term sleep disorders caused by physical or emotional stress (e.g. serious illness, anxiety before surgery, unfamiliar surroundings); treatment should last no longer than three weeks because of the high risk of dependency

HEADACHES

Complaints

Most people get occasional headaches; for some they are frequent, or even regular, occurrences. Headaches can happen anytime and range in intensity from mild to unbearable. They also occur in connection with visual or other disorders (see Migraines, p. 225); some headaches are chronic.

Causes

A sign of physical or psychological stress, headaches are triggered by various physical causes (see Headaches, in Signs and Symptoms, p.91) or mental or emotional tension.

All the "Stress Factors" listed on p. 186, if not corrected, can lead to headaches.

Each of us experiences pain differently. Emotional, social and childhood experiences influence how acutely we react to pain. If, as a child, you were comforted when injured, you probably tend to take pain more in stride than someone who was yelled at for crying. Anxiety and depression can magnify pain, as can stress.

Possible Aftereffects and Complications

Headache pain that doesn't respond to treatment, or whose causes are not addressed, may become chronic. The pain itself then becomes the illness requiring treatment (see Migraines, p. 25).

However, reaching for a pill every time your head aches can be risky: The medication may be suppressing or masking the symptoms of a serious illness, or may even eventually cause the headache as you come to depend on a specific level of medication. This in turn might cause liver and kidney damage over the long term (see Analgesics, p. 660).

Prevention

Headaches can be prevented by doing everything possible to keep your life and environment in a healthy balance (see Health and Well-Being, p. 182).

When to Seek Medical Advice

If headaches occur regularly or are long-lasting, consult a health-care provider to find out whether a physical ailment is at fault. If pain persists, visit a clinic or center that specializes in chronic pain management.

Self-Help
— Take a fresh-air walk, or a warm relaxing bath.
— Lie down and tune out outer and inner noise.
— Apply cold or hot compresses on forehead and nape

of neck; massage painful areas with ice.
— Rub earlobes vigorously.
— Brush hair forward and in different directions to stimulate scalp.

See Relaxation Methods, p. 694
See Massages, p. 686
See Hydro Therapy, p. 692

Treatment

In order to treat acute headaches effectively, a cause—whether physical or not—must be determined. To get to the root of the problem, you may need to do some investigating into psychological tensions or conflicts. Sometimes this is easier with professional help (see Counseling and Psychotherapy, p. 697).

Acute, temporary headaches can be eased with analgesics (see p. 660); some people with recurring or long-lasting headaches find relief through alternative methods including acupressure (see p. 680) and acupuncture (p. 679).

MENTAL HEALTH DISORDERS

If you're suffering from a physical illness, help and support flow easily from family and friends. A psychiatric illness, however, is a different story. You may experience a variety of common reactions from family, friends, and community: Embarrassment, being unsure of what to do or how to help, denial, or complete avoidance.

Almost everyone experiences feelings and thoughts that can be similar to the symptoms of psychiatric illness. This fine line between illness and "normalcy" can be a source of fear and anxiety. Mental health disorders are at one end of the continuum of endless variations of human thoughts, feelings, and behavior. At some point in our lives, almost all of us have suffered (or will suffer) to some degree from a neurotic or psychosomatic disorder (see Health and Well-Being, p. 182).

NEUROTIC BEHAVIOR

Human beings develop in a series of phases. The most important phases of our development are usually considered to be childhood and youth, since it is during these periods that we establish lifelong behavior patterns, attitudes, and coping mechanisms. In later years we fall back on these learned patterns, often finding them effective in a variety of situations, such as problem-solving and forming relationships.

When such a pattern is not successful but we keep trying to apply it anyway, we may speak of a neurosis. Most of us live with some degree of so-called neurotic disorders; usually they are neither complex nor highly noticeable. They may manifest as a compulsion, a particular anxiety, or a tic, varying in degree and duration. They influence our choice of partners, professions, and daily choices; our lives are usually configured in such a way as to minimize the appearance of the neuroses.

Complaints

When past patterns of learned behavior can no longer help us cope with an overwhelming situation in the present, the neurosis becomes a complaint. At this point, psychological energy is being expended not to solve the problem at hand, but to suppress the stress engendered by the inability to cope.

Classic neurotic disorders include personality disorder, anxiety disorders, phobias, tics, and borderline disorders.

Personality Disorder

This category refers to behavior unsuited to the reality of a situation. For example,
— Hypochondria though enjoying good health
— Compulsive neatness even in orderly environments
— Compulsive hoarding amid abundance
— Inappropriate obsession with being on time, resulting in being way ahead of time
— Constant self-doubt amid many accomplishments
— Compulsive "sleeping around," though having many relationships is unsatisfying
— Depression
— Exaggeratedly fearful behavior, childlike dependence

Like personal characteristics or idiosyncracies, personality disorders have endless variations.

Compulsions

Compulsions are different from personality disorder in that they manifest only in very specific situations. A compulsion is a repetitive behavior pattern of which we are aware but over which we have no control. For example,
— Obsessive bodily washing in spite of being thoroughly clean
— Obsessive housecleaning in spite of a spotless home
— Compulsive orderliness, collecting, or stealing (kleptomania)

Mild compulsions are almost always easily integrated into our lives. When they begin to interfere with normal daily life, however, they become problems. An example of this is constantly checking that the front door is locked and finally being unable to leave the house.

Phobias

Phobias are intense yet unjustifiable feelings of fear. Between 200 and 250 varieties have been identified, dealing with different objects and situations. For example,
— Arachnophobia (fear of spiders); other animal phobias also exist, for example fear of mice, rats, or snakes
— Agoraphobia (the inability to cross wide open spaces)
— Claustrophobia (fear of enclosed spaces such as small rooms, elevators, and subways for fear of getting trapped)

— Fear of flying (out of proportion to the relatively small actual risk of a plane crash)

People with phobias realize their fears are not reality-based, but seem unable to control them. The phobias may intensify into panic attacks. Usually people learn to live with phobias by avoiding situations that trigger them, but this avoidance can obviously become restrictive.

Anxiety Disorders

Those affected are overwhelmed with general, uncontrollable anxiety and have no idea what triggers it. The anxiety can become so great and intense it turns into a panic attack. Often, an anxiety disorder is based on an exaggerated hypochondria or fear for one's own body, e.g., fear of heart failure, AIDS, or cancer.

Many people can live a relatively normal life even with an anxiety disorder. When they feel an attack coming on they withdraw, try to relax, or take sedatives and wait it out. If this does not work, such attacks can develop into severe neurotic fears with an extreme impact on the quality of life.

Tics

Tics are uncontrolled, unmotivated body reactions that may or may not have an organic cause. Examples are eye-twitching, head-shaking, making faces, or tongue-clicking. Such overt behavior constitutes a problem when it starts alienating other people. Tourette's syndrome, in which movement and speech are impaired, is well known. It begins in childhood with excessive nervousness, attention deficit, and typical compulsive behavior.

A variety of mild tics, especially in children, are caused by specific situations — e.g., rapid blinking when agitated. Often these types of tics will disappear on their own.

Borderline Disorders

The term *borderline* refers to personality disorders similar, but not equivalent, to psychotic disorders. About 5 to 10 percent of the population fall into this category. Borderline personalities are often sensitive, have a fragile ego, and are distrustful and easily irritated. They suffer from severe self-doubt and feelings of inferiority, and sometimes exhibit strong aggression toward themselves and/or others. Many tend toward over-sensitivity, dependency, irritability, distrust, and sometimes apparently crazy impulses.

Borderline personalities change relationships frequently, risking involvement in violent or degrading situations. They inflict pain on themselves, some injure themselves—with knives or lit cigarettes, or scratching till blood is drawn—for reassurance of self.

Depending upon the severity of the disorder, treatment may include a period of residency in a clinic or long-term psychotherapy (see p. 699).

Causes

Neurotic disorders such as anxieties, tics, obsessions, phobias, personality disorders, or borderline disorders usually have a long history. They can stem from

— A history of being overprotected, psychologically suffocated, or controlled—or neglected in a situation lacking sufficient attention, care, and love.
— Ongoing mental and emotional stress or injury.
— Ambivalent situations and decisions. Living with contradictions and ambivalence is one of the hardest tasks in life. Very few individuals can live with a simultaneous experience of love and hate. Almost everyone denies a part of his or her emotional life to dampen the potential anguish caused by the constant presence of ambivalence.
— Traumatic experiences such as divorce, death, all forms of physical and mental abuse, sexual abuse, rape, torture, war, being a refugee, prisoner, or concentration camp survivor.

Who's at Risk

When we are confronted with a potential crisis, we can approach it in a healthy way or a neurotic way—and the more stressful the situation, the higher the risk of the neurotic option. This can happen at any time of life. Possible triggering situations include puberty, leaving home, starting a family, breaking up a family, suddenly losing a job, experiencing other losses, or suffering from health problems.

Possible Aftereffects and Complications

Complications result when the neurotic behavior can no longer be made to fit in with "normal" life and it becomes impossible to work and maintain relationships. Many neurotic behaviors, particularly anxieties and compulsions, can become chronic and have a profound, lifelong impact.

Prevention

The most effective prevention against neurosis is, in a word, openness. The more freely you can talk about your feelings, thoughts, wishes, hopes and fears, the less likely you are to react to potential conflicts in a neurotic way (see Health and Well-Being, p. 182).

When to Seek Medical Advice

Seek medical help if the neurotic behavior is causing extreme suffering and distress in both the victim and the family. General practitioners are usually not of great help in these situations, although they can rule out any physical causes. Seek support and counseling from professionals in the field (see Counseling and Psychotherapy, p. 697).

Self-Help

Self-help is rarely feasible in the case of neuroses, as the causes usually lie in the unconscious. Sometimes, however, it is possible to get close to the real issues when confiding and talking as openly as possible to others.

Treatment

The odds of spontaneous healing are good, and such healing can come about under various circumstances. It may happen with the beginning of a new relationship, a change in lifestyle, or a new outlook on life. However, the longer the suffering, the greater the risk of chronic neurosis and the smaller the chance of spontaneous healing.

Neurosis can be overcome through psychotherapy (see p. 699); phobias, tics and obsessions can be brought under control. Often after only approximately thirty sessions, life can already return to normal, for the most part. The more serious the problem, of course, the longer it will take to resolve (see Counseling and Psychotherapy, p. 697).

In the case of an acute crisis or a severe attack, antidepressants can effectively treat anxiety, destructive mania or depression, thereby paving the way for the beginning of psychotherapy. Tranquilizers should be avoided as they are potentially addictive (see Sedatives, p. 189; Medication Summary, p. 657).

Affective Disorders

We are all familiar with mood swings—highs and lows, euphoria and joy as well as sorrow and self-doubt. These feelings become extreme and uncontrollable in people with affective emotional disorders: sadness turns into depression, euphoria into mania. The depressed person withdraws, sometimes to the point of paralysis, while the manic person becomes a whirlwind of hyperactivity. When such extremes are reached, it is often hard to tell what triggered the behaviors, so the causes remain unknown. Metabolism may play an important role in balancing extreme behavior.

DEPRESSION

As medically defined, the term *depression* is rather narrow, referring to people who feel "down" and heavy-hearted, with serious feelings of inferiority and self-reproach. The condition usually has its origin in a reaction to a traumatic event, experience, or phase of life (see Neurotic Behavior, p. 195). Depression can range from mild to severe. Milder forms are usually easily diagnosed and may occur following the death of a loved one, for example. More serious depression is harder to diagnose. Severe depression may be accompanied by delusions, including disproportionate feelings of guilt, neediness or destructiveness. Severe depression can cause the total inability to move (depressive stupor) and include suicidal tendencies.

Masked and Chronic Depressions

Masked Depression (Atypical Depression)
Some forms of depression can be detected only through changes in disposition. The person does not feel emotionally "depressed," but feels physically sick and exhausted, with sleeping disorders and mild symptoms of stress. Many doctors believe that chronic fatigue syndrome (CFS) is really a form of depression expressed as chronic physical exhaustion (see Health and Well-Being, p. 182). Sometimes depressions manifest directly as somatic disorders; for example, constant stomach problems: In these cases it is as if psychological suffering were simply projected or transferred onto the body (see Functional Disorders, p.186; Psychosomatic Disorders, p. 186).

Chronically Depressed Mood (Dysthymia)

When life is utterly bereft of joy and desire, and the prevailing moods are sadness and dissatisfaction, chronic depression (dysthymia) may be the cause. This disposition, which often cannot be relieved by medication, is common among refugees or exiles who, having lost their roots and cultural orientation, get through daily life with no apparent abnormalities but are simply unable to experience happiness. This condition is also not uncommon among people who have experienced traumatic events such as the death of a child.

Complaints

— Melancholy mood and withdrawal into self
— Shutting oneself off from the outer world; preoccupation with self-doubt, feelings of inferiority, delusional tendencies, depending on severity of depression
— Feelings of emptiness and worthlessness, often connected with anxiety, exhaustion, sleep disorders (including excessive sleep), loss of appetite and weight, or food cravings and weight gain
— Inability to concentrate; apathy and immobility
— Suicidal thoughts or death wish, developed to a greater or lesser degree

Causes

Depressed individuals often suffer from unconscious aggressive feelings directed at no one in particular. Sorrow, rage, anger, doubt, and disappointment cannot find an outlet and are turned on the self, since the individual has apparently lost the ability to express painful feelings.

Physical factors may also be at fault. Diseases of the liver, intestines, thyroid, or anemia can all cause depression, as can chronic diseases such as arthritis and cancer, or metabolic changes (see Biorhythms, p. 183).

Depression accompanied by fatigue, loss of appetite, and headaches may also be the result of environmental influences on the central nervous system: Exposure to heavy metals (lead, mercury, thallium), synthetic-based materials such as acrylamide, benzene compounds or solvents, or volatile hydrocarbon and organophosphate compounds (e.g. insecticides).

Who's at Risk

Depression usually manifests between the ages of 30 and 40, or between 50 and 60. The World Health Organization (WHO) estimates 3 to 5 percent of the global population is affected; U.S. figures indicate 5 to 10 percent. Two thirds of those suffering from depression are women. Due to differences in childrearing practices, girls tend to learn to internalize conflicts, unlike boys. Because aggressive feelings do not match our culturally acceptable images of women, they are often hidden, denied, and finally turned in on the self. In addition, women are at higher risk of developing depression due to a variety of external factors such as poverty, loneliness, isolation, unsatisfying relationships and/or single parenting, particularly of young children requiring large amounts of care, time, and energy.

Possible Aftereffects and Complications

Physical consequences: The depressed person usually neglects bodily care, exhibits listlessness and immobility, and may not eat enough or correctly. Vitamin deficiencies and circulatory disorders may result.

Social consequences may include total withdrawal into self and complete immobility. The depressed person is self-absorbed and no longer interacts with family, friends, or partners. Particularly with those exhibiting delusional behavior, unfamiliar people are usually unable to make contact.

Prevention

We all have depressive tendencies. The more aware we are of this fact, the better we will be able to cope in times of crisis. The following points may help:
— Examine your daily life and ask yourself whether everything you're dutifully taking the time to do is really essential. Many things we may feel obliged to accomplish aren't necessary.
— Don't denigrate yourself; acknowledge your strengths and successes. We all fear failure; being able to talk about your fears is key. The more you withdraw from others, the greater the risk of depression.
— Grief, pain, separation anxiety, and aggressive feelings are all parts of life that must be lived. The more you can process these feelings and get them off your chest, the better your chances of preventing depression.

Sharing with others really helps (see Balance is Possible, p. 185).

When to Seek Medical Advice

Professional intervention becomes necessary when tendencies toward apathy and withdrawal begin to manifest and affect your life. A psychotherapist is the best person to talk to. In cases of severe depression, psychiatric help is imperative, either from a therapist in private practice or the outpatient services of a psychiatric hospital. The risk of a suicide attempt is high in depressed people, particularly in severe cases. Family members should act as soon as possible by getting treatment for the person, even against his or her will.

Self-Help

Self-help cannot be effective in overcoming depression, since the desire to solve one's problems in isolation is one of the causes of the depression. Instead, the depressed person must learn to turn to others, talk to them, and trust them. It is advisable for depressed people to stay active, both socially and professionally; withdrawal and solitude only exacerbate this illness.

Treatment

Mild forms of depression are usually alleviated by counseling, helpful advice, and talking things through (see Consultation and Psychotherapy, p. 697). More serious cases require professional treatment, preferably com-

Suicide

It is estimated that about 20 percent of severely depressed individuals commit suicide during a critical phase of their disease. Statistics don't tell the whole story, however, since car "accidents" and "accidental" drug and alcohol overdoses often disguise suicides. Almost all those who commit suicide, however, give warnings before attempting the act.
— Pay attention to these warnings, even if you don't believe the person really means anything by them. Take seriously all conversational references to suicide or death wishes.
— Serious, truthful conversations and sincere offers for help are the only way to build the trust necessary to reestablish a suicidal person's connection to the world. If you don't take the person's suffering seriously, you will only deepen his or her hopelessness.
— Suicides by depressives are often so well planned that they are nearly impossible to prevent.
— People who carefully plan suicides can rarely be dissuaded from following through with their plans. About 10 percent of suicides occur while patients are under psychiatric care.

Medications for depression

Antidepressants are very effective, with a wide range of potencies and applications. They can alleviate suffering, often enabling the patient to begin psychotherapy, but don't treat the causes of depression. Medications should not be prescribed without concurrent psychotherapy. Antidepressants that act as stimulants get rid of listlessness and apathy very quickly; they take another 1 to 3 weeks to dispel the depression itself. But because the apathy was preventing action, this interim period is dangerous: with the ability to act upon one's intentions restored, the patient may commit suicide during the crucial 1 to 3 weeks.

The most commonly prescribed antidepressants are Tricyclics: amitriptyline, amoxapine, desipramine, doxepin, imipramine, nortriptyline, pritriptyline, trimipramine

Selective serotonin reuptake inhibitors: fluoxetine, sertraline, paroxetine

Others: buproprion, venlafaxine

Most common side effects: Dry mouth, urine retention, visual disturbances when changing focus, disorders of nerve endings, especially in the heart.

Warning—Combination Medications: It is not advisable to take antidepressant medications containing antipsychotics or sedatives because of the increased risk of side effects. Also, those containing sedatives can lead to dependency (see Sedatives, p. 189). Because long-term use is necessary, the risk of dependency is extremely high (see Medication Summary, p. 657).

bining medications and psychotherapy. Depending on individual cases, relaxation (see p. 693), light therapy, or other therapies affecting biorhythms may be helpful.

If there is an acute danger of suicide, hospital admission is necessary. In this case it is advisable to contact a psychiatrist or psychiatric clinic for evaluation.

MANIA

Mania is the opposite of depression. Instead of an inferiority complex, delusions of grandeur and omnipotence prevail. Manic people usually feel great, euphoric and "high."

Complaints

Since manic people feel their disorder is normal behavior, one cannot really speak of "complaints" in the traditional sense. People suffering from this disease consistently "push the limits" of acceptable behavior,

frequently acting outrageously in public.
— They may appear relaxed, cheerful, and witty, or defensive and irritated.
— They race through a variety of activities at top speed, leaving chaos in their wake.
— Because they are oversensitive to their surroundings and can't tune out stimuli, they are constantly distracted, unable to think things through or finish the innumerable projects they start.
— People in the manic phase outdo themselves: Everything seems possible, doable, easily accomplished. They run up enormous debts, buy property, start companies or relationships, and dissolve them again.
— Physical achievements can be amazing as manic people rush through the day with incredible energy. They hardly need sleep, "forget" to eat, and feel no pain.
— When the manic phase subsides, it is almost always followed by depression (see p. 197) and self-destructive tendencies.

Causes
Biochemical changes in the brain are believed to cause mania.

Psychologically stressful situations can also be triggers, although the connection is usually no longer apparent by the time the mania is diagnosed; the disease appears gradually, and may simply look like an unusually high level of activity at first.

In rare cases, infections, stroke, or brain injury can cause this illness.

Who's at Risk
Individuals prone to manic depression are at risk during periods of change or upheaval in their lives (see Depression, p. 197).

Possible Aftereffects and Complications
Physical consequences: Chronic lack of sleep, lack of attention to the body's warning signs, and life in the "fast lane" can all lead to total exhaustion.

Social consequences: Manic people make great demands on their families. They can be tactless and ruthless as well as charming. Their exaggerated confidence and self-centeredness make them ride roughshod over all conventions, leaving in their wake wrecked personal relationships, divorces, and abandoned children. The

Lithium
Taking lithium as part of a regular, carefully monitored treatment program can enable manic depressives to lead a relatively normal personal and professional life, in the short or long term. The effect of lithium is to stabilize the emotions, restoring life's equilibrium.

incredible energy unleashed during the manic phase destroys social contacts and may lead to financial ruin.

Prevention
Preventing the onset of mania is not possible; once the illness has been diagnosed, lithium, carbamazepine and valproic acid can be beneficial.

When to Seek Medical Advice
Seek help immediately when unusually high-energy activities lead to chaotic behavior with no apparent thought to consequences. Because manic people don't acknowledge their illness as such, it is up to family and friends to get them into therapy. If they refuse help, intervention by social services may be necessary.

Self-Help
Not possible.

Treatment
Medical treatment is the first line of action; psychotherapy can also help sufferers evaluate the disorder realistically and learn to live with it.

Psychoses
Until recently, psychotic disorders and altered perceptions, especially schizophrenia, were considered untreatable. Today we know that the right combination of medication and psychotherapy can help. Psychotic patients can live relatively normal lives outside the psychiatric clinic when supported appropriately by outreach programs, outpatient clinics, group homes, and/or crisis intervention.

Disorders acquired at an early age play an important role in the development of this illness. Definitive factors may include organic disorders, stressful life situations, or schizophrenic parents; family and social circumstances may then trigger the manifestation of the disease.

The psychotic state of mind is best described as an inability to protect oneself against the onslaught of impressions and sensations. Under normal circumstances, only 10 percent of the countless stimuli constantly bombarding us make it into our consciousness; if we become aware of 20 percent, we're on the verge of a nervous breakdown (see Acute Stress Disorders, p. 182); at 30 percent we become overwhelmed and psychologically ill, unable to judge what is going on or deal with other people.

None of us is immune from this. It is relatively easy to provoke psychotic states or hallucinations even in "healthy" persons; chronic sleep deprivation can, for example, trigger psychotic epidodes and perceptual changes after only a few days.

SCHIZOPHRENIA

In the vernacular, schizophrenia has come to imply "split personality," but this is rarely a true representation of the illness.

In general, schizophrenia is understood as a disconnectedness in one's thoughts and feelings. The boundaries between self and environment are lost, and it becomes impossible to tell what is important and what isn't, which things belong together and which don't; in effect, the schizophrenic loses touch with reality.

Schizophrenics are usually hypersensitive, extraordinarily creative people whose heightened perceptive abilities make it hard for them to live a normal life. They are often able to "see through" other people, but are unable to integrate this information properly.

This heightened perceptiveness can lead to distorted perception, delusions, and hallucinations.

Complaints

There are three types of classic schizophrenic behavior.

Hebephrenia is characterized by juvenile, inappropriate, bizarre and unpredictable behavior, in which laughter and tears follow each other with no apparent rhyme or reason.

Catatonia is characterized by tense, cramped and agitated behavior. The sufferer may freeze into statue-like immobility, or act out wildly and uncontrollably.

Paranoia is the most common form of schizophrenia, usually accompanied by hallucinations:
— Perceptive disorders prevail, accompanied by agitation and the inability to differentiate between reality and fantasy.
— Unrelated events are arbitrarily associated, and hallucinations convince the sufferer he or she is being manipulated, shadowed by stranger, or threatened by bizarre plots.
— Hallucinations may involve all the senses. The schizophrenic sees unusual things, smells and tastes strange foods, hears voices, and behaves as though these perceptions are real.

Causes

Alcohol, drugs and medications can cause schizophrenic episodes.

Changes in brain processes are almost always discovered in schizophrenics.

Their causes are unknown, although metabolic disorders and enzyme deficiencies are believed to play a role.

Hereditary factors are involved. Although the incidence of schizophrenia is 0.8 percent in the general population, among children of a schizophrenic parent it stands at 5 to 10 percent, and 8 to 14 percent among siblings of schizophrenics.

Patterns of schizophrenic behavior can run in families; the behavior tends to manifest in the presence of aggravating social and psychological factors.

Who's at Risk

About 1 percent of the population has a schizophrenic episode requiring psychiatric treatment during these individual's lifetime; 80 percent of these take place before age 40. (So-called "senile schizophrenia" sets in after age 60.) Women are usually affected after age 30, men before.

Paranoid schizophrenia is almost always triggered by a psychologically extremely stressful situation.

Possible Aftereffects and Complications

Paranoid schizophrenics are almost always at high risk for suicide, especially at the onset or end of a crisis. Social isolation frequently results from schizophrenic behavior, leading to the loss of job, friends, and relationships. Schizophrenic episodes often recur repeatedly, costing the sufferer tremendous amounts of energy and accelerating his or her social alienation.

Prevention

Children with one schizophrenic parent require special attention from the healthy parent; the risk of learned (induced) aberrant behavior is high.

When to Seek Medical Advice

Seek help as soon as altered or distorted perception becomes apparent.

Self-Help

Schizophrenics can help themselves only if they recognize that they are suffering from an illness. Friends, family and others can help by not abandoning the sufferer, and by convincing him or her that psychotherapy and medical treatment could spell freedom from the disease.

Many communities offer support groups for persons living with schizophrenia.

Workshops and informative seminars are also available in many areas; contact your local hospital or community center for further information.

Treatment

Psychiatric and medical therapies are the most effective, making it possible for the schizophrenic gradually to bring thoughts, feelings, and perceptions under control. Following the acute phase, psychotherapy is beneficial; unfortunately, relatively few psychotherapists are willing to undertake the years of patience and commitment required to work with a schizophrenic. Medication helps prevent relapses and shortens acute attacks.

Whereas countless schizophrenics spent their lives in psychiatric institutions in the past, today they can live relatively normal lives with the help of medication, therapy, and support groups. Schizophrenia is not a life sentence; it can even go into complete remission. The understanding and love of others is indispensable if this is to occur.

Eating Disorders

Individuals with eating disorders aren't necessarily grossly overweight or underweight. The "disorder" is in their relationship to food: eating becomes an obsessive focus, and is often an expression of psychological strife. Eating disorders are classified as psychosomatic illnesses (see p. 185).

Neuroleptics (Antipsychotics)

The most common treatment for schizophrenia is neuroleptic medications, which suppress delusions and hallucinations, alleviate the constant feeling of being threatened or followed, and reduce anxiety. Unfortunately, neuroleptics have numerous side effects. The most common are
— Indifference to outside stimuli; slowed reactions
— Listlessness and lethargy, to the point of apathy
— Eye and tongue cramps, trembling, restlessness, dry mouth, and impaired intellectual ability
— Tardive dyskinesia, developing into movement disorders, for example facial contortions that can become permanent
The most commonly prescribed neuroleptics are
Tricyclics: Phenothiazines: chlorpromazine, triflupromazine, mesoridazine, thioridazine, acetophenazine, perphenazine, trifluoperazine, fluphenazine
Thioxanthines: chlorprothixene, thiothixene, loxapine
Nontricylics: Dihydroindolone: molindone Butyrophenones: haloperidol, droperidol
Recently introduced neuroleptics
Clozapine suppresses delusions and hallucinations without leading to apathy and indifference. However, it must be administered only under strict medical supervision, including weekly blood testing, as it carries a high risk of decreasing the white blood cell count (agranulocytosis).
Risperidone also has lower risk of extrapyramidal effects and does not have increased risk of agranulocytosis.

ANOREXIA NERVOSA AND BULIMIA

Though they manifest differently, these disorders are related and have the same root causes; sufferers often alternate between them.

Complaints of Anorexia

Sufferers are usually pubescent girls who are often unaware of their condition. Parents should learn to recognize the symptoms, which include
— Careful monitoring of food intake; constant calorie-counting
— An obsession with not eating; constant attempts to lessen food and calorie intake
— Excessive sports activities (e.g., running a marathon), or the use of laxatives and appetite suppressants, in some sufferers
— Distorted body image, "feeling fat" in spite of being

extremely thin, with no recognition of the extent of the disorder; ingestion of no more than 200 calories a day for long periods

— In many anorexics: periodic binges, during which enormous quantities of food are ingested, only to be followed by induced vomiting (bulimia); family members may notice nothing until the refrigerator or pantry shelves are suddenly found nearly empty

Complaints of Bulimia

In bulimia, large quantities of food—up to 30,000 calories at a time—are ingested, in a kind of frenzy. The food is immediately vomited. The time actually spent eating is the only moment of calm in the bulimic's life: At all other times, food is the obsessive focus ("When can I buy more, and what will I buy?"). An excessive amount of money is spent on food.

The process of eating and vomiting involves secrecy and guilt. Bulimics usually have normal body weight and are aware of their illness, although it is seldom evident to other people.

Causes

Eating disorders usually stem from childhood experiences (see Neurotic Behavior, p. 195) and manifest in puberty, when it becomes important to establish one's own identity as separate from the family.

Anorexic girls have a distorted relationship to their bodies, not perceiving them as they actually are. Unconsciously, many are trying to distance themselves from their mothers and to deny their impending womanhood. The fact that they lack the feminine characteristics of fleshy breasts, buttocks, hips and thighs, and often do not menstruate, gives them the illusion of having overcome their own gender. Conquering hunger imparts a sense of independence, and intense hunger turns into a euphoric high after a few days.

In anorexic boys the issue is less one of sexual identity and more the desire for independence.

Women suffering from bulimia are also in a crisis of identity and self-confidence. However, rather than making them feel powerful and in control, their addiction to bingeing and vomiting leads to constant depression. Bulimics know they are sick and feel too guilty to talk about it. They usually try to get a handle on their illness for long periods before giving up and seeking professional help.

Who's at Risk

Girls and women are statistically more affected by eating disorders than men, although this is changing as men become increasingly weight-conscious.

It is estimated that about 2 percent of girls between the ages of 15 and 18 are anorexic. An increasing number of women are becoming anorexic at about age 30. The statistics for bulimia are much less clear, but it is estimated that 4 to 6 percent of girls are affected.

The risk of eating disorders increases when experimenting with diets and fasting (see Body Weight, p. 727).

Possible Aftereffects and Complications of Anorexia

— Metabolic and hormonal changes; cessation of ovulation and menstruation (see Menstrual Disorders, p. 103, 508).

— Extreme emaciation and dehydration; general weakness; heart and kidney damage; edema.

— Final metabolic breakdown and loss of electrolyte function as a result of long-term starvation. Of all the organs, the brain is supported longest; when it can no longer function, psychosis sets in.

— About 10 percent of all anorexics die. Twenty percent remain at risk, shuttling between clinics for years, with relatively normal periods between episodes. Thirty percent have food issues for the rest of their lives, but can stabilize their situation without further clinical treatments. The rest of those affected by anorexia during puberty outgrow it.

Possible Aftereffects and Complications of Bulimia

Bulimia is usually not life-threatening. Frequent vomiting can disrupt bodily water and electrolyte levels and lead to chronic inflammations of the esophagus and stomach.

Self-Help Groups for Eating Disorders
Overeaters Anonymous: Check newspapers or contact your local hospital or community center.

Social Consequences

These are dramatic in both forms of the illness. Anorexics often lose social contacts, have no close relationships or sex lives, and live in isolation. People with bulimia usually try to live apparently normal lives, but are under constant financial pressure due to their enormous food bills and may be debt-ridden; stealing may result.

Prevention

The example set by parents is important; the less pressure the child feels to eat certain foods or particular amounts, the less likely the danger of developing eating disorders later on. Eating disorders, particularly anorexia, are a form of rebellion.

When to Seek Medical Advice

Seek help as quickly as possible with anorexia, since it calls for careful monitoring. With bulimia, medical intervention is not as important since physical well-being is seldom at risk; immediate psychotherapy is much more beneficial (see Consultation and Psychotherapy, p. 697).

Self-Help

Talking and sharing with others can help greatly. Support groups for individuals with eating disorders are widespread, and are often run by professionals.

Treatment

Anorexics in critical condition are almost always admitted to a hospital for intravenous and/or tube feeding, weight gain, and stabilization.

Psychotherapy should begin at this time, as well. Usually treatment in a clinic specializing in psychosomatic illnesses or eating disorders is followed by 1 to 2 years of counseling (see Counseling and Psychotherapy, p. 697).

SITOMANIA (OVEREATING)

This is the least common eating disorder, characterized by chronic, binge-like and addictive devouring of food. People with this condition are obsessed with food; unlike those with bulimia, however, they gain lots of weight, which puts them at risk for cardiovascular diseases, diabetes, high blood pressure, metabolic disorders, joint illnesses, and arthritis. Life expectancy is also drastically reduced.

In those suffering from this disorder, the natural sensations of hunger and satiety are distorted and eventually lost due to continuous food consumption, causing confusion in the corresponding brain centers. In effect, sufferers lose touch with their bodies and feelings. They are often acutely aware that they are hiding problems underneath their weight, and that by losing weight they would have to get in touch with their bodies and deal with these issues. Psychotherapy and support groups are advisable (see Counseling and Psychotherapy, p. 697).

Surgery should be used only as a last resort. Options are
— Removing part of the stomach to make it smaller
— Altering the digestive tract to absorb fewer calories from food
— Inserting a bag into the stomach to reduce its capacity.

Addictions and Dependencies

Hankering for a special thrill, a moment of intense happiness, or an experience of deep relaxation doesn't necessarily mean you have the makings of an addict. What places you at risk, however, is losing the ability to choose freely whether or not to indulge. For example, if you can no longer do without your nightly cigarette and in fact crave more than one, you are no longer free to either smoke or not.

Dependencies don't only involve nicotine, alcohol or drugs (see Mood-Altering Substances and Recreational Drugs, p. 754). They may also result from a craving for intense sensations like the euphoria generated by playing sports hard, or working non-stop, or fasting (see Eating Disorders, p. 202). Withdrawal symptoms are emotional as well as physical, leaving the person wanting more.

Psychological dependency refers to the strong desire to repeat the addictive experience, which may alleviate anxiety, solve problems, lessen pain, or simply make you feel good.

Physical dependency refers to increasing levels of tolerance by the body, necessitating ever-higher dosages to produce the desired effect.

ALCOHOLISM
(See also Alcohol, p. 756)

Complaints
The symptoms of alcoholism include the following:
— You need to drink a certain amount in order to feel good and relaxed.
— You think you can deal with stressful situations only with the help of alcohol.
— You drink in order to forget your anger, worries, or problems.
— You believe you can handle increasing amounts of alcohol.
— Your first drink of the day keeps getting earlier and earlier, until finally it's the first thing in the morning.
— You feel nervous and distraught if there's no alcohol around.
— You lie to yourself and everybody else about how much and how often you drink.
— You suffer from sleeplessness and disorders of the libido.
— You have a secret stash of alcohol.

Causes
Alcoholism is caused by a combination of individual, psychological, and social factors (see Alcohol, p. 756). Drinking is a learned behavior, and children are influenced by their parents' patterns. In youth groups, drinking helps young people feel that they "belong," or helps them feel grown-up or "cool." Such imitation can lead to excess, misuse, and dependency.

The main reason people drink, however, is alcohol's primary effect: relaxation and alleviation of anxiety. This instant, positive feeling brings with it the temptation to escape from any and all problems, conflicts, or stressful situations with an alcohol high.

Who's at Risk
In Western society, the risk of alcohol addiction is extremely high.

Alcohol is easily available, it's affordable, and it occupies an established niche in our culture; and its status as a legal drug keeps alive the illusion that one can simply drink troubles away.

Advice and Help
Alcoholics Anonymous (AA) and Al-Anon: These support groups are found everywhere.

Possible Aftereffects and Complications
Alcoholism has serious consequences for the drinker, his or her family members, and society as a whole.

Mental and Emotional Consequences
These include disorders of long-term memory, lowered concentration, increased fatigue, impaired judgment, euphoria alternating with depression, feelings of mistrust or paranoia.

Alcohol Delirium and Delirium Tremens
This disorder involves loss of orientation, delusions, anxiety attacks, irritability, euphoria, and infantile behavior. Left untreated, it usually lasts 4 to 10 days, with a death rate of 15–30 percent.

Wernicke-Korsakow Syndrome
This disorder of the nervous system shows up in 3 to 5 percent of all alcoholics. They are unable to direct their vision and are unsteady on their feet. They may lose their memory, may be incapable of remembering new things to fill the gap, may lose their powers of concentration, and may hardly be able to orient themselves. Imagining something and putting it into words becomes nearly impossible.

Physical Consequences
— Undernourishment and vitamin deficiency, since alcohol is supplying most of the body's calories
— Massive diarrhea and occasional gastric bleeding
— Cirrhosis of the liver (see p. 396)
— Pancreatitis (see p. 400)
— Frequent vomiting, causing deep fissures where the esophagus joins the stomach, which may bleed;
— Numbness in feet and legs, tingling in lower legs, calf pains and unsteady walking, muscle weakness (polyneuropathy)
— Disorders of the heart muscles, leading to congested lungs
— Susceptibility to infectious illnesses like pneumonia (see p. 310) and tuberculosis (see p. 311)

Social Consequences

Alcoholics often lose their partners and friends; these circumstances frequently lead to violence, job loss, and/or debts. The economic consequences—insurance and health-care costs, automobile and workplace accidents, and loss of productivity—are incalculable.

Prevention

If you like to drink, don't underestimate the dangers of crossing the line into alcohol abuse. Under no circumstances should you use alcohol as a solution to your problems or to bolster you against anxiety or stress.

When to Seek Medical Advice

Check out the list of symptoms under the "Complaints" heading. If you recognize yourself, more than likely you are an alcoholic or are close to becoming one, and should seek professional help.

Self-Help

Alcoholics have a broad and supportive network of self-help groups and organizations at their disposal (see Advice and Help, p. 205).

Treatment

Detoxification: This first step usually takes place in a "detox" or "dry-out" clinic run by medical professionals in conjunction with therapy.
Withdrawal Phase: After detox, withdrawal therapy begins. The alcoholic and professional team decide together which route to choose; choices include rehabilitation centers, halfway houses, and psychotherapy on an outpatient basis. Treatment usually takes several months (see Consultation and Psychotherapy, p. 697).
Follow-Up Care: This important component is supplied by substance-abuse clinics, support groups, or social service centers.

MEDICATION DEPENDENCY

In Western industrialized society, after alcohol, medications are the addiction of choice. They include:
— Strong painkillers, including morphine and its relatives, and methadone derivatives. Most potent painkillers are habit-forming and quickly become addictive. With time, they are also capable of causing personality changes.
— Strong cough medicines, often containing codeine

Codependency

Codependent people form a bond with their partner's alcoholism, in effect, by trying to control and stop his or her drinking patterns. What starts out as caring support turns into increasing isolation and self-neglect, while the alcoholic continues to drink.

In most cases it is women whose entire thoughts, feelings and actions come to revolve around dealing with the alcoholic spouse: "How can I help him? What can I do to make him stop? How can I keep others from noticing? What can I do to prevent him losing his job?"

Codependencies exist for every type of addiction. Codependents often contribute unconsciously to the dependency by keeping up a front and trying to deny the problem. Support groups for codependents can help (see Advice and Help, p. 205).

or related substances that, depending on amounts and dosage, are also habit-forming and addictive. Prescription cough medicine with codeine is especially prone to abuse and can lead to perceptual disorders, confusion, and memory loss.
— Simple pain and migraine medications: Over-the-counter products combining analgesics and caffeine are frequently abused (see Medication Summary, p. 657).
— Sleep medication and sedatives: Almost all are potentially addictive, especially those containing benzodiazepines; chronic use can cause confusion, concentration difficulties and emotional changes.
— Tranquilizers: Includes the most commonly abused medications, the benzodiazepines (see Sedatives, p. 189). Used regularly over long periods of time, even "normal" doses can become addictive, causing perceptual and emotional changes, sleep disorders, and impaired consciousness.
— Alcohol: Many cough syrups and so-called "tonics" contain up to 20 percent alcohol (some as much as 79 percent).
— Stimulants: Most consist of amphetamines or similar substances, or in combination with an analgesic. Long-term use can cause psychotic symptoms.
— Appetite suppressants: chemically similar to amphetamines and ephedrine. Long-term misuse can cause perceptual disorders.
— Laxatives: Chronic use can lead to dependency (see Constipation, p. 44, 406).

Complaints

When a medication becomes indispensable—for example, if you try to discontinue its use, only to find that the original symptoms return stronger than ever—suspect dependency. "Low-dose" dependency refers to cases in which you don't need to increase your dose, but still can't do without the medication. Watch for these signs of dependency:

— You pack extra medication whenever you leave the house.
— The thought of skipping a day's medication makes you anxious.
— You start to hurt, physically and psychologically, upon discontinuing medication.
— You go to more than one doctor and pharmacist to obtain your medication.
— You lie to yourself, your family, friends and doctor about the amount of medication you take .

Causes

Prescriptions: Nearly three-quarters of all medication dependency starts in the doctor's office. Huge quantities of benzodiazepines—tranquilizers, sleep aids, sedatives—are prescribed annually; about two thirds of these are taken for more than three weeks, long enough to establish the cycle of dependency (see Sedatives, p. 659).
Self-medication: People suffering from chronic pain are at high risk for developing dependencies. Often, pills seem (deceptively) to be the only way of getting through daily life without pain. Chronic abuse of appetite suppressants or laxatives (mostly by women) is a dangerous, although widespread, method of weight loss.
Social and personal conflict: See Health and Well-Being, p. 182 and Mental Health Disorders, p. 195.
Combining medications: Analgesics and sedatives, stimulants and appetite suppressants are also used to intensify the effects of alcohol and other drugs.

Who's at Risk

Medication dependency, especially to tranquilizers, is not uncommon. Two thirds of people with medication dependency are women receiving analgesics and psychopharmaceuticals, making women more at risk.

Possible Aftereffects and Complications

The physical and mental consequences of constant abuse depend on the medication. One example of physical damage is kidney failure from years of ingesting analgesics (see Kidney Failure, p. 425).

— Decreased, disturbed, or altered reaction abilities increase the risk of accidents in the workplace, car, or home.
— Chronic use of tranquilizers can cause personality changes, emotional, and perceptual disorders (see Psychoses, p. 200) and long-term brain damage.
— General malaise, poor nutrition, and/or vitamin or protein deficiencies are symptoms of almost all medication dependencies.
— Social consequences include loss of relationships or jobs and criminal behavior, as the abuser resorts to obtaining drugs by theft and prescription forgery.

Prevention

Individual prevention starts early: Before you take any medication, find out what it can do, both in positive and negative terms (see Medication Summary, p. 657). It is also important that you be made aware of all side effects and possible risks before taking the medication. If it has been prescribed and you become physically ill without having been informed of possible side effects, you may have recourse to legal action.

When to Seek Medical Advice

Seek help at the first sign of complications or dependency.

Self-Help

Information about support groups and counseling is available through your local health centers or hospitals. It is dangerous to go through withdrawal on your own; some medications have severely adverse affects when you stop taking them.

Treatment

The phases of treatment for medication dependency are the same as for alcoholism, depending on the severity and nature of symptoms (see p. 206). Depending on the medication, withdrawal may be implemented either by the abrupt "cold turkey" method, or by gradually decreasing the dosage. Problems with partners and families are often contributing factors in medication dependency, so it is advisable to seek therapy as well (see Consultation and Psychotherapy, p. 697).

ADDICTION TO ILLEGAL DRUGS

In addictions to illegal drugs, it is important to differentiate between the drugs in question and between primarily physical or primarily psychological addictions. Only heroin and crack cocaine have been documented to develop a rapid, powerful physical addiction; in the cases of hashish, "Ecstasy," and cocaine, the addiction is more of a psychological nature.

Causes

The first step in drug experimentation almost always happens in youth, and results from a strong desire to "belong." If your friends are smoking, sniffing, and shooting up, there is a great temptation to find out what it's like. Drugs like heroin often require only one "hit" to start an addiction; many first-time users need a second hit the same day, thus starting the cycle.

Contributing factors to drug addiction include
— The kinds of people you hang out with
— The availability of drugs
— Your degree of curiosity about the unknown and the illicit
— The pressure to be "cool," and/or imitate role models or pop idols

The presence of personal problems or crises, from which drugs are used as an escape, may contribute to the likelihood of addiction, but is not necessary for experimentation with drugs.

Who's at Risk

The risk of drug addiction depends on the degree of personal insecurity of the user, the degree of peer pressure, and the availability of drugs on the black market.

Possible Aftereffects and Complications

The serious health consequences of drug abuse stem from life in the drug subculture rather from the drugs themselves.
— The addict's life is one of squalor, insolvency, prostitution, and crime, because of the exorbitant prices of illegal drugs.
— Life at the margins of society generally involves poor health and low immunity to disease (because of poor nutrition, poor sleep, and poor hygiene).
— Bacterial and viral infections (e.g., AIDS) from dirty needles and adulterated heroin are part of the addict's everyday life, as are infections of the blood

(bacteremia), heart (endocarditis), liver, kidneys, and lungs, etc.
— Overdoses usually result from adulterated heroin or from trying to make it through a heroin-free phase by using alcohol and/or medications. After a period of abstinence, what used to be a normal dose can easily become an overdose.

Methadone Programs

Programs run by medical facilities for controlled dispensing of oral medications, such as methadone, make illegal aquisition of drugs unnecessary, and decrease the spread of HIV by reducing the need to share/use potentially infected needles.

Psychotherapy and counselling are important aspects of methadone programs.

Relapse is less likely in long-term programs than with short-term treatment protocols.

Prevention

The fact that these drugs are illegal is largely at fault for their health and social costs, especially among youths who are tempted by anything forbidden. Legalizing drugs might help prevent the crime and physical and social ramifications engendered by the illegal drug subculture (see Illicit Drugs, p. 759).

Individual susceptibility begins in the family and at school. Generally speaking, the more secure a teenager feels in the process of growing up, the more he or she is protected against addictions of any sort.

When to Seek Medical Advice

Seek help immediately.

Self-Help

Only in rare cases is self-help possible. The optimal response is to go to the closest drug intervention center or health center for information.

Treatment

Treatment is like that described for alcoholism (see p. 206). The patient's commitment to "kicking the habit" is the critical element in treatment, whether or not medications are used in treatment. Going "cold turkey" requires immediate abstinence. Fear of the physical pain and effects of withdrawal scares most addicts away from this radical method, leaving them to choose the medical support route—that is, methadone. This morphine-like substance, itself addictive, is used in withdrawal treatment programs in major cities:

— On an outpatient, short-term basis while waiting for a slot to open in a long-term therapy program. Doses are gradually reduced under medical supervision

— In intermediate-term treatments to prepare the addict for a long-term program leading to abstinence. The dose is gradually reduced. This treatment should definitely be supplemented with psychotherapy

— In long-term treatments, especially for individuals addicted for years who have lost all motivation to "kick the habit." A constant dose of methadone is administered regularly over a long period, to help get the addict out of crime and help establish a less ruinous lifestyle.

Advice and Help
Information about drug rehabilitation centers is available through health or crisis intervention centers as well as many community centers or social service agencies.

BRAIN AND NERVE DISORDERS

The nervous system is the most varied and complex part of the body. It is divided into the central nervous system (CNS), consisting of the brain and the spinal cord, and the peripheral nervous system, which connects all other nerve pathways.

Brain

All of our thinking, emotions, sensations, and the dealings between them take place in the brain (cerebral hemispheres). Many unconscious body functions, such as breathing or maintaining balance, are regulated by the brain as well.

Twelve pairs of cranial nerves originate in the brain and send and receive impulses to and from various body regions. Three layers of tissue (the meninges) contain and surround the brain: the two inner layers are soft, and the outer layer, which protects the brain and connects it to the bones of the skull, is harder. An inflammation of these tissues is called *meningitis.*

Hollow spaces inside the brain are filled with cerebrospinal fluid, as is the space between the two soft meninges. The soft mass of the brain floats in this fluid, which helps it retain its form as well as protecting and cushioning it; the fluid surrounds the entire CNS and is also found in the spinal cord.

In the event of a disorder of the brain or meninges, the composition of the cerebrospinal fluid changes; diagnoses can be performed by examining fluid extracted between lumbar vertebrae via a lumbar puncture.

Spinal Cord

The spinal cord may be seen as an extension of the brain, reaching down the spine to the lumbar area, and surrounded by cerebrospinal fluid and meninges.

The spinal cord does not go the full length of the spine, ending at the third lumbar vertebra. Through openings between the vertebrae, spinal nerves branch out from the spinal cord into all areas of the body.

Peripheral Nervous System

The peripheral nervous system connects the CNS with the various tissues of the body. It transmits sensations and perceptions from inside or outside the body to the CNS, and it transmits commands from the CNS to

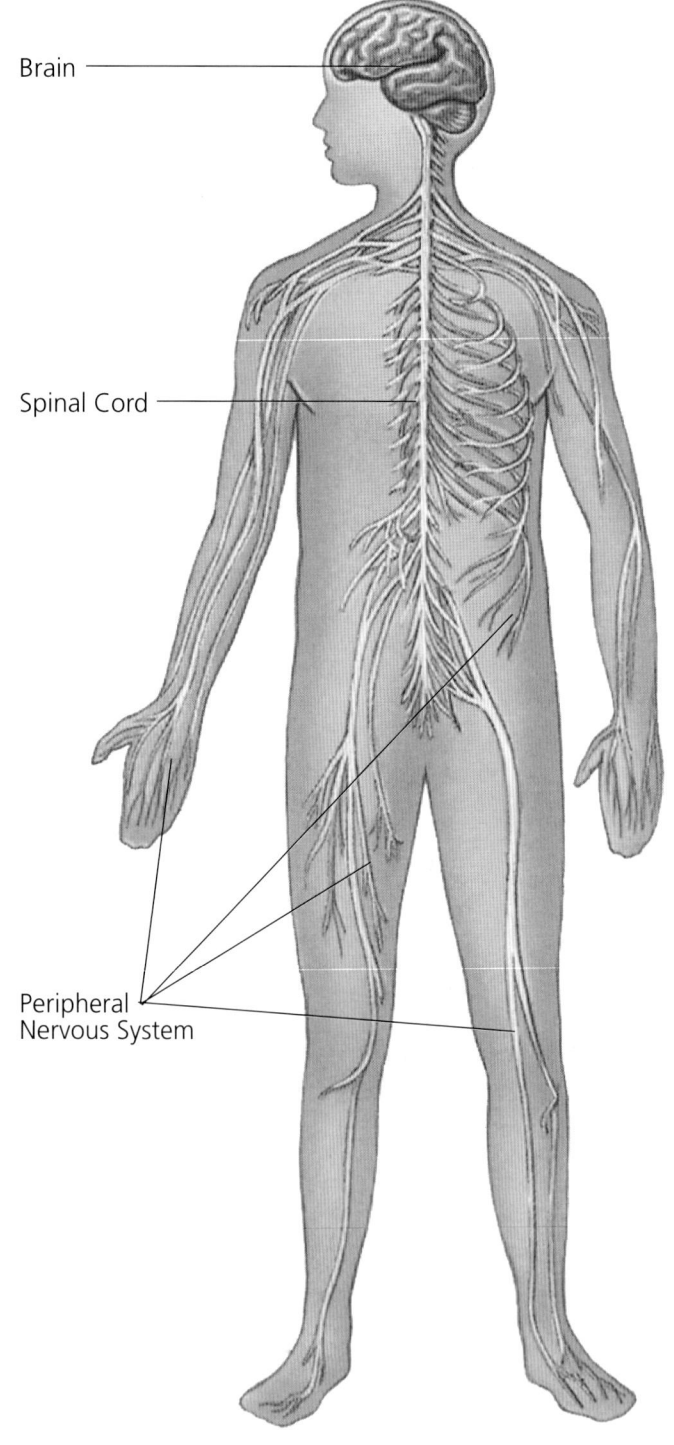

Brain

Spinal Cord

Peripheral
Nervous System

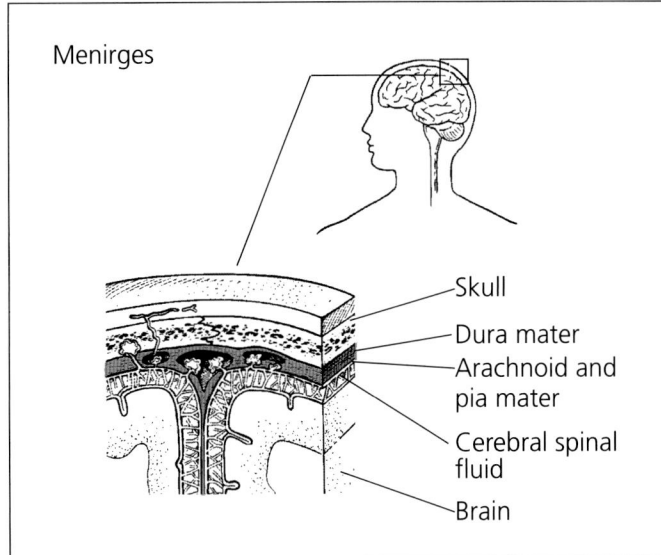

Menirges

Skull
Dura mater
Arachnoid and pia mater
Cerebral spinal fluid
Brain

muscles and organs.

Information is transferred between nerve cells by small electrical impulses or chemical reactions. The CNS then connects and coordinates various information.

Autonomic Nervous System

The autonomic nervous system works independently and is not influenced by our volition. Without our awareness, it regulates every single body function—from the tensing of a muscle in order to move or speak, to breathing, heartbeat, and digestion.

Two main nerve areas within the autonomic nervous system have opposite and complementary functions. The sympathetic nervous system is responsible for activity, exertion, and energy consumption, while the parasympathetic nervous system is responsible for relaxation and energy conservation.

The autonomic nervous system is not the only arbiter of seemingly "automatic" behavior, however. Reflexes like snatching your hand away from a hot stove, or walking upright, which have become unconscious long before adulthood, were originally learned with the aid of the brain and central nervous system.

CONCUSSION

Complaints

An accident may cause loss of consciousness for a few seconds or several minutes. This is usually followed by a phase of partial consciousness, often accompanied by vomiting, headaches and/or dizziness. The victim is often left with no memory of the seconds immediately preceding the accident.

If the period of unconsciousness lasts longer than 15 minutes, or the phase of partial consciousness lasts over an hour, there is reason to suspect the damage is more than just a simple concussion (see Cerebral Contusions, p. 212; Intracranial Hemorrhage, p. 214).

Causes

Concussions are caused by a forceful impact to the head and indicate that nerve cell function has been temporarily disturbed, but without permanent damage to the tissue.

Possible Aftereffects and Complications

Headaches, dizziness, and difficulty concentrating may persist for months after the accident. Only very seldom do hemorrhages occur 2 to 4 weeks after the initial injury (see p. 214). In these cases, headaches commonly worsen and paralysis is a possibility.

Prevention

Wearing a helmet when riding a bicycle or motorcycle, or when doing heavy construction work, is extremely useful for protecting the head and reducing impact.

When to Seek Medical Advice

Anyone who is unconscious or vomiting after a head injury should be brought to the hospital immediately. Depending on the intensity of the symptoms, either observation or diagnostic tests, such as a computed tomography (CT) scan, may be necessary (see X rays and Electroencephalogram (EEG), p.646).

Self-Help

Once it is established that there are no other damages besides a concussion, 12 hours to 2 days of bed rest are sufficient for recovery.

Treatment

For prolonged unconsciousness and recurrent vomiting, a hospital stay for purposes of observation is recommended.

CEREBRAL CONTUSIONS

Complaints
Common symptoms are unconsciousness, often lasting longer than 15 minutes, severe headaches, stiff neck and vomiting. Less common symptoms are partial paralysis and disorders of speech, vision, and breathing. Usually symptoms appear immediately following the injury; in rare cases, from 1 to 4 days later.

Causes
Severe impact to the head can cause damage to internal blood vessels. A blow that would result in a black-and-blue bruise on a leg may have serious consequences when applied to the head, as pressure from blood and tissue fluids damage the brain.

Possible Aftereffects and Complications
Consequences of a cerebral contusion depend on its distention and position. They range from frequent headaches, seizures, and memory disorders to severe paralysis, behavior disorders, or coma.

When to Seek Medical Advice
The above symptoms necessitate immediate hospitalization.

Self-Help
Not possible.

Treatment
Patients are hospitalized until they are symptom-free. In the event of severe hemorrhage, the blood must be aspirated or removed surgically. Depending on the extent of damage, either physiotherapy, speech therapy or other therapy may be indicated.

SKULL FRACTURES

Complaints
See Concussion, p. 211. Additional complaints include a bluish swelling around one or both eyes, and possibly a clear discharge from the nose.

Possible Aftereffects and Complications
Complications may arise because of bleeding or fluid buildup in the brain.

When to Seek Medical Advice
Immediate referral to the hospital is necessary when a skull fracture is suspected. X rays or a CT scan may reveal the damage.

Treatment
Skull fractures will heal without complications if nothing other than the bone was damaged. For the treatment of hemorrhages, see p. 215. Leakage of cerebrospinal fluid should be treated with antibiotics to prevent infection.

MENINGITIS

Complaints
Over the course of a few hours, the patient may develop a headache, fever, light sensitivity, neck stiffness, and occasional vomiting. In serious cases, loss of consciousness may occur. Small children show these symptoms only rarely, however, usually developing instead seizures or a stomach ache. Children are susceptible to a very serious form of meningitis, characterized at its onset by fever and dark spots on the skin.

Babies are in particular danger of undiagnosed meningitis, since its symptoms may manifest only as shrill crying (irritability), listlessness or the diminished ability to suck.

Causes
Meningitis is a bacterial or viral infection of the meninges, caused by agents either transported by the blood from an affected organ or transmitted directly from an ear or sinus infection.

Who's at Risk
Children are at high risk of contracting meningitis.

Prevention
The proper treatment of ear infections and sinusitis can inhibit the spread of organisms responsible for meningitis. A vaccination also exists for *Haemophilus influenzae type B*, a common cause of one form of bacterial meningitis in children.

Possible Aftereffects and Complications
In severe cases meningitis may result in mental retardation or even death.

When to Seek Medical Advice

If you suspect meningitis, see a doctor or go to the hospital immediately. A lumbar puncture (spinal tap) will be performed to check for infections or other causes of illness.

Self-Help

Not possible.

Treatment

Hospitalization is almost always necessary in the event of meningitis. If the cause is bacterial, antibiotics should be administered intravenously. If the cause is viral, all one can do is give supportive care and hope the patient's body is stronger than the disease.

ENCEPHALITIS

Complaints

Depending on severity, the symptoms range from fever, headaches, and exhaustion to paralysis, visual disorders with double vision, seizures, and unconsciousness.

Causes

Encephalitis is almost always the result of a viral infection such as flu, measles, German measles, or mumps. Viruses transmitted by ticks may also trigger such infections.

Who's at Risk

Babies and elderly people are at higher risk for developing encephalitis following a viral infection.

Possible Aftereffects and Complications

Very mild cases of encephalitis accompanying the flu often go unrecognized, and disappear together with the flu symptoms. Viruses such as herpes simplex may lead to a serious illness requiring weeks of hospitalization and causing long-term paralysis and speech disorders. In rare cases, Parkinson's disease may develop after encephalitis (see p. 218).

Prevention

Vaccinations protect against certain viral infections from developing into encephalitis (see Immunizations, p. 667).

When to Seek Medical Advice

Seek help if encephalitis is suspected. Examination of blood and cerebrospinal fluid may be required, as may an EEG (see p. 646).

Self-Help

Mild cases of encephalitis do not require self-help; in serious cases it is not possible.

Treatment

Severe cases of encephalitis require hospital treatment to help prevent further complications such as loss of consciousness or seizures. If a herpes simplex virus is suspected to have triggered the encephalitis, intravenous acyclovir may prove beneficial.

BRAIN ABSCESSES

Complaints

Symptoms include paralysis; numbness in arm or leg; occasionally speech disorders, fever, headaches, and delirium.

Causes

In a brain abscess, pus buildup causes pressure on specific areas of the brain. The culprit is a nearby bacterial infection—either a bacterial meningitis or an ear or sinus infection.

Increased Risk Factors

The risk of a brain abscess increases
— When an ear or sinus infection is left untreated
— In individuals with cyanotic heart defect (see p. 344)

Possible Aftereffects and Complications

If the abscess is treated in time, there are no untoward consequences. A large abscess exerting pressure on the brain may lead to permanent paralysis.

Prevention

Prompt treatment of bacterial infections with antibiotics.

When to Seek Medical Advice

See your health-care provider or local hospital immediately if a brain abscess is suspected.

Self-Help
Not possible.

Treatment
Sometimes use of intravenous antibiotics is sufficient. In severe cases the accumulation of pus must be removed surgically.

TRANSIENT ISCHEMIC ATTACKS (TIA)

Complaints
The symptoms of this cerebral circulatory disorder vary, according to the part of the brain whose blood flow is blocked. The symptom will usually occur in the body part for whose functioning that part of the brain is responsible. For example, one arm, one leg, or one half of the body may become numb and/or paralyzed; in other cases, visual or speech disorders, confusion, or loss of consciousness may be the only symptoms. Symptoms may last anywhere from a few minutes to several hours.

Causes
In this disorder, a brain artery—often already constricted due to hardening of the arteries—becomes blocked by a blood clot, which has either formed there or traveled from another blood vessel (often the carotid artery). The resulting lack of oxygen to one area of the brain impairs brain function.

In a transient ischemic attack, the blood clot dissolves within a few minutes, circulation is restored, and the system returns to normal.

Who's at Risk
Those factors that increase the risk of calcification of the arteries also increase the risk of cerebral circulatory disorders: obesity, high blood pressure, smoking, diabetes, and old age (see Arteriosclerosis, p. 318).

Possible Aftereffects and Complications
Cerebral circulatory disorders may recur repeatedly until the blockage finally fails to dissolve, possibly resulting in a stroke.

Prevention
Avoid all possible factors that contribute to arteriosclerosis (see p. 318). In those individuals who have already experienced more than one cerebral circulatory disorder, it may be worthwhile to start taking clot-inhibiting medication, or, in rare cases, undergo surgery.

When to Seek Medical Advice
Call an ambulance immediately when
— An arm or leg suddenly becomes numb and/or paralyzed
— Visual or speech disorders, or loss of consciousness, suddenly appear

The site of the blockage may be located by various means: Ultrasound, EEG, blood analysis, CT or magnetic resonance imaging (MRI) scans, or angiograms. Most of these tests are available only in a hospital setting.

Self-Help
Anything that helps reduce the risk of arteriosclerosis can help prevent transient ischemic attack (see Arteriosclerosis, p. 318).

Treatment
Depending on the cause of the illness, it may be beneficial to take medication to lower blood pressure or thin the blood. In rare cases, surgery of the carotid artery may be indicated.

INTRACRANIAL HEMORRHAGE

Complaints
During an intracranial hemorrhage, a particular area of the brain is deprived of oxygen. The symptoms are similar to those of a stroke (see p. 215); their type and severity vary depending on the size and location of the affected area.

Suspect intracranial hemorrhage if, following an accident, the victim starts losing consciousness, or if a person unaccountably loses consciousness for over 15 minutes. In the advanced stages, the pupil of the eye is fixed in a wide-open position.

Causes
Intracranial hemorrhage is caused by a blood vessel bleeding into the brain. Depending on the volume of blood, the affected part of the brain is subjected to excessive pressure. The broken blood vessel may be caused by high blood pressure, calcification, aneurysm (see

p. 331), or head injury.

Who's at Risk
Ten percent of all strokes are caused by acute bleeding. Strokes, because of intracranial hemorrhage, are more common in younger adults than in older people.

Possible Aftereffects and Complications
Untreated accumulations of blood or fluid in the brain may cause death. However, even after appropriate treatment, lasting damage may remain, depending on the cause of the stroke and the location of the affected area of the brain.

Prevention
Not possible.

When to Seek Medical Advice
Immediate hospitalization is recommended for anyone who has lost consciousness after an accident and whose condition deteriorates. A CT scan can determine the exact location and extent of the bleeding, and distinguish between bleeding and fluid accumulation.

Self-Help
Self-help would be life-threatening.

Treatment
Blood accumulations in the brain should be surgically removed as soon as possible. High doses of corticosteroids or medications to reduce swelling may also be used.

STROKES

Complaints
During a stroke, the cerebral blood flow is compromised. Symptoms vary according to the location of the affected artery and the function of the corresponding area of the brain. Often one arm, one leg, or one half of the body becomes numb and/or paralyzed; in other cases, visual or speech disorders, confusion, or loss of consciousness may be the only symptoms.

Symptoms frequently occur upon awakening in the morning. Unlike transient ischemic attacks, the symptoms of a stroke usually last longer than 24 hours.

Stroke
By slow, progressive hardening of the blood vessels, it becomes more and more difficult for the blood to flow to supply the brain with oxygen and nutrients. Blood clots can occlude an already narrowed blood vessel more rapidly, meaning that the brain area supplied by the occluded vessel receives no more blood supply.

Causes
Most strokes are caused by blockage of an artery in the brain. Occasionally they are caused by bleeding into the brain (see Intracranial Hemorrhage, p. 214).

Who's at Risk
About 80 percent of strokes are due to insufficient blood circulation in the brain. All factors that increase the risk of arterial calcification also increase the risk of a stroke (see Arteriosclerosis, p. 318).

Possible Aftereffects and Complications
About one third of all stroke patients recover completely within a few weeks or months; another third are left with speech and visual disorders or paralysis; the remaining third do not survive.

Even when there is no permanent damage, a stroke is an alarm signal that more—and more serious—strokes are possible down the line.

Prevention
Lower your risk factors as much as possible (see Arteriosclerosis, p. 318). Anticoagulants, or in rare cases surgery on the brain's blood vessels, may help.

When to Seek Medical Advice
When a stroke is suspected, hospitalization is recommended. The site of the blockage may be located by various means: ultrasound, EEG, blood analysis, CT or MRI scans, or angiogram.

Self-Help
Stroke-induced speech and movement disorders can be overcome by way of therapy, if the patient is strong and has a strong desire to live. Stroke victims can regain independence through regular exercise and hard work. Family members and caregivers should keep in mind

that even though stroke victims may be unable to speak or move, they can usually hear and understand what is said in their presence.

Treatment

The initial treatment of a stroke patient requires hospitalization. Although starting physical therapy as soon as possible in the hospital would significantly increase patients' chances for rehabilitation, this does not happen in most cases. Ideally, insurance coverage of hospital treatment should include early rehabilitation procedures.

Depending on the cause of the stroke, medication for lowering blood pressure or for thinning the blood may be beneficial. In some cases an operation on the carotid artery may be necessary. The hospital will supply information on subsequent mandatory or optional therapies, rehabilitation centers, and support groups.

EPILEPSY

Complaints

There are several types of seizures.

Grand mal (generalized) seizures may be preceded by days of headaches, nausea, restlessness, and depression. During the seizure itself, the victim suddenly loses consciousness, falls down, and becomes rigid; arms and legs twitch or jerk uncontrollably, and breathing may become irregular. This phase usually lasts a few minutes, after which the victim falls into a deep sleep and wakes feeling groggy. Usually urine is released involuntarily; less often, a bowel movement.

— In petit mal (smaller) seizures, the victim does not fall down. In young children the only symptoms of a petit mal seizure may be a momentary interruption in activity and a blank stare straight ahead. Afterwards the child often has no idea of what has happened, so seizures of this nature are often mistaken for periods of daydreaming.

— In temporal lobe seizures, the victim often does not lose consciousness, but has a few minutes of peculiar behavior: laughing inexplicably, fumbling, and smacking the lips.

— In focal seizures, one half of the face or one hand starts twitching, and the twitching gradually spreads over half the body.

— In status epilepticus, epileptic attacks follow each other in rapid succession for a prolonged period.

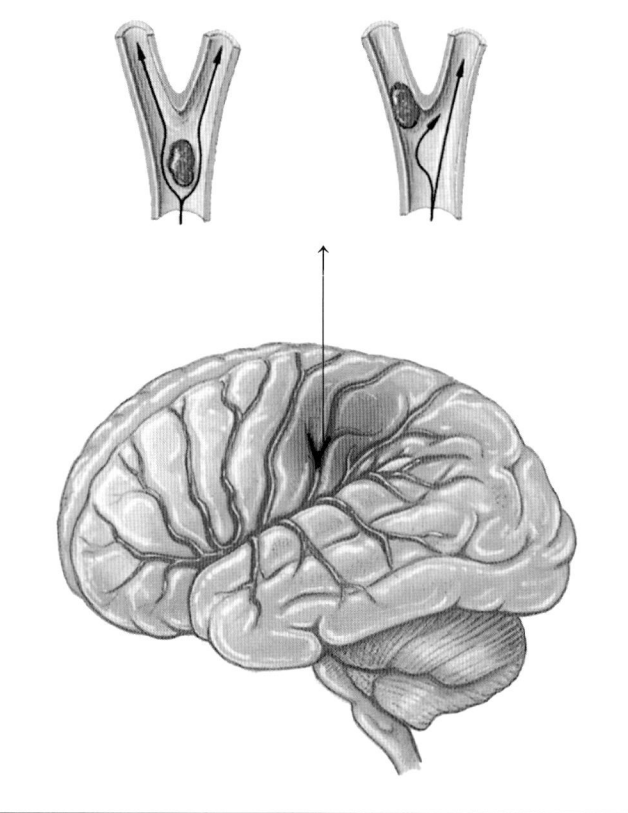

Stroke

By slow, progressive hardening of the blood vessels, it becomes more and more difficult for the blood to flow to supply the brain with oxygen and nutrients. Blood clots can occlude an already narrowed blood vessel more rapidly, meaning that the brain area supplied by the occluded vessel receives no more blood supply.

The term *epilepsy* is used only when seizures recur. A febrile seizure in a child, or a seizure in a diabetic experiencing a sugar low, has nothing to do with epilepsy.

Causes

Seizures are caused by abnormal electrical impulses in nerve cells in the brain. These may be caused by damage during birth, brain infections, deteriorating brain processes, metabolic illnesses, brain injury, brain tumors, or intoxication (notably alcohol). Often the cause of epilepsy is unknown.

Who's at Risk

Individuals with some brain damage, such as a tumor or the results of a serious head injury, are at greater risk

What to Do if You Witness a Seizure
— Move all potentially harmful objects out of the way.
— Move the victim only if absolutely necessary (for example, if he or she is lying on a flight of stairs).
— Do not hold the victim or try to stop the twitching.
— Do not insert anything between the victim's teeth.
— Unbutton the victim's collar.
— Though the victim's breathing may be irregular, don't give mouth-to-mouth resuscitation—it is neither necessary nor advisable.
— When sleep comes following the attack, turn the victim on his or her side and let him or her sleep.
— Call a physician immediately if the seizure lasts longer than 3 minutes, or if another attack follows soon afterwards.

for epilepsy. So are children who underwent oxygen deprivation at birth. Some types of epilepsy seem to be inherited family traits.

Possible Physical Consequences and Complications
The danger of injury is greater in a grand mal seizure than in other types because the victim falls unconscious. Bitten tongues are common.

All seizures are potentially harmful to the individual and others, especially, for example, if the seizure occurs while the victim is driving an automobile. Several attacks in rapid succession constitute a life-threatening emergency.

Epilepsy can only rarely be cured. Some children outgrow epilepsy, but we are as yet unable to predict which ones will and which ones won't.

Possible Social Consequences and Complications
To this day, epilepsy remains a mysterious illness surrounded by prejudice and fear. Unconscious fear makes many people withdraw when they find out someone is an epileptic. Because of this, epileptics suffer needlessly.

Their social lives depend on the controllability of seizures, and possible side effects, through medication. According to the country they live in, a driver's license may be obtainable only after specific requirements are met and no seizure is experienced in two to three years. Epileptics who wish to have children should con-

sult a specialist about the possible risk of passing the disease along to their children. The following guidelines should be followed:
— Women who have been seizure-free for several years should, if possible, stop taking their medication before getting pregnant.
— Epileptics on medication have a 90 percent chance of delivering a healthy baby. The risk of abnormality in the child is increased two to three times as a result of the mother's epilepsy and/or treatment.
— Women who seek medical advice only after the first trimester should not automatically be advised to terminate their pregnancy. They should make a choice only after they and the child have been examined and experts have been consulted.
— The risk of birth defects varies by medication and phase of pregnancy. It is not advisable to switch medications during pregnancy.
— Discontinuing epileptic medication during pregnancy may trigger seizures, harming both mother and child.
— Possible effects on the baby of low doses of medication in breast milk are not known.

Children with epilepsy should be raised as normally as possible, but their choice of profession should not include any in which they could harm themselves or others during a seizure.

Prevention
There is no prevention for epilepsy; medication can help reduce the incidence of seizures.

When to Seek Medical Advice
Seek help in the event of a seizure. Depending on the kind of seizure and the circumstances, blood and sometimes cerebral fluid should be tested and an EEG (see p. 646) or CT scan (see p. 649) performed. Based on the description of a seizure, medical personnel are often able to tell whether or not epilepsy is involved.

Self-Help
A lifestyle that consciously minimizes risk factors and avoids triggering situations can reduce the incidence of seizures. Alcohol consumption and lack of sleep trigger seizures for many epileptics.

Treatment

Successful treatment by experienced medical personnel can put an end to seizures in 50 to 60 percent of epileptics, and substantially improve the condition of another 20 to 30 percent.

If possible, only one medication per patient should be used to control epilepsy. Finding the right medication and dosage may take months, as every patient reacts differently. Hospitalization is sometimes advisable during this period of adjustment, especially for children; standard procedures include EEGs and monitoring of blood medication levels. Any unauthorized changes in dosage may negatively affect treatment and undo past gains. When taking medication for epilepsy, patients should be vigilant about any other substances ingested: Anticonvulsants may react with other medications and with alcohol in a variety of unwelcome ways.

After two to three seizure-free years, the health-care provider may attempt to decrease the medication gradually over a period of 6 to 12 months, while closely monitoring the patient's progress, with the goal of stopping the medication altogether. However, it may also be necessary to continue medication for the rest of the person's life.

It is sometimes possible to identify the part of the brain that triggers seizures and intervene surgically. Such stereotactic operations have successfully ended seizures in about 55 percent of those suffering from temporal-lobe epilepsy, and have reduced the number of seizures in another 30 percent.

Behavioral therapy techniques such as biofeedback (see p. 695) are often used to help patients control seizures.

Effective Medications for Epilepsy

Phenytoin (Dilantin)	Primidone
Carbamazepine (Tegretol)	Clonazepam
(Klonopin)	
Phenobarbital	Felbamate
Valproic Acid (Depahene)	Gabapentin
(Neurontin)	
Ethosuximide	

PARKINSON'S DISEASE

Complaints

Parkinson's disease often begins with a slight trembling when the patient is at rest, which then disappears during movement or sleep. Another typical symptom is rubbing the index finger and thumb together, so-called "pill-rolling." In some cases a particular movement suddenly becomes difficult or impossible.

Depression often accompanies the movement disorders, and speech and cognitive abilities slow down.

Over time, the ability to walk, move the arms and blink the eyelids slows down and decreases progressively. Initiating movement becomes extremely difficult, and the patient's steps are small and shuffling. It becomes difficult to maintain one's balance because the arms can no longer move easily. The face tends to grow rigid, the patient speaks in a monotone and is hard to understand, and handwriting gets smaller and less legible. Muscles become increasingly stiff and very painful.

Causes

The nerve cells that produce the neurotransmitter dopamine gradually die, which disrupts the chemical balance necessary for the proper functioning of the nervous system. It is not known why these cells die in some people. Occasionally the disease can be traced to exposure to neurotoxins, carbon monoxide or methanol, or to some forms of brain infection. Neuroleptic medications used in the treatment of schizophrenia can temporarily produce the same symptoms as Parkinson's disease.

Who's at Risk

When not caused by brain infections or exposure to toxins, Parkinson's disease usually shows up in individuals over age 50. In occasional very severe cases it can begin much earlier. The disease seems to run in families to some degree.

The Parkinsonism caused by neuroleptic medications disappears when the neuroleptic is discontinued. If this is not advisable, the symptoms may be counteracted by another medication (e.g., biperiden [Akineton]).

Possible Aftereffects and Complications

The slowly advancing movement disorders of Parkinson's disease make daily life increasingly difficult. Severe cases may be accompanied by psychological breakdown and depression. However, with appropriate treatment, many patients are able to lead fairly normal lives.

Prevention

Not possible.

When to Seek Medical Advice

The gradual onset of trembling in an elderly person is not in itself a cause for concern. However, if movement suddenly becomes difficult or there are changes in the patient's speech, medical advice should be sought.

Early diagnosis can help make lifestyle adjustments and medical treatment less invasive and easier to handle.

Self-Help

Avoiding stress and overwork will allow you to lead as normal a life as possible. Practical aids such as stair railings, chairs with high arm rests, or shoes with velcro instead of laces can help a lot. Many Parkinson's sufferers find that joining a support group can be a first step out of the isolation caused by this disease.

Treatment

Parkinson's medications contain an ingredient which the brain processes into dopamine, the missing neurotransmitter. In advanced stages of the disease, when all the affected nerve cells have died, the L-dopamine dosage is increased until it no longer has any effect.

Effective Medications for Parkinson's Disease

Dopaminergic Agents
Pramipexole (Mirapex)
Amantadine
Bromocriptine Mesylate (Parlodel)
Levodopa
Carbidopa/levodopa (Sinemet)
Pergolide (Permex)
Selegiline (Eldepryl)
Anticholinergic Agents
Benzotropine (Cogentin)
Biperiden (Akineton)
Procyclidine (Kemadrin)

Especially at high dosages, this medication can cause the patient's involuntary movements to become highly exaggerated; while the patient may find this a small price to pay for the alleviation of the disease, other people may be put off by the behavior. Occasionally, hallucinations occur as a result of medication.

An extremely important factor in treatment is physical therapy, in which cramped muscles are moved both passively and actively.

Recent medical research has shown that the rate of dopamine depletion can be slowed by monoamine oxidase (MAO) inhibitors, such as selegiline; and medications that can stimulate dopamine production.

Beta-blockers (see p. 324) can sometimes alleviate severe trembling.

Research into implanting embryonic dopamine-producing cells into diseased brains is still at the experimental stages.

ALZHEIMER'S DISEASE

Complaints

The dementia typical of Alzheimer's disease takes two forms, one appearing between 40 and 65 years of age, the other after age 65.

The patient becomes increasingly forgetful, misplacing objects and repeating questions that have already been answered. Logical thinking, knowledge, and many abilities are lost; the patient's speech becomes deficient and monotonous in tone. In the advanced stages, the patient is no longer able to function in daily life and no longer recognizes familiar people; in the final stages, control of bodily functions is lost.

Sensations and emotions remain intact for a long time in Alzheimer's patients, who are quite aware of their gradual loss of faculties, and of the reactions of those around them. This often leads to depression or increasingly aggressive behavior.

Causes

In Alzheimer's disease, nerve cells in the brain die and form clumps. The production of neurotransmitters, the brain's "messengers," which are responsible for transmitting information between nerve cells, drops lower and lower.

Why this occurs in some people and not in others is unknown. Hereditary and/or genetic factors are known to play a role, as Alzheimer's disease tends to run in families. Environmental influences may also be factors; however, neither nutrition, stress nor excess aluminum intake have emerged as decisive factors.

People who have ever suffered a brain injury are at greater risk for Alzheimer's disease.

Who's at Risk
Alzheimer's disease is the major cause of progressive dementia in the elderly. Its frequency increases with age; 40 percent of those over age 90 are affected.

Possible Aftereffects and Complications
This illness may take a variety of forms, but the more it advances, the more dependent on others the patient becomes. Over the course of 5 to 10 years, complete physical and mental degeneration results, eventually ending in death.

Prevention
Not yet possible.

When to Seek Medical Advice
Seek help at the first suspicion of this disease. Other possible causes of the symptoms must first be ruled out. Even then, it is often difficult to tell whether the patient is exhibiting symptoms of Alzheimer's disease, or merely of old age.

Self-Help
The support and encouragement of family and friends can help Alzheimer's patients deal with their increasing disabilities as long as possible.

Accurate information about the disease and its course can help care-givers find creative ways of dealing with it. Support groups are very beneficial in this regard.
— Continue demonstrating warmth and support.
— If at all possible, keep the patient in familiar surroundings and routines.
— A large clock, a calendar, and labels on objects in the patient's surroundings can help them stay oriented.
— Let the patient perform as many daily tasks and duties as possible.

Treatment
Although medications cannot heal this illness, they can influence its course. Cholinesterase inhibitors like Tacrine (Cognex) for example have proven effective, but involve many side effects. Tacrine is one of the few medications that lessen the symptoms of Alzheimer's disease. Donepezil (Aricept) is also helpful. Neuroleptics (see p. 202) may counteract sleep disorders and periods of anxiety or restlessness.

Forms of treatment that utilize the patient's remaining intellectual capabilities without overloading them can also have a beneficial effect on the course of the disease.

In the final stages of the disease, living at home may no longer be an option. Visiting nurses, home health aides, or a nursing home may be the next step.

MULTIPLE SCLEROSIS

Complaints
The symptoms of multiple sclerosis (MS) vary greatly and may be only sporadic at the onset of the disease: weakness in arms or legs, numbness, trembling, slurred speech, and visual disorders. Usually the symptoms disappear, occasionally for good; often, however, they recur repeatedly after pauses of a few months or years. Some of them may not subside completely each time, resulting in increased disabilities following each new episode.

Causes
In MS, the myelin sheath insulating the nerves becomes damaged in spots in a process known as demyelination, limiting nutrients to the nerves and interfering with their ability to transmit impulses. The damage may occur in various parts of the brain or spinal cord, and may subside spontaneously. If damage occurs to the nerve itself, some symptoms will remain. It is not clear what causes demyelination: one possibility is low-level viruses acting over the course of many years.

Who's at Risk
Multiple sclerosis generally appears in people aged 20 to 40 and is more common in women than men.

Possible Aftereffects and Complications
For many people, the course of this disease is slow and moderate, and individual episodes are separated by years. Because the symptoms increase during pregnancy, female MS patients are advised not to become preg-

nant.

Prevention
Not possible.

When to Seek Medical Advice
If multiple sclerosis is suspected, a neurologist should be consulted. A positive diagnosis may be made by examining cerebrospinal fluid. Sometimes a MRI (see p. 650) or EEG (see p. 646) may also be necessary.

Self-Help
Stay as active as possible. Support groups can be a great help. Relaxation exercises can help ease cramps in paralyzed muscles.

Treatment
There is no cure for multiple sclerosis. Physical therapy is extremely important in managing the disease, and occupational therapy can help MS sufferers cope better with daily life. During a flare-up, high-dose intravenous corticosteroids (see pa. 665) may alleviate symptoms; however, corticosteroids have numerous serious side effects and their effectiveness is reduced with long-term use. Sometimes muscle relaxants are beneficial; in other cases they worsen the symptoms.

BRAIN TUMORS
See also Cancer, p. 470.

Complaints
Symptoms vary greatly depending on location and size of the tumor. Headaches made worse by lying down are common; sudden vomiting without previous nausea may also indicate a tumor, as well as weakness or paralysis on one side of the body, numbness, balance disorders, visual disturbances, or epileptic seizures.

Causes
As with other bodily cancers, brain tumors form when brain cells grow beyond their normal rate (see Cancer, p. 470).

Especially in adults, brain tumors can be initiated by invading cancer cells from a metastasizing breast or lung tumor.

Who's at Risk
The risk of developing a brain tumor is relatively low.

Possible Aftereffects and Complications
Since space inside the skull is limited, even a small tumor exerts a lot of pressure on the brain. For this reason, even a benign tumor may cause death if not treated in time. Rarely, tumor cells from the brain can lead to a spinal cord tumor.

Prevention
Not possible.

When to Seek Medical Advice
Seek help if symptoms include paralysis, long-term numbness, or frequent headaches that are made worse by lying down or are accompanied by sudden vomiting. Through comprehensive examinations and use of CT scans (see p. 649), MRI (see p. 650), and EEGs (see p. 646), a definitive diagnosis of brain tumor can be made. Sometimes an angiogram of the brain is also necessary.

Self-Help
Not possible.

Treatment
Often all or most of the tumor can be surgically removed, followed by a course of radiation therapy if necessary. In some cases, however, the most that can be done is to ease symptoms temporarily. Medications for relieving seizures or increased pressure on the brain may also be indicated.

SPINAL CORD INJURIES

Complaints
Spinal cord injuries always cause temporary or permanent numbness or paralysis. Which parts of the body are affected depends on the location of the injury. Injuries to the cervical vertebral column may affect arms and legs, digestion, elimination, sexual organs, and breathing. Injuries to the upper thoracic spinal cord affect the legs and often the organs of elimination as well, but not always the arms and hands. Spinal cord injuries to the lower vertebra area may paralyze both legs.

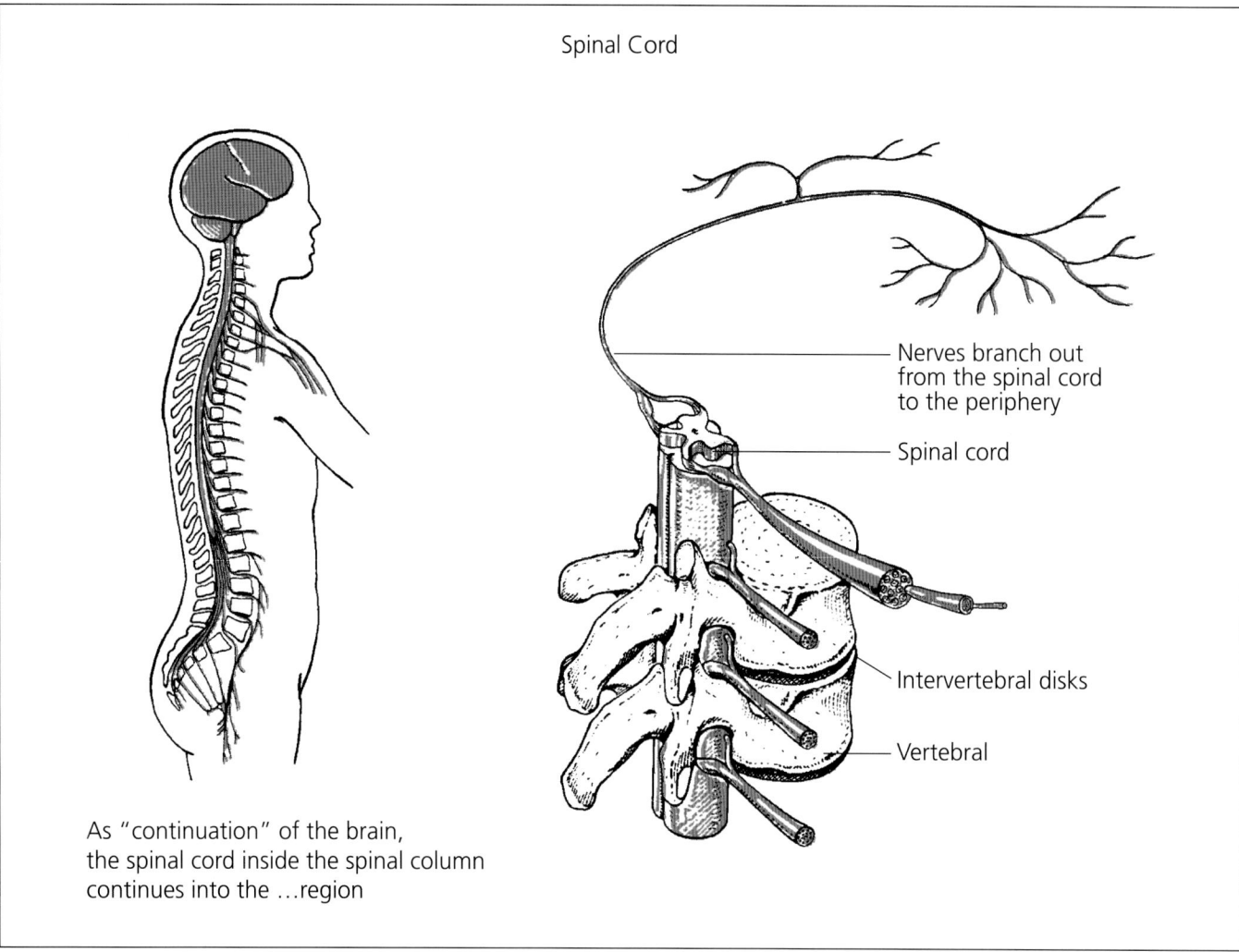

Spinal Cord

Nerves branch out from the spinal cord to the periphery

Spinal cord

Intervertebral disks

Vertebral

As "continuation" of the brain, the spinal cord inside the spinal column continues into the …region

Causes

A swelling in the spinal cord may be caused by an impact or distraction injury, bleeding, or severing of the spinal cord.

Who's at Risk

Injuries to the spine do not automatically result in spinal cord injury; only about 10 to 20 percent of those with spine injuries suffer from spinal cord injuries.

Experts estimate that about half of those who end up as paraplegics suffered additional damage to the spinal cord as a result of improper transportation after an accident.

Possible Aftereffects and Complications

Spinal cord injuries have a huge impact on victims' lives. Lengthy initial hospitalization is followed by years of rehabilitation, with unpredictable results.

Many paraplegics become dependent on other people. They may be confined to a wheelchair; some

may have access to a car with hand-operated controls, improving their means of getting around. A paralyzed bladder may lead to urinary tract infections which often go unnoticed and result in pyelonephritis (infection of the kidneys). Often the body's functions of circulation, sweat production, and temperature regulation are compromised.

When to Seek Medical Advice

Call an ambulance immediately if you suspect a spinal cord injury: such injuries require professional treatment according to strict protocol, and it is better not to move someone with a spinal injury than to attempt it and risk doing it improperly. The victim should be transported on a hard, flat surface (see First Aid/Injury of Bones, p. 709) by professionals only; speed is second in priority.

Self-Help

Not possible.

Treatment

Treatment requires hospitalization, followed by reha- bilitation, and depends on the nature of the injury. There is much information available to help victims and their families cope with all the issues involved with a spinal cord injury.

POLIO

Complaints

Ninety percent of all polio infections go unnoticed and result in the person's future immunity to the disease. These "silent" infections are found mainly in underde- veloped countries, in infants infected while still under the protection of the mother's antibodies from pregnancy. The symptoms of this illness appear in the following order, but some people exhibit only the first stage, some only the first two stages:
— Two to 5 days of fever, nausea, back and joint pain, hoarseness, constipation, diarrhea
— Two to 3 days later: very high fever, headache, muscle and back pain, vomiting
— Muscle weakness, changing gradually into paralysis

Causes

Polio is caused by the polio virus, which invades the grey matter of the spinal cord.

Who's at Risk

The older a person is when infected with the polio virus, the higher the risk of developing the symptoms of disease. Adults traveling to countries where polio is still common are at increased risk for contracting the illness if they do not get a booster shot before traveling (see Immunizations, p. 667).

Possible Aftereffects and Complications

Polio can result in irreversible paralysis in the limbs, the bladder muscles, and the muscles used for breathing.

Prevention

Prevention of polio is possible through vaccination (see p. 667).

When to Seek Medical Advice

Seek help if polio is suspected.

Self-Help

Not possible.

Treatment

There is no cure for polio.

LYME DISEASE

Complaints

About a week after being bitten by a tick, which may not necessarily have been noticed, the patient develops a red "bull's-eye" circular rash around the bite. The rash may be accompanied by fever and joint pains.

Two to 6 weeks later, intense joint pains may ensue, and taste and hearing may be affected. Often half the facial muscles are paralyzed (Bell's palsy).

Fever and various degrees of heart block may indicate the presence of heart inflammation (carditis), often accompanied by joint pain, headaches, and neck pains. Carditis occurs rarely.

If the disease goes untreated, the third stage involves pain in the knees or other large joints after a period of months or years. Nerve damage may also occur.

Causes

Lyme disease is caused by a bacterial infection trans- mitted by the bite of a tick.

Who's at Risk

Ticks are more likely to carry Lyme disease than viruses. The risk of contracting Lyme disease depends on geographic regions (most cases are reported in the Northeast), and on the length of time the tick is attached. Animal studies indicate that transmission re- quires 24 to 48 hours of tick attachment.

Possible Aftereffects and Complications

Damage to the cranial nerves, heart, and large joints may be permanent if the disease goes unrecognized and is not treated in time.

Prevention

The only way to prevent Lyme disease is to avoid being bitten by a tick. It is sensible to use a tick repellent and/ or wear appropriate clothing when outdoors, to prevent ticks from gaining access to the skin. Daily skin inspection for ticks should be done, especially if in an area where Lyme disease is common.

When to Seek Medical Advice

Seek help as soon as symptoms appear. Since they are not specific, however, make sure to let your health-care provider know you've been bitten by a tick. Usually a blood test will indicate the cause, although a cerebrospinal fluid test is also sometimes necessary.

Self-Help

Not possible.

Treatment

Amoxicillin, cephalosporin or doxycycline (for adults only) (see Antibiotics, p. 661) taken for about 2 weeks will suppress further development of the disease and counteract any damage.

PERIPHERAL NERVE DISORDERS

Complaints

Symptoms include "pins and needles" on palms of hands and soles of feet. Body parts slowly become insensitive to touch and pain; common reflexes disappear and muscles weaken.

Causes

Nerve inflammations may be caused by bacterial or viral infections or other agents; additional causes may include
— Alcoholism (see p. 205)
— Toxic chemicals such as thallium (used in the metal industry and in some rat poison), arsenic (in insecticides), or lead (in the paint, metal, and battery industries)
— Numerous medications
— Diabetes
— Liver and kidney disorders
— Hormonal disorders
— Metabolic disorders

Who's at Risk

The first four causes listed above account for about three quarters of all nerve disorders in adults. They are rare in childhood.

Possible Aftereffects and Complications

Most damage from nerve disorders is the result of lowered sensitivity to temperature and pain: Wounds and illnesses do not heal because they are not recognized and therefore not treated.

Prevention

Diabetics, see p. 483.

Be especially careful when handling heavy metals or solvents.

When to Seek Medical Advice

Seek help if experiencing pain or numbness.

Self-Help

Not possible.

Treatment

While actual nerve disorders cannot be treated, the underlying illness may be: Diabetes, p. 483; Alcoholism, p. 205; Health in the Workplace, p. 789.

NEURALGIA

Complaints

Symptoms of neuralgia usually include sudden, stinging bursts of pain lasting for only a few seconds, but possibly recurring up to 100 times a day. Sometimes these attacks are triggered by pressure or contact on a specific part of the body, or by a particular movement. *Trigeminal neuralgia:* usually involves pain in the upper and lower jaw area.
Intercostal neuralgia: involves pain in the rib area.

Causes

A variety of factors can irritate nerves to the point of pain—inflammations, tissue growths, or scars, for example. When there are no physical causes for nerve pain, psychological clues should be sought (see Health and Well-Being, p. 182).

Who's at Risk

Older individuals are affected more frequently than young people.

Prevention

Not possible.

When to Seek Medical Advice

Seek help when painful attacks start.

Self-Help

Not possible.

Treatment

Acupuncture (see p. 679), transcutaneous electrical nerve stimulation (TENS) (see p. 691), and other therapies may be beneficial.

A simple analgesic containing only acetaminophen (Tylenol), is seldom effective enough. Severe neuralgia may have to be treated with the anticonvulsant carbamazepine (Tegretol) or stronger pain medication.

If the pain is constant and unbearable, an option may be to sever the nerve in question, but this should be considered only after all other possibilities, including psychosomatic factors, have been ruled out.

MIGRAINES

Complaints

Migraines are severe, recurring headaches that come on relatively suddenly. They usually begin on one side of the head and slowly spread to other areas.

Vomiting, light sensitivity, and visual disturbances frequently precede a migraine, as may a tingling or weakness in one arm, or a ringing in the ears.

Causes

During a migraine, blood vessels in the brain first constrict, and pain is caused by the resulting lack of oxygen in the tissues; later the arteries expand, causing more pain. These circulatory changes trigger a series of biochemical processes which, in turn, cause pain.

Predispositions to migraines seem to be congenital. Many migraine sufferers can learn to identify triggering factors, which may include red wine, chocolate, certain cheeses, alcohol, physical stress, bright light, winds such as the Santa Ana in California, hormonal changes during menstruation, birth-control pills, or pregnancy.

Who's at Risk

Migraines often begin after puberty, but seldom after age 40. They are more prevalent in women than in men, by a ratio of 4 to 3. The risk is higher in people with relatives who are affected.

Cluster Headaches

These are a specific type of headache, that affect men more commonly than women. The pain begins on one side of the head, often accompanied by teary eyes and a runny nose. Often the pain starts in the middle of the night, lasts a few hours, stops and begins again. These headaches may recur frequently, or disappear for years. Causes and treatment are the same as for migraines.

Possible Aftereffects and Complications

Migraines are harmless from a medical point of view, but they can cause great suffering. If you take analgesics to stop the pain, you run the risk of addiction or kidney or liver damage (see Analgesics, p. 660).

Prevention

Leading a balanced life in harmony with oneself and one's environment may prevent migraines (see Health and Well-Being, p. 182).

Individual attacks may be prevented by carefully observing one's eating, sleeping, and living habits, determining what triggers the headaches, and then changing or avoiding the cause. Early recognition of an impending attack can lead to a preemptive strike; sometimes a cup of strong coffee is all it takes, possibly with lemon, or an analgesic taken as soon as possible (see Analgesics, p. 660).

Prevention with Medication

Stress management via biofeedback (see p. 695) is beneficial in preventing attacks of migraine. For those suffering more than two attacks per month, prophylactic prescription medication may be helpful.
— Relatively beneficial are beta-blockers containing propranolol (e.g., inderal), atenolol (tenormin), or metoprolol.
— Methysergide can have severe side effects. It should only be taken as a last resort, for no more than three months, at the lowest effective dose.

Other medications such as some tricyclic antidepressants (especially nortriptyline, amitriptyline and doxepin) are also known to be effective in preventing migraines.

After about 6 months on medication, you should try to phase it out slowly.

When to Seek Medical Advice

Seek help if you have never suffered from migraines in the past and suddenly experience severe headaches, possibly accompanied by visual disorders.

Self-Help

Lying down in a darkened room in peace and quiet will bring some relief. A gentle massage along the shoulders and spine may help.

Relaxation exercises (see p. 693) help in coping with the attacks and, when done regularly, may help lessen the frequency of attacks.

Treatment

Many nontraditional treatment methods are very effective for migraines, acupuncture (see p. 697) tops the list. Also effective are behavioral counseling, biofeedback (see p. 695) and TENS (see p. 691). Homeopathy (see p. 684) also helps in easing migraines. Prescription medications for the various symptoms of migraines include:

— Metoclopramide (Reglan) or intravenous chlorpromazine (Thorazine) or prochlorperazine (Compazine), for nausea and vomiting. If taken 10 minutes prior to an analgesic, it will speed up its effect.

— Two tablets of aspirin or acetaminophen (Tylenol) (see Analgesics, p. 660) for pain.

— Ergotamine, such as dihydroergotamine or ergotamine/caffeine (Cafergot) to shorten the attack. Caution: Never take more ergotamine than prescribed; excessive quantities may result in increased headaches.

— Sumatriptan (Imitrex) will also shorten an attack.

Since migraines can develop into a chronic illness, it is advisable to seek treatment at a specialized center (see Headaches, p. 193).

FACIAL PARALYSIS (BELL'S PALSY)

Complaints

Depending on the form of illness, different muscles on one half of the face are paralyzed; bodily movements are accompanied by facial distortions. The paralysis appears over the course of a few hours and usually disappear after a few weeks.

Causes

Facial paralysis is often a secondary symptom of infections, e.g., Lyme disease (see p. 223).

Sometimes facial paralysis occurs as a result of an ear operation in which nerves were inadvertently damaged.

In idiopathic Bell's palsy, one of the facial nerves becomes swollen, often for unknown reasons.

Who's at Risk

Those undergoing ear operations are at increased risk.

Possible Aftereffects and Complications

In some people the paralysis dissipates after 4 to 6 weeks; in others it may take several months. Only rarely is it permanent.

Facial paralysis may be disfiguring. The patient needs compassion and understanding in order to be able to heal without suffering psychological damage as well.

When the eyelid muscle is affected, the eye cannot close completely during sleep, causing the cornea and conjunctiva to dry out. This may result in corneal damage.

Prevention

Not possible.

When to Seek Medical Advice

Seek help if facial paralysis appears.

Self-Help

Nothing can be done for the paralysis. If the eyelid cannot close, artificial tears (see Eyestrain, p. 228) can help keep the cornea moist; the eye may have to be taped shut at night.

Treatment

If idiopathic Bell's palsy is suspected, a short burst of high-dose corticosteroids (see p. 665) may be beneficial. If Lyme disease is suspected, treatment should be with antibiotics, in addition to corticosteroids (see Lyme disease, p. 223). Surgeons may try to repair damaged nerves by transplanting healthy ones.

EYES

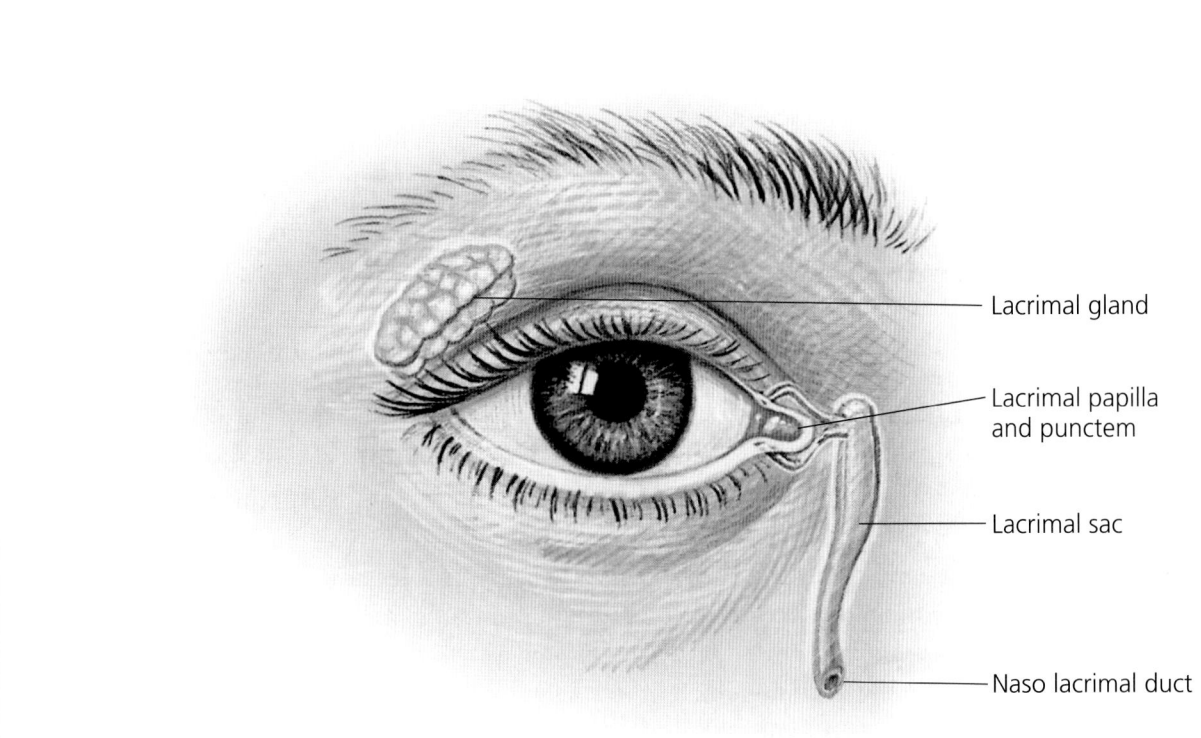

Lacrimal gland

Lacrimal papilla and punctem

Lacrimal sac

Naso lacrimal duct

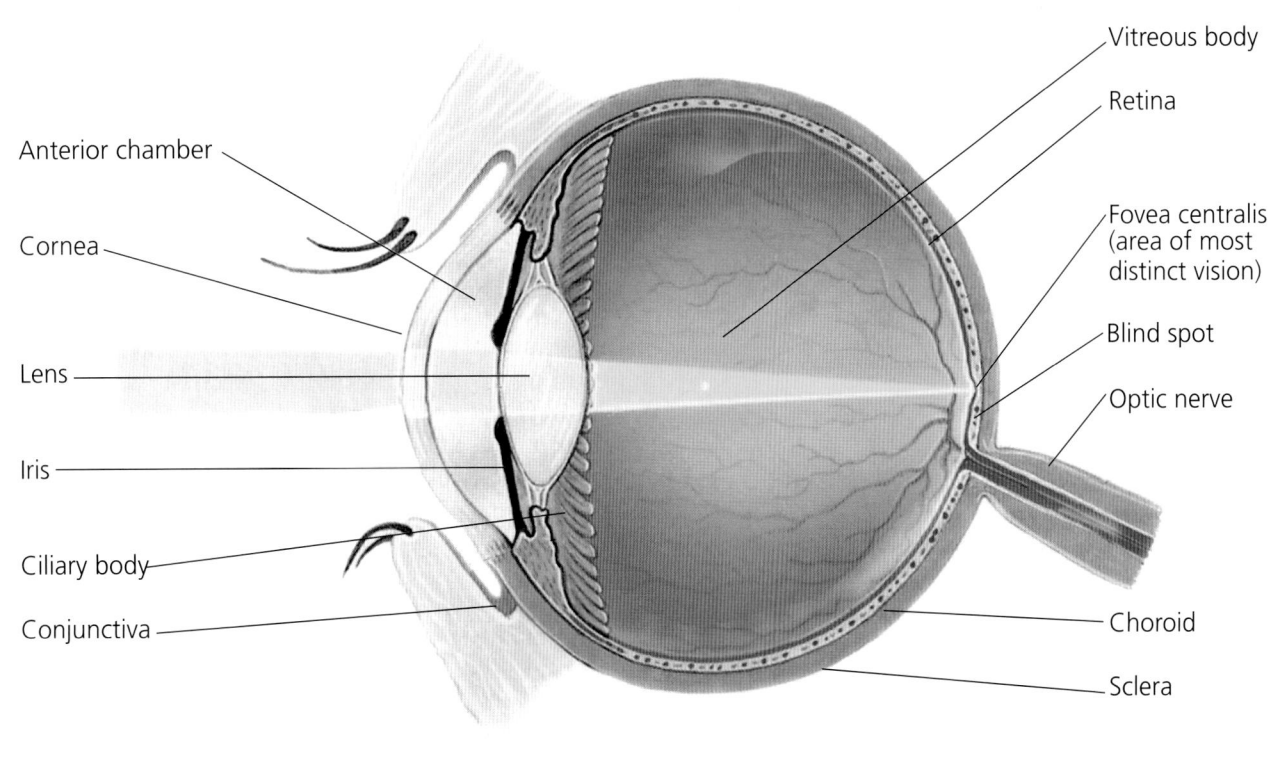

Anterior chamber

Cornea

Lens

Iris

Ciliary body

Conjunctiva

Vitreous body

Retina

Fovea centralis (area of most distinct vision)

Blind spot

Optic nerve

Choroid

Sclera

The eyes have been called the mirrors of the soul; they serve as our windows on the world. The sense of sight intertwines with all human activities, and the eye is constantly working in harmony with the whole person.

The eye can turn in every direction, thanks to six muscles in the socket that give it mobility. Every time we blink, the eyelid ensures the even distribution of tears from the tear ducts. The conjunctiva, the delicate membrane lining the eyelids and eyeball, protects the eye from germs. It has three layers: The hard sclera, with an opening into which the transparent cornea fits like a watch crystal; the choroid; and the retina, extending from the rear of the eyeball around the iris. At the center of the iris is the opening known as the pupil, and behind this sits the lens.

Two fluid-filled chambers regulate the eye's internal pressure and maintain its form. The ciliary muscle changes the lens shape so that incoming rays of light are refracted into a sharp image on the retina; the visual cells transmit the image—in shades of gray if light levels are low, in bright color by daylight—through the optic nerve to the brain. Here the images from both eyes are coordinated into one visual impression.

The amount of light received by the retina also determines our circadian rhythms and influences our moods.

EYE STRAIN

The eyes are always primed for maximum performance without recharging; however, their capacities are temporarily diminished under stress and exhaustion.

Good lighting is a prerequisite for good vision, especially when reading or doing detailed work, for the eyes compensate for insufficient visual contrast by the process known as accommodation, which can result in eye fatigue over time. The need for light increases with age. Regardless of the type of work you do, the best lighting is a steady, nonflickering source behind you, illuminating your work. When watching television or working at a computer, make sure lighting is not reflected in the screen or shining into the eyes (see Health in the Workplace, p. 789).

Self-Help for Tired Eyes
— Have eyes checked regularly; have faulty vision corrected.
— If eyes are tired and burn or smart, and vision is diminished, relaxation (see p. 693) can help: Lie down for 15 minutes, covering closed eyes gently with palms or a warm compress.
— People who wear glasses may find it relaxing to remove them when reading (unless they have presbyopia).
— Focus your gaze on a distant point for a few minutes.
— Using fingertips, gently massage forehead, cheeks, temples, and eyebrows, applying pressure at bridge of nose.

Self-Help for Dry Eyes
Overheated rooms, tobacco smoke, perfumes, and aerosol sprays can cause itchy, stinging, and painful eyes. Ozone from smog, laser printers, and copiers may thin the eye's lacrimal fluid. Car fans and air conditioners scatter dust and bacteria. The result is a drying of the lacrimal fluid that bathes the eyes.
— Turn off ventilation if possible.
— Make sure air is sufficiently moist. During heating season, damp cloths hung around the room are helpful. Avoid electric humidifiers.
— Take breaks during work and blink more frequently.
— "Artificial tears" and eyedrops can help, but if they contain preservatives, they may irritate eyes over time.
— Do not rinse eyes with teas. This can worsen irritation and invite infections.
— Do not use vasoconstricting drugs; they only dry eyes further and make complaints worse.

Self-Help for Foreign Object in Eye
Dust particles and small objects are usually flushed out by tears; you can help by running clear water over the eye and wiping the object towards the inside corner of the eye. If this does not seem to help and the eye hurts, the cornea is probably injured: See an eye doctor (see Corneal Ulcers, p. 242).

The following artificial tears are effective with short-term use:
Liquifilm
Tears Plus
Tears Naturale
Lacrilube

Self-Help for a Black Eye

A black eye can be soothed by cold compresses (see Cold Treatments, p. 685). Taking vitamin C and papaya can help speed the healing process. If pain lasts beyond a reasonable time, see an eye doctor. Contusions can severely damage the inner eye.

FAULTY VISION

Faulty vision is not an illness. Deviations of up to 3 diopters (the units in which eyesight is measured) are normal. Farsightedness is more common than nearsightedness; presbyopia, a form of farsightedness, affects everyone in their forties, and eye disorders also become more common at this age, so it is wise to have your eyes checked every year or two once you reach 40.

One out of every 10 adults lacks spatial perception, due to partial or total vision loss in one eye as a result of undiagnosed eye disorders in early childhood. This could be averted by preventative care including early eye and vision examinations for children.

Indications of Faulty Vision

A child complains of headaches, dizziness, and tiredness when looking at things close up. One of his or her eyes may turn in a little, the child blinks, and often squeezes his or her eyes shut; tilts his or her head when looking at something, stumbles and bumps into things, reaches next to what he or she wants, rubs his or her eyes, and has trouble staying on the line he or she is trying to follow with a pencil.

What Accounts for Variations in Vision

The eye delivers sharp images when its refractive power and axis length (distance from cornea to retina) are in correct relationship. Refractive power is the eye's ability to focus incoming light rays; it is measured in diopters. One diopter corresponds to the refractive power of a lens focusing light at a distance of 1 meter. The eye adjusts its refractive power according to the distance of an object by the process of accommodation: When the object moves closer the pupil contracts, and the curvature of the lens increases. In dim light or at a greater distance, the pupil widens and the lens curvature lessens.

When the eye's axis length and refractive power are not in correct relationship, the focused light rays will not fall exactly onto the retina. If the focused image is in front of the retina, we are nearsighted, and distant objects appear blurry. If the focused image is behind the retina, we are farsighted.

FARSIGHTED VISION (HYPEROPIA)

Complaints

Things at a distance are seen clearly, but close up they appear out of focus.

Causes

Usually, farsighted persons are born with "short" eyeballs, causing the image to appear behind the retina, not on it. Depending on the individual, this defect may correct itself.

Who's at Risk

About 55 percent of the population is farsighted, but corrective glasses are not necessary in all cases.

Possible Aftereffects and Complications

Young eyes can compensate for farsightedness, but this places a strain on the lens muscle which can quickly lead to tiredness, headaches, eye pain, and temporary inward turning eye(s) (strabismus). If corrective glasses are not worn in time, strabismus may persist throughout life. As a result, one eye may lose strength of vision. People with farsightedness frequently develop glaucoma (see p. 244) in old age.

Prevention

Preventive measures include early examinations by an ophthalmologist, and glasses or contact lenses when indicated.

When to Seek Medical Advice

Seek help as soon as inward turning of eye(s) is noticed, or the abovementioned symptoms appear. Early diagnosis is especially important in children.

Self-Help

Not possible.

Treatment

An eye doctor can recommend glasses with convex lenses (see Glasses, p. 235), which make objects appear bigger and closer, but tend to flatten space. Contact lenses (see p. 236) may also be used for farsightedness, although they do not affect its development.

NEARSIGHTED VISION (MYOPIA)

Complaints
Nearsighted people can see clearly up to 15 feet in front of them; beyond that, they see a blur.

Causes
In nearsightedness the image falls in front of the retina instead of on it, usually because the eyeball is too long, occasionally because the cornea and lens are excessively curved.

There are two types of nearsightedness. In "students' myopia" nearsightedness increases among young people up to age 25 and stays under - 6 diopters. The second type is genetic degenerative nearsightedness, which occurs only rarely, and involves the continuous lengthening of the eyeball with the passing of years.

Who's at Risk
Nearsightedness may temporarily increase in the presence of physical or psychological stress, insufficient lighting, or unfavorable working conditions. It may also appear temporarily when caused by medications such as sulfonamides or acetazolamide, contusions, or high blood-sugar levels. Hormonal changes during pregnancy can also permanently worsen nearsightedness.

The gradual clouding of the lens associated with aging can cause nearsightedness. Farsighted people may temporarily be able to read without glasses again as this form of nearsightedness progresses.

Possible Aftereffects and Complications
Nearsighted people often don't see well in the dark (night blindness) and should avoid driving at night. Because in nearsighted individuals the eyeball's shape is long, the retina is stretched, and retinal defects become more common in the range between 6 and 8 diopters. In genetic nearsightedness, retinal detachment and bleeding may impair vision if not treated promptly.

Prevention
Avoid working at night and in artificially lighted rooms.
— Always make sure your workplace is adequately lighted.

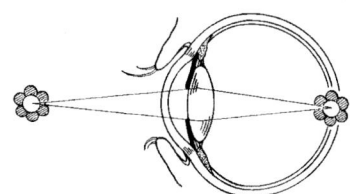

Normal vision

Light rays meet on the retina.
The image is clear

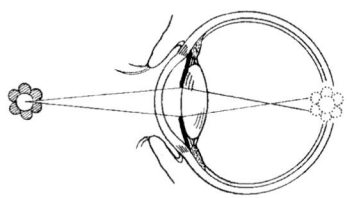

Near sightedness

Light rays meet in front of the retina.
The image is unfocused.

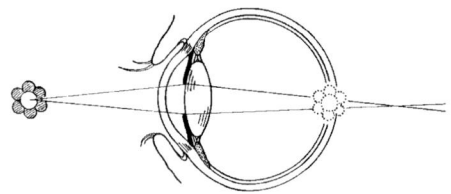

Far sightedness

Light rays meet behind the retina.
The image is unfocused.

— Keep your eyes at a proper distance from your work: for reading, 14 to 16 inches; for computer monitors, 20 inches (see Health in the Workplace/Computer Screens, p. 790).
— Avoid straining your eyes with too much detailed work. When your eyes are tired, take a break.
— Very nearsighted people should not do hard physical work: Vitreous hemorrhages could result.

Most nearsighted people are light-sensitive and should wear sunglasses outdoors. Indoor glasses should be only slightly tinted, if at all.

When to Seek Medical Advice

Seek help if you find it necessary to squint in order to see clearly at a distance. Nearsighted children are often unaware of their problem. Regular visits to the eye doctor will help in early detection of changes in the retina, assisted by a biomicroscopy of the retina and choroid. This procedure is relatively uncommon.

Self-Help

Up to about 0.75 diopters of nearsightedness, many people don't bother wearing glasses, even though they can't see clearly at a distance. When driving a car, however, optimal vision is a requirement, both for one's own safety and that of others.

Physical and mental relaxation takes the pressure off the eyes and may alleviate nearsightedness; breathing exercises (see p. 693) and muscle relaxation (see p. 693) are especially effective.

Treatment

Nearsightedness is corrected by glasses with concave lenses (see Glasses, p. 235): Objects appear smaller, space has more depth, and the floor looks closer than it is. When seen through the outer rim of the lens, straight lines appear curved—increasingly so, the greater the nearsightedness. The brain learns to correct this distortion. However, if you switch to larger or stronger glasses or contact lenses, the brain needs time to adjust, and a distorted image, headaches, and/or dizziness may persist for a few days until this occurs.

Wearers of contact lenses do not experience such peripheral distortion.

SURGERY
Radial Keratotomy

Radial incisions in the cornea can correct nearsightedness of up to - 6 diopters in 90 percent of all cases, although visual clarity may vary. Light-sensitivity and scarring may result from this surgery.

Laser Surgery

Photorefractive keratectomy (PRK) reshapes the cornea through use of a laser. Most often used to correct nearsightedness, it is sometimes used to treat farsightedness and astigmatism, as well. Though many are happy with the results, complications may include infection, under- or overcorrection, slow healing, and the development of astigmatism. Laser in situ keratomileusis (LASIK) is a similar, more recent procedure that slices the cornea from the side and reshapes the tissue of the inner layer of the cornea.

Corneal Transplants

A donated, specifically cut and fashioned, cornea is surgically attached to the cornea. This procedure has been successful in treating extreme nearsightedness, missing lenses, and extremely protruding corneas (keratoconus) with few complications.

ASTIGMATISM

Complaints

In astigmatism, vision is distorted as it is underwater; a single point may appear as a distorted line. Astigmatism often accompanies near- and farsightedness.

Causes

Astigmatism is a curvature of the cornea and is probably genetic in origin. Changes in the cornea (e.g., scarring following injuries or infections) may develop into astigmatism.

Who's at Risk

Astigmatism resulting from injuries, infections, or ulcers may deteriorate further.

Possible Aftereffects and Complications

If the defect is not corrected, eyes may hurt and redden when doing detailed work.

Prevention

Not possible.

When to Seek Medical Advice

Seek help when symptoms appear.

Self-Help

Usually not possible. Only rarely do specific relaxation techniques (see p. 693) alleviate astigmatism.

Treatment

Glasses with specifically cut lenses can correct for astigmatism. If near- or farsightedness are also present, glasses need to balance both conditions.

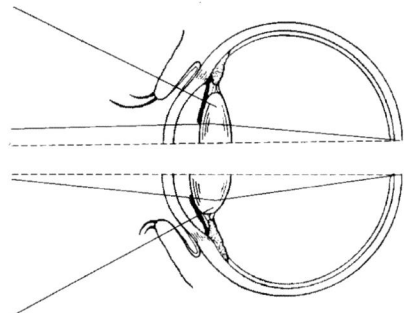

Accommodation of the Lens

The lens is relaxed when looking into the distance, it stretches, the power of refraction is decreased.

The lens contracts when looking at close objects, it curves, and refraction increases.

Hard contact lenses (see p. 236) are especially effective in correcting for astigmatism.

Severe distortion of the cornea can be corrected with a corneal transplant (see p. 231).

PRESBYOPIA

Complaints
After age 40, closeup vision becomes increasingly blurry.

Causes
The lens of the eye hardens with age, diminishing the eye's ability to adjust its curvature to see well at close range.

Who's at Risk
Presbyopia sets in for everyone in their fifties, as changes in the lens slowly increase.

Possible Aftereffects and Complications
Focusing at close range becomes increasingly difficult, and eyes tire easily when reading or doing closeup work.

Prevention
Not possible.

When to Seek Medical Advice
When focusing up close becomes difficult. After age 40, eyes should be checked annually.

Self-Help
Not possible.

Treatment
Glasses should compensate for the eye's failing ability to accommodate at close distances (e.g., 14 to 16 inches when reading). Those who also need to be able to focus at further distances (e.g. for work) should consider an additional pair of glasses. The more detailed your work, the more precise your prescription needs to be.

Narrow reading glasses (the ones you can look over to see further away) have only a small field of vision. If faulty vision already exists, additional corrections are necessary to adapt for close-range vision.

Presbyopia can occasionally correct for nearsightedness, but only affects close-range vision. The presbyopic requires two different prescriptions: one pair of glasses (or contacts) for long-range vision, one pair for short-range. Because switching back and forth can be a nuisance, bifocals, with both prescriptions ground into a single lens, have become popular.

— If a line separates the two prescriptions, it will distort the image slightly; this requires a few weeks of getting used to.

— The short-range lens may also be seamlessly incorporated into the long-range lens.

Trifocals also exist: they correct for nearsightedness, farsightedness, and an additional in-between zone. The size of the short-range lens area is adjustable according to the wearer's requirements. If the differences between the three prescriptions are not too great, these glasses are easy to get used to. However, they are not indicated for use when driving, because the long-range field of vision is too small.

Multifocals combine several prescriptions into one pair of glasses without dividing lines. Disadvantages include the fact that the mid-range field of vision is very narrow, and beyond the short range, the image appears curved and seems to move when you move your head. Possible reactions include headaches and dizziness to the point of nausea. Multifocals are expensive, and because presbyopia is progressive, you will need new glasses about every two years.

Multifocals are indicated if
— Presbyopia is not yet pronounced.
— They correct defective vision.
— They are worn constantly.
    Multifocals are not indicated if:
— You require optimal clarity in mid-range vision, and there is a big difference between your short- and long-range vision.
    Multifocals may cause problems if:
— Your work or lifestyle requires constant shifting between visual ranges (e.g., teachers or construction workers)
— You drive.
    In these cases you should either get two separate pairs of glasses, or bifocals.

STRABISMUS (CROSSED-EYES)

Being cross-eyed doesn't only affect our physical attractiveness; it affects vision as well. Even if the deviation from parallel vision is only minimal, sight in both eyes suffers as a result. About 4 percent of the adult population suffers from this condition, which in many cases could have been corrected by early intervention.

Strabismus is the most common childhood vision disorder and should be treated as soon as possible. There are various forms of strabismus:
— The eyes may deviate horizontally, either inward or outward. In rare cases they may deviate vertically.
— The angle of deviation may be constant; one eye is either always leading, or they alternate.
— One eye may only occasionally deviate while the other focuses ("wandering eye").

PHORIA (MILD FORM OF STRABISMUS)

Complaints
In this disorder, the eyes occasionally deviate from their normal positions; this becomes noticeable only when one eye is covered. Results may include so-called asthenopic symptoms: Burning or easily tired eyes, difficulty focusing, sensitivity to glare, double vision, eyelid infections, and headaches.

Causes
The eye muscles are not synchronized, so they neither work nor rest at the same time. One eye deviates from the line of sight (usually outward). This condition begins in childhood.

Who's at Risk
Tiredness, illness or the influence of alcohol tend to make hitherto unnoticed phoria apparent.

Possible Aftereffects and Complications
Phoria may develop into permanent strabismus.

Prevention
Avoid alcohol and stress.

When to Seek Medical Advice
As soon as the condition is noticed. Often parents and doctors don't notice phoria or take it seriously, but it should be checked for during all eye examinations, particularly when reading problems exist.

Self-Help
Try this focusing exercise: With outstretched hand, move your index finger in toward the eyes and focus on it as long as possible. Repeat this several times; then close your eyes and relax.

Treatment
Eye training (see p. 234) may remedy phoria in children. Only if eye exercises do not help should prismatic glasses be introduced; ground glasses are better than laminated ones. This treatment is also possible for adults.

PERMANENT STRABISMUS

Occasional instances of cross-eyedness in children is seldom noticed, yet it may lead to permanent strabismus.

Complaints
The condition becomes obvious and pronounced, and spatial perception is impaired.

Causes
— Heredity, or a possible consequence of measles, pertussis, or scarlet fever, among other diseases
— Farsightedness
— Asymmetrical refractory error
— Psychological crises
— Tumors, concussions

— Eye-muscle weakness or paralysis
— Total or partial misalignment of the optic tract
— Injury; clouding of one lens

Who's at Risk

Faulty eyesight should be treated early so permanent strabismus will not develop.

Possible Aftereffects and Complications

The fixed eye may remain permanently weaker even though it is not defective, or the patient may alternate which eye is doing the seeing, in which case vision stays intact in both eyes.

In both cases, depth perception is affected and the risk of losing the good eye in an accident is increased threefold.

Prevention

Preventive measures include regular eye checkups for early detection.

When to Seek Medical Advice

Seek help as soon as the condition is noticed.

Children up to age 5 should be given a "shadow test," which involves putting a 0.5 percent atropine solution into the eyes twice a day for 4 days to numb the lens muscle and disrupt the process of visual accommodation. This allows the doctor to determine whether vision is faulty and whether one eye is in danger of becoming weak (see p. 233).

Self-Help

Not possible.

Treatment for Children

Specialized eye clinics are recommended for treatment. Have your specialist describe the treatment in detail. It should concentrate on strengthening the weak eye, programming the retina correctly, and correcting the short- and long-range line of vision for each eye.

One in three children with permanent strabismus requires two to three operations to correct the condition. Sometimes follow-up treatment is necessary; the child, parents, and professionals must work together patiently to ensure optimal results. Usually these efforts pay off and the corrections are permanent; sometimes

depth perception remains defective.

Treatment by Glasses and Occlusion

When early farsightedness is the cause of strabismus, treatment begins with the prescription of glasses. This is feasible even in the first year of life: The child needs to wear the glasses all the time, except when sleeping. Success is possible only when this is implemented consistently.

This is followed by occlusion treatments, in which the eyes are covered alternately, with the dominant eye covered longer than the other one. This is done either by
— bandaging the eye, or
— taping over one lens of the glasses, or
— dilating the pupil with eyedrops

Occlusion treatments may take months or years and the doctor's instructions should be followed strictly. Do not be discouraged if the strabismus reappears together with improved eyesight; this can be corrected with additional treatment.

Eye training should be done by a specialist. Currently, the most promising treatment is based on stimulation of the weak or "lazy" eye. The good eye is taped over, and the patient learns to follow the movements of the specialist with the weaker eye, thus training and strengthening its muscles. This training may be necessary before or after surgery.

Surgical Treatment

Nearly one in two children with strabismus requires surgery to correct the outer eye muscles. This entails either a shortening of the muscles, or realignment so they are as straight as possible. Depending on the disorder and preceding treatments, this operation may have to be performed several times.

Congenital strabismus, pronounced strabismus, eye tremors, and strabismus involving cocking of the head are treated surgically as early as age 2; otherwise surgical treatment is done at age 5. One-sided strabismus must first be changed into alternating strabismus. If strabismus appears later it should be operated on as soon as possible.

Treatment for Adults

Contact lenses improve depth perception.

Surgery for strabismus usually serves a purely cosmetic purpose in adults. The patient risks developing double vision, or retaining non-parallel vision. Consult an experienced specialist before embarking on this course. If you have worn prismatic lenses and experienced double vision as a result, you should not undergo this operation: Chances for success are slim.

AMBLYOPIA

Complaints
In this disorder one eye is weaker than the other, although this is barely recognizable.

Causes
Weakness in one eye is probably caused by an undetected childhood developmental disorder. The following conditions may trigger the symptoms: Eyelid disease, strabismus, clouding of the lens, farsightedness, eye tremors, disorders of the visual centers, inherited or acquired disorders of the optic tract, or extended atropine treatment.

Who's at Risk
Weak vision in one eye occurs in about 10 percent of the population below the age of eight. If the aforementioned conditions are not ruled out, the risk increases.

Possible Aftereffects and Complications
Weak vision in one eye disqualifies the patient from all jobs requiring depth perception—for instance, working with intricate mechanisms or rapidly rotating machinery, piloting a plane or locomotive, or performing surgery. This condition also causes the risk of losing the good eye in an accident to increase threefold.

Prevention
Prevention requires regular eye exams from age 3 on. Children's eyes should be checked periodically, but especially in the event of crossed eyes, or if the child starts to stumble and reach next to (not directly for) an object. A simple diagnostic test (Lang) is available.

Treatment
Specific eye exercises may help (see p. 234).

NIGHT BLINDNESS

Complaints
If there is difficulty in adjusting visually to dark conditions, night blindness is diagnosed, even if shapes remain identifiable.

Causes
Severe night blindness can be hereditary. It may also occur in connection with nearsightedness, vitamin A deficiency, as a side effect of jaundice, with age, and when a light-refracting part of the eye is clouded.

Possible Aftereffects and Complications
These include lack of confidence when moving around in the dark, and increased danger and risk of accident when driving at night.

Prevention
Prevention is possible only if the cause of the night blindness is vitamin A deficiency (see Vitamin A, p. 740).

When to Seek Medical Advice
Seek help as soon as you notice symptoms.

Self-Help
Not possible. Be extremely careful when driving at night.

Treatment
Treatment is possible only if the cause is vitamin A deficiency.

GLASSES
Prescriptions for new glasses should preferably be written in conjunction with a complete eye examination, which can reveal the early stages of eye diseases and disorders, especially after age 40. However, opticians can also take the necessary measurements for fitting glasses.

The quality of materials used for frames and glasses is standardized. When buying inexpensive glasses, it is important to establish whether they conform to the industry standard. Glasses from a cut-rate supplier should not be used even as spares, since they may not be properly adjusted either to your eyes or your head shape.

Frames

Frames should fit well and not obstruct the field of vision.

Metal frames last longer than plastic ones, but when metal allergies (e.g., nickel allergy) are involved, plastic frames should be used instead.

Farsighted individuals with high-diopter prescriptions should opt for a lighter frame for easier-to-wear glasses.

Nearsighted individuals with high-diopter prescriptions should go with a thicker frame, so the thicker lenses won't be as noticeable. Smaller frames have the advantage of minimizing distortions at the edge of the field of vision, reducing the appearance of thickness, and weighing less.

Lens Materials
Glass

Glass makes for heavy, thick lenses in cases of severe nearsightedness, and puts a lot of pressure on the nose. Special high-refraction lenses are thinner, but also significantly more expensive.

Synthetics

With synthetic lenses the injury rate from breakage is low. They are also much lighter than glass, but can be very thick in cases of extreme nearsightedness. They scratch easily, which may interfere with good vision. Some high-refraction synthetic lenses are coated with quartz to increase durability and wear.

Glare-Resistant Glasses

Both glass and synthetic glasses can be tinted to various degrees to reduce glare, enhance perception of contrasts, and improve vision under poor light conditions.

Sunglasses

Eye damage from ultraviolet (UV) rays is on the rise. To protect the lens and retina, it is advisable to wear sunglasses when your eyes are exposed to the sun, especially:
— For children under age 2
— In the presence of bright, glaring light from snow, water or sand—e.g., when skiing, surfing, sailing, or on safari—and on car and plane trips
— If you have corneal scarring or a clouded or missing lens

Tips for People with Glasses
Because glasses scratch easily, especially synthetic ones, you should
— Always keep glasses in a large case.
— Never set glasses with lenses face down.
— Clean them with soap and warm water (or have an optician do a general cleaning) .
— Keep a second pair of glasses on hand when you're driving, when you're playing sports, or if you're very nearsighted.

Make sure any sunglasses you purchase carry a guarantee that the product filters out UV rays. It is also advisable to buy glasses that do not distort color values; they should be tinted brown, a 65 percent tint for normal use, a 100 percent tint for use under extreme conditions. How dark your glasses are has nothing to do with their degree of UV protection; to be on the safe side, have your optician measure their UV-filtering capacity.

If you choose sunglasses with changeable lenses, keep in mind that when you're driving at night, the glasses shouldn't be filtering out more than 15 percent of the light hitting them. These type of glasses darken in the presence of UV rays. If you wear them constantly, they should not be highly glare-resistant or tinted more than 10-15 percent. They are not recommended for indoor use, especially if the wearer is nearsighted.

CONTACT LENSES

Unlike eyeglasses, contact lenses don't break when in place, fog up, put pressure on the nose, feel bulky, get in the way, or distort or limit the field of vision. They are nevertheless a foreign object in the eye, and the following precautions should be taken:
— The contacts and cleaning solution should not irritate the eyes.
— Lacrimal fluid should be sufficient to keep the contacts moist.

Do not use contacts if you have chronic eye illnesses, nasolacrimal duct (tear duct) illnesses, corneal infections or ulcers, allergies or dry eyes. Sometimes older people need to start using contact lenses following cataract surgery.

Lens Materials

Contact lenses come in various types:

— Hard, nongas-permeable
— Stable, slightly gas-permeable
— Flexible, highly gas-permeable
— Soft, water retaining
— Soft, highly water absorbable

As a general rule, the harder the lens, the smaller it is, the more alien it feels to the eye, and the longer it takes for the eye to get used to it. The softer the lens, the larger it is, and the more easily the eye adjusts to it. The choice of lens material depends on individual prescriptions, needs, and preferences.

Hard Lenses

Hard lenses are relatively inexpensive and last a long time. During the initial adjustment phase they are worn only a few hours a day, with the length of time gradually increasing. If this adjustment period is interrupted, it needs to be started over. Changing from contact lenses to glasses also involves an adjustment period: Things will look a bit blurry at first.

Gas-Permeable Lenses

Permeable lenses are easy to tolerate because they "breathe," allowing oxygen to reach the cornea. Although more expensive than hard lenses, they are more comfortable. They last about 2 years.

Soft Lenses

These are made of a water-based synthetic that adjusts itself to the eyeball shape. After a short adaptation period, they can be worn all day long. These lenses must be cleaned carefully to avoid damage to the conjunctiva and cornea. They must also be replaced yearly. After years of using soft lenses, the wearer runs a higher risk of eye damage than with hard lenses.

Extended-Wear and Disposable Lenses

Permanent lenses can be worn constantly, day and night. They are recommended only for those born without a lens in an eye, for older people following cataract surgery, or for disabled patients. They must be checked, fitted and cleaned every 3 to 4 weeks.

Wearing disposable lenses increases the risk of corneal ulcers by a factor of 14 and may also damage eyesight.

Contact Lens Tips

— Put on your contacts half an hour after getting up in the morning.
— Always wash your hands before handling lenses.
— Handle each lens separately so as not to mix the two lenses up.
— Take good, regular care of your lenses.
— Never sleep with lenses on (except permanent lenses); give the cornea much-needed rest.
— Always carry the contact lens case and a pair of glasses with you (on trips, take along a complete care kit).
— Use water-soluble cosmetics. Always spray lenses before putting them on.
— Dried-out soft lenses can be put into dishwashing liquid to soften (careful, they break easily!). Disinfect before using.
— When a lens slips under the upper eyelid, lift eyelid and pull down lens with a finger. Don't worry, the conjunctiva prevents the lens from ever sliding behind the eyeball.
— Wear protective glasses when playing ball sports. Swim without lenses if possible: The soft ones may absorb chlorine, and the hard ones get lost easily.
Important: Take out lenses before using eyedrops and before any eye operation.
Important: If you experience stinging, itching, mucus, red eyes, worsening vision, or pain, remove lenses immediately (use eyedrops to facilitate this, if necessary) and make an appointment with your eye doctor.

Tinted Contact Lenses

Because tinted lenses restrict the amount of available light, they may pose a hazard at twilight and when driving.

Lens Fitting

Contact lenses are fitted by eye doctors and opticians who have undergone special training. The fitters take detailed information on lifestyle, work situations, possible allergies, current medications, and eye problems. After a thorough examination the appropriate lenses are selected, tried, and checked until they fit perfectly. During the fitting, the wearer learns how to care for the lenses, for how long to wear them, and what to do when problems arise. The price of contact lenses usually covers cleaning and care materials and check-ups for the first 6 months. Usually contact lenses come with a free 3-month trial period.

Lens Care

Care and cleaning supplies, including a storage case with a fluid well, are usually provided at your fitting. For soft lenses a storage solution and protein remover may be provided as well.

Never mix products from different manufacturers.

Additives may cause problems: Use the preservative-free kind available in single-dose packets.

Lenses should be taken out and cleaned daily. This is done by rubbing with cleaning solution, rinsing thoroughly, and then disinfecting in the storage solution to kill off any bacteria, viruses, and fungi.

If wearing your contact lenses becomes a problem, have your eyes as well as your contacts checked. Other possible problems may involve
— Aging of lenses.
— Incompatibe cleaning solutions (eyes may redden and sting).
— Illness, pregnancy, stress (all can change the lacrimal fluid. Short-term use of artificial tears may be helpful—see p. 228).
— Smog, cigarette smoke, and air conditioners (gas-permeable lenses are more appropriate in dry, dusty environments and for concentrated work, e.g., at a computer monitor).
— Gaseous substance absorption by soft lenses.
— Medications: Diuretics, hormones, and drugs for allergies, depression, and high blood pressure can all change the lacrimal fluid.

Eye Disorders

STYES

Complaints
A stye is an inflamed, swollen, pus-filled, very painful lump on the eyelid with a reddened conjunctiva.

Causes
Styes are caused by an infection of the sweat gland on the edge or inside of the eyelid by pus-forming bacteria.

Who's at Risk
Styes recur in people with weakened immune systems, chronic eyelid infections, or poor hygiene.

Prevention
Wash hands before and after touching eyes.

When to Seek Medical Advice
Seek advice if symptoms do not clear in 5 to 8 days.

Self-Help
Warmth is good for styes: Expose the closed eye to a heat lamp or a warm compress for as long as it's comfortable. Repeat several times.

Treatment
A health-care provider may lance the stye and prescribe an antibiotic salve.

CHALAZION (TARSAL CYST, CYST OF THE EYELID)

Complaints
A *chalazion* is a small, painless lump that develops on the eyelid and often lasts for weeks. Typically, the skin over the lump can be moved easily, which differentiates a chalazion from potentially malignant mass.

Causes
Chalazions are caused by secretions of the oil (sebaceous) glands of the skin.

Who's at Risk
Those with secretory disorders are at higher risk for developing chalazions.

Possible Aftereffects and Complications
Chalazions can become infected, causing the eyelid to swell painfully.

Prevention
Not possible.

When to Seek Medical Advice
Seek help if painful inflammation on the eyelid develops.

Self-Help
Small chalazions usually disappear after a few weeks. You can speed up the process by gently massaging the eyelid.

Treatment

Larger chalazions may require surgical removal on an outpatient basis.

EYELID INFLAMMATION (BLEPHARITIS)

Complaints

In this disorder, the eyelids are red and they itch and sting. Scales form between the eyelashes; the lashes may fall out. Pus and scabs form and may feel like a foreign object in the eye. During sleep the eyelids are stuck together by dried secretions.

Causes

Causes may include irritation due to smoke, dust, cosmetics (e.g., eye shadow), air conditioning, or a bacterial infection.

Who's at Risk

Those exposed to the abovementioned irritants are at increased risk.

Possible Aftereffects and Complications

Eyelid inflammations may recur indefinitely.

Prevention

Avoid the irritants listed above. If you wear glasses, have the prescription strength checked regularly.

When to Seek Medical Advice

Seek help if symptoms persist longer than a few days.

Self-Help

Discomfort can be alleviated by a cold compress.

Treatment

Eyelid inflammations may be tenacious; usually only antibiotic salves will clear up the problem. Before treatment, however, the inflammation should be checked for the presence of bacteria. General antibiotic use tends to lead increasingly to corneal fungal infections.

Treatment lasts 1 to 2 weeks. If long-term corticosteroid (see p. 665) use is included in treatment, the internal pressure of the eyeball must first be checked.

EYELID TUMORS (BENIGN AND MALIGNANT)

(See also Cancer, p. 470.)
A variety of benign growths—fatty tumors, blood vessel growths, chalazions, or warts—may appear on the eyelid; malignant tumors may also develop.

Complaints

Usually there are no complaints.

Causes

The causes of cancers of the eyelid are unknown. They may be triggered by various tissue growths, or chronic inflammations of the sebaceous glands.

Who's at Risk

Flattened tumors with rough edges (basal cell tumors), usually appearing in the inner corner of the eye, are relatively rare.

Possible Aftereffects and Complications

Basal cell tumors rarely metastasize. Early diagnosis of eyelid cancer can lead to surgery and 100 percent recovery. If untreated the cancer may spread into the eye socket and jeopardize vision.

Prevention

Not possible.

When to Seek Medical Advice

See a dermatologist or eye doctor immediately if wartlike growths or crusty tumors appear. Often eyelid cancer begins with recurring crusts or scales on the eyelid.

Self-Help

Not possible.

Treatment

Small benign tumors often disappear on their own after a few months. If not, they can be removed surgically, usually on an outpatient basis, often without anesthesia.

ENTROPION AND ECTROPION

Complaints

An *entropion* is an inward curling of the eyelid in which the lashes rub against, and irritate, the conjunctiva and cornea. An *ectropion* is an outwardly turned eyelid, in which the conjunctiva, cornea and inside of the lid dry out, causing pain.

Causes

With advancing age, the eyelid tissues slacken. Ectropions may arise as a complication of cosmetic surgery.

Who's at Risk

The risk of developing these disorders increases with age.

Possible Aftereffects and Complications

The dry eyes and constant irritation associated with these disorders may cause conjunctival and corneal diseases.

Prevention

No prevention is possible.

When to Seek Medical Advice

Seek help if the symptoms cause distress.

Self-Help

Rinsing the eye with water or artificial tears (see p. 228) may ease irritation.

Treatment

The condition can be corrected with a minor, relatively painless operation, usually done on an outpatient basis with local anesthesia.

NASOLACRIMAL DUCT OBSTRUCTION (BLOCKED TEAR DUCT)

Complaints

In children: Eyes tear up continuously.
In adults: Often there are no complaints; occasionally poor eyesight or pain.

Causes

The tear ducts or their openings may become blocked following chronic colds or a conjunctival infection. Or they may be blocked from birth.

Who's at Risk

This disorder is relatively common in newborn babies.

Possible Aftereffects and Complications

If the tear ducts remain blocked, the lacrimal sac may become infected and swollen, and a dangerous ulcer may develop on the cornea.

Prevention

Not possible.

When to Seek Medical Advice

Seek help if the above symptoms appear.

Self-Help

A congenital blockage often clears up by itself, up to the age of 6 months. This may be stimulated by massaging the tear duct toward its opening.

Treatment

An eye doctor should probe and rinse out the tear duct. This can be done under brief local anesthesia at an eye clinic, followed by a few days' regimen of eyedrops to reduce swelling of the mucous membrane.

CONJUNCTIVITIS

Complaints

In conjunctivitis, the conjunctiva gets red, swollen, occasionally itchy and painful, and produces secretions so that the eye is sealed shut when awakening in the morning.

Causes

— Allergic reactions (see Allergies, p. 360), e.g., to pollen or eye makeup.
— Stress due to irritating gases (e.g.: ozone, fumes from dry cleaning and other solvents, tobacco smoke), especially in conjunction with use of contact lenses.
— Irritation from a foreign object or ultraviolet rays (even in a tanning salon).
— Bacterial infection, characterized by the secretion of mucus or pus, usually affecting both eyes.
— Chlamydia infection (see p. 546), transmitted by

contact to the eye.

—Viral infection, characterized by pus-filled, watery secretions, usually affecting one eye first and the other after a few days. In the event of epidemics involving the whole family, school class, etc., additional symptoms include headaches, exhaustion, and swollen glands in the jaw area.

Who's at Risk
Conjunctivitis is the most common eye illness. The risk of infection is increased by the use of eye makeup, dirty towels, or swimming pools with insufficient hygiene; by rubbing the affected eye with dirty fingers; or by sunbathing without sunglasses, including using a tanning salon.

Possible Aftereffects and Complications
The infection may spread to other areas of the eye, notably the cornea and sclera. Sometimes allergic conjunctivitis may develop into hay fever or asthma.

Prevention
Avoid the above risk factors.

When to Seek Medical Advice
Seek help if symptoms persist for more than 3 days.

Self-Help
Because of the risk of further infection, don't use "eye baths" and be careful to use only your own towel.

Treatment
The cause of infection should be diagnosed by an eye doctor.

Allergic conjunctivitis can be treated with eyedrops containing cromolyn, levocabastine (Livostin), olopatadine (Patanol), naphazoline (Albalon, Vasocon, Naphcon), naphazoline and pheniramine (Naphcon-A) as soon as possible.

Bacterial conjunctivitis can be treated with antibiotic eyedrops and ointments, available by prescription. The widespread, all-purpose use of antibiotics can lead to chronic fungal infections in the eyes. Corticosteroids (see p. 665) should not be prescribed until the cause of the conjunctivitis is determined. In the presence of the herpes simplex virus, the therapeutic use of corticosteroids may cause severe corneal damage.

Viral conjunctivitis (except in the case of herpes simplex virus) will clear up on its own after a few weeks. A short-term course of corticosteroids may be advisable (except with herpes) to decrease the chances of the cornea being affected. Treatment with viral medication may also be tried (e.g., acyclovir [Zovirax]).

KERATITIS (CORNEAL INFLAMMATION)

Complaints
The symptoms of keratitis may almost escape notice: The eye is red and slightly painful, with eyesight somewhat affected.

Causes
Keratitis is frequently caused by irritation due to exposure to ultraviolet light, e.g., while playing outdoor sports, welding, or using a photocopier. In rare instances the inflammation is caused by herpes viruses.

Who's at Risk
Individuals who use corticosteroid preparations inappropriately in the eye area are frequently at high risk for corneal herpes infections.

Possible Aftereffects and Complications
Scars on the cornea may weaken eyesight.

Prevention
Wear protective glasses when exposed to ultraviolet rays over extended periods, or when welding. Avoid looking at the light in the photocopier.

When to Seek Medical Advice
Seek help as soon as possible.

Self-Help
Take time out to relax and rest your eyes.

Treatment
For minor corneal inflammations, cold compresses on the closed eyes are helpful (make sure to use a clean cloth).

For snow blindness and "flash blindness," eyedrops are indicated to decrease mucous membrane swelling, as are local painkillers. During this period the patient's ability to work is reduced.

If the infection is fungal, an antifungal medication should be prescribed.

Viral infections are diagnosed based on the condition of the cornea and should be treated accordingly with an antiviral medication such as acyclovir (Zovirax). Treatment usually takes a long time.

CORNEAL ULCERS

Complaints
Corneal ulcers are usually whitish-grey to greenish-yellow, in the center of the cornea. Eyesight is impaired and severe pain causes cramping of the eyelid. Pus may develop in the eye.

Causes
Ulcers can develop from small corneal abrasions or, less frequently, following a bacterial or viral infection.

They may also develop because the eyelids do not close, because the patient wears soft contact lenses, or because a vitamin A deficiency or a fungus is present.

Who's at Risk
Individuals with scratched or injured corneas, or those who wear contact lenses continuously, are at increased risk.

Possible Aftereffects and Complications
Corneal ulcers always occur in conjunction with a corneal inflammation. Ulcers are one of the most dangerous eye diseases because of the attendant risk of anterior uveitis, softening of the cornea, or glaucoma (see p. 244). Even with continual treatment the eye may be irretrievably damaged.

Prevention
Regular eye examinations for wearers of soft contact lenses.

When to Seek Medical Advice
Immediately, if symptoms arise.

Self-Help
Not possible.

Treatment
Initially, the eye will be treated with antibiotic drops or ointments, often supported by antibiotic injections.

Only if these methods are ineffective will the ulcer be cauterized.

After healing, residual scars can distort vision; this may be improved by the use of contact lenses.

ANTERIOR UVEITIS (IRIDOCYCLITIS—INFLAMMATION OF THE IRIS AND THE CILIARY BODY)

Complaints
With uveitis, the eyeball is very red and mildly painful; eyesight is impaired and the pupil is constricted.

Causes
— Allergies to the blood-borne protein of a bacteria or virus from an infection somewhere else in the body.
— Consequence of a general illness such as rheumatoid inflammation, toxoplasmosis, tuberculosis, or syphilis; or as a consequence of injuries, or of corneal and retinal diseases.

Who's at Risk
Those who have an infection, rheumatism or an eye injury are at increased risk.

Possible Aftereffects and Complications
Pressure inside the eyeball may rise (see Glaucoma, p. 244) as a result of the iris adhering to the lens. Further complications may arise if the ciliary body is affected, including opacity or milkiness of the vitreous body, and pressure fluctuations in the eye, which can endanger eyesight.

Prevention
Not possible.

When to Seek Medical Advice
Seek help immediately if mild eye pain is accompanied by impaired vision.

Self-Help
Not possible.

Treatment
Causes must be diagnosed and treated. Prescription

eyedrops containing atropine are used twice daily to dilate the pupil, preventing the iris from becoming sealed shut and also decreasing the inflammation. Uveitis must often be treated with high doses of corticosteroid medication, orally and/or topically (see p. 665).

CATARACTS

Complaints

A cataract causes a gradual loss of visual clarity over the course of months or years, until things appear foggy. The eye also becomes sensitive to glare.

Causes

— Natural aging of the lens. Cloudiness begins either at the edge or the center of the lens. If only the center is clouded, the patient may be able to read without glasses again for a short time. Surgical intervention is contraindicated.

— Cataracts are occasionally acquired before birth, either by heredity or due to an illness during pregnancy (mumps, measles, German measles, chicken pox, polio, hepatitis). Babies can be operated on in the first year of life.

— Aftereffect of diabetes, tetanus, or neurodermatitis.

— Aftereffect of extended corticosteroid treatment. The cataract will subside after medication is discontinued.

— Elevated levels of UV-B rays in sunlight, due to the hole in the earth's ozone layer.

— Exposure to lightning, fire, or X rays.

— Contusions, injuries, and infections in the eye.

Who's at Risk

The risk increases in persons identified by the above factors.

Possible Aftereffects and Complications

Eyesight may deteriorate until the patient can distinguish only light and dark, but is not completely blind.

Prevention

Prevention is possible only if you avoid the final four factors listed above. Wear sunglasses that filter out UV light (see p. 236, 685) when spending long periods outdoors or when sunbathing, hiking, or engaging in water sports or similar activities. Wear protective glasses if work requires it, and shield your eyes during X rays.

When to Seek Medical Advice

Seek help if symptoms appear.

Self-Help

Make sure your living and working spaces are well lit; do detailed work during daylight hours; choose lamps with shades to protect against glare. Protect eyes with a visor or hat when out in the sun; when reading, place a dark page over the book with a slit cut into it so only a limited portion of the text is visible at a time.

Treatment

Medications are ineffective against cataracts. Surgery should not be considered until the cataract is fully developed. In general, an eye that is still able to read should not be operated on. If you feel your quality of life is being compromised, however, it's time to discuss options with your eye doctor. The best choice may be a synthetic lens replacement.

Cataract Operations

Today, the safest technique for older people is microsurgery usually performed under local anesthesia. The cataract is destroyed by ultrasound, removed, and replaced with a synthetic lens, and the patient can see immediately after the bandage is removed. Usually only a day's hospitalization is necessary. After 3 months all normal duties can usually be resumed; a pair of eyeglasses is necessary for closeup work.

When the operation is performed by an experienced surgeon, complications are rare. Astigmatism sometimes develops from the small scar, but it subsides after a few months when the scab has healed.

Correction of Eyesight

In cases in which synthetic lens replacement is not an option, thick glasses (10 to 20 diopters strong) are necessary after surgical removal of the cataract. Two pairs are required, one for long-range and one for short-range vision.

Objects seen through such glasses appear one third larger, and if the other eye is still seeing normally, this may require a difficult adjustment. Usually in such cases, the operated eye is covered with an opaque lens until an operation on the second eye is necessary, finally making equal vision with both eyes possible.

The operated eye may also be covered with a contact lens, possibly a permanent lens, which lessens the difference in vision between the two eyes, making adjustment easier. In any case, reading glasses will be necessary.

Glasses or contact lenses for the eye missing its lens must contain UV filters to protect the retina.

GLAUCOMA

In glaucoma, the pressure inside the eyeball is increased; normal pressure is from 8 to 30 mmHg. With acute glaucoma, intraocular pressure may be as high as 70 mmHg. The pressure inside the eyeball is independent of blood pressure.

Complaints
Chronic glaucoma can go unnoticed for years. Patients experience occasional blurry vision and headaches, and need new glasses more often. Eventually they notice a loss of vision in the center of the field of vision.

Acute glaucoma affects only one eye and is characterized by sudden pain in the eye and forehead accompanied by nausea, vomiting, shivering, feeling faint, and fever.

Because the relatively minor symptom of a red eye is often overlooked, a common misdiagnosis of epigastric illnesses is made. Eyesight is impaired, light is experienced as blinding, the eye is teary, and the eyeball hard as a rock.

Warning signals of glaucoma are occasional foggy vision, or rainbow rings seen surrounding light sources.

Causes
The pressure inside the eye rises because drainage from the eye's anterior chamber is blocked. This happens with age and may also be a belated consequence of retinal vein thrombosis, an injury or long-term use of corticosteroid medication.

Narrow-angle glaucoma: in some people the iridocorneal angle of the eye is too narrow, leading to symptoms similar to the warning signals of acute glaucoma, followed by pain in the eye and head, frequently at night.

Acute glaucoma attacks are usually triggered by excitement and darkness (e.g., watching a thriller on television), unaccustomed physical stress, drinking large quantities of liquids, or overconsumption of coffee, alcohol, or nicotine. Medications that dilate the pupils (like some used for depression) may also cause them.

Who's at Risk
Four percent of the population develops glaucoma, usually after age 40. In some families it occurs more frequently.

Possible Aftereffects and Complications
Vision is jeopardized because the pressure in the eye increasingly damages the optic nerve. In most cases, however, treatment can prevent the disease from worsening and causing blindness.

Prevention
Yearly eye examinations are recommended after age 40, including an examination of the optic nerve and determination of the field of vision. If the eyes are at risk simply because of their structure, they may be operated on as a precautionary measure (see Glaucoma Operations, p. 245).

When to Seek Medical Advice
Seek help at the first indication of foggy vision, and if you see rainbows surrounding light sources.

Seek immediate medical treatment at the first sign of visual disorders accompanied by red eyes, headaches and nausea. Repeated glaucoma attacks accelerate the destruction of the optic nerve.

Self-Help
Chronic glaucoma: avoid drinking large quantities of liquids. Avoid smoking, which restricts blood flow to the optic nerve. Avoid physical and emotional stress.

Normally strenuous activities like sports, sex, and air travel are not harmful. In some cases bicycling three times a week for half an hour will lower eye pressure.

Your health-care provider will inform you if your eyesight is adequate for driving.
Acute glaucoma: Pressure can be lowered as a first-aid measure by a swig of brandy or vodka.

Treatment of Chronic Glaucoma

The correct combination of medications must be found to equalize the pressure in the eye. A hospital stay is necessary so the pressure can be measured every 4 hours around the clock, taking individual blood pressure fluctuation rhythms into account. The appropriate medications are then prescribed. If this approach is unsuccessful, surgery is necessary.

Medications

Pilocarpine to contract the pupil is administered in eyedrops every five to six hours. During the night an ointment may be used. If pilocarpine cannot be tolerated, other topical glaucoma medications are prescribed. Years of use of pupil-contracting medication may lead to eyesight disorders and allergic reactions in the eye.

Blood-pressure medications (beta-blockers) are effective for 12 hours and can be used up to twice daily. They do not cause visual disorders, although in rare cases they may contribute to optic nerve damage in the elderly.

In most cases, a combination of pilocarpine and beta-blockers will stabilize internal eye pressure effectively. Sometimes additional medication is needed to inhibit production of the aqueous fluid; the most effective is dipivefrin (Propine) eyedrops, used twice a day. This medication may also lead to optic nerve damage.

If these combinations are insufficient, oral medications such as acetazolamide (Diamox) may be taken to inhibit production of eye fluids. Long-term treatment, however, can lead to potassium deficiency (see p. 744).

Glaucoma Operations

Operations should be considered only when medication does not arrest the development of chronic glaucoma.

Laser Treatment

This method is often successful. The connective tissue around the ciliary body is subjected to laser treatment, enabling the fluid to drain and lowering the pressure. It is neither painful nor risky and can be done on an outpatient basis.

With surgical widening of the chamber angle, the success rate is 80 percent. As a last resort, an artificial valve can be implanted to help drain the eye.

Problems can arise with any of these approaches. In

Topical Glaucoma Medications
Pilocarpine (Pilocar, Isopto Carpine)
Apraclonidine (Iodipine)
Brimonidine (Alphagan)
Dipivefrin (Propine)
Echothiophate iodide (Phospholine Iodide)
Latanoprost (Xalatan)

Topical Beta-Blockers for Glaucoma
Betaxolol (Betoptic)
Carteolol (Ocupress)
Levobunolol (Betagen)
Timolol (Timoptic)

Carbonic Anhydrase Inhibitors
Brinzolamide (Azopt)
Dorzolamide (Trusopt)

a third of all cases, a cataract may develop more quickly as a result of the operation.

Following surgery, 2 weeks of rest are necessary; a return to hard physical work is possible after two months. Regular monitoring of internal eye pressure continues to be important, and after surgical widening of the chamber angle, disinfectant eyedrops must be used in perpetuity.

Treatment of Acute Glaucoma

The dramatic symptoms of acute glaucoma are alleviated by medications to reduce the pressure and calm the patient. Thereafter, laser surgery is performed, if possible. The eye must not be opened for this procedure.

Iridectomy: A small piece of the iris is removed so the fluid can drain into the anterior eye chamber. Since the other eye is usually in danger of a glaucoma attack as well, it is wise to operate on both as a precaution.

Two weeks after surgery, the patient can resume normal life.

If you have glaucoma
— Always use eye medication at the same time each day.
— Always wipe off excess eyedrops.
— Always have a good supply of eye medication. Do not use eyedrops if they've become cloudy. Write down the name and concentration of your medication in case of an emergency.

— Do not use medications containing corticosteroids.
— If you feel stressed by your chronic ailment, psychotherapy may help (see Behavior Therapy, p. 700).
— Many eye medications elevate eye pressure, so be sure to ask your doctor or pharmacist whether what you are taking is appropriate for someone with glaucoma.

MACULAR DEGENERATION

Complaints
When the macula, or central spot of the retina, deteriorates, the eyes lose their ability to focus clearly. This may occur in both eyes simultaneously, or one after the other. Often this goes unnoticed until the patient can no longer read. Eyesight is better in dim light.

Causes
Hereditary predisposition; arteriosclerosis; circulatory diseases; metabolic disorders; high cholesterol levels; diabetes.

Who's at Risk
Five percent of the population can expect degenerating clarity of vision after age 60.

Possible Aftereffects and Complications
Over time the patient may see less and less sharply, although the colors of the landscape will still be discernible. In a specific type of macular degeneration, peripheral vision remains intact, enabling the patient to stay oriented and lead a normal life.

Prevention
Have regular eye exams at least every other year after age 40.

When to Seek Medical Advice
Seek help as soon as you notice a blurry spot in the middle of your field of vision, which grows larger over time.

Self-Help
— Quit smoking immediately; drink only moderate amounts of alcohol.
— Make sure you're getting good nutrition (see p. 722).
— Get a good rest at night; take afternoon naps.
— Build cardiovascular fitness through regular physical activity (see p. 762).

Treatment
There is no effective medication for this illness. It has been conjectured, but not yet proven, that circulation-enhancing medications can slow the deterioration of the macula.

In a less common form of macular degeneration, the edge of the macula will respond to laser treatment, making possible the formation of new blood vessels. This painless treatment is performed at specialized clinics without anesthesia.

The procedure does not improve vision already lost.

Visual Aids
There is no visual aid for improving long-range vision; and although stronger reading glasses enlarge the image, reading becomes extremely strenuous because of the close range. Not only is the text enlarged, but so is the empty spot in the field of vision.

Appropriate visual aids, e.g., bifocals that magnify up to four times, depend on the individual and must be fitted individually. Opticians sometimes loan these glasses for trial periods.

In rare cases a magnifying reading instrument may improve reading ability. This is a camera which magnifies a text up to 25 times and displays it on a screen.

BLOOD VESSEL DISORDERS OF THE RETINA

Complaints
In acute disorders:
— Sudden blindness in one eye without warning.
— Sudden missing areas in the field of vision in one eye (rarely both), as if obscured by a black curtain. The eye doesn't hurt.
— Significant deterioration of vision.
In chronic blood vessel disorders:
— Slowly deteriorating vision.

Causes
— Closure of central artery of the retina; or acute blood vessel disorder of the optic nerve due to an inflammation of the blood vessels (see Chronic Rheumatoid Arthritis, p. 455).

— Closure of blood vessel branches in the retina.
— Closure of the retina's central vein.
— High blood pressure, hardening of the arteries.

The specific cause of the disorder can only be determined by an examination of the rear of the eyeball.

Who's at Risk

The older you are, the greater the risk of this disorder. Blood-clotting disorders, high blood pressure, stress, and nicotine add to the risk.

Possible Aftereffects and Complications

Closure of the retina's central artery and the blood vessels supplying the optic nerve often leads to unavoidable blindness.

Massive bleeding after a venous thrombosis in the retina leaves eyesight extremely limited, and bleeding may recur even after treatment. In rare cases, glaucoma may develop.

Prevention

With blood-clotting disorders, treatment with aspirin may be a worthwhile precautionary measure.

When to Seek Medical Advice

Seek immediate professional treatment if parts of your field of vision are missing.

Self-Help

Not possible.

Treatment

Acetylsalicylic acid (aspirin) treatment is important because it reduces clumping of platelets in the blood. The medication may have to be taken for months, depending on circumstances. Blood-thinning medications (e.g., anticoagulants containing coumarin or heparin) seldom make sense and are risky.

Laser treatment may slow the formation of new blood vessels in the diseased retinal area; the procedure can be performed without anesthesia on an outpatient basis. Information about this technique is available at eye clinics. A period of rest is necessary following treatment.

RETINAL DETACHMENT

Complaints

Persons suffering from a detached retina report seeing flashes of light; the air crawling with "bugs"; later, a rising black wall or a descending dark curtain. Thereafter, vision is distorted and blurry, or restricted to impressions of light.

Warning Signals

Flashes of light and foggy and blurry vision, especially in the dark, are symptomatic of the detachment of the vitreous body in one eye, which could in turn be followed by retinal detachment.

Causes

The tendency to develop a retinal detachment is genetic. What actually occurs is that the vitreous body detaches from the retina, causing the two retinal layers to detach from each other and tearing a hole in the retina. Fluid from the vitreous body seeps between the two retinal layers. If not treated, this situation can lead to total blindness as the entire retina detaches.

An accident or a cataract operation may cause retinal detachment as well.

Who's at Risk

The risk is increased
— In people whose nearsightedness measures between 6 and 8 diopters;
— In older people;
— In accident victims.

Prevention

If one eye is already affected, it is crucial that the other one also be checked regularly. To prevent retinal fissures, portions of the retina can be reattached via laser treatments. Despite this, however—or possibly as a complication—retinal detachment can still result.

Possible Aftereffects and Complications

Vision can be severely impaired, to the point of total blindness.

When to Seek Medical Advice

Seek professional treatment immediately if the above symptoms appear.

Self-Help

Not possible.

Treatment

Medications are of no use in this disorder. Cryotherapy, performed by specialists, is indicated as soon as possible. Under local anesthesia, the two retinal layers are reconnected again: A supercooled metal instrument is inserted into the tissue, effectively gluing together the retinal fissures. This complex operation may take hours.

Following surgery, a 1-week hospital stay is necessary. After this period, the eyes still need rest, including avoiding any quick eye movements (while reading, e.g.,). Watching television is not harmful.

The earlier the operation, the greater the chance of restoring vision to previous levels. The 10 percent failure rate rises to 30 percent if the operation is done too late; a more difficult operation is then indicated. However, without surgery, the eye will definitely become blind.

RETINITIS PIGMENTOSA (HEREDITARY RETINA DISORDERS)

Complaints

The first symptoms of this disorder include night blindness, inability to adjust to changes in light, and light sensitivity. Progressive loss of peripheral vision, often in the form of an expanding ring scotoma or concentric contraction of the field, is usual.

Causes

Retinitis pigmentosa is an inherited illness. Its cause is unknown.

Who's at Risk

Retinitis pigmentosa may occur at any age. If onset is within the first 10 years of life, it often leads to blindness in mid-life; onset in old age leads to increasingly impaired vision.

Possible Aftereffects and Complications

Blindness.

Prevention

Not possible.

When to Seek Medical Advice

Seek help at the first symptoms of illness.

Self-Help

Support groups may make life with this disability easier and are good sources of information.

Treatment

To date there is no effective method for treating this illness. High-tech measures such as the implantation of chips are still in the experimental stages.

EARS

The ears make us aware of sound and also help us maintain balance. The parts of the ear are the outer, middle, and inner ear, and the auditory nerve with the central auditory pathways.

Outer Ear

The outer ear consists of the cartilaginous auricle and the external auditory canal, which is about an inch long and borders the eardrum. The outer ear serves to carry sound to the eardrum and to protect the middle ear.

Middle Ear

The middle ear consists of the eardrum, the tympanic cavity, the auditory ossicles, the eustachian tube (a canal connecting ear and nasopharynx), muscles, and the air chambers behind the ear (the mastoid process).

The middle ear's function is to convert sound vibrations in the eardrum into pressure, or mechanical vibrations, and to transmit these to the inner ear. The eardrum is a soft membrane a half-inch in diameter that vibrates in response to external sounds and trans-mits the vibrations along the ossicles—the hammer, anvil and stirrup. The eustachian tube helps to balance pressure inside and outside the head. The air chambers apparently serve to muffle internal noises, such as chewing.

Inner Ear

The inner ear consists of the actual hearing organ (the cochlea) and the vestibular system, which functions as the organ of balance. The snail-shaped cochlea converts the mechanical vibrations received by the stirrup into electrical impulses. The vestibular system consists of two vesicles and three fluid-filled tubes, the semicircular canals.

Auditory Nerve and Central Auditory Pathways

These pick up the electrical impulses produced by the cochlea and transmit them to the brain, at which point we "hear" the sound.

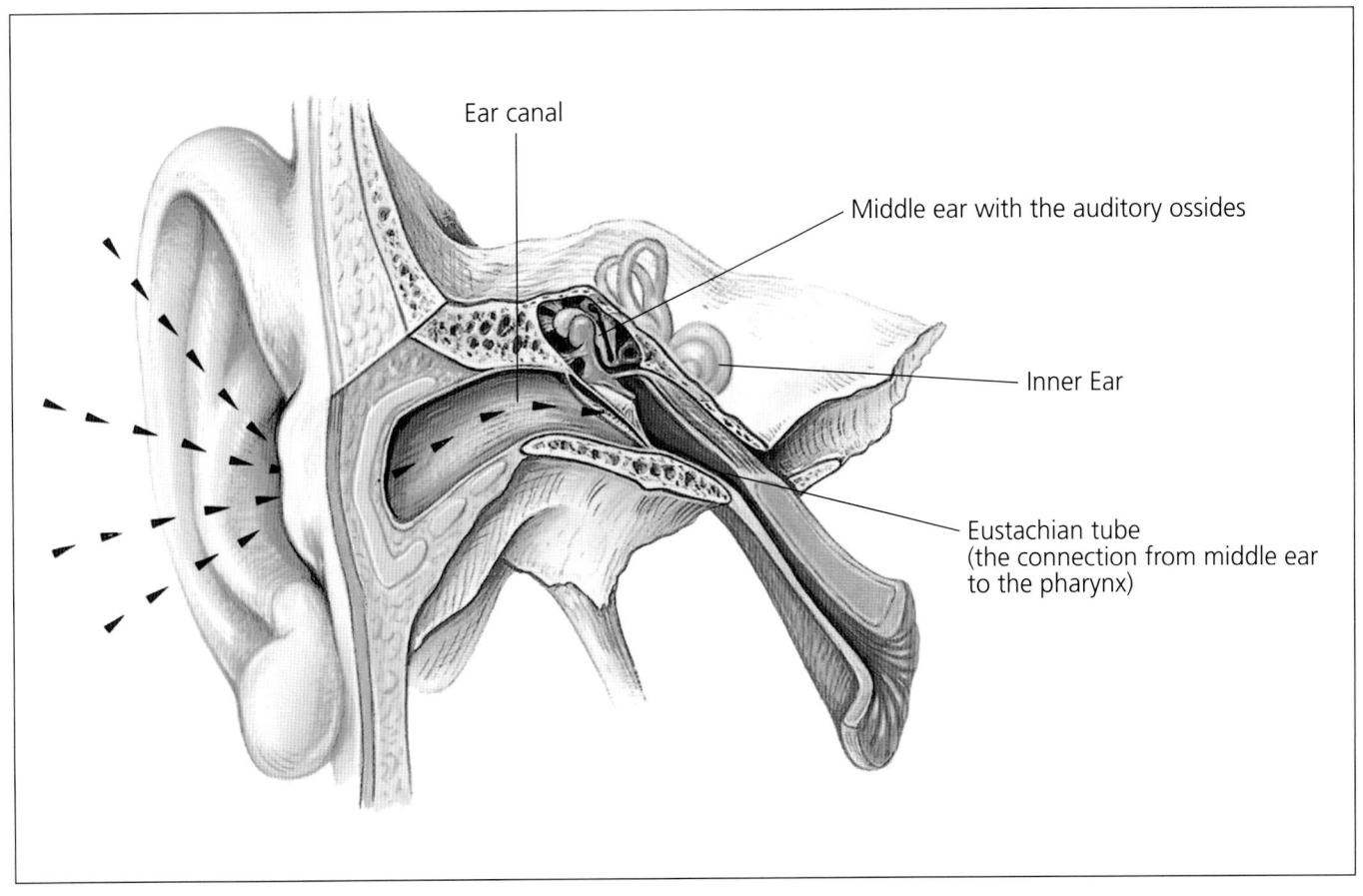

Ear canal

Middle ear with the auditory ossides

Inner Ear

Eustachian tube
(the connection from middle ear
to the pharynx)

HEARING LOSS (IMPAIRED HEARING)

Complaints
— Inability to hear a ticking clock.
— Constant difficulty hearing over the telephone.
— Needing to sit in the front rows at the movies or theater to hear well.
— Difficulty following conversations involving more than one other person.
— Hearing an oncoming car only at the last minute.

Causes
There are two different types of hearing loss: Conductive hearing loss and sensorineural hearing loss.

Conductive hearing loss stems from damage to the external auditory canal, eardrum, or middle ear. This type of hearing loss is caused by cerumen or earwax (see p. 253); closure of the auditory canal by foreign bodies in the ear or an inflammation (see p. 254); malformations of the outer and/or middle ear; consequences of injuries or eustachian tube disorders (see p. 254); acute (see p. 255) and chronic middle ear infections (see p. 256); or otosclerosis (see p. 259).

In many cases, conductive hearing loss can be treated successfully or improved through medical or surgical intervention.

Sensorineural hearing loss occurs when the fine hair cells in the inner ear are damaged, or transmission to the brain is impaired. This type of hearing loss, by far the most common, is caused by noise. There is a danger of permanent hearing loss when the ears are exposed to 85 decibels (dB) (equivalent to loud dance music) or more on an ongoing basis. A heavy truck passing within a few yards can register 90 dB; rock concerts usually reach 100 dB; construction workers operating air compressors without ear protection (110 to 120 dB) will definitely suffer hearing loss.

Further causes of sensorineural hearing loss include hereditary conditions; injuries; reactions to medication; chronic middle ear infections (see p. 256); encephalitis; inner ear infections; meningitis; certain brain tumors; Ménière's disease (see p. 258); malformations of the inner ear; aging of the cochlea; sudden deafness (see p. 260); and multiple sclerosis (see p. 220).

Who's at Risk
Older people suffer from hearing loss more frequently than younger ones.

The risk of hearing loss is increased for those who
— work in a noisy environment.
— frequently go to a discotheque.
— frequently use a personal listening device with the volume on high.
— live on a busy street.
— live near an airport.

Loudness—measured in decibels (dB)—does not increase in a linear manner, but subjectively doubles every 6 dB. Therefore, 120 dB is not twice as loud as 60, it's approximately 10 times as loud.

Long-term exposure to sound levels of about 85 dB or more can damage hearing. Noise exceeding 120 dB causes earaches. The noise of an explosion registering 125 dB may result in permanent damage to hearing.

Prevention At Work
Try to avoid exposure to noise over 85 dB for long periods of time. Because this limit is often not observed in the workplace, personal hearing protection is recommend.
— Regular cotton is cheap, comfortable and effective up to 100 dB.
— Flexible synthetic ear plugs are more effective than cotton, although they may be less comfortable.
— Foam ear plugs combine cotton with synthetics and are relatively effective and reusable.
— Ear flaps are practical when only occasional protection is needed.

Noise Levels in Decibels

Ticking watch:	20
Ambient noise in home at night:	30 to 35
Quiet living room:	40
Ambient noise in home, daytime:	40 to 45
Normal conversation:	60
Office:	70
Noisy restaurant:	70
Loud music or busy street:	80
Truck at five yards:	90
Lawnmower:	90 to 100
Average loudness of a walkman:	95
Rock concert or disco:	100 to 110
Accelerating motor vehicle:	110
Jackhammer at about one yard:	100 to 120
Jet engine at 30 yards:	120 to 130

Get information from your union or occupational health and safety administration on means of reducing noise levels in the workplace.

Discos and Personal Listening Devices
Many young persons suffer hearing loss due to loud music in discos and on personal listening devices.

Jet Engines
Studies have found that low-flying military planes registering up to 130 dB are especially damaging to children's hearing.

Possible Aftereffects and Complications
Hearing loss can profoundly impact professional opportunities as well as social life. Severe hearing loss due to workplace noise can be grounds for litigation.

When to Seek Medical Advice
Seek help as soon as you notice hearing loss.

Self-Help
The best option is to prevent hearing loss in the first place.

Information on problems connected with hearing loss is available from a wide variety of sources.

Tips for the deaf or hard-of-hearing during social interactions:
— Inform those with whom you are communicating of your hearing loss.
— Always have your hearing aid with you and visible.
— Encourage people to turn toward you when speaking; they don't need to shout, just speak clearly.
— Make sure you can see the face and mouth of persons you are talking with.
— Speak calmly and clearly so others will speak to you in the same way.
— Be patient and ask to have something repeated if you didn't understand it.
— Don't claim to have understood something when you haven't: It only perpetuates misunderstandings.
— If you have trouble hearing, first check your hearing aid to see if it is adjusted correctly or needs a new battery. Proper use of hearing aids can prevent frustration.

Treatment
If hearing loss is caused by medication, discontinue medication immediately, after consulting your doctor.

In cases where hearing loss can be corrected by a hearing aid, the aid should be selected by a doctor or audiologist.

Hearing loss is not simply the inability to hear sounds: It also involves the range of sounds heard. Older people often have a hard time hearing higher-frequency sounds. This is why hearing aids must be adjusted to each individual.

DEAFNESS

Complaints
A person is diagnosed as deaf when all hearing ability is gone.

Causes
Children are born deaf every year, and some become deaf as a result of meningitis.

Later in life, factors that would merely have caused hearing loss earlier can cause deafness (see p. 250).

Who's at Risk
Risk is increased by the same factors as described for hearing loss (see p.250).

Prevention
Deafness at birth is not yet a preventable disorder. For noise levels harmful to hearing, see Hearing Loss, p. 250.

Possible Aftereffects and Complications
Children born deaf may be delayed in their development; many learn speech late, or not at all. Deafness has a major impact on social contact and professional opportunities.

When to Seek Medical Advice
Seek help as soon as you notice significant hearing loss.

Which Hearing Aid?

The body (pocket) aid: This is a battery-operated microphone connected by a wire to a molded plastic earpiece. Because it is relatively bulky, it is usually kept in a pocket. Used by those with profound hearing loss.

Behind-the-ear hearing aid: A tiny microphone amplifies and transmits sounds by means of a small plastic tube to the ear canal. This device can also be attached to eyeglasses. Used for mild to extreme hearing loss.

Auricular aid: The audiologist takes an impression, creates a mold and implants the hearing aid into the external ear. The advantage of this aid is that sound is heard at the natural site of hearing. Reproduction of higher frequency sounds is better with this aid, as is directional indication. Not as easy to use as other aids. Appropriate for mild to moderate hearing loss.

Ear-canal device: This fits into the ear canal and is practically invisible. Quality of hearing and sound reproduction is similar to the auricular aid; however, its use requires some skill. Beneficial for mild to moderate hearing loss.

Self-Help

Lip-reading may become necessary and useful. If it is insufficient, a language for the deaf such as American Sign Language may be helpful. It is, of course, best if your friends and family learn sign language simultaneously.

Treatment

For completely or profoundly deaf individuals, cochlear implants may be indicated. There are various types of implants, all of which basically consist of internal and external coils, electrodes, a speech processor that picks up sound and transmits it directly to the brain. The critical requirement for a cochlear implant is a functioning auditory nerve.

Children born deaf should receive implants between the ages of 2 and 3 so that speech can develop; after age 8 this is no longer possible.

Likewise, cochlear implants in adults are effective if the patient already has speech.

TINNITUS (RINGING IN THE EARS)

Complaints

Symptoms include continuous or sporadic ringing, humming, whistling, or other noises in the ear, audible only to the patient.

Causes

— Damage caused by loud noise or explosion
— Earwax (see p. 253)
— Foreign object in outer ear
— Otosclerosis (see p. 259)
— Eardrum injury (see p. 257)
— Head injury
— Circulatory illness
— Hyperthyroidism (see p. 496)
— Stress
— Side effects of medication (rarely)
— Poisoning from lead, carbon monoxide, mercury
— Ménière's disease (see p. 258)

Who's at Risk

This disorder is common in individuals exposed to noise or constant stress.

Prevention

Not really preventable—except by avoiding general hearing damage.

Possible Aftereffects and Complications

Compromised well-being, sleeping disorders, depression, anxiety, social withdrawal. Tinnitus does not lead to hearing loss.

When to Seek Medical Advice

Seek help if symptoms do not disappear after a short time.

Self-Help

If the tinnitus is not too loud, low-volume background music may be soothing, especially upper-register music for strings with little or no bass. Music has been composed specifically for tinnitus sufferers (e.g., tone therapy). Relaxation exercises may also bring some relief (see p. 693).

Treatment

Get a general physical and specialized ear examination so that possible causes may be identified. Although tinnitus is often incurable, its symptoms can be alleviated. Only acute tinnitus can be healed in the first few hours or days, using medication to stimulate blood flow. If the tinnitus is determined to be caused by an illness, the illness should be treated; if by medication, the medication should be discontinued. If the tinnitus persists, there are possible medications to alleviate the condition.

Soft laser or oxygen-pressure therapies are often expensive and of questionable worth. Stress management programs including yoga, music, and support groups can help you cope with the constant presence of tinnitus.

If symptoms persist following treatment, a small device like a hearing aid that produces noise to drown out the symptoms of tinnitus may be helpful.

PROTRUDING EARS

Complaints
Ears that stick out may negatively impact appearance and self-image.

Self-Help
So-called home remedies, like taping the ears to the head at night in the hope of changing their position, are ineffective.

Treatment
The only successful treatment option is an operation requiring a one- or two-day hospital stay, in which cartilage is removed from the ear and the ear is pulled back and sutured into a less prominent position.

This procedure is not recommended for children under five, in whom outer ears are not yet fully developed, but it is advisable to schedule the operation before the child becomes too self-conscious.

CERUMEN (EARWAX)

Complaints
In the presence of impacted cerumen, the ears feel clogged and hearing ability suffers. In rare cases, noises are heard inside the ear.

Causes
We each produce varying amounts of earwax; at times the wax builds up and clogs the ear canal.

Who's at Risk
Many people each year go to the doctor complaining of earwax. Individuals that work in extremely dusty environments or produce large amounts of earwax are at greater risk of developing impacted cerumen.

Possible Aftereffects and Complications
Impacted cerumen is harmless.

Prevention
Wear ear protection when working in dusty environments.

When to Seek Medical Advice
Seek help if impacted cerumen can be felt in the ear canal.

Self-Help
Earwax buildup must be removed by a doctor. Do not attempt this with cotton-tipped swabs or sharp utensils.

Treatment
If the eardrum is intact, a health-care provider will use lukewarm water to flush the ear, removing the cerumen.

If this is unsuccessful or the eardrum is injured, the cerumen is removed by using a small hook, or by suction.

FOREIGN OBJECTS IN THE EAR

Complaints
Symptoms include the feeling of a foreign body in the ear; pain or pressure; noises in the ear; decreased or disturbed hearing, if the object is in the ear canal.

When to Seek Medical Advice
Seek help in all cases and have whatever it is—e.g., an insect, a pea, a pencil eraser, a wad of cotton—removed professionally.

Self-Help
Having an insect in your ear can be very uncomfortable. For first aid, place a few drops of oil into the ear canal. This usually kills (or at least quiets) the insect. Then seek medical care.

Treatment
If the eardrum is not injured, your health-care provider will usually rinse the canal with lukewarm water. If this is unsuccessful, the foreign body must be removed with instruments (in small children, this is usually possible

only under sedation). If the ear canal is extremely swollen, it must first be treated with alcohol or ear drops, then rinsed with water.

INFLAMMATION OF THE EAR CANAL (OTITIS EXTERNA)

Complaints

Symptoms include an itchy outer ear that is frequently painful as well. In a serious infection, yellowish-green pus emerges from the ear, hearing is limited, and head movements are painful.

Causes

The whole canal may be infected, or only part (as in a furuncle or abscess). Causes of infection are usually bacterial or viral, occasionally fungal. Outer ear infections may be caused by scratching, poking with sharp objects, hair spray, dirt, dust, or contact with polluted water (swimmer's ear).

Who's at Risk

The outer ear canal naturally cleans itself as the topmost layer of skin grows toward the opening, taking earwax with it. This self-cleaning mechanism is disturbed when cotton-tipped swabs are used to clean the ears.
    The risk of infection increases in the presence of
— Moisture in the ears after bathing, swimming, or diving
— A warm, moist environment
— Skin diseases
— Injuries from cleaning the outer ear.

Possible Aftereffects and Complications

If the infection remains untreated, it may spread to the cartilage and bone as well as the middle ear.

Prevention

Avoid scratching or poking in ears with cotton-tipped swabs or anything else: the ears normally clean themselves.
    Before swimming or diving, protect ears with oil-soaked cotton.

When to Seek Medical Advice

Seek help as soon as you suspect trouble in the outer ear, or there is evidence of infection.

Self-Help

Avoid the use of eardrops; seek professional treatment instead.

Treatment

Your health-care provider may
— Clean the ear canal by rinsing it out.
— Apply alcohol strips to reduce swelling.
— Apply antibiotic and/or corticosteroid eardrops.

EUSTACHIAN TUBE DISORDERS

Complaints

Symptoms include pressure and a clogged sensation in the ear; disturbed hearing; at times, noises in the ear.

Causes

Blockage of the eustachian tube is usually caused by inflammations in the nose and throat area, sudden changes in air pressure during air travel or when diving (see Barotrauma, p. 257), or nose or throat tumors.

Who's at Risk

This disorder occurs frequently in children.

The eustachian tubes connect the ear and pharynx

Possible Aftereffects and Complications

If a eustachian tube disorder goes untreated, a thick discharge builds up in the middle ear which may lead to permanent hearing disorders.

Prevention

To prevent eustachian tube disorders, inflammatory illnesses of the nose and throat area should be treated, especially in children.

When to Seek Medical Advice

Seek help as soon as possible if symptoms occur.

Self-Help

Not possible.

Treatment

Nose drops can significantly reduce swelling (see p. 298). To restore air circulation to the middle ear, the following techniques may be helpful:

— With mouth closed, the patient holds the nose closed and carefully breathes out against the closed nostrils.
— If this procedure doesn't help, the health-care provider may use a blower bulb to blow air into one nostril while closing the other one; simultaneously the patient is asked to speak, which lifts the soft palate, closes the nose/throat area, and forces air into the eustachian tubes.
— If this procedure is still unsuccessful, the nasal mucous membrane is anesthetized and a catheter inserted through the nose into the eustachian tube.
— If there is fluid in the middle ear, it must be drained under local anesthesia by making a small incision in the eardrum and suctioning.
— Maintaining sufficient air flow to the middle ear is critical for the health of the eustachian tubes. This may mean surgical removal of adenoids (see Nasal Polyps, p. 301); treatment of nose or sinus inflammations; or the insertion of ear tubes (tympanostomy tubes) into the eardrum for several months.

ACUTE OTITIS MEDIA (ACUTE EAR INFECTION)

Complaints

Symptoms include a sensation of fullness in the ear, followed by throbbing pain that may worsen at night. These may be followed by hearing disorders and high fever, and in young children perhaps accompanied by nausea and vomiting.

Very young children may communicate an earache merely by screaming.

Middle ear infections create pressure which, over a few days, causes rupture of the eardrum, releasing pus and, on occasion, a bloody discharge. This instantly eases the pain, followed by a decrease in fever. In the final healing phase, pus formation stops, the eardrum heals over, and hearing normalizes.

Causes

Middle ear infections are caused by bacteria, usually following a viral infection of the upper respiratory tract, such as a cold, flu, or measles.

Who's at Risk

Acute middle ear infection is a common problem. About half of these patients are children below age 11.

The risk of illness is greater in individuals with colds, recurring adenoid (see Nasal Polyps, p. 301), nose and throat inflammations, and in those who have recently had measles, mumps, and scarlet fever.

Possible Aftereffects and Complications

Delayed or incorrect treatment of acute middle ear infection may lead to chronic middle ear infection. If the infection spreads into the bone behind the ear (see Mastoiditis, p. 256), there is an even greater health risk; in this case, surgery is necessary to remove the infected bone. Meningitis is another serious complication of acute middle ear infection (see p. 212).

When to Seek Medical Advice

Seek help as soon as possible when symptoms occur.

Self-Help

Self-help measures include bed rest, a hot water bottle or hot, damp cloth on the ear, and perhaps an analgesic for the pain. Treatment with eardrops is ineffective.

Treatment

Treating the infection with antibiotics is the first step (see Antibiotics, p.661); additional options include nose drops, antihistamines, and analgesics.

During the healing phase it is essential that the middle ear receive adequate air circulation. This may be accomplished by using a bulb to blow air into one nostril while closing the other one, and simultaneously speaking; this lifts the soft palate and forces air into the eustachian tubes.

When pain is caused by immense pressure in the middle ear, a small incision in the eardrum is necessary to release the pus. In small children, this procedure is performed under local anesthesia in the hospital. The injured eardrum will heal over within a week or two.

CHRONIC OTITIS MEDIA (CHRONIC EAR INFECTION)

Complaints
Symptoms include constant or recurring pus discharges from the ear and limited hearing, frequently accompanied by noises in the ear or the sensation of water in the ear.

Causes
The following factors contribute to chronic bacterial or viral middle ear infections:
— Inappropriate or sloppy treatment of an acute middle ear infection.
— Hereditary susceptibility of the middle ear mucous membrane.
— Innate or acquired changes in the middle ear and eustachian tube.
— Resistant bacteria or persistent viruses.

Who's at Risk
Chronic middle ear infections are most common in children aged 1 to 5 and adults after age 40.

Possible Aftereffects and Complications
These include hearing disorders caused by a punctured eardrum or damaged auditory ossicles.

The limited hearing caused by chronic middle ear infections may hinder speech development in children so they are unfairly judged to be clumsy or slow. The severest complication of chronic middle ear infections is meningitis (see p. 212).

Prevention
Correct treatment of acute middle ear infections (see p. 255) can help prevent chronic infections.

When to Seek Medical Advice
Seek help as soon as possible when symptoms occur.

Self-Help
Keep ears clean and dry. Wipe pus or discharge from ear with a clean cloth. Avoid getting water into ears.

Treatment
The ears are cleaned and dried with eardrops; antibiotics are prescribed. Mastoiditis (see below) requires surgery. Damaged auditory ossicles can be replaced by artificial ones, which often improve hearing.

MASTOIDITIS
Mastoiditis is an inflammation in the mastoid process, the prominent bone behind the ear.

Complaints
Mastoiditis should be suspected if, during an acute middle ear infection with pus being discharged from the ear, the patient's temperature rises; the ear aches; there is pain when tapping around the ear; the ear protrudes excessively from the head; and the patient becomes increasingly hard of hearing.

Causes
If the pus arising from an acute middle ear infection cannot drain, it will spread into the surrounding bones.

Who's at Risk
Individuals with acute middle ear infections are at risk of developing mastoiditis as a complication.

Possible Aftereffects and Complications
With appropriate treatment, mastoiditis can heal with no lasting hearing loss.

Prevention
Treatment of acute middle ear infections with antibiotics will decrease the risk of mastoiditis.

When to Seek Medical Advice

Seek help as soon as possible when symptoms occur.

Self-Help

Not possible.

Treatment

X rays, or a computed tomography (CT) scan (see p. 646), are necessary to diagnose mastoiditis. Intravenous antibiotics are the standard treatment. If the infection has progressed to the point of developing a red swelling behind the ear, immediate surgery is necessary to remove the infected bone.

EARDRUM INJURY

Complaints

Symptoms include severe pain in ear, sometimes followed by bleeding and impaired hearing.

Dizziness indicates that the inner ear is also injured.

Within a few days, pus may drain from the ear as a result of an infection, especially if water gets into the middle ear.

Causes

Injuries to the eardrum are caused by the insertion of objects (cotton-tipped swabs, pencils, etc.) into the ear; serious middle ear infections; severe blows to the ear; explosions; diving or water-skiing accidents.

Who's at Risk

The outer ear canal naturally cleans itself as the topmost layer of skin grows toward the opening, taking earwax with it. This self-cleaning mechanism is disturbed when cotton-tipped swabs are used to clean the ears.

The risk of eardrum injury increases in the presence of
— Impact injuries to the ear
— Blasting noise when ears are unprotected
— Injuries incurred while cleaning ears (even with cotton-tipped swabs)

Possible Aftereffects and Complications

Eardrum injuries may develop into middle ear infections. There are no further problems once the eardrum is healed; usually, hearing is only slightly affected.

Prevention

Avoid scratching or poking in ears with cotton-tipped swabs or anything else.

When to Seek Medical Advice

Seek help as soon as possible when symptoms occur.

Self-Help

Temporary use of analgesics will alleviate severe pain (see Analgesics, p. 660). A hot-water bottle or warm compress on the ear is soothing.

Treatment

To prevent infections, antibiotics and eardrops (to reduce swelling) are used. Under local anesthesia the eardrum may be covered with a thin sheet of plastic to speed the healing process. It usually takes 2 weeks to heal.

If the eardrum doesn't heal over within 2 months, surgery is necessary to replace it (tympanoplasty, myringoplasty).

BAROTRAUMA

Complaints

Severe ear pain, throbbing noises in the ear, a clogged feeling in the ear, and diminished hearing are all symptoms of barotrauma; dizziness may also occur.

Causes

During a cold, the eustachian tube may constrict or close completely. When flying, diving, using a ski lift or cable car, pressure inside and outside the middle ear is normally equalized through this tube. When the tube is blocked, the pressure differential between the middle ear and the outer canal stretches the eardrum, possibly causing it to tear.

Possible Aftereffects and Complications

Big differences in pressure may cause bleeding in the middle ear. With proper treatment, no hearing loss should result.

Prevention

Avoid flying, diving, ski lifts, and cable cars if you have a cold and are experiencing clicking in your ears or discomfort due to pressure changes. During an airplane landing, babies should be held upright so their eustachian tubes don't close.

During a plane flight, chew gum or open your mouth wide as if to yawn. If this doesn't help, close your mouth, press your nostrils shut and try to breathe out strongly through the nose. This forces air into the eustachian tube and equalizes the pressure. Applying nose drops (the kind used for colds) before takeoff and landing can help by reducing swelling in the surrounding tissues.

When to Seek Medical Advice
Seek medical advice if symptoms persist more than 3 to 5 hours.

Self-Help
See "Prevention" above.

Treatment
If the procedures described under "Prevention," above, don't ease the pain, a health-care provider can aerate the middle ear by inserting a catheter through the nose into the eustachian tube, after anesthetizing the nasal mucous membrane.

If there is still no improvement, a small incision may be made in the eardrum and ear (tympanostomy) tubes implanted. The eardrum will usually heal within 2 weeks.

CHOLESTEATOMAS
Cholesteatomas are benign growths of the ear's top skin layer.

Complaints
Symptoms include slight to severe hearing loss, sometimes accompanied by a foul-smelling discharge from the ear, headaches, earaches, and dizziness.

Causes
Cholesteatomas usually develop after eardrum injury due to chronic middle ear infection. Occasionally they are congenital or caused by long-term disorders in the air circulation of the middle ear.

Who's at Risk
Middle ear infections that extend to the edges of the ear canal may result in damage to the eardrum.

Possible Aftereffects and Complications
Untreated cholesteatomas may spread and destroy the auditory ossicles, resulting in permanent hearing disorders. Cholesteatomas recur after surgery in one out of five patients; this is dangerous only if not treated immediately.

Prevention
Correct treatment of chronic middle ear infections can prevent the occurrence of cholesteatomas.

When to Seek Medical Advice
Seek medical advice as soon as symptoms appear.

Self-Help
Not possible.

Treatment
Cholesteatomas require surgery. In the advanced stages, the auditory ossicles must be replaced by metal, ceramic, or bone prostheses. In about 20 percent of cases, the illness recurs after surgery.

MÉNIÈRE'S DISEASE

Complaints
Symptoms of this disorder include occasional dizzy spells (vertigo), lasting minutes or hours, that strike anywhere from every other week to every other year, accompanied by ringing in the ears, feelings of constriction or anxiety, nausea, vomiting, breaking into a sweat, and decreased hearing, especially in the lower ranges. Sometimes the sensation of pressure in the ear precedes a spell.

The disorder may also be more or less constant, in which case the spells diminish in intensity and hearing remains limited. In 70 percent of cases, hearing is permanently lost in only one ear.

Causes
Fluid builds up in the labyrinth, the part of the inner ear that regulates balance; the resulting pressure damages the sensitive membrane walls, disturbing the sense of balance. The cause of the fluid buildup is unknown.

Who's at Risk
The onset is most frequently in the fifth decade of life.

Possible Aftereffects and Complications
Often the symptoms are minimal. Seriously affected individuals, on the other hand, often suffer from anxiety and migraines as well.

In rare cases the illness may lead to complete hearing loss, with its attendant drawbacks and negative impact on well-being and social life (see Deafness, p. 251).

Prevention
A low-sodium diet can decrease the risk of recurrent spells of Meniere's disease (see Nutrition, p. 722).

When to Seek Medical Advice
Seek medical advice as soon as symptoms appear. For a precise diagnosis to be made, tests of equilibrium and hearing are necessary, as are a neurological exam, X rays, and examination of the hearing center in the brain.

Self-Help
At the first sign of an attack, lie down and remain as still as possible.

Restrict salt and fluid intake.

Treatment
Medication can alleviate the symptoms, but not cure the disease.

Treatment of Acute Spell
Treatment includes bed rest and intravenous medications for nausea and vomiting.

Long-Term Treatment
Tranquilizers are effective in treating the anxiety, paranoia, and profuse sweating associated with this disorder.

Surgery
If medication doesn't help, surgery is necessary. This involves drilling a hole through the bone of the middle ear to release pressure built-up in the inner ear. In about 70 percent of cases, this eliminates the dizzy spells. The symptoms tend to return after some time, however.

OTOSCLEROSIS

Complaints
Symptoms include ringing in the ear, often described as being similar to a cricket's chirping, and increased hearing loss, affecting one ear more than the other.

Causes
In otosclerosis, the bony labyrinth of the inner ear calcifies. The illness often affects the area between the stirrup of the middle ear and the oval window of the inner ear. This causes the stirrup to become immobilized and lose its ability to transmit sound properly. Why this calcification occurs is unknown; heredity may play a role.

Who's at Risk
Otosclerosis mainly affects older people.

Possible Aftereffects and Complications
In many cases, surgery can improve hearing lost to otosclerosis. However, the more affected the ear, the greater the hearing loss, even in the event of successful surgery.

Prevention
Not possible.

When to Seek Medical Advice
Seek medical help as soon as you suspect otosclerosis.

Self-Help
Not possible.

Treatment

If the inner ear is still functional, the middle ear's stirrup can be surgically replaced by an artificial one. Only 1 percent of patients experience complete hearing loss following surgery.

In cases where surgery is not possible, a hearing aid can help restore some hearing.

SUDDEN DEAFNESS

Complaints

Symptoms include sudden partial or total hearing loss in one ear, often accompanied by dizziness, noises and pressure in the ear, and severe anxiety. In about 10 percent of cases, both ears are affected.

Causes

Circulatory disorders in the inner ear, viral infections, and certain medications are suspected to cause sudden deafness. In rare cases, the cause may be cancer or neurological disorders. Stressful life conditions may also be a factor (see Health and Well-Being, p. 182).

Who's at Risk

Those affected are usually over age 40.

Possible Aftereffects and Complications

Sudden deafness is a medical emergency and must be treated immediately. Usually hearing will spontaneously return.

Prevention

Not possible.

When to Seek Medical Advice

Seek help immediately.

Self-Help

Not possible.

Treatment

Treatment includes immediate hospitalization and intravenous administration of low-molecular-weight dextran, circulatory stimulants, vitamins, and procaine, followed by oral medication.

SKIN

The skin is the largest organ, measuring over 2 square yards and weighing a total of almost 4 pounds. It is our boundary with the outside world and has several functions:

The skin is the organ through which we sense touch, pain and warmth. It is of primary significance in our contacts with other people, as well as our personal well-being. The skin protects our bodies from physical impacts and friction, and regulates the body's temperature by way of an outer insulating layer containing hairs, a fatty layer, a cooling system involving blood vessels, and sweat glands. The epidermis or top layer of skin is dry and acidic to help protect against germs; it also protects us against the sun's harmful ultraviolet (UV) rays by darkening and thickening. As a barrier between organism and environment, the skin keeps the body from drying out and protects it from all manner of external influences.

Because the skin is such a visible organ, skin disorders usually affect psychological well-being. For example, having acne, a frequent medical problem in young people, may influence a teenager's personal development. Rashes, skin discolorations, and birthmarks may be so prominent as to be offensive to others. The variety of cosmetic products available shows us the importance of skin and hair for our self-image.

The skin can also serve as an organ of expression, a mirror of the soul. Fear makes us sweat or grow pale; shame or embarrassment make us blush; situations that "get under our skin" may result in a rash.

SKIN CARE

Regular care of the skin keeps us clean, helps prevent disease, and generally improves our sense of well-being. Which skin-care regimen is right for you depends on your skin type (dry, normal, or oily—though your face

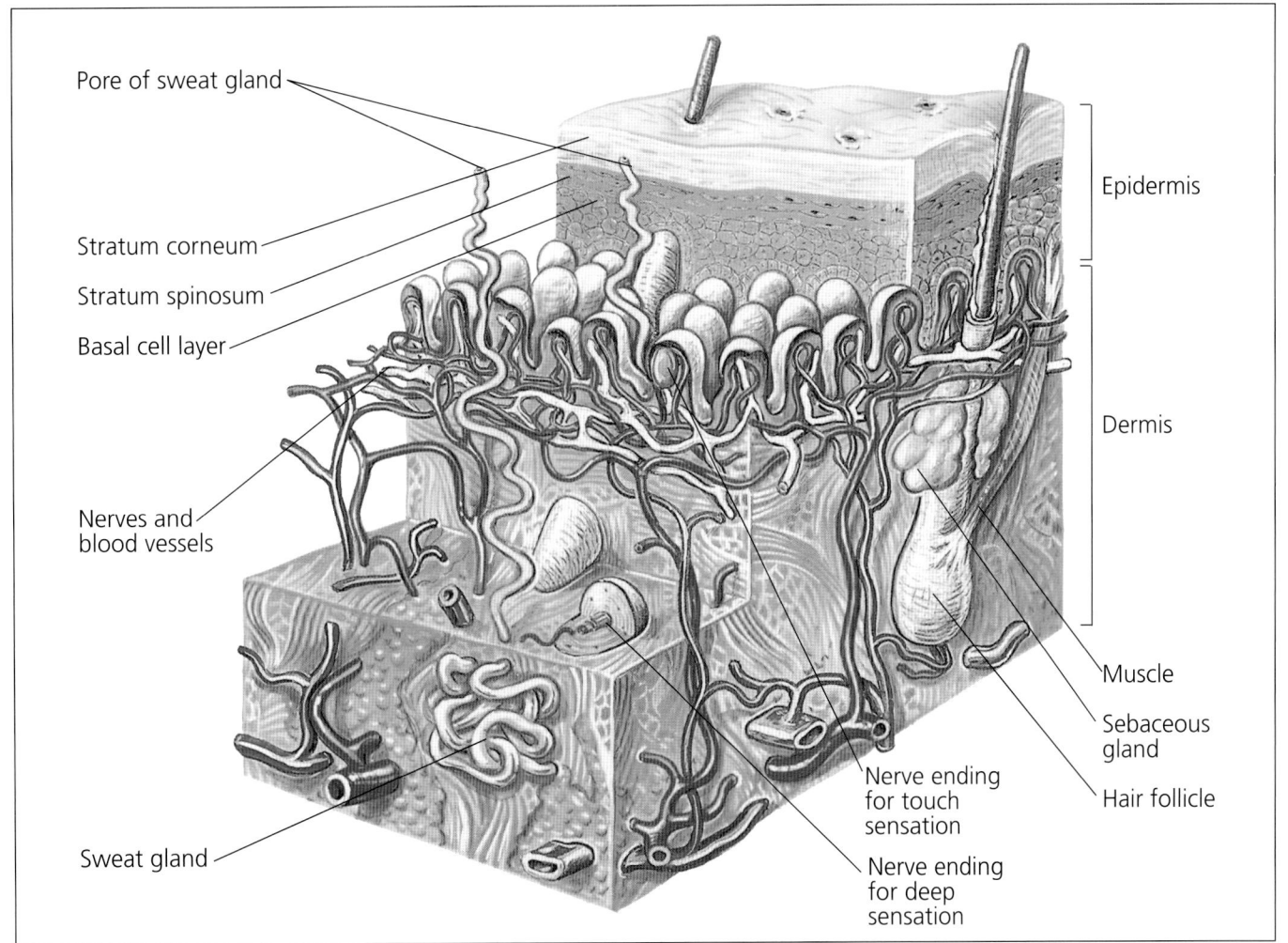

Pore of sweat gland

Stratum corneum

Stratum spinosum

Basal cell layer

Nerves and blood vessels

Sweat gland

Epidermis

Dermis

Muscle

Sebaceous gland

Hair follicle

Nerve ending for touch sensation

Nerve ending for deep sensation

may be a combination), the season (skin is dryer in winter than summer), hormonal levels, and general state of health.

There are different skin preparations such as ointments, creams, lotions, and solutions.

Ointments, or salves, are oily and contain little or no water. They provide a layer of oil and are especially effective on moistened skin.

Creams are emulsions, or stable oil/water mixtures. There are two kinds: Water-in-oil emulsions, which are quite oily and spread less easily; and oil-in-water emulsions, which are less oily, spread easily, and are absorbed quickly.

Lotions are a mixture of oil, water, and powder. They go on easily and have a soothing, cooling, drying effect on inflamed or blistered skin.

Solutions consist of water or alcohol with dissolved solids; like lotions, they dry the skin.

Skin Cleansing

Even rinsing with water, but especially washing with soap, removes dirt, grease, scales, and moisturizing substances from the skin, leaving it dry and rough. Healthy skin normally replenishes lost oils within a short time; in addition, most skin cleansers also contain moisturizers.

Too much washing without replenishing oils can cause dry, flaky skin.

Soaps, synthetic detergents, cleansing milks, astringent lotions

Synthetic detergents resemble soaps, but contain slight acidity, matching the skin's natural pH of 6 more closely than soap, which is more alkaline with a pH of 10.
— Synthetic detergents remove oil extremely efficiently, so they are recommended for oily skin.
— Soap is better for dry skin, especially if it has a high fat content (as in baby soap, for example).
— Healthy skin tolerates soap just as well as the more expensive synthetic detergents; both can cause harm if overused.
— Baby skin care products should be additive- and fragrance-free.
— Hard soaps and synthetic detergents contain no preservatives, unlike cleansing lotions.
— Cleansing milks are thin oil-in-water emulsions that

are applied and then rinsed off with water. They are especially gentle and are recommended for makeup removal.
— Astringent facial cleansers contain alcohol; in spite of their stimulating and revitalizing action, they are not recommended because of their drying effect.

Dry Skin

Dry skin tends to look dull, feel tight and flaky, and wrinkle sooner than other types.

Dry skin often appears in
— older people, due to relatively underactive sebaceous glands
— persons who spend time in heated or air-conditioned environments
— persons that use strong oil-removing soaps or bath or shower gels

Frequent bathing isn't good for dry skin. Also, the hotter the bath or shower, the more moisture it removes from the skin. After washing, bathing or showering, a cream or lotion should be applied to help keep dry skin moist. Care products for dry skin tend to be oily.

Choosing Skin Care Products

The best way to find the most effective skin care product for you is by testing it on your skin. If your skin feels dry shortly after application, try an oilier product (usually a water-in-oil emulsion); but if a sticky sheen is the result, your skin is oversaturated and an oil-in-water emulsion is enough.

Unfortunately, manufacturers of all-purpose skin creams seldom list which emulsion type they contain. Most so-called day creams are oil-in-water emulsions, while night creams are usually water-in-oil emulsions.

Normal Skin

Normal skin is coated with a water-and-oil layer that usually requires no special care. Normal skin quickly replenishes oils lost in cleansing. After age 25 the sebaceous glands become less productive, meaning skin becomes increasingly drier with age.

The best day skin creams
According to tests, the most expensive and/or most famous brand names are not necessarily the best.

Oily Skin

In oily skin the sebaceous glands are over-productive, expanding the pores. Oily skin may appear shiny and oily, or dry if oil has dried in the hair follicles. Many people have both types of oily skin, with an oily forehead, nose, and chin and dry cheeks, for example.

Care products for oily skin are oil-free and contain oil-removing ingredients. They should be applied twice a day.

SUNBURN

The body protects itself from the sun's ultraviolet (UV) rays by darkening and thickening. The skin's deeper basal-cell layer produces melanin, a black substance that spreads through the epidermis and gives skin its color. In the presence of UV rays, melanin production is increased, causing overall darkening, and cell production in the epidermis is stimulated, causing skin to thicken.

Complaints

Sunburn manifests as red, hot, sensitive skin, sometimes swollen as well. Blisters develop in serious cases.

Causes

Sunburn is inflammation of the skin from overexposure to the sun. Because of the thinning of the earth's protective ozone layer, we are exposed to more UV radiation today than we were even a few years ago; therefore, sunburns take less time to develop. Even on cloudy days or in the shade, reflected sunlight can cause a burn; it's easy to underestimate the sun's power if we don't notice its heat.

Who's at Risk

Those with naturally pale skin are at higher risk for sunburn, as are people who spend time in hot climates or high in the mountains.

Possible Aftereffects and Complications

Regular tanning over the years causes skin to age prematurely and lose its elasticity. Above all, sunburn increases the risk of skin cancer (see p. 286).

Prevention

Wear a hat and protective clothing. Up to 20 percent of UV rays can penetrate clothing; wet clothes let more rays through than dry clothes, and light-colored clothes let more through than dark colors.

When swimming, keep in mind that 60 percent of UV rays penetrate as far as 20 inches below the water's surface.

When sunbathing, make sure the length of your tanning session matches your skin type and sunscreen rating; a slow tan will look more even and last longer. Keep in mind, however, that wearing sunscreen does not guarantee protection from either sunburn or skin cancer. Studies have shown that sunscreen users are just as susceptible to skin cancer as nonusers.

Tanning Tips

Each skin type has its own sunburn rate. Sunscreens' sun protection factor (SPF) numbers indicate how long those wearing sunscreen can expect to stay in the sun without burning. For example, a person with type III skin (see chart, p. 264) will burn after about 20 minutes without protection; using a SPF 6 sunscreen, he or she can expect to start burning only after six times the exposure, or about 2 hours.

Warning: SPF numbers should only be taken as guidelines, as protection rates vary widely between individuals. Sun protection factors also vary from product to product, and SPF ratings are not standardized in all countries.

Many people don't realize that sunscreens take about 20 minutes after application to work properly. Deodorants, cosmetics or perfumes should not be used while tanning, as permanent skin discoloration may result.

Remember to apply sunscreen to ears and behind ears.

Some sunscreens are water-resistant so they won't wash off easily while swimming.

Sunscreen lotions and creams, suntan oils, tanning products

— Sunscreen lotions are applied to the whole body. Tests show that inexpensive products work just as well as expensive ones, and products with higher SPF numbers are usually (though not always) more effective than those with lower ones.

— Sunscreen creams are oilier than sunscreen lotions and harder to spread on the skin, therefore used more on the face.

— Suntan oils offer hardly any protection and are primarily used to keep skin moist and oily.

SkinTypes

Type	Skin	Freckles	Hair	Nipples	Sunburn	Minutes before Burning
I	Very light	Lots	Reddish/	Very light/	Always very painful	5–10
II	Light	Occasional	Blond/ brown	Light	Always very painful	10–20
III	Light/ light brown	None	Dark blond/ brown	Darker brown	Occasional, mild	20–30
IV	Light brown/ olive	None	Dark brown	Dark	Hardly ever	40

— Pre-tan products supposedly stimulate skin cells to produce more color, but this is disputed by experts.

— Self-tanning products contain dihydroxyacetone (DHA), which dyes the top skin layer a brown that does not necessarily resemble the color of a natural tan. These products are not a substitute for sunscreen. The color lasts about a week and carries no health risks.

— Ultraviolet sensors have been touted as aids in sunburn protection, but their effectiveness has not been proven. They are not recommended.

When to Seek Medical Advice

Seek medical advice if sunburn is very painful, if fever and nausea are present, or if blisters form.

Self-Help

Sunburn pain can be relieved by moist compresses; change them frequently. Apply a skin care product to red areas. Aspirin will help reduce pain and inflammation (Analgesics, p. 660).

Treatment

Your health-care provider may prescribe an anti-inflammatory medication containing a corticosteroid (see p. 665).

BURNS

(see also First Aid, p. 704)

When to Seek Medical Advice

Seek medical advice if burns are not improving, and in any case if over 5 percent of a child's skin surface has been burned: In babies and small children, this amounts approximately to a lower arm, or a quarter of the head surface. Adults should seek advice if over 20 percent of the skin has been burned. The degree of the burn is less important than the surface area affected.

Self-Help

Immediately immerse affected area in cold water, or hold under cold running water, or cover with cold compresses, until the pain subsides. This can take anywhere from a few minutes to half an hour. This procedure usually helps to prevent blisters and inflammations. Make sure to drink plenty of liquids if burns are extensive.
Tip: Do not apply powder, flour, cream, or oil to wound. Only sterile bandages should be used as a covering.

Treatment

Depending on the degree and extent of burns, hospitalization may be necessary.

COLD INJURIES (FROSTBITE)

(see also First Aid, p. 704)

Complaints

The symptoms of cold injury differ according to its stage of advancement.
First degree: redness
Second degree: redness and blisters

Tanning Salons

Modern tanning salons filter out aggressive UV-B rays and use mostly UV-A rays. Though this results in a tan, the skin doesn't thicken, so it can still burn when exposed to sunlight. Make sure you use only clean, high-quality tanning salons.

Adhere to the following guidelines:
— Don't wear sunscreen.
— Don't sunbathe and visit a tanning salon on the same day.
— Wear protective glasses.

As a rule, the number of tanning salon visits and sunbathing sessions should not total more than 50 per year.

Third degree: white, stiff, numb areas of skin; after thawing, black, leathery, dry, dead areas of skin.

Causes
Cold injury results when unprotected body parts are exposed to cold temperatures for too long.

Who's at Risk
People suffering from arteriosclerosis (see p. 318) or taking beta blockers are at higher risk for cold injury.

Tiredness, alcohol use, or a lack of oxygen at high elevations can lead to an inability to recognize the impending danger of cold injury. Children are often oblivious to the risk.

Possible Aftereffects and Complications
Complications depend on the degree of injury. If frostbite is treated promptly, chances are no complications will result. Severe injury, on the other hand, may require amputation of the frozen body part.

Prevention
Cold injuries can be prevented by sufficient protection against the cold, especially of the ears, hands, and feet, and even the nose.

When to Seek Medical Advice
Seek medical advice if self-help is not effective.

Self-Help
Tip: Do not massage frozen areas, rub with snow, or heat directly with heating pads, electric blankets, or hair dryers. Drink hot beverages, but not alcohol.

Do not walk around on frozen feet.

To warm frozen body parts, follow this procedure:
— Hold frozen hands under armpits or immerse in lukewarm water.
— With hands in dry mittens or gloves, cover facial areas until normal color returns.
— Elevate frozen toes or feet and keep them warm, or immerse in lukewarm water. Move the warmed areas with care.

The warming period may be very painful and take 45 minutes to an hour. Analgesics may help relieve pain (see Analgesics, p. 660).

Warning: Repeated freezing and thawing will cause extensive tissue damage. Performing this warming procedure is only advisable once the affected individual is able to stay out of extreme cold for an extended period.

Treatment
Surgery may be necessary in extreme cases.

ATHLETE'S FOOT

Complaints
Symptoms of athlete's foot usually appear between the toes, but may also appear on the soles, edges of the soles, or toe tips. Skin becomes red, then oozes, itches, peels, and smells unpleasant. Painful fissures may also develop.

Causes
Athlete's foot is a contagious fungal infection.

Who's at Risk
Athlete's foot is a very common disorder; it is more likely to develop in skin softened by water or sweat— for example, if areas between toes are not thoroughly dried after swimming.

Possible Aftereffects and Complications
Athlete's foot is harmless. Although the fungi are contagious, people with healthy skin and immune systems are less susceptible to infection, even from fungi present on their own bodies.

Prevention
Always dry between your toes after bathing or swimming, using your own towel. Wear socks and shoes made of natural materials. Go barefoot frequently (but not on hotel carpets or bathmats).

When to Seek Medical Advice
Seek medical advice if self-help is ineffective.

Self-Help
If there is no inflammation or it has already subsided, an antifungal medication is advisable.

Important: The medication must be used for at least 2 to 3 weeks, even after symptoms disappear, to prevent recurrence.

Severely inflamed feet should first be bathed in a

disinfectant (potassium permanganate solution) or brushed with a lotion containing zinc oxide, talc, glycerine, and water, to cool and dry affected areas.

Do not use formaldehyde-containing disinfectants; they often cause contact eczema.

Treatment

In young people, athlete's foot often heals itself the first time around, provided self-help and preventive measures are followed and aggressive treatment, which may dampen the body's own healing abilities, is avoided. Reinfection is unlikely in these individuals, who develop a kind of immunity.

If toenails are affected, treatment usually takes several months and involves a prescription antifungal medication, taken orally.

CORNS

Complaints

Corns are painful calluses on the feet, usually where shoes press the most.

Causes

Corns are usually caused by tight and/or high-heeled shoes.

Possible Aftereffects and Complications

Corns can be very painful.

Prevention

Wear comfortable, roomy shoes (see Feet, p. 443).

When to Seek Medical Advice

Seek medical help if self-help measures prove ineffective.

Self-Help

Wear shoes with plenty of room.

Wear a corn plaster, available in drugstores.

Treatment

Corns can be removed surgically if all else fails.

FRICTION BLISTERS OF THE FEET

Prevention

— Wear new shoes for only a half hour at a time to break them in slowly, switching to more comfortable shoes at other times.
— Rub your feet with petroleum jelly.
— Acrylic socks are the best protection for blisters. Ill-fitting socks increase the risk of blisters.

Self-Help

Pricking the blister and squeezing out the fluid will relieve the discomfort.

To do this, press the fluid into one side of the blister and prick it horizontally with a needle which has been sterilized by dipping it in alcohol or boiling water, or holding it briefly over a flame. Do not remove the skin. Cover with an adhesive bandage.

CALLUSES

Complaints

Calluses are thickened areas of skin, found mostly on soles of feet and hands.

Causes

Calluses are caused by repeated rubbing or pressure on the affected areas.

Possible Aftereffects and Complications

Painful skin lacerations may result.

When to Seek Medical Advice

Medical treatment is not necessary.

Self-Help

Soften calluses by soaking (in a bath, for example), then rub with a pumice stone and apply petroleum jelly.

CRACKED LIPS

Causes

Dry and cracked lips are caused by wind and dry indoor air, most common in the winter months.

Some toothpastes, candies, and chewing gums contain allergenic substances that may cause cracked lips.

They can also be caused by exposure to UV rays in sunlight.

Self Help

— Avoid running your tongue over your lips; this only makes them drier.
— Use humidifiers indoors.
— Drink plenty of liquids.

Lip balms containing glycerine cause lips to dry out still further.

When to Seek Medical Advice

Seek medical advice if cracks at the corners of mouth don't heal; these are usually caused by bacterial or fungal infections.

WARTS

Complaints

Warts are raised, horny, usually skin-colored (but not always) lumps that may appear anywhere on the body. Warts themselves don't hurt, but may cause pain depending on their location—for example, on the soles of the feet.

For genital warts, see p. 547.

Causes

Two conditions are necessary for warts to develop:
— A wart virus (human papilloma virus) must be present.
— The virus must be able to penetrate the skin.

Wart viruses are transmitted not only by direct skin contact, but also in swimming pools and gyms. The average incubation period between the contact and the appearance of the wart is 3 to 4 months.

Who's at Risk

Many people see a doctor for warts every year. Warts may appear at any time in life, but are most prevalent in children and adolescents, seldom in older people.

Possible Aftereffects and Complications

Warts are harmless, but can spread over the entire body, which may influence appearance and well-being (Health and Well-Being, p. 182).

Prevention

Prevention is theoretically possible by avoiding skin contact with someone who has warts. Always dry off well, using your own towel, at pools and saunas. In general, wear shoes in communal surroundings.

When to Seek Medical Advice

Seek help if
— your warts are extensive
— your well-being is negatively affected
— you have warts on the penis or labia
— you are over 45 (to rule out skin cancer)
— self-help measures prove ineffective

Self-Help

There are numerous folk remedies for warts, from "talking them away" to mysterious herbal tinctures. Scientists suspect that "talking warts away" stimulates the immune system so much that it removes them.

In any case, many warts disappear on their own within 6 months.

The American Board of Health recommends using a wart plaster containing salicylic acid. The plaster is changed every three days until the wart turns white; this may take up to three months. The softened wart is then filed down or cut off. This treatment does not prevent the recurrence of warts.

Treatment

Treatment depends on the warts' type, location and quantity. Usually the first step is to try removing warts by using solutions and plasters containing salicylic acid, podophyllum or retinoic acid.

Medications

— Plantar warts (on soles of feet) and so called common warts are usually treated with salicylic acid solutions or plasters.
— Flat warts on the face and hands can be treated daily with retinoic acid, which is used to treat acne and in most instances causes the warts to peel off and detach.

Surgery

If treatment with medications is ineffective, warts can be removed surgically in several ways:

— Cryotherapy with liquid nitrogen. Local anesthesia is not necessary. The wart is frozen, creating a blister which is removed and then treated with antibiotics; the process may cause discomfort. Although there are no scars, the procedure must usually be repeated several times for common warts.

— Cauterization: Under local anesthesia, the wart tissue is burned out by a high-frequency current, then removed. Often, painful scars remain. In about a third of these operations, warts regrow.

— Under local anesthesia, warts can also be removed using a carbon dioxide laser. This causes no bleeding and only slight discomfort.

INSECT BITES AND STINGS

Complaints

The telltale mark of an insect bite or sting is a red, itchy, swollen wheal.

Causes

The culprits are gnats, flies, mosquitoes, wasps, bees, hornets, spiders . . .

Possible Aftereffects and Complications

Stings or bites are usually harmless. In some cases, bee, wasp, or hornet stings and spider bites can set off a life-threatening allergic reaction, characterized by severe itching on the scalp and tongue, large areas of reddened skin, difficulty breathing, vomiting, stool expulsion, rapid pulse, and eventually unconsciousness.

Swelling caused by bee, wasp, and hornet stings in the mouth area can also be life-threatening.

Prevention

Sleep under a mosquito net, or use screens in windows.

Insect Control

Insect strips: Some active ingredients may have negative side effects. Pay attention to label warnings about using strips in sickrooms, bedrooms, children's or babies' rooms, campers, or tents.

Insect sprays should be avoided for two reasons:
— Studies show that some users may suffer from side effects including breathing difficulties, feeling sick, nausea, headaches.
— The propellants are harmful to the environment.

Electric vaporizers that plug into outlets are effective, but a health risk: Everyone in the room is exposed to their toxic emissions.

Ultrasound insect repellents: Their ultrasound waves are harmless to people, but also unfortunately to insects. They are useless.

Ultraviolet insect zappers: This supposedly amazing weapon has two distinct disadvantages: Biting and stinging insects are rarely attracted to the light, so instead countless useful and harmless insects are killed.

Insect repellents are effective for 6 to 8 hours after application to skin; so far, no harmful health effects have been documented.

When to Seek Medical Advice

Seek medical advice if an insect sting or bite causes an allergic reaction.

Seek help immediately for stings or bites in the mouth and throat area.

Self-Help

A bee stinger may remain stuck in the skin and must be removed carefully so as not to release more venom into the wound. Wash affected area with water and soap. Apply ice (not directly) or a cold compress.

Treatment

Seriously inflamed insect stings and bites can be treated with prescription medications containing corticosteroids (see p. 665).

LICE

Lice are blood-suckers.

Complaints

Head lice: Symptoms include an itching head, an eczema-like irritation at the hairline behind ears and at nape of neck, and whitish, dandrufflike nits that stick to hair.

Body lice: Symptoms include small itching pimples, welts, and oozing pus on the trunk and limb. Often 2 to 3 red pimples also appear on the back.

Crab lice: Symptoms include an eczemalike irritation and small, very itchy blue spots (bites) in pubic-hair and underarm regions, on breasts, sometimes on eyelashes. Crab lice are yellowish-grey and about $\frac{1}{16}$ of an inch long. The eggs appear as tiny dots on pubic hairs.

Causes

Head lice usually measure under ⅛ inch and are often found in hair on back of head and behind ears. They are usually the same color as the hair, making them difficult to spot. In their 30-day life span they lay 50 to 150 small, transparent eggs (nits) which adhere to hair close to the scalp.

Head lice neither jump nor fly, but run extremely fast. They are transmitted between persons by way of hair-to-hair contact, shared personal items such as combs, scarves, or hats, or contact with a fallen hair containing nits.

Body lice live in clothes and are between ⅛- to ¼-inch long.

Crab lice are round and flat and measure under ⅛ inch in diameter. They are transmitted by way of sexual contact, clothing, and bed linen, where they can survive up to 4 days.

Who's at Risk

Contrary to popular belief, cleanliness and neatness are no guarantee against infestation with lice. The recent resurgence of lice epidemics has little to do with family hygiene and more to do with lifestyles that encourage shared clothes, close contact in crowded buses, overcrowded lockers in schools and gyms, and runaway lice lying in wait on headrests, pillowcase, and so on.

Possible Aftereffects and Complications

Louse bites may become infected. Several family members or close friends are usually affected simultaneously.

Prevention

Avoid bodily contact with people who have lice. Don't lend or borrow combs, brushes, hats, scarves, towels, or bed linens.

When to Seek Medical Advice

Seek medical advice if you suspect you (or your child) have lice.

Self-Help

Fear and embarrassment are one reason lice infestations continue to spread. Your child's kindergarten or school should be informed immediately if you see signs of lice, as should your child's friends' parents. It's usually impossible to tell who infected whom, but with some determined effort it is possible to avoid having lice as house pets.

Children should return to school only after they have been treated and checked by a health-care professional to make sure they are free of lice.

Head lice die at temperatures exceeding 150°F, so brushes, combs, towels, barrettes, hairbands, and bed linens should be washed in extremely hot water. Lice infesting other items can be starved by placing the items in a plastic bag, closing it tightly, and storing it for at least 2 weeks in as warm an environment as possible.

Head lice and nits can be disposed of promptly by cutting hair as short as possible.

Body lice: Wash all clothing, bed linens, and towels in the hottest water available, or have them dry cleaned.

Crab lice: Wash underwear, pajamas and bed linen in the hottest water available.

Treatment

Do not use lice medications for prevention: Some are potentially toxic. Use lice medications as directed, repeating treatment in a week to 10 days if lice reappear. Babies and small children should be treated with medication only under the supervision of a health-care provider. Be especially careful to avoid applying medication to wounds or scratches.

Head lice: After successful treatment, only empty nits will remain. Rinsing hair with vinegar water makes it easier to comb out nits with a fine-toothed comb.

Lice Medications

Head or crab lice: 1 percent gamma benzene hexachloride shampoo, 1 percent permethrin shampoo, or 0.3 percent pyrethrin shampoo applied for 10 minutes, and then rinsed out results in an 80 percent cure rate. Gelatinous nits need to be mechanically removed with a fine-toothed comb (nit comb).

Body lice: 1 percent gamma benzene hexachloride lotion is applied to affected skin areas for 12 to 24 hours.

FLEAS

Complaints

Flea bites produce red, itchy raised areas with a dot in the middle (the bite). Often the bites seem to be grouped in threes.

Who's at Risk

Individuals living in unhygienic conditions, or in close contact with house pets, are at increased risk for flea bites.

Possible Aftereffects and Complications

Flea bites are uncomfortable because they're so itchy, but are harmless and will heal in several days.

Prevention

Avoid close contact with pets.

When to Seek Medical Advice

Seek medical advice if itching becomes unbearable.

Self-Help

Fleas live unseen in fabrics, coming out only when they need a blood meal. Flea sprays will kill them where they live: Beds, upholstery, carpets, curtains, and clothing.

Pets and their bedding should also be treated. The effectiveness of flea collars is uncertain.

If your efforts to eliminate fleas prove unsuccessful, contact a professional exterminator.

Treatment

Severe itching may be treated with insect bite medications.

SCABIES

Complaints

The symptoms of scabies are small, red, itchy raised lines like dashes on the sides of fingers, insides of wrists, ankles, buttocks, and genital area. Itching tends to worsen shortly after going to bed. This condition is easily misdiagnosed as allergies or eczema, and topical corticosteroids are often mistakenly prescribed as a result.

Causes

Scabies is caused by mites that burrow through the skin like moles in earth. Scabies is transmitted by direct contact (sexual, for example) or, contact with infested bed linen or clothing. Itching begins 3 to 4 weeks after infestation. Scabies can be contracted even under the most hygienic conditions.

Who's at Risk

The risk of contracting scabies increases in those living in close quarters.

Possible Aftereffects and Complications

Usually an entire family will be infested with mites. The severe itching often results in scratches, which can become infected.

Prevention

Not possible.

When to Seek Medical Advice

Seek medical advice as soon as you suspect you have scabies.

Self-Help

Wash all potentially infested clothing and bed linen in the hottest water available. If this is not feasible, avoid contact with these items for at least 4 days, after which time all mites will have died.

Treatment

People in close contact with each other should be treated together.

Whole-body application of medications containing 1 percent gamma benzene hexachloride lotion (lindane) can be used. However, pregnant women and infants should not be treated with these medications because of the potential toxicity.

Preferred treatment is with a 5 percent permethrin cream (Elimite), applied from head to foot for 8 to 14 hours, which produces a 98 percent cure rate. This should not be used in infants under 6 months of age.

Infants with hundreds of lesions may require several retreatments.

In any infant or toddler, covering the hands with clothing to prevent licking the medication from the skin is recommended.

CONTACT DERMATITIS
(see also Allergies, p.360)

Complaints
Symptoms of contact dermatitis include red, swollen patches of skin, usually combined with itching and blisters. In the advanced stages, blisters may burst, ooze and crust over; scaly skin is left when the inflammation subsides. In chronic cases, the skin thickens and forms calluses.

Contact dermatitis may appear anywhere on the body and may also spread to other areas of the body.

Causes
Contact dermatitis is caused by
— Direct contact with irritating or harmful substances. Strong irritants such as acids, alkalis or phenol cause visible skin changes within minutes; the effects of milder irritants may take a few days to manifest (see Healthy Living, p. 772).
— An allergic reaction to a substance with which initial contact was made anywhere from a few days to a few years earlier. When contact is renewed, a sudden eczema outbreak results—even though the substance may have caused no allergic reaction in the past (see Allergies, p. 360).

Identifying the cause is complicated by the fact that contact dermatitis sometimes develops only when sunlight is factored into the potential effect of an irritant or allergen (phototoxic or photoallergic contact dermatitis). The development of an allergic condition usually also implies some psychological concerns (see Health and Well-Being, p. 182).

Who's at Risk
The following are at higher risk:
— Persons prone to allergies.
— Persons in constant contact with potential allergens, e.g., construction workers, hairdressers (see Health in the Workplace, p. 789).
— Persons experiencing stress.

Possible Aftereffects and Complications
Long-term, direct exposure to the irritant or allergen may cause the dermatitis to spread over the whole body. As long as the skin is affected, and even after it heals, it will remain hypersensitive.

Possible Causes and Locations of Contact Dermatitis
Scalp: All cosmetics, including coloring agents, shampoos, conditioners, etc. The scalp is especially resistant to allergens, so allergic reactions caused by these substances often show up on lashes, ears, neck, face, or hands.
Eyelids: All substances applied to hair, face, or hands, especially nail polish, contact lens fluid, etc.
Forehead: Substances used in making hats (chromium compounds and some synthetics).
Face: All cosmetics used in and around the face, as well as substances transferred to the face by hands or present in the air.
Between eyebrows, behind ears: Substances used in making eyeglasses (cobalt compounds) or hearing aids.
Earlobe: Metal earrings, especially nickel.
Nose: Nasal ointments, drops, or sprays: perfumes; mentholated tissues.
Lips, mouth area: Toothpaste, mouthwash, citrus fruits, preservatives, lipsticks, lip balms, cigarette and cigar tips, cigarette holders.
Neck: Perfumes, cosmetics, dyes used in clothing (especially black), jewelry.
Underarms: Deodorants and antiperspirants, depilatories, perspiration guards sewn into clothing, dyes used in clothing, perfumes.
Hands, forearms: Soaps, detergents, adhesives, jewelry.
Palms of hands: Plastic or dye from steering wheels.
Backs of fingers: Rubber gloves.
Index finger: Eyeglass frames; keyboards; using finger to insert suppositories or apply creams; onions, garlic, tomatoes, carrots; any number of other substances.
Upper body: Clothing, bath gels or oils, soaps, massage oils.
Genital area: All materials and substances used for birth control, intimate products, perfumes, medications.
Abdomen: Buttons, zippers, etc.
Buttocks: Toilet seats, cushion or seat covers.
Anus: Hemorrhoid suppositories and creams, foods consumed, laxatives.
Thighs: Girdles or garter belts, contents of pants pocket, detergent residue in underwear.
Legs: Materials and dyes used in socks or stockings, treatment of leg ulcers.
Feet: Materials used in shoes: leather, synthetics, adhesives, shoe polish, fungus medications, antiperspirants, disinfectants containing formaldehyde.

Skin damaged by dermatitis may become easily infected by bacteria or fungi. Contact dermatitis is not contagious.

Prevention

If you are able to identify a substance as having caused your dermatitis, avoid it. If possible, avoid using cosmetics. Wear cotton gloves under polyvinyl chloride (PVC) gloves when doing housework or using potentially allergenic substances. Rubber (latex) gloves can cause contact dermatitis.

When to Seek Medical Advice

Seek medical advice as soon as symptoms appear.

Self-Help

To help alleviate itching: Several times a day, apply a plastic bag containing ice cubes to a cloth covering the itchy area.

For oozing contact dermatitis, dip a clean cloth into cold milk and apply to area for about three minutes; repeat two or three times, then rinse milk residue off with cold water to avoid odor. Avoid irritants and allergens wherever possible; cosmetics with ingredients listed on packaging make this task easier. If you have hand contact dermatitis, wash with mild soap or cleanser. Always dry hands well, and apply fragrance-free hand cream several times a day.

Wear cotton gloves under PVC gloves for all cleaning jobs.

Treatment

Since contact dermatitis can resemble other skin diseases (for example fungal conditions), a careful diagnosis is required before treatment is begun. Finding the correct cause may be difficult, but incorrect treatment will be ineffective at best, and may cause the ailment to recur. The examination process should include questions about lifestyle, profession, hobbies, activities, habits, clothing, medications, and so on. Special patch tests are performed only after the acute stage of illness is over (see Allergies, p. 360).

Acute contact dermatitis is treated with corticosteroid creams, which should usually be used for no more than three weeks because of possible side effects (see Corticosteroids, p. 665).

If itching is severe, antihistamines can help (see Allergies, p. 360).

In cases of severe and extensive contact dermatitis, corticosteroids may be administered intravenously.

ECZEMA (ATOPIC DERMATITIS)

Complaints

This chronic, extremely itchy inflammation can have various symptoms and courses:
— Infantile eczema: Babies of three months or more may have red skin, blisters, and scales on cheeks, entire face, or scalp (cradle cap).
— Atopic dermatitis in children and adults: Usually this condition shows up symmetrically on the face, neck, elbows, or behind knees as red, thickened, scaley, ragged patches of skin that are extremely itchy and have discolored areas.

Causes

The exact cause of eczema is not known; it frequently appears in babies and is an indicator of hereditary tendencies toward specific allergies. Four out of five children stand a chance of outgrowing eczema in puberty.

This ailment tends to appear and recur especially in individuals undergoing emotionally stressful experiences (see Health and Well-Being, p. 182).

Newer research claims that certain foods such as milk products, egg whites, and citrus fruits, can cause red, itching skin; however, most medical texts question such a causal connection.

Other factors such as extreme fluctuations in temperature, wearing wool or silk clothing, ingesting certain oils and fats, or contact with chemical allergens may also trigger this disorder.

Immersion in fresh water may make this condition worse, whereas sea water has no such effect.

Who's at Risk

About 7 to 10 percent of babies and children are affected by eczema. It often appears in people with a family history of hayfever, asthma, or conjunctivitis.

Possible Aftereffects and Complications

Eczema typically involves severe itching that comes in waves and causes serious scratching. The scratching often leads to serious skin damage, with the additional danger of infections.

This condition is usually extremely stressful both for the sufferer and his or her family. The itching can be especially bad at night in children, which can make life difficult for the whole household. The resulting emotional stress only worsens the condition, and can even trigger it, and according to some doctors, a vicious circle with both physical and psychological effects.

Parental behavior may unconsciously encourage the condition when a child is showered with attention during eczema attacks; the child may interpret this as a reward (see Health and Well-Being, p. 182). This is not to say children suffering from dermatitis should be neglected; they need loving care, but also careful observation.

Eczema may eventually lead to insecurity, withdrawal and depression requiring psychotherapy (see p. 699).

Prevention
Breastfeeding babies for as long as possible may prevent early contact with potentially allergenic substances. Some specialists recommend that children from "atopic families" be fed hypoallergenic-prepared baby foods if they are not breastfed. The benefits of such a regime have not been completely proven.

When to Seek Medical Advice
Seek medical advice if self-help measures are ineffective, or if the condition is severe.

Self-Help
Since eczema is rarely "cured" and treatment usually leads only to an easing of symptoms, numerous support groups exist for people with this condition. The various recommendations discussed in such settings may include unusual-sounding treatments as well as more mainstream ones. Some patients respond favorably to therapy of any kind, be it a different diet, relaxation exercises, homeopathic remedies, or others. Most proponents of different treatments would agree with the following guidelines:
— Create as stable an emotional environment as possible. Relaxation techniques (see p. 683) may help you deal with stress and learn how to keep from scratching every itch. If you feel unable to cope with problems on your own, get professional help (see

Counseling and Psychotherapy, p. 697).
— Avoid extremely humid or extremely dry climates.
— Use a humidifier in extremely dry rooms.
— Avoid clothing made of wool or rough synthetics; cotton is best.
— Try to avoid washing your skin with cleansers as much as possible. Often plain water will suffice.
— Use bath oil instead of bubble bath; use warm water instead of hot.
— After washing, apply moisturizing lotions, creams, or ointments.
— Make sure clothes are rinsed well after washing. Don't use fabric softeners; a good substitute is a tablespoon or two of vinegar added to the final rinse.
— If eczema is a problem on feet, avoid footgear that doesn't let feet "breathe," like rubber boots. Instead of felt or fur slippers, wear open leather or linen ones.
— Warmth increases itching.
— Treat all skin infections promptly.
— Avoid all foods to which you may be sensitive. These often include citrus fruits (including orange juice), cow's milk, fish, eggs, nuts (including almonds), peas, and chocolate. Children especially can be seriously stressed by the wrong diet.
— Spend some weeks in a climate that's healthy for skin, either by the ocean or in high mountains. This will not prevent relapses once you return home, however.

Treatment
If self-help measures fail or symptoms are unbearable, physicians will usually prescribe a corticosteroid cream or ointment. This does not cure the ailment, but brings temporary relief from the inflammation. Unfortunately, symptoms often reappear with renewed vigor after the corticosteroid is discontinued. Various side effects may result (see Corticosteroids, p. 665).

Although eczema may last for months or years, corticosteroids should not be used for this long under any circumstances; they should be reserved for emergencies or acute situations.

Antihistamines can help relieve severe itching especially at night (see Allergies, p. 360). In chronic cases, medications containing tar may be beneficial.

ACNE

Complaints

The symptoms of acne are blackheads (open comedones), whiteheads (closed comedones), and red pustules or pimples (inflamed comedones). Serious cases may leave pits, lumps, and scars on the skin.

Causes

Acne is due neither to poor hygiene nor a particular hairstyle, but to hormonal changes, usually during puberty, when the body is trying to achieve a balance between male and female hormones. The male hormone testosterone stimulates the sebaceous (oil) glands to increase production. Excess oil is blocked from flowing out onto the skin's surface, and the resulting mixture of oil and cell debris thickens, hardens, and turns black, producing a blackhead. If the blackhead or whitehead becomes inflamed, pimples or pustules result; if the skin's deeper layers are also affected, the condition is known as acne.
Acne may worsen in psychologically stressful situations.

Medications containing corticosteroid, iodine, bromine, lithium, and vitamins B^6, B^{12} and D^2, as well as antiepileptic medications, may also cause acne. This type of acne is characterized by its sudden appearance in people not undergoing puberty, and its unusual locations (trunk, arms, legs).

Acne can also be caused by poisoning from polychlorinated hydrocarbon compounds (e.g.,dioxin).

Some acne develops due to long-term skin contact with tar, pitch, or oils; this type usually appears at contact points, for example on the thighs, due to oil-drenched pants.
Very greasy skin creams may also help acne develop.

Who's at Risk

Many people a year seek medical help for acne. Most are between the ages of 12 and 20, when the body's hormones are establishing equilibrium, so almost everyone goes through a phase of having to deal with it. In women acne is usually more prevalent during the second half of the menstrual cycle.

Acne usually improves during the summer months due to increased exposure to the sun's ultraviolet rays, which kill bacteria.

Possible Aftereffects and Complications

Acne appears at a turbulent, self-conscious time for teenagers during which they are establishing their own identities; worrying about one's appearance can cause additional suffering.

If acne is not treated correctly, permanent scars may result.

Prevention

Not possible.

When to Seek Medical Advice

Seek medical advice if self-help proves ineffective.

Self-Help

— Wash affected areas twice daily with a mild cleansing lotion. An all-purpose acne cream such as Clearasil may be applied after washing to maintain the skin's clean environment.
— Synthetic detergents are recommended for washing because of their strong oil-removing properties (see p. 262).
— Use an oil-free skin cream or makeup base.
— Preparations containing benzoyl peroxide soften callused skin, reduce oil production, and inhibit bacterial growth.
— The best approach is to leave pimples alone or have them removed by a cosmetician. If this is not possible, squeeze the pimple the right way (see box below) so as not to make matters worse.
— Sunlight disinfects and dries the skin.
— A connection between acne and certain foods has not been proven.

The right way to squeeze a pimple:
— Apply a hot compress for 10 minutes to soften the skin.
— Disinfect affected area with 70 percent isopropyl alcohol.
— Wrap fingers in a clean cloth.
— Pull apart the skin surrounding the pimple, then squeeze from underneath.
— Prick pus-filled head with a single-use injection needle; squeeze out completely.
— Finally, apply a mud pack or chamomile extract to stabilize and heal skin.

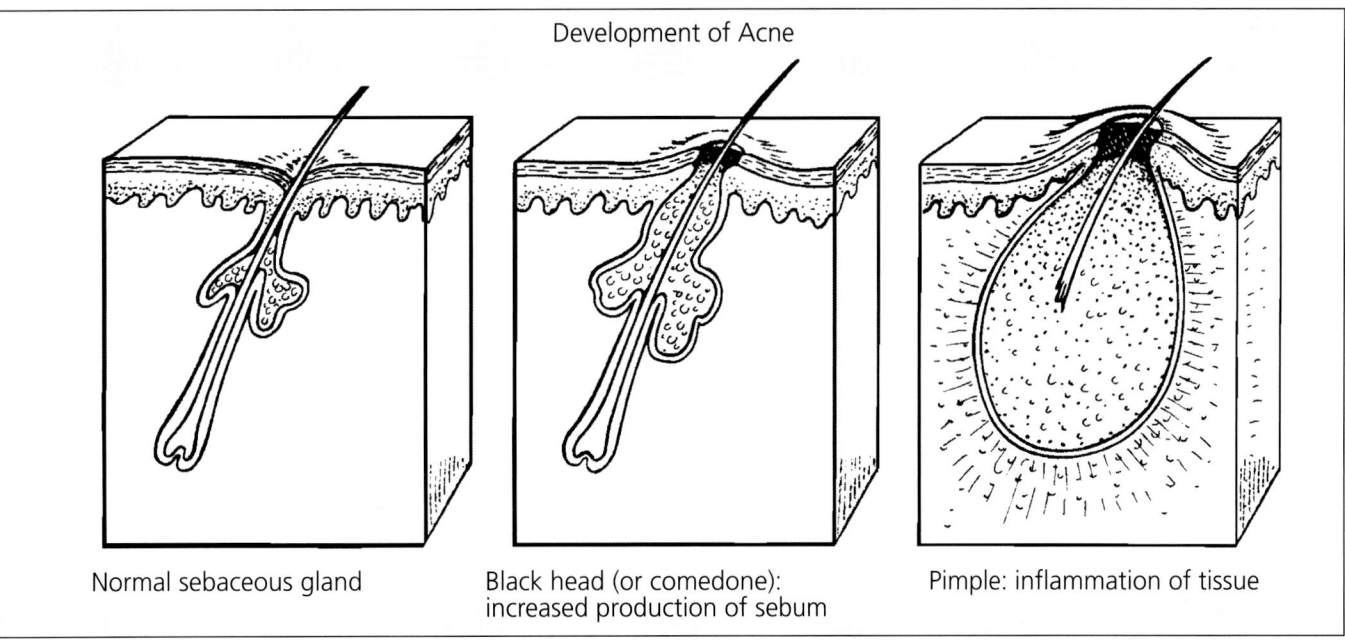

Development of Acne

Normal sebaceous gland | Black head (or comedone): increased production of sebum | Pimple: inflammation of tissue

Treatment

Acne almost always disappears on its own once hormone levels stabilize. If it is extensive or extremely severe, however, medical treatment may be appropriate.

Topical Treatment

Treatment with retinoic acid is effective, but very aggressive. The acne may initially worsen with treatment, but then improves visibly within two months at the latest.

Internal Treatment

If external treatment alone is not effective, supplementary internal treatment is indicated.
—The antibiotic tetracycline inhibits bacterial growth in the sebaceous glands. Taken both internally and externally in an ointment, tetracycline will usually improve acne by 40 percent after two months, 60 percent after four months, and 80 percent after six months. Pregnant women should not take tetracycline.
—When other measures have failed, pronounced acne has responded favorably to isotretinoin. This medication has side effects detrimental to the skin and mucus membranes, however, and can also cause birth defects. If there is even a remote chance of pregnancy, it should not be taken, and rigorous contraception must be practiced when taken. If taking isotretinoin, contraceptive measures should be used for at least 1 month before beginning therapy, should be used during therapy, asnd should be used for 1 month after discontinuing therapy.

HYPERHIDROSIS (EXCESSIVE SWEATING)

Complaints

Perspiration is a normal bodily reaction to warmth, exertion, or tension; the accompanying odor may be unpleasant. Some people perspire so profusely under stress that "rivers of sweat" flow.

Causes

Sweating helps regulate the body's temperature. Excessive sweating over the entire body may be caused by fever, an overactive thyroid gland (see p. 496), hormonal imbalances, or medications (e.g., corticosteroid).

Psychologically stressful situations may cause palms, soles, and underarms to sweat profusely (see Health and Well-Being, p. 182).

Who's at Risk

Especially profuse sweating occurs in
— extremely overweight people
— youths during puberty
— hairdressers who handle certain chemical products often develop sweaty hands, resulting in eczema.

Advisable external treatment with benzoyl peroxide and/or retinoic acid
Side effects: Skin irritations that increase with higher doses without improving effectiveness.

Possible Aftereffects and Complications

Although excessive perspiration is harmless, it may be uncomfortable, and the accompanying odor may be embarrassing.

Wet skin due to perspiration is more susceptible to irritations and infections.

Prevention

Wear clothing of natural fibers such as cotton, silk, and linen, which absorb moisture. Avoid coffee, tea, and alcohol, which induce sweating. Lose excessive weight. Wear gloves when handling certain chemical hair products.

When to Seek Medical Advice

Seek medical advice if self-help proves ineffective.

Self-Help

— Washing helps prevent perspiration odor.
— Sage tea inhibits sweat production.
— Increased sweating caused by stress or fear may be relieved by relaxation methods (see p. 693).
— Deodorants contain alcohol, fragrance, and "deodorizers." Alcohol dries the skin and imparts a fresh feeling; fragrance covers perspiration odor; deodorizers supposedly kill the bacteria that break down perspiration and cause odor. All deodorants work the same way, the only differences being price and fragrance. Skin irritations may result from deodorant use. For ecological reasons, pump-sprays, roll-ons, and sticks are preferable to aerosol sprays.
— Antiperspirants can reduce heavy sweat production by 20 to 50 percent. They contain aluminum salts that constrict the sweat glands and kill bacteria. After long-term use the glands become partially inactive. Antiperspirants may cause skin irritations and inflammations.
— Baking soda (not talcum powder) may be used as a good, inexpensive alternative to antiperspirants; it absorbs sweat without irritating skin.

Treatment

— So-called anticholinergic medications like atropine block the sympathetic nervous system, which regulates sweat production. They have significant side effects, however, which may appear even before sweat production is reduced.

— Surgical procedures, such as removal of sweat glands or severing the nerves stimulating sweat production, should be evaluated carefully as they involve extensive risks and side effects.

SEBORRHEIC DERMATITIS

Complaints

Mild seborrheic dermatitis manifests as greasy, yellowish flakes on the scalp and, in adults, possibly also on eyebrows, eyelids, and nose. Red, itchy, scaly skin may also appear in folds and wrinkles on the face and under the chin. In men, seborrheic dermatitis sometimes spreads to the beard area and hairs on the chest and back.

Symptoms often appear in childhood; frequent recurrences are common.

Causes

The causes of this disorder are not yet known. It is suspected that a predisposition to this condition is hereditary, with outbreaks then precipitated or aggravated by a stressful situation (see Health and Well-Being, p. 182), extremely low temperatures, or insufficient air humidity (e.g., in overheated rooms).

Who's at Risk

Seborrheic dermatitis is a common disorder.

Possible Aftereffects and Complications

Although this condition is not contagious, it may spread over the entire body, resulting in extensive red, scaly patches.

Prevention

Not possible as yet.

To minimize body odor
— Avoid eating onions, garlic, fish, or curry. Several hours after eating, their odors are still noticeable in perspiration.
— Shaving underarms doesn't stop perspiration, but may lessen the odor.
— Wash feet and change socks daily.
— Use a deodorant.

When to Seek Medical Advice

Seek medical advice if condition doesn't improve or is severe.

Self-Help

Not possible.

Treatment

Usually corticosteroid ointments will help alleviate symptoms, but they should not be used for more than 3 weeks. Permanent skin damage may result from longer use (see Corticosteroids, p. 665).

A very effective medication is the antifungal medication ketoconazole.

ICHTHYOSIS (SEVERE DRY SKIN)

Complaints

Symptoms of ichthyosis begin in early childhood and include rough, dry skin and white or grey, tight, fine-meshed scales ("lizard skin"). Arms and legs are affected more than the torso or face, and the skin on palms and soles is thick and callused.

Causes

This disorder is inherited and is caused by excessive production of a layer of the skin (hyperkeratosis).

Who's at Risk

About .3 percent ($3/1000$) of the population, of both sexes, suffers from inherited ichthyosis.

There is also an extremely rare form that affects only men.

Possible Aftereffects and Complications

This disease is neither contagious nor painful. Treatment cannot cure it permanently, but can significantly improve appearance and symptoms.

Prevention

Prevention is not possible.

When to Seek Medical Advice

Seek help as soon as possible.

Self-Help

Cold weather usually aggravates the disease, so dress warmly and wear gloves.

It is important to keep the skin soft, so
— use soap sparingly
— take brief (10-minute) baths to help skin absorb moisture, then apply petroleum jelly (vaseline).

Treatment

Ointments containing lactic acid, citric acid or ammonium lactate are used to remove scaly skin and to help the skin store moisture for longer periods.

The synthetic retinoids given orally, used for treating acne, are very effective in treating ichthyosis, but women especially should evaluate risks carefully before undergoing treatment because these medications can cause birth defects (see Acne, p. 274).

PITYRIASIS ROSEA

Complaints

This condition usually appears first as one or more large, red or pink scaly patches on the torso, and spreads over the next few days to the entire torso, thighs, and upper arms. Face, hands, and feet are usually spared; symptoms usually last between 4 and 12 weeks.

Causes

Although the exact cause of pityriasis rosea is not known, it is believed to be a viral infection.

Who's at Risk

The characteristic rash may appear at any age, but is most prevalent in women between the ages of 12 and 40. Most cases occur in the spring and fall.

Possible Aftereffects and Complications

Pityriasis rosea is not contagious and heals on its own in 4 to 6 weeks. Recurrences are uncommon.

Prevention

Not possible.

When to Seek Medical Advice

Seek medical advice as soon as symptoms appear, so other diseases with similar symptoms may be ruled out.

Self-Help

The disease is often tenacious in people who wash

frequently. Those with severe symptoms should avoid hot baths, showers, sweating, saunas, and massages.

Treatment

Special treatment is not necessary. If rash and itching are severe, a corticosteroid ointment may be prescribed, but is of limited value and should not be used for more than three weeks because of possible side effects (see p. 665).

PSORIASIS

Complaints

The symptoms of psoriasis include bright red, raised patches of skin (psoriatic plaques) covered with silvery scales. Itching is usually not present. The plaques may be as small as dots, or as large as coins or small plates. They appear most frequently on knees, elbows and scalp, and above the tailbone, and occasionally on underarms, chest, genitals, and anus.

Psoriasis on hands and feet commonly appears as sharply defined red areas with painful cracked skin or blisters.

In a third to a half of psoriasis sufferers, fingernails are also affected: They become thickened and develop "pits," and may turn yellowish-white, with the nail's edge resembling an oil spot. Nails also grow faster than normal and become slightly detached from the nail bed. The frequency, intensity, and duration of psoriasis flare-ups vary from person to person.

Causes

Psoriasis is probably caused by an inherited disorder that raises the rate of skin-cell production to abnormal levels. It may be triggered by
— Infections, such as flu and bronchitis
— Medications, such as lithium for treatment of depression, antimalarial medications and beta blockers for treatment of cardiovascular illnesses;
— Emotional stress (see p. 182)
— Skin injuries

Who's at Risk

About 2 percent of the population suffers from this disease, but the risk of psoriasis in children increases to 25 percent if one parent has psoriasis, and to 60 to 70 percent if both parents have it.

Possible Aftereffects and Complications

Psoriasis may last a lifetime, although about two thirds of sufferers experience increasing periods of near-dormancy of the disease.

Psoriasis is not contagious, but many sufferers feel ostracized during visible flare-ups. This can result in feelings of inferiority and social withdrawal. Support groups and professional help are available for those whose well-being is seriously affected (see Counseling and Psychotherapy, p. 697).

Those with visible psoriasis on the hands may have an especially difficult time on the job because the creams and ointments used to treat the disease are greasy and leave marks everywhere.

In rare cases psoriasis may lead to complications that are difficult to treat effectively:
— Erythroderma (when the psoriasis plaques spread over the entire body)
— Pustular psoriasis (when pustules are present in the plaques)
About one-fifth of psoriasis sufferers also experience disorders of the joints (see Psoriatic Arthritis, p. 458).

Prevention

Not possible.

When to Seek Medical Advice

As soon as possible.

Self-Help

This disease is not affected by diet.

Sunbathing usually improves symptoms, but sunburn aggravates them.

The skin should be kept soft by
— Periodic baths to which a glass of milk and 2 teaspoons of olive oil have been added, and/or
— Regular application of oily body lotions
Shave areas affected by psoriasis with an electric razor. The small nicks and cuts caused by razor blades increase the risk of flare-ups.

A more relaxed attitude toward life may lessen the frequency of flare-ups (see Relaxation, p. 693).

Treatment

Although topical treatments are uncomfortable and time-consuming, all possibiliies should be exhausted before internal treatment is considered.

Topical Treatment
— Salicylic acid medications help dissolve scaly skin.
— Shampoo containing tar should be used when washing hair.
— Tar-containing medications have a beneficial effect on the skin, though it may take 2 and 8 weeks to become evident. These medications have a strong smell, however, and tend to leave blotches.
— In especially stubborn cases of chronic psoriasis, tar-containing medications may be combined with timed exposure to ultraviolet rays. Two or 3 times a day the skin is coated with a tar preparation, which is removed before exposure to the rays. Treatment takes 4 to 6 weeks; improvement is usually visible after about three weeks.
— Although corticosteroid ointments quickly produce dramatic results, the disease usually returns with increased intensity after medication is stopped. For side effects of corticosteroids, see p. 665.
— Anthralin has proven effective in treating psoriasis, but dyes clothing and healthy skin yellow-brown so its use is practical only during a hospital stay. Three to 8 weeks of daily treatment are required.

Internal Treatment
— Psoralen plus ultraviolet-A (PUVA) therapy is considered the most effective internal treatment. A medication containing methoxsalen is taken orally, followed by exposure to UV-A radiation. The combination prevents cell division, thus hindering the development of psoriasis plaques.
— Because PUVA therapy is time-consuming (radiation four times a week), eventually causes skin damage, and increases the risk of skin cancer, it is usually reserved for the most severe psoriasis cases.
— Only if all other therapies fail, methotrexate treatments may be considered. Methotrexate is a cancer medication with serious side effects (see Chemotherapy, p. 476).
— Some forms of psoriasis are treated with oral retinoids. Results may appear in 4 to 6 weeks. Side effects usually include a dry mouth and cracked lips, and sometimes temporary hair loss, nosebleeds, and itching. Because these medications also cause birth defects, pregnancy must first be ruled out, and strict contraception practiced both during and after treatment.
— Oral corticosteroid medications should not be taken for psoriasis.

STRIAE (STRETCH MARKS)

Complaints
Stretch marks are stripes on the skin of different lengths and widths, either parallel or radiating, and most commonly found on hips and breasts, but also on thighs, shoulders, abdomen, and buttocks. Initially red or bluish-red, they eventually become lighter than the surrounding skin.

Causes
Elevated levels of adrenocortical hormones in the blood over an extended period cause the skin's elastic fibers to become overextended (see Corticosteroids, p. 665).

Who's at Risk
Stretch marks may appear
— During pregnancy
— During puberty
— In extremely overweight people
— As a result of overproduction of adrenocortical hormones (see Cushing's Syndrome, p. 503)
— As a result of corticosteroid treatment

Possible Aftereffects and Complications
Although stretch marks are harmless, they may cause discomfort because they don't correspond to generally accepted aesthetic norms.

Prevention
Stretch marks caused by hormonal changes, such as those in puberty or pregnancy, cannot be prevented. For those caused by corticosteroid treatment, see p. 665.

When to Seek Medical Advice
Seek medical advice if you are worried about your stretch marks.

Self-Help
Body brushing and periodic massage are sometimes recommended for stretch marks, but the effectiveness of either has not been proven.

Treatment
Effective treatment is not possible.

PIGMENTATION DISORDERS (CHLOASMA)

Complaints
Pigment disorders usually manifest as yellowish-brown spots, symmetrically distributed on forehead, temples and cheeks.

Causes
Possible causes of pigment disorders include:
— Hormonal changes due to pregnancy or oral contraceptives.
— Sunlight increases discoloration; exposure to sunlight while using skin products containing petroleum jelly.
— Exposure to sunlight while using certain fragrances (e.g., bergamot oil).

Who's at Risk
Pigment disorders occur 5 to 10 times more frequently as a result of using cosmetics and skin-care products than as a result of hormonal changes.

Possible Aftereffects and Complications
Pigment disorders are harmless and not contagious; once the cause is removed, they usually disappear on their own.

Prevention
Either don't use cosmetics or perfumes before sunbathing, or check to make sure the product you're using does not contain bergamot oil.

Avoid exposing the face to prolonged sunlight, or use a high-sun-protection factor (SPF) sunscreen (see Sunburn, p. 263).

When to Seek Medical Advice
Seek medical advice if pigment disorders are causing you problems.

Self-Help
Cover affected areas with makeup.

Treatment
— Darker spots may be bleached with specific creams.

It is advisable to test any such products behind the ear for a week before use, as they may trigger an inflammation or bleach skin excessively.
— A physician can also freeze the spots with liquid nitrogen. The resulting scabs will fall off in 8 to 10 days, and in about 3 weeks normally pigmented new skin will be in place.

VITILIGO

Complaints
Symptoms of vitiligo include white, sharply defined skin patches, often with darker edges. They are especially obvious on tanned or dark skin. They tend to become gradually larger over time, and often appear in babies and small children.

Causes
The cause of vitiligo is unknown, but it is believed to be a disorder of the general immune system.

Who's at Risk
Vitiligo is commonly found in people with diabetes, thyroid disorders, or immune disorders.

Possible Aftereffects and Complications
Although the patches are harmless and noncontagious, their appearance may cause psychological discomfort to the vitiligo sufferer. The white patches are extremely susceptible to sunburn.

Prevention
Prevention is not possible.

When to Seek Medical Advice
Seek medical advice if white patches are extremely noticeable.

Self-Help
The visual contrast between white patches and surrounding skin can be lessened by avoiding exposure to sunlight or using a high-SPF sunscreen (see Sunburn, p. 263).

White patches may also be covered with makeup or darkened with self-tanning products (see Sunburn Prevention, p. 263).

Treatment

— Localized photochemotherapy: psoralen is applied to small areas of skin, which are then exposed to sunlight or UV-A rays. This will sometimes darken white skin patches.
— PUVA therapy, as used for psoriasis (see p. 279): This treatment takes a lot of effort, months or years may be required to achieve the desired skin color, and the risk of skin cancer is increased.
— Instead of darkening the whitened skin, another option is bleaching the rest of the skin on face and hands to achieve a uniform tone (see Pigmentation Disorders, p. 280).

TINEA VERSICOLOR

Complaints

In body areas with high concentrations of sebaceous glands, such as the chest and middle of the back, various dirty yellow or brownish skin patches may appear. The skin on them is usually flaky and scaly.

An unusual form of the disease (pityriasis versicolor alba) causes white spots.

Causes

Tinea versicolor is caused by a harmless, superficial, noninflammatory fungal infection. The fungus causes affected skin areas to lose their pigment over time and makes surrounding skin appear darker, especially after tanning, which is probably why the condition is more noticeable in the summer.

Who's at Risk

This is a common disorder. People who perspire profusely are at increased risk; wearing sun lotions and creams stimulates fungal growth.

Possible Aftereffects and Complications

This condition is harmless and barely contagious. As with all diseases affecting appearance, it may negatively influence self-image and psychological well-being (see Health and Well-Being, p. 182).

Prevention

Prevention consists of regular washing and rubbing the skin thoroughly with a massage brush.

When to Seek Medical Advice

Seek medical advice if patches are causing you to worry.

Self-Help

Not advisable without correct diagnosis.

Treatment

Affected areas are treated regularly for 1 to 2 weeks with antifungal medication. Because the scalp is often invisibly affected as well, a shampoo containing selenium sulfide should be used simultaneously (e.g., Selsun).

A dermatologist may also prescribe special tinctures.

If external treatment is unsuccessful and the condition is extensive and keeps recurring, taking ketoconazole orally is helpful. This medication must be taken for about 2 weeks; liver damage is a rare but serious side effect.

After the fungal infection is treated, discolored patches may remain until they are exposed to sunlight enough to blend with surrounding skin.

ROSACEA

Complaints

Symptoms of rosacea include an initial redness of the large-pored skin areas, primarily on the nose, forehead and cheeks, which later develops into lumps and pustules. This condition may recur periodically over many years, or be constantly present. It usually affects light-skinned people between the ages of 30 and 50.

If rosacea is untreated, a characteristically bulbous nose (rhinophyma) may develop, almost exclusively in men.

Causes

Many factors are suspected to cause rosacea, e.g., a hereditary predisposition and internal ailments. Contrary to a long-held belief, alcohol plays no role in the development of this "red nose." Various irritants may trigger the reddening effect, including excitement, emotional stress, heat, spicy foods, or hot drinks. According to many specialists, the composition of the sebum (oil produced by the sebaceous glands) plays a decisive role in the development of this disease.

Who's at Risk
Women are affected slightly more often than men.

Possible Aftereffects and Complications
Although this ailment is harmless and noncontagious, it does affect the individual's well-being because of its appearance (Health and Well-Being, p. 182).

In cases where eyes are also affected by rosacea, conjunctivitis may develop.

Prevention
Prevention is not possible.

When to Seek Medical Advice
Seek medical advice when symptoms appear.

Self-Help
As with acne, clean skin is important: Clean affected areas with a mild cleanser twice a day. Use only creams or lotions prescribed or recommended by your health-care provider.

Treatment
Treatment of rosacea is similar to treatment for acne and includes careful skin cleansing, a course of antibiotics (such as tetracycline) for several weeks, and, in serious cases, the use of retinoic acid.

If corticosteroid medications are used, rosacea may worsen after discontinuing the medication.

Enlarged blood vessels may be cauterized with a fine needle in a relatively painful procedure known as electrodesiccation. Several sessions are required; results are usually good, but symptoms may recur.

A bulbous nose can only be corrected surgically. It will heal quickly, but new growths may develop in time.

HIVES (URTICARIA)
(see also Allergies, p. 360)

Complaints
"Urticaria" comes from the Latin word for "nettle," and hives make you look as if you had just touched stinging nettles. It is characterized by fleeting, raised red or white itchy spots on the skin. In serious cases, whole body parts such as face, hands, feet, joints, or neck may swell (angioneurotic edema). If the rash is caused by a medication, it will usually start on the torso and spread down toward the feet, and may last 2 to 3 weeks.

Hives resulting from medication or insect bite allergies are usually accompanied by nausea, headaches, shortness of breath, sweating, stomach cramps, and a severe drop in blood pressure. In rare cases these symptoms can trigger a life-threatening anaphylactic shock (see Allergies, p. 360).

Causes
Hives are often, but not always, caused by allergies. The rash may be a reaction to
— Foods (often fish, eggs, grain, cow's milk, crustaceans, shellfish, nuts, berries)
— Food additives (e.g., quinine in tonic water, menthol in peppermint flavoring and toothpaste, yellow food coloring (see Taste-Enhancing Substances, p. 733)
— Residue of chemical sprays used on fruit and vegetables, or medications in meat (see Hazardous Substances in Food, p. 729)
— Medications taken orally (especially penicillin or salicylates like aspirin)
— Ointments and suppositories
— Metals in the body, such as amalgam used in tooth fillings or metals used in surgery
— Insect bites or stings, especially from wasps and bees
— Emotional stress
— Skin contact with plants
— Skin contact with animal hair
— Sunlight, X rays
— Pressure on the skin, especially the soles of feet and buttocks
— Extreme fluctuations in temperature, extreme cold
— Acute pus-generating infections, e.g., of the sinuses
— Viral infections

Who's at Risk
Hives are an extremely common disorder. About twice as many women are affected as men.

Possible Aftereffects and Complications
Allergic skin rashes are uncomfortable, but usually not dangerous. In some cases, however, life-threatening conditions may result that require immediate medical treatment.

Prevention
Avoid all factors that might cause hives.

When to Seek Medical Advice
Seek medical advice if symptoms cause discomfort or occur frequently.

Self-Help
Moist compresses can help cool affected body parts. Pinpointing the exact cause of the allergy may prove difficult because most foods today contain artificial chemical additives or preservatives.

Healthy nutrition (see Balanced Nutrition, p. 723) will avoid most triggers caused by preservatives and additives.

Allergic reactions often diminish or disappear on their own after a while.

Treatment
For questions about desensitization, see Allergies, p. 360. The acute symptoms of hives usually disappear on their own within a day to a week. Antihistamines may help relieve symptoms (see Allergies, p. 360).

Life-threatening allergic reactions are treated with corticosteroids and adrenalin, administered by injection.

IMPETIGO

Complaints
This disorder is characterized by small blisters, usually around nose and mouth, that dry up after a short time and develop a honey-colored crust almost like brown sugar. Impetigo causes itching and is spread by scratching.

Causes
Impetigo is a highly contagious bacterial skin infection.

Who's at Risk
Most impetigo sufferers are children.

Possible Aftereffects and Complications
Normally this ailment is relatively harmless, but if left untreated it may spread over the whole body and become life-threatening to very small children. Appro-

priate treatment usually nips it in the bud. Afterwards, the affected skin appears a little lighter than the surrounding area, but it soon darkens to its normal color. No scars remain.

In rare cases, streptococcal bacteria are involved, and the kidneys may be affected.

Prevention
Avoid contact with persons suffering from impetigo.

When to Seek Medical Advice
Seek help as soon as you suspect this illness.

Self-Help
Remove scabs and crusts carefully with soap and water; apply a cream recommended or prescribed by your health-care provider.

The soap and towels used by the impetigo sufferer should be rigorously separated from others.

Children with impetigo should not go to school or kindergarten until they have recovered.

Treatment
Scabs and crusts are normally removed by an oily antibiotic ointment. If extensive blisters are present, antibiotics should be taken orally. To make sure kidneys are not affected, a urine sample should be taken 3 weeks and 5 weeks after the infection disappears.

ERYSIPELAS

Complaints
Symptoms of erysipelas include sharply outlined, painful, red swollen areas with flame-shaped extensions. Sometimes blisters of various sizes appear in affected areas, usually the lower leg and face. The skin condition is accompanied by chills and high fever.

Causes
Erysipelas is caused by streptococcal bacteria which are introduced into the body through damaged skin (e.g., athlete's foot, a lower-calf ulcer, or skin lesions around the nostrils) and spread through the lymphatic system.

Who's at Risk
All age groups are susceptible to this disease.

Possible Aftereffects and Complications

Chronic, recurring erysipelas may lead to destruction of the lymphatic tracts. This may result in swelling of various body parts and thickened skin, especially in the legs; worsening infection of the cellular tissue (phlegmon); blood infection (sepsis).

Prevention

Promptly treat any skin damage through which erysipelas could develop.

When to Seek Medical Advice

Seek help as soon as you think you may have erysipelas.

Self-Help

Not possible.

Treatment

Treatment consists of bed rest and high doses of antibiotics such as penicillin or erythromycin.

BOILS AND CARBUNCLES

Complaints

These are deep, inflamed, painful lumps with a center of pus, caused by inflammation of the hair follicles. Boils develop around hair follicles in places often bathed in sweat or subjected to friction, such as the neck, face, underarms, and buttocks. An especially large boil, or several close together, are called a carbuncle. A boil on the eyelid is called a stye (see p. 238).

Causes

Boils and carbuncles are staphylococcal bacterial infections of the hair follicles.

Who's at Risk

The risk is increased in persons with generally poor health, poor hygienic habits, or diabetes.

Possible Aftereffects and Complications

In some people, boils and carbuncles recur repeatedly over a long period of time.

In rare cases, the infection may spread over a large part of the body; it is then referred to as phlegmon.

Prevention

Good bodily hygiene can do much to help prevent boils and carbuncles.

When to Seek Medical Advice

Seek help if:
— Boils do not heal within 2 weeks
— Boils keep recurring
— Carbuncles are present
— Fever is present
— A boil appears on the face.

Self-Help

Most boils form a head and burst within two weeks. Moist, hot compresses changed every couple of hours can speed up the maturing process.

Because bacteria from the boil may be spread by hands into food and cause food poisoning, you should wash hands carefully before handling food if you are suffering from boils. Shower instead of bathing when possible, to lessen the chance of spreading bacteria over the entire body. Make sure to change towels often.

Treatment

When the boil is mature it will burst on its own. Your health-care provider may also make a small incision to drain the pus.

Antibiotics are only necessary if the boil or carbuncle is in the nose or on the face; if fever is present; if the infection spreads to the surrounding tissue; or if boils keep recurring.

SHINGLES

Complaints

Shingles can appear anywhere on the body, but show up most frequently on one side of the torso or face. The affected areas are painful and red with blisters. The blisters appear gradually along nerve pathways, then scab over and disappear in 2 to 3 weeks, leaving tiny scars. The stinging pain may persist for weeks or months, however. (In rare cases, pain may persist for years.)

Before the rash appears, the skin often begins to hurt, and the patient often feels nauseous and exhausted.

Causes

Shingles is an infection caused by the varicella zoster virus, which also causes chickenpox. After the infection disappears, the virus remains latent in the spinal ganglia; a weakening of the body's immune system can suddenly reactivate it.

Who's at Risk

Shingles may appear at any time in life, but are most common in people over age 50 and in those with weakened immune systems.

Possible Aftereffects and Complications

Shingles are contagious as long as there are blisters. Adults who haven't yet had chickenpox often come down with chickenpox if exposed to shingles.

Usually shingles heal within 2 to 4 weeks without permanent damage, in some cases, remain painful for years.

Facial shingles may cause temporary paralysis. If eyes are affected, there is the danger of conjunctival and corneal damage, leading to loss of eyesight.

Prevention

Prevention is not possible, but early intervention can limit the disease significantly. Shingles only appear once in a lifetime in people with healthy immune systems.

When to Seek Medical Advice

Seek medical advice at the first signs of shingles. If the face is affected, see an eye doctor as soon as possible.

Self-Help

Avoid drafts and cold or damp environments. Warmth has a soothing effect on shingles. If eyes are affected, get lots of rest. An analgesic may help relieve distress (see p. 660).

Treatment

Creams with a high oil content can help loosen scabs. The affected areas can be covered with a bandage.

In pronounced or extremely painful shingles outbreaks, acyclovir (Zovirax) taken either orally or intravenously will help lessen and shorten the illness. Acyclovir does not alter the possibility of lasting pain, however.

HERPES SIMPLEX

Complaints

Fever blisters, the common name for herpes simplex, are painful blisters on the lips or mucous membranes of the mouth, often preceded by itching, tightness and tingling. The clear liquid in the blisters becomes cloudy and then dries, forming brownish scabs which fall off after a few days. Symptoms usually last no longer than 10 days.

Causes

Herpes simplex virus infections often occur, unnoticed, beginning in early childhood. The virus is transmitted from person to person by direct skin contact. After an infection has subsided, the virus becomes latent, remaining imperceptibly in the body until the next outbreak is triggered by some form of stress or irritation: An illness involving fever, intense sunlight, dental work, abrasions on the lips, food allergies, or hormonal changes during the menstrual cycle.

Who's at Risk

Almost everyone is a carrier of the herpes simplex virus.

Possible Aftereffects and Complications

Although fever blisters are contagious, they will not develop in people with healthy immune systems. Only rarely do scars remain. Those prone to the infections will usually experience repeated outbreaks in the same areas.

In people with serious immune disorders, the illness may spread and become life-threatening (see Encephalitis, p. 213). Herpes infections of the cornea endanger eyesight (see Keratitis, p. 241).

Prevention

Preventive application of antiviral medications, e.g., during exposure to strong sunlight, will not prevent blisters from forming but may lessen the severity of the outbreak.

When to Seek Medical Advice

Seek medical care if the outbreak is extensive or has not improved after several days.

Self-Help
Not possible. For blisters inside the mouth, rinsing with sage tea may bring relief (see Stomatitis, p. 379).

Treatment
Lotions with drying and disinfectant action will help relieve this condition.

Applying virus medications (topical Zovirax) to affected skin areas as soon as an outbreak is noticed can prevent further spreading, but the virus can only be counteracted effectively by the body's defenses.

If fever blisters appear frequently and outbreaks are severe, acyclovir can also be taken orally or intravenously.

MOLES (NEVI)

Complaints
Moles come in all different sizes. They may be a light flesh color, yellowish-brown, or black, and their surfaces may be smooth, hairy or lumpy, raised or flat.

Although moles cause no organic problems, they may negatively affect appearance.

Causes
Usually the tendency to develop moles is inherited. Exposure to sunlight may stimulate their development.

Who's at Risk
Moles are rarely found on newborns, but over the years most people develop at least a few.

Possible Aftereffects and Complications
Moles are almost always harmless. Occasionally, however, they develop into skin cancer (see Skin Cancer, below); the gradual transformation from mole to cancer can often be observed. Skin cancer is suspected if numerous moles appear over a short time, or if one mole
— grows larger
— changes color
— becomes rough, scaly or lumpy
— hurts, itches, bleeds, or becomes inflamed

About 40 to 50 percent of malignant skin cancers develop from the pigment cells of moles.

Prevention
Prevention is limited to avoiding exposure to sunlight.

When to Seek Medical Advice
Seek medical care if moles are negatively affecting your quality of life or if you suspect you are developing skin cancer.

Self-Help
Not possible.

Treatment
Unattractive or potentially cancerous moles can be removed under local anesthesia.

A benign mole cannot become cancerous once surgically removed.

SKIN CANCER
(see also Cancer, p. 470)

Complaints
Indications of a precancerous skin condition include
— changes in skin spots or moles
— new moles
— scaly moles and lumps, usually in the face, especially around eyes and nose, that bleed and increase in size
— changes in genitals or nipples (wartlike formations, whitening or reddening, thickening)

Causes
Skin cancer is caused by malignant cell growth. Skin that has already undergone some damage (especially from sunburn, but also from existing tumors, tight scars, exposure to X rays) is especially susceptible to cancer.

Who's at Risk
Skin cancer has become one of the most common forms of cancer, due in part to the thinning of the earth's ozone layer, and in part to the fact that having a tan is considered attractive. To achieve the desired skin color, many people spend too much time in the sun and in tanning salons. Most skin cancer develops in people over age 50, in the areas most exposed to the sun.

Possible Aftereffects and Complications

There are three types of skin cancer:

— Most common skin cancers are basal cell carcinomas. They grow very slowly, are only occasionally malignant, and do not metastasize (see Cancer, p. 470).
— Squamous cell carcinomas usually go deeper and are more apt to metastasize.
— Malignant melanomas grow quickly and metastasize early on.

With early treatment, almost all forms of skin cancer can be healed; without treatment, cancer cells can spread throughout the body.

Prevention

Avoid excessive exposure to sunlight and indoor tanning rays. In any case, avoid sunburn (see Sunburn, p. 263).

With early diagnosis, almost all skin cancers can heal, so vigilance and regular monitoring are important. If you are between the ages of 20 and 30, you should thoroughly examine your skin, especially the parts regularly exposed to the sun, once a month. If you note any suspicious changes, see your health-care provider as soon as possible. If you are over 30, have your skin examined by a health professional once a year.

When to Seek Medical Advice

Seek medical advice as soon as you notice any unusual skin changes. Most usually prove harmless, but a professional should be consulted nonetheless.

Self-Help

Not possible.

Treatment

After a thorough examination of the affected skin area, possibly including a biopsy and lab tests, the cancerous tissue is surgically removed. Usually this does not require a hospital stay.

After treatment, regular checkups are required so any recurrences may be detected early.

LEG ULCERS

Complaints

The symptoms of this disorder consist of lower leg wounds that won't heal, especially around ankles.

Causes

Lower leg ulcers are almost always caused by disrupted blood flow in the leg veins (see Phlebitis, p. 329; Deep Vein Thrombosis, p. 330).

Causes may also include
— Arterial circulatory disturbances
— Diabetes
— Bacterial or fungal infections
— Skin cancer
— Syphilis
— Certain types of anemia

Who's at Risk

Lower leg ulcers are extremely common, and the risk increases with age.

Possible Aftereffects and Complications

With correct treatment, ulcers will heal quickly. Untreated, or treated incorrectly, ulcers may develop contact dermatitis as well as bacterial and fungal infections.

Prevention

Prevention is possible if venous stasis is avoided:
— Move your legs frequently.
— Avoid standing for long periods.
— Put your feet up as often as possible.
— Wear support hose.
— Get appropriate treatment for varicose veins (see p. 328), phlebitis (see p. 329), and deep vein thrombosis (see p. 330).

When to Seek Medical Advice

Seek medical advice as soon as symptoms appear.

Self-Help

Avoid applying creams or topical medications. This condition leaves skin especially sensitive to irritation.

Treatment

Crusty or oozing ulcers should be cleaned with moist compresses.

Ulcers will heal only when the venous blockage is removed. This is achieved by wearing a pressure bandage extending from above the toes to below the knee.

The pressure should be strongest on the foot and ankle, decreasing toward the knee. This creates lower pressure in the direction of the heart, which supports the blood flowing back to the heart.

The pressure bandage must be applied every morning upon arising. Make sure you learn this procedure from a professional so you or a family member can do it at home.

BEDSORES (DECUBITUS ULCERS)

Complaints
Continuous pressure on the same area of the body, e.g., being bedridden for a long time or confined to a wheelchair, can cause bedsores. These begin as reddened, swollen areas, with toughened skin. In advanced stages, skin and muscle tissue may decompose; in extremely serious cases, bone disintegration and blood infection result.

Causes
The continuous, long-term pressure blocks the circulation, leading to a lack of oxygen in the body's tissues. The result is the decomposition of skin and underlying tissue.

Who's at Risk
Persons who are required to stay in bed for long periods of time and have lost some sensitivity to pain often suffer from bedsores, which develop quickly in the presence of friction and irritation from roughness or folds in bed linens or clothing. Moisture from perspiration or urine or bowel incontinence contributes to bedsore development.

Possible Aftereffects and Complications
If decubitus ulcers are not treated promptly, permanent muscle and bone damage may result.

Prevention
Bedridden people should change position at least every 2 hours. Those unable to do this on their own should be turned by another person (see bed positioning, p. 612). Special silicone or water mattresses help distribute weight evenly. A sheepskin bed pad is also beneficial.

Persons in wheelchairs should change position every 5 to 10 minutes, even when using a pressure-reducing cushion.

Skin should be kept clean and dry, and bed linens changed frequently. Any kind of activity is beneficial, even when lying down.

It is of utmost importance to check skin thoroughly every day, otherwise serious tissue damage may occur within a short time.

When to Seek Medical Advice
Seek help as soon as possible if bedsores develop.

Self-Help
If they are detected while in the early stages, decubitus ulcers can be nipped in the bud. The affected areas should be kept dry, uncovered and free of any pressure. Inflatable rubber tubes and other devices are available expressly for this purpose. Gentle massage can help stimulate circulation.

Treatment
Bedsores should be cleaned by a health professional, and damaged tissue removed surgically when necessary.

HAIR

Hair is a determining factor in our appearance, and therefore in our sense of well-being. Hair consists of keratin cells that are slowly pushed out of the follicles. A healthy hair will grow for 2 to 6 years, at a rate of about 0.014 inches (0.35 millimeters) a day. This growth is followed by a rest period of approximately 3 months; finally the hair falls out, and after some time a new hair appears in the same location.

The human scalp contains approximately 100,000 to 150,000 hairs, of which about 30 to 60 fall out each day. Losing up to 100 hairs a day is still considered normal, however.

HAIR CARE

Beautiful hair is so important to many people that they spare no effort or money to attain it.

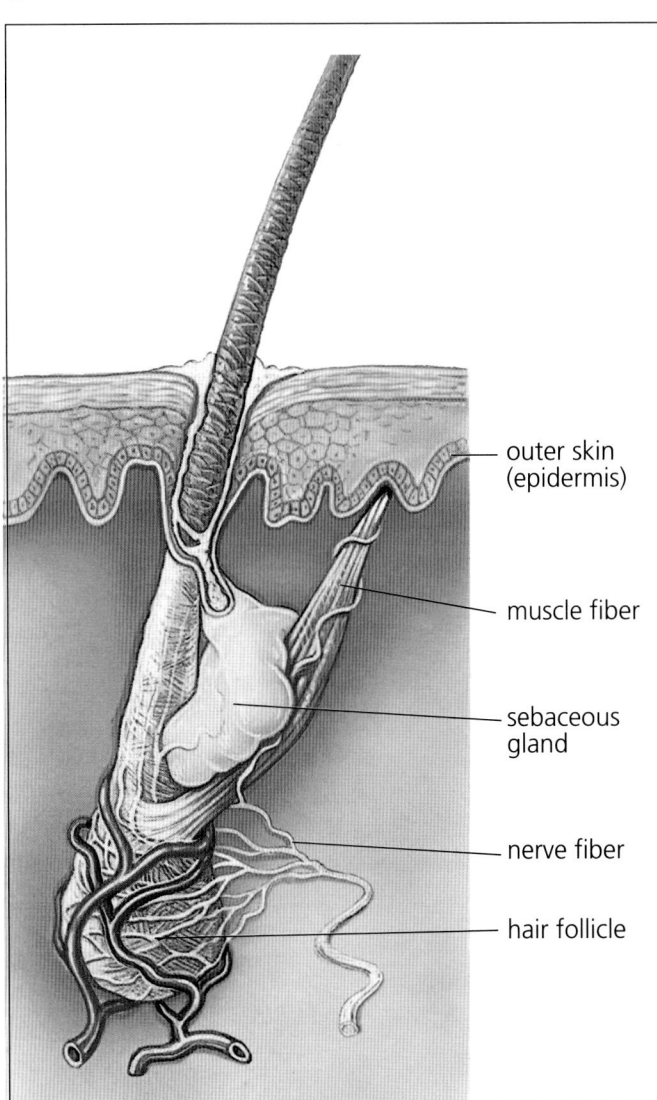

outer skin (epidermis)

muscle fiber

sebaceous gland

nerve fiber

hair follicle

Shampoo

Because the keratin cells comprising each hair are dead, the vitamins, proteins, and other nutrients contained in many hair-care products are wasted. Proper hair care simply means regular washing. There is almost no difference in the effectiveness of different shampoos, although they vary significantly in price and fragrance.

Coloring

Artificially coloring hair is quite harmful to it. For the color to penetrate the hair shaft, the hair must first be prepared by applying a harsh alkaline agent.

It is thought that some hair coloring products can enter the bloodstream through the skin, creating a favorable environment for cancer to develop.

Frequent use of hair color can also lead to allergies, a common ailment of hairdressers.

A more favorable alternative to chemical hair colors are natural dyes such as henna, walnut leaves, or tea.

Permanent Waves

The process of permanent waving involves first relaxing the hair with one chemical and then curling it with another. When done professionally, a permanent will not harm the scalp. Permanent waving, and bleaching, too frequently can lead to split ends, which can only be eliminated by cutting them off.

Conditioners and Gels

The use of conditioners and gels entails no health risk and does not harm the hair. Conditioners make hair more easily manageable after shampooing and give hair a smoother, thicker appearance; they coat each hair with a thin film consisting mostly of oils, emulsifiers, and waxes.

Shaving Cream

Aerosol shaving creams are widely used even though the propellants they contain escape into the atmosphere and accumulate there. A more ecologically sound solution would be the use of soap or nonaerosol cream.

DANDRUFF

Complaints

Dandruff is principally a cosmetic problem. For flaky skin elsewhere on the body, see Skin, p. 261, and Psoriasis, p. 278.

Causes

The scalp is constantly shedding dead cells. What is called "dandruff" occurs when more cells than usual are shed, due to various causes including seborrheic dermatitis (p. 276) or psoriasis (p. 278). Dandruff is not caused by faulty nutrition or affected by diet.

Prevention

Prevention of dandruff is not an option given current levels of medical knowledge.

Possible Aftereffects and Complications

Dandruff is harmless.

When to Seek Medical Advice

Seek medical advice if dandruff becomes severe, or if less severe outbreaks do not respond to self-help.

Self-Help

You can decrease dandruff formation by:

— Specially formulated dandruff shampoos contain sulfur or tar compounds. Dandruff shampoos become effective after 3 or 4 weeks of use. You may need to try several shampoos until you find one that works for you. After each washing, rinse hair well. Washing hair too often and blow-drying at high temperatures can irritate the scalp and encourage

Hairwashing Tips

— Washing hair daily will not harm hair or hasten oil buildup.
— Choose a mild shampoo. Shampooing once per washing is sufficient.
— Rinse hair well (about five times longer than shampooing time).
— Shampoo prices have nothing to do with product quality.
— The listing of pH on shampoo labels is just advertising. All shampoos are formulated to correspond to the scalp's pH.
— Air-drying your hair is best. High-temperature blow dryers can damage hair.

dandruff formation.

— If dandruff becomes severe, wash with a selenium sulfide shampoo, e.g., Selsun. Results should become evident within a few weeks. Side effects may include faster oil buildup and, if hair has been insufficiently rinsed, a yellow tinge to hair.

HAIR LOSS, BALDNESS

Complaints

Partial or complete loss of hair.

Causes

Starting at about age 25, everyone experiences some thinning of hair.

In men, baldness is almost always part of the natural aging process. The extent of the hair loss is hereditary, determined by the mother's or father's genes.

Many women experience increased hair growth during pregnancy; about three months after giving birth, hair may become thinner than usual, returning to normal thereafter. Thinning of hair is a universal symptom after menopause. These changes are caused by changes in estrogen and male sex hormones.

Hair loss can also be caused by tight ponytails or similar hairstyles pulling on the roots.

Sudden temporary hair loss may be caused by acute serious illness, operations, stress, anemia (see p. 345), or discontinuing oral contraceptive use. Cancer chemotherapy is often accompanied by hair loss (see Cancer, p. 470); vitamin A, beta-blockers, and medications for high cholesterol, arthritis, and stomach ulcers can also cause hair loss.

Who's at Risk

Hair loss is normal in men.

Prevention

Prevention of hair loss is not an option given current levels of medical knowledge.

Possible Aftereffects and Complications

Hair loss is harmless, but can strongly affect feelings of self-worth.

When to Seek Medical Advice

Seek medical advice if you feel your hair loss is not due to natural aging factors.

Self-Help
If you are unwilling to accept your thinning hair, buying a wig or hairpiece is an option. The effectiveness of the many "wonder drugs" on the market for baldness has not been proven.

Treatment
Eighty to 90 percent of users of a 2 percent minoxidil solution (Rogaine) rubbed into the scalp twice a day have experienced a termination of hair loss. Perhaps half of the users experience new hair growth. After treatment is discontinued, hair loss may resume as before.

Similarly, many men have experienced an increase in hair growth through the use of Propecia, a pill typically taken once a day.

Hair transplants from elsewhere on the head have proven effective on a temporary basis. The transplanted hair may fall out after a few years. Eventually, the original hair surrounding the transplants may fall out, leaving islands of transplanted hair on an otherwise bare scalp.

Transplants are performed under local anesthesia; small sections of scalp containing 10 to 15 active hair follicles are removed and implanted into the desired area, where skin has been removed. Between 10 and 40 sections are transplanted at a time. For best cosmetic results, 100 to 200 such operations are necessary; large-scale transplants can be costly. Hair will never grow again in the places where the transplants originated.

FOLLICULITIS

Complaints
Characterized by pustules surrounded by a reddened area, pierced by a hair, frequently found on the torso or in the beard area.

Causes
Pus-filled inflammations of the upper follicle frequently have no known cause. During shaving, beard hairs may bend and reenter the skin, causing inflammation.

Prevention
Prevention is not an option. To avoid beard inflammation, pluck ingrown hairs with tweezers.

If ingrown beard hairs are a frequent problem, growing a beard will stop the complaint.

Who's at Risk
Superficial folliculitis occurs in all humans, but ingrown beard hairs only in men.

Possible Aftereffects and Complications
Superficial folliculitis can develop into boils or carbuncles (see p. 284).

When to Seek Medical Advice
Seek medical advice if symptoms are bothersome.

Self-Help
Change your shaving methods. Avoid dampness, heat, sweating, and oily ointments.

Treatment
Swab affected areas with antiseptic or antibiotic preparations.

ALOPECIA AREATA

Complaints
Sudden hair loss in circular patches on head or in beard area.

Causes
Unknown.

Who's at Risk
This ailment may affect anyone at any age; it is often seen in children.

Prevention
Not possible.

Misconceptions About Hair and Hair Loss
— Hair loss is not caused by dandruff or frequent shampooing.
— Pulling out hair will not cause permanent local baldness.
— Frequent haircuts will not hasten hair growth.
— Frequent haircuts or shaving will not cause hair to grow in more thickly.
— Good scalp circulation does not result in increased hair growth.

Possible Aftereffects and Complications

About one third of cases will clear up in a few months; one third will persist, with permanent hair loss in those areas; one third will spread into permanent hair loss all over the body.

When to Seek Medical Advice

Seek medical advice if hair loss is proceeding rapidly.

Self-Help

Cover affected areas with hairpieces, kerchiefs ,or hats.

Treatment

The effectiveness of corticosteroid injections under the scalp has not been proven. Artificially irritating the scalp to produce contact dermatitis to stimulate new hair growth involves lengthy treatment and its effectiveness is uncertain.

NAILS

Nails are made of keratin, a horny material that grows slowly out of the nail bed. Fingernails grow more quickly than toenails, and an average thumbnail grows about four-thousands of an inch per day.

Hardly any other body part is as susceptible as the nails to the minor injuries caused by work- or weather-related impacts, chemical irritations, or extremely cold or wet conditions.

The effects of numerous general illnesses can be traced in the nails, for instance, slowed growth, thinness or brittleness, deformations, or discolorations (see Misshapen Nails in Signs and Symptoms section, p. 114).

Nails may split when, as a result of excessive exposure to water, soap and detergents, the top layers detach and splinter off. As a preventive measure, rubber gloves should be worn when handling alkaline solutions such as soaps or detergents, possibly with cotton gloves underneath them.

Brittle or soft nails are usually an indication of general ill health; this should be investigated further. Massaging nails with nail cream or olive oil will improve their condition.

Grooves, pits or blotches on the nails are considered normal, unless pits are extensive: This may indicate psoriasis (see p. 278) and requires medical attention.

Furrows in the nails develop as a result of minor injuries to the nail bed and disappear without treatment.

Bluish nails indicate bleeding under the nail due to an impact or compression. They are often painful. This condition may disappear without treatment.

Yellowish nails usually result from wearing nail polish and are harmless.

White spots on the nails indicate minor injuries to the nail and are harmless.

Some skin disorders may affect the nails, e.g., fungal infections (see Athlete's Foot, p. 265).

NAIL CARE

— Cut nails regularly; short nails don't tear or split easily.
— If toenails are cut straight across instead of rounding the edges, they damage the surrounding skin less easily.
— After washing hands, push cuticles back with a towel or the other thumb. Do not cut cuticles.
— If nail polish chips, it's better for the nail to apply polish to the chipped portion than to redo the whole nail.
— To keep nails from becoming soft and brittle, don't use nail polish remover more than once a week.
— Immerse dry, brittle nails frequently in a plant oil such as sunflower or olive.
— Older people and those suffering from diabetes should always seek medical advice for nail-bed infections. If possible, those with impaired sensation should have someone help them with foot care.

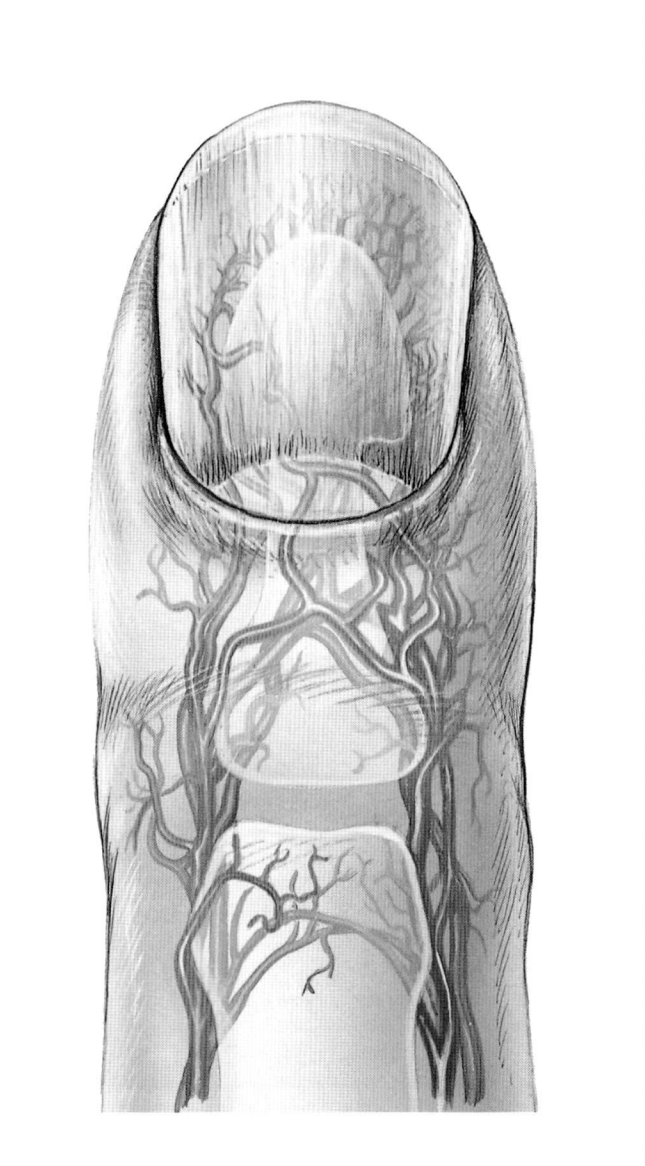

PARONYCHIA

Complaints
Symptoms of paronychia include a red, swollen, inflamed nail bed, often quite painful, with pus-filled surrounding tissue.

Causes
Paronychia is usually the result of a nail-care injury becoming infected by bacteria or fungi. Bacterial infections are usually acute; fungal infections develop more slowly.

Who's at Risk
People with diabetes and those whose hands are frequently immersed in water develop paronychia more readily than others.

Prevention
Wear polyvinyl chloride (PVC) gloves over cotton ones when working in water. Take good care of nails.

Possible Aftereffects and Complications
If the nail root is inflamed, deformations and discolorations often result.

When to Seek Medical Advice
Seek medical advice if you exhibit the symptoms of paronychia.

Self-Help
Not possible.

Treatment
If the infection is caused by bacteria, it is treated with antibiotics. If it is caused by a fungus, the infected areas are treated with a topical (or oral) antifungal medication for several months; the medication should not be forced under the nail. If treatment proves ineffective, an antifungal may be given orally. These medications occasionally cause serious side effects.
Important: All fungal medications, whether topical or oral, must be taken for as long as they are prescribed, even if this means months and even if all signs of disease have disappeared; the fungus may still be present in the tissues.

INGROWN TOENAILS

Complaints
An ingrown toenail is one—usually on the big toe—whose corners have grown into the surrounding soft tissue, causing pain and inflammation.

Causes
Ingrown toenails are caused by cutting nails too short at the corners.

Who's at Risk
Wearing excessively tight shoes encourages ingrown toenails.

Prevention
Cut toenails straight across so the corners extend over the skin.

Possible Aftereffects and Complications
Painful inflammations.

When to Seek Medical Advice
Seek help if the surrounding tissue becomes inflamed, or if you are diabetic.

Self-Help
If surrounding tissue is not yet inflamed, a thin piece of cotton cloth may be inserted under the corners of the affected nail to enable it to grow without digging into the flesh. Change the cloth twice a day and wear loose, comfortable socks and shoes.

Treatment
It may be necessary to remove the ingrown toenail by minor surgery.

RESPIRATORY SYSTEM

We breathe by using the respiratory muscles of the chest and diaphragm to inflate the lungs. Air is taken in through the nose and passes through the pharynx, larynx, and bronchial tubes. It is filtered, warmed, and moistened in the nose, and, like food taken in through the mouth, passes through the pharynx. At the larynx, air and food go their separate ways: When we swallow food, the flap of skin called the epiglottis blocks the trachea and food enters the esophagus. During an in-breath, the epiglottis is open and air travels through the trachea into the bronchi.

Like the branches of a tree, the bronchi are a system of tubes transporting air through finer and smaller passages to the alveoli of the lungs.

A dense network of capillaries surrounds each alveolus, working to change the makeup of the blood. Oxygen breathed in with the air enters the bloodstream; carbon dioxide produced in the body travels through the blood into the alveoli where it is then expelled from the lungs. When we exhale, the respiratory muscles relax and the thorax collapses, forcing the air out. The vocal cords in the larynx vibrate with the exhalation, making speech possible.

The various airways from the nose into the smallest bronchioles have a slippery membrane, the pleura, which keeps the passages moist and elastic through the continuous secretion of mucus by numerous tiny glands. With the help of numerous small cilia (also a part of the membrane), the mucus transports foreign substances such as dust and soot back into the mouth cavity.

When the membrane becomes inflamed, it swells and produces even more mucus—e.g., the fluid from the nose and the mucus coughed up in bronchitis.

Constant irritation to the airways from smoking or air pollution may permanently damage the mucous membranes. During excess mucus production, the number of cilia decreases, irritating the bronchi and making it harder to expel any mucus.

Nose

The nose is not simply our organ of smell: it is also the first stop for air on the way to the alveoli of the lungs. As it enters the nose, air is filtered by fine hairs, then moistened by the mucous membranes and warmed by delicate capillaries before it proceeds to the pharynx. Passages connect the nose with the nasolacrimal duct,

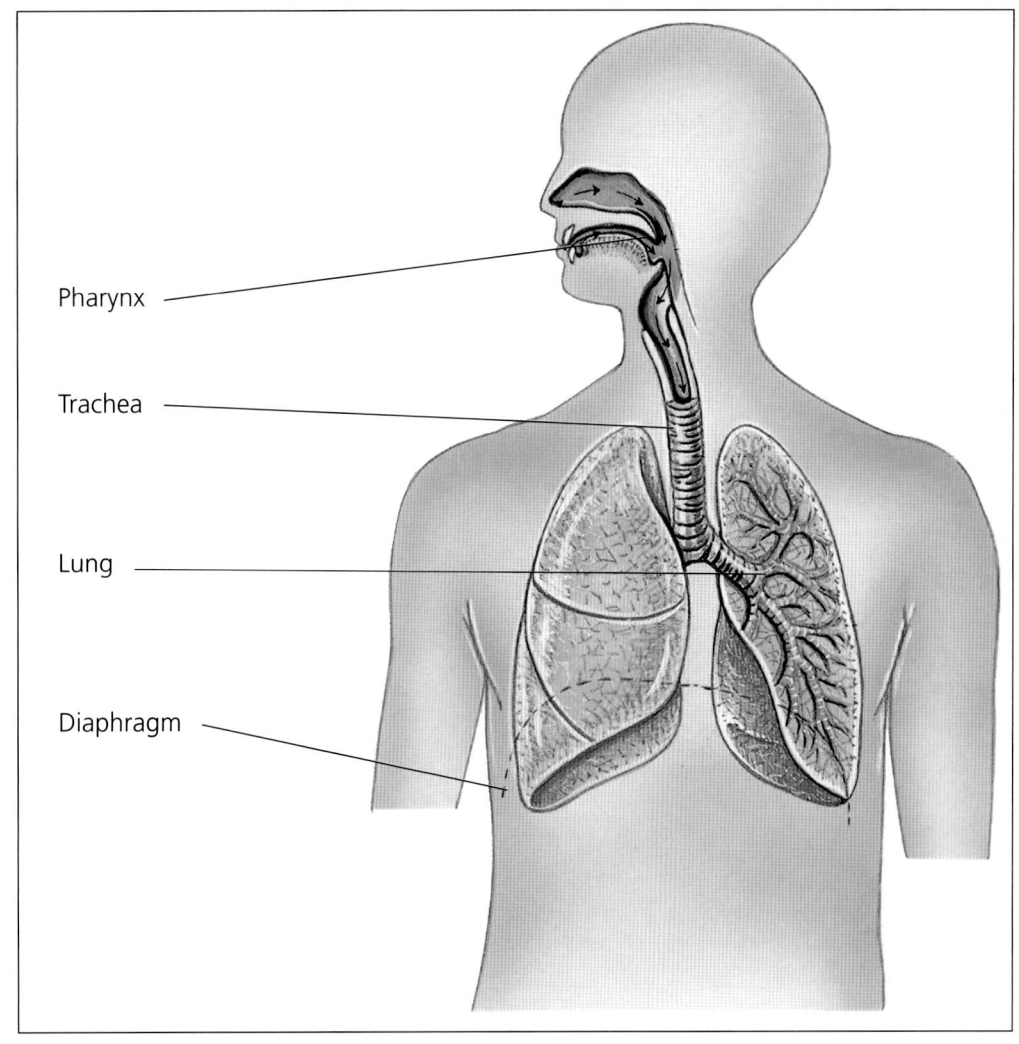

Pharynx

Trachea

Lung

Diaphragm

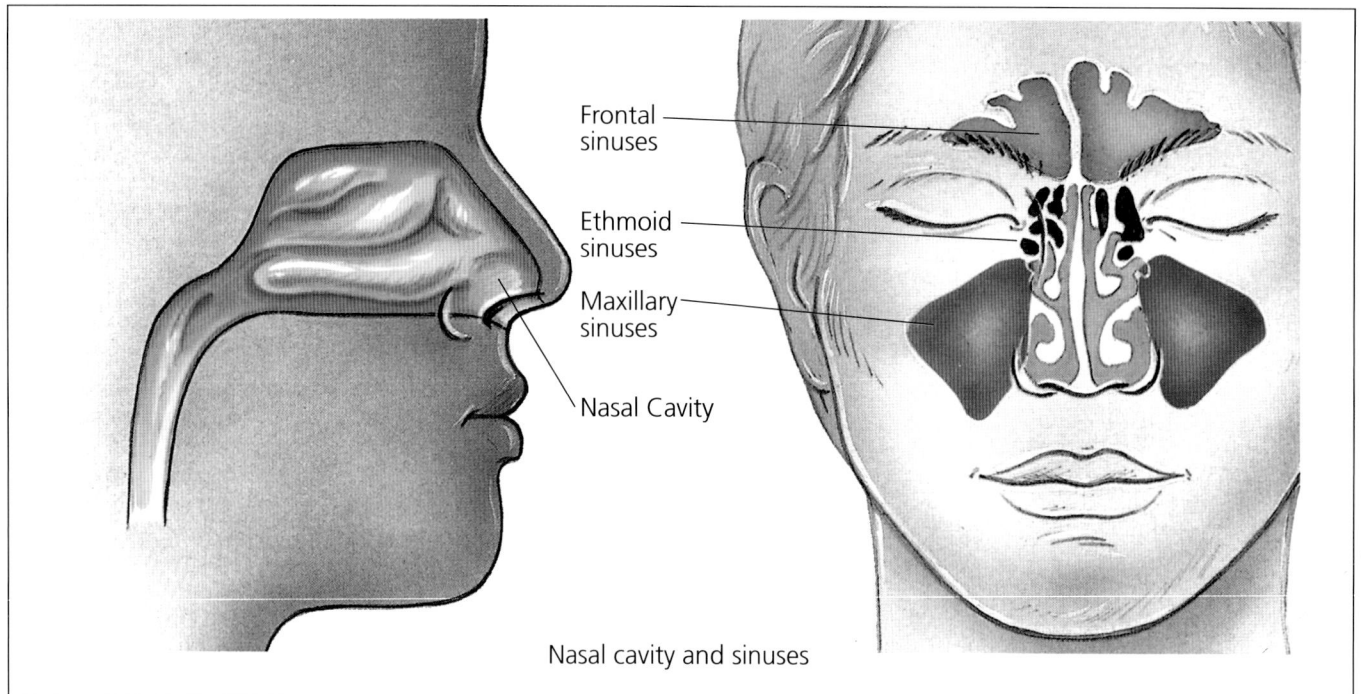

Frontal sinuses

Ethmoid sinuses

Maxillary sinuses

Nasal Cavity

Nasal cavity and sinuses

the sinuses, and the middle ear. The sinuses, mucous membrane-lined chambers in the facial bones, also warm the inhaled air.

INJURIES, NOSEBLEEDS

Nose injuries can be open, visibly apparent and bleeding, or they can occur inside the capillaries of the mucous membrane.

The nasal bone or cartilage may be injured in accidents.

Complaints

A nosebleed is evident from its symptoms.

A fractured nasal bone is recognizable by a deformed nose and the ability to move the nose in unusual directions or to an unusual degree, accompanied by pain.

Causes

Nose injuries are usually caused by a fall or sudden impact.

Nosebleeds occur when the capillaries, especially those in the front of the nose, are injured by impact or frequent nose-blowing, or when the mucous membrane is dried out. Some people have chronic nosebleeds for no apparent reason.

Who's at Risk

People especially prone to nosebleeds include those with high blood pressure, arterial sclerosis, or blood clotting disorders.

Possible Aftereffects and Complications

Nosebleeds: Although often alarming, they are usually harmless and can easily be stopped. Only rarely does a nosebleed lead to serious blood loss; this is possible in conjunction with a blood clotting disorder.

External injuries: As with all open injuries, there is a risk of infection.

Internal injuries: Sometimes a nasal bone fracture or dislocation of the nasal cartilage may block or constrict air flow to the nasal cavity or the sinuses. In rare cases, this can result in blood clot (hematoma) and infection.

Prevention

Those prone to nosebleeds should keep nasal membranes from drying out. Dry air, especially in heated rooms, should be kept humid. Avoid blowing the nose forcefully.

When to Seek Medical Advice

Seek medical help if:

—You are unable to control a nosebleed or nosebleeds occur frequently and are not attributable to a cold or injury.

— You have an open wound—a cut or tear; serious injuries should be stitched under local anesthesia.

— You have an injury to the nasal bone or cartilage; X rays will reveal any fracture, and treatment options will be explored.

Self-Help
Immediate aid for a severe nosebleed: Bend head forward and firmly pinch the nostrils shut for 5 to 10 minutes. A cold washcloth or ice placed at the nape of the neck can also help. Cold constricts the capillaries. If possible, avoid blowing nose for 12 hours following a nosebleed so the blood vessels can heal.

Injuries: Open wounds in the nasal area should be covered with a clean, dry cloth until you get to a doctor. With injuries to the nasal bone or cartilage, no self-help is possible.

Treatment
Nosebleed: For a severe nosebleed that cannot be stopped by manual pressure, the doctor applies a gauze strip that presses on the ruptured blood vessel and remains in place for 12 hours. In rare cases, silver nitrate is used to seal the ruptured blood vessel.

If nosebleed is caused by an illness (high blood pressure or blood clotting disorder) the illness should be treated (see High Blood Pressure, p. 321; Thrombocytopenia, p. 349).

External injuries: The wound should be cleaned and disinfected (and stitched as needed) professionally.

Internal injuries: If the nasal bone is fractured and needs setting, it can usually be set later under local anesthesia in adults.

Dislocated nasal cartilage in the front part of the nose does not require treatment as long as breathing is not affected. However, if after an injury of this kind breathing becomes difficult or sinus infections increase, surgical intervention may be indicated.

THE FLU

Complaints
A cold is often the first and only symptom of a flu. Sore throat, slight cough, headaches, joint pains, exhaustion, and fever may also be present.

Causes
The flu is a viral infection of the upper airways, easily transmitted from one person to another through sneezing or coughing. It is highly contagious, causing many people to become infected one after the other.

The virus manifests first in the mucous membranes of the nose and pharynx, causing swelling and increased mucus production; the virus can then spread to the bronchi or sinuses.

Who's at Risk
Children frequently get the flu as their immune systems adapt to the many different viruses to which we are all exposed.

Flus are more common in winter than other times of the year, probably because people spend more time indoors in close contact with each other, enabling the viruses to be spread easily by way of tiny droplets in the air.

Possible Aftereffects and Complications
Flus cause discomfort but are harmless, clearing up after 3 to 5 days.

Sometimes, particularly in the case of the influenza virus, the infection may spread to the lungs, brain, or heart. Only when an influenza virus is involved is the illness a "bona fide" flu.

With all flus, additional bacteria may settle in the mucous membranes, causing secondary infections. This is of particular concern in young children, the elderly, and those with immune systems weakened by disease or medications; occasionally a flu may end in death.

Prevention
The flu is extremely contagious; the only way to prevent infecting others is to stay home when sick.

"Flu shots" offer protection from only a small number of viruses (see Immunizations, p. 667), and many can trigger the illness itself.

Taking additional vitamins does not decrease the chances of catching a flu (see Healthy Nutrition, p. 722).

When to Seek Medical Advice
Seek medical help if the flu lasts longer than 7 days, or if the infection spreads and self-help measures are not effective after 3 days. Signs of a worsening flu include: Fever exceeding 102.2°F; severe sore throat or earache; dry, painful cough; breathing difficulties; severe headache.

Self-Help

Stay in a warm (but not overheated) environment. Rest. Soothe the infected mucous membranes and lessen irritation by humidifying the air.

If you have no appetite, don't force yourself to eat, but make sure to drink plenty of liquids.

Fever is an important defense mechanism of the body, killing many viruses at high temperatures. A temperature up to 105.8°F is not considered harmful if the body is not weakened by other illnesses. For a high fever, tepid compresses may be helpful (see Compresses, p. 692). Sweating may also be beneficial (see Heat Baths, p. 691).

Treatment

Try to relieve the symptoms (see below; Pharyngitis, p. 302).

Medications containing acetaminophen (e.g. Tylenol) or ibuprofen (e.g., Motrin, Advil) (see Analgesics, p. 660) may help to bring down fever, relieve headaches, and make sleep easier .

Be cautious of so-called "flu medications" containing several active ingredients: Their therapeutic effectiveness is doubtful and some combinations can also be harmful.

COLDS

Complaints

A congested nose is usually the first, often the only, symptom of the common cold. The nose runs, breathing through it becomes more difficult, the voice sounds hoarse or congested and the sense of smell is impaired. The clear, watery discharge may later thicken and turn greenish-yellow.

Causes

Colds are usually triggered by viruses transmitted from one person to another through airborne droplets. (This is not the case with allergic colds such as hayfever—see p. 299). The illness causes the mucous membranes of the nose to get red, swollen, and produce a discharge. Sometimes bacteria also settle in the inflamed nasal passages. If you have already taken nose drops for an extended period, see Colds from Cold Medications, p. 299.

Who's at Risk

Children are at increased risk for colds because their bodies are still building immune defenses against the large variety of cold-causing viruses.

Possible Aftereffects and Complications

In most cases, a cold is harmless and clears up after 3 to 5 days.

If the infection spreads to the sinuses, the illness may last longer (see Sinusitis, p. 300).

A cold may create problems for infants when they attempt to drink. In small children, a clogged nose can easily lead to infection of the middle ear.

Prevention

Not possible.

When to Seek Medical Advice

Seek help if
— The cold lasts longer than 5 to 7 days.
— The cold has spread to the sinuses or lower respiratory system. Symptoms include: Fever of over 102.2°F; severe sore throat or earache; dry or painful cough; breathing difficulties; pain in forehead or under eyes.

Some effective short-term use nose drops and sprays

Phenylephrine (Neo-Synephrine)
Oxymetazoline (Afrin)

Important side effects: After the effect of the medication wears off, it is often followed by increased swelling of the mucous membranes and, after prolonged use, the condition known as "medication cold" may develop. Infants may develop impaired breathing, unconsciousness, or agitation.

Recommendation: Use for a maximum of 2 to 3 days.

Natural and Homeopathic Remedies for Colds

There are many different kinds available.

Not recommended: "Cold Medications"

Some of these medications contain antihistamines, which do not affect cold symptoms and may cause drowsiness. Other products can elevate blood pressure to undesirable levels, and some may even make colds worse.

Saline rinses: helpful and harmless

Dissolve 1 part salt to 100 parts water. Drip into nose as you would nose drops. For small children, administer 1 to 2 drops in each nostril five times a day. A solution with no more than 1 percent salt will cause no harm; the nose may sting after treatment, however.

There are numerous over-the-counter saline products available as nose drops, sprays, and gels.

Self-Help

— Drink plenty of liquids to keep discharge watery.
— Keep your environment warm but not hot. Avoid further irritation to the nasal mucous membranes by humidifying the air—either by using a humidifier or hanging up moist towels.
— Use saline-solution nose drops.
— Inhaling warm steam will clear a stuffy nose and help reduce swelling in the nasal passages. Sniffing saline solution, taking a warm shower or steam bath, or going swimming can also help.
— Blow the nose properly: Close one nostril and blow air through the other. If you close both nostrils at the same time, some of the mucus may be forced up the nasal passages, increasing the risk of sinus infection.

Treatment

One can only ease a cold's symptoms, not cure it. If self-help measures fail, vasoconstricting medication is the next option. Depending on the product, effectiveness may last 3 to 9 hours. These products may make drinking easier for infants with colds.

Colds from Cold Medications

If nose drops are used for more than 2 to 3 days, discontinuing the medication may cause marked swelling and the condition known as "medication cold." If nose drops are begun again to combat the symptoms, the process can turn into a vicious circle leading to a chronic medicated cold and causing serious damage to the nasal mucous membranes.

For this reason cold medications should not be taken for more than 3 days, followed by a 10-day break.

For those who have used nose drops for an extended period of time, withdrawal can be hard. These tips may help:

— Use nose drops in one nostril only until the swelling has subsided in the other, so you can always breathe through at least one nostril.
— Instead of medicated nose drops, try saline solution (see pink box opposite).

HAY FEVER

(see also Allergies, p. 360)

Complaints

An "allergic cold" is one symptom of an allergic reaction and is characterized by nasal discharge (usually watery and clear), frequent sneezing, and, usually, itchy, watery eyes.

Causes

Predisposition to allergic reactions is probably congenital, although the triggering of an allergic reaction depends on many factors (see Allergies, p. 360). Individual psychological conditions and stress levels help determine when and how the body finally reacts to one or more of the many potential irritants in the environment.

Hay fever results when the nasal mucous membranes respond to allergens such as pollen from certain blossoms, dust mites, or dander from pets.

In an allergic cold, the nasal mucous membranes swell and produce excessive amounts of discharge.

Who's at Risk

— Those prone to allergic reactions, skin rashes, or asthma are at increased risk for hay fever.
— The risk also increases with prolonged contact with the allergen.

Possible Aftereffects and Complications

Those suffering from allergic colds are frequently susceptible to sinusitis (see p. 300).

Hay fever may develop into asthma over time.

Prevention

Prevention is possible only if you determine what triggers allergies and then try to avoid the cause. Symptoms during spring and early summer are usually caused by pollen. If you can find out which pollen is affecting you, you can avoid it, perhaps by taking a vacation during the blooming season: There is hardly any pollen above altitudes of 6,000 feet and by the ocean. During peak season, the media report levels and movements of certain windborne allergens (pollen, smuts, and mold).

If animal hair or dander cause allergies, you may have to get rid of your pets. For controlling house dust mites, see Allergies, p. 360.

When to Seek Medical Advice

Seek help if you suspect your cold is caused by allergies.

Self-Help for Pollen Allergies

— Wash your hair at night.
— Keep windows closed at night.
— Don't mow lawns or prune shrubs when pollen count is highest.
— Certain allergy nose drops (e.g., NasalCrom) and other cold medicines are available without prescription.

Treatment

Because your psychological condition can affect the development of allergies as well as their intensity, it is wise to choose a health-care professional trained in treating psychosomatic illness.

It's preferable to treat an allergic cold by preventing or avoiding the cause rather than treating the runny nose. By asking specific questions, the doctor may be able to identify what triggers the allergy.

Desensitization (see Allergies, p. 360) is most successful when hay fever is triggered by only a few different kinds of pollen.

Treatment with Medication

Hay fever may be treated with medications containing cromolyn sodium. These take effect over a few days, and may be preventative.

Nose drops to reduce swelling associated with colds may also ease the symptoms (see Colds, p. 298).

Hay fever may also be controlled with antihistamines taken orally (See Allergies, p. 360).

SINUSITIS

The sinuses are hollow cavities in the facial bones located next to, behind, and above the nose (in the forehead, they are called frontal sinuses). They connect to the nasal cavity and are lined with mucous membranes.

Complaints

Sinus infections are indicated by headaches, pains, and the sensation of pressure in cheekbones or above eyes a few days after the onset of a cold. Usually the nose has stopped running. The pains are especially strong on getting up or bending over.

Causes

During a cold, bacteria or viruses enter the sinuses and cause swelling in the mucous membranes of the interconnecting canals, preventing normal drainage.

Sinuses may also be affected by an allergic cold (see Hay Fever, p. 299).

Who's at Risk

The risk of sinusitis is increased in
— Persons with nasal polyps (see p. 301)
— Persons with a deviated septum, which further constricts the passages of the sinuses
— Those suffering from allergic colds

Sometimes frequent sinusitis is the only symptom of an allergy.

Possible Aftereffects and Complications

When bacterial sinusitis is recognized early and treated properly, there are seldom serious consequences. Left untreated, it may in rare cases spread to the brain.

Prevention

When you have a cold, drink lots of fluids, keep the air moist and inhale steam (or saline solution) several times a day. This helps with colds and also aids in preventing sinusitis. Proper, frequent nose-blowing will also help (see Colds, p. 298).

If you frequently suffer from sinusitis, use a saline solution and nose drops (if your doctor approves) when you have a cold to help decrease swelling in the mucous membranes (see Colds, p. 298).

For those who frequently have sinusitis caused by nasal polyps or a deviated septum, a doctor can recommend whether to remove the polyps or correct the septum. Frequent sinusitis sufferers should also be investigated for allergies (see p. 360).

When to Seek Medical Advice

— Seek help if symptoms last longer than 3 days or are accompanied by high fever.
— If you frequently suffer from sinusitis.

Self-Help

Often sinusitis will subside on its own after 2 to 3 days. To relieve symptoms, treat as for a cold with warmth, humidity, and inhalations (see Colds, p. 298).

Treatment

Nose drops should reduce swelling in the mucous membranes and reopen the connecting passages between the nasal cavity and sinuses (see Colds, p. 298). If the source is a bacterial infection or the condition lasts longer than 3 days, antibiotic treatment is necessary (see Antibiotics, p. 661).

Occasionally, surgery is recommended to open a passage between the nasal cavity and sinuses.

NASAL POLYPS

Complaints

Nasal polyps only rarely cause problems. However, they may make breathing through the nose difficult, causing the voice to sound "nasal." People with nasal polyps tend to breathe through the mouth and, because they do this while sleeping, often snore.

Causes

Nasal polyps most often are benign growths of the nasal mucous membrane.

Who's at Risk

People with allergic colds are at increased risk of developing nasal polyps.

Possible Aftereffects and Complications

Nasal polyps may make it difficult to breathe through the nose, causing increased mouth breathing, especially during sleep. Mouth breathing does not allow pathogens in the air to be filtered by the nose, making upper respiratory infections more likely.

A polyp may block a sinus connection, causing frequent sinusitis.

In children nasal polyps are often the cause of middle ear infections.

Prevention

Not possible.

When to Seek Medical Advice

Seek help if
— Breathing through the nose is obstructed, your voice is nasal, and you snore.
— You frequently have sinusitis.
— Children have frequent middle ear infections. Using an illumination device, doctors can determine whether nasal polyps are at fault.

Self-Help

Not possible.

Treatment

Nasal polyps do not require treatment as long as they cause no problems; in fact, many people have them without knowing it. However, if they cause frequent sinusitis they can be surgically removed in a relatively easy operation.

Throat and Pharynx

After inhaled air has been filtered, moistened and warmed by the nasal cavities and sinuses, it passes through the pharynx and into the trachea. Look in a mirror, open your mouth wide and press down the tongue: on either side of the back of your throat you see a rounded mass. These are the tonsils, a part of the body's immune system, which swell when an infection is being fought. When we inhale, the epiglottis opens to let air pass by the vocal cords and trachea, and on into the bronchi.

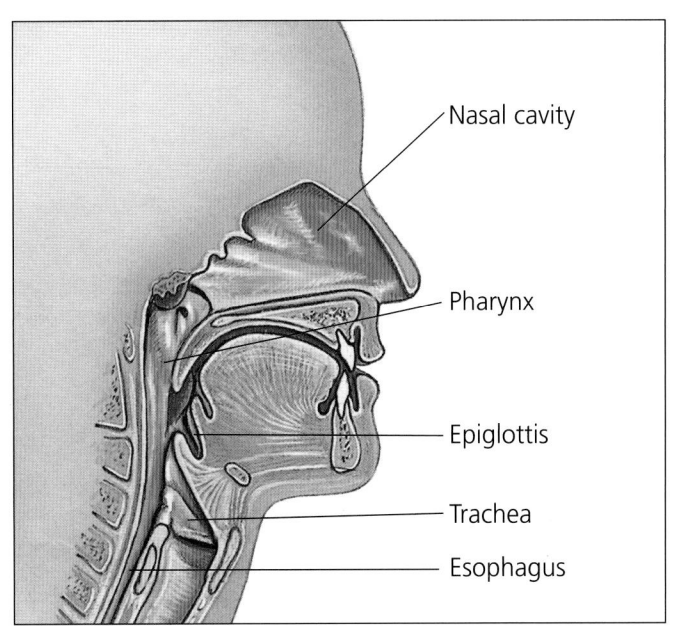

Nasal cavity

Pharynx

Epiglottis

Trachea

Esophagus

In the larynx, exhaled air in conjunction with the vibrating vocal cords makes speech possible. All parts of the pharynx are lined with mucous membranes.

TONSILLITIS

Complaints

Symptoms of tonsillitis are sore throat, difficulty swallowing, fever, and headaches. In the pharynx, the tonsils are visibly red and swollen, often coated with small white dots.

Causes

Tonsillitis is often caused by a streptococcal bacterial infection transmitted between people on airborne droplets. Sometimes a viral infection in the pharynx causes tonsils to become red and swollen.

Who's at Risk

Tonsillitis occurs frequently during childhood and only rarely in adults.

Possible Aftereffects and Complications

Strep infections during childhood may cause serious heart illnesses or kidney problems later on if they are not treated promptly with antibiotics.

Prevention

If a family member has tonsillitis caused by strep, it may be advisable to take penicillin as a precaution.

When to Seek Medical Advice

Seek help if tonsillitis is suspected and symptoms don't improve within 2 days.

Self-Help

Stay in bed, keep warm, and take only soft or liquid nourishment. Drink plenty of fluids but avoid fruit juices, which irritate the throat (cold milk is often soothing).

Treatment with Medication

If the cause is bacterial, the treatment is penicillin (see Antibiotics, p. 661). Viral tonsillitis is treated like pharyngitis (see below).

If fever and headaches are present and sleep is difficult, a mild analgesic with acetaminophen (e.g., Tylenol), acetylsalicylic acid (e.g., aspirin) or ibuprofen (e.g., Motrin, Advil) may be appropriate to control pain and lower temperature (see Analgesics, p. 660).

Surgery

Children should retain their tonsils, which serve an important immune function, for as long as possible. Tonsils should be removed only if they are enlarged and causing breathing difficulties (recognizable by loud snoring, or interruption of regular breathing), or if tonsillitis recurs despite treatment (in children, four cases of pharyngitis in a year would be the benchmark).

PHARYNGITIS

Complaints

Symptoms of pharyngitis (infection in the upper pharynx) include sore throat, difficulty swallowing and possible fever. The back of the pharynx becomes red and swollen.

Causes

Pharyngitis is usually viral and often accompanies or follows a flu. Occasionally it is caused by streptococcal bacteria. Long-term sinusitis may also spread into the pharynx.

Who's at Risk

A compromised mucous membrane makes it easier to contract pharyngitis. Excessive alcohol consumption, cigarette smoke, industrial and automotive pollution, and irritants or hazardous substances in the workplace can all increase susceptibility to pharyngitis.

Possible Aftereffects and Complications

Pharyngitis may last for weeks or months or become chronic in smokers, in people who consume excessive alcohol, or in people frequently exposed to airborne irritants.

Pharyngitis caused by sinusitis may also become chronic and clear up only when the original cause is treated.

Prevention

Avoid substances irritating to the mucous membranes.

When to Seek Medical Advice
Seek medical advice if symptoms don't improve within 2 to 3 days.

Self-Help
The most important thing you can do is protect your irritated pharynx:
— Stay in a warm—but not hot or smoke-filled—environment, preferably a humidified one. Hanging up wet towels is one way to increase ambient humidity.
— Drink plenty of fluids but avoid fruit juices, whose acids irritate the throat.
— If symptoms are severe, take only soft nourishment or liquids, if possible.
— Gargling, or sucking on candy, can help moisten the pharynx.

Treatment
Try gargling with chamomile or sage tea, or a 1 percent saline solution.

Prolonged infection of the pharynx resulting from another illness (e.g., sinusitis) can be cured only by treating the original illness.

Gargling with medicated solutions is not recommended: These liquids may contain unnecessary (or even harmful) ingredients.

Lozenges containing antibiotics, antiseptics and/or local analgesics are also not advisable: Saliva dilutes their therapeutic properties. Tests have shown that for treating pharyngitis, lozenges are merely expensive candy and may even have a negative effect: Those that contain antibiotics can give rise to resistant strains of bacteria. It is more beneficial and cheaper to suck on sugar-free bonbons or salt tablets, which work to stimulate the flow of saliva.

In the case of a bacterial infection, antibiotics may be prescribed.

LARYNGITIS, VOCAL CORD INFLAMMATION

Complaints
During pharyngitis, the lower parts of the throat (the larynx, epiglottis, and vocal cords) frequently become affected as well. Difficulty swallowing, hoarseness, and pain in addition to the already sore throat result in what is known as laryngitis. This may also cause breathing problems and a barking cough, mainly in children (see Croup, p. 596) because their airways are narrower.

Causes
Laryngitis often accompanies a cold or flu and is usually triggered by a virus; only rarely is it bacterial in nature. A long-lasting case of sinusitis may also spread to the larynx and vocal cords.

Excessive alcohol consumption, cigarette smoke, industrial and automotive pollution, and workplace toxins that irritate the mucous membranes can all cause laryngitis. If primarily the vocal cords are affected, the cause may be loud or prolonged talking or singing.

Who's at Risk
A previously damaged laryngeal mucosa is more susceptible to illness. Smokers or people exposed to airborne irritants are at higher risk.

Possible Aftereffects and Complications
Laryngitis can become life-threatening in children (see Epiglottitis, p. 597; Croup, p. 596).

In adults the symptoms are similar to laryngeal cancer; care must be taken to ensure a proper diagnosis.

Prevention
Avoid substances that irritate the mucous membranes.

When to Seek Medical Advice
— If there is shortage of breath, go to the hospital immediately.
— Seek medical advice if symptoms such as hoarseness, pain when speaking, or sore throat last longer than three days.

Self-Help
It is most important to let the irritated larynx and vocal cords rest.
— Keep warm, but avoid smoky or overheated environments. Try to keep air moist, for example, by hanging wet towels on radiators.
— Give your voice a rest.
— Gargle with saline solution.

Treatment
In the rare cases that laryngitis is found to be caused by

bacteria, antibiotics may be prescribed; take orally, never as lozenges or for gargling.

VOCAL CORD POLYPS, NODULES, AND LARYNGEAL CANCER
(see also Cancer, p. 470)

Complaints
Tumors in the larynx can be either benign (polyps on the vocal cords) or malignant (cancer of the larynx). Early symptoms are usually gradual changes in the voice, hoarseness, sore throat, pain when speaking, and swallowing difficulties; breathing problems may develop later.

Causes
Benign tumors (nodules) may be caused by excessive stress to the vocal cords (frequent loud speaking or singing), irritants in the air (cigarette smoke, industrial pollution), or viruses.

Who's at Risk
The risk increases in those who smoke or consume excessive alcohol.

Possible Aftereffects and Complications
Failure to treat any tumor, whether malignant or benign, can result in serious breathing problems.

After removal of a cancerous larynx the patient can learn to speak with an artificial glottis. Rehabilitation with the help of a trained specialist in phoniatrics is highly recommended. Because speech is invariably affected, everyday life may become more stressful; join a support group for people in the same situation.

Prevention
After an episode of nonmalignant tumors of the vocal cords, taking good care of the voice can prevent a recurrence. Malignant tumors may possibly be prevented by a lifestyle as free of stress as possible.

When to Seek Medical Advice
Seek help
— If you intermittently or constantly have a hoarse voice, without accompanying cold or flu symptoms
— If, in conjunction with a cold or flu, symptoms of sore throat, hoarseness, and difficulty swallowing last longer than 4 days

With a specialized instrument, a doctor can check the larynx for the presence of a tumor. A biopsy can determine whether it is benign or malignant.

Self-Help
Not possible.

Treatment
Benign tumors can easily be removed surgically, often under local anesthesia.

With early recognition, a malignant tumor can sometimes be treated with radiation. However, laryngeal cancer usually calls for surgical removal. If the cancer has spread, a new opening for breathing will be created below the larynx. The patient then learns to speak using artificial vocal cords, while the opening is held shut.

Bronchi
After air is inhaled and passes through the larynx, it travels through the bronchi, a system of progressively smaller branching tubes, into the alveoli of the lungs.

The process of warming, moistening, and filtering the inhaled air, begun in the pharynx, continues in the bronchi. The bronchi are lined with a slippery membrane lining which constantly produces mucus that traps foreign material (dust, pollen, bacteria), and is then transported by the cilia into the trachea and pharynx, where it is swallowed.

The mucous membrane lining is sensitive to repeated irritation from tobacco smoke, air pollutants, or infection. Such irritants may damage the cilia, making it increasingly difficult to transport dust and mucus out of the lungs. Coughing is the body's attempt to rid itself of this matter by other means. The irritated lining becomes increasingly susceptible to infection, giving rise to more frequent attacks of bronchitis and pneumonia.

Like the nasal mucous membrane, the lining can also be the site of allergic reactions. Allergic asthma is a narrowing of the bronchi.

Finally, constant irritation of the lining can also cause malignant tumors—e.g., cancer of the bronchi.

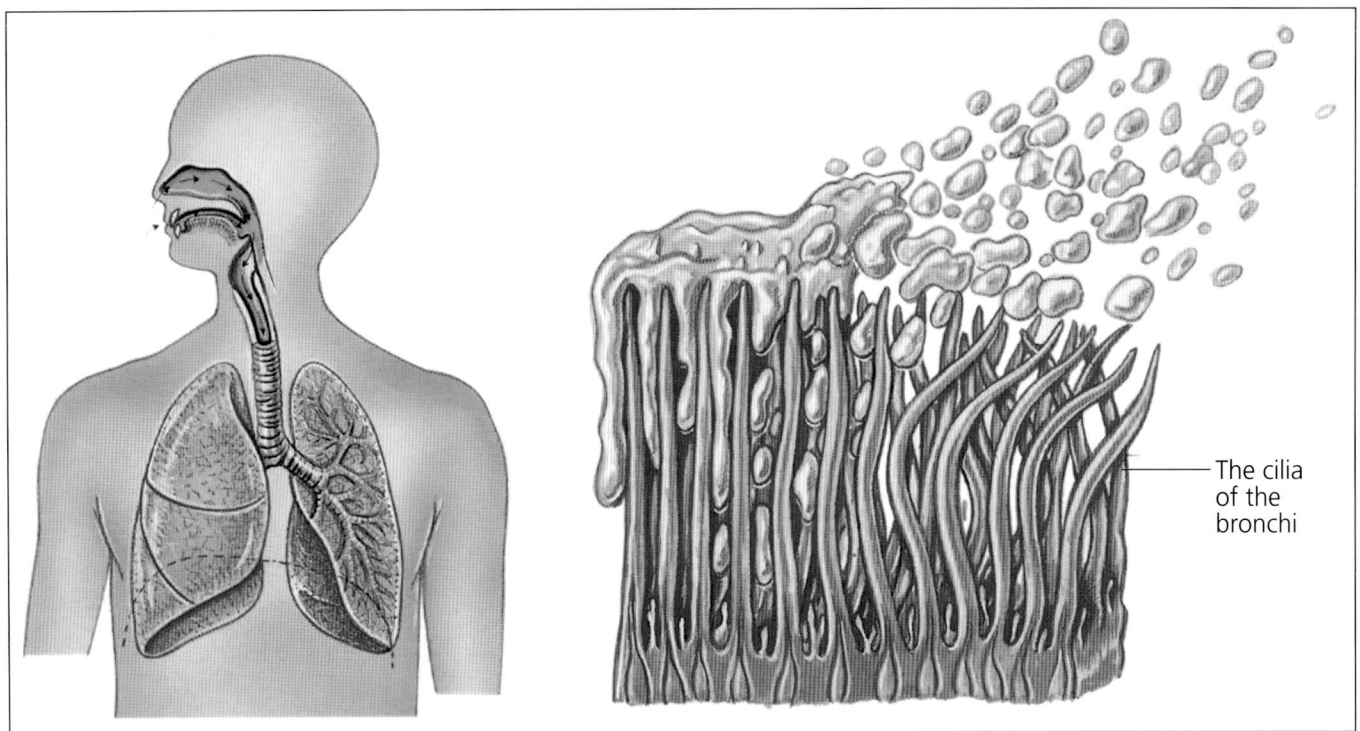

The cilia of the bronchi

ACUTE BRONCHITIS

Complaints

Acute bronchitis usually occurs in conjunction with a common cold. After 2 to 3 days, the bronchitis starts with a painful cough and, frequently, yellowish-white drainage. These symptoms are often accompanied by fever, occasionally by breathing difficulties. For bronchitis in children, see Bronchiolitis, p. 597.

Causes

The same viruses that cause the common cold can infect the bronchial lining; occasionally bronchitis is caused by bacteria invading a damaged bronchial lining.

Who's at Risk

The risk of acute bronchitis is increased in:
— Smokers (see Smoking, p. 754).
— People exposed to severe air pollution (see Air Pollution, p. 783; Healthy Living, p. 772).
— People with heart diseases and lung problems (asthma, emphysema, bronchiectasis).
— Children by virtue that they have colds more frequently than adults.

Possible Aftereffects and Complications

Pneumonia may develop following bronchitis in older people, or in those with weakened immune systems.

Those suffering more than one case of bronchitis a year are at risk of permanent damage to the bronchial lining.

Prevention

Try to reduce stress in life; avoid breathing polluted air; most importantly, do not smoke.

When to Seek Medical Advice

Seek help if:
— Bronchitis does not clear up after 2 to 3 days.
— Symptoms include a temperature of 102.2°F or more.
— You cough up blood.
— You have difficulty breathing.

Self-Help

Avoiding smoke- or steam-filled environments, as well as air pollution, will reduce irritants to the airways.

Stay warm but avoid overheated rooms; get plenty of rest.

Humidity in the air helps prevent additional irritation; hang damp cloths in your room. Make sure you drink plenty of liquids to keep mucus fluid. In the event of a fever, the body needs even more liquids.

Warm water compresses may reduce high fever (see Compresses, p. 692).

Cough-calming teas can be therapeutic.

Treatment

Simple bronchitis does not require medical treatment. For those who need it, a simple analgesic will relieve pain or fever (see p. 660).

Cough Remedies

Many cough remedies contain cough suppressants, particularly codeine. They are usually not beneficial because they suppress the coughing up of mucus and slow the natural process of healing.

Other products have a mucus-thinning or expectorant effect, making it easier to cough. Although these remedies appear effective, there is no conclusive evidence.

Antibiotics

In the rare cases that the cause of bronchitis has been identified as a bacterial infection (possible symptoms include a tenacious cold and greenish sputum), antibiotics may be appropriate (see Antibiotics, p. 661).

CHRONIC BRONCHITIS

Complaints

The symptoms of chronic bronchitis are the same as for acute bronchitis: Painful cough, often combined with yellowish-white sputum; occasional fever and breathing difficulties. The symptoms appear ever more frequently until they last year-round. Smokers often mistake the cough, which usually occurs in the morning, for "smoker's cough." Over the course of time the cough worsens and sputum thickens, usually leading to shortness of breath in the later stages.

For bronchitis in children, see Bronchiolitis, p. 597.

Causes

Recurring acute bronchitis causes permanent damage to the bronchial lining, leading to more frequent infections. The bronchial walls thicken, producing excessive mucus that is harder to cough up. The cough becomes chronic, accompanied by excessive sputum and shortness of breath.

Who's at Risk

The risk of chronic bronchitis is increased in people who
— Smoke (see Smoking, p. 754)
— Are exposed to air pollution (see Air Pollution, p. 783)
— Are frequently exposed to hazardous materials (see Health in the Workplace, p. 789)
— Live in substandard conditions. Economically disadvantaged people are six times as likely to suffer from chronic bronchitis as those living in clean, safe environments
— Live in foggy areas
— Were exposed to environmental pollution as children

Possible Aftereffects and Complications

Chronic bronchitis can go undetected for a long time and its severity is often underestimated; changes in the bronchial lining may continue until the situation becomes life-threatening. Other complications include changes in the lungs (see Emphysema, p. 309), constant shortness of breath, and insufficient oxygen supply. Constriction of blood vessels in the lungs can also weaken the heart, and the risk of developing pneumonia increases.

Since the symptoms of chronic bronchitis and malignant tumor are similar, early detection of cancer in smokers is often missed.

Prevention

Reduce stress in your life; avoid breathing polluted air; most importantly, do not smoke.

When to Seek Medical Advice

Seek help if you suffer an attack of bronchitis more than once a year. Discuss your life and work situations with your doctor, who may recommend X rays, an electrocardiogram (EKG), and a test of lung function. People with chronic bronchitis need regular medical care.

Self-Help

Self-help is especially important with bronchitis.
— Smokers should consider chronic bronchitis an alarm signal and quit smoking immediately (see Smoking p. 754).
— Avoid smoke-filled environments.
— If you are exposed to toxins in the workplace, change jobs.
— Avoid contact with people who have colds. A cold that is easily fought off by a healthy person can be

life-threatening for those with chronic bronchitis.
— Avoid excessive physical exertion; regular, moderate outdoor activities and sports can be beneficial (see Physical Activity and Sports, p. 762).

Treatment

Treatment for bronchitis is primarily aimed at slowing its progress. Expectorants may be prescribed (see Acute Bronchitis, p. 305).

Bronchodilators

If chronic bronchitis causes occasional or constant breathing difficulties, it may be necessary to take bronchodilators either as inhalers or orally (see Asthma, p. 307).

Corticosteroid Inhalants

Corticosteroid inhalants may be prescribed (see Asthma, p. 307). An important side effect of inhaled corticosteroids is that they may lower the body's resistance to infections, possibly resulting in a fungal infection of the mouth (see Thrush, p. 380). To prevent this, rinse your mouth with water extremely well after use.

Antibiotics

Bacterial infections of the bronchi should be treated immediately with antibiotics; identifying the bacteria before prescribing the antibiotic is optimal but not always possible (see Antibiotics, p. 661). Whether administration of a constant low dose of antibiotics prevents serious infection is still being debated.

ASTHMA

Complaints

The symptoms of asthma are usually fits of coughing and shortness of breath which, in contrast to bronchitis, occur as attacks and subside quickly when treated.

An asthma attack usually begins with an irritating, worsening cough, combined with serious shortness of breath. Exhaling becomes especially difficult and is accompanied by a characteristic whistle/wheeze, audible in mild cases only by putting an ear to the patient's chest. Eventually, thick, clear mucus is produced. Desperate efforts to inhale more air prove futile and only cause the lungs to become more distended. After the attack, the lungs return to normal.

Causes

In asthmatics, the bronchial lining is hypersensitive. During asthma attacks, the lining is swollen and the muscles of the bronchial walls constrict, further narrowing the bronchi. Fluid builds up in the pleura and thick mucus plugs the bronchial opening. This level of sensitivity is probably congenital. Several conditions need to be met for someone to react to triggers with a full-blown asthma attack (see Allergies, p. 360).

In about half of asthma sufferers, the triggers are infections of the airways. About 20 percent of asthmatics suffer from allergy induced asthma, most commonly triggered by pollen, animal hair, dust, chemicals, and medications, particularly analgesics like acetylsalicylic acid (see Allergies, p. 360). Stress-induced asthma, caused by physical exertion, affects some people. In some cases the cause of the attacks is not known.

Who's at Risk

The risk of asthma increases in
— People exposed to smoke, polluted air, fog, or toxins in the workplace (see Health in the Workplace, p. 789)
— Those who suffer from frequent bronchitis.
— Those prone to allergies, or with allergies in the family
— Children, most often between ages 5 and 10; asthma often disappears after puberty

Possible Aftereffects and Complications

The frightening experience of an asthma attack may cause anxiety about future attacks. Fear and stress can, in turn, trigger subsequent attacks or make them worse. This psychological component may become an increasingly important factor in the course of the illness.

In half of all cases, asthma changes the lungs permanently. After several years, chronic asthma can develop, severely affecting one's productivity. A side effect of long-term asthma is recurring bronchial infections.

An untreated asthma attack can cause death from suffocation, particularly in old and infirm persons.

The overall condition and well-being of an asthmatic can alter rapidly, necessitating changes in treatment which should be monitored by a health professional. However, asthmatics also need to be familiar with symptoms and know when and how to treat them.

Continuous dependence on doctors, emergency

services and hospitals can be a great strain on asthmatics and their families; support groups can help.

Prevention

While asthma itself cannot be prevented, the frequency and severity of attacks can be controlled. For asthma triggered by allergies it is important to determine, and then avoid, the source. In the case of pollen allergies, desensitization may help (see Allergies, p. 360). For preventing attacks, see Self-Help, below.

When to Seek Medical Advice

Seek help as soon as you suspect asthma. Your health-care provider can make a definitive diagnosis by listening to your lungs and taking a detailed history. Sometimes additional testing is necessary, including X rays, EKG or lung function tests (see p. 646).

If you are already in treatment for asthma, seek help if

— You find yourself severely debilitate
— You wake up at night short of breath
— Asthma symptoms are still present 20 minutes after taking the prescribed medication
— You need medication more frequently than every 4 hours to stay symptom-free

Self-Help

Asthma can be treated successfully only when patient and doctor work together closely. You can do several things to prevent or control an attack, including:
— Find out what the triggers are and try to avoid them (see Allergies, p. 360).
— Quit smoking (see p. 755).
— Avoid smoke-filled environments.
— If at all possible, avoid irritants such as strong odors, kitchen fumes and pollution in the air and at work.
— Be physically active (see Physical Activity and Sports, p. 762). Swimming is highly recommended. If your symptoms are triggered by exertion, take medication before activity.
— If cold air triggers your asthma, cover your mouth and nose with a scarf before going out.
— Learn autogenic training; this may only ease symptoms a bit, rather than preventing an attack. Yoga, when practiced regularly, has also proved beneficial for asthmatics.

Treatment

The approach to asthma treatment differs for adults and children, and is determined by type, medication dosage, frequency, and severity of attacks.

A chronically inflamed bronchial lining will undergo irreversible changes. The priority in treatment is to curb the inflammation as effectively as possible, and to suppress side effects. In adults this is achieved primarily with corticosteroid inhalers. Cromolyn sodium may also be prescribed. This drug acts to prevent the body from producing substances that trigger asthma attacks. The reverse order of treatment is sometimes recommended for children, since the effects of corticosteroid inhalers in children are not fully known.

In acute asthma attacks, inhaling a fast-acting bronchodilator relaxes the muscles around the bronchi so they don't constrict when irritated. Asthmatic children can also use inhalers that release premeasured doses.

If symptoms occur several times a day and the patient's functioning is impaired, additional bronchodilators need to be given regularly and/or longer-lasting medications inhaled.

With severe asthma, continuous doses of corticosteroids may not be avoidable; this can have far-reaching side effects (see Glucocorticoids, p. 665).

An important aid for asthmatics is the peak flow meter, which measures the pressure of air released by the lungs during forceful exhalation. The result of this "home lung function test" determines which medication needs to be used for acute cases. Peak flow measurements are recorded daily in a log book.

Warning: Asthmatics should not take certain medications (e.g., beta blockers or acetylsalicylic acid). Even if asthma attacks are triggered by infections, treatment with antibiotics will not reduce the frequency or severity of attacks.

Patient Education

Asthma treatment works best when the patient is able to assess his or her situation and react accordingly. In a few weeks' time, competent doctors can teach patients to do this. The program should cover causes, effects, understanding the illness, monitoring breathing volume, use of appropriate medications in different situations, and possibly autogenic training and/or psychotherapy.

Medical treatment of asthma is successful only when the asthmatic knows exactly what to do and why. Ask

Asthma Medications

Inhaled Corticosteroids
Beclomethasone Dipropionate (Vanceril, Vanceril Double Strength DS, Beclovent)
Budesonide (Pulmicort Turbuhaler)
Flunisolide (AeroBid, AeroBid-M)
Fluticasone Proprionate (Flovent)
Triamcinolone Acetonide (Azmacort)
Possible side effects: fungal infections of mouth or pharynx (Thrush, p. 595). Try to prevent this by thoroughly rinsing mouth with water after use of inhaler.

Beta-Agonists
Albuterol (Proventil, Ventolin)
Bitolterol (Tornalate)
Albuterol/Ipratropium (Combivent Inhalation Aerosol)
Isoetharine (Bronkometer, Bronkosol)
Metaproterenol (Alupent)
Pirbuterol (Maxair)
Sameterol (Serevent)
Terbutaline (Brethaire, Brethine, Bricanyl)
Possible side effects depending on medication class: gastrointestinal disturbances, sleep disorders, shaking, restlessness, chest pain, palpitations.

Leukotriene Inhibitors
Montelukast (Singulair)
Zafirlukast (Accolate)
Zileuton (Zyflo)
Note: to be taken regularly, not for acute exacerbations

Methylxanthines
Aminophylline
Theophylline (Elixophyllin, Slo-bid, Slo-Phyllin, Theo-Dur, Theo-24, Uniphyl)

your doctor as many questions as you need to, until you are sure you understand everything.

Part of asthma management includes keeping a daily log of peak flow measurements along with a record of medications and the status of the airways. This keeps both patient and doctor aware of daily fluctuations in the disease, and helps identify the most effective medications with the fewest side effects.

Additional Treatment Possibilities

Because the appearance of asthma, and the intensity of attacks, can also have an impact on your emotions, counseling may be appropriate. Relaxation (see p. 693) may help ease the fear of an attack; many studies have shown the benefits of practicing yoga. Acupuncture and homeopathy have also been successful in supplementing, and reducing the need for, conventional medical treatment.

Lungs

Air travels through the bronchi into the lungs, where three hundred million alveoli, equivalent in area to the surface of a tennis court, take up the air and supply its oxygen to the blood. In exchange, carbon dioxide (or "used air") is removed from the blood and exhaled. Various lung diseases may disrupt this exchange of gases.

EMPHYSEMA

Complaints

Emphysema develops slowly, as do its symptoms. Because the deterioration is so slow, taking months or years, it is often not recognized in time to intervene.

Physical capabilities decrease slowly and shortness of breath occurs more quickly during bodily exertion. There may be difficulty in breathing while lying flat, or a whistling sound as in asthma.

Some patients suffer from cough symptoms similar to those of bronchitis, including coughing up whitish-yellow mucus on waking.

Emphysema sometimes becomes noticeable only when it affects the heart muscle, giving rise to edema, or swelling, in the legs and feet.

Causes

Emphysema is usually the result of chronic bronchitis, which has irritated the bronchi and caused the bronchial lining to swell. Because of this increased pressure, the alveoli become stressed and eventually die; they are insufficiently replaced, decreasing the net surface area through which the exchange of gases takes place. Over time, this causes the lung tissue to stiffen, causing the heart to work harder to pump blood through the lungs. All factors contributing to chronic bronchitis (see p. 306) can also cause emphysema. Asthma seldom causes it.

Who's at Risk

The risk of emphysema is very high in people suffering from chronic bronchitis. Those exposed to severely polluted air are also at increased risk.

Possible Aftereffects and Complications

Because fewer alveoli are present, the body no longer gets enough oxygen, leading to constant shortness of breath.

The increasingly hardened lung tissue places too much stress on the heart. Severe emphysema may lead to heart failure and death.

Prevention

All factors that prevent chronic bronchitis also prevent development of emphysema (see p. 309).

When to Seek Medical Advice

Seek help if symptoms of chronic bronchitis worsen, your activities are curtailed, and your lung capacity diminishes.

Those who know they have emphysema should see a doctor for every cold, any suspicion of a bronchial infection, and any sudden turn for the worse.

Self-Help

Most important: Lead as stress-free a life as possible.
— Quit smoking immediately (see Smoking, p. 755).
— Avoid smoke-filled environments.
— If you work in a polluted environment, change jobs.
— Stay away from people with colds. A cold any healthy person can handle may be life-threatening to someone with emphysema.
— Avoid excessive physical exertion. However, regular, moderate outdoor activities may be helpful.

Treatment

Changes in the lungs caused by emphysema are irreversible, but symptoms can be eased and progression of the illness prevented.

All infections of the bronchi or lungs should be treated; frequently antibiotics are necessary. Often medications that thin the mucus can offer relief (see Chronic Bronchitis, p. 306). If wheezing begins, asthma medications may help (see Asthma, p. 307).

People with emphysema often need oxygen, either occasionally during the course of an infection, or always. Sometimes they also need to take medications to strengthen the heart (see Congestive Heart Failure, p. 337) and diuretics (see Hypertension, p. 321).

PNEUMONIA

Complaints

The symptoms of pneumonia vary depending on its cause. Often a high fever and chills are combined with exhaustion, joint pains and headache. Usually the cough

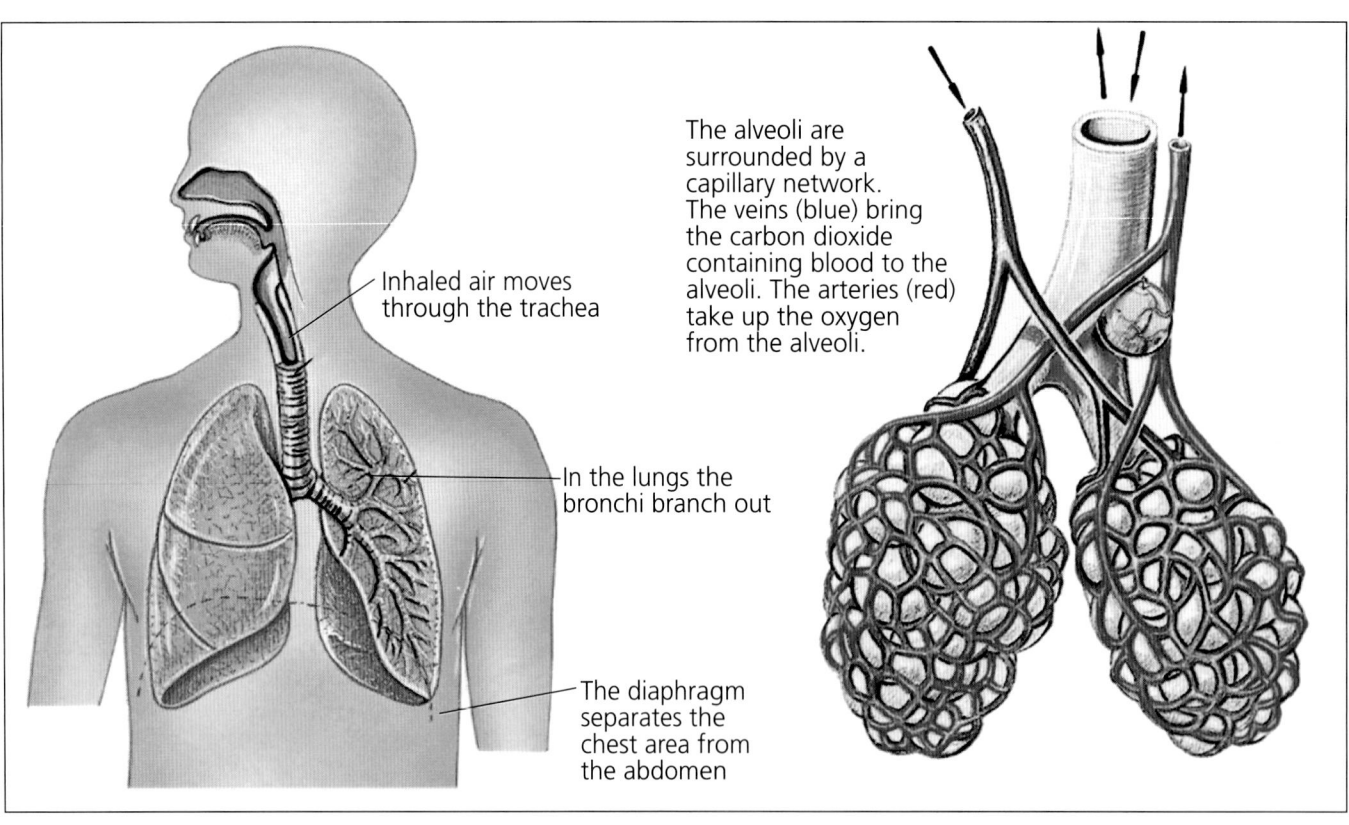

Inhaled air moves through the trachea

In the lungs the bronchi branch out

The diaphragm separates the chest area from the abdomen

The alveoli are surrounded by a capillary network. The veins (blue) bring the carbon dioxide containing blood to the alveoli. The arteries (red) take up the oxygen from the alveoli.

is dry and painful. Traces of blood may be found in the sputum. In severe pneumonia, breathing is always rapid. Patients may barely be able to breathe when lying flat. Lips and fingernails may turn bluish, indicating a lack of oxygen.

Causes

Pneumonia can be caused by bacteria, viruses, fungi, chemical irritants, or a foreign body (e.g., food) in the airway. The most delicate parts of the lung tissue become inflamed. Both lungs, or only one lobe or part of a lobe may be affected.

Who's at Risk

The following are at increased risk of contracting pneumonia:
— Children under the age of 2 or 3.
— Children living with a smoker.
— The elderly.
— Smokers.
— Those with weakened immune systems.

Possible Aftereffects and Complications

In an otherwise healthy person, pneumonia treated with antibiotics will heal within 2 to 3 weeks with no negative consequences, though some people feel tired and weak for a few weeks thereafter. For the elderly or those already weakened by another illness, pneumonia can be life-threatening.

Pleural Effusion, Lung Abscess

Sometimes during a bout with pneumonia, the delicate membranes between the lung and rib cage become infected. Fluid may accumulate between the membranes and pressure may build, making it difficult to breath. To facilitate breathing or to make a diagnosis, some of this fluid may have to be removed.

If pneumonia is caused by a foreign body or bacteria, the resulting pus-filled infection can develop into a lung abscess.

Prevention

There are no general preventive measures.

When to Seek Medical Advice

Seek help if
— Cough and high fever last longer than 2 days

— Breathing and coughing cause pain
— There are brown traces (old blood) in the sputum. Seek medical attention immediately
— If breathing becomes rapid even when resting, or shortness of breath occurs

Doctors can diagnose pneumonia simply by listening to and tapping on the lung area. Sometimes X rays must be taken as well (see Chest X Ray, p. 649). Blood and saliva tests can also be diagnostic.

Self-Help

Not possible.

Treatment

Pneumonia is almost always treated with antibiotics (see Antibiotics, p. 661). Although antibiotics cannot help a viral infection, they may prevent a secondary bacterial infection. If the infection has spread to a large part of the lung, hospital treatment is necessary. Medications are given intravenously and supplemental oxygen may be needed.

TUBERCULOSIS

Tuberculosis usually begins in the lungs and, if not treated, spreads by degrees to other organs. The symptoms arise from the body's reaction to inflamed spots in the affected organs, which destroy the tissue and may later seal themselves off.

Complaints

The initial symptoms of tuberculosis are not what one would necessarily associate with the disease: Slight temperature, general malaise, and weight loss. The more characteristic symptoms, which might not appear for up to 2 years, include cough with yellowish-green mucus, coughing up blood (particularly in the mornings), chest pain, and intermittent fever.

Causes

This disease is caused by *Mycobacterium* tuberculosis, a strain of bacteria. Persons infected with the bacteria are contagious, passing them on through direct contact or via airborne droplets. The bacteria are hardy enough to survive for days without water in a sealed room. The disease may also be contracted by drinking unpasteurized milk from infected cows.

Older children and adults with healthy immune

systems seldom get tuberculosis even when infected with the bacteria: they produce antibodies that help prevent onset of the disease.

Who's at Risk

The risk of tuberculosis is increased by
— Poor nutrition and high-density living quarters
— Contact with those who either have tuberculosis, or had it and were not treated
—Weakened immune systems and weakened resistance to infections

Although the incidence of tuberculosis in the industrialized world has been drastically reduced since the nineteenth century thanks to improved hygiene and public health policy, it has risen again in recent years due in part to the deterioration in living conditions of parts of the population.

Possible Aftereffects and Complications

If tuberculosis is not treated promptly, it may spread to other organs and lead to death.

Prevention

Vaccinating against tuberculosis is not advisable except in very rare cases (see p. 670).

Preventive treatment with tuberculosis medication is recommended for people who meet all three of the following conditions: High risk of illness, insufficient antibody levels, probable recent exposure to tuberculosis bacteria (e.g., while traveling).

Tuberculosis testing (with purified protein derivative [PPD]) can establish whether antibodies are present.

When to Seek Medical Advice

Seek help if:
—You think you have had, or will have, contact with a person who has tuberculosis, especially if your immune system is weakened by illness or medications.
—You have the symptoms of weight loss, fatigue, and cough productive of yellowish-green phlegm. A chest X ray or sputum examination will facilitate diagnosis.

Self-Help

Not possible.

Treatment

Tuberculosis is always treated with specialized medications. According to the stage of the disease, it may be necessary to take two to four different medications concurrently. Treatment can take months or years.

The disease should be treated with several different medications at the same time so as to lessen the risk of the bacteria developing a resistance to one of them, resulting in the loss of effectiveness of that medication. The recent upsurge in the number of resistant strains of tuberculosis bacteria is due in part to the fact that such threefold or multiple-drug regimens were not completed.

Following 2 weeks of treatment, tuberculosis is no longer contagious. In the past, patients were isolated; today this is necessary only at the beginning of treatment or if there are complications. A thorough examination of each family member and/or persons sharing living quarters with a tuberculosis patient is essential.

PULMONARY EMBOLISM, PULMONARY INFARCTION

Complaints

In these disorders, breathing suddenly becomes rapid and difficult, leading to panic. A dull pain under the rib cage, cough, or fever may also be present.

Antitubercular Medications

Important: Successful treatment depends upon taking the medications daily for the prescribed time. The medications should not be stopped, except if you are advised to do so by your health-care provider, even if you no longer feel ill. While taking antitubercular medications, you should also be taking multivitamins.
Medications:
Isoniazid (INH)
Possible side effects: dizziness, headache, liver toxicity, gastrointestinal, blood, and nerve disturbances.
Rifabutin (Mycobutin)
Rifampin (Rimactane)
Possible side effects: liver toxicity, gastrointestinal disturbances, dizziness, headache. Birth control using oral contraceptives may be unreliable.
Ethambutol Hydrochloride (Myambutol)
Possible side effects: occasionally visual disturbances, constipation, rarely gout.
Ethionamide (Trecator-SC)
Pyrazinamide

These symptoms, however, are by no means restricted to pulmonary embolism. They may also indicate other illnesses.

Causes

Blood clots form in a vein, usually in the lower body, and are transported to the lung, where they block one or several blood vessels. In rare instances this can cause a pulmonary infarction in which circulation is cut off to a whole section of the lung tissue, which then dies.

Who's at Risk

The risk of these disorders increases in
— Persons at risk for blood clots, including those who have been bedridden for a long time or have phlebitis (see p. 329) or some forms of cancer
— Women who are pregnant or take birth control pills.
— Overweight persons
— Persons with chronic lung or heart disease
— Persons with a prior pulmonary embolism that went untreated

Possible Aftereffects and Complications

Any lasting effect of pulmonary embolism depends on the size and number of blood vessels involved. Blocked blood circulation to large sections of the lung can cause lack of oxygen, forcing the heart to work harder to pump blood into the lungs. Lack of oxygen also progressively weakens the heart muscle and can lead to congestive heart failure.

Pulmonary embolism is always potentially life-threatening, but may also resolve without complications.

Prevention

In order to prevent blood clots from forming, those patients who are able are encouraged to walk as soon as possible after undergoing surgery.

High-risk patients or those confined to bed may get injections of heparin.

When to Seek Medical Advice

Pulmonary embolism can be treated only in a hospital setting. To identify the illness, numerous procedures are involved (blood tests, EKG, X rays and lung perfusion scans).

Self-Help

Not possible.

Treatment

Surgery is rarely necessary because blood clots can usually be dissolved with specific medications.

Pulmonary embolism may require additional medication for strengthening the heart and aiding circulation, as well as analgesics and/or oxygen. Follow-up medication should be prescribed for the prevention of future blood clots (see Phlebitis, p. 329).

PULMONARY EDEMA

Complaints

Symptoms of this disorder include serious breathing difficulties: gasping, rapid breathing, the sensation of suffocation or not getting enough air. Pallor and outbreaks of sweating frequently accompany the above. Lips and nails may turn blue as a sign of oxygen deprivation.

Causes

In pulmonary edema, fluid seeps from the blood vessels into the alveoli and surrounding areas, making it difficult or impossible for inhaled oxygen to be taken up into the bloodstream.

The cause is usually a heart too weak to pump blood out of the lungs and back into circulation (see Congestive Heart Failure, p. 337).

Breathing poisonous gases (e.g., fluorine or chlorine) can also cause pulmonary edema.

Who's at Risk

The risk of pulmonary edema is increased in people with serious or untreated problems in the left ventricle of the heart (see Congestive Heart Failure, p. 337).

Possible Aftereffects and Complications

Pulmonary edema always results in oxygen deficit, which should be remedied as quickly as possible. If not recognized and treated in time, it may be fatal.

Once the cause of the edema is treated, it quickly subsides, leaving no lasting damage to the lung.

Prevention

Treatment for congestive heart failure (see p. 338).

When to Seek Medical Advice

Pulmonary edema should be treated in a hospital as soon as possible. The patient is transported in as upright a position as feasible, to facilitate breathing.

Self-Help

Not possible.

Treatment

Usually pulmonary edema can be treated with oxygen, medications to strengthen the heart, and diuretics.

PNEUMOTHORAX (COLLAPSED LUNG)

Complaints

Symptoms vary according to the degree of illness. They may range from curtailed activity and an unwell feeling to serious shortness of breath and circulatory collapse. Frequently there are stabbing pains in the chest, shoulder, or upper stomach, and occasionally a dry cough.

Causes

In a collapsed lung, air leaks from the alveoli and collects in the delicate membranes surrounding the lung, so that part of the lung can no longer inflate when air is inhaled.

In tension pneumothorax, a particularly severe kind of collapsed lung, the amount of air between the lung membranes increases with each breath until the lung can no longer expand.

Pneumothorax may be caused by an external injury. Alveoli may also burst in conjunction with emphysema (see Emphysema, p. 309), cystic fibrosis (see p. 598), a lung abscess, or tuberculosis (see p. 311).

Who's at Risk

Those suffering from cystic fibrosis or emphysema are at much higher risk for pneumothorax than the average population.

Possible Aftereffects and Complications

Small air pockets in the lungs usually disappear on their own after a few days. Serious shortness of breath or tension pneumothorax must be treated in a clinical setting.

Pneumothorax may or may not recur, depending on the cause.

Prevention

If large blisters of emphysema are the cause of recurrent pneumothorax, surgery may be necessary.

When to Seek Medical Advice

Seek help if you suspect a collapsed lung.

Self-Help

Not possible.

Treatment

To treat pneumothorax, a tube is inserted between the lung membranes and left there for several days to suction out the air. Surgery may be necessary, depending on the cause.

LUNG CANCER

(see also Cancer, p. 470)

Complaints

Usually the initial symptoms of lung cancer are similar to those of chronic bronchitis: Cough with whitish-yellow mucus, shortness of breath or wheezing during physical exertion, sometimes stabbing pain while inhaling, or a constant mild pain in the rib cage.

If these symptoms are not recognized, cancer cells may spread to other organs such as the skin, bones, liver, or brain.

Causes

Ninety percent of all lung cancer patients are former smokers. Chronic smoker's bronchitis and its effects on the bronchial cells probably contribute to the development of cancer. Even in smokers, however, a genetic predisposition to lung cancer may be necessary. Psychological factors may also contribute to the development of cancer. The second highest cause of lung cancer, after tobacco, is high indoor radon levels (see Healthy Living, p. 772). Many other air pollutants may also be involved in its development (see Air Pollution, p. 783; Health in the Workplace, p. 789).

Who's at Risk

The risk of contracting lung cancer increases with every cigarette smoked, and also depends on the age at which smoking began: People who started smoking regularly at age 15 are 5 times more likely to get lung cancer than people who started smoking at age 25. Persons who smoke up to 10 cigarettes a day are 5 times more likely to get lung cancer than a nonsmoker; those who smoke over 35 cigarettes a day are 40 times more likely.

Tests have shown that nonsmoking women whose living partners smoke are 33 percent more likely to get lung cancer than women whose partners don't smoke. Cigar and pipe smokers are four times as likely to get lung cancer as nonsmokers.

Possible Aftereffects and Complications
Fewer than 1 in 10 lung cancer cases can be treated successfully with surgery, radiation, and/or chemotherapy, even with early detection.

Prevention
Don't start smoking. If you already smoke, quit. After 15 years of abstention, the risk to former smokers of contracting lung cancer is the same as for those who have never smoked.

When to Seek Medical Advice
Seek help if symptoms appear.

Self-Help
Not possible.

Treatment
If lung cancer is detected early, the affected part of the lung can be removed, followed by radiation treatment and possibly chemotherapy. When surgery is not possible, both radiation and chemotherapy are used. Both have serious and long-term side effects.

The type of treatment used depends on the type of cancer and how far it has spread.

HEART AND CIRCULATION

It pumps, and pumps, and pumps . . . . The heart beats tirelessly from birth to death, 100,000 times a day, 2½ billion times in the course of a 70-year life.

Whether we're working or sleeping, our hearts automatically adjust to different workloads and provide the entire body with blood. As the heart contracts, it pushes blood into the arteries leading to the lungs or to the rest of the body. The arteries branch into ever narrower vessels, down to the arterioles; these branch still further, down to the tiny blood vessels called capillaries. In the capillaries, blood releases oxygen and nutrients for the tissues and picks up waste products, especially carbon dioxide, an end product of metabolism that colors the blood dark. The dark blood is collected in the veins and transported back to the heart, which pumps it into the lungs for oxygenation.

THE HEART

The heart is separated into halves by a wall of muscle. Each half consists of an atrium (auricle) and a ventricle, which are connected by a set of muscular flaps called the atrioventricular valves. The right atrium and ventricle pump oxygen-depleted blood; the left atrium and ventricle pump oxygenated blood. To ensure that the blood flows in only one direction, the atrioventricular valves prevent the return of blood from the ventricles to the atria, and another set of valves, the semilunar valves, prevent the return of blood from the arteries back into the ventricles.

Efficient blood flow through the heart also requires coordination of the contractions of the four chambers, by electrical impulses conducted from sinus node in the right atrium through other nodes and fibers and on to the heart muscles.

The pumping of the heart follows this sequence:

1. The atria fill with blood: Carbon dioxide-loaded blood flows out of the systemic circulation into the right atrium, while oxygenated blood from the lungs flows into the left atrium.
2. The atria contract, causing the atrioventricular valves to open, and the blood is squeezed into the ventricles.
3. When the ventricles are full, they contract; the atrioventricular valves close, and the semilunar valves into the aorta and pulmonary artery open. The carbon dioxide-containing blood from the right ventricle is pumped into the lungs, and the oxygenated blood from the left ventricle goes into circulation through the rest of the body.

Because the left ventricle has to do the most work, its muscles are the strongest part of the heart.

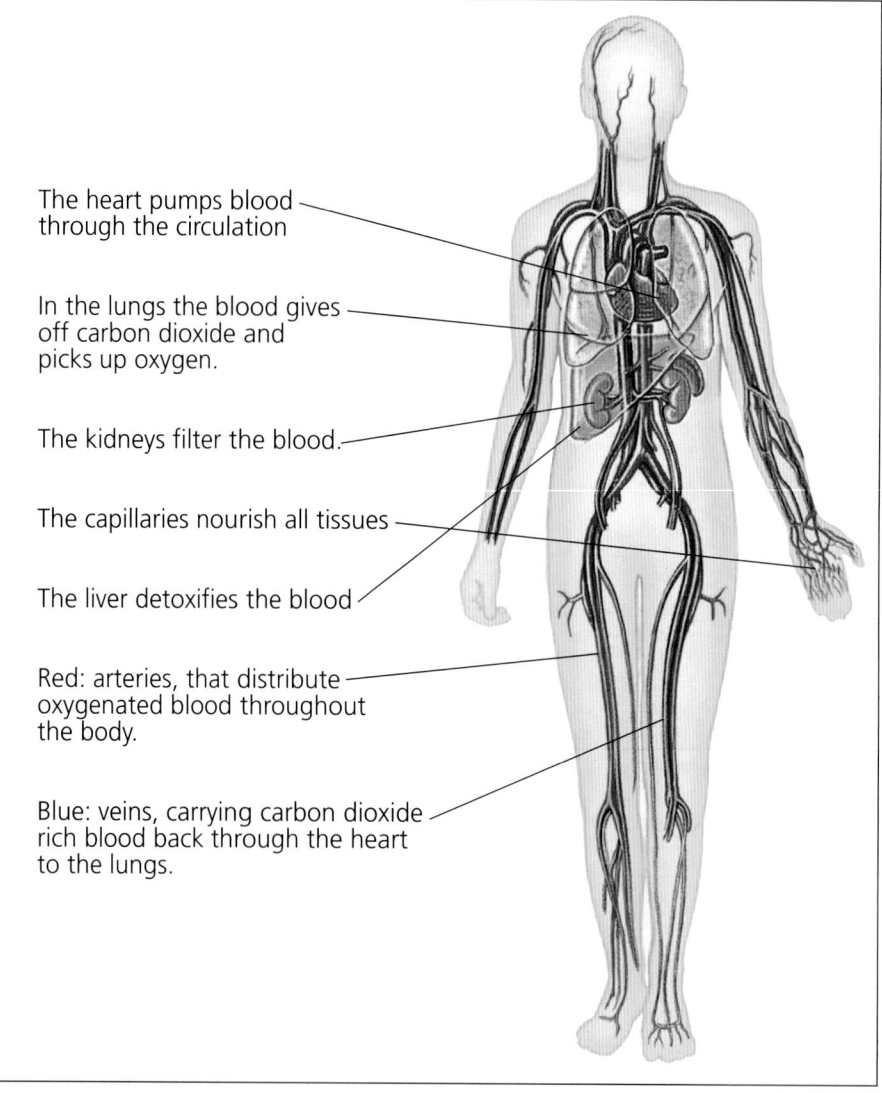

The heart pumps blood through the circulation

In the lungs the blood gives off carbon dioxide and picks up oxygen.

The kidneys filter the blood.

The capillaries nourish all tissues

The liver detoxifies the blood

Red: arteries, that distribute oxygenated blood throughout the body.

Blue: veins, carrying carbon dioxide rich blood back through the heart to the lungs.

The heart itself is not directly nourished by the blood passing through it, but has its own system of blood vessels, the coronary vessels.

The inside of the heart muscle (myocardium) is covered with a thin layer called the endocardium. The outside of the heart muscle is surrounded by a double-walled sac called the pericardium. The inner layer of this sac is fused to the heart muscle (epicardium); the outer layer provides a mobile linkage between the heart and the rib cage, backbone and esophagus. The inner and outer layers of the pericardium are separated by a fluid.

CIRCULATION

The total length of all the blood vessels in the body is approximately 60,000 miles. Blood moves through them in two separate circulations, the pulmonary and systemic.

In the pulmonary circulation, venous blood is pumped from the heart to the lungs, where it releases carbon dioxide and absorbs oxygen. Then the blood is returned to the heart, which pumps it out into the systemic circulation.

The vessels leading away from the heart, the arteries, need to be able to withstand the high pressures generated by each heartbeat, so their muscle layer is thicker than that of the veins. Veins are also less elastic than arteries.

When our bodies move, our muscles contract; this exerts pressure on the veins, pressing the blood back toward the heart. The one-way flow of blood through the veins is ensured by built-in valves.

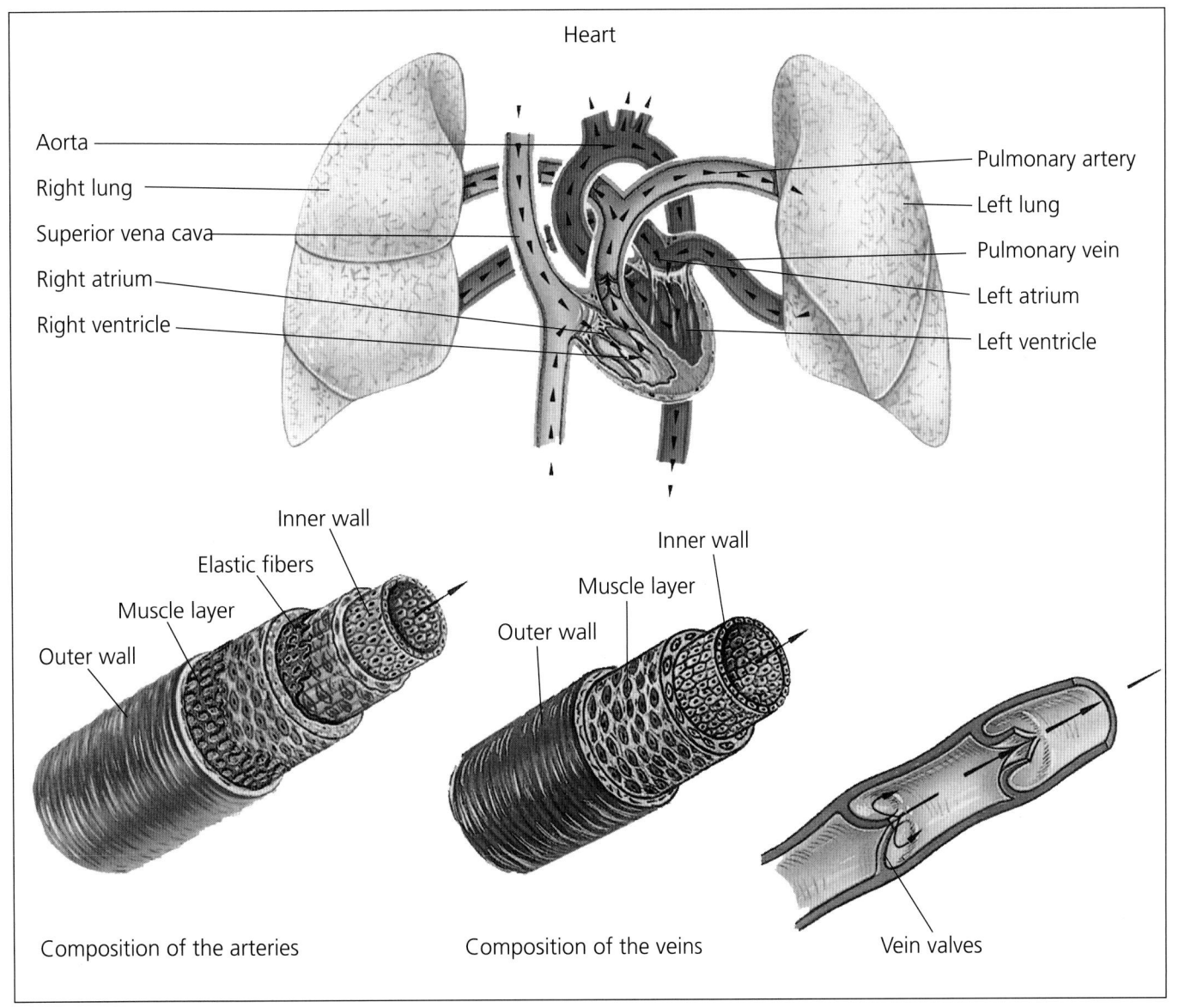

Heart

Aorta

Right lung

Superior vena cava

Right atrium

Right ventricle

Pulmonary artery

Left lung

Pulmonary vein

Left atrium

Left ventricle

Inner wall

Elastic fibers

Muscle layer

Outer wall

Composition of the arteries

Inner wall

Muscle layer

Outer wall

Composition of the veins

Vein valves

RISK FACTORS

Many factors can contribute to coronary and circulatory diseases, primarily hypertension (high blood pressure), too much fat in the blood (high blood cholesterol and triglyceride levels), unfavorable composition of the cholesterol (too much "bad" cholesterol in the blood), smoking, diabetes, and obesity. Men are at greater risk than women. Additional risk factors include lack of exercise, advanced age, and a family history of early atherosclerosis.

The more risk factors that apply to you, the greater your chances of developing heart or circulatory disease.

CORONARY ARTERY DISEASE

The most common form of heart disease is coronary artery disease, also called ischemic heart disease (ischemia—inadequate blood supply in muscle tissue). The term includes a variety of diseases, all caused by narrowing of the coronary arteries (see Arteriosclerosis, p. 318):
— Angina Pectoris (see p. 333)
— Heart Attack, or Myocardial Infarction (see p. 335)
— Congestive heart failure (see p. 337)

The risk of contracting coronary artery disease is higher for people who
— Smoke (see p. 754)
— Have high blood pressure (see p. 321)
— Have diabetes (see p. 483)
— Have unfavorable ratios of various kinds of cholesterol in the blood (see p. 319)
— Have gout (see p. 454)

It is also suspected that people who are overweight or under constant stress are at higher risk of coronary artery disease (see Health and Well-Being, p. 182).

ARTERIOSCLEROSIS

Complaints

Arteriosclerosis is a natural aging process, which by itself produces no symptoms. It becomes noticeable only when secondary diseases appear.

Causes

Healthy arteries are elastic and muscular, adapting to differences in pressure by expanding and contracting. In the presence of hypertension, excessive blood cholesterol, and arterial wall damage, however, fatty substances ("atheroma") can begin to build up on the interior arterial walls. Gradually, the fat deposits increase; other substances, such as calcium, are added to the sites. The arterial walls harden, inhibiting blood flow, until one day the body's tissues are no longer receiving enough blood. Physicians call this progressive calcification of the vessels "arteriosclerosis."

Who's at Risk

The risk of arteriosclerosis is higher in
— Those with very high blood cholesterol levels (see atherosclerosis, below)
— Men
— Smokers
— Physically inactive people
— People with diabetes, weak kidneys, or hypertension

Possible Aftereffects and Complications

— Poor Circulation (intermittent claudication; see p. 326)
— Kidney Failure (see p. 425)
— Angina Pectoris (see p. 333)
— Heart Attack (see p. 335) and secondary diseases such as congestive heart failure and cardiac arrhythmia
— Stroke (see p. 215)

Prevention

Stop smoking. Nonsmoking dramatically reduces the risk of heart attack, and quitting is beneficial at any age (see Smoking, p. 754).

Treatment

The treatment depends on the secondary disease (see Possible Aftereffects and Complications, above).

ATHEROSCLEROSIS

(Elevated Blood-fat Levels)

Complaints

Even with unusually high levels of cholesterol and triglycerides in the blood (and what constitutes "normal" levels is still a subject of debate), no symptoms are detectable except by blood tests (see p. 636).

Most nutritionists agree that an elevated blood-

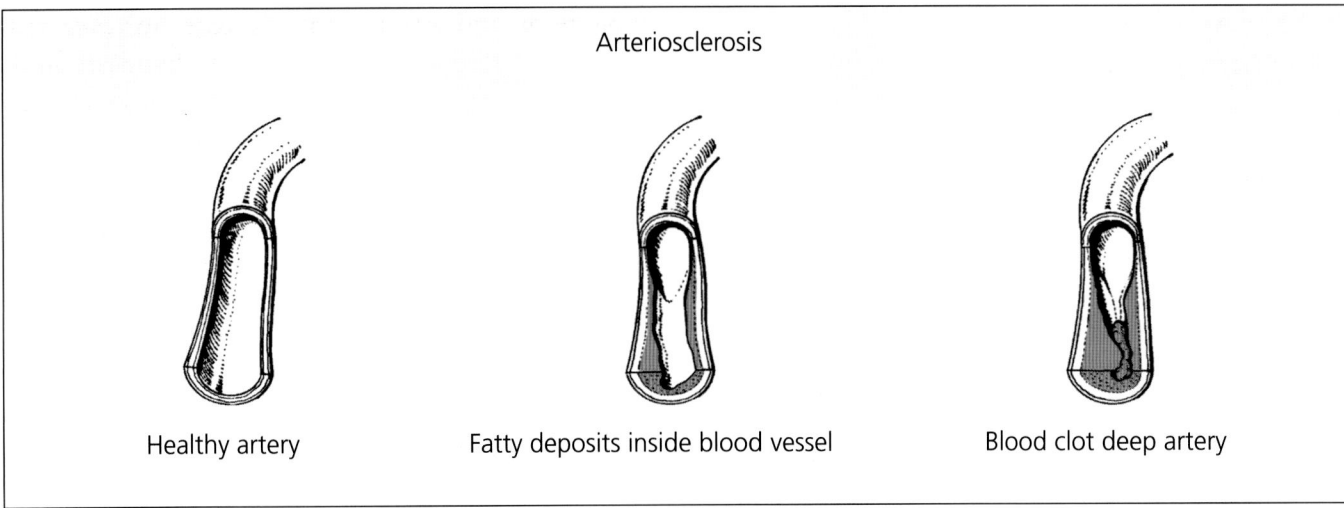

Arteriosclerosis

Healthy artery   Fatty deposits inside blood vessel   Blood clot deep artery

cholesterol level contributes to the development of arteriosclerosis (see p. 318), and thus to diseases such as coronary artery disease, heart attack, stroke, circulatory problems, etc. However, there is no agreement as to when a decrease in cholesterol level actually has a positive effect on arterial disease; the question of when drugs should be used is even more contentious.

It has not been demonstrated that triglycerides play a role in the development of arteriosclerosis. Elevated triglycerides in people with diabetes are taken as a definite indicator of elevated risk for arterial disease. If the level of triglycerides is over 10 times higher than normal, the pancreas is endangered.

Causes

There are two sources of body cholesterol. Most of it is produced by the liver, and it is also ingested in animal foods.

A fatty diet, diseases of the liver, thyroid, or kidneys, and diabetes can all lead to elevated blood cholesterol. However, the condition can also be hereditary.

Various Fats

What is determined as "blood fats" in the laboratory is the sum of several different kinds of fat: cholesterol, triglycerides, phospholipids, and free fatty acids.

The fats ingested in food are not soluble in blood, so there is a special transport system for them. The carriers of these fats are specific proteins called lipoproteins.

Different lipoproteins have different roles in the hardening of arteries: The "good" lipoproteins are the high-density lipoproteins (HDL), which probably pro-

tect the arteries from arteriosclerosis. A number of studies have shown that coronary artery diseases, such as angina pectoris, are only about half as frequent when HDL values increase from 30 to 60 mg/dl.

The low-density lipoproteins (LDL) are "bad," in that high levels of LDL increase the probability of arteriosclerosis. About two thirds of the fats in the blood are transported in the form of LDL, one third as HDL.

Triglycerides are the "classic" fats consumed as part of food. It is debated whether higher blood triglyceride levels can lead to arteriosclerosis. However, elevated triglyceride values are believed to be less dangerous to health than high cholesterol values. Triglyceride values are raised by high-fat or high-carbohydrate diets, alcohol, diabetes, kidney diseases, hypothyroidism, certain medications, and heredity.

Who's at Risk

Atherosclerosis is a common disease problem in the United States.

Possible Aftereffects and Complications

Over long periods of time, elevated cholesterol levels can accelerate the process of arteriosclerosis, reducing life expectancy. On the other hand, there are also indications that low blood-cholesterol levels, including those attained through medical treatment, may increase the risk of other diseases which affect neither heart nor circulation.

Prevention

Just how high blood-cholesterol levels can get without increasing risk of disease is disputed.

The American Heart Association recommends the following:

— Cholesterol levels up to 200 mg/dl are not dangerous.
— If levels read above 200 mg/dl, repeat the test in a few weeks to exclude the possibility of error.
— If the reading is between 200 and 239 mg/dl and there are no symptoms of heart muscle disease such as angina pectoris, or fewer than two accompanying risk factors (smoking, diabetes, high blood pressure, overweight, or male gender), test again in a year and monitor nutrition (see Self-Help, below).
— If there are signs of heart muscle disease, more than two risk factors are present, or the cholesterol reading is above 240 mg/dl, a blood test should be made to determine all lipoproteins. If the LDL value is above 160 or the HDL value is below 35, the diet should be changed (see Self-Help, below).

When to Seek Medical Advice
Elevated cholesterol levels are usually discovered by chance. Adults over 20 years of age should have their cholesterol checked every five years. This is a normal part of routine physical exams (see Checkups, p. 629).

False-Positive Results
A recent study indicated that because of inaccurate measurement techniques, more than half of all reported fat levels were false. A diagnosis of high cholesterol levels can stand only if at least three blood tests at intervals of one or several weeks show elevated levels. The patient should fast for 12 to 16 hours before a test and consume no alcohol the night before. Cholesterol levels change so greatly during weight-reduction diets, during serious disease, and after surgery that testing at such times is pointless—wait at least 6 weeks after these conditions before testing cholesterol levels.

Cholesterol Levels During Pregnancy
During the last trimester of pregnancy, cholesterol levels normally rise by 35 percent, regardless of diet.

Self-Help
— Quit smoking (see Smoking, p. 754).
— Physical exercise increases HDL levels, which protect against arteriosclerosis.
— Stick to a balanced diet (see Nutrition, p. 722).

There is some indication that dietary changes can reduce cholesterol deposits that have not yet become calcified. This would mean that the process of arteriosclerosis can at least be retarded, up to an age of 60 or 70 years.

Treatment
In general, people who have reached 65 without developing coronary artery disease no longer need to worry about their cholesterol levels, as long as they aren't extremely high.

Treatment Without Medications
If high blood-fat levels are the result of poorly regulated diabetes, or liver or kidney disease, treatment of the primary disease will normalize them. Otherwise, the main treatment consists of normalization of body weight.

Many experts are skeptical about making specific nutritional recommendations for the general public; changing your diet makes sense only as the result of an individual nutritional analysis and consultation. Meanwhile, dietary recommendations keep changing: e.g., just a few years ago, oils like sunflower or corn oil were unconditionally recommended, but this is no longer necessarily the case. (For warnings concerning transfatty acids formed in the manufacture of margarine, see p. 725.)

In general, it has been found that a Mediterranean-type diet consisting largely of bread, vegetables, fruit and olive oil, with fish usually replacing meat, increases the life expectancy of people at high risk for heart and circulatory diseases—even when the diet has no effect on serum cholesterol levels. In any case, it's wise to limit consumption of meats (especially fatty meats), milkfat, and egg yolks.

However, in some people high blood-fat levels do not respond even to a rigorous diet.

Treatment with Medications
Medications make sense only in combination with a diet, and then only if the diet alone has not been successful.
— Cholestyramine (Questran, Questran Light) is a useful medication, prescribed only rarely due to gastrointestinal side effects and because it is complicated to take. The same is true for colestipol (Colestid), a similar medication.

— Lovastatin (Mevacor), pravastatin (Pravachol), simvastatin (Zocor), fluvastatin (Lescol), and atorvastatin (Lipitor) inhibit an enzyme needed for the synthesis of cholesterol in the body. However, because they can damage the liver, treatment must be monitored by laboratory tests. Rarely, muscle damage can also occur, in which case the medication should be discontinued immediately.
— Gemfibrozil (Lopid) and niacin (vitamin B³) are also prescribed.

All other medication used for treatment of elevated fat levels are considered controversial.

HYPERTENSION (HIGH BLOOD PRESSURE)

Complaints

High blood pressure has almost no symptoms unless it is extremely high, in which case it can produce headaches, heart palpitations, and a general sick feeling.

Blood-pressure measurement is part of all routine physical exams, so high blood pressure is usually discovered by chance on such occasions.

Causes

The cause of high blood pressure can be discovered in only 5 to 10 percent of patients, usually individuals with diseases of the kidneys, glands, or heart. This condition is known as secondary hypertension.

One frequently overlooked cause of high blood pressure is as a side effect of medications containing phenylpropanolamine, formerly found in many over-the-counter cold medications. These were especially risky in combination with caffeine-containing stimulants and could, in healthy people, lead to a diastolic (lower value) blood pressure of 105 mm Hg or more.

In 90 to 95 percent of cases, the cause of high blood pressure is unknown and the condition is called essential or primary hypertension.

Experts recognize that high blood pressure can result from overly stressful lifestyles (see Health and Well-Being, p. 182). Another possible explanation is excessive adrenal hormone production.

Who's at Risk

The risk of high blood pressure increases with age. In people under 35, about 1 in 10 is affected, but in those over 65, about 1 in 4. Of those with high blood pressure, only 1 in 8 receives treatment that returns the blood pressure to a normal range.

A variety of studies have shown that several factors contribute to primary hypertension:
— High blood pressure is twice as frequent in overweight individuals.
— In some people, high salt intake causes blood pressure to rise.
— Alcohol is a "calorie bomb" and, over the long term, causes metabolic changes that may lead to obesity and high blood pressure.
— Insufficient exercise can promote obesity, leading to high blood pressure.
— People with diabetes often have high blood pressure.
— Blood pressure rises for a short time in response to acute stress. It is suspected that chronic stress leads to chronic high blood pressure (see Health and Well-Being, p. 182).
— Constant loud noise levels from low-flying planes, traffic, or machinery apparently contribute to high blood pressure (see Deafness, p. 251).
— From studies on twins, it has been concluded that heredity plays some role in high blood pressure.
— Countless medications can raise blood pressure as a side effect, e.g., oral contraceptives, some cough medicines, corticosteroids, eyedrops, cold remedies, etc. The same is true for licorice in large quantities.

Possible Aftereffects and Complications

If blood pressure remains high over a long period, the

Caution! The following medications may elevate blood pressure:

Cold remedies:
Actifed
Dimetapp
Contac
Entex
Naldecon
Triaminic
Among others
Weight-loss drugs:
Dexedrine
Among others

risk of stroke, heart disease, kidney problems, and retinal damage increases, and life expectancy decreases correspondingly. This is particularly true when other damaging factors such as smoking, obesity, high blood-cholesterol levels, or lack of exercise are present.

Prevention
— Lose weight if you are obese (see Body Weight, p. 727).
— Engage in sports regularly. Endurance sports like cross-country skiing, jogging, cycling, and hiking are best (see Physical Activity and Sports, p. 762).
— Get enough sleep, and make sure it's restful. Avoid stress overload, and reduce or remove sources of noise.

When to Seek Medical Advice
To avoid secondary diseases, high blood pressure should be treated as soon as possible. Blood pressure can be measured at a doctor's office or public screening campaign.

Measuring Blood Pressure
In general, blood pressure is measured by wrapping the upper arm in a rubber cuff which is pumped up until blood can't flow through the artery in the arm; this is determined by listening with a stethoscope on the inside of the elbow. The pressure in the sleeve is gradually released until the heart is able to force blood through the artery.
— The pressure at which the first sound of blood passing the artery is heard is called the upper (systolic) value; it is measured as the heart contracts and squeezes blood into the arteries. This pressure wave can also be felt as the pulse at the wrist.
— When the blood flow no longer makes a sound because the constriction has been released, the lower (diastolic) value is observed. The heart is now relaxing and filling with new blood.

The blood pressure is usually given as a fraction, such as 140/90 mm Hg (millimeters of mercury; this refers to the height of a mercury column under the given pressure). Both the upper and lower values are of interest in evaluating blood pressure, but the lower (diastolic) value is of greater significance.

Blood pressure varies considerably during the day, depending on activity level and degree of nervous tension. A diagnosis of high blood pressure is made only when several measurements, taken on different days while the patient is at rest, give upper (systolic) values greater than 160 and lower (diastolic) values greater than 95. Values between 140/90 and 160/95 are considered borderline.

Errors in Measurement
A number of studies have shown that mistakes are often made in measuring blood pressure. Usually, errors arise because:
— Patients are nervous during the test. This causes the blood pressure to rise automatically. An approximately "correct" value can be obtained from self-measurement (see p. 323), or if the health-care provider takes three or four measurements over a period of 10 minutes, and only uses the last one.
— Narrow, short rubber cuffs are often used on people with large upper arms, resulting in readings that are too high by 10 to 15 mm Hg.
— If blood vessel walls are thickened and rigid, actual blood pressure may be much lower than the measured value. This situation can be detected by feeling the pulse at the wrist while blood pressure is being measured. When the pressure in the sleeve is higher than the upper (systolic) blood pressure, one can usually feel neither pulse nor artery. However, if the arterial wall is thickened, one can still feel the artery, but not the pulse. If this is the case, it can be assumed that the measured blood pressure is 10 to 60 mm Hg too high.
— In older people, blood pressure may be elevated when seated, but normal when standing; therefore it should be measured while standing.
— Many technical errors can occur in the measurement process: Stethoscope placed incorrectly, air let out of the sleeve too quickly, incorrect hearing of sounds, pressure misreading, or faulty equipment.

Self-Help
If your health-care provider has determined that you have high blood pressure, it is worth considering buying your own measuring device. Testing your blood pressure in a relaxed atmosphere may show normal levels, in which case no treatment is required.

If you are taking medications to reduce blood pressure, self-measurement is useful to monitor treatment; but do not change dosages without consulting your physician.

Testing Your Own Blood Pressure

— Before buying the apparatus, have a health professional explain its use in detail.
— Do the test sitting and standing, after 5 to 10 minutes of rest.
— If possible, do the test between 8 and 10 a.m. and whenever you aren't feeling well.
— Always test on the same arm.
— Use a cuff that fits your arm. The cuff width should cover two thirds of the length of your upper arm.
— Place the cuff about two finger-widths above the elbow.
— Pump the cuff up to about 30 mm Hg above the expected upper value (about 170 mm Hg).
— Hold your arm still.
— Let the air out so that the pressure sinks by 2 to 3 mm Hg per second.
— Before repeating the test, wait at least one minute and deflate the cuff completely.
— Write down the measurements, along with the date, time and situation (whether you're sitting or lying, etc.) and any unusual stresses.
— If you don't have an automatic device and always get results different from those obtained by a health professional, you should consider the possibility that your hearing may be impaired.

Treatment Without Medications

Most people with high blood pressure have only slightly elevated levels, with diastolic values between 90 and 105 mm Hg. In these cases, most experts recommend treatment without medications, at least to begin with:
— Lose weight if you're overweight (see Body Weight, p. 727).
— Laughter is indeed the best medicine! Laugh a lot— it's relaxing, which helps reduce blood pressure. Keeping a pet can also help you relax.
— Reduce alcohol consumption. Sometimes this alone will normalize blood pressure; it also makes weight loss easier.
— Take up a sport.
— Learn and regularly practice relaxation techniques (see Relaxation, p. 693).

— Take a look at your lifestyle. Take care to get enough restful sleep, and if possible, cut down on commitments.
— If possible, stop using medications that can elevate blood pressure: Oral contraceptives, rheumatism medicines, corticosteroids, stimulants, some nose drops and appetite depressants.
— Stop smoking. Smoking is much more dangerous to your heart and circulation than high blood pressure, although it contributes only slightly to hypertension.
— Moderate amounts of coffee, tea, cocoa, and cola are permissible.

Low-salt diets, which used to be recommended, have turned out to be nearly ineffectual and are now prescribed only for elderly patients.

Treatment With Medications

Medications are indicated only if treatment without medications has been unsuccessful, blood pressure has not been reduced sufficiently, or the patient simultaneously has kidney or heart disease.

If the lower (diastolic) blood pressure is above 115 mm Hg, the danger of a stroke or heart attack almost always necessitates medication. However, the self-help measures discussed above should always accompany treatment.

There are many medications for high blood pressure. It is advisable to follow a graduated plan, as follows:

Step 1: In patients older than about 60, treatment begins with a diuretic, and in younger patients, a beta blocker. (If for any reason one of these is contraindicated, the above may be reversed.)

Step 2: If the medication used in Step 1 does not produce a sufficient drop in blood pressure, a second medication (ideally, the other one from Step 1) is added. If this is not possible, other medications may be combined, such as vasodilators like hydralazine, prazosin, methyldopa or clonidine, with a diuretic. This is one of the few cases in which combination medications make sense.

Step 3: If two different types of medication together do not bring down the blood pressure, a combination of three is used.

Beta Blockers

These medications inhibit or block the effect of the sympathetic nervous system on the heart and blood vessels so that the heart beats more slowly and blood pressure is lower, both at rest and under stress. Beta blockers affect other organs as well, which explains their various side effects. Dizziness, confusion, and slowed pulse occur relatively frequently. Beta blockers can also cause constantly cold feet, lively dreams, depressive moods, loss of potency, and dry eyes. Fat metabolism may be negatively affected (the "good" HDL level drops and triglyceride levels rise).

There are now innumerable beta blockers.

Diuretics

Diuretics cause the kidneys to excrete more water and sodium. This reduces the amount of liquid in the blood vessels, and the blood pressure drops. When used over a long period, diuretics reduce tension in the blood vessels, which also contributes to a drop in blood pressure.

A number of diuretics increase potassium excretion as a side effect. To preserve the body's supply of this important substance, potassium sparing diuretics are often prescribed. Some medications also contain a precise ratio of potassium sparing to potassium excreting diuretics. The symptoms of excessive potassium loss are unusual fatigue, weak legs, cramps in the calves, constipation, and disturbed heart rhythm. Diuretics can also interfere with fat metabolism.

When diuretics are begun, the need to urinate becomes more frequent, but after a few days the frequency returns to normal.

Calcium Channel Blockers

Calcium channel blockers inhibit the effect of calcium on the muscular walls of the blood vessels, causing them to relax and the vessels to dilate. As a result, blood pressure drops.

These medications may produce the following side effects: Headaches, flushed face, pounding heart, swollen ankles, or rashes.

The most commonly used beta blockers are

acebutolol, atenolol, betaxolol, bisoprolol, carteolol, carvedilol, esmolol, labetalol, metoprolol, nadolol, penbutolol, pindolol, propranolol, sotalol, timolol

Alpha Blockers (e.g., Prazosin, Terazosin)

These medications dilate the smaller blood vessels, causing blood pressure to drop.

Possible side effects include: Headaches, feeling hot, and rapid heartbeat. In addition, the body retains salt and water, so these medications are usually taken with a diuretic. Prazosin has a very strong effect on blood pressure and may cause weakness, pallor, or collapse at the beginning of treatment.

Reserpine

The possible side effects of this medication (depression, stomach ulcers, etc.) are so severe that it should only be prescribed if other medicines are contraindicated or insufficiently effective.

Clonidine and Methyldopa

These two medications have similar effects and side effects: they can impair reaction times, cause dry mouth, and cause impotence. Because they lead to increased salt and water retention, they should be prescribed only in combination with a diuretic.

Angiotensin-Converting Enzyme (ACE) Inhibitors

These medications (captopril, enalapril, etc.) interfere with the action of the hormone that keeps blood vessels constricted and blood pressure high.

They are quite well tolerated, though they often cause coughing and sometimes rashes, and may interfere with taste. Serious side effects, such as interference with blood-cell formation and kidney damage, are rare; regular laboratory testing is necessary for their early diagnosis.

Reducing Side Effects

For about 3 weeks at the beginning of treatment, all patients feel worse as their bodies get used to lower (normal) blood pressure.

The following can usually prevent or lessen the severity of side effects:

— Tell your health-care provider about all the medications you're taking, and about any side effects of medicines you've taken in the past.
— Take to heart the "Treatments Without Medications," p. 323. If you follow them, you will need fewer medicines.

Diuretics

Diuretics—Loop
Bumetanide (Bumex)
Ethacrynic acid (Edecrin)
Furosemide (Lasix)
Torsemide (Demadex)

Diuretics—Potassium Sparing
Amiloride (Midamor)
Sprironolactone (Aldactone)
Triamterene (Dyrenium)

Diuretics—Thiazide Type
Chlorthiazide (Diuril)
Chlorthalidone (Hygroton)
Hydrochlorothiazide (Esidrix, HCTZ, HydroDIURIL, Microzide, Oretic)
Indapamide (Lozol)
Methyclothiazide (Aquatensen)

Metolazone (Mykrox, Zaroxolyn)

Diuertics—Carbonic Anhydrase Inhibitors
Acetazolamide (Diamox)

Calcium Channel Blockers— Dihydropyridines
Amlodipine Besylate (Norvasc)
Felodipine (Plendil)
Isradipine (DynaCirc)
Nicardipine (Cardene)
Nifedipine (Adalat, Procardia)
Nisoldipine (Sular)

Calcium Channel Blockers— Other
Bepridil (Vascor)

Diltiayam (Cardizem)
Verapamil (Isoptin, Calan)
Antiadrenergic Agents
Clonidine (Catapres)
Doxazosin (Cardura)
Guanabenz (Wytensin)
Guanadrel (Hylorel)
Guanethidine (Ismelin)
Guanfacine (Tenex)
Methyldopa (Aldomet)
Prazosin (Minipress)
Reserpine (Serpasil)
Terazosin (Hytrin)

ACE Inhibitors
Benazepril (Lotensin)
Captopril (Capoten)
Enalapril Maleate (Vasotec)
Fosinopril Sodium (Monopril)
Lisinopril (Prinivil, Zestril)

Moexipril (Univasc)
Quinapril (Accupril)
Ramipril (Altace)
Trandolapril (Mavik)

Antihypertensives— Miscellaneous
Diazoxide (Hyperstat)
Epoprostenol (Flolan)
Hydralazine (Apresoline)
Minoxidil (Loniten)
Nitroprusside sodium (Nipride)
Phenoxybenzamine (Dibenzyline)
Phentolamine Mesylate (Regitine)
Tolazoline (Priscoline)

— If possible, begin treatment with a medication containing only one active ingredient.
— Begin treatment with the lowest possible dose, so your circulation can adapt gradually. The effect of many medicines becomes noticeable only after a few days.
— If you experience side effects, inform your healthcare provider at once.

When to Stop Taking Medications

Half of all patients with slightly elevated blood pressure return to normal within 6 months, without medicines. This applies especially to those who limit alcohol consumption and lose excess weight. However, the higher the blood pressure and the longer it remains high, the less likely it is to normalize spontaneously.

If your blood pressure returns to normal when you take medication, after several months you can discuss with your doctor the possibility of slowly reducing the dose, or of stopping the medication altogether.

High Blood Pressure During Pregnancy

Caution: During pregnancy, the thresholds for treatment of high blood pressure are lower. High blood pressure in pregnancy is a health risk for both mother and child. Pregnant women should first attempt to reduce their blood pressure without medication; often rest alone is sufficient—for example, lying down for several hours each day. If medications are necessary, either beta blockers or methyldopa should be used, as they will not damage the fetus.

HYPOTENSION (LOW BLOOD PRESSURE)

Complaints

Low blood pressure is not always noticeable. As long as it produces no symptoms, it is almost a blessing: People with low blood pressure have above-average life expectancies.

The most common symptoms of hypotension are dizziness and faintness right after getting up in the morning, or irregular or rapid heartbeat. General indicators include outbreaks of sweating, chills, sensitivity to weather, sleep disturbances, difficulty getting started in the morning, limited physical capacity, impaired vision, difficulty concentrating, a tendency to dizziness, and blacking out of vision when standing up from a sitting or lying position.

In children, low blood pressure may manifest as lack of appetite at breakfast, headaches, or stomachaches, difficulty concentrating, or tiredness.

Causes

This disorder is caused by faulty distribution of blood in the body. Eighty-five percent of the body's blood is found in the venous circulation. In persons with low blood pressure a large proportion of the blood remains in the leg veins, and there is a temporary shortage of blood returning to the heart.

Possible causes of low blood pressure:
— Constitutional predisposition: Tall, slender people are often affected.
— Psychic stress, combined with exhaustion and resignation, can reduce blood pressure (see Health and Well-Being, p. 182).
— Loss of blood or liquids, through vomiting, internal bleeding, or diarrhea.
— Various diseases of the heart and circulatory system.
— Long confinement to bed.
— Infectious diseases.
— Neurological diseases.
— Side effects of medications, e.g., diuretics and medications for hypertension, angina pectoris, psychoses, and depression.

Who's at Risk

Low blood pressure is not an uncommon finding.

Possible Aftereffects and Complications

Low blood pressure can be unpleasant, but it is almost never dangerous. However, dizziness can lead to falls and serious injuries, especially in older people.

Low blood pressure during pregnancy can lead to lower birth weight in the baby.

Prevention

The following improve circulation:
— Sufficient restful sleep
— Alternating hot and cold showers
— Exercise (see p. 327)
— Beginning the day slowly in the morning

When to Seek Medical Advice

Seek help if you find symptoms oppressive and self-help measures don't help.

Self-Help

The most important therapy is intensive physical training: Treading water, hot and cold showers, breathing exercises, and regular participation in sports. Swimming is one of the best sports for circulation.

The following are also useful:
— Take your time while getting up in the morning.
— A cup of coffee or black tea is a reliable method of increasing blood pressure.
— Take a walk after eating.
— Drink 6 to 8 glasses of liquid each day.

Treatment

Your health-care provider should first determine the cause of the symptoms, and treat any other diseases which may be present, such as infectious or heart diseases.

Only if the above self-help procedures prove inadequate should medications be tried, and then only for a short time. They are no substitute for lifestyle changes, and in some cases may actually make matters worse.

Before prescribing medication, the doctor should determine the type of low blood pressure. After a period of lying down, the patient stands up and the doctor measures pulse and blood pressure while the patient stands quietly. The results indicate which of the following medication types should be used:
— If both upper and lower blood pressure-values fall and the heart does not beat faster, so-called sympathomimetics are used. These drugs constrict the blood vessels in the arms and legs.
— If only the upper blood-pressure value falls while the lower one rises and the heart beats faster, the active ingredient dihydroergotamine is effective. This medication increases the flexibility of the veins; however, its action develops only after several days.
— In some cases, a combination of a sympathomimetic and a dihydroergotamine may be beneficial. Popular but ineffective products include vitamins, adenosine, nicotinic acid, hawthorn, balm mint and salicylic acid.

Note: You should not take low-blood-pressure medication for more than a few weeks.

POOR CIRCULATION (INTERMITTENT CLAUDICATION)

Complaints

The symptoms of this disorder most often affect the legs, and there are various levels of severity.

1. Pain when carrying heavy loads; occasional limping. The patient can walk only short distances without pain. After a rest of 1 to 5 minutes, he or she can walk a bit further, until the pain recurs. (This is sometimes known as "window-shopping disease.")
2. Severe pain in legs and toes, even at rest; the pain worsens when legs are lifted.
3. Damage to skin and muscle tissue, tissue necrosis.

Causes
This disorder is caused when hardened, thickened arteries can no longer deliver enough blood to the muscles. Arteriosclerosis is caused mainly by
— Natural aging
— Too much fat in the blood (see p. 318)
— Smoking

Who's at Risk
The risk of disease increases
— With age
— In people with diabetes
— With obesity
— With high blood pressure
— With high uric-acid levels in the blood (gout)
— With lack of exercise

Possible Aftereffects and Complications
In the final stages of this disease, ulcers develop on the toes, heels, and legs. The muscles shrink, and tissue dies (necrosis) and may decay (gangrene). In order to keep the products of this decay from poisoning the entire body, the leg must be amputated.

Prevention
Stop smoking (see p. 755), exercise (see p. 327), eat a low-fat diet (see Antherosclerosis, p. 318) and lose weight (see p. 727).

When to Seek Medical Advice
You should see a physician as soon as you suspect that your circulation is impaired. Using a Doppler ultrasonic instrument, a health-care provider can measure the systolic blood pressure in the arm and leg, and determine how good the circulation is.

Self-Help
Self-help measures can slow or even stop the progression of the disease. These include

— Stopping smoking (see p. 755).
— Losing weight (see p. 727).
— A low-fat diet (see Atherosclerosis, p. 318).
— Treatment of high blood pressure (see p. 323).
— Careful treatment of diabetes (see p. 486).
The following can lessen symptoms:
— The most important treatment for intermittent limping is walking training: Count how many steps you can go before the pain begins. Walk three fourths of this distance with a brisk stride. Wait a couple of minutes before walking the same distance again. Train for one hour each day in this manner. Each week, again measure how far you can go without pain, and lengthen the distance you walk between rests accordingly. As time goes on, you will be able to walk farther and farther without pain.
— Raise the head of your bed by 4 to 6 inches.
— Do not use a hot water bottle or electric blanket.
— Check the soles of your feet daily for pressure sites, cracks, ulcers, and corns. To do this, lay a large hand mirror on the floor.
— Wash your feet daily in lukewarm water with mild soap; dry them carefully and well.
— If the skin on your feet is very dry, frequently rub in hand or body lotion.
— Wear shoes with enough room for your toes.
— Never go barefoot.

Treatment with Medication
If necessary, you can ease the pain for a short time with a painkiller containing acetylsalicylic acid (see p. 661). A daily dose of 150 to 300 mg of acetylsalicylic acid can also prevent blockage of the arteries.

Daily exercises for better circulation
— Stand about 1 yard in front of a wall. Keeping your feet flat on the floor, lean forward and place your hands on the wall. Bend your arms, keeping your back and legs straight, and then push yourself back upright. Repeat 10 times.
— Sit on a chair, then stand up with folded arms. Repeat 10 times.
— Stand with feet flat, then rise to your toes and return to your starting position. Repeat 20 times.
— When standing, lift first one heel and then the other, keeping the opposite heel down.
— Do 10 deep knee bends with your back straight, holding onto the back of a chair so you don't fall.
— Use stairs instead of elevators. While you are climbing the stairs, frequently go on tiptoes.

Treatment of poor circulation by medication only makes sense if the distance you can walk remains very limited, in spite of walking training, or if you experience pain even while resting. In this case, you should take so-called vasodilators (vessel-dilating drugs). After a period of at most three months, your health-care provider should determine whether further treatment is indicated.

Treatment with Surgery

In cases of pronounced impairment of circulation, the arteries can be stretched with a balloon catheter; the procedure is known as percutaneous transluminal angioplasty and often improves the situation.

Another procedure consists of bypassing the highly constricted arteries in the leg using a prosthetic piece, or a piece of transplanted skin vein. This method greatly reduces the symptoms for most patients, and in some cases can stave off the need for amputation.

Relatively recent blockages can still be dissolved by drugs, but this treatment should only be carried out in a hospital.

VARICOSE VEINS

Complaints

Varicose veins are visibly swollen, convoluted veins, usually in the legs; they are sometimes painful.

People with varicose veins often have swollen, tired feet even after standing for a short while or after shopping. At the end of the day, their shoes seem too small. In women, these symptoms are usually more pronounced a few days before menstruation begins. In severe cases, the skin acquires a brown discoloration, usually near the ankles, because of the limited blood circulation.

Causes

The heart's pumping action alone is not enough to make blood return to the heart. Blood in the veins is also pressed towards the heart by muscle contractions. To prevent blood from flowing in the wrong direction, the veins contain flap-like valves. If for any reason these valves are not functioning properly, some of the blood that should be flowing back to the heart is pressed into the veins lying on muscle surfaces. Because veins, unlike arteries, have only a relatively thin muscular wall,

they expand and bend: a varicose vein has developed.

Genetic factors probably play a role in the development of varicose veins, as do large body size, lack of physical activity, overweight, work done mainly in a standing or sitting position, and a diet lacking in fiber.

Who's at Risk

The risk of developing varicose veins increases with age, and women are more frequently affected than men.

Possible Aftereffects and Complications

Varicose veins are usually a primarily cosmetic issue: Many people find the bluish, convoluted lines along the legs unsightly. In pronounced cases of varicose veins, the skin on the legs acquires a brownish discoloration. Dermatitis, lower leg ulcers, edema, and venous thromboses (p. 330) are possible complications.

Prevention

It may be possible to reduce the risk of developing varicose veins through the following measures:
— Eat plenty of fiber (see Nutrition, p. 722).
— Maintain a normal weight (see Body Weight, p. 727).
— Get enough exercise (see Physical Activity and Sports, p. 762).
— Avoid standing still for prolonged periods of time.
— Put your feet up as often as possible.

When to Seek Medical Advice

If you wish to have varicose veins removed, or if symptoms become unpleasant, see your health-care provider. If varicose veins or lower leg ulcers begin to bleed, seek medical attention at once.

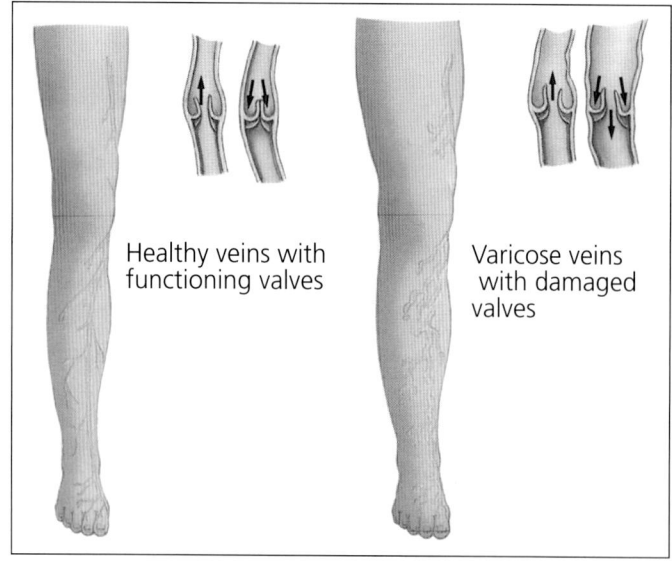

Healthy veins with functioning valves

Varicose veins with damaged valves

Self-Help

In addition to the measures listed above under "Prevention":

Wear elastic support hose all day, every day. They should be bidirectional tension compression hose, such as are available in a surgical supply store. Ordinary "support hose" are not effective. Put them on before you get out of bed.

Treatment

Varicose veins are not improved by rubbing in lotions or taking so-called "vein tonics."

There are only two effective methods of treatment: sclerosing or stripping the veins. In either case, you should wear compression hose for 3 to 6 weeks after the surgery and exercise as much as possible. However, new varicose veins may develop after the operation.

Sclerosing Varicose Veins

Varicose veins are most often sclerosed if the small skin veins (spider veins) are affected, or if both the main skin veins and their side branches are enlarged. Sclerosing does not require hospitalization. Because of the danger of thrombosis, women should not take oral contraceptives for 6 weeks before the operation.

Veins are sclerosed by injecting a solution into them which causes an inflammation. Then the leg is bandaged, which presses the veins together and causes them to stick. The bandages must be worn for about 3 weeks, during which it is important to continue normal activities and walk a great deal. If varicose veins on both legs need this procedure, the operations will be scheduled for different days.

Risks: If the physician accidentally injects the solution outside the veins, it can cause ulcers and painful inflammation of the surrounding tissue. In some cases, the skin acquires a brownish discoloration. In rare cases, there is an allergic reaction. On average, one in 10,000 patients dies as a result of this procedure.

Stripping Varicose Veins

If the large veins of both legs have become varicosed, the most reliable treatment is to remove them. This requires hospitalization for about a week.

First the physician will check whether the deep leg veins are open, using ultrasound or an X ray procedure called phlebography in which a contrast material is injected into the veins at the back of the foot.

If the deep veins are open, small incisions are made, under general anesthesia, at the ankle, back of the knee, and groin and the veins are pulled out.

After the operation, a pressure bandage is used to prevent heavy bleeding. To prevent formation of clots, the patient should stand up and walk around, if possible on the same day as the operation.

Risks: In about 20 percent of cases, the main nerves in the ankle region are injured, causing loss of sensation in the affected areas. Heavy bleeding, infections, and injury to the arteries or deep thigh veins occur rarely. On average, 1 in 5,000 patients dies.

SUPERFICIAL PHLEBITIS

Complaints

Symptoms of this disorder include tension and pain in the muscles of the lower leg; swollen legs; in severe cases, reddening, itching, and a hard, stringlike swelling in the area of the affected veins; in some cases, low-grade fever. Phlebitis is especially likely to occur in the area of varicose veins (see p. 328).

Causes

The veins usually become inflamed through infection or injury. The inflammation inhibits blood flow through the vein, and as a result, clots can develop and adhere to the walls of the inflamed veins. The condition is called thrombophlebitis.

Who's at Risk

The risk of disease is increased by
— Varicose veins (see p. 328)
— Veins damaged by injections, infusions, or catheterizations
— Increased tendency of the blood to form clots, e.g., because of oral contraceptives or certain types of cancer
— Blood stagnation after childbirth, surgery or prolonged periods of bed rest in patients with chronic diseases

Possible Aftereffects and Complications

Phlebitis is usually not dangerous.

Prevention
— Maintain normal weight (see Body Weight, p. 727).
— Get plenty of exercise (see p. 762).
— Put your feet up as often as possible.
— Eat plenty of fiber (see Nutrition, p. 722).
— On long car trips, stop often. On plane or train trips, stand up often and walk around. Drink plenty of liquids so the blood does not thicken.

When to Seek Medical Advice
Seek help as soon as you notice the symptoms described above.

Self-Help
Get a pair of compression hose fitted by a specialist, put them on, and walk a lot. A word to the wise: Bandages applied incorrectly can cause more damage than good. The pain can be relieved by acetylsalicylic acid (see Simple Analgesics, p. 661). Do not massage painful areas unless your health-care provider specifically recommends it: Massage can release a clot (thrombus) and cause an embolism.

Treatment
Treatment includes:
— Compression bandages
— Anti-inflammatory drugs such as indomethacin.
    With appropriate treatment, symptoms will disappear within a few weeks.

DEEP VEIN THROMBOSIS
(Inflammation of the Deep Veins)

Complaints
Symptoms of this disorder include swollen, painful calves or ankles, and bluish or reddish discoloration of the skin. The inflamed veins cannot usually be seen or detected by palpation. Sometimes, by pressing on the back of the lower leg, one can feel a hard strand deep down.

Causes
Blood clots form in the deep veins of the legs and block the return of blood to the heart.

Who's at Risk
About 90 percent of all vein thromboses are located in the legs and pelvis, and about 4 percent are found in

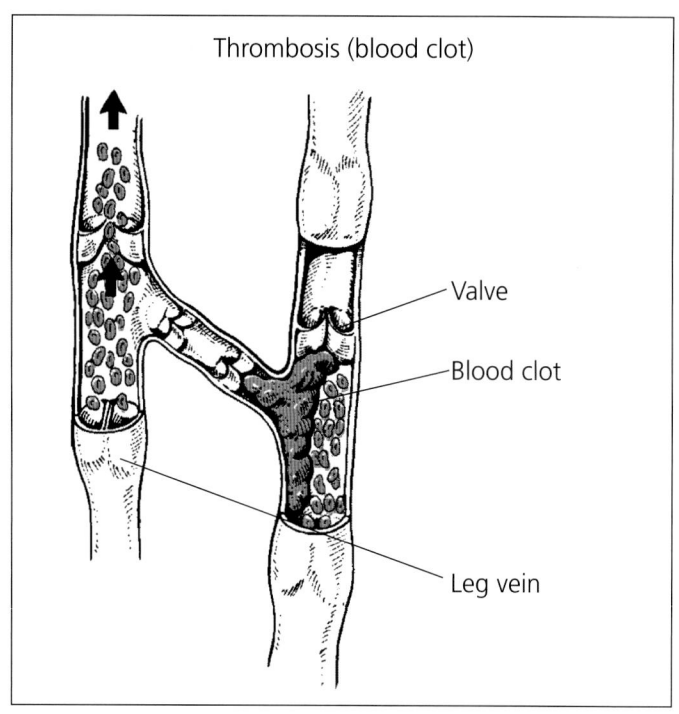

Thrombosis (blood clot)

Valve

Blood clot

Leg vein

the arms and shoulders. The remainder are spread over the rest of the body.

Deep vein thrombosis occurs most often after severe injuries or major surgery. It affects approximately one in three patients over the age of 40 who undergo such surgery.

However, long trips in buses, cars or planes can also cause deep vein thrombosis, due to the restriction of physical activity.

The following factors also increase the risk of thrombosis: cancer and diabetes, a weak heart, obesity, varicose veins, pregnancy, heart attack, paraplegia, and smoking. Even a plaster cast on a leg increases the risk.

There is also a congenital form of defective clotting (antithrombin III deficiency) which produces an increase in thromboses.

Possible Aftereffects and Complications
If a blood clot is released from one of the veins in the lower legs, it is carried in the blood stream into larger and larger veins, and eventually into the pelvic veins. From there, it is carried into the inferior vena cava and then into the heart. Since the arteries leading away from the heart and into the lungs branch and become smaller and smaller, the clot will eventually get stuck in one of the lung arteries, and block it. The lung tissue which depends on this artery will suddenly be deprived of blood; this is a pulmonary embolism (see p. 312), which

is a life-threatening condition. It is the greatest risk engendered by deep vein thrombosis.

Prevention

Because of the danger of life-threatening pulmonary embolisms, prevention is very important:

—Women over the age of 35, especially if they smoke, should use contraceptive methods other than oral contraceptives.

— Stop smoking (see p. 755).

— If you are confined to bed for a long period, you should repeatedly contract your leg muscles and move your ankles and toes to stimulate blood circulation.

— In situations where the danger of thrombosis is acute, e.g., after operations or while a limb is in a cast, heparin is injected. This is an clot inhibitor, and patients can learn to inject it themselves.

— If the treatment is prolonged, the doctor may prescribe warfarin (Coumadin) to be taken orally. These medications do not take effect for 1 or 2 days, however.

When to Seek Medical Advice

Seek help immediately, as soon as the above symptoms occur.

Self-Help

Not possible.

Treatment

An acute deep vein thrombosis must be treated immediately and in a hospital. There the legs are elevated, and heparin infusion is begun.

Attempts are made to dissolve existing clots, if possible, with medications such as urokinase and streptokinase. Once the swelling in the affected leg has gone down, the patient must wear support hose to prevent pain, skin discoloration, renewed swelling, and ulcers.

In some cases, the clot must be surgically removed.

To prevent a recurrence of the thrombosis, the patient should take clotting inhibitors such as Coumadin. During this time, regular blood tests are required to make sure clots can still form if the patient is injured, to prevent excessive bleeding.

ANEURYSMS

Aneurysms are bulges in damaged arterial walls.

Complaints

Symptoms can vary considerably, depending on which site in the body is affected and the size of the aneurysm.

—Aneurysm in the aorta can cause constant coughing, hoarseness, difficulty breathing, and chest pains.

—The chest pain, which is similar to that felt in a heart attack, can be caused by a dissecting aortic aneurysm. In this condition, the wall of the aorta is separated into several layers, and the blood is forced, under high pressure, between these layers.

— Aneurysms in the brain region can cause severe headaches.

— In the abdominal region, the symptom may be a visibly pulsating lump on the descending aorta, sometimes coupled with a loss of appetite and weight.

Causes

There are basically three causes of aneurysms

— Congenital weakness of the muscular layers of the arteries

— Inflammations that weaken the arterial walls

— Degeneration of the arterial walls due to arteriosclerosis (see p. 318) and high blood pressure (see p. 321)

Who's at Risk

The risk increases as one ages, as most aneurysms occur as a result of arteriosclerosis in connection with high blood pressure.

Possible Aftereffects and Complications

Depending on where they occur and how extensive they are, aneurysms are life-threatening under some circumstances.

Prevention

If the blood pressure is elevated, it should be brought back to normal (see high blood pressure, p. 321). Otherwise, the usual measures to prevent or inhibit arteriosclerotic processes also may prevent aneurysms (see Arteriosclerosis, p. 318).

When to Seek Medical Advice

Seek help as soon as you suspect you have an aneurysm.

Self-Help

Not possible.

Treatment

If a thorough examination using X rays (angiograms), ultrasound, computed tomography, or magnetic resonance imaging reveals an aneurysm, and if it is either painful or dangerous, medications are prescribed to bring down the blood pressure (see p. 323), and/or an operation may be needed.

RAYNAUD'S DISEASE AND RAYNAUD'S PHENOMENON

Experts make a distinction between Raynaud's disease and Raynaud's phenomenon, depending on the cause of the condition.

Complaints

Symptoms include sudden discoloration of the fingers or toes, which first turn white, then bluish, and finally reddish. The affected limbs feel numb for minutes or hours, or they experience a prickling sensation, but they are not painful. Over the long term, Raynaud's disease may cause the skin of the fingers to become smooth, shiny, and stiff.

Causes of Raynaud's Disease

For unknown reasons, the small arteries react with unusual sensitivity to cold or emotions by contracting. The result is an inadequate supply of blood to the muscle tissue and, occasionally, deterioration of the skin and tissues.

Causes of Raynaud's Phenomenon

The above complaints may result from a variety of diseases, such as
— Autoimmune diseases (see Scleroderma, p. 461, Rheumatoid Arthritis, p. 455)
— Diseases of the arteries.
— Toxic medications containing ergot alkaloids or methysergide.
— Side effects of medications for high blood pressure (e.g., beta blockers or clonidine) or headach remedies containing ergotamine
— Chronic damage caused by years of working with power saws or jackhammers.

Who's at Risk

Raynaud's disease is about four times as common in women as in men; young women are most often affected.

Possible Aftereffects and Complications

The poor blood supply to the tissues can eventually impair the sense of touch.

Raynaud's disease progresses very slowly, while Raynaud's phenomenon worsens rapidly. Raynaud's phenomenon can shrink the affected tissue and cause ulcers to form.

Prevention of Raynaud's Disease

None is known.

Prevention of Raynaud's Phenomenon

The condition could often be prevented if workers were not required to work regularly, over many years, with power saws or jackhammers.

When to Seek Medical Advice

Seek help if symptoms do not improve in spite of self-help measures.

Self-Help

— Always keep hands and feet dry and warm.
— Do not wear tight shoes.
— Stop smoking; it impairs circulation still more (see p. 755).
— Avoid spending time in the cold.
— Do relaxation exercises (see p. 693).

Medications for Raynaud's Disease:
Nifedipine
Pentoxifyllin
Prazosin Hydrochloride—orally at bedtime

Medications for Raynaud's Phenomenon:
Pentoxifyllin
Phenoxybenzamine Hydrochloride
Reserpine
   Treatment should be directed at identifying the underlying disorder, and minimizing tissue loss if present.

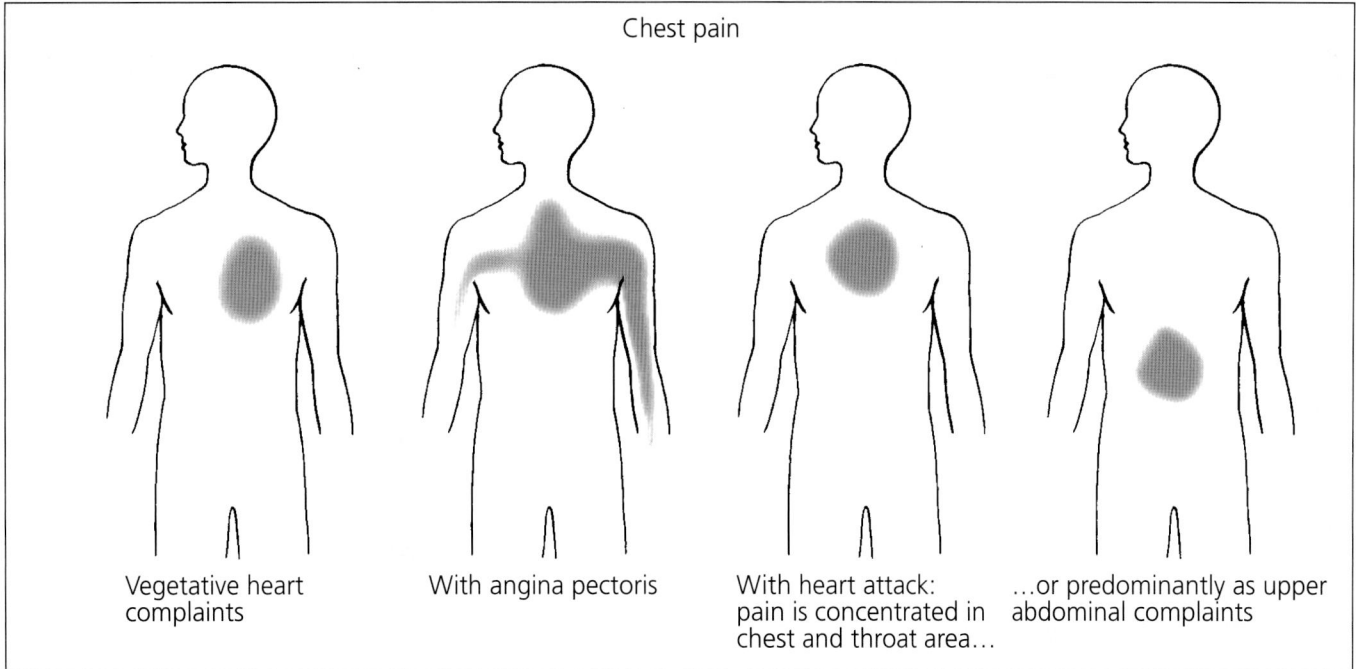

Chest pain

Vegetative heart complaints

With angina pectoris

With heart attack: pain is concentrated in chest and throat area...

...or predominantly as upper abdominal complaints

Treatment with Medications

If self-help measures are not sufficient, medications that dilate blood vessels can help, but they should only be used for a short time.

Operations

If Raynaud's phenomenon or disease become worse and make the patient an invalid, surgical intervention may be useful under some circumstances. The operation, called a sympathectomy, consists of removing certain nerves. It only improves symptoms for 1 to 2 years, however.

ANGINA PECTORIS

Complaints

The symptoms of angina usually include tightness, difficulty breathing, and pains in the middle of the chest, which may expand to the neck, chin, back, and arms. In rare cases, the pains occur only in the arms, wrists, or nape of the neck. The symptoms can vary widely, depending on the direction in which the pains radiate; as a result, angina pectoris symptoms are sometimes misinterpreted as tooth, stomach, or wrist pains.

The pain is dull yet strong, characteristically occurs during physical exertion, often lasts only a few minutes, and ceases when the patient rests. The attacks are often accompanied by severe anxiety and the sensation of the chest being clamped in an iron ring.

Angina attacks can occur as often as several times a day, or as infrequently as every few months or years. They may become increasingly frequent, or disappear completely. If the number of attacks changes, or if the attacks last longer than usual, occur when the patient is at rest, or occur during slight exertion, the condition is called unstable angina.

Causes

In angina pectoris, the arteries supplying the heart muscle with blood are constricted. The three large coronary arteries are only slightly interconnected, so if one artery is constricted, the others cannot compensate.

During physical exertion, the heart must pump more blood. The constriction in the arteries prevents the heart from receiving enough oxygenated blood, resulting in typical angina pectoris pains.

Who's at Risk

Angina pectoris is one of the most common diseases of old age. The risk increases with the following factors:
— Increasing age
— Smoking
— Diabetes
— High blood pressure
— Too much cholesterol in the blood
— Too much uric acid in the blood (gout)

Debate continues as to whether lack of exercise, obesity, and heavy stress at home or work increase the risk of angina pectoris (see Health and Well-Being, p. 182).

Possible Aftereffects and Complications

Self-help measures and treatment permit many people with angina pectoris to lead normal lives, but they still run an increased risk of heart attack or sudden heart stoppage. Life expectancy depends on the degree of damage to their coronary arteries. Medications, bypass operations, and stretching of the constricted arteries can help many patients live without symptoms for many years.

Prevention

Not possible.

When to Seek Medical Advice

Seek help if you suspect that you have angina pectoris.

Coronary Angiography

For this procedure, the patient is given a sedative, but not complete anesthesia. The physician inserts a catheter into the artery in the arm or groin, injects an X ray contrast medium into the coronary arteries, makes an X ray exposure, and can then see exactly which arteries are damaged and the extent of damage.
Risk level: Life-threatening situations arise in 1 per 1,000 patients as a result of an angiography.

Self-Help

— Stop smoking (see p. 755). If you are able to stop smoking for more than 2 years, your risk will drop to the same level as that of someone who never smoked.
— Reduce if you are overweight (see Weight, p. 727).
— Let a physician treat your high blood pressure; this is absolutely necessary (see p. 323).
— Bring down your cholesterol level if it is too high (see p. 318).
— Get exercise. Jogging is especially helpful, but have a medical exam first (see Exercise and Sports, p. 762).
— Avoid foods that seem to burden your stomach.
— Avoid psychological stress, sudden exertion, and sudden major changes in temperature.

The following medications will interrupt an angina attack or help with short-term prevention:

Nitroglycerin (sublingual or oral spray during acute attack; transdermal patch, topical ointment, or oral long-acting as preventative)

Beta blockers such as:	*Calcium channel blockers such as:*
Atenolol	Amlodipine Besylate
Metoprolol	Bepridil Hydrochloride
Nadolol	Diltiazem
Timolol Maleate	Felodipine
	Isradipine
	Nicardipine
	Nifedipine
	Verapamil Hydrochloride

Treatment with Medications

The treatment of angina pectoris with medications has two goals:
1. To interrupt or temporarily prevent acute attacks.
2. To prevent further attacks.

Attacks of angina pectoris may be interrupted by taking a capsule of nitroglycerin (under the tongue) or nitroglycerin spray orally. This treatment has been used for decades, and it can prevent attacks for about 20 to 30 minutes. The most common side effect of nitroglycerin is headaches.

The drug Nifedipine has also proved useful in treating acute attacks; again, the capsule must be taken under the tongue to stop the attack.

Over the long term, further attacks can be prevented either by nitrates, beta blockers, or calcium channel blockers.

Bypass Operation

If neither self-help measures nor medications offer sufficient improvement, an angioplasty or a bypass operation may help. An examination with EKG, stress EKG, isotope injections, or coronary angiography will show the surgeon exactly which regions of the heart muscle are not receiving enough blood. This information will determine whether a bypass or an angioplasty is more likely to succeed. If two or three coronary arteries are partially blocked, a bypass operation may be life-saving.

However, if only one or two vessels are affected, surgery is usually attempted only if the symptoms are very intense.

Coronary Artery Bypass

In a bypass operation, a piece of vein is removed from the lower leg and inserted as a "bypass" between the aorta and coronary artery so the blood can flow unobstructed. Alternatively, one or more arteries from the inside of the rib cage are transplanted into the coronary artery past the constricted section. The operation lasts several hours, and patients usually remain in intensive care for several days; the hospital stay is about two weeks.

In 85 percent of bypass patients, symptoms either disappear or are significantly improved; yet the disease may continue to progress anyway. In patients in whom the narrowing of the coronary arteries was starving large regions of the heart muscle of blood, the operation definitely lengthens life expectancy.

Level of risk: About 1 out of every 300 patients dies as a result of coronary artery bypass surgery.

Angioplasty or Dilatation

These operations are ideal for patients in whom only one or two vessels are partially blocked near the heart.

In angioplasty, the surgeon first anesthetizes a site on the arm or leg where a catheter can be introduced into the artery. The catheter, with a balloon at the end, is pushed through the artery to the constricted point near the heart; the balloon is then blown up and stretches the artery. The procedure lasts about 45 minutes.

Experienced surgeons using this procedure can improve circulation to the heart in about 80 percent of patients; in about 20 percent, the blood vessels become clogged again within days or weeks of the operation. Sometimes bypass surgery must be initiated during the angioplasty.

In dilatation, several different techniques are used. The clogged arteries are opened with drill bits, lasers, or small rotating knives, and tubular artery prostheses are introduced. This operation is successful about 90 percent of the time; however, in 30 to 50 percent of patients, the arteries become clogged again.

Level of risk: Fewer than 1 percent of patients die from this operation.

HEART ATTACK (MYOCARDIAL INFARCTION)

Complaints

The symptoms of an acute heart attack are usually similar to those of an angina pectoris attack: Breathing is difficult and there are deep, dull pains in the center of the chest, which may spread to the neck, chin, back, and arms. The patient becomes anxious about dying, breaks out in a cold sweat, and has a racing pulse.

On the other hand, in about one in five cases, a heart attack may manifest as a sudden loss of consciousness with vomiting, but without pain; vague symptoms in the upper belly or an inexplicable shortness of breath; or slight pressure in the middle of the chest, with inexplicable pains in one arm or in the jaw.

Unlike angina pectoris, the symptoms of a heart attack do not clear up when the patient takes a nitroglycerin capsule or rests for a few minutes. In fact, heart attacks can occur while the patient is at rest. Most occur in the early morning.

Causes

The cause of heart attacks is the same as the cause of angina pectoris: The heart is deprived of oxygen because it is not receiving an adequate supply of blood. This can be the result of coronary arteries narrowed by arteriosclerosis. The attack is often precipitated by a blood clot lodged in the constricted artery. The difference between a heart attack and angina pectoris is that in the former, oxygen depletion in a section of heart muscle is so severe that the tissue dies, unless the constricted artery is unclogged within about 6 hours.

Who's at Risk

Ischemic heart disease is the leading cause of death among adults in the United States. Nearly 1 million deaths annually are due to heart attacks in the United States. Heart attacks are more common in men under 50 than in women that age; however, since women live longer on average, the total number of heart attacks is greater in women. In addition, the frequency of heart attacks in men has decreased in recent years, while it has risen slightly in women.

For many years, women were incorrectly thought to be less susceptible to heart attacks than men, and their risk factors were largely ignored. Only in the last few years have physicians routinely begun to consider a diagnosis of heart attack when a woman presents the symptoms.

The following factors increase the risk of a heart attack:
— Smoking (increases risk two- to fivefold)
— High blood pressure (see p. 321)
— Diabetes (see p. 483)
— Elevated blood-cholesterol levels (see p. 318)
— Gout (see p. 454)

It is thought that overweight and over-stressed people are also at greater risk of a heart attack (see Health and Well-Being, p. 182).

Possible Aftereffects and Complications

About 85 percent of heart attacks are fatal. In those who survive, part of the heart muscle is permanently damaged, which means that the heart's capacity to tolerate stress is reduced. Regular physical training can increase this capacity, but because hardening of the arteries increases with age, there is always the danger of another heart attack. Appropriate preventive measures can reduce this risk.

Prevention

— Stop smoking (see p. 755). A person who succeeds in quitting for more than 2 years has the same risk as someone who never smoked.
— Lose weight if obese (see Weight, p. 727).
— Treat high blood pressure without fail (see p. 321).
— Bring down your cholesterol level if it is too high (see p. 318).
— Get exercise. Jogging is especially helpful, but first have a medical exam (see Exercise and Sports, p. 762).
— Avoid foods that burden the stomach.
— Avoid psychological stress, sudden exertion, and sudden major changes in temperature.
— Arrange your life so it contains appropriate amounts of both tension and relaxation (see Health and Well-Being, p. 182).

When to Seek Medical Advice

A heart attack can happen anytime, anyplace: At the movies, at home, while playing tennis, and so on. Most people die within an hour of noticing the first symptoms—so the first hour determines your chances of survival.

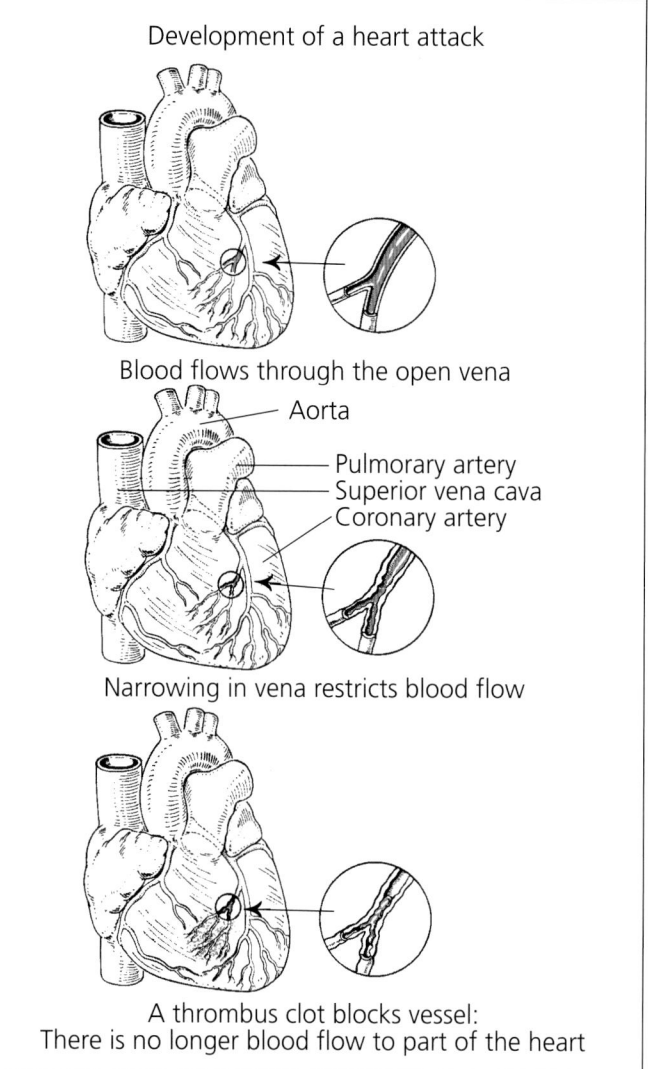

Development of a heart attack

Blood flows through the open vena

Aorta
Pulmorary artery
Superior vena cava
Coronary artery

Narrowing in vena restricts blood flow

A thrombus clot blocks vessel:
There is no longer blood flow to part of the heart

If you suspect you are having a heart attack, have someone take you to a hospital immediately. Half of those who die of heart attacks would survive if they had received timely medical treatment.

Self-Help

The most important lifesaving action you can take is to call an ambulance immediately—provided you or those around you recognize the symptoms of a heart attack and lose no time.

If you suspect you are having a heart attack, lie down at once, take an aspirin, and avoid physical activity or excitement.

Treatment

If a heart attack is suspected, the heart's activity is monitored. Medications are given intravenously to reduce pain and anxiety, to reduce stress on the heart, and to allow it to recover its rhythm.

During the first hour after symptoms appear, doctors can still try to dissolve the blood clot in the artery with medications, to limit damage to the heart muscle. Most survivors of heart attacks suffer from depression after a few days, which should also be treated (see Depression, p. 197).

Any patient confined to bed for a long time is at risk of a lung (pulmonary) embolism; heparin (clot inhibitor) injections can prevent this.

Coronary Artery Bypass

Depending on the condition of the coronary arteries, a bypass operation following a heart attack may increase the patient's life expectancy (see Coronary Artery Bypass, p. 335).

After Leaving the Hospital

Heart attack patients are usually kept in the hospital for 2 to 3 weeks, then moved directly to a rehabilitation center, where their physical activity is gradually increased. (Studies have shown that women are much less frequently offered such rehabilitation; they should demand equal treatment.) The rehabilitation program is tailored to the individual, factoring in such variables as the patient's age, profession, and personal expectations, the extent of damage, possible arrhythmias, and the possible presence of congestive heart failure.

If possible, enroll in an outpatient support group; you can ask for an address in the cardiology department of the hospital.

About 6 weeks after a heart attack, if your heart is working well, you can usually expect to be leading a normal life again. However, to prevent further attacks and improve your chances for enjoying life a good while longer, preventive measures must be strictly observed.

Avoid sexual activities for 3 to 4 weeks after the attack. Small amounts of alcohol are permissible.

Medications to Prevent Further Heart Attacks

Aspirin: Many experts recommend a daily aspirin tablet to prevent further attacks, but make sure you take only specially formulated aspirin that will not irritate the stomach.

Clotting inhibitors such as Coumadin: The medical profession has debated for decades whether such medications prevent heart attacks. They should certainly be used if clots are lodged in the heart in the region of the attack; ultrasound can help determine whether this is the case. *Beta blockers:* A number of studies show that beta blockers increase the survival rate.

CONGESTIVE HEART FAILURE (CORONARY INSUFFICIENCY)

Complaints

Congestive heart failure can affect either the left or right side of the heart, as indicated by the symptoms.

The symptoms of left-side insufficiency include dyspnea (shortness of breath) and tachycardia (racing heart) during heavy physical effort. In the advanced stages, the patient is short of breath even while resting, especially in the evening. Gasping and wheezing are also symptoms. When lying flat, the patient needs more air and must either sit up completely or lean against several pillows. The attacks of dyspnea usually last no longer than an hour and may awaken the patient from sleep. In severe cases, symptoms include chest pains and coughing up blood.

The symptoms of right-side insufficiency include swollen ankles, feelings of fullness in the neck and stomach, and tiredness.

Causes

Congestive heart failure is so called because the weakened heart, unable to pump adequate amounts of blood, draws in too little blood from the vena cava and pulmonary vein, with the result that blood backs up in these veins. Its pressure gradually forces liquid out of the veins into the surrounding tissues, leading to edema.

Possible causes of congestive heart failure include coronary heart disease, and secondary diseases such as heart attack and angina pectoris; high blood pressure; defective heart valves; all other diseases of the heart muscle (such as cardiomyopathy); lung embolisms; and acute rheumatic fever.

Who's at Risk

Congestive heart failure is one of the most common diagnoses in general medicine. Approximately 3 million people in the United States have the condition, and approximately 400,000 new cases are recognized each year. Its prevalence increases directly with age.

Possible Aftereffects and Complications

Untreated, congestive heart failure can cause cardiac arrhythmias (see p. 339). Untreated left-side insufficiency can lead to life-threatening accumulations of fluid in the lungs (see Pulmonary Edema, p. 313). The edema caused by right-side insufficiency can damage the skin and subdermal layer of the legs. The congestion can also damage the liver, gastric mucosa, and kidneys.

Prevention

If you suffer from high blood pressure, have it treated.

When to Seek Medical Advice

Seek help as soon as you suspect that you have congestive heart failure.

Self-Help

— Get as much rest as possible. Sit rather than lying down. Limit physical activities, but don't stop moving completely, as movement stimulates blood circulation.
— Eat a low-sodium diet. Your body will retain less water, reducing the danger of edema.
— After about 5 p.m., drink fewer liquids.
— If you are overweight, lose weight (see p. 727).

Treatment

Before beginning treatment, your health-care provider should determine whether another disease is causing the congestive heart failure, in which case the primary disease should be treated first. There are several ways to treat congestive heart failure:
— Self-help measures
— Medications that improve the heart's pumping ability
— Diuretics
— Medications that dilate the blood vessels, which ease the heart's workload (ACE inhibitors)

Heart-Strengthening Medications (Cardiac Glycosides, e.g., Digoxin)

Correctly used, these medications are a blessing. However, because the margin between a therapeutically effective dose and a toxic dose is rather small, there is a danger of overdose. Also, these medications often tend to be prescribed unnecessarily.

The effective dose of heart-stimulating medications differs from one patient to the next, and even varies for the same person. The health-care provider must determine the correct dose, taking into account age, body weight and any damage present in various organs. It can take 1 to 4 weeks before the tablets are effective. The proper dosage can be determined only by careful observation of the patient, and not by blood tests alone.

Symptoms of Toxicity May Include:

Loss of appetite, nausea, or vomiting, pain in the lower abdomen, diarrhea, unusual weakness, low or irregular pulse rate, visual disturbances (colored halos seen around objects), dizziness, confusion or depression, headaches.

If you suspect you may have overdosed on your heart-stimulating medicine, see your doctor immediately.

A 3- to 6-month course of this medication is often sufficient. Because of the danger of cardiac arrhythmia, patients should not discontinue use on their own, but should slowly taper off the therapy under the care of a physician.

Diuretics

A low-sodium diet in conjunction with diuretics reduces the amount of fluid in the body, which is important for the long-term treatment of congestive heart failure. For the effects and side effects of diuretics, see Hypertension, p. 321.

Vessel-Dilating Medications (ACE inhibitors)

These medications reduce strain on the heart by widening the blood vessels so the heart has less resistance to overcome. Frequent checkups and laboratory tests are necessary during treatment, because as a side effect these medications reduce blood pressure and may interfere with kidney function (see Hypertension, p. 321).

Medications useful in Treatment of Congestive Heart Failure:

ACE inhibitors	Epinephrine
Amrinone	Furosemide
Beta blockers	Morphine
Digoxin	Nitroglycerin
Dobutamine	Nitroprusside
Dopamine	

Heart Transplants

If the heart continues to weaken in spite of self-help measures and medications, the only remaining possibility is a heart transplant. These operations have become routine at special centers, and their success rate is high: 2 years after surgery, about 80 percent of patients are still alive.

The greatest problem in all organ transplants is the body's rejection of the foreign tissue. The immune system reacts as if the transplanted organ were an invading pathogen, and produces high levels of white blood cells and antibodies. The transplanted organ rapidly loses strength under the onslaught. To prevent this reaction, organ-transplant patients must take immunosuppressants for the rest of their lives, and these medications have major side effects.

CARDIAC ARRHYTHMIAS (ABNORMAL HEART RHYTHMS)

The heart works only if it continually receives impulses generated in its so-called "pacemaker" nerve center, the sinus node, located in the right atrium. The pacemaker generates about 70 impulses per minute, which are carried through the heart via a system of nerve cells. The stimuli cause individual muscle cells to contract at precisely determined intervals, carrying out the heart's pumping activity. When this complex system is not functioning perfectly and its synchrony is interrupted, an arrhythmia results. There are many possible causes, including
— Emotional and physical stress
— Excessive consumption of alcohol, tobacco, or caffeine
— Side effects or overdoses of medications
— Toxic substances (anything that damages nerves can irritate the cardiac nerves; see p. 773)
— Secondary symptoms of heart or circulatory disease, such as angina pectoris, heart attack, rheumatic heart disease, etc.
— Secondary symptoms of other serious diseases and injuries
Cardiac arrhythmias that have organic causes must be medically treated.

ECTOPIC BEATS

Complaints

Symptoms of this disorder are experienced as extra heartbeats or skipped beats. A pause results when one beat comes too soon, and the heart rests for a beat to hold the pulse rate constant.

Causes

Ectopic beats can start either in the atrium or ventricles of the heart.
Atrial ectopic beats are common
— In completely healthy people
— During periods of nervousness
— With the consumption of alcohol or coffee
— In untreated cases of congestive heart failure (the atrium is stretched and irritated by the congested blood)
— During or after myocarditis, which is often not recognized
— In people with hyperactive thyroids
Ventricular ectopic beats are common
— In completely healthy people
— In people with coronary heart diseases (see p. 337), especially during or after a heart attack.
— In congestive heart failure
— In patients with congestive heart failure who take excessive doses of digoxin
— During or after myocarditis

Who's at Risk

The feeling of one's heart occasionally skipping a beat is extremely common.

Possible Aftereffects and Complications

In most cases, ectopic beats are harmless. Whether treatment is needed depends on the symptoms, and also on the presence of heart disease. If ectopic beats are too common (such as every other beat), the heart's pumping ability will be diminished. Under some circumstances, ectopic beats can lead to tachycardia (see p. 340).

Prevention

If you are aware of the factors that lead to ectopic beats (alcohol or coffee consumption, e.g.), you can try avoiding them.

When to Seek Medical Advice
Seek help if your heart repeatedly skips beats.

Self-Help
Limit alcohol, coffee and cola consumption.

Treatment
Treatment is usually not necessary, but under some circumstances, the doctor may prescribe beta blockers, digoxin, calcium channel blockers, or special rhythm-influencing medications. A heart specialist should be consulted in these cases. Nearly all medications used to control ectopic beats can also cause the beats, as a side effect.

TACHYCARDIA

Complaints
The symptoms of tachycardia are extremely rapid heartbeats, leading in some cases to weakness, faintness, feelings of confinement, and pounding heart, combined with a sharp pain in the region of the heart.

Causes
There are two types of tachycardia.

The first type is caused by excitement, anxiety or physical exertion (sinus tachycardia). The pounding of the heart experienced in these situations is normal and harmless. Sometimes the rapid heartbeat can lead to shortness of breath, faintness or pain in the heart, with the heart nevertheless remaining completely healthy (see Health and Well-Being, p. 182).

The second type of tachycardia comes on unexpectedly, lasts a few beats or several hours, and usually ends suddenly. The heart races at about 180 beats a minute, causing blood pressure to drop; the patient feels dizzy, weak and hemmed in, and is fearful. Usually this form of tachycardia begins in the atrium (supraventricular tachycardia). The causes are the same as in atrial ectopic beats (see p. 339). Much less often, the second type of tachycardia begins in the ventricle (ventricular tachycardia); this rarely occurs except in hearts which have been damaged. In this case, the patient may lose consciousness because the pumping capacity of the heart is extremely limited.

Who's at Risk
The form of tachycardia caused by excitement and exertion (sinus tachycardia) is common. Supraventricular tachycardia is rare, and ventricular tachycardia is extremely rare.

Possible Aftereffects and Complications
Type 1: This is not dangerous and ceases when the stressful situation ends. However, if life experiences produce such massive physical reactions in someone, it can be expected that other organs will also be damaged by the chronic stress (see Health and Well-Being, p. 182).

Type 2: Supraventricular tachycardia can be oppressive, as the patient is incapable of doing anything during the attack, and may faint.

Ventricular tachycardia caused by disease can sometimes be life-threatening, in that it interrupts circulation.

Prevention
Prevention consists of treatment of any disease that can cause the tachycardia (see above).

When to Seek Medical Advice
Seek help if you have repeated episodes of inexplicable or frightening tachycardia, or a single severe attack. Using an EKG, and other tests, your health-care provider can determine the exact cause.

Self-Help
Cutting down on the amount of coffee you drink is a good idea.

If the tachycardia is produced by psychosocial stresses, you should attempt to reduce these stresses, or better manage them. If you are unable to do this alone or with the help of relatives or friends, seek professional help (see Counseling and Psychotherapy, p. 697). Relaxation exercises may also be helpful (see p. 693).

Supraventricular tachycardia can often be relieved by stimulating the vagus nerve, which can slow the pulse. This may be accomplished by bearing down as if to expel a stool; drinking ice-cold water; or vigorously massaging only one of the carotid arteries (have your health-care provider show you how).

Treatment

If a doctor determines that the tachycardia has an organic cause such as myocarditis, congestive heart failure, etc., the treatment will be based on this cause. If the tachycardia is caused by psychosocial stress and self-help measures do not bring adequate relief, medications such as beta blockers or sedatives may be prescribed.

Supraventricular tachycardia does not require treatment if the episodes are infrequent and short. Otherwise, medications such as digoxin, calcium channel blockers, and special rhythm regulators can be helpful.

Ventricular tachycardias are treated in the hospital, through rhythm-regulating medications or a heart operation. In a few cases, a type of pacemaker is implanted.

HEART BLOCK

Complaints

Symptoms include slowing of the pulse, combined with dizziness, faintness, visual blackouts or temporary unconsciousness, and intermittent gasping breaths. Sometimes the pulse is normal, but some heartbeats are missing. This condition can be differentiated from so-called ectopic beats only by an EKG (see EKG, p. 646).

Causes

In a heart block, the conduction of impulses in the heart is interrupted at some point. This can be caused by
— Rheumatic or arteriosclerotic heart diseases
— Overdoses of heart-stimulating medicines (see p. 338)
— Acute rheumatic fever (see p. 458)
— Cancer
— Syphilis (see p. 548)
— Heart attack (see p. 335)
— Aging of the system that conducts heart impulses

Who's at Risk

A heart blockage can occur in conjunction with any of the heart diseases, and is therefore a relatively common condition.

Possible Aftereffects and Complications

The attack can be fatal if it stops the circulation for more than 3 to 4 minutes.

Prevention

Not possible.

When to Seek Medical Advice

Seek help as soon as possible.

Self-Help

Not possible. Give first aid until an ambulance arrives.

Treatment

If the impulse-conducting system is permanently damaged, a pacemaker can provide a normal heartbeat.

Pacemakers

These devices deliver small pulses of electric current to the heart in the desired rhythm. They are implanted in the wall of the chest or abdomen, and connected to the heart by a thin cable.
Level of Risk: Surgical techniques have been refined to the point that the risk is slight; fatal complications have been markedly reduced. The life expectancy of people with pacemakers depends only on the underlying illness.

Pacemakers last several years. About every 6 months, the patient and device should be examined. The remaining charge in the battery can be determined at this time, using an external electronic device.

A person with a pacemaker can drive a car with no problems. Modern pacemakers are protected against external interference (e.g., from airport metal detectors, electric razors, or cordless telephones) by metal capsules. Even so, these devices should not be held too close to the pacemaker.

HEART INFLAMMATIONS: MYOCARDITIS, ENDOCARDITIS, AND PERICARDITIS

Complaints

Myocarditis and endocarditis: The symptoms can be quite varied and nonspecific, including fever, tachycardia, feelings of constriction, shortness of breath, tiredness, pallor, and low blood pressure.
Pericarditis: Fever, tachycardia, and chest pains.

Causes

Heart inflammations are usually initiated by inflammatory processes in other organs. They may occur

— As a result of general infections, such as flu, diphtheria or scarlet fever
— Following difficult operations
— As a result of rheumatic fever (see p. 458)
— As a result of centers of infection in the body, such as chronic tonsilitis
— Following dental work
— As a result of using nonsterile needles, e.g., by drug addicts.

The inflammation is caused by pathogens or toxins carried by the blood.

Myocarditis is an inflammation of the heart muscle itself; endocarditis affects the inner membranes of the heart, and pericarditis is an inflammation of the pericardium, the sac around the heart.

Who's at Risk

Endocarditis acquired by infection usually affects people between the ages of 15 and 60. Men are about twice as likely to suffer it as women.

Myocarditis is a rare disease that may occur as a complication of severe infection. Mild forms of pericarditis are common, but they usually cause no complaints; severe forms, which cause pain, are relatively rare.

Possible Aftereffects and Complications

Endocarditis, if untreated, is usually fatal. If treated, it ordinarily responds within a few days. The heart valves may be damaged as a complication of endocarditis; weakened by the inflammation, the valve flaps shrink, stick together, or cannot function properly.

Myocarditis: Severe forms can cause death by cardiac arrest.

Pericarditis is usually not life-threatening. However, if it spreads and causes a discharge in the pericardium, this may exert dangerous pressure on the heart.

Prevention

Endocarditis: For patients with certain diseases of the heart valves, preventive doses of antibiotics are recommended before surgery or dental work.
Pericarditis and myocarditis: There are no preventive mea-

sures. However, myocarditis is often a mild, unnoticed complication of a cold. Therefore, one should wait a week after a cold before engaging in heavy physical activity.

When to Seek Medical Advice

Seek help as soon as you suspect you have a heart inflammation.

Self-Help

Self-help is not feasible.

Treatment

Because symptoms can vary, it is often difficult for health-care providers to determine if an inflammatory heart condition is present. Usually X rays, blood tests, and an EKG are necessary for diagnosis. The treatment includes strict bed rest, and probable hospitalization.

Medications

If the inflammation is caused by bacteria, antibiotics are necessary, and also possibly painkillers and anti-inflammatory medications such as corticosteroids (see p. 665).

Surgery

Pericarditis: In cases of acute inflammation, the fluid must sometimes be removed from the pericardium by tapping it with a needle.
Endocarditis: Sometimes the infection must be removed immediately by surgery on the heart valves (see p. 344); at times this will be necessary only years later.

DISEASES OF THE HEART MUSCLE (CARDIOMYOPATHIES)

Certain congenital or acquired diseases of the heart muscle are called cardiomyopathy:

Hypertrophic cardiomyopathy: The heart muscle is thickened.

Dilated cardiomyopathy: The heart muscle is weak and thin, for unclear reasons, and it does not pump effectively.

Restrictive cardiomyopathy: The walls of the heart chamber are stiff and inelastic.

Complaints

Cardiomyopathies often cause complaints similar to those of congestive heart failure (see p. 337) or other heart diseases. The symptoms of different types of cardiomyopathies are different.

Hypertrophic cardiomyopathy: Difficulty breathing, angina pectoris symptoms (see p. 333), ectopic beats.

Dilated cardiomyopathy: Congestive heart failure (see p. 337) and cardiac arrhythmia.

Restrictive cardiomyopathy: Difficulty breathing, rapid tiring, congestive heart failure (see p. 337).

Causes

The causes of cardiomyopathy are often unclear, but some factors may be: Genetic predisposition; inflammation of the heart muscle caused by bacteria or viruses; alcohol; medications (e.g. certain cancer medications (cytostatics), antidepressants, etc.); heart tumors; and various nutritional deficiency diseases, such as beriberi.

Who's at Risk

Dilated cardiomyopathy is the most common form and affects mainly men.

Restrictive cardiomyopathy is extremely rare.

Possible Aftereffects and Complications

Cardiomyopathy is often a very serious illness that greatly decrease, the patient's life expectancy. However, the disease can stop progressing at any stage, and may even improve.

Prevention

Not possible.

When to Seek Medical Advice

Seek help as soon as possible.

Self-Help

Get sufficient rest and avoid stress. People with dilated cardiomyopathy should avoid all alcohol.

Treatment

A diagnosis of cardiomyopathy is usually based on extensive testing, including EKG and X rays, so the physician can rule out other possible causes for the symptoms (hypertension, valvular heart disease, heart attack, etc.). Treatment is often very difficult and requires extensive specialized information. A number of medications are used, including ACE-inhibitors, diuretics, heart rhythm stabilizers, digitalis, etc. In some cases, a heart transplant is needed (see p. 339).

HEART VALVE DISORDERS

Complaints

The four heart valves regulate blood flow, and if they do not work properly, the same symptoms arise as in congestive heart failure (see p. 337). General signs are a tendency to tire easily, shortness of breath, and pounding of the heart after physical exertion. In severe cases, these symptoms occur even when the patient is at rest.

Causes

— Endocarditis (see Heart Inflammations, p. 341)
— Rheumatic heart damage
— Older age
— Heart attack (see p. 335)

Who's at Risk

Heart valve defects become more common with increasing age.

Possible Aftereffects and Complications

Without treatment, the patient's life expectancy decreases. Untreated heart valve defects can lead to coronary insufficiency (see p. 337), cardiac arrhythmia (see p. 339), pulmonary edema (see p. 313), and other life-threatening illnesses.

Prevention

Prevention includes proper treatment of rheumatic fever (see p. 458) and endocarditis (see Heart Inflammations, page 341).

When to Seek Medical Advice

Seek help as soon as symptoms of the disease are noticed.

Self-Help

Not possible.

Treatment

If the defect is not severe, treatment with heart stimulants or diuretics is often sufficient. If it is severe, surgery is the only effective treatment. Before the operation, the heart must be examined by catheterization: A thin tube, to measure heart chamber conditions, is introduced into the heart through a vein or artery.

Heart Valve Operations
In this surgical operation, the damaged heart valve is removed and replaced. There are four choices for the replacement:
— Metal and plastic valves
— Specially prepared pig-heart valves
— Plastic surgical reconstruction of tissue from another site
— Specially prepared human heart valves
   The patient is connected to a heart-lung machine for the duration of the operation, which lasts 2 to 4 hours. The recovery period in the hospital is about 2 weeks, and after an outpatient recovery time of several more weeks, 80 percent of all patients are able to lead normal lives. However, they need to take clot inhibitors (e.g., Coumadin) for the rest of their lives.

CONGENITAL HEART DEFECTS

Complaints
Shortness of breath and pallor indicate a so-called "pink" defect, while a bluish cast indicates "cyanotic" heart defects. The blue coloration arises because the defective heart is permitting oxygen-rich arterial blood to mix with oxygen-poor venous blood in the heart.

Causes
The cause of this defect is incorrect development of the heart in the womb. In some cases, a specific cause can be determined, such as genetic damage or the mother's having a rubella infection during pregnancy. However, the defect can also arise as a side effect of certain medications.

Who's at Risk
Congenital heart defects occur in about 1 of every 120 births.

Possible Aftereffects and Complications
Mild heart defects have only a slight effect on the pumping capacity of the heart, and may not require surgery. Babies with severe heart defects may die shortly after birth.

Prevention
Not possible.

When to Seek Medical Advice
Heart defects are normally discovered during routine examinations after birth or during infancy.

Self-Help
Not possible.

Treatment
The only possible treatment is an operation. Cyanotic heart defects are corrected very early, often in the first 2 years of life, while "pink" heart defects are corrected somewhat later.
Level of Risk: The surgical risk is extremely low for "pink" defects, somewhat higher for cyanotic defects (depending on severity, the risk of death may reach 15 percent).

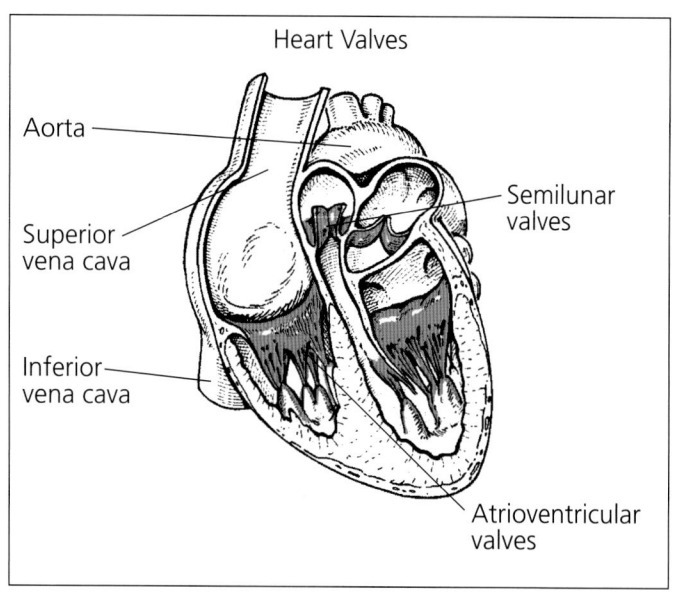

Heart Valves

Aorta

Superior vena cava

Inferior vena cava

Semilunar valves

Atrioventricular valves

BLOOD

Blood has two important functions:

1. Distribution: The red blood cells transport oxygen to the tissue cells and in turn take up carbon dioxide, a waste product of metabolism, which they then return to the lungs to be breathed out. Blood also distributes nutrients from the intestinal tract to the entire body, and carries vital substances such as enzymes, hormones, antibodies, etc. from their sites of production to anywhere they are needed.

2. Clotting: When skin or other tissues are injured, blood has the essential task of clotting and sticking the edges of the wound back together. A number of blood components work together in an extremely complicated, step-like process to accomplish this.

An adult's body contains about 11 pints of blood, the main components of which are red blood cells (erythrocytes), white blood cells (leucocytes), platelets (thrombocytes), and liquid plasma.

Blood diseases are organized into three main categories:
— Anemias
— Clotting deficiencies (e.g., hemophilia)
— Leukemias (blood cancers)

ANEMIA: IRON DEFICIENCY

Complaints

Tiredness, uneasiness, pallor, dry skin, hair loss, brittle and fragile fingernails, fissures in the nasal mucous membrane.

Causes

Iron is an essential nutrient. The adult female body contains about 15 mg of iron per pound of weight, and the adult male body about 20 mg. Sixty to 70 percent of the body's iron is bound up in hemoglobin, and the

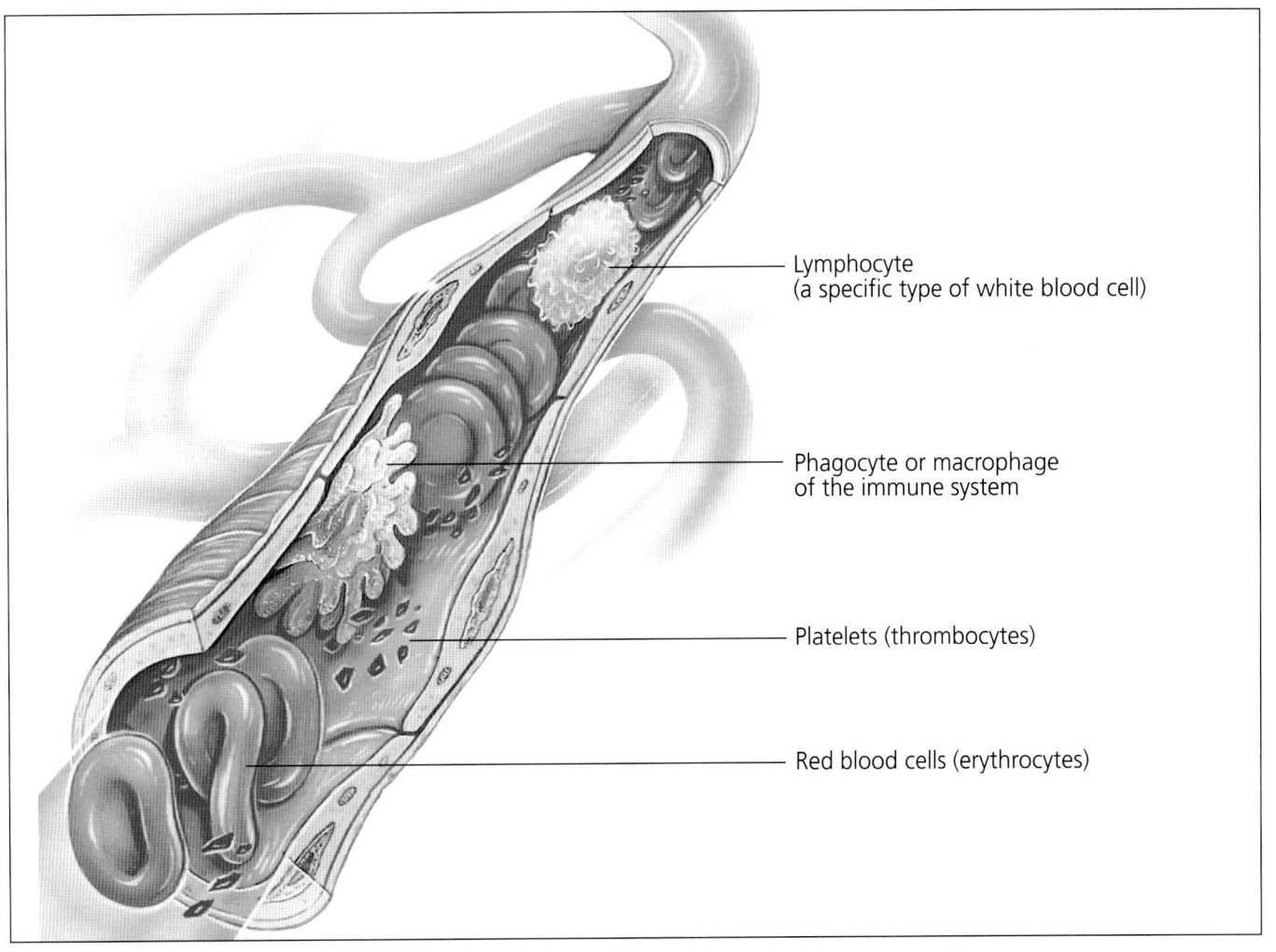

Lymphocyte
(a specific type of white blood cell)

Phagocyte or macrophage
of the immune system

Platelets (thrombocytes)

Red blood cells (erythrocytes)

rest is stored in the liver, spleen, and bone marrow.

The most common causes of iron deficiency are:

— Severe loss of blood, e.g., due to heavy menstruation, gastritis, ulcers or cancers in the gastrointestinal area, hemorrhoids, or tapeworms. A number of medications can cause bleeding leading to iron deficiency anemia; these include acetylsalicylic acid (e.g., aspirin), indomethacin (a nonsteroidal antiinflammatory drug), drugs for high blood pressure (such as reserpine), sex hormones, cancer chemotherapeutic agents, and corticosteroids.

— Iron poor diets can cause problems, especially in young children and in adults on restricted diets.

— The gastrointestinal tract may be incapable of absorbing iron, e.g., after a stomach operation.

Who's at Risk?

In developed nations about 1 child in 3 and 1 woman in 10 suffers from iron deficiency. Pregnant women have increased iron requirements.

Blood Groups

Blood cannot be randomly transfused or donated between people; a severe allergic reaction may ensue if this is attempted, as the antigens present in one person's blood react with the antibodies in the other person's blood, resulting in agglutination, or clumping of blood cells. To prevent this reaction, blood is tested beforehand for the presence and type of antigens. The four main types of antigens give the four blood groups their names: A, B, AB, and O.

The relative frequencies of these groups vary in different human populations. Type O blood contains neither A nor B antigens, and may safely be transfused into persons of any group. Type AB blood contains both A and B antigens and no antibodies against them, so people with type AB blood can receive blood from any of the four groups. However, it is now the practice to transfuse only blood of the same type as the recipient's own.

In addition to the A-B-O blood typing system, there are several minor systems, of which the rhesus (Rh) factor is best known. Human blood may be either Rh-positive or Rh-negative, and blood for transfusion must be matched for this factor. During pregnancy, an Rh-negative woman carrying an Rh-positive child may have problems.

Possible Aftereffects and Complications

Iron-deficiency anemia weakens the body, but is not normally life-threatening.

Prevention

A normal diet will provide sufficient iron. Iron from animal sources is assimilated by the body 10 to 20 times better than iron from plant sources. Fish and meat are good sources of iron (see Iron, p. 746), but vegetarians need not worry about iron deficiency if they eat enough dairy products, green leafy vegetables, and whole-grain products.

When to Seek Medical Advice

Seek help if you suspect you have the symptoms of iron deficiency.

Self-Help

Self-help is not possible if the iron deficiency is already established.

Treatment

If you are not getting enough iron from your diet, your body will first use up its stored iron. Anemia arises only after these reserves are depleted and red-blood-cell formation is impaired. Iron deficiency is detectable by a blood test.

Treatment of iron-deficiency anemia has two goals:

— Removing the cause of iron deficiency

— Replenishing iron reserves

It usually takes about 2 months of iron supplements before iron levels in the blood return to normal, but it takes at least 6 months to replenish iron stores.

Iron deficiency is best treated with medications containing divalent iron, such as ferrous sulfate. Supplements combining iron with vitamins and other metals are usually unnecessary and expensive. Other additives are also unnecessary, as are iron products that are absorbed very slowly from the gastrointestinal tract.

Any iron supplement can occasionally cause nausea, stomachache, vomiting, diarrhea, or constipation. It should therefore be taken either an hour before or two hours after eating, with half a glass of water. Black bowel movements are normal when taking iron.

PERNICIOUS ANEMIA

Complaints

Symptoms of pernicious anemia include pale, slightly yellowish skin and eyes, loss of appetite and energy, and stomach and digestive troubles. Sometimes the tongue and inside of the mouth are inflamed. After an extended vitamin B^{12} deficiency, neurological symptoms may appear, such as difficulty with locomotion or some loss of sensation of vibration in the limbs.

Causes

The cause of pernicious anemia is usually a vitamin B^{12} deficiency, very rarely a folic acid deficiency. Treatments for the two disorders differ considerably, so it should first be established which one is causing the symptoms.

Vitamin B^{12} Deficiency

In order for the body to absorb vitamin B^{12} from food, a substance known as the intrinsic factor must be present. The intrinsic factor is formed by the gastric mucosa. If not enough of the mucosa is present, e.g., due to partial removal of the stomach or a deterioration of the mucosa, insufficient intrinsic factor is produced and the body cannot absorb enough vitamin B^{12}.

Folic Acid Deficiency

This condition is rare, but it is sometimes seen in malnourished alcoholics.

Who's At Risk?

The risk of developing pernicious anemia is increased by partial or total removal of the stomach or small intestine; severe intestinal diseases; increasing age; alcoholism; and eating a very unbalanced diet over a long period of time.

Possible Aftereffects and Complications

Once treated, pernicious anemia has no long-term aftereffects. Untreated, it can lead to spinal cord damage and permanent neurological disorders.

Prevention

A varied diet (see p. 722) can prevent pernicious anemia, but only if the body is producing enough intrinsic factor to make vitamin B^{12} available the blood. Vitamin B^{12} is found in meat, fish, milk, egg yolk and cheese.

Vegetables and other plant foods do not contain vitamin B^{12}, with the exception of those pickled with lactic acid, e.g., sauerkraut (see Vitamin B^{12}, p. 742).

When to Seek Medical Advice

Seek help as soon as you suspect you have a vitamin B^{12} or folic acid deficiency. If someone in your family has pernicious anemia, mention this to the doctor.

Self-Help

Self-help is not possible for an existing vitamin B^{12} deficiency. A mild folic acid deficiency can be corrected through diet (see Folic Acid, p. 742).

Treatment

If the vitamin B^{12} deficiency is caused by lack of intrinsic factor, the vitamin must be administered by injection (if taken orally, it is simply eliminated without being absorbed). Several shots a week are usually required initially; later, a single monthly injection is usually enough, but treatment often continues for the rest of the patient's life.

Folic acid deficiency is treated by a change in diet and oral or injected folic acid supplementation.

HEMOLYTIC ANEMIA

Complaints

Symptoms include pallor, fatigue, shortness of breath, and pounding or fluttering of the heart, especially during exertion. Sometimes skin turns yellowish and urine looks darker than normal. If the condition lasts a long time, gallstones may form.

Causes

— Hereditary (in this case, symptoms appear at birth or soon thereafter).

— Infectious diseases.

— In so-called autoimmune hemolytic anemia, the body forms antibodies against its own blood cells. The causes of this have not yet been determined.

— Chemicals (see Hazardous Substances in Food, p. 729) or medications (acetylsalicylic acid, e.g. aspirin; sulfonamides and other antibiotics). These may suddenly trigger hemolytic anemia in susceptible persons.

— Blood transfusion (the body may produce anti-

bodies against the foreign red cells).
— After surgical insertion of artificial heart valve.
— Snakebite.

Who's At Risk?
People with the aforementioned conditions or factors are at increased risk.

Possible Aftereffects and Complications
The disease is seldom fatal, but sometimes is difficult to treat.

Prevention
Avoid chemicals that trigger the condition.

When to Seek Medical Advice
Seek help immediately if you suspect you have hemolytic anemia.

Self-Help
Not possible.

Treatment
The type of treatment depends on the cause of the disease. If it is the side effect of a medication, the patient must discontinue any medications that could be at fault. If the patient works with chemicals that can cause hemolytic anemia, he or she should change jobs if possible.

If the disease is caused by antibodies, medications that may limit their production and activity should be used.

Surgically removing the spleen may lead to significant improvements in the patient's condition or even complete recovery, especially in hereditary cases of hemolytic anemia.

HEMOPHILIA

Complaints
The symptoms of hemophilia usually appear during childhood and include bruises on knees and elbows simply from crawling; lengthy bleeding from cuts and scratches; internal bleeding, swollen limbs, and pains in the joints from a simple fall.

Causes
Factor VIII, which is required for blood clotting, is missing from the blood. In about 75 percent of cases, hemophilia is inherited. The hemophilia gene can be transmitted by both males and females, but the disease affects almost exclusively males.

Who's At Risk?
One hemophiliac in the family may be a sign that others carry the gene. Men or women who are related to hemophiliacs and want to have children can seek genetic counseling about their chances of having a hemophiliac child. The disease is not passed on to every child, and tests during early stages of pregnancy can determine whether the fetus will develop it.

Possible Aftereffects and Complications
Modern treatment methods have considerably reduced the chances of disability or premature death. However, major injuries can still be life-threatening. Hemophiliacs and their families live with the reality of omnipresent dangers and constant dependency on medical help.

Prevention
Timely injection of factor VIII after an injury can prevent permanent damage to the joints.

When to Seek Medical Advice
Seek help if you suspect your child's blood is not clotting properly.

Self-Help
Avoid dangerous sports. Don't take medications that increase the risk of bleeding, such as aspirin.

Hemophiliacs usually learn to inject themselves with factor VIII in specific situations.

Treatment
If the patient is bleeding seriously, factor VIII should be administered intravenously as soon as possible. Depending on the severity of bleeding, it may be necessary to repeat this procedure several times over the next 5 to 10 days.

THROMBOCYTOPENIA

Complaints

Symptoms include a skin rash consisting of small dots, bright or dark red in color, marking tiny blood flows under the skin. The rash may appear anywhere on the body but usually begins on the legs. Nosebleeds and bleeding under the skin are frequent, and cuts bleed longer than normal.

Causes

At times the body forms antibodies that destroy platelets, either as a result of an infection or for unknown reasons.

The platelet count may also diminish as a side effect of cancer treatments, or as a result of leukemia.

In addition, almost all medications can cause platelet deficiency as a rare side effect.

Who's At Risk?

The risk of thrombocytopenia is increased in persons with any of the aforementioned conditions or factors.

Possible Aftereffects and Complications

If the disease is left untreated, severe and ultimately fatal internal bleeding may result. Occasionally, bleeding in the brain may lead to paralysis.

Prevention

At present, prevention is not possible.

When to Seek Medical Advice

Seek help as soon as symptoms appear.

Self-Help

Not possible.

Treatment

Your health-care provider may take you off all nonessential medications, since thrombocytopenia may be an unwanted side effect.

If the platelets are being destroyed by antibodies, corticosteroids may slow the process considerably. Symptoms may improve within a few weeks or disappear entirely. If corticosteroids are ineffective, large quantities of immunoglobulins may be injected, or the spleen may be surgically removed.

If the bone marrow cannot produce sufficient quantities of platelets, transfusions may be necessary.

LEUKEMIAS

There are four types of leukemia: acute lymphocytic leukemia (ALL), acute myelocytic leukemia (AML), chronic lymphocytic leukemia and chronic myelocytic leukemia (see also Cancer, p. 470).

Complaints in Acute Leukemias

The first symptoms are fatigue, loss of energy, shortness of breath, weight loss, infections especially in the mouth and throat, fever, night sweats, pains in the bones and joints, and ulcers on lips and mouth. Later symptoms include bleeding from the skin and mucous membranes, swollen lymph nodes, and enlarged spleen and liver.

Complaints in Chronic Leukemias

Chronic leukemias often produce no symptoms for a long time and are discovered by chance during a blood test.

The first symptoms are loss of appetite and weight, usually accompanied by fever, night sweats, an enlarged spleen that feels like a swelling in the upper left abdomen, and signs of anemia: Pale skin and generalized weakness.

Causes

Leukemia results when mutations of unknown origin cause white blood cells in the bone marrow to proliferate uncontrollably and enter the blood.

Elevated exposure to radiation (e.g., after the nuclear reactor accident in Chernobyl) is known to cause leukemias, as is exposure to gasoline fumes. There is also evidence that dioxin can cause leukemia.

Who's at Risk for Acute Leukemia?

Acute lymphocytic leukemia is more common in younger people, especially children, while acute myelocytic leukemia is more common in older people.

Who's at Risk for Chronic Leukemia?

The older you are, the higher the risk. The chronic lymphocytic form is 2 to 3 times more common in men than in women. The frequency of the chronic myelocytic form is approximately the same in men and women.

Aftereffects and Complications of Acute Leukemia

If untreated, the disease can be fatal within a short time. If treated, children have a very good chance (70 percent) of cure. About 20 to 40 percent of adults can be cured, or at least given a symptom-free remission period of several years.

Aftereffects and Complications of Chronic Lymphocytic Leukemia

Average life expectancy after the first symptoms appear is about 7 years. Because the body's immune defenses are impaired, infections are frequent and are the most common cause of death in chronic lymphocytic leukemia patients.

Aftereffects and Complications of Chronic Myelocytic Leukemia

Average life expectancy after the first symptoms appear is 3–4 years.

Prevention

There is no known way to prevent leukemia.

When to Seek Medical Advice

As soon as you suspect you have leukemia.

Self-Help

Not possible at present.

Treatment of Acute Leukemias

Treatment requires hospitalization, if possible at a specialized leukemia center. It consists mainly of cancer chemotherapy using cytostatic medications, which destroy the leukemia cells. Both the disease and its treatment make patients extremely susceptible to infection and to bleeding, so antibiotics and transfusions of red blood cells and platelets are often necessary.

An additional method of treatment is a bone marrow transplant. In certain cases, bone marrow can be removed from the patient before treatment with cancer chemotherapeutic agents, "purified" of the cancerous cells, and then reintroduced after the chemotherapy. In this way, the bone marrow's functions of red-blood cell production and defenses against disease are preserved.

Treatment of Chronic Lymphocytic Leukemia

If a leukemia that is causing no symptoms is discovered by chance, no treatment is needed, only regular checkups for observation. Many patients live symptom-free for years.

The appearance of symptoms such as swollen lymph nodes, spleen or liver; low platelet count; fever; weight loss or anemia, necessitate cancer chemotherapy. Radiation therapy can help reduce an enlarged spleen or lymph nodes. Anemia should be treated with blood transfusions, and infections with antibiotics.

Treatment of Chronic Myelocytic Leukemia

The goal of treatment for most patients is to ease symptoms and bring blood counts within the normal range. Cancer chemotherapy is usually prescribed, to be administered intravenously at a hospital on an outpatient basis. Sometimes radiation is also used. If the patient is anemic, blood transfusions are necessary.

IMMUNE SYSTEM

The term "immune system" actually refers to several different systems working together to keep the body healthy and protect it from illness. As long as we feel no obvious sensations of illness, we are unaware of the battles raging within our bodies; only when our defenses are under attack—from viruses, bacteria, fungi, foreign proteins, protozoa, toxins—do we notice the effects of the battle (pain, fever, sweat, inflammation), and feel sick. The immune system is not an isolated mechanism but rather the constant, complex interaction of the blood, nervous and hormonal systems.

Psychological conditions are known to affect the immune system. Exactly how this works is not completely understood, although it is known that stress can cause the onset or outbreaks of some infectious diseases (e.g., herpes). Sometimes the reverse is also true: Psychological conditions can prevent disease. Therefore, how you cope with stress is critically important (see Health and Well-Being, p. 182).

While there is as yet no proof that stress causes allergies, cancer, and autoimmune illnesses, it definitely contributes to their intensity. There is also no evidence that certain personality types are predisposed to allergies, cancer, or autoimmune diseases.

Immune Response Throughout Life

From the moment of birth, the immune system is constantly coping with foreign organisms that enter the body through food or drink, in the air, or by way of injuries. The efficiency of the immune system varies over the course of our lives.

In small children, the immune system evolves its immunity and defenses, producing greater numbers and different kinds of defense cells with each bout of illness.

The system's capabilities diminish in old age as its components work together less efficiently; the elderly are therefore more susceptible to illness. This applies to cancer as well, because the immune system is also fighting cancer cells wherever and whenever they may develop throughout our lives.

ORGANS OF THE IMMUNE SYSTEM

The cells that constitute the immune system circulate throughout the body but are concentrated in the lymph nodes, spleen, bone marrow, thymus, and tonsils. Broadly speaking, the skin, the mucous membranes, and the blood–clotting process are also part of the immune system.

Thymus

The thymus gland has a central function in the development of T cells, a special kind of white blood cell. The thymus, located behind the rib cage, grows until puberty and then progressively shrinks while still functioning as part of the immune system.

Lymph Nodes

These round or bean-shaped knots of tissue, measuring up to an inch in diameter, can be felt in different parts of the body—under the arms, in the groin, and on both sides of the neck. The tonsils and appendix are also part of the lymph tissues, all of which can enlarge in the event of inflammations or infections.

Lymph nodes are centers of lymph circulation. They also act as filters for foreign substances and waste products.

Spleen

The spleen is involved in lymphocyte formation, blood filtration, and the breakdown of red blood cells.

Anticoagulant System

When defender cells come in contact with microbes, enzymes activate the anticoagulant system, which is the body's way of trying to isolate the affected tissue.

Skin and Mucosa

The skin is the body's first line of defense against foreign organisms. Additional protection comes from the lactic and fatty acids in sweat and sebum, which make the skin acidic and an inhospitable environment for germs.

The body's large openings (mouth, nose, eyes, urethra, anus, vagina) are further protected by skin or mucus secretions that deny access to invasive organisms. Additionally, foreign cells are expelled by coughing or sneezing, as well as by the continual outbound movement of the top layer of the mucosa.

Tears, saliva, and urine have a similar function, and

contain substances that kill bacteria. Stomach juices contain acid for this purpose; sperm contain spermine and zinc; tears, nasal secretions, and saliva contain the enzyme lysozyme.

The bacteria colonizing the body's surface are also of vital importance, preventing other microbes (e.g., fungi) from settling there.

THE WORKINGS OF THE IMMUNE SYSTEM

The body's defense system consists of two very different elements: Cell-mediated immune response, and humoral antibody defense.

Phagocytosis

So called phagocytes, or "eating cells," are cells that can ingest and destroy microbes completely. This process is referred to as "phagocytosis." Phagocytes are white blood cells of two types, granulocytes and macrophages, that originate in the bone marrow.

The life cycle of granulocytes is 2 to 3 days; they are found primarily in the blood but also in inflamed tissues, usually fighting pus-forming bacteria.

Macrophages have a longer life and are present mainly in the lungs, liver, spleen, and lymph nodes, but also in connective tissue and small blood vessels. They can usually be found fighting microorganisms hiding in the body's cells.

The onset of phagocytosis sets off a chain reaction of chemical processes.

Complement

The liver-based defense system known simply as "complement" involves some 20 different proteins working together with increasing intensity to fend off foreign organisms.

The complement system has three basic functions:
— It works in concert with macrophages. Various parts of the complement system surround the foreign organism, making it easier for the phagocytes to find them.
— Single-protein components of the complement system dilate the capillaries so they can distribute defenses to the body's tissues more effectively. This causes skin to become red and swollen.
— Some components of this system kill invading cells outright by fatally damaging their cell walls.

— When the threat is removed, the complement system deactivates; without this self-neutralizing mechanism, the body would itself be harmed.

Immune Mediators

When the body registers an infection or tissue damage, it quickly produces great quantities of immune mediators that work together with the complement system. These include the interleukin-1 and -2, fibrinogen, etc.

E.g.,, interleukin-1 increases the defense readiness of T and B cells, raising the body's temperature (inducing fever) to kill microbes more quickly.

Interferons

These proteins work specifically against viruses. They are produced by the T cells (see Thymus, p. 351), among others. Synthetic interferon is also produced and used in certain treatments.

Body cells attacked by a virus start producing interferon which surrounds neighboring, uninfected cells, creating a barrier. In addition, interferon can also influence the activity of other defensive cells.

Killer Cells

The natural killer cells are large white blood cells specialized to defend against viruses and cancer cells. Various interferons work closely with the natural killer cells, increasing their effectiveness.

Cellular and Humoral Immunity

This second element of the body's defense consists of the T and B cells. Barely present at birth, it develops through contact with foreign organisms.

There are about 1,000 billion of these cells in an adult body, of which 1 billion are renewed daily.

Lymphocytes circulate constantly throughout the body, but are concentrated in the spleen, lymph nodes, and intestinal lymph tissues.

T and B cells store information about antigens encountered in the past. When an invader reappears, they "remember" it, ensuring that all defenses are alerted; as a result, the body is effectively immune to reinfection. This type of immunity develops to most childhood diseases (measles, mumps, German measles, chicken pox), provided one has had either the illness itself or the corresponding vaccination (see p. 667).

B Cells

These lymphocytes form in the bone marrow and travel to the peripheral lymphoid tissue (stomach/intestinal area, airways, urogenital tract) where they come in contact with foreign cells (antigens) and as a result of this contact, change their form.

B cells are covered with 100,000 antibodies (immunoglobulins), ready to be passed on to the body's fluids.

Antibodies recognize and kill foreign and abnormal cells (e.g., cancer cells) by working in concert with other processes of the immune system.

Like a key to a lock, each antibody perfectly matches a specific type of foreign cell. Millions of types of foreign cells exist, however, so the body must either have the appropriate antibodies on call, or have the ability to produce them.

When a foreign cell is identified, all B cells carrying that specific antibody start producing the antibody continuously and in huge quantities (at a rate of 2,000 per second) until the invading organism has been fought off successfully. This process usually lasts several days and causes the person to feel sick.

Each antibody has the following capabilities:
— It can differentiate between endogenous (familiar) and exogenous (foreign) cells.
— It can recognize invading cells (antigens).
— It can attach itself to antigens.
— It can rally the complement system.
— It can rally phagocytes.
— Antibodies treat cells that have been altered by an illness as if they were foreign organisms.

T Cells

These cells form in the bone marrow but get their immune power from the thymus. They specialize in fighting invaders that have crept into "familiar" cells—mainly viruses that cannot multiply outside these cells.

T cells can be found throughout the lymphatic system, primarily in the peripheral lymph tissues.

A sub-group, called helper T cells, targets disguised invaders and marks them with a "kiss of death" so other cells can exterminate them. With help from the interleukin protein group, helper T cells can also activate natural killer cells. Another subgroup of T cells then collects and stores information about the enemy.

Like the B cells, T cells are activated on contact with antigens, changing their function from cell multiplication to munitions production, so to speak.

IMMUNE SYSTEM DISORDERS

Illness is always caused by stress to the defense capabilities of the immune system. Some illnesses, however, specifically affect the defense system.

Autoimmune Diseases

When the immune system loses the ability to differentiate between its own and foreign cells, or between healthy and sick cells, it suddenly starts to attack its own healthy cells, resulting in autoimmune (from the Greek "autos" meaning "self") diseases. These include Rheumatoid Arthritis (see p. 455), Scleroderma (see p. 461), Systemic Lupus Erythematosus (see p. 460), Type-1 Diabetes (see p. 484), Graves' Disease (see p. 496), Myasthenia Gravis (see p. 438), Multiple Sclerosis (see p. 220) among others.

The self-destructiveness of autoimmune diseases can be stopped only through outside intervention. Highly effective medications include corticosteroids (see p. 665), immune suppressors (see Rheumatism, p. 449), interferons and interleukins. Psychotherapy can also be of significant value in helping patients fight certain autoimmune diseases.

Allergies

Allergies are hypersensitivity reactions of the body to repeated contact with foreign substances such as pollens, medications, animal dander, chemicals, etc. Extreme defense reactions can manifest as rashes, mucous membrane inflammation (as with asthma) or whole-body (systemic) reaction (as can happen in an allergic reaction to penicillin). For general allergies, see p. 360.

Immunodeficiency Disorders

If the body cannot supply enough efficient defense cells, its condition is referred to as immunocompromised. This disorder can be congenital or acquired. Diseases such as acquired immunodeficiency syndrome (AIDS), leukemia, and nephrotic syndrome, and medical treatments such as chemotherapy or radiation therapy, can cause immunocompromise. Burns can also cause immunocompromise.

IMMUNOTHERAPY

A strong immune system can provide effective defense against illness. Various medications and procedures strengthen the immune system.

Immune System Strengthening, Immune Modulation

Formerly known as "toughening," the purpose of these procedures is to strengthen the immune system by exposing the body to cold, warmth, baths, saunas, high altitudes, physical activities, sports, particular diets, relaxation, fasting, various herbal remedies, antibiotics (taken orally or injected), and more. For more information on this approach, see Natural Healing and Alternative Medicine, p. 679.

A new field of research, psychoneuroimmunology, examines connections between psychological conditions and the health of the immune system. Little of substantive value has emerged from this field to date.

LYMPHATIC SYSTEM

The lymphatic system consists of lymph vessels, lymph nodes, and the spleen. Lymph vessels drain the body's tissues. The network of tiny lymph vessels absorbs fluid and small particles from the tissue and transports it, with the aid of a valve system like that of the veins, into larger vessels. The major lymph vessels empty into a vein in the upper chest cavity, returning the lymphatic fluid to the bloodstream.

The lymphatic system is a major component of the body's system of defenses. The lymph nodes trap microbes, foreign substances, and wandering cancer cells and attempt to neutralize them. To this end they produce lymphocytes, a special type of white blood cell.

INFECTIOUS MONONUCLEOSIS

Complaints
Symptoms resemble those of the flu, with a moderate temperature for 1 to 2 weeks, accompanied at times by a sore throat and cold. Swollen lymph nodes are evident in the throat and neck area, and possibly the groin and underarm as well. Head and neck movements may be painful. A skin rash may be present.

The symptoms can be so similar to those of flu or strep throat, that "mono" often goes unrecognized; a blood test will rule out other disorders.

Causes
Mononucleosis is caused by infection with the Epstein Barr virus, which is transmitted by close contact, such as mouth-to-mouth contact (hence the name "kissing disease"), but possibly also by sharing cups or utensils.

The virus may lie dormant, to be activated only when the body's defenses are down.

Who's at Risk
Mononucleosis is most prevalent in adolescents and young adults. Up to 7 weeks may elapse from the moment of infection to the time symptoms appear.

Possible Aftereffects and Complications
Symptoms normally disappear completely after two to three weeks. Sometimes, however, weeks or even months of fatigue, weakness, and depression may follow the illness.

Changes in the immune system may make the body more susceptible to secondary infections. The spleen may become dangerously enlarged with blood. Bleeding in the intestinal tract and airways is also possible.

Prevention
Not possible.

When to Seek Medical Advice
Seek help if a throat inflammation is accompanied by painful, swollen lymph nodes.

Self-Help
Use cold compresses to reduce fever; use compresses to soothe a sore throat.

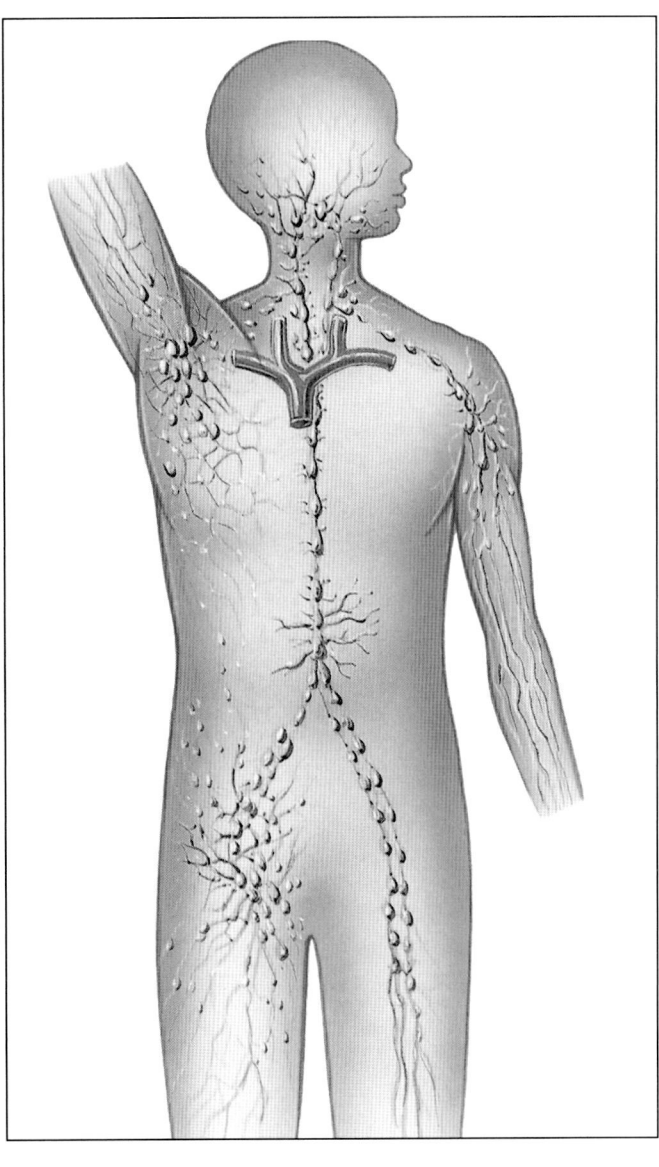

Treatment

Treatment will not speed recovery. Symptoms may be relieved with simple pain and fever medications (see p. 29). Secondary bacterial infections can be treated with penicillin or other antibiotics.

HODGKIN'S LYMPHOMA

See also Cancer, p. 470.

Complaints

The initial symptoms of this form of cancer are swollen lymph nodes in the throat, under the arms, or in the groin. Other symptoms include fever, outbreaks of sweating, fatigue, spells of weakness, weight loss, and itching skin.

Causes

Hodgkin's lymphoma is caused by lymph cells suddenly becoming malignant. Recent research suggests that this tendency is acquired, rather than innate.

Who's at Risk

The disease rarely occurs before age 5. Peak incidence is between ages 15 to 34, with a second peak occurring after age 50.

Possible Aftereffects and Complications

If left untreated, Hodgkin's lymphoma is almost always fatal. Depending on the stage of the disease, 60 to 90 percent of those treated can be cured.

Prevention

Not possible, to date.

When to Seek Medical Advice

Seek help as soon as you suspect this disease.

Self-Help

Not possible.

Treatment

The majority of cases respond to radiation and chemotherapy.

In some situations, however, serious side effects may appear up to 20 years after treatment and remission. Depending on the type of treatment, side effects such as sterility, heart damage, lung and thyroid cancer, or other types of secondary tumors may result.

NON-HODGKIN'S LYMPHOMA

See also Cancer, p. 470.

Complaints

The first symptoms of this ailment are usually swollen lymph nodes; subsequent symptoms might include general malaise, loss of appetite, weight loss, fever and night sweats.

Causes

The cause is unknown; a viral infection is suspected.

Who's at Risk

Lymphomas can occur at any age, but are more common in older people.

Possible Aftereffects and Complications

There are benign and malignant lymphomas. Benign lymphomas may require no treatment for a long period of time. Malignant lymphomas, if untreated, are fatal. With treatment, about a third of all cases can be cured.

Prevention

Not possible, to date.

When to Seek Medical Advice

Seek help if lymph nodes in the neck area are swollen, but no infection is present.

Self-Help

Not possible.

Treatment

If not all the lymph nodes are affected, the disease is usually treated with radiation, possibly followed by chemotherapy.

If the disease is already widespread, it is treated primarily with cancer chemotherapeutic agents.

AIDS

When acquired immunodeficiency syndrome (AIDS) was first identified in the early 1980s, it was thought to affect only homosexuals and intravenous drug users. Some viewed it as "God's punishment" for the amorality of our times.

When heterosexuals and small children also became infected, a new angle was exploited: It was predicted that the AIDS epidemic would spread exponentially, far faster than current methods of care could keep up, and that the entire medical system would collapse under the burden. Since then, there are indications that the epidemic has leveled off in some parts of the world; in others it continues to spread rapidly (e.g., areas of Africa and Asia).

Complaints

A few days after infection with the human immunodeficiency virus (HIV), flu-like symptoms may develop.

However, the HIV infected person usually remains clinically healthy for the next few months or even years. Symptoms that suggest the progressive development of AIDS include bouts of fever, weight loss, diarrhea, swollen lymph nodes, general weakness, headaches, episodes of confusion or altered awareness, skin rashes, or infections in the mouth or throat area.

These nonspecific symptoms may subside, with months or years elapsing before a full-blown case of AIDS is diagnosed with the following possible symptoms:

— Shortness of breath, dry cough, and fever (indicating pneumonia)
— Severe diarrhea
— Difficulty swallowing (indicating fungal infections of the esophagus)
— Fever blisters (herpes simplex), especially in the anal region
— Cancer (Kaposi's sarcoma or non-Hodgkin's lymphoma)
— Tuberculosis
— Skin rashes
— Personality changes, forgetfulness, loss of energy, or seizures (these may be symptoms of progressive brain damage, or AIDS-related dementia caused by the virus)

Causes

AIDS is caused by the human immunodeficiency virus (HIV). As a result of infection, a specific type of white blood cell decreases slowly over the years. These cells are part of the body's advance guard against cancer and other pathogens. The deterioration of these cells means the body can no longer protect itself sufficiently.

There are only three ways to get infected with HIV.
1. Unprotected sexual intercourse: Where risk is increased due to existing disease and infections.
Men and women practicing anal sex without condoms are especially at risk. Cells infected with the virus are transmitted by direct contact or through fissures in the intestinal mucous membrane.
2. Cross-contamination with HIV-infected blood: Especially at risk are addicts who share needles. Until a few years ago, those with blood diseases were unknowingly placed at very high risk by receiving transfusions of contaminated blood. Reliable screening of the blood supply for HIV now practically eliminates the danger of receiving infected blood or blood products.
3. Transmission from an infected mother to her baby. About 20 to 30 percent of babies born to HIV-positive mothers are infected either before or during birth; the rest remain healthy. AZT (Zidorudine; Retrovir) therapy during pregnancy can cut the number of HIV-positive newborns down to 8 percent.

AIDS is NOT transmitted by

— Shaking hands or embracing. HIV-positive people need touching and compassion at least as much as uninfected people.
— Normal day-to-day contact in the workplace.
— Door handles, telephone handsets, towels, work tools, coughing, sneezing, or casual contact.
— Mosquitoes or other insects.
— Swimming in public pools, even if a cut or scrape is present.
— Sharing a toothbrush with someone who is HIV-positive. There is no record of AIDS being contracted in this manner. However, sharing a toothbrush is not a good idea, for reasons of general hygiene.
— Using public toilets.
— Sharing utensils or eating off the same dish with someone who is HIV-positive.

— Scissors and razors at the hairdresser's or barber's.
— Dental equipment (as long as it is sterilized after each patient).
— Light kissing. Theoretically, deep kissing resulting in direct blood-to-blood contact (from minor mouth injuries or bleeding gums) can cause infection; however, saliva is an unlikely source of transmission.

Possible Aftereffects and Complications

It has been shown that living with HIV infection, even for long periods of time, does not necessarily lead to AIDS and death. In about 2 percent of all HIV patients, the immune system remains intact for 10 years or more, apparently effectively preventing the spread of the virus. Recently, an apparently "harmless" form of HIV—one that does not attack the immune system—was discovered. In addition, the immune systems of some HIV-positive individuals are somehow able to keep the virus in check.

Research also indicates that some individuals are apparently immune to HIV; despite repeated contact, they do not become infected.

Usually several years pass between initial infection and the appearance of the first symptoms.

After the onset of the disease, appropriate treatment can prolong life expectancy.

Prevention

To avoid infection with AIDS:
— If you are a drug user, investigate needle-exchange drug programs, which eliminate the reuse of needles and thereby the resulting risk of infection. Never share needles; utilize single-use needles.
— If you have various sexual partners, make sure you use condoms and practice sex that does not involve exchanging bodily fluids. This also applies to those in steady relationships where there is even the remote possibility of sexual contacts outside the relationship. The risk of infection is very low (though not zero) when using a condom. Unprotected sex is risky, especially with prostitutes, and especially in Africa or Asia where many prostitutes are HIV-positive.

When to Seek Medical Advice

If you suspect you have been infected with HIV, see your doctor or go to an AIDS clinic.

To determine the presence of HIV, a routine examination is followed by a two-part blood test on a single blood sample. If both parts of the test reveal the presence of HIV antibodies, the diagnosis of HIV infection is confirmed.

A negative test does not necessarily mean you are not infected, however. The antibodies in question take between 4 and 12 weeks to develop after exposure, so they may simply not be showing up yet.

Self-Help

Do not get tested for HIV before consulting a doctor you trust, or getting AIDS counseling.

HIV tests cannot be performed without the individual's consent, even in hospitals. Prior to surgery, you may be pressured into having your HIV status determined to protect hospital personnel who may be exposed to the virus during the operation.

By law, all HIV test results must be kept confidential. This law has been repeatedly disregarded, however, with serious social and professional repercussions for those testing positive.

Many life- and health-insurance companies include negative HIV test results in their prerequisites for coverage.

If HIV infection is determined, the following protocol is recommended:
— Have regular checkups to keep tabs on your situation. Checkups are free of charge at AIDS clinics, where you can usually also find referrals to other doctors such as dentists or gynecologists who guarantee anonymity and are prepared to treat patients, no questions asked.
— Maintain as healthy a lifestyle as possible: Limit alcohol and nicotine consumption, eat a balanced and varied diet, avoid prolonged exposure to sun light, do sports in moderation.
— Avoid traveling to the tropics, where you may be exposed to obscure pathogens and hard-to-treat diseases.
— Treat any infections promptly and thoroughly. An AIDS clinic can answer your questions confidentially and at no charge, and provide
   — Information, clarifications, and health/sex education
   — Professional advice on medical, psychological, or sexual issues, in person or over the phone

— HIV testing

— Counseling for HIV-positive persons and their families

— Legal advice; discussion and support groups; help from social workers; visiting nurse and home health-aide programs for AIDS patients at home or in the hospital; hospice services; emotional support ("buddy") systems

Treatment

The progress of AIDS can be slowed by taking combinations of various drugs such as AZT, ddC, ddI, among others. The decreasing number of deaths due to AIDS in the industrialized world may be due to this type of "drug cocktail" therapy. Effective prevention and treatment exists for almost all types of infections associated with AIDS-related complex (ARC). To date, no effective HIV vaccination has been developed; it is unclear when this will happen.

ALLERGIES

Allergies are reactions of the immune system (see Immune System Disorders, p. 353). There are various types of allergic reaction. A food allergy may affect only the digestive mucous membranes of one patient, while another experiences swelling over the entire body.

The term *allergy* can mean either: A sudden onset of hypersensitivity in a specific organ or whole body, or a condition developing gradually over time.

How Allergies Work

The body's immune defense system reacts to foreign substances (antigens) by making antibodies. Antigens and antibodies interact with each other and activate designated white blood cells.

Normally, these cells protect us against infections and other harmful processes and substances; in an allergy, however, the immune system interprets normally harmless substances—particular foods, fabrics, airborne matter, etc. as being foreign and dangerous, and goes on the attack. Unusually high levels of antibodies are found in the blood, and the white blood cells go into over-drive, emitting tissue compounds such as histamines. These compounds then cause severe reactions in the various mucous membranes of the body, especially the digestive tract, skin, eyes, nose, and bronchial tubes.

Once the immune system has undergone such a reaction, it "remembers" the supposed antigen from then on. In the future, whenever it encounters these substances, it will react defensively much more quickly than it did initially.

Complaints

Certain allergic symptoms are familiar: The sudden onset of a runny nose with hayfever (see p. 299); the teary eyes of conjunctivitis (see p. 240); the itchy skin of hives (see p. 282) and the sudden, unexpected onset of allergic asthma (see p. 307).

Anaphylactic reactions—whole-body allergic reactions that can cause serious results if untreated—are sudden in onset. Pharmaceutical products and poisonous insect bites are two examples of substances that can cause such "shock reactions." Examples of gradually developing whole-body allergic reactions are contact dermatitis (see p. 271) and food allergies.

Anaphylactic Shock

Anaphylactic shock can occur within 15 minutes of exposure to the allergen, causing itching, skin reddening or pallor, whole-body swelling, difficulty breathing, a drop in blood pressure and, sometimes, nausea and vomiting.

First aid for anaphylactic shock consists of laying the patient flat, elevating the legs higher than the head and calling for immediate medical assistance.

Causes and Triggers

Allergic reactions appear to be hereditary; however, many factors have to work together to make a person allergic.

One of these factors is surely our increasingly chemical environment. Hundreds of thousands of chemical substances are in use, and hundreds more are added every year. Additionally, it seems that certain toxins such as heavy metals, airborne soot particles, pesticides, etc. aggravate the effects of particular antigens. Defending the body against all these factors overtaxes the immune system in many individuals.

The connection between general well-being and immune function is generally accepted nowadays (see Health and Well-Being, p. 182). Psychological factors have been shown to strengthen or weaken the body's defenses against allergens. In principle, any substance can function as an allergen, but certain categories of substances consistently cause frequent allergies in a large part of the population.

Many substances don't even cause allergic reactions directly; they pave the way for allergies by damaging the skin and mucous membranes, enhancing their permeability to allergens. The pollutant sulfur dioxide can either cause an immediate allergic asthma attack or damage the bronchial membranes so that an eventual allergy to birch pollen results.
— Healthy Living, p. 772;
— Air Pollution, p. 783;
— Health in the Workplace, p. 789.

Who's at Risk

Allergies have increased to an alarming degree in the industrialized nations.

Aftereffects and Complications

Life can be very difficult for those suffering from allergies, requiring frequent visits to doctors or hospitals in attempt to identify the causes. If the allergens are identified, one can try to arrange one's life so as to avoid them; if they haven't been identified, one's entire life is affected by the ensuing illnesses and treatments. Year-round or seasonal allergies alike can tarnish one's image as an efficient and well-functioning worker; frequent absences caused by illness may cause constant anxiety over the possibility of losing a job.

An allergy sufferer may experience psychological drawbacks as well as physical effects, e.g., if co-workers obviously find an allergic rash distasteful and tend to avoid contact with him or her. Other factors can damage the sufferer's self-confidence as well.

Allergy treatments often cause physical symptoms that are almost as unpleasant as the allergies themselves.

Allergies have the unfortunate characteristic of changing their location and/or severity without warning, as when hayfever develops into asthma.

Organs weakened by allergies often develop other illnesses more easily.

Anaphylactic shock can be fatal.

Prevention

Gaining control over one's external and internal daily environments can help minimize the negative effects of allergies. Factors include a diet carefully selected to exclude unhealthy foods as far as possible; carefully controlled living and working environments; regular exercise, participation in sports, or other physical activities to increase health and well-being; and striving for a proper balance between activity and relaxation, for both body and mind.

Newborn babies who are only breastfed are protected from allergies by mothers' milk for about 6 months. Mothers who wish to breastfeed and have a family history of allergies should insist that their babies not be fed any other milk products from birth on. Cows' milk given during the first few days of life probably encourages allergies, even if the baby begins to nurse afterward. If mothers' milk is not available and there is a history of allergies within the family, certain hypoallergenic formulas should be tried in order to decrease the risk of allergies (e.g., Nutramingen).

The custom of piercing little girls' ears and inserting nickel-plated earrings can encourage the development of a nickel allergy.

When to Seek Medical Advice

If allergies are suspected, you should seek medical help. However, general practitioners are not trained in the detective work of identifying allergens; an allergist should be consulted.

After a thorough physical exam, you will be asked a series of detailed and comprehensive questions to help identify possible allergens. Keeping an "allergy diary" can help you answer questions like the following:
— What are the complaints and symptoms?
— When do they occur: during the day, at night, or both?
— Do outbreaks occur in connection with particular seasons, weather, tasks, places or environments, or persons?
— Are the symptoms intensified under specific circumstances?
— Where do symptoms occur: In closed rooms, only in certain rooms, at work, at home, or outdoors?
— Are outbreaks associated with certain foods, clothing or jewelry, activities such as cleaning or contact with chemicals?
— Are you taking any medications?

Descriptions of your place of work, home, and daily habits are also needed.

Since we are never entirely conscious of all our daily activities, keeping a diary of anything that seems relevant for a while will be helpful.

Once a search direction has been identified, the allergist can expand the search by way of various medical tests.

Skin Testing

In a skin test, the skin on the back or lower arm is scratched with a needle and a series of suspected allergens is applied to the scratch or, in some cases, injected under the skin. In the presence of an allergy, the skin becomes raised and red. However, since the eyes, nose, lungs, or intestines may react entirely differently from the skin, these tests do not provide conclusive evidence. Tests with substances known to cause severe allergic shock reactions should not be performed unless the appropriate first-aid remedies are on hand.

Provocation Testing

In these tests, the suspected allergen is brought into direct contact with the reacting organ. For instance, an extremely diluted pollen solution is dropped into the eyes or nose of a hayfever sufferer, or, in the case of allergic asthma, inhaled.

If a food allergy is suspected, a reverse form of this test is often attempted by first eliminating all suspected foods and then reintroducing them one by one, while observing the reactions. Concentrated solutions of various foods can also be tested on the skin.

Self-Help

After the allergen has been identified, effective treatment is not always simple. It's not always easy to avoid certain substances completely. Reading all product labels carefully is a good beginning. Getting rid of a beloved pet is difficult; changing your job or profession is harder; avoiding household dust is virtually impossible—yet these are the only really effective treatments available.

Other suggestions follow:

For pollen allergies during peak season:
— Avoid spending time outdoors.
— Keep windows and doors closed.
— Schedule vacation time for these periods. At altitudes higher than 6,500 feet and by the ocean, the air is almost entirely pollen-free. See Hayfever, p. 299.

For household dust and dust mite allergies:
— Dust mites don't like synthetic fabrics, so switching from natural to synthetic home furnishings is a good idea.
— Remove all dust collectors from your home (drapes, carpets, slipcovers, throws, knick-knacks).
— Replace any featherbeds or horsehair mattresses with synthetic-fiber ones and have them washed or dry-cleaned every 6 to 8 weeks.
— Remove wallpaper; paint rooms instead.
— Replace carpets with seamless, washable flooring.
— If this isn't feasible, vacuum everything daily, including bedding.
— Buy a vacuum cleaner especially adapted for removing common household dust allergens.
— Consider purchasing special indoor paints containing a substance toxic to dust mites.

— In spring and fall, use a product that kills dust mites and brings together their excrement for easier vacuuming.

For mildew:
— Disinfect all damp walls and floors.
— Change wallpaper.

Treatment

For specific treatment of allergies in particular organs, see the listings for the respective illnesses.

Desensitization

This procedure attempts to make the patient less sensitive to an allergen by injecting or administering orally an extremely diluted solution of the allergen. As treatment progresses, the solution is gradually strengthened. Ideally, the body develops a certain tolerance to the allergen so it can eventually withstand concentrations that would previously have caused an outbreak.

In order for desensitization to be successful, one must be certain that the allergen in question is indeed the one causing the reaction; a skin test alone is not a sufficient basis for making this determination. It is also important that not more than one or two substances be injected; solutions containing six or seven allergens are usually not effective. Treatment usually lasts at least 3 years—unless a marked improvement occurs sooner.

Desensitization doesn't make sense for substances that can easily be avoided in everyday life.

Side Effects: Desensitization is not without risks; since antigens are introduced directly into the body, there is a relatively high risk of anaphylactic shock. Therefore, this treatment should only be undertaken if
— Symptoms are severely impairing the patient's functioning and cannot be alleviated by other medical therapies
— The allergic condition has existed less than 5 years
— The patient is under 50 years old
— The patient is able to make frequent office visits

Desensitization should only be undertaken by specialists with the ability to treat possible emergencies that may result. Patients should remain under medical observation for at least 30 minutes following each injection; thereafter, they should be instructed to seek medical help at the first sign of nausea or breathing difficulties.

Acupuncture

Acupuncture can have a positive effect on allergies, particularly slight or moderately severe ones. Even in cases where acupuncture cannot prevent an allergic reaction, it can reduce the need for medications (see Acupuncture, p. 679).

Treatment by Medication

Cromolyn sodium (Intal) and nedocromil sodium (Tilade) are two kinds of preventive medications that, if taken on a regular basis, inhibit the white blood cells from releasing substances that trigger allergic reactions.

Antihistamines

Antihistamines inhibit the effects of the histamines, or tissue hormones, that trigger uncontrolled allergic reactions; in the process, they relieve itching but often cause drowsiness. Applied to the skin, antihistamines can themselves trigger allergies. Antihistamines should only be taken when absolutely necessary, and only when a topical treatment (like applying eye or nose drops) is not possible.

Corticosteroids

Intravenous or injected corticosteroids are part of emergency treatment of life-threatening anaphylactic reactions. Corticosteroids may also be used to treat long-lasting allergies that don't respond to other medications (see p. 665).

Medications that are Preventative:
For the eyes:
Cromolyn sodium

For the nose:
Cromolyn sodium

For asthma:
Cromolyn sodium (Intal)
Nedocomil (Tilade)

Side effects: Inspiration of medicine may result in cough and shortness of breath.
Oral Antihistamines—sedating
Brompheniramine maleate (Dimetane)
Chlorpheniramine (Chlor-Trimeton)
Tavist
Diphenhydramine (Benadryl)
Hydroxyzine (Vistaril)
Warning: because these medications are sedating, see how you react to the medication before you drive, operate machinery, or do any tasks that require careful attention.
Oral Antihistamines—nonsedating or low-sedating
Astemizole hydrochloride (Hismanal)
Cetirizine (Zyrtec)
Fexofenadine hydrochloride (Allegra)
Loratadine (Claritin)
w
Warning: Astemizole hydrochloride and terfenadine are not to be taken concurrently with cisapride, erythromycin, itraconazole, ketoconazole, mibefradil, nefazodone medications.

DENTAL CARE

The teeth are supported by the jaws, which consist of the upper and lower jawbones (maxilla and mandible) and are joined at the rotating temperomandibular joints. The tooth buds for both sets of teeth are completely formed at birth, although the milk (baby) teeth do not normally begin to erupt for several months.

By the time a child is 18 months old, all 20 milk teeth have usually erupted and are visible. There are 28 to 32 permanent teeth, which replace the milk teeth as those are shed. By the time children are 13 or 14 years old they usually have two incisors, a canine tooth, two premolars and two molars on each half of each jaw.

The third molar, the last in the row, usually comes through at about age 21, but in about one third of the population, these "wisdom" teeth never erupt.

For teeth to align properly, the muscles of the tongue, cheeks and lips must be in proper relationship to each other from childhood onward. Habitual sleep positions, thumbsucking, and genetic factors all influence the bal-ance between these muscles and help determine the way the jaws fit together, including the presence of overbite, underbite, or crossbite. Poorly positioned or missing teeth can cause problems in the tempero-mandibular (jaw) joints or make chewing difficult.

Modern eating habits don't give jaws enough of a workout. Soft, sugary foods have caused an increase in tooth and gum diseases in industrialized countries; fortunately, good dental care can greatly reduce the ill effects.

TOOTH CARE

Toothbrushes

The most important factors in good dental health are a low-sugar diet and complete removal of plaque. The toothbrush is the most important dental tool. It should be small and maneuverable enough to reach into all the corners of the mouth. Its bristles should be straight

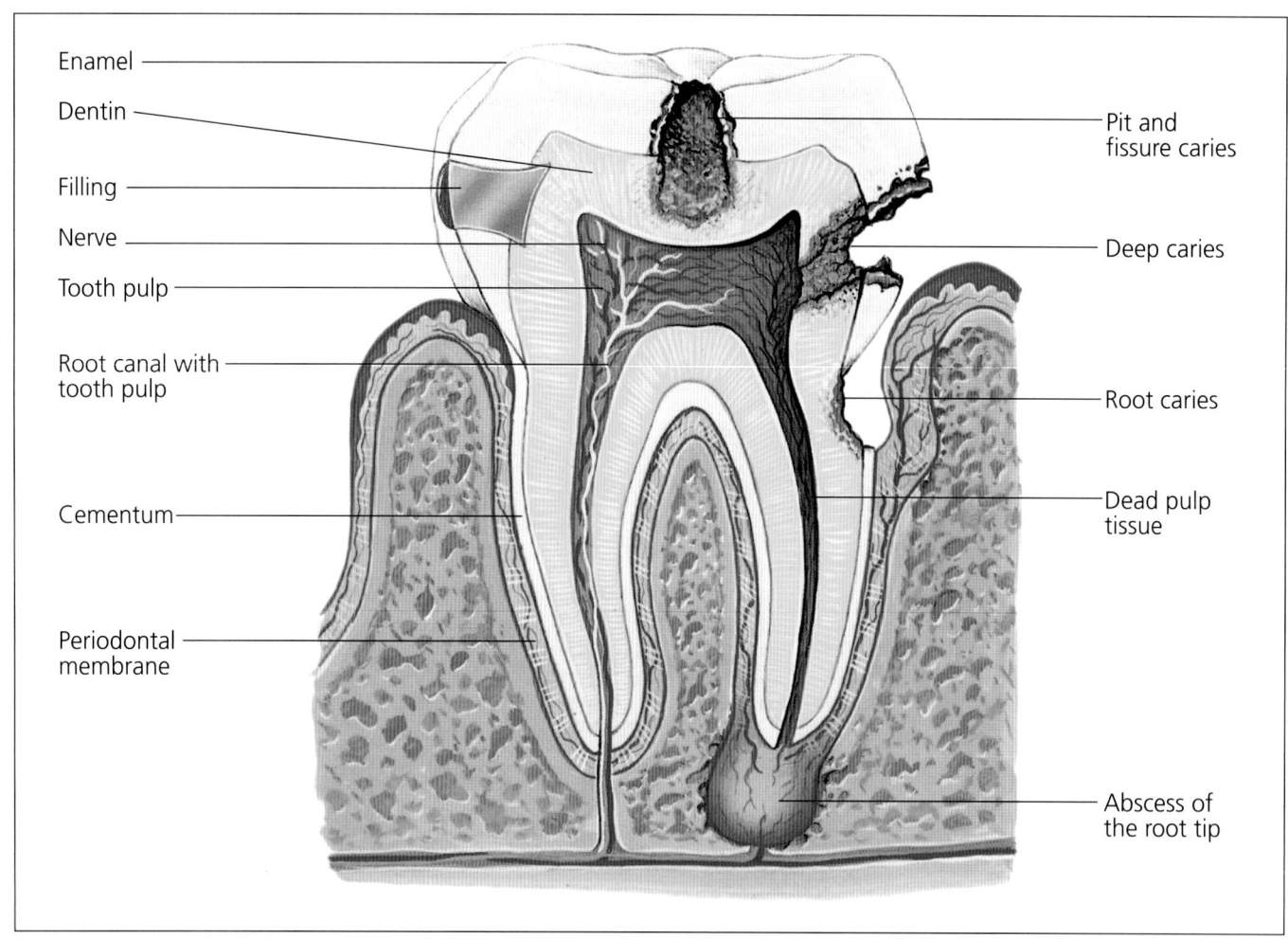

Enamel

Dentin

Filling

Nerve

Tooth pulp

Root canal with tooth pulp

Cementum

Periodontal membrane

Pit and fissure caries

Deep caries

Root caries

Dead pulp tissue

Abscess of the root tip

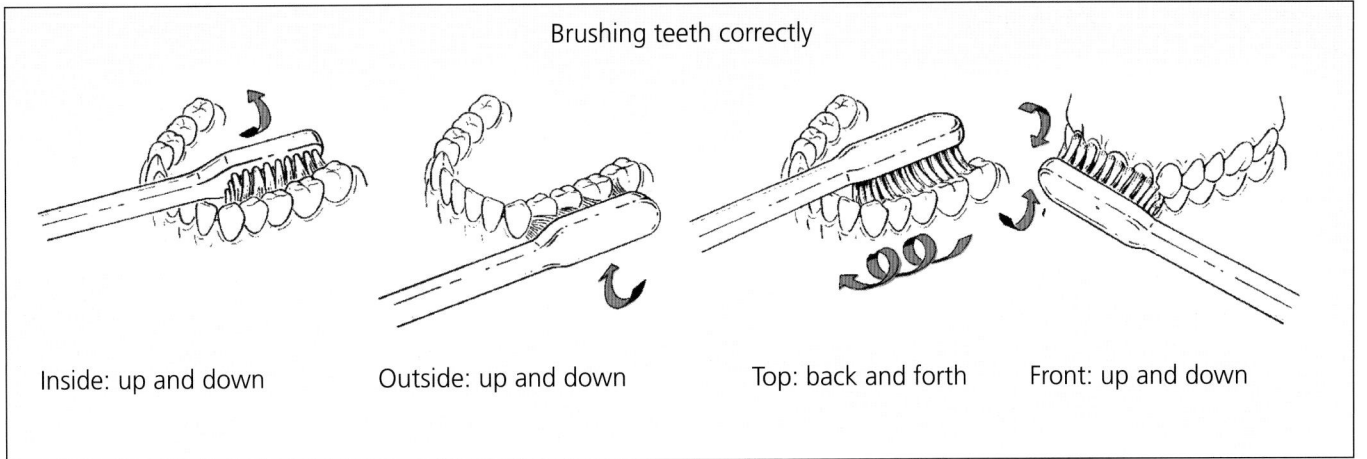

Brushing teeth correctly

Inside: up and down   Outside: up and down   Top: back and forth   Front: up and down

and all the same length, and made of plastic soft enough not to injure the gums.

When brushing teeth, move brush from the gums to the tips of the teeth, making sure the bristles slide into all the interstices. Each tooth should be brushed on its inner surface, its outer surface, and its chewing surface. Brushing also massages and stimulates the gums. If gums have receded, it is important to keep the spaces between them free of food residues with a special brush.

Electric toothbrushes are appropriate for people who are unable to use a manual toothbrush properly—e.g., those who are bedridden or physically disabled.

The jet of water produced by a water pick is no substitute for manual brushing; it should only be used to supplement brushing. In the presence of gum disease, jets of water can force dead cells or bacteria deeper into the tooth sockets. Simply rinsing the mouth out with water after brushing teeth, and swishing it forcefully between the teeth several times, works fine.

A thorough cleaning of the teeth takes at least 3 minutes. It is helpful to have a well-lighted mirror at eye level (especially for children) to check how well you've brushed, as well as a small mouth mirror and egg timer.

Dental Floss

Because tooth decay usually starts at the contact points between teeth, teeth should be kept plaque-free with the help of dental floss. Unwaxed floss is best. Wind the ends around your fingers or stretch the floss across a forked floss holder; then slide it carefully between the teeth and down the side of each tooth. Floss should also be used to clean thoroughly under dentures; special tools exist for threading floss into these areas.

Toothpaste and Mouthwash

Toothpastes aren't medications; they are simply lubricants that supposedly impart "freshness" to the mouth. Toothpastes often contain chemical additives—disinfectants, or detergents like sodium lauryl sulfate—that may damage the gums. It has been shown that brushing teeth with pure water is just as effective as brushing with toothpaste, without the side effects.

It has not been proven that herbal additives or vitamins in toothpaste strengthen gum tissue, nor that certain additives remove plaque or prevent its formation. Plaque forms spontaneously between brushings, and only vigorous brushing will remove it from tooth enamel.

Fluoride additives are said to harden tooth enamel, but this only happens while the toothpaste is actually touching the tooth. Toothpaste formulas are not supervised by any regulatory agency.

As a rule of thumb, the less foamy a toothpaste is and the less sweet it tastes, the better it works. Basically, the less toothpaste you use and the longer you brush, the better.

Mouthwash is not a requirement for oral hygiene; it just covers up the results of inadequate tooth care. If it contains alcohol, it can damage the lining of the mouth; if it contains disinfectants, it can disturb the beneficial microorganisms that help keep the mouth healthy.

FEAR OF THE DENTIST

If you are afraid to go to the dentist, the best approach is not to take a sedative, but to discuss your apprehensions directly with the dentist. He or she should be able to explain in detail what your pain-reduction options are and what procedures and steps will be involved in your treatment. If your anxiety is so severe that you are unable to go through with it, you may want to consider behavioral therapy (see p. 700).

Here are some tips for helping a child reduce fear of the dentist:
— Prepare for the visit by playing "dentist"; examine the child's mouth with a mirror.
— Take the child along for your own dental appointment (unless you yourself are obviously anxious about it!)
— Find a dentist who will take the time to win the child's trust.
— Don't promise the child that It won't hurt; instead, appeal to his or her ability to cooperate.

Accidents

A broken jaw, loose teeth, or a split lip should be given first aid at a dental clinic, and brought to a dentist for follow-up care.

A tooth that has been knocked out can be surgically reinserted into the jaw, especially in young people, and survive for several years.

On the way to the dentist or oral surgeon, the tooth should be placed in a tooth preserving system (TPS) containing Hank's solution. If this is not possible, immersing the tooth in milk will allow the living parts of the tooth to survive for about an hour.

Small children often fall onto their mouths. If a tooth is loosened or pushed into the bone, take the child to a dentist immediately. The pulp may die as a result of such an injury, in which case the tooth will darken. Sometimes the underlying developing permanent tooth is also damaged.

If a child's front teeth are knocked out, a dentist can bridge the gap with a temporary denture. Installation of a permanent bridge is not advisable until the patient is about 20 years old.

CAVITIES (DENTAL CARIES)

Complaints

Cavities make a tooth sensitive to cold, heat, and sour and sweet foods. Cavities don't hurt until they penetrate the tooth enamel and have reached the dentin layer. Yellowish or brown discoloration of the enamel are the first signs of a developing cavity.

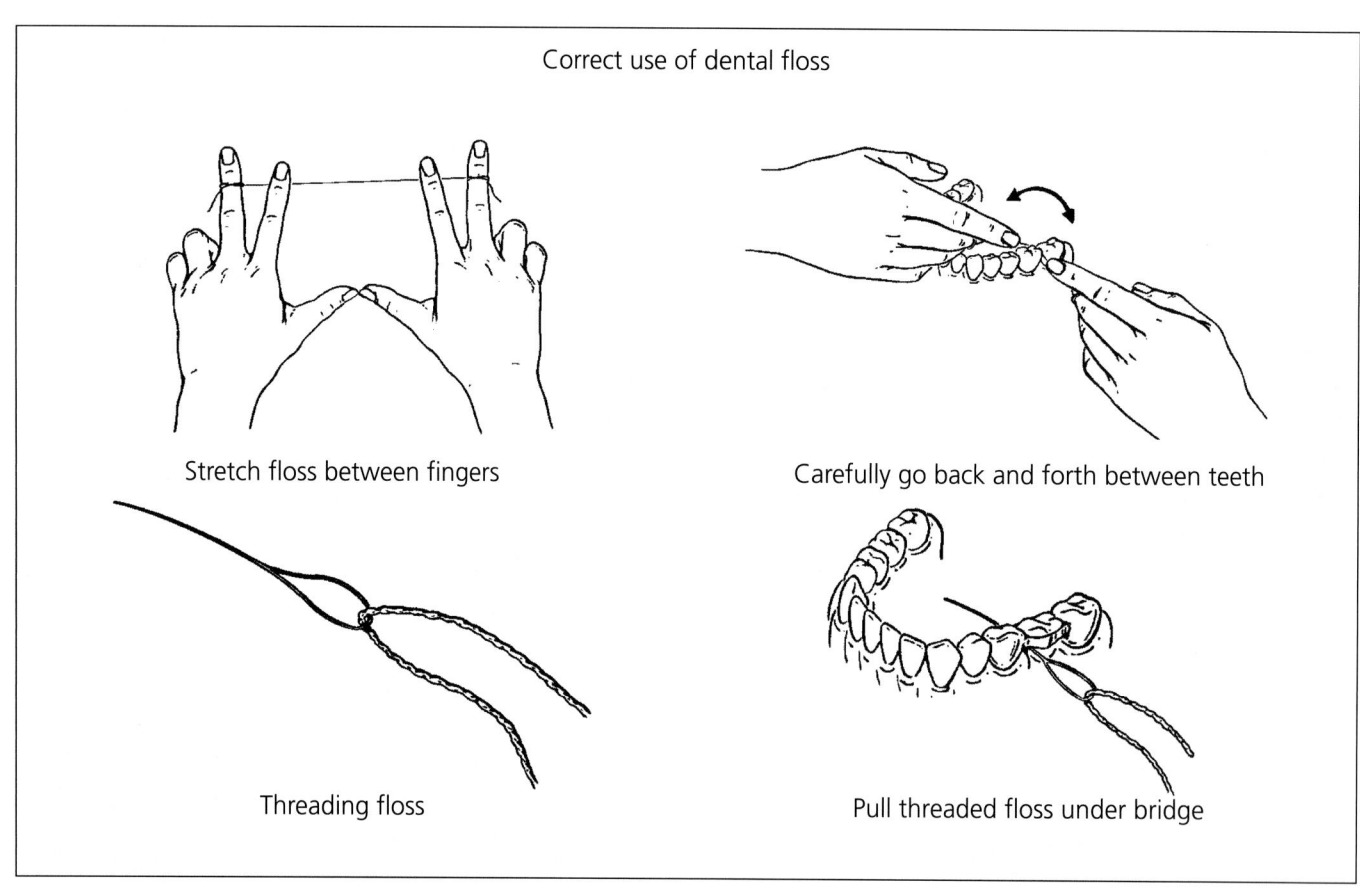

Correct use of dental floss

Stretch floss between fingers

Carefully go back and forth between teeth

Threading floss

Pull threaded floss under bridge

Causes

Cavities are caused by plaque, which consists of sticky microorganisms that live on sugars and convert them to acids. The acids dissolve the enamel, allowing bacteria or fungi to enter the tooth. If the enamel is dissolved all the way through, the cavity begins to eat into the dentin. Plaque is promoted by
— All types of sugar, including fructose and honey, and starches
— Inadequate tooth care (see p. 364)
— Working in very dusty environments or in the presence of acidic or alkaline fumes

Who's at Risk

The risk of dental caries is increased by inadequate tooth care, frequent snacking, and lack of prompt treatment of damaged teeth.

Prevention

Cavities can largely be prevented by a sugar-free diet and careful, regular care of the teeth: Brushing twice a day and always rinsing the mouth with water after eating sweets or drinking sugar-containing beverages (see Tooth Care, p. 364).
Important: Get two dental checkups a year. The dentist should check your brushing techniques and oral hygiene each time.

Preventing Caries with Fluoride

When taken orally or applied directly to teeth, fluorides can harden tooth enamel.

Water should not be fluoridated, however, and neither should milk or salt. The reason for this is that fluorides are already abundantly present as environmental pollutants in our air and food. It has not been proven that fluoride tablets prevent cavities. It is also inadvisable to give children fluoride tablets as a preventive measure because this may contribute to an uncritical attitude toward taking pills in later life.

Fluorides should only be given to children and young people who are especially prone to cavities and have poor dietary habits. They should be applied directly to teeth by the dentist in the form of a liquid or gel.

Tablets containing a combination of vitamin D and fluoride appear to be of little value.

Tooth Sealing

Tiny depressions in the chewing surfaces of the teeth can be protected by sealing them with a layer of composites, which can stop caries in the early stages. Before applying the composite, the site must be cleaned thoroughly.

Possible Aftereffects and Complications

Previously unnoticed cavities may suddenly begin to hurt during a drop in pressure, e.g., while at high altitudes, while on a plane, or while diving.

An untreated cavity may continue to deepen, eventually resulting in a tooth pulp infection, which can expand into the jaw, sinuses, and muscles. The tooth may have to be extracted. Neighboring teeth may then move out of alignment, making chewing more difficult.

When to Seek Medical Advice

See a dentist twice yearly for checkups; toothaches usually appear too late in the game to be an effective early warning signal.

Self-Help

Not possible. Home remedies such as alcohol or cloves should not be applied to a toothache, since they can damage pulp and gums. A visit to the dentist is the most effective painkiller. Dentists make emergency appointments for patients in pain.

While waiting to see the dentist, you can reduce tooth pain as follows:
— Firmly rub the acupuncture point on the outer corner of the nail of your index finger.
— Briefly place a cold, wet cloth on the cheek.
— For a short time, take a simple analgesic. Taking pain medication for a longer period makes diagnosis more difficult. Use analgesics containing acetaminophen (e.g., Tylenol) as the active ingredient.

Medications containing acetylsalicylic acid (aspirin) promote bleeding, and are suitable only when no dental surgery (such as tooth extraction) is anticipated (see Analgesics, p. 660).

Only in exceptional cases, if pain is extremely severe, should a dentist prescribe a combination of aspirin or acetaminophen and codeine (e.g., Tylenol #3).

Other combination painkillers should be avoided (see Analgesics, page 660).

Useful for toothaches: acetaminophen
Tylenol
Panadol
Tempra
Most important side effects: If taken frequently over a period of years, they may damage kidneys. Overdoses may damage the liver.

Useful for toothaches: salicylates
Aspirin (Ecotrin, Empirin, Bayer, ASA)
Salsalate (Salflex, Disalcid)
Diflunisal (Dolobid)
Most important side effects: stomach pains, nausea, tendency to bleed, faintness, ringing in ears

Treatment

A dentist should drill out the cavity to remove all decayed material, using a local anesthetic if necessary to numb the tooth. Local anesthetics may interfere with your concentration for several hours, however, so do not drive a car or use heavy machinery during this time.

Before filling the cavity, the dentist will protect the tooth pulp with a subfilling of cement. If the cavity is large, he or she may place a small ribbon of metal or plastic around the tooth, to prevent the filling from spilling over and damaging the gum.

If food particles often become lodged between your teeth, have your dentist investigate.

After filling any cavity, a dentist should check the bite and adjust the filling until it feels no different from the natural bite. If this is not done, you will have trouble chewing and jaw problems, so, if necessary, encourage the dentist to keep working until your bite feels normal.

Avoid different metals in fillings, especially in teeth that touch when you bite down. Two different metals in contact may act as a battery and generate electric currents, promoting corrosion of the fillings.

Laser Treatment

Laser drilling of teeth, a supposedly painless procedure, is not legally approved in the United States. Laser treatment of gums is possible, but incorrect application of this technology can cause irreversible damage. Laser equipment manufacturers are responsible for educating dentists in the correct use of the equipment.

PULPITIS (INFLAMMATION OF THE TOOTH PULP)

Complaints

Symptoms of inflammation of the tooth pulp include a constant toothache with penetrating, throbbing, or dull pain, extending over the face and jaw. Cheeks and lymph nodes in the lower jaw and neck may swell.

Causes

The tooth pulp is inflamed or infected.

Who's at Risk

People with untreated cavities are at highest risk.

Prevention

Regular tooth care and semiannual dental checkups.

Possible Aftereffects and Complications

The affected tooth may die; the infection may spread into the jaw. The dead tooth may become a focus of infection, reducing the patient's resistance to other diseases, especially chronic ones, and promoting allergic reactions.

Fillings

There is no ideal material for fillings, and recent studies have shown that all available filling materials can cause allergies. The best filling is a healthy tooth!

Tooth-Colored Composites

These materials harden with exposure to light and are suitable for filling in visible sites in the teeth. The more they are polished after hardening, the better they resist plaque. Composites are not strong enough to be used on chewing surfaces of molars. They may also release toxins.

Gold Alloys

Gold alloys are expensive, and require more of the tooth to be removed than for amalgam fillings. After drilling, an impression of the tooth is used to create a mold. Gold is poured into the mold in the laboratory, then cemented into place in the tooth. If the edges of the filling are improperly sealed, plaque can get through. "Onlays" cover the entire chewing surface and protect the whole tooth; "inlays" are suitable only for small defects in the tooth.

Ceramic Inlays

These have rough edges that fit less exactly than gold inlays and may break.

Amalgam Fillings

Amalgam is a mixture of silver, copper, other metals, and mercury. Some of the mercury from the filling is absorbed by the body. These fillings last a long time and release less mercury if
— The dentist uses non-gamma-2 amalgams, taps the filling firmly, and polishes it at least 1 day later
— The amalgam does not come into contact with other alloys in the mouth
— You take good care of your teeth and avoid extremely hot foods

Like gold and other alloys, amalgam can cause allergic reactions in the oral mucosa and skin elsewhere on the body. Headaches, inability to concentrate, and nervousness may also result from amalgam fillings, though they are extremely rare.

Mercury Poisoning

Although it has been suspected for years, there is still no proof that mercury from fillings causes psychosomatic complaints such as migraines, asthma, back pain, and depression, let alone diseases such as connective tissue disorders or cancer. Depending on the number of fillings, the body may absorb about six times as much mercury from fillings as it does from foods. The mercury accumulates mainly in the kidneys, brain, and liver. So far as is now known, it does not cause health problems. However, to prevent future problems, it is recommended that pregnant or nursing women and small children under age 6 not be given new fillings, nor have old fillings drilled out. Drilling old fillings releases mercury vapor, causing higher exposure.

The amount of mercury in the body should be measured in a 24-hour urine sample.
Caution: Many examiners recommend extensive work on "mercury-poisoned" jaws. Before you decide on such treatment, get a second opinion.

When to Seek Medical Advice?

Have a dental checkup every 6 months. If you have even slight tooth pain, see a dentist at once.

Self-Help

Not possible. For pain relief, see Cavities, p. 366.

Root Canals

Teeth with infected or dead pulp can still be retained. Root canals can lead to higher risks in a few types of systemic illnesses. In these cases, and also in the following situations, the tooth should be extracted:
— if there is advanced inflammation of the gum and the tooth is loose,
— if roots are crooked and a root canal seems unlikely to succeed,
— if the tooth is broken deep in the crown or in the root, or
— if the tooth is not important for chewing, esthetically, or as an anchor for a false tooth. Anytime a dentist suggests pulling a tooth, you should ask why this is necessary.

Root canals may require several appointments. First, the dentist must drill into the tooth and remove the pulp. Pulp should not be killed chemically, e.g., with arsenic. Any infected dentin must also be removed. This operation often requires an anesthetic.

Before treatment, an X ray will reveal how deep the treatment needs to go. Afterward, another X ray will reveal whether the root has been successfully filled. Ask to see these X rays and have them explained.

Materials for Root Fillings

There is no optimal material for filling roots. Usually the composition of the materials used is unknown; the jawbone may be affected if the filling leaks out of the root. The dentist should be careful to apply the filling paste and pin only to the root tip. However, there is a residual risk of a root tip inflammation (see p. 370).

Certain filling pastes can help reduce existing inflammations.

Anchoring with Dental Screws

Within a few months after a root canal, the tooth is provided with a filling or a crown. If the crown of the tooth is too severely damaged, the filling or crown can be anchored in the dentin with screws. The ideal metal for these screws is titanium, which does not corrode. Teeth with filled roots may discolor with time and become brittle, so in many cases an anchored crown is advantageous.

INFLAMMATIONS OF THE ROOT TIP: ABSCESSES, GRANULOMAS, FISTULAS, CYSTS

Complaints

Teeth with inflamed root tips become sensitive to tapping or pressure; pain in the area throbs in time with the pulse and becomes progressively worse.

An abscess can spread into cheeks, tongue, gums, or sinuses. In children, abscesses usually burst spontaneously.

If pus spreads into soft oral tissues, it can cause swelling in the cheek, floor of the mouth, jaw, or gums. The swelling does not always hurt, but is sometimes accompanied by fever.

Sometimes, especially in children, the inflammatory process forms a fistula tract in the oral mucous membrane through which the pus drains to the outside. Usually this does not hurt.

Causes

Root-tip inflammations are caused by untreated cavities (see p. 366).

Who's at Risk

Those with untreated cavities are at risk.

Prevention

Inflammations can be prevented by consistent care of the teeth and a sugar-free diet. Semiannual dental checkups are important.

Possible Aftereffects and Complications

The inflammation may become chronic. The focus of inflammation at the tip of the root may encapsulate and become the source of chronic illness in the body. A jaw cyst may form, and the jaw sinuses may become infected.

When to Seek Medical Advice?

Seek help as soon as possible if symptoms appear.

Self-Help

Heat or warm, moist compresses (see Compresses, p. 692) make abscesses mature more quickly.

Treatment

Abscesses that don't burst spontaneously should not be opened until they are mature.

If a root canal operation cannot heal a root tip inflammation, the root tip should be removed (root tip resection). An X ray and local anesthetic are used to prepare for this treatment. After the root tip is removed, the dentist cleans out the hollow to remove infected tissue and pus. Sometimes the tip of the root is filled; amalgam should not be used, however. Finally, the wound is stitched closed and cared for until it heals.

This operation is relatively simple for front teeth, but is not always possible for molars.

Cysts in the jaw are removed in a similar operation and will usually result in a larger hole. If surgery is successful, however, the hollow will gradually be filled in by bone tissue.

If the inflammatory process is far advanced, the tooth may have to be pulled. In young people, it is sometimes possible to implant the tooth again after cleaning out the abscess.

GINGIVITIS (GUM INFLAMMATION)

Complaints

The inflamed gum becomes very sensitive to touch. Its usual pale pink color turns bluish-red. It swells between the teeth and bleeds easily, especially during toothbrushing.

Causes

Gingivitis is caused by plaque and tartar above, and especially below, the gum line, by poorly fitting prostheses, vitamin deficiencies, diabetes, liver diseases, allergies, hormonal changes during pregnancy, and side effects of anticonvulsant medications. Working with lead can also cause gingivitis; in this case, the gum line turns black.

Who's at Risk

The risk of gingivitis is increased by the factors listed above and also by inadequate tooth care, the presence of tartar (tartar should be removed by a professional), and gums irritated by toothpaste, mouthwash, or denture adhesives or care products.

Possible Aftereffects and Complications

Chronic gingivitis promotes periodontal disease (see p. 371, below).

Prevention

Practice regular oral hygiene, get a dental checkup every 6 months, and have tartar removed professionally.

A low-sugar diet will also prevent the disease. Fiber-rich foods strengthen the gum tissue by providing massaging action during chewing. Massaging gums with a clean finger several times a day will produce a similar effect.

When to Seek Medical Advice?

Seek help if gums bleed.

Self-Help

Incipient gum problems can be stopped by brushing teeth thoroughly (see Tooth Care, p. 364) three times a day. The effectiveness of so-called gum-strengthening toothpastes or mouthwash has not been proven.

Treatment

There is no medical treatment for gingivitis. Part of every dental visit should include removal of tartar, especially tartar located under the gumline, which irritates the gum. In addition, your dental professional should demonstrate proper tooth care.

GUM DISEASE: PERIODONTITIS, PERIODONTAL DISEASE, TRENCH MOUTH

Complaints

Periodontitis: Pus collects in deep pockets in the gums. Late in the disease, a mildly painful tension develops in the gum; sometimes teeth are sensitive to pressure. Teeth become loose.
Periodontal Disease (atrophy of the gums): Perhaps as a result of periodontitis, the jaw bones atrophy. Periodontal disease becomes more common with advancing age.
Trench Mouth: Is a rare, tissue-destroying form of gum inflammation that occurs mainly in young people and is extremely painful.

Causes

Periodontitis is a result of gingivitis.

The causes of periodontal disease have been completely identified, but inadequate oral hygiene, poor dental work and changes in blood circulation due to stress or smoking are contributing factors.

Trench mouth is an infection promoted by inadequate dental hygiene.

Who's at Risk

The risk of these ailments is increased in people who practice inadequate dental hygiene.

Prevention

Regular care of the teeth (see p. 364).

A dental professional should regularly remove tartar above and below the gumline, because tartar promotes gum disease. Specialized cleaning, including the use of hand tools, should be automatically done at every visit to the dentist, although this is unfortunately not always the case.

After tartar is removed, the tooth enamel should be polished with a cleaning paste and rotating brushes or rubber pads to remove discolorations caused by drinking tea or smoking.

Possible Aftereffects and Complications

Periodontitis and periodontal disease: The jaw bones atrophy, and teeth become loose and fall out.
Trench mouth: The patient's overall health is seriously impaired.

When to Seek Medical Advice

Seek help if
— Gums bleed
— There are swollen pockets at the bases of teeth
— Pus is present
— The mouth has a rotten odor
— There is a pulling sensation on the teeth
— Teeth are sensitive to pressure
— Gums or oral mucosa hurt

Self-Help

Not possible.

Treatment

There are no effective drugs or homeopathic remedies for diseases of the periodontal region. Surgery followed by proper mouth care is the only option.

Several appointments are necessary. In the course of these, existing fillings are polished and the patient is taught optimal oral hygiene. Inflamed tissue is removed surgically and the root of the tooth is evened out (curettage). This causes discomfort and is therefore performed under local anaesthesia. The gums bleed profusely during this treatment.

The teeth remain hypersensitive for several weeks after treatment. Teeth will also appear longer because gums have receded; however, the gum tissue will strengthen, holding loosened teeth more firmly.

If this operation is to be successful, it must be followed by regular toothbrushing and the use of dental floss. A dental professional should teach the patient proper oral hygiene techniques and schedule checkups every 3 to 6 months.

To prevent recurring inflammation, teeth should be cleaned regularly.

There is no effective cure for atrophy of the jawbone and loss of teeth caused by periodontal disease. These occur most frequently in older people, in about 5 percent of cases.

DISORDERS OF THE TEMPEROMANDIBULAR JOINT

Complaints

Symptoms include an aching jaw, with pain radiating to the neck and head; possibly a "popping" jaw; inability to open the mouth all the way; cramps in the chewing muscles; headaches; muscle pains extending into shoulder.

Causes

— Usually these symptoms are caused by tension-releasing habits such as clamping jaws or grinding teeth. The latter is especially common at night and in stress situations.
— Fillings that stick out too far, prostheses, or malocclusion of the jaw bones may place so much stress on the temperomandibular joint that it is damaged.
— The temperomandibular joint may be inflamed.

Who's at Risk

Inflammations in the joints are more common in people over age 50 because of increased wear and tear.

Possible Aftereffects and Complications

The mobility of the joint may decline. Habitual clenching of the teeth may also leave you more vulnerable to jaw problems (see Health and Well-Being, p. 182).

Prevention

Have a dentist check your mandibular arch, fillings, and dental prostheses to be sure they allow a proper bite.

When to Seek Medical Advice?

Seek help if above symptoms are present.

Self-Help

Moist, warm compresses can ease pain. Eat soft foods and avoid moving your jaw.

Treatment

An uneven or malformed bite should be corrected, e.g., by wearing a retainer at night.

For treatment to be successful over the long term, you'll need to learn how to handle stress without tooth-clenching or grinding (see Counseling and Psychotherapy, p. 697; Relaxation, p. 693), reducing the need for painkillers and sedatives.

Finally, opening and stretching exercises for the jaw are important so the joint can retain its mobility. These are also needed in cases of rheumatic joint inflammations (see Rheumatoid Arthritis, p. 455).

UNEVEN BITE

Hardly anyone has a perfect bite. Minor misalignments and tooth rotations are common and can give the smile a personal touch or contribute to someone's special charm.

After the jaw has grown to its adult size, treatment is indicated only if the misalignment impairs chewing, speech, and/or the general health of the gums. Severe overbite or underbite often require surgery. The decision to operate should be made by the orthodontist and the patient together.

Disadvantages: Usually treatment is comprehensive and can take years, representing a major psychological stressor. Braces are visible on the teeth and may interfere with professional and domestic life. There have been few studies on the long-term success rates of such treatments. Any gum diseases should be treated before braces are fitted. The danger of cavities and loss of calcium from enamel is high. If there were problems with speech before the treatment, speech therapy is usually needed afterwards. Wisdom teeth often cause problems; e.g., they may grow in sideways, allowing the formation of gum pockets where infections can lodge, or they may not grow in all the way and may need to be extracted. If their roots are badly bent, complications may result (see If the Tooth Can't Be Saved, below).

Obviously, there are many factors to weigh before deciding on treatment (see Baby Teeth, p. 376).

IF THE TOOTH CAN'T BE SAVED

Extracting a tooth should always be the treatment of last resort. Even if the pulp is dead, the tooth should only be pulled if
— Its root canals are crooked and impenetrable, and a root tip inflammation cannot be treated by root-tip resection
— The tooth is loose because of a gum inflammation, or if the patient has a chronic illness such as connective tissue disorders, kidney inflammation, heart disease, or iritis
— A cavity extends into the root of the tooth
— The tooth is tipped on its side or badly misaligned and frequently gets inflamed (e.g., a wisdom tooth).

Pulling Teeth

The dentist injects a local anesthetic, then loosens the gum tissue around the tooth. The next step is to pull the tooth with dental pliers. Even when great care is used, parts of the crown or root may break off; broken pieces must be carefully removed, and inflamed tissue should carefully be cut out.

The initial heavy bleeding after a tooth is pulled is staunched by biting on a wad of gauze, but it actually aids the healing process to have the opening in the bone filled with fresh blood.

Normally, no painkiller is needed after a tooth is extracted. The injected anesthetic will keep working for a while, and after that a cold pack on the cheek will help relieve the pain.

If you do take a painkiller, make sure it doesn't contain aspirin (see Cavities, p. 366), which promotes bleed-

ing. Analgesics containing acetaminophen (e.g., Tylenol) are better.

Many dentists prescribe oral antibiotics, although topical treatment should be sufficient. If you receive a prescription for oral antibiotics, you should ask why. They are justified only if
— A local infection threatens to spread, e.g., when there is further swelling, lymph nodes are involved, or there is fever
— The body's resistance is weakened
— There are fresh injuries in the jaw area and infections need to be prevented

Don't use antibiotic salves that are applied to the oral mucous membrane—they reduce the body's resistance to microbes.

After Oral Surgery

— Get plenty of rest. Keep your tongue away from the wound. Don't talk much, and eat only liquid or mushy foods. Avoid stimulants such as cola, tobacco, or coffee.
— Don't use gargles, rinses, or mouthwash: They will interfere with the healing process.
— If bleeding recurs, rinse your mouth and bite on a clean, folded cloth. If bleeding does not stop within an hour, have the dentist check the situation.
— If you have severe pains 2 to 3 days after the tooth extraction and the hole is filled with a grayish-yellow, foul-smelling coating instead of clotted blood, the wound needs to be cleaned out again and the area disinfected.

CROWNS

An artificial crown or cap should be applied only if a tooth is no longer capable of anchoring a filling.

If the tooth is loose and the root tip is infected, it should not be crowned. Misaligned teeth should not be ground down for aesthetic reasons. Crowned teeth have a shorter life expectancy than others.

Preparation for a Crown

No pain will be felt while the tooth is being ground down because a local anesthetic will be administered beforehand. Only the part of the tooth above the gumline should be ground, after which a temporary crown will be installed.

Mild pain is normal at this point; if it becomes

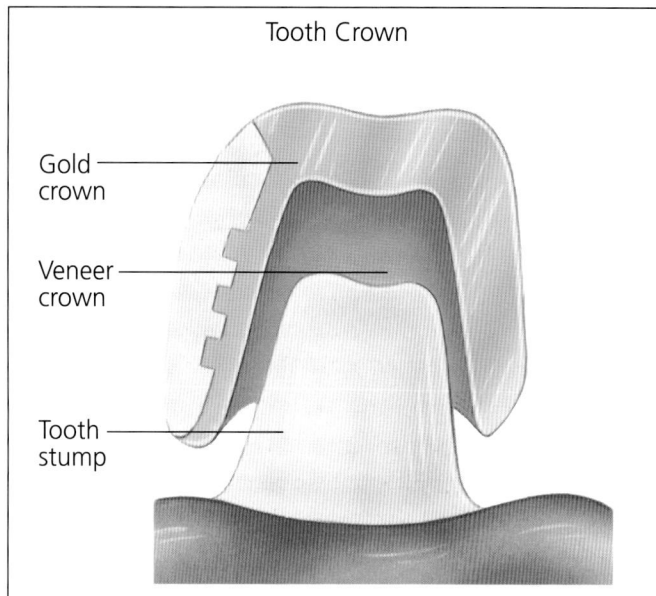

Tooth Crown

Gold crown

Veneer crown

Tooth stump

intense, tell your dentist.

The permanent crown should not be glued on until it is certain that

— The edges of the crown lie smoothly on the tooth.
— There is sufficient contact with the neighboring teeth.
— Nothing is interfering with the bite, or impeding chewing.

Irritability of the tooth should stop after a few days, but sensitivity to temperature may last longer. If the procedure was performed incorrectly, symptoms include

— A sharp increase in pain when eating or brushing teeth
— Swollen, bleeding gums
— Food residue getting caught
— The crown falling out

A properly installed crown should last 10 years. However, a long-term study showed that procedures are incorrectly performed in half of all crown operations, decreasing the crown's life span.

Crown Materials

The best crowns are made only of pure metal, but for cosmetic reasons, metal-alloy crowns are often covered by a porcelain layer in the visible places, with the color of the porcelain matched to the other teeth. Plastic coatings wear off rapidly. There is debate over the merit of coating even the chewing surfaces with porcelain. Crowns made entirely of porcelain or plastic do not fit

as well, or wear out quickly. Computer-aided crown fitting is not yet as successful as hand fitting.

BRIDGES

Sometimes gaps between the teeth don't interfere with tooth function. On the other hand, a bridge is indicated to span the gap if

— The neighboring teeth begin to loosen or tip into the gap, or if pockets form in the gum tissue.
— The opposite tooth grows into the gap.
— The gap interferes with biting and chewing, or the jaw or its joints begin to hurt.

Types of Bridges

Ideally, a bridge should consist only of the two anchoring teeth and one false tooth. A bridge made of a metal alloy and covered with porcelain to blend in with the other teeth works best. The support teeth need to be filed down and crowned; the ends of the bridge are then fastened to the crowns. A bridge can carry more than one tooth only if the two anchor teeth are healthy.

The bridge should not touch the gum where the tooth is missing, to prevent damage to the gum tissue, unless the missing tooth is an incisor. In this case, one point of the false tooth will touch the gum, to make it look natural.

Only if chewing pressure is light, a Maryland bridge may be used. Its two ends are glued to the backs of the anchor teeth, which have been filed slightly. Such bridges usually don't last long.

Preparation for a Bridge

The anchor teeth should be filed, as described for crowns (see p. 373).

The bridge is set in temporarily, until it is certain there are no problems with crowns and no irritation of the mucous membranes under the bridge. Only then is the bridge permanently cemented in place.

The dentist should check the fit and contact with the gum tissue carefully.

Treatment should include a good explanation of the use of a special "interdental" toothbrush and dental floss.

PARTIAL DENTURES

If not enough anchor teeth are available, or a bridge is too expensive, the remaining option is partial dentures.

The transition from one's own teeth to the remov-

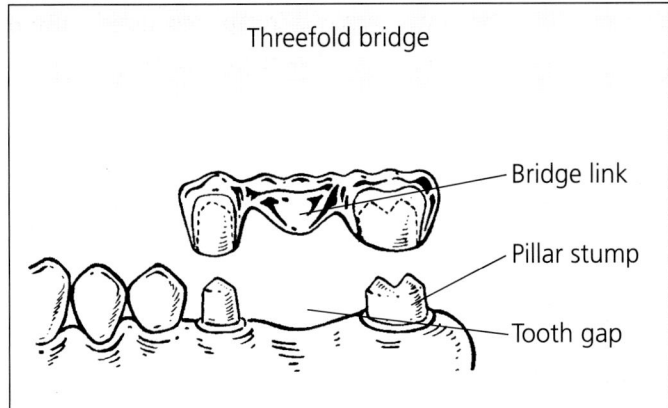

Threefold bridge

Bridge link

Pillar stump

Tooth gap

able denture is not always easy. It may be weeks before the tongue, cheek, and mouth muscles get used to the denture. Don't be discouraged. If the denture fits, these initial difficulties will soon pass, as long as you maintain a relaxed attitude.

Problems with Dentures

Laughing, coughing, sneezing, speaking and chewing will seem difficult at first, and your sense of taste will seem slightly off. You can help yourself by practicing patiently. Eat only soft foods at first, and practice speaking in front of a mirror.

The dentist should regularly check the placement of your prosthesis. Because bones and mucous membranes change position over time, a lining may need to be placed on the underside of the denture.

You should not, under any circumstances, do this yourself. The American Dental Association gives this warning about glues and inserts for dentures: "Poorly fitted dentures can be hazardous to your health." If your dentures hurt, see your dentist.

Denture Care

Taking good care of your dentures is extremely important, because the large areas of jaw and gums they cover cannot be reached by saliva for cleaning purposes. Food particles can easily become lodged between mouth and dentures, causing bad breath as they decay. Dentures, gums, and remaining teeth should be thoroughly cleaned, preferably with a brush and household soap.

Chemical denture cleansers may irritate the mucous membranes and roughen the soft lining on the underside of the dentures. To remove calcium deposits, soak dentures in vinegar occasionally. Sonic cleaners, available in medical supply stores, also remove tea and

tobacco stains. Before replacing dentures in your mouth, rinse them well with water.

Materials for Partial Dentures

Partial dentures made of plastic should only be temporarily worn (and have direct contact with the oral mucous membrane), while the site of a tooth extraction is healing.

Permanent partial dentures are cast from metal alloys and the false teeth are mounted on the metal base. The removable denture is clamped onto anchor teeth, which support it. Since cavities can easily form under the clamps, and because daily removal of the denture can damage the enamel of the anchor teeth, it is wise to crown them.

Anchors that slide like snaps into the crowns of the supporting teeth are expensive and difficult to manufacture. Have your dentist explain, with the aid of printed information, which solution he or she prefers and why.

Fitting Partial Dentures

After an impression is made, partial dentures are fabricated in the laboratory. The color and material can be selected with the help of your dentist. Before the impression is made, the remaining teeth should be cleaned, and any gum diseases should be treated.

When new, partial dentures may cause some discomfort where they touch the gum. Your dentist can easily correct this. If you develop a chronic runny nose soon after receiving new dentures, you may be experiencing an allergic reaction to cobalt, chromium, or nickel in the metal alloy; you should inform your dentist of this problem.

If the prosthesis is too loose, and if friction or pains in the residual teeth develop, these may indicate substandard work.

The dentist should

— test the placement of the prothesis as long as necessary to insure that normal chewing is possible.

— show you exactly how to insert and remove the prothesis.

— check at regular intervals whether the saddle of the denture needs an underlining. (*Warning:* Do not attempt this procedure yourself.)

— teach the patient proper mouth and denture care (see Denture Care, p. 375, at left).

DENTURES

Solid, cavity-free teeth should be retained in the mouth as long as possible. They are important as anchors for false teeth and cushions for the pressure of chewing. This function is especially important in the lower jaw.

If several teeth, or the last remaining teeth, must be pulled, the final set of dentures cannot be inserted until the jaw is completely healed. This usually takes a few months, during which time one can live with a temporary set of dentures. Temporary dentures are usually inserted immediately after the teeth are pulled, while the local anesthetic is still active. Because the affected area and the jaw may change position, it may be necessary to correct the placement of temporary dentures several times.

Plastic is the best material for dentures. The teeth should be made of abrasion-resistant plastic. Although porcelain teeth look almost identical to real ones, they are more likely to break than plastic teeth, and often make a clicking sound when biting.

TOOTH IMPLANTS

Pins made of metal or other materials can be implanted into the jaw, and either crowns cemented onto them, or false teeth anchored to them.

There are various implantation systems, and all of them are expensive. If the implant does not grow properly into the jaw, it can make matters much worse than they originally were. The main problem with implants is the fact that bacteria can move along them into the bone, which they then proceed to destroy, causing a problem much worse than missing teeth.

Although the popularity of tooth implants is growing, a rule of thumb is to resort to implants only if removable dentures are out of the question.

BABY TEETH

The best way to prevent future problems with teeth is to breastfeed your baby (see Nursing, p. 584). Breastmilk has exactly the right composition for proper mineralization of the developing teeth. In addition, sucking on the breast promotes proper jaw formation.

Teething

In many babies, the gums are painfully tense. A rubber teething ring or hard crust of bread will help, and will promote chewing ability as well.

So-called teething remedies, on the other hand, should be avoided because their sweet taste creates a craving in the child for the number one tooth menace: Sweets.

Cavities in Baby Teeth

Sweets, especially sticky ones, should be given to children as seldom as possible. If they do eat snacks, they should learn to brush their teeth immediately afterward (see Tooth Care, p. 364).

Baby teeth are small, so cavities can destroy them much more quickly than permanent teeth. Baby teeth play an important role as placeholders for permanent teeth, helping them to grow in straight. Unfortunately, parents and dentists often don't take baby teeth seriously enough, because they do fall out.
Warning: Take your child to the dentist immediately if baby teeth are sensitive to sweets, heat, or cold; if enamel is discolored (white or brownish); if food particles often lodge between teeth; if parts of the enamel are broken off; or if fillings break.

Uneven Bite

Misalignment of teeth and jaws can be hereditary, or it may be promoted by the early loss of baby teeth or habits like tongue-pressing, nail-biting, or sucking on lips or fingers. Slight misalignments are not a problem and may be outgrown, if the uneven tooth is filed down a bit by the dentist. A purely cosmetic orthodontic treatment should not be undertaken lightly.

Deciding on Treatment

Orthodontic treatment is advisable if
— Teeth are so far out of line that gaps between them promote tooth decay or gum disease.
— Speech and chewing are impaired.
— The child cannot close lips and breathes primarily through the mouth.

Risks

Orthodontic intervention in a complicated system may unleash an avalanche of changes if the braces or retainer are not used properly. The treatment may last for years and take its toll on the entire family. It can impair the jaw joints, and may promote cavities and gum disease.

Relapses and setbacks are not uncommon.

Tips If You Wear a Retainer

— The feeling of a foreign body in the mouth will subside after a few days. Reading aloud will help for difficulty in speaking.

— Thoroughly clean the teeth and retainer three times a day. Don't soak them in cleanser; rinse well with water. Do not eat between meals if you can avoid it.

— Hold the retainer by the plastic part while inserting it, so wires don't get bent.

— When not wearing the retainer, keep it in a rigid container and protect it against breakage.

— If the retainer won't stay in place, go to the orthodontist at once.

Tips If You Wear Braces

— Brush your teeth very carefully after every meal, using a special "interdental" brush as well as a regular toothbrush, and possibly a mouthwash. Some dentists suggest rinsing the mouth with a fluoride solution or using fluoride gel or liquid.

— Each time they are adjusted, the braces will press on your teeth for several days. This is normal. However, if parts of the braces press, stick, or hurt immediately after the adjustment, the dentist should be told so that the mucous membranes are not injured.

— Every evening, after brushing your teeth, check with a fingernail to feel whether any bands or brackets have come loose. If they have, they should be tightened as soon as possible, so your treatment program isn't extended for weeks.

The results will be satisfactory and lasting only if the orthodontist plans the treatment carefully and the child cooperates fully.

Planning Orthodontic Treatment

The orthodontist should discuss the treatment with parents in great detail, including pointing out the deviating teeth, describing their potential for trouble if not treated, describing the goals, steps and duration of the treatment, and explaining the various hardware (braces, retainers) involved.

Treatment usually doesn't need to start until the child is eleven. It may begin as early as age 9, but only in acute cases involving the temporomandibular joints, or deviations or misalignments that are causing problems with speech, biting, or closing the lips. If you and your child are uncertain whether to begin treatment, get a second opinion.

Orthodontic treatment should be taken seriously in the child's life. The parents and dentist should make it clear that the child will have to assume some responsibility for himself or herself and his or her health, but that they will be there to help. A few days of not wearing the braces can undo the work of months.

With the help of a written treatment program, parents and child can track progress. This may help motivate the child to keep going all the way to the end of the treatment.

Certain important points in the treatment should be performed by the orthodontist, not an assistant: Placing the braces on the teeth, cementing the bands in place, gluing the brackets, bending and fitting wires, and all checkups.

It is important that the orthodontist or assistants regularly remind the child about proper tooth care, and that the child continue to visit the dentist twice a year to check for cavities.

After Braces Are Removed

When the teeth have finally reached the desired position, it may be hard for a child to understand that the treatment isn't over yet. After braces are removed, the mouth's mechanisms for keeping teeth in place (gums, mucosa, tongue, lips, and chewing and facial muscles) need to adapt to the new arrangement, and during this period there is a high risk of teeth moving back into their old positions. Therefore, this phase of the treatment should be taken seriously.

Various retention devices are available for postbrace treatment. An ideal solution is a retainer made of elastic material, which is worn around the clock for a week, and thereafter only at night.

A plaster model and X ray, and/or a photograph of the "new" teeth can document the conclusion of treatment and make possible a comparison with the original positions.

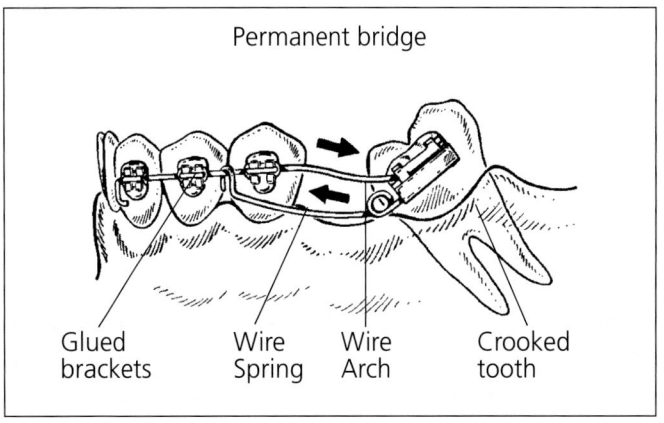

Permanent bridge

| Glued brackets | Wire Spring | Wire Arch | Crooked tooth |

DIGESTIVE SYSTEM

The gastrointestinal tract, which is lined with mucous membranes, begins with the mouth and ends at the anus. The process of breaking down food begins with mastication by the teeth. At the same time that food is chewed, it is mixed with saliva, which begins the process of chemical breakdown. In the remainder of the gastrointestinal tract, the slurry of food is reduced to its components: Carbohydrates are broken into simple sugars, proteins into amino acids, and fats into glycerol and fatty acids. Larger molecules than these cannot pass through the intestinal wall into the blood. The chemical building blocks are then recombined by the body into its own products: Hormones, enzymes ,and other proteins, fats, sugars, and starch.

The moistened, chewed food passes through the throat and esophagus into the stomach, where it is further broken down by hydrochloric acid and protein-digesting enzymes. From there, it passes into the duodenum, the first part of the small intestine. The pancreas and gallbladder also open into the duodenum; pancreatic juice neutralizes the mixture and adds enzymes which break down carbohydrates and fats, while bile from the liver serves as both a detergent and a neutralizing agent.

Most of the digestive process occurs in the small intestine, which is between 16 and

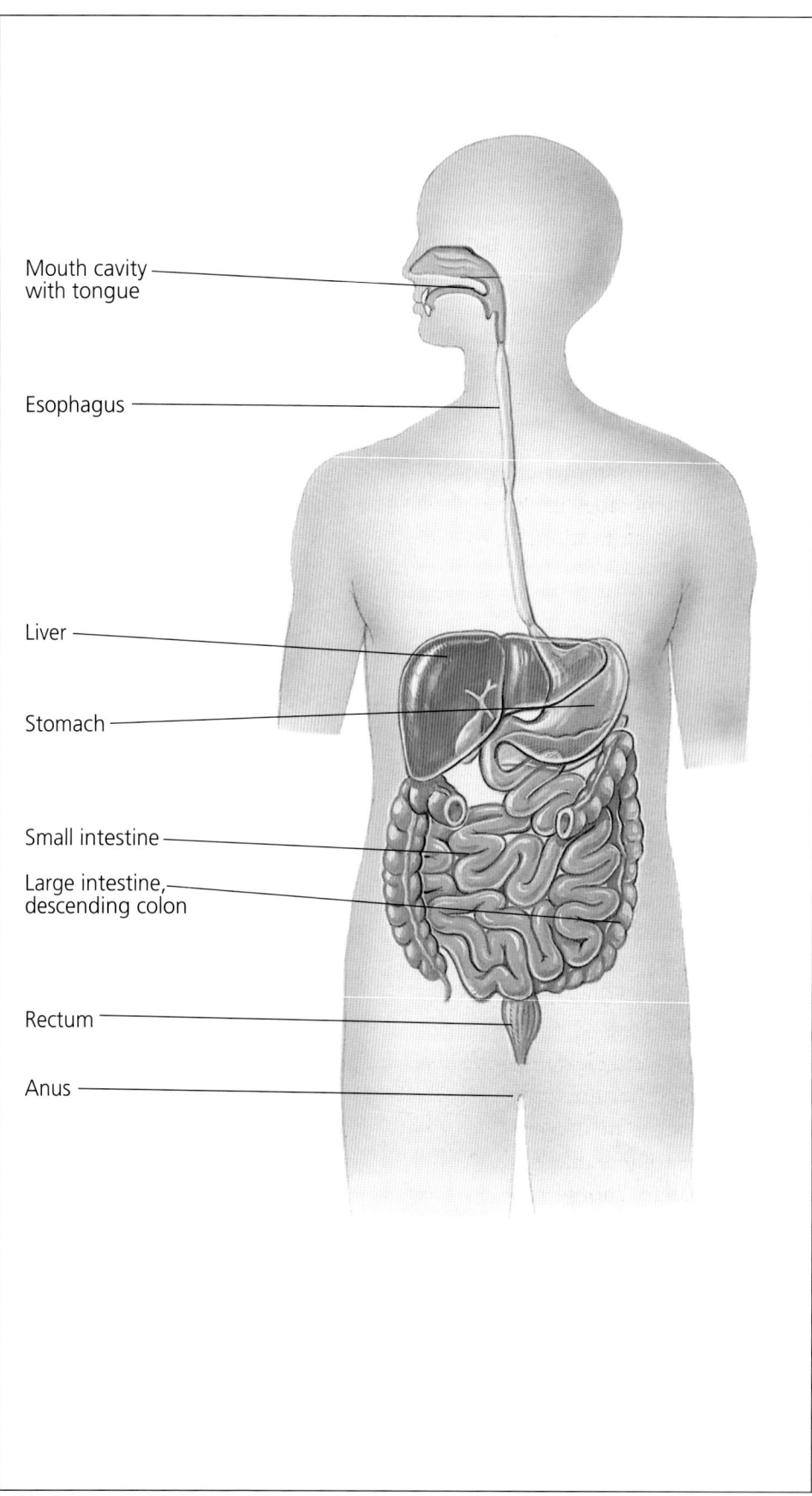

Mouth cavity with tongue

Esophagus

Liver

Stomach

Small intestine

Large intestine, descending colon

Rectum

Anus

26 feet in length. It is lined by tiny projections, the villi, which absorb nutrients and pass them on to the blood. The veins from the intestine feed into the portal vein, which leads directly to the liver. There, the nutrients are processed further.

The appendix is a short, dead-end piece of the small intestine just past where it opens into the large intestine. It is 2 to 3 inches long and has no known function in humans.

The slurry of food, from which by this time nearly all nutrients have been extracted, passes from the small intestine into the large intestine. As it passes through the ascending, transverse and descending colons (see large intestine), water is continuously extracted from it. Finally, the remaining indigestible mass enters the rectum and then passes out through the anus as stool (see Feces, p. 404). The stool also contains shed cells from the mucous membranes, minerals, and bacteria that have helped process the food. Its brown color comes from the bile pigments.

Mouth (Oral) Cavity

The oral cavity is surrounded by the lips, cheeks, tongue, gums, jaws, joints, chewing muscles, teeth, and the floor of the mouth. This entire system is involved in the articulation of speech. The tongue carries the taste buds and helps manipulate food. Food is shredded and ground in the mouth, as well as moistened and lubricated by saliva, which also dissolves some of its components.

Three pairs of salivary glands open into the mouth: the submaxillary, sublingual, and parotid glands. Other glands are scattered throughout the oral mucosa, which lines the oral cavity.

Saliva rinses and cleans the oral cavity; many bacteria, fungi, and other microorganisms live in it, in equilibrium. Changes in the mucous membrane and the surface of the tongue may indicate internal illness; pronounced changes should always prompt a visit to the doctor or dentist.

STOMATITIS (ORAL MUCOUS-MEMBRANE INFLAMMATION)

Complaints

Symptoms of stomatitis include pain or a burning sensation in the lining of the mouth, which is red and swollen. The mouth may feel dry even when it is bathed in saliva. Sometimes blisters or even ulcers form. The tongue may be coated and turn yellowish to dark red. It is painful to eat solid foods, and the sense of taste is impaired. There may be a rotten smell to the breath, combined with a mild fever.

Causes

Stomatitis is caused by inadequate oral hygiene in addition to injuries from sharp edges of teeth, bite wounds, irritations from tobacco smoke, allergic reactions to plastic and metal parts of dental prostheses, deficiencies of vitamins B or C or iron, bacterial infections, blood diseases, working at high temperatures, lye vapors, or heavy metal poisoning (see Health in the Workplace, p. 789).

Who's at Risk

The risk of stomatitis is increased by
— Poor oral hygiene
— Smoking
— Allergenic dental prosthesis parts and cleansers
— A diet deficient in vitamins (see Nutrition, p. 722), often caused by unfamiliar foods and poor sanitary conditions encountered on vacation
— Weakened immune defenses due to other illnesses

Possible Aftereffects and Complications

— Shrinkage of the gums
— Loss of appetite
— Severe physical impairment

Prevention

Correct oral hygiene is important (see Tooth Care, p. 364). Avoid oral contact with people who have a mouth inflammation. Give up smoking (see Smoking, p. 755).

When to Seek Medical Advice

Seek help if
— Swelling, redness, and pain persist beyond a few days in spite of self-help measures
— Breath smells strongly and fever is present
— Pressure marks caused by false teeth remain even when false teeth are removed
— Ulcers develop

Rinses that bring relief:
— Three percent hydrogen peroxide, diluted 1:1 with water. Use for no more than 7 days.
— Sage or chamomile tea (see Healing with Herbs, p. 688)

Self-Help

Clean teeth with great care. Avoid coarse foods, and avoid smoking.

Treatment

Have teeth cleaned daily by a professional using hydrogen peroxide solution. Sometimes antibiotic treatment is indicated. Dentists advise against treating inflammations of the oral mucous membranes with gargles, lozenges, sprays, or salves, all of which have side effects and don't treat the underlying cause.

Medications for short-term use only:
Topical anesthetics should be used only for a short time; they may cause allergic reactions.

THRUSH

Complaints

Symptoms of thrush include pain in the entire mouth, and creamy white spots that bleed when scraped. The lymph nodes in the neck may be swollen.

Causes

Thrush is a fungal infection.

Who's at Risk

The risk of contracting thrush is increased by antibiotic use, corticosteroid inhalation (e.g., for asthma), and insufficient saliva production; also following radiation therapy.

Possible Aftereffects and Complications

The fungus may spread throughout the entire body.

Prevention

Use antibiotics only for specific infections (see Antibiotics, p. 661). Rinse mouth thoroughly with water after inhaling corticosteroids.

When to Seek Medical Advice

Seek help as soon as symptoms appear.

Self-Help

Not possible.

Treatment

The physician should prescribe appropriate antifungal medication.

CANKER SORES

Complaints

Canker sores are painful sites on the lips and insides of the cheeks, sometimes on the tongue as well. They are usually round and white, with red rims.

Cause

Canker sores are caused by infection by a virus usually present in most human bodies; the disease breaks out when the patient's resistance is low.

Who's at Risk?

People under stress or with weakened immune systems are at increased risk for canker sores.

Possible Aftereffects and Complications

Loss of appetite.

Prevention

A healthy and balanced lifestyle will help prevent outbreaks.

When to Seek Medical Advice

Seek help if you suspect you have canker sores.

Self-Help

Allow yourself time to relax.

Treatment

Topical anesthetics can temporarily relieve symptoms (see Stomatitis, p. 379). They are applied to the sores with cotton swabs. In severe cases, medications containing acyclovir can bring relief.

If canker sores recur frequently and are extremely bothersome, gamma globulin injections may be given to help boost the immune system.

PAROTITIS (SALIVARY GLAND INFLAMMATION)

Complaints

In parotitis, the salivary glands swell painfully. Salivary ducts may become inflamed and filled with pus.

Cause

Bacteria in the glandular ducts may initiate the inflammation. Other causes may include stomatitis (inflammation of the oral mucous membranes), salivary stones, benign or malignant tumors, or radiation therapy.

Who's at Risk

The risk of disease is increased by low saliva production, intestinal diseases that cause mucous membranes to dry out, and liver infections. Parotitis may also be a late complication of mumps in childhood.

Possible Aftereffects and Complications

The outlet ducts of the salivary glands in the lower jaw are fairly frequently blocked by stones. These may become purulent and break through to the outside.

Prevention

Not possible.

When to Seek Medical Advice

Seek help if pain is severe.

Self-Help

Eating a lemon or chewing gum can help stimulate saliva flow.

Treatment

Antibiotics are used to combat the infection. Sometimes the gland must be surgically removed. Salivary stones are removed under a local anesthetic.

GLOSSITIS (TONGUE INFLAMMATION)

Complaints

In glossitis, the tongue becomes smooth and dark red and may swell, burn and hurt.

Causes

— Irritation by sharp edges of teeth, ill-fitting prostheses, alcohol, tobacco, pungent spices, mouthwash, burns, or mechanical injury
— Vitamin B or iron deficiency
— Various skin diseases, diabetes, syphilis
— Psychological conditions

Who's at Risk

The risk of contracting glossitis is increased by inadequate oral hygiene and smoking.

Possible Aftereffects and Complications

Difficulty in eating or breathing.

Prevention

Regular mouth care (see Tooth Care, p. 364).

When to Seek Medical Advice

Seek help if inflammation continues for several days in spite of self-help measures. It may be an early symptom of pernicious anemia (see p. 347), or a sign of celiac disease (see p. 411), or iron deficiency anemia (see p. 345).

Self-Help

Rinse mouth with 3 percent hydrogen peroxide solution, or sage or chamomile tea.

Treatment

The cause of the inflammation should be determined and treated.

LEUCOPLAKIA (WHITE AREAS IN MOUTH)

Complaints

Leucoplakia manifests as bluish-white spots on the edges of the tongue and the mucous membranes of the mouth, which become rough and horny.

Causes

This disorder is probably caused by chronic tongue irritation by teeth, tooth fillings, pipe smoking, or habits like pressing the tongue against the gums or sucking in the cheeks.

Who's at Risk

This ailment occurs most often in men between the ages of 25 and 55. The risk is increased by the presence of cadmium and radioactive substances in cigarette smoke (see Smoking, p. 754).

Possible Aftereffects and Complications

Cancer may develop, especially in smokers.

Prevention

Don't smoke (see Quitting Smoking, p. 755).

When to Seek Medical Advice

If the typical signs of this ailment appear, see a dermatologist or dentist.

Self-Help

Not possible.

Treatment

The cause should be treated, and it may be necessary to remove the spots surgically.

Oral Cancers (Cancer of the Mouth Area)

(see also Cancer, p. 470)

Complaints

The symptoms vary: burning, the feeling of a foreign body in the mouth, numbness underneath dentures, blood in the saliva. Any knots, lumps, or hardened areas of the tongue are suspicious (except for Canker Sores, see p. 380), as are persistent sores.

Causes

Smoking is the primary cause of mouth cancers. Tumors of the tongue and oral mucous membranes can also be promoted by broken teeth, excessively prominent fillings or dentures that don't fit. Benign tumors of the tongue may also become cancerous.

Who's at Risk

The risk is higher in men over age 45 and in those who smoke a pack of cigarettes daily, or chew tobacco, and drink alcohol regularly. People who work in galvanizing or metal polishing plants are at additional risk.

Possible Aftereffects and Complications

Tumors under $2/5$ inch in diameter can usually be healed. However, cancer cells spread quickly to the numerous lymph nodes in the mouth and neck areas. In a third of cases, these may lead to formation of another tumor in the mouth, throat, larynx, esophagus, or lungs.

Prevention

Stop smoking (see Smoking, p. 755) and have your teeth checked by a dentist twice a year.

When to Seek Medical Advice

Seek help at the first signs of hardening, small lumps, or reddish-colored ulcers, especially on the floor of the mouth, underside of the tongue, soft palate, or insides of cheeks. Cancer cells can be detected early by doing a smear of the area.

Self-Help

Do things that you enjoy and are good for you; this can positively affect the course of disease.

Treatment

There is no treatment using medications or alternative medication. Any cancer in the mouth region must be removed surgically. Often parts of the jawbone, face or neck must also be removed. In advanced cancers, chemotherapy followed by radiation treatment is useful. Even in cases where extensive surgery is required, disfiguration of the face can be avoided. Plastic surgery using tissues and bones from other areas of the body or prostheses can rebuild the face.

This reconstruction should begin as soon as possible after the first operation. Patience and cooperation on the part of the patient are required in any case. If rehabilitation is offered, it's a good idea to take advantage of this. Psychotherapy can help the patient adjust better to the disease and the prostheses.

Esophagus

The esophagus is a muscular tube that connects the mouth to the stomach. Its muscular wall moves everything that we swallow to the opening of the stomach. At this point, a sphincter (ring-shaped) muscle and flaps of mucous membrane prevent the contents of the stomach from flowing back up. The esophagus is lined with a mucous membrane that is not protected against acid.

ACID REFLUX

Complaints

In this disorder, the contents and acid of the stomach repeatedly come up, accompanied by burning, pressing pains behind the breastbone (heartburn). The symptoms may repeatedly occur at the same interval of time after eating; the interval will vary from one person to the next.

Causes

— Weakness in the muscle that closes the lower esophagus
— Overweight (see Body Weight, p. 727)
— Pregnancy (see p. 565)
— Diaphragmatic hernia (see p. 439)

Who's at Risk

People who smoke and drink large amounts of alcohol and coffee often suffer heartburn. During pregnancy, tight clothing, weight gain, and pressure against the stomach increase the tendency for heartburn.

Possible Aftereffects and Complications

— Painful swallowing; while eating, the feeling of something stuck in the throat.
— Inflammation of the esophagus (see below).

Prevention

— Avoid smoking and drinking coffee or alcohol (see Mood-Altering Substances and Recreational Medications, p. 754)
— Avoid fatty foods and sweets. Keep the evening meal light, and do not engage in midnight snacking. Eat in an upright position, and swallow several times in succession.
— Avoid excessive weight gain, tight clothing, and continuous sitting. Don't bend forward after eating.
— Raise the head of your bed.

When to Seek Medical Advice

Seek help if sour stomach contents repeatedly come up and symptoms persist.

Self-Help

Lose weight (see Losing Weight, p. 728).

Treatment

Treatment of gastroesophageal reflux corresponds to treatment for inflammation of the esophagus (see p. 384).

ESOPHAGITIS (ESOPHAGEAL INFLAMMATION)

Complaints

When the esophagus is inflamed, burning pain and pressure (heartburn) develop behind the breastbone, usually after mealtimes or when the patient is lying down. The pain may extend up to the throat, and sometimes undigested food and stomach acid come up. Coughing at night, breathlessness, or hoarseness are additional symptoms.

Swallowing cold or hot foods is difficult.

Causes

— Abuse of alcohol or cigarettes.
— Heartburn
— Irritation by medications; capsules especially may remain stuck in the esophagus. The dangerous medications include pain relief tablets with aspirin or indometacin, iron, beta blockers, and tetracycline (see Medication Summary, p.657).
— Fungal infections of the esophagus.
— Diaphragmatic hernia (see p. 439).
— Injuries (e.g., from fish bones) or burns (e.g., from acids or alkali).

Who's at Risk

The risk is increased by smoking and misuse of alcohol.

Possible Aftereffects and Complications

Scars, constrictions, and bleeding ulcers may form.

Prevention
— Avoid smoking cigarettes and drinking alcohol (see Smoking, p. 754; Alcohol, p. 756).
— Always take medications with a large glass of water while standing up. A couple of bites of banana may help lubricate its passage.

When to Seek Medical Advice
Seek help immediately if pain is severe, if difficulty swallowing becomes worse, or if there is bloody vomit. These are also warning signs of cancer of the esophagus. To determine whether there is a tumor, the physician will examine the patient using an endoscope (see A Look Inside, p. 651).

Self-Help
— Avoid cigarettes, citrus fruits, and alcohol.
— Lose weight if you are overweight.
— Eat sitting upright, chew well, and swallow small bites. The last meal of the day should be the smallest.
— Raise the head of your bed.

Treatment with Medications
Acid-binding medications (see Antacids, p. 391) can help soothe burning pains and inflammation. H^2-blockers are considered optimal (see Stomach and Duodenal Ulcers, p. 389). Fungal infections are treated with antifungal medications.

Treatment by Surgery
Surgery is indicated if medications prove inadequate and the esophageal inflammation is caused by a diaphragmatic hernia. The operation can be performed using a laparoscope inserted through a small incision in the abdomen. Usually only a 3-day stay in the hospital is needed.

ESOPHAGEAL POUCHES (DIVERTICULA)

Complaints
Esophageal pouches produce feelings of pressure and the sense of a foreign body in the esophagus and difficulty swallowing. Undigested stomach contents come up repeatedly. A noticeable gurgling is heard when the patient speaks.

Causes
The mucous membranes lining the esophagus develop sac-like bulges that fill with food remains. The muscular wall becomes thinner. These type of pouches don't necessarily produce symptoms.

Who's at Risk
Esophageal pouches are relatively uncommon.

Possible Aftereffects and Complications
Severe inflammations of the esophagus are possible. Also, the food slurry can accidentally get into the trachea and lungs, leading to a lung abscess.

Prevention
Not possible.

When to Seek Medical Advice
Seek help if symptoms appear.

Self-Help
Eat small portions, chew well, and swallow carefully.

Treatment
Esophageal pouches must be removed surgically. This is a relatively complicated operation, performed under general anaesthesia.

ESOPHAGEAL STENOSIS (NARROWING)

Complaints
In this disorder, swallowing produces strong spasms with feelings of pressure, and a strangling sensation. Breathing hurts and may be partially blocked.

Causes
Scars from ulcers or burns of the mucous membranes can cause narrowing of the esophagus. In rare cases, diseases like scleroderma (see p. 461) may be the cause. Cauterizing varicose veins in the esophagus (see Cirrhosis of the Liver, p. 396) can also leave scars.

Who's at Risk
Esophageal stenosis is rare. The risk is increased by burns or ulcers.

Possible Aftereffects and Complications
There may be chronic difficulty swallowing. The gastric slurry may enter the trachea and lungs, causing a lung abscess. Eating difficulties can lead to weight loss.

Prevention
Not possible.

When to Seek Medical Advice
Seek help if swallowing difficulties do not subside.

Self-Help
Chew well, swallow carefully.

Treatment
Physicians can stretch the esophagus using an endoscope which has metal "olives" attached. This makes the esophagus functional for a long time.

If scarring is present, or the narrowing is due to a burn, an operation is often needed to remove the damaged piece of the esophagus and replace it with a piece of the large intestine (colon interposition). This is a difficult, risky intervention.

ESOPHAGEAL CANCER
(see also Cancer, p. 470)

Complaints
The early stages of esophageal cancer produce no symptoms. Later, swallowing becomes difficult and may become impossible. Other symptoms are weight loss, bad breath, nausea, vomiting, and pains behind the breastbone.

Causes
It is not known why cancers develop.

Who's at Risk
Esophageal cancers usually appear only after age 60, and 80 percent of them are in men. At increased risk are
— People who drink large amounts of distilled liquor and who smoke (see Alcohol, p. 756).
— People with esophageal ulcers

Possible Aftereffects and Complications
The tumor may spread rapidly and form metastases in the lung(s) and liver.

Prevention
Use moderation in smoking and drinking.

When to Seek Medical Advice
Stubborn difficulty in swallowing is a warning signal for esophageal cancer; see your health-care provider as soon as this appears. An endoscope may be used to check for cancer (see A Look Inside, p. 651).

Self-Help
Doing things you enjoy, and which are good for you, can have a positive influence on the course of disease.

Treatment
It is nearly impossible to operate on a cancer in the upper third of the esophagus. In the middle third, a combination of surgery and radiation may help. Tumors in the lower third of the esophagus must be removed surgically. One patient in four can be healed.

Laser treatments can immediately widen a narrowed esophagus, without surgery. Swallowing difficulties can be greatly reduced by radiation therapy.

You should discuss with the treating team which measures are necessary and helpful, and design a program to ease the symptoms.

Psychotherapy can support the healing process. Self-help groups can help the patient come to terms with the illness. Alternative medicine may improve the patient's outlook, but there is no evidence that it inhibits the growth of tumors.

Stomach

The stomach is a muscular bag with a volume of over 1 quart. It collects food, adds gastric juices, and begins the process of digestion. Carbohydrates remain in the stomach for about an hour, proteins somewhat longer, and fats the longest. The pyloric valve, a ring-shaped muscle at the base of the stomach, allows the food slurry to enter the duodenum.

The autonomic nervous system, which is sensitive to moods and psychological states, directs the muscle motions with which the stomach churns the food slurry. The autonomic nervous system is also responsible for the production of gastric juices and the hormones

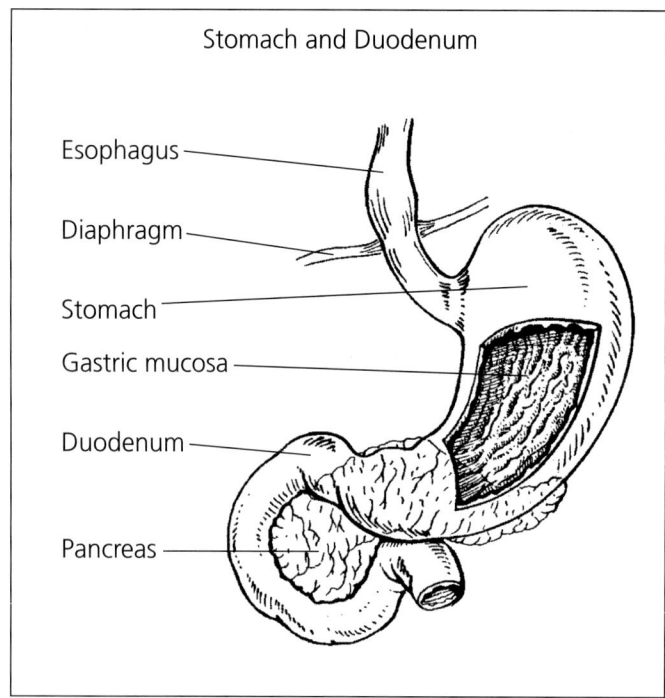

Stomach and Duodenum

Esophagus

Diaphragm

Stomach

Gastric mucosa

Duodenum

Pancreas

histamine, prostaglandin, and gastrin, which, in turn, direct the process of digestion. Patients with stomach complaints should therefore also be on the lookout for psychological causes and discuss them with their treating physician (see Health and Well-Being, p. 182).

NERVOUS STOMACH

Complaints

Symptoms occur periodically or occasionally; sometimes individually, sometimes together; and sometimes on an empty stomach, but often during or after eating. Many people mistakenly believe that the symptoms are caused by food:

— Burning, spasmodic pains in the upper abdomen
— Nausea, vomiting
— Heartburn, eructation (belching)
— Feelings of pressure or fullness
— Flatulence
— Lack of appetite
— Dry mouth, burning tongue and/or difficulty swallowing

The symptoms are often accompanied by a depressed mood, anxiety, restlessness, sleeplessness, feeling overwhelmed, tingling in the mouth, constricted breathing, heart symptoms, or trembling of the limbs.

Causes

— A hectic lifestyle and irregular eating patterns can "hit you below the belt" and interfere with emptying of the stomach.
— Situations that cause anxiety or distaste can lead to nausea. The body thus clears what is "making it sick," such as conflicts at school which are unbearable for a child. Disgust is also a cultural phenomenon, however, and people learn to be disgusted by certain things.
— Crises or major life changes, such as puberty, marriage, birth of children, mid-life crisis or job changes, may all contribute to a nervous stomach, as may
— Psychological stress, conflicts in relationships, loss of a life partner, work, nationality, etc.
— Work on an assembly line, heavy labor or shift work

Who's at Risk

Stomach complaints are common, accounting for one out of every ten visits to a physician. Stress, both emotional and physical, increases the risk.

Possible Aftereffects and Complications

If symptoms occur repeatedly, it should be determined whether there is an organic cause.

Prevention

— Do not smoke cigarettes on an empty stomach. Better, give up smoking (see Smoking, p. 755), and avoid concentrated alcohol.
— Avoid stress, excitement, anger and anxiety. Deliberate relaxation (see p. 693) and deep breathing help prevent stomach upset.
— After consulting with a physician, stop using all medications that upset your stomach.

When to Seek Medical Advice

Seek help if symptoms recur repeatedly. If they persist longer than 4 weeks, the gastric mucosa should be examined by endoscopy (see Gastroscopy, p. 652). This can rule out a diagnosis of gastritis, which is frequently made in error.

Self-Help
— "Tune out" and relax. Consciously relaxing the muscles can help (see p. 693).
— A hot water bottle, a warm and moist or cool compress (see Compresses, p. 692), hot and cold showers and warm baths with calming herbs (see p. 688) can all help ease pains.
— If the empty stomach hurts, a small snack can help: Fiber-rich snacks, bananas or apple juice.
— If the stomach aches after eating, an Alka Seltzer should help; for children, a carbonated drink. Wait for half an hour before undertaking renewed activity, or take a walk.
— Don't drink very hot or cold liquids, avoid hot and cold foods that are hard to digest, and don't eat in the late evening.
— A special diet is not needed. Eat what tastes good to you, and avoid things that disagree with you. Eat and drink slowly, and chew your food well. Your diet should contain lots of vegetables, fruits and whole grain products (see Nutrition, p. 722).
— Various kinds of tea can help, even through the ceremony of preparing them (see Stomach Teas, p. 388).
— Acupressure (see p. 680), learned from an experienced masseur or masseuse and practiced by your partner, or even yourself, can help.

Treatment
— Massage (see p. 686) can help you relax.
— Relaxation training (see p. 693) and breathing techniques can also help you relax (see Breathing Therapy, p. 681).
— Acupuncture (see p. 679) may be able to interrupt the vicious cycle of symptoms.
— Some people find homeopathic treatment (see p. 684) helpful.
The best advice is to try these methods out and find which are most pleasant and effective for you.

Medications
Choosing a medication depends on the cause of the symptoms:
— Infection with *Helicobacter pylori* bacteria requires a threefold therapy (see Stomach and Duodenal Ulcers, p. 389).
— Excess acid can be buffered with antacids and acid blockers.

— Nausea and a full feeling can be relieved by medications containing metoclopramide, but only for a short time (see Acute Gastritis, below). Other medications and combinations are less useful.
— Flatulence is caused by increased gas formation in the gastrointestinal tract. It is doubtful that the preparations sold for this purpose are effective, but if they seem to help, it does no harm to take them for a short time.
— The effectiveness of appetite stimulants is open to debate.
— Sedatives are often prescribed for people with stomach problems, but they have many side effects and can lead to dependency. In situations of acute stress, a single prescription of a beta blocker is defensible. You should not take neuroleptics if you have acute stomach pains.
Psychotherapy (see p. 699) may be helpful in finding the deeper psychological causes of stomach pains and then working them out.

ACUTE GASTRITIS
The term *gastritis* is often applied incorrectly to an irritated stomach (see Nervous Stomach, p. 386). Actually, gastritis is an acute inflammation of the gastric mucosa caused by poisoning (e.g., by spoiled food or poisonous mushrooms).

Complaints
The symptoms differ, depending on the cause: Sudden intense stomach pain accompanied by general weakness, headache, feeling of fullness, nausea and perhaps vomiting, possibly bad breath, coated tongue, fever. Usually these symptoms disappear spontaneously in the course of a day.

Causes
— Abuse of alcohol
— Medications that irritate the gastric mucosa (e.g., painkillers, overdoses of heart preparations containing digoxin, corticosteroids, antibiotics, or c a n c e r medications)
— Acid or alkali burns
— X rays used in radiation therapy
— Foods spoiled by the toxin of the Clostridium botulinum bacteria, which grow in spoiled meat, sausage, canned vegetables, etc. Botulism is extremely

dangerous and may begin with paralysis of the eye muscles (double vision), difficulty swallowing, nausea, and cold sweat, followed by intestinal paralysis and constipation.

—Viral infections.

— Spoiled or poisonous mushrooms usually cause temporary diarrhea, sometimes with vomiting.

Who's at Risk

Those who abuse alcohol or can identify with any other causes listed above are at increased risk.

Possible Aftereffects and Complications

Damaged gastric mucosa may bleed, causing the patient to vomit blood or have a dark-colored stool. *This can be life-threatening. Get medical help at once.*

— Only a few species of poisonous mushrooms are dangerous. E.g.,, the *Gyromitra* interfere with the nervous system and can cause seizures, abdominal pain, nausea, vomiting, liver and kidney failure, weakness, and death in 15 to 40 percent of cases. The *Amanitas* can cause liver damage and death in up to 60 percent of cases.

— Untreated botulism is fatal within a week.

Prevention

—Avoid excess alcohol (see Alcohol, p. 756) and medications that can damage the stomach.

—Throw spoiled food away.

— Never leave cleansers and cleaning fluids where children can reach them.

— If you have collected mushrooms and are not sure of the species, let an expert check them. You should eat fresh mushrooms within 30 hours.

When to Seek Medical Advice

First aid for poisoning: see p. 708. Go to a hospital if you suspect botulism.

Go to a doctor immediately if you have bloody vomit or stool.

You should also get medical help if you do not know the cause of the symptoms, or if you suspect poisoning.

Self-Help

Symptoms of gastritis usually disappear on their own after a day or two in bed, during which the patient eats nothing. The stomach pain can be eased by a warm

Soothing Stomach Teas

Slowly drink freshly prepared warm herbal teas between meals three to four times daily.

Peppermint Tea
Pour 1 cup hot water over 1 tablespoon peppermint leaves, steep for 5 minutes, then strain leaves.

Chamomile Tea
Pour 1 cup boiling water over 1 tablespoon chamomile flowers, steep for 10 minutes, then strain.

Yarrow Tea
Use 2 teaspoons of yarrow tea, prepare as you would for chamomile tea.

Stimulating Stomach Teas
Drink these teas half an hour before meals, to stimulate secretion of stomach juices. They taste spicy to bitter.
Possible side effects: occasionally may cause headaches in people who are sensitive to bitter substances.

Centaury Herb Tea
Pour 1 cup boiling hot water over 1 to 2 teaspoons of centaury herb, steep for 15 minutes, then strain.

Stomach Tea Blend
Pour 1 cup boiling hot water over 2 teaspoons of tea blend, steep for 10 to 15 minutes, then strain. Blend consists of: 1 ounce centaury, 1 ounce wormwood, $\frac{2}{3}$ ounce gentian root, $\frac{2}{3}$ ounce bitter-Seville orange peel, and $\frac{1}{3}$ ounce cinnamon.
Warning: Don't use if you have stomach or peptic ulcers.

compress, a hot water bottle, or black, peppermint or chamomile tea (see Nervous Stomach, p. 386).

Treatment

Treatment is normally not required unless there is bleeding. In this case, an endoscopy will determine its source. If symptoms are caused by medications you absolutely need to take, consult your health-care provider about ways your stomach might be spared.

Medications

— Hycosamine (Bentyl) and dicyclomine (Levsin) can be given for acute stomach cramps, either by injection or orally. Most antispasmodics contain a number of active ingredients and carry a high risk of side effects.

— Chronic vomiting in adults can be relieved by metoclopramide (Reglan) or cisapride (Propulsid).
— Herbal remedies and other alternatives are not effective.

CHRONIC GASTRITIS

Complaints
Often there are no symptoms, but sometimes pain, pressure, or a bloated feeling after meals are symptoms of chronic gastritis.

Causes
The gastric mucosa becomes inflamed and atrophies, sometimes completely. It is suspected that the causes are
— Infection by *Helicobacter pylori* bacteria. This is detected by a gastroscopy and biopsy (see p. 652).
— Age-related factors, influenced by individual circumstances.
— Changes in blood supply to the gastric mucosa.
— Bile reflux after a stomach operation.

Who's at Risk
Half of all people are infected with *Helicobacter pylori* bacteria. The risk of atrophy of the gastric mucosa increases with age.

Possible Aftereffects and Complications
The most advanced stage of chronic gastritis, which is rare, is called atrophic gastritis and can lead to iron deficiency and pernicious anemia (vitamin B^{12} deficiency). It also increases the risk of cancer. Therefore, people in whom atrophy of the gastric mucosa has been diagnosed should have an endoscopic and histological exam every year.

Prevention
Avoid alcohol (see p. 756), extremely cold or hot drinks, hot spices, and medications that irritate the stomach.

When to Seek Medical Advice
Seek help if symptoms appear. Often chronic gastritis has no symptoms and is discovered in the course of an endoscopic exam for some other problem; in this case, no treatment is needed.

Self-Help
Not possible.

Treatment
If a *Helicobacter pylori* infection with ulcers is detected, proton-pump inhibitors (see p. 391), combined with antibiotics, can heal the inflammation in a few days and eliminate the bacteria.

Regeneration of the mucosa cannot be hastened. Antacids (see p. 391) can help treat secondary symptoms. If there is a deficiency of iron or vitamin B^{12}, supplements should be taken.

STOMACH AND DUODENAL ULCERS
An *ulcer* is a defect in the mucous membrane of the stomach or duodenum. It may penetrate the muscular wall, bleed, or perforate the wall. Ulcers are common.

Complaints
Signs of a stomach ulcer are pressure and a bloated feeling in the region of the stomach immediately after a meal.

The sign of a duodenal ulcer is pain on an empty stomach. The pain is extremely sharp, often between the navel and the middle of the curve of the rib, and is usually felt 2 hours after a meal or at night. It is often accompanied by vomiting.

Both types of ulcer cause a loss of appetite. One person in three who have ulcers will experience a burning sensation in the pit of the stomach and symptoms resembling those of a nervous stomach. Half of all ulcers produce no symptoms. Therefore, bleeding in the stomach and perforation can happen without forewarning. If they do, medical treatment should be sought immediately.

Seek Immediate Medical Treatment for
Stomach bleeding: nausea, vomiting blood and bloody, black stools with a peculiar smell. If the quantity of blood lost is large, the patient can rapidly go into shock.
Stomach perforation: knifelike pains in the belly, profuse sweating, rapid pulse. After about 6 hours, the patient goes into shock.

Causes
— Ninety percent of all ulcer patients are infected with *Helicobacter pylori*.
— It seems that persons with a genetic predisposition to ulcers form them in reaction to stress at work or in relationships, hectic lifestyles, nicotine, and alcohol.
— Pain medications containing acetylsalicylic acid (aspirin) promote the formation and retard the healing of ulcers. Other medications that promote ulcers include corticosteroids (see p. 665), some preparations for bronchitis, asthma, vomiting, infections (antibiotics), and high blood pressure; some blood thinners, and some medications for allergies, diabetes, circulatory disease, and some antifungals.
— Severe accidental injuries or operations may start ulcers within a few hours (stress ulcers).

Who's at Risk
Two people out of every hundred have ulcers at some time in their lives. The risk of disease increases in the presence of
— Irregular meals.
— Shift or assembly-line work, hard or stressful work, work in chemical plants, the metal and transportation industries or handling of toxic or hazardous substances.
— Smoking increases the risk that a new ulcer will form after healing.,

Possible Aftereffects and Complications
— Scars may cause the outlet of the stomach to become narrowed (stenosis), leading to bloated feelings, loss of appetite, and extensive weight loss.
— An untreated ulcer can perforate the stomach wall and bleed. This is life-threatening and requires immediate surgery.
— Repeated stomach ulcers increase the risk of stomach cancer.

Prevention
— Do not take pain medications except when medically prescribed.
— Consume alcohol, coffee, tea, nicotine, and citrus fruits sparingly.
— If possible, avoid stress, anxiety and conflicts.

When to Seek Medical Advice
If vague pains in the upper belly, and other symptoms, occur repeatedly.

Self-Help
— Stop smoking (see p. 755)
— Avoid alcohol.
— Avoid medications that damage the stomach (see above) if possible. Keeping a diary of symptoms can help you keep track of the effects and side effects of medications.
— Stomach pains can be relieved by chamomile, balm mint, or peppermint teas (see p. 388).
— Warm, moist compresses and bindings where symptoms are felt (see Compresses, p. 692) help moderate the pain.
— Acupressure (see p. 680) also eases pain.
— Eat what agrees with you, and avoid foods that you have found do not sit well. A diet consisting of a variety of nutritionally sound foods is an advantage (see Nutrition, p. 722). If you have a stomach ulcer, you may continue to consume the usual three meals a day. For duodenal ulcers, divide meals into several smaller portions and avoid eating in the late evening.
— Do some thinking about your life situation, and make changes where appropriate. Avoid anger, anxiety, and excitement. Learning relaxation techniques (see p. 693) can be the first step; behavioral therapy (see p. 799) or treatment in a psychosomatic clinic are useful supplements.

Treatment with Medications
More than a third of ulcers heal spontaneously.

All treatments have two goals: To heal the ulcer and to prevent recurrence.

Acid-inhibiting medications (H^2-receptor blockers) rapidly relieve pain; in nine of ten cases, they allow the ulcer to heal within 8 weeks at most. When they are taken over the long term, they can prevent recurrence of the ulcer. All H^2-blockers are equally effective.

Proton pump inhibitors, like omeprazole, are considered reserve medications for short-term, acute treatment but can be risky over the long term.

If acid-inhibiting medications cannot be taken because of their side effects, preparations including sucralfate, which protect the mucous membranes, are a good alternative. These are taken in the morning and evening, half an hour before a meal.

Medications that inhibit the formation of gastrin, can also help.

Antacids are effective at relieving pain and healing the ulcer, but not at preventing recurrence. These are taken three times a day, between meals. More than fifty different combinations have been tested; of these, those which contain aluminum and magnesium have the fewest side effects.

If the ulcer is caused by infection with *Helicobacter pylori*, the most rapid healing is obtained with bismuth medications combined with antibiotics like tetracycline, clarithromycin, and metronidazole and proton-pump inhibitors.

If the bacteria are successfully eradicated, there are hardly ever any recurrences.

Treatment by Surgery

Modern medication treatment is so successful that surgery is rarely needed.

— If the ulcer bleeds or perforates, or if it is a stress ulcer, an operation is usually needed.
— An operation is needed if ulcers recur in spite of efforts to control them by medications and regular application of relaxation techniques.
— If a stomach ulcer is not completely healed within 3 months, surgery should be considered to rule out any suspicion of cancer.

There are several surgical techniques:

— Removal of part of the stomach (partial resection). The particular name of the procedure will indicate how much of the stomach is removed, and how the remainder is connected to the duodenum. These operations carry a number of risks: Diarrhea, vomiting and diarrhea shortly after eating, loss of weight, reflux and degeneration of the gastric mucosa (this is frequent after the Billroth II method).
— Cutting the vagus nerve (vagotomy). In selective vagotomy, only those nerve branches are cut which control production of stomach acid. This is considered the best method for treating duodenal ulcers and stomach ulcers near the pyloric valve.

After the Operation

It will take a while before the patient can resume normal life. This time can be put to good use by learning relaxation techniques (see p. 693). In principle, recovering surgery patients can eat and drink anything that appeals to them except alcohol, which should either be avoided or drunk in strict moderation.

After a vagotomy, there may be difficulty swallowing and a feeling of fullness; but these symptoms disappear spontaneously after a while.

After a partial resection, it is helpful to eat small portions several times a day.

STOMACH CANCER

(see also Cancer, p. 470).

Complaints

During its long initial phase, stomach cancer remains confined to the gastric mucosa, but then suddenly begins to grow rapidly. If there are any symptoms, they resemble those of a nervous stomach. The only signal unique to cancer is a distaste for meat. The sensations of pressure and bloating may become more intense; loss of appetite and rapid weight loss occur later. The patient may vomit dark blood, or pass a bloody, dark stool with a peculiar odor—as in the case of a bleeding ulcer.

Causes

The causes are not fully known. It is known, however, that smoking and alcohol abuse increase the risk of stomach cancer.

Recommended Antacids:
Aluminum hydroxide (Alternagel, Amphojel)
Aluminum and magnesium hydroxide (Maalox, Mylanta)
Calcium carbonate (Tums)
Magaldrate (Riopan)

Recommended Acid Inhibitors (H$_2$ Blockers):
Cimetidine (Tagamet)
Famotidine (Pepcid)
Nizatidine (Axid)
Ranitidine (Zantac)

Recommended Proton Pump Inhibitors:
Lansoprazole (Prevacid)
Omeprazole (Prilosec)

Some Other Antiulcer Medications:
Cisapride (Propulsid)
Misoprostol (Cytotec)
Sucralfate (Carafate)

Nitrosomines, used in smoked foods, and toxins formed in burning fats (polycyclic aromatic hydrocarbons) can initiate stomach cancer. Aflatoxins, which are secreted by molds into spoiled foods, are also potent carcinogens. It is likely that Helicobacter bacteria also contribute.

Who's at Risk

Stomach cancer is one of the most common cancers. It usually appears after age 40. The risk is increased by
— Hereditary tendencies
— Stress
— Degeneration of the gastric mucosa (atrophic gastritis)
— Stomach ulcers

Possible Aftereffects and Complications

If stomach cancer is detected early and removed promptly, the patient's life expectancy is not decreased. However, if the tumor is removed only at an advanced stage, the chances of survival are dramatically reduced. Unfortunately, stomach cancer is often not recognized and surgery is performed too late.

Prevention

— Don't smoke, and limit your consumption of alcohol (see p. 756).
— Avoid obesity and limit your consumption of meat, poultry, and fatty foods (see Nutrition, p. 722).
— Avoid smoked, preserved, and grilled meat; these are "cancer suspects." When frying foods, do not let the oil get smoking hot.
— Do not eat any food on which you see mold, except for the molds used to make cheese. Molds on nuts are hard to see. Store nuts in the refrigerator.

When to Seek Medical Advice

— If the symptoms of a nervous stomach last longer than 4 weeks, you should have an endoscopic examination, possibly including a biopsy (see Gastroscopy, p. 652).
— If you have atrophic gastritis or a stomach ulcer, regular endoscopic checkups are necessary.

Self-Help

Do things you like to do. Anything pleasant and beneficial will improve your quality of life and strengthen your resistance to disease.

Treatment

Immediate surgery is necessary. Depending on the size of the tumor, a larger or smaller section of the stomach will be removed; the remaining part is then connected to the small intestine. This is a major operation, but even with the entire stomach removed, a normal life is still possible afterwards. It may be months before small amounts of normal foods can be eaten and digested, however. If your diet during the recuperation period is lacking in vitamins, minerals, or other nutrients, these can be supplied as medications.

After the operation, smoking, alcohol, and other stimulants are forbidden (see Stomach Surgery, p. 391).

Patients should discuss how to reestablish a bearable everyday life with the treatment team, and design a program to relieve symptoms. Psychotherapy can support the healing process, and self-help groups can help the patient come to terms with the disease. Alternative medication may improve the patient's outlook, but there is no evidence that it inhibits tumor growth.

Liver, Gallbladder, Pancreas

The largest part of the liver sits in the upper right section of the abdomen, in front of the stomach. The left lobe is behind it, and the pancreas sits behind that. The liver has various functions.
— Digestion: The liver produces up to a quart of bile per day, which is stored in the gall bladder and passes through the bile duct into the duodenum. Bile acids help to break down fats in food, so that, along with fat-soluble vitamins, they can be absorbed by the intestinal mucosa.
— Circulation: Before birth, red and white blood cells are produced in the liver. During our entire lives, the liver is the site where old red blood cells are broken down and the iron in them is stored.
— Metabolism: The liver "checks" the blood for toxins and detoxifies it. It also absorbs digested nutrients from the blood and uses them to synthesize the body's proteins. It stores sugar and releases it as needed to the rest of the body. Urea, the product of protein decomposition, is transported by the blood to the kidneys, where it is excreted.
— Hormone balance: The liver synthesizes the starting materials for sex hormones and the body's fats.

An organ with so many vital functions is essential to life. For this reason, the liver has an astonishing capacity to regenerate. Even if two thirds of it are removed, the remainder, if healthy, can take over the functions of the entire organ. If the liver is completely destroyed, the only hope is a liver transplant—an extremely difficult operation.

The pancreas, like the liver, produces digestive juice containing enzymes that empty into the duodenum through a duct it usually shares with the gallbladder. For the function of the pancreas as an endocrine gland, see Diabetes, p. 483.

JAUNDICE

Jaundice is not a disease, but an indication of various diseases, usually of the liver or the bile. The skin, mucous membranes, and whites of the eyes become yellowish in color, and the patient usually suffers severe itching.

The shade of yellow is an indicator of the underlying illness:
— Reddish yellow indicates liver damage (see Hepatitis, p. 395; Cirrhosis of the Liver, p. 396).
— Greenish yellow indicates biliary congestion (see Gallstones, p. 398; Liver Cancer, p. 397).

LIVER FAILURE

Complaints

When the liver is damaged by alcohol or medications, no symptoms appear for a long time; eventually jaundice develops (see above).

After consumption of poisonous mushrooms, the signs of jaundice appear suddenly; but in the case of deadly *Amanitas*, they appear no sooner than 24 hours after ingestion.

Who's at Risk

Poisoning is the most common disease of the body's "detox center," the liver.

Causes

Alcohol (see Cirrhosis of the Liver, p. 396)

Medications

Medications are an important cause of liver disease. If doses are too high, medications may be directly poi-

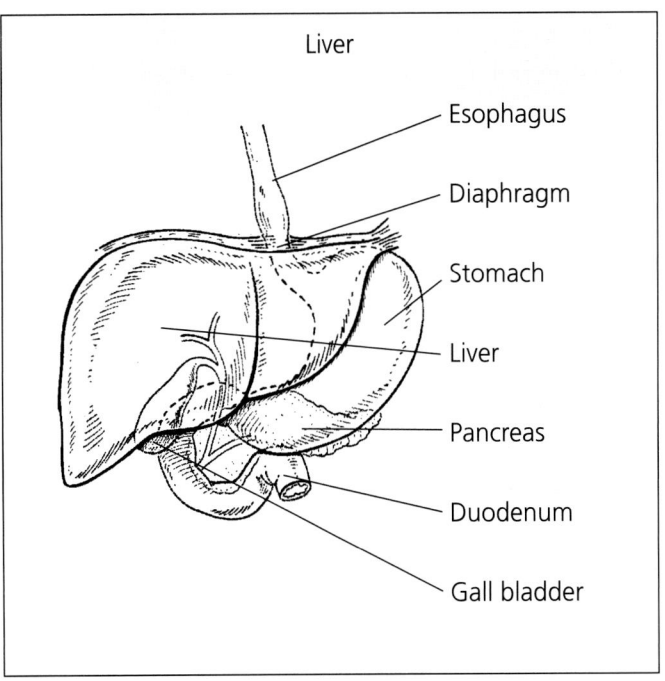

sonous; however, someone with a sensitivity to the medication can suffer liver damage independently of the dose. Painkillers (simple analgesics) cause the most liver damage.
— Painkillers: Acetaminophen in high doses can lead to acute or chronic liver damage.
— Antipsychotics (phenothiazines), antidepressants (tricyclic antidepressants).
— Rheumatism medications (phenylbutazone) and certain antibacterial agents (erythromycin) can cause damage that resembles cirrhosis, but can heal again completely.
— Birth control pills may cause benign liver tumors and thus lead to biliary congestion.
— General anesthetics (halothane, enfluran) may, after repeated use, cause severe liver inflammation several days after application. In some cases, the inflammation is fatal.
— The tuberculosis medication isoniazid may cause a clinical picture similar to hepatitis even a year after use.

Some medications can interfere with liver function. These include: acetylsalicylic acid (aspirin), tetracycline, sulfonamides and other antibiotics, heartbeat stabilizers (quinidine), sedatives (chloral hydrate), diuretics, heart-circulation medications (calcium channel blockers), medications for gout (allopurinol) and epilepsy (valproic acid), and cancer medications.

Toxins

Carbon tetrachloride (used in the plastics and metal industries, and in dry cleaning) can damage or destroy liver tissue.

The toxin from *Amanita* mushrooms also causes liver function to break down, and thus leads to death.

Prevention

Drink only moderate amounts of alcohol.

Use medications only when symptoms cannot be eased in any other way, or when they are prescribed.

Follow protective regulations when working with toxic substances (see Health in the Workplace, p. 789).

Let an expert examine mushrooms you have gathered, or else eat them only if you are completely certain about the species.

When to Seek Medical Advice

Go to a hospital immediately if signs of jaundice appear (see p. 393).

Self-Help

Not possible.

Treatment

Treatment as for fatty liver (see below) can reverse most of the damage caused by acute alcohol or medication poisoning. If poisoning is chronic, the liver will remain damaged. In cases of poisoning by other substances, chances of survival depend on intensive medical intervention. In *Amanita* poisoning, penicillin and silibinin may be helpful.

FATTY LIVER

Complaints

Although a fatty liver is always enlarged, its symptoms are otherwise barely noticeable. At times, one feels full or has mild nausea. Occasionally, pain might be felt under the ribs on the right side.

Causes

Fatty infiltration of the liver has nothing to do with consumption of fatty foods. The causes of this disease are

— Alcoholism (see p. 205)
— Poisoning by any of a large number of chemicals and medications
— Diabetes
— A few rare, hereditary diseases of fat metabolism
— Pregnancy
— A monotonous diet rich in carbohydrates and low in fats
— Obesity

Consumption of large amounts of alcohol over a long period of time interferes with the liver's ability to metabolize fats. It can no longer break them down, and stores them in its cells instead.

Who's at Risk

The risk of this disease is increased by frequent consumption of large amounts of alcohol and by an unbalanced diet rich in carbohydrates.

Possible Aftereffects and Complications

Fatty liver is usually harmless, and may spontaneously revert to normal. The liver can be further damaged, however, if the cause is poisoning. Acute forms of infiltration can be life-threatening in the presence of excess alcohol.

Prevention

Switch to a more healthful lifestyle, including a balanced diet, little alcohol, and use of medications only when necessary. Avoid contact with chemicals. Participate in a sport.

When to Seek Medical Advice

Seek help if you suspect this disease is present.

Self-Help

Reduce the amount of carbohydrates you consume by half. Strict avoidance of alcohol may permit the fatty liver to heal completely.

These measures can be supported by warm compresses and massage (see p. 686).

Treatment

Treatment with medications is not necessary, except in cases of hereditary defects of fat metabolism.

HEPATITIS

Complaints

The early warning signal of hepatitis is pain under the ribs on the right side.

Hepatitis begins like the flu: Fatigue, headache, sometimes pain in the joints, frequently nausea and vomiting, and a distaste for fat, meat, alcohol, and nicotine. Constipation, diarrhea, and flatulence follow. Because the liver becomes somewhat enlarged, there are pains under the right rib cage. There is often a mild fever and an itching rash resembling bee stings.

In the second phase of the disease, the skin and eyes acquire a reddish-yellow cast, and urine becomes dark. The fever subsides; stool becomes pale. Sometimes the lymph nodes swell, and the spleen becomes enlarged. The pulse may become slower, and the blood pressure elevated. Usually jaundice becomes more pronounced in the first 3 weeks.

Viral infections often produce no symptoms, and for this reason the risk of contagion is high.

Causes

Viruses, bacteria, parasites, medications. However, the causes are often unknown.

Infection with hepatitis viruses: The viruses known to cause hepatitis are denoted by the letters A, B, C, D, E, F, and G. In some cases, these viruses take a long time to become established and cause disease:

Type A (travel or HAV hepatitis) from about 6 to 50 days.

Type B (HBV hepatitis) up to 6 months.

Types C, D, and other viruses are not yet sufficiently well known.

Other viruses, including mumps virus, Epstein Barr virus of mononucleosis, herpes simplex, and varicella all can cause hepatitis.

There are two main routes of infection.

Hepatitis A is transmitted by oral contact with water, beverages, or food, especially seafoods, contaminated by infected urine or feces; or by close contact with infected individuals (by way of eating utensils, dishes, toilets). Flies can also transmit the pathogens.

Hepatitis B and C are transmitted through the blood. Microscopically small openings in skin are sufficient to allow entry of the viruses in infected saliva, urine, feces, vaginal secretions, semen, blood or blood plasma. In spite of this, infection through ordinary contact or sex is rare. Medical or dental procedures are much more effective routes of infection; similarly, nonsterile needles used in tattooing or acupuncture, or instruments used for manicures and pedicures, may transmit these viruses. Blood products were formerly the main route for hepatitis C infections, but they are now routinely tested for the presence of these viruses.

People who have been infected can infect others before they notice any symptoms. Infectious particles may still be present in the blood for as long as 3 months after recovery.

Who's at Risk

Hepatitis A: The risk increases for travelers (see Immunization, p. 669)

Hepatitis B: Drug addicts, prostitutes and dialysis patients are at relatively high risk. People who frequently receive transfusions and blood products (e.g., hemophiliacs) are no longer at such high risk, since these products are now screened for hepatitis B viruses. The risk is high for medical personnel who must handle blood, blood products, or stool samples, and for the personnel in dialysis and cancer units.

Because more and more people carry the hepatitis B virus, the risk of infection for sexually active persons is increasing (see Immunization, p. 667). In Southeast Asia, sub-Saharan Africa and in the Amazon region, hepatitis B is widespread.

Possible Aftereffects and Complications

Acute hepatitis: In rare cases, an acute case of hepatitis can become dramatically worse; extreme sleepiness is followed by confusion, then loss of consciousness. Death follows in a few days. The causes are not yet known. Alcoholics are more frequently affected.

Chronic hepatitis: In 10 to 15 percent of patients, HBV hepatitis becomes chronic. For the HCV form, four out of five cases become chronic. Hepatitis A never becomes chronic.

Chronic hepatitis often progresses without jaundice, and may continue for years. If it is caused by medication, it may disappear as soon as the offending medication is no longer taken. The forms caused by HBV and HCV may progress to cirrhosis of the liver (see p. 396) or liver cancer. The aggressive form of chronic hepatitis, in which jaundice breaks out repeatedly and rarely heals, is due to defects in the immune system. This form usually leads to liver failure and/or cirrhosis.

Prevention

Hepatitis A: Cleanliness in handling food and beverages, and bodily hygiene (see Travel, p. 717). This is especially important on trips to countries in which standards of hygiene are low. An immunization against hepatitis A is available (see p. 675).

Hepatitis B: An immunization is available, and is highly recommended for all medical personnel (see p. 675).

Hepatitis B and C: Medical procedures and transfusions should be undertaken only when necessary; it may be advisable to donate one's own blood for later use if an operation is planned. Condoms protect against infection during sexual intercourse. Avoid tattooing and do not inject drugs.

When to Seek Medical Advice

Seek help if your general health is impaired and you notice a yellow coloration of urine, skin, and eyes. Suspected hepatitis must be confirmed by a blood test. Even in the early stages, the various types of hepatitis can be distinguished.

Self-Help

As soon as the disease is recognized, avoid intimate contact with others to prevent transmission. Extreme cleanliness is important, since urine, feces, saliva, and blood can transmit the disease. Washcloths, towels, and bed linens should be boiled. If you are living with a sexual partner who has hepatitis B in his or her blood, you must reconcile yourself to the danger of infection during intercourse, which is greater than that of AIDS transmission. You should either use condoms for the rest of your life, or be immunized and have your antibody titer checked regularly to make sure you are still protected. Remember your booster shots on time if needed!

Treatment

Usually the acute stage passes spontaneously after 4 to 6 weeks. Bed rest is not necessary. Allow yourself to rest until the fever has subsided and your doctor has determined that your blood values have improved; then you may return to work.

In 9 out of 10 cases, HBV hepatitis heals completely within 3 to 4 months. Hepatitis A patients always recover without aftereffects. Hepatitis B and C can be treated with interferons.

Diet

The lack of appetite in the early stages of the disease passes after a few days, and a special diet is not necessary. Contrary to what was formerly thought, the second phase of the disease is shortened by foods rich in fat and protein.

CIRRHOSIS OF THE LIVER

Complaints

People suffering from cirrhosis of the liver frequently look and feel fine most of the time, with only occasional spells of weakness, anemia, and a feeling of illness.

However, symptoms may include
— Tingling and numbness in feet and fingers, and tiny blood vessels (spider veins) showing on the skin.
— Facial pallor, with a slightly dirty look.
— Loss of appetite and weight.
— Men may develop breasts. This happens because the liver is no longer able to break down the small quantities of female sex hormones normally produced by the male body, and their concentrations increase. The testes shrivel, and both sex drive and potency decrease.
— In the advanced stage of the disease, underarm and pubic hair fall out.

In the early stages of the disease, the liver is enlarged (see Fatty Liver, p. 394), but later it may atrophy.

Symptoms usually do not appear until after age 30, and severe damage not until after age 40, if the liver has suffered for a very long time.

Causes

— Years of alcohol abuse, in which case jaundice is often present. Alcohol can also intensify cirrhosis caused by other agents.
— Anesthetics, cleaning fluids, and medications.
— A complication of hepatitis B or C, congestive heart failure, or an inflammation of the bile ducts.
— Hereditary diseases of iron, copper or fat metabolism.

Who's at Risk

One-half to one-third of all men who consume a daily average of 2 to 3½ ounces of pure alcohol for 20 years or more will develop cirrhosis of the liver. This corresponds to 4 to 7 bottles of beer, 1 bottle of wine, or a fifth to a pint of distilled liquor a day. The risk for women is the same, only for them the damage threshold is lower: 1 to 1½ ounces of alcohol daily.

Alcoholics believe they can tolerate large amounts of alcohol. This belief is just as mistaken as that they are less sensitive to sedatives and antibiotics. Such medications can actually damage their livers still further.

Possible Aftereffects and Complications

— Bleeding from the esophagus. Congestion in the portal vein leads to the formation of varicose veins in the esophagus (esophageal varices), which may burst if subjected to too much pressure. Bleeding from the esophagus (bright red vomit) is an emergency, and the esophageal varices must immediately be cauterized in a hospital. Thirty to 50 percent of those with cirrhosis die of variceal bleeding with subsequent collapse of all liver functions (liver coma).
— Fluid in the abdomen (ascites) collects because of congestion in the liver circulation and disturbances in the body's fluid balance. The symptoms are swelling of the belly, difficulty breathing, and pressure pains.
— Altered states of consciousness and anxiety (delirium tremens)
— Hemorrhoids (see p. 417)
— Liver cancer (see below)

If untreated, cirrhosis of the liver is fatal. The proximate cause of death is liver coma, severe variceal bleeding or kidney failure.

Prevention

A healthy lifestyle is the best way of preventing cirrhosis of the liver: little alcohol, medications only when absolutely necessary, avoidance of contact with chemicals.

When to Seek Medical Advice

Seek help at the first signs of liver disease.

Blood tests will determine the cause and extent of liver damage. If you wish to have the condition of your liver tested, you can have liver enzymes determined (see GOT, GPT, and GGT, p. 642, in the Diagnostic Tests/Procedures section).

Self-Help

If you are at risk, abstain completely from alcohol. A diet low in fat but rich in vitamins and other nutrients will support recovery of the liver.

Treatment

Liver cells that have died are gone forever. However, if the disease is recognized before the destructive process has begun, and if the patient immediately stops drinking any alcohol, the liver can regenerate.

Cirrhosis caused by hepatitis B or C can be treated with interferon. Otherwise, only the secondary complaints can be treated: A mild liver coma can be helped by intravenous administration of nutrients, and mild variceal bleeding can be halted by surgery. Accumulation of ascites and electrolyte imbalances are treated with diuretics (see High Blood Pressure, p. 321).

Progressive cirrhosis is life-threatening. The remedy of last resort is a liver transplant, but this is a complicated operation and is done in only a few places. Its success depends on the cause of the disease.

LIVER CANCER

(see also Cancer, p. 470)

Complaints

Liver cancer has few typical symptoms. Possible signs include loss of weight, loss of appetite, pains in the upper right part of the abdomen, deterioration of the general condition, and low-grade fever. The liver feels hard and enlarged and hurts when pressed.

Causes

— Usually, a complication of cirrhosis of the liver
— Aflatoxin, the metabolic product of a mold found in some kinds of spoiled food
— A complication of hepatitis B or C
— Rarely, the malignant transformation of a benign liver tumor formed in response to birth control pills

Who's at Risk

Liver cancer is rare in industrially developed countries; more common in Africa and Southeast Asia. Chronic hepatitis B increases the risk by a hundredfold.

Possible Aftereffects and Complications

Because liver cancer is often discovered late, it is usually fatal within a few months of diagnosis. In the rare case of a specific liver carcinoma, which occurs in younger people who have not previously suffered a liver disease, the chance of survival is better.

Prevention

Only a few of the factors that cause liver cancer can be avoided by preventive measures. Don't eat moldy food; avoid working with polyvinyl chloride, protect yourself from hepatitis B by using a condom during sexual intercourse or, if you are especially at risk, by immunization.

When to Seek Medical Advice

Seek help if you suspect you have a liver disease.

Cancer is diagnosed with the help of ultrasound, computer tomography, MRI, angiography, and a liver biopsy (see Diagnostic Tests/Procedures, p. 635).

Self-Help

Not possible.

Treatment

Only rarely is liver cancer discovered while it is still small and contained enough to be removed surgically. Radiation and cancer chemotherapy often do not improve the situation.

Liver transplants are usually not feasible for liver cancer.

Patients should discuss with their treatment team what measures are reasonable and necessary, and design a program to relieve symptoms. Anything that you enjoy and that contributed to your well-being will increase your quality of life and your resistance to the disease.

Psychotherapy may be a useful support measure. In particular, behavioral therapy can reduce stress and anxiety associated with cancer. Support groups can also be useful in helping one to come to terms with the illness. Alternative medicine may improve the patient's outlook, but has not been shown to inhibit tumor growth.

GALLSTONES

Complaints

Gallstones may be present for years without causing any symptoms. Only occasionally, often after a fatty meal, vague pains might be felt in the upper abdomen along with nausea, perhaps spreading into the back area.

Then, one day, there is a sudden severe colic: violent, almost unbearable cramps in the upper abdomen, possibly extending to the shoulder, together with vomiting, sweating, dizziness, and often fever and chills.

The colic may disappear spontaneously within 3 days, only to reappear suddenly, days or months later.

Causes

Metabolic disorders in the liver can lead to the formation of solid cholesterol or calcium stones in the bile. These may be as small as grains of sand, as large as gravel, or even larger. If the stones lodge in the duct leading from the gallbladder to the duodenum, or in the bile ducts, they cause colic.

The main causes of gallstones are overeating and overweight. Gallstones are
— Common in women who have had several pregnancies, use birth control pills
— Common in those with chronic inflammation of the gallbladder (see p. 400), diabetes (see p. 483) or cirrhosis of the liver (see p. 396)
— Less common after Crohn's Disease (see p. 412) and Ulcerative Colitis (see p. 411).

Who's at Risk

Gallstones are among the most common illnesses, affecting 20 percent of women and 10 percent of men. They usually do not occur before age 30, and half of those who have them never experience any symptoms. They are frequently discovered by chance during an X ray or ultrasound examination.

Possible Aftereffects and Complications

Each episode of colic increases the risk of complications. If gallstones lodge in the gallbladder or bile ducts, they may cause jaundice and/or
— Inflammation of the gallbladder and/or bile ducts (see p. 400)
— Suppuration (pus formation) in the gallbladder, possibly followed by perforation of the gallbladder

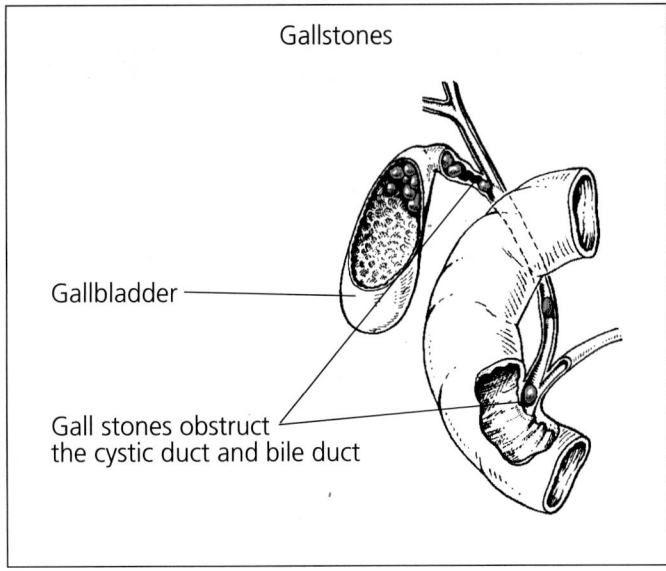

Gallstones

Gallbladder

Gall stones obstruct
the cystic duct and bile duct

and peritonitis (see p. 409)
— Biliary congestion with subsequent damage to the
 liver
— Pancreatic inflammation (see p. 400)
— Intestinal obstruction (see p. 407)
— Cancer of the gallbladder or bile ducts (see p. 400)

Prevention
Avoid obesity (see Body Weight, p. 727).

When to Seek Medical Advice
Seek help if you suffer repeated acute or chronic forms
of colic, high fever, and jaundice.

Self-Help
Chronic or acute pains can be eased by a hot-water
bottle, or a hot or cold compress, on the gallbladder
area (see Compresses, p. 692).

Sipping water will also help. An antispasmodic
suppository can help make the time spent waiting for
medical help more bearable.

Treatment
After an injection of painkiller, the cause of the colic
must be determined.

Ultrasound and cholecystography are the most
reliable means of locating gallstones (see p. 398).

Mineral water cures and hydropathic treatment can
ease inflammation caused by gallstones, but surgery is
the most reasonable treatment method to preclude the

need for emergency surgery in case of acute complications (see Gallbladder Inflammation, p. 400).

Surgery
Gallbladder Surgery: A gallbladder filled with stones
should be completely removed, especially if it is
inflamed and suppurated. The risks of gallbladder
surgery are lowest during symptom-free periods, so
surgeons usually wait 6 weeks after an acute attack of
colic. Surgery is usually performed laparoscopically.
Starting the day after the operation, the patient should
stand up for short periods and can drink liquids. By the
third day, he or she can tolerate soft foods and may go
home.

Bile Duct Surgery: If stones have formed in the bile ducts,
they can be removed by an operation that will keep the
ducts intact. In another method, an endoscope is inserted (see A Look Inside, p. 651) and used to widen
the opening of the bile duct (papillotomy). Stones are
then removed using a special instrument.

The symptoms and postsurgical advice are the same
as for a gallbladder removal. Sometimes new gallstones
form in the bile ducts, in which case another operation
is required.

Pulverization of Gallstones
Only in certain cases stones can be pulverized by ultrasound. This is easiest for stones in the gallbladder, and
more difficult if they are in the bile ducts. However, no
surgery is required for this procedure.

Diet for Gallstone Patients
A diet of cooked cereal, zwieback and tea is required
only in acute episodes. Limiting your fat intake will
not prevent further episodes of colic; you can eat anything that tastes good to you, even fried foods, and
drink small amounts of alcohol. (If fatty and fried foods
don't agree with you, however, cross them off your
menu.) Avoiding gas-producing foods like onions,
cabbage, etc. is a good idea.

Divide your daily food intake into five small portions so as to avoid large meals.

Any symptoms such as intestinal gas, nausea, a
full feeling, constipation or diarrhea are probably not
caused by the operation; only in 7 percent of postoperative gallbladder patients does the surgery cause
discomfort and problems such as scarring or damage
to nerves or blood vessels.

Medications

If gallstones are not over three quarters of an inch in diameter and do not contain calcium, they can be dissolved by medications containing bile acids. This treatment takes months, and should only be chosen if an operation is ruled out. It is not appropriate for patients who are overweight or pregnant, or have a liver or bile disease.

There are over 200 products on the market that claim to aid in liver and gallbladder protection or ease gallbladder pains, but their effectiveness in both areas has not been proven.

CHOLECYSTITIS (GALLBLADDER INFLAMMATION)

Complaints

Symptoms include the sudden onset of colic-like pains in the right side below the ribs, preceded by frequent vague pains in that area, and accompanied by fever, chills, vomiting, discolored stool, and temporary jaundice. The belly is hard and sensitive to pressure.

Causes

Inflammations of the gallbladder (cholecystitis) or inflammation of the bile ducts (cholangitis) are usually provoked by gallstones. Occasionally, inflammations, e.g., in the intestine, are responsible. Gallbladder inflammations without stones can also be the result of severe accidents, burns, and operations.

Who's at Risk

Anyone who has gallstones may experience repeated gallbladder inflammations.

Possible Aftereffects and Complications

— If a gallstone blocks the bile ducts during a gallbladder inflammation, the result can be jaundice, inflammation of the pancreas, chronic liver damage, or peritonitis.
— In the course of many years of repeated inflammations, gallbladder cancer may develop. Gallbladder cancers account for 5 percent of all cancerous tumors. They tend to metastasize, mainly to the liver. Gallbladder cancers are usually discovered late, and therefore only one third of patients survive.

Prevention

If the inflammation is caused by gallstones, it is a good idea to have them removed as a cancer-preventive measure.

When to Seek Medical Advice

Seek help if you have colic pains.

Self-Help

Not possible.

Treatment

An acute episode of gallbladder inflammation may subside on its own after two to three days, and disappear within a week. If there is no particular risk from another disease that would contraindicate surgery, the gallbladder should be removed as soon as possible. The operation is simple (see Gallstones, p. 398). It is now also possible to remove the gallbladder laparoscopically, inserting instruments through two small incisions in the abdomen. After a few days in the hospital and a few weeks of recovery, one can lead a normal life again. For questions concerning diet, see Gallstones, p. 398.

The colic usually does not recur after surgery. If it does, small gallstones in the bile duct may have been overlooked, or the outlet of the bile duct may not be functioning properly. In these cases, a second operation is needed. An endoscope is used to cut into the outlet so that the stones can be removed (see A Look Inside, p. 651).

PANCREATITIS (PANCREAS INFLAMMATION)

Complaints

An acute pancreatic inflammation is life-threatening. Alarm signals include
— Pain in the middle of the upper abdomen, occasionally gradual but usually sudden. Pain may radiate to both sides and the back, or to the lower abdomen. Anxiety and fear of death frequently accompany the pain. In 20 percent of cases, the abdominal surface is hard.
— Usually, vomiting of large amounts of bilious gastric juice.
— In the first days, fever up to 103°F.
— In severe cases, a flushed face, racing pulse, and rapid

breathing.

— A life-threatening state of shock may soon follow: Facial pallor, cold sweat, loss of blood pressure, tachycardia, respiratory distress.

A chronic inflammation may continue for years and include the pains described above—usually strongest after eating or drinking alcohol, or when lying down— or no pain may be present. Stools may be fatty and massive; the pancreatic tissue is destroyed by the constant inflammation.

Causes

— Existing inflammations (e.g., gallstones or duodenal disorders), or stones in the pancreatic ducts. When these ducts are blocked, digestive enzymes in pancreatic secretions destroy the pancreatic tissue itself.
— Chronic alcohol abuse (see Alcohol, p. 756)
— Abdominal surgery
— Other possible causes: disorders in fat metabolism; hyperthyroidism; vitamin D overdoses; hormone supplements; probably autoimmune diseases

Who's at Risk

If any of the aforementioned causes apply to you, you are at increased risk.

Possible Aftereffects and Complications

Although acute inflammations are life-threatening, 95 percent of patients with mild inflammations survive them. Severe inflammations, however, are fatal in 20 percent of cases.

Chronic inflammations may produce lifelong diabetes (see p. 483) and inadequate digestion with deficiency symptoms (see Pancreatic Insufficiency, see below). The risk of acquiring pancreatic cancer is elevated.

When to Seek Medical Advice

Seek help as soon as possible after alarm signals appear.

Self-Help

In acute inflammations, immediately stop eating and drinking.

In chronic inflammations, there is an absolute prohibition on alcohol.

Treatment of Acute Pancreatitis

Severe acute inflammations should be treated in an intensive care unit.

Patients with pancreatitis must be fed intravenously, as they cannot eat or drink until symptoms have eased— often for as long as 8 weeks. If vomiting continues, a tube in the stomach should be used to suck out gastric juice. Severe pains can be managed by strong painkillers.

In some cases, surgery cannot be avoided. The pancreas must be partially or completely removed if there is no improvement after three days, if stones are blocking the release of pancreatic juices, or if there is an abscess. Patients whose entire pancreas has been removed must inject insulin from then on (see Diabetes, p. 483).

Treatment of Chronic Pancreatitis

Treatment begins with absolute abstinence from alcohol.

Because the digestion of fats depends on pancreatic enzymes, which are insufficiently produced during inflammations, plant and animal fats must be largely removed from the menu. They may be replaced by coconut oil, which does not require pancreatic enzymes for digestion.

The missing enzymes must also be taken as dietary supplements.

Pain from chronic pancreatitis is often severe and long-lasting. Because painkillers don't do the job completely, the danger of painkiller addiction is high (see Medication Misuse, p. 658).

If diabetes develops during chronic pancreatitis, insulin must be injected (see p. 483).

If pancreatitis recurs repeatedly although no more alcohol is consumed, and the patient's general condition does not improve, it may be necessary to remove the entire pancreas.

PANCREATIC INSUFFICIENCY

Complaints

Massive, fatty stools with a consistency of cooked cereal; general weakness.

Causes

A weakened pancreas secretes insufficient amounts of the enzymes needed to digest fats and proteins, which also enable absorption of fat-soluble vitamins from food. Pancreatic insufficiency is a result of chronic pancreatitis (see below) or pancreatic cancer (see p. 402).

Who's at Risk
This disease is rare.

Possible Aftereffects and Complications
Underweight conditions and vitamin deficiencies are the most common results of pancreatic insufficiency:
— Muscle atrophy because of lack of protein absorption
— Degeneration of solid bone because of vitamin D deficiency
— Night blindness because of vitamin A deficiency
— Slow or impaired clotting of blood because of vitamin K deficiency
— Skin changes because of vitamin E deficiency

Prevention/Self-Help
Not possible.

When to Seek Medical Advice
Seek help if the aforementioned symptoms appear.

Treatment
Treatment is the same as treatment for chronic pancreatitis (see p. 401).

Pancreatic Cancer
(see also Cancer, p. 470)

Complaints
Pancreatic cancer produces no symptoms until it is has reached a late stage. Symptoms differ depending on the location of the tumor. Tumors at the tip of the pancreas cause vomiting, loss of appetite, weight loss and gradually progressive, painless jaundice. Tumors in the body of the pancreas cause nagging pains in the upper abdomen, extending into the back, that worsen after meals or when the patient is lying down.

Causes
The only known cause is a pancreatic inflammation.

Who's at Risk
Pancreatic cancer usually occurs after age 60 and is not rare: it accounts for 3 percent of cancer fatalities. In 90 percent of patients, the cancer has metastasized by the time it is discovered, usually to the liver or lungs.

Possible Aftereffects and Complications
Two percent of those affected survive longer than 5 years.

Prevention
Not possible.

When to Seek Medical Advice
Pancreatic cancer is usually discovered during ultrasound examinations performed for some other reason. The diagnosis can be confirmed by computer tomography and biopsy (see Diagnostic Tests/Procedures, p. 635).

Self-Help
Not possible.

Treatment
If the tumor is restricted to the pancreas, the organ should be removed completely. This gives 10 percent of patients a chance of survival; however, they have now become diabetic and must inject insulin (see Diabetes, p. 483).

In all other cases, surgery is not possible. A combination of radiation and cancer chemotherapy (see p. 474) can prolong life.

Psychotherapy and self-help groups can support the patient's efforts to cope with the illness. Alternative medicine can improve the patient's outlook, but there is no evidence that it can stop growth of the tumor.

Intestines

No other bodily function is so variable and so dependent on external influences as the bowel movement. The composition and consistency of the stool depend on age, eating habits, mood, and social and cultural factors, as does the frequency with which the bowels are emptied. Some people have two or three movements a day, others only two or three a week. Some people hardly think about their digestion, others enjoy the process of relieving themselves, while still others repeatedly have problems with it.

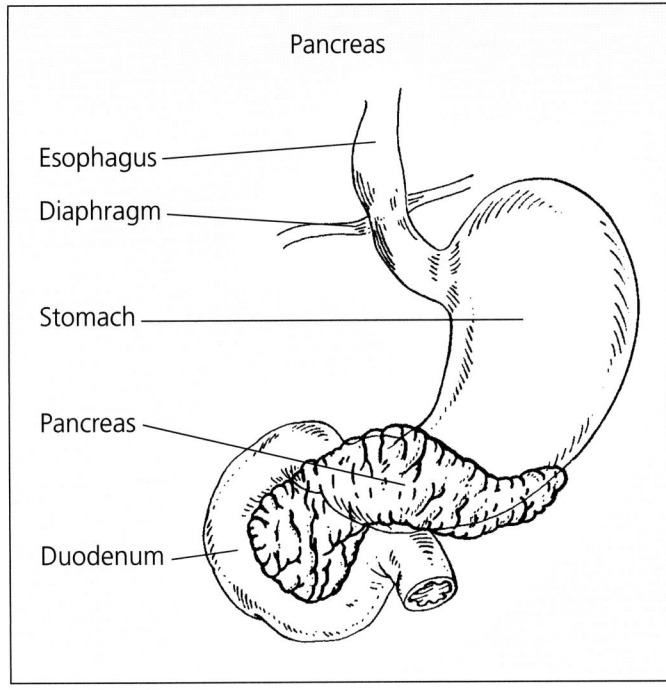

Pancreas

Esophagus

Diaphragm

Stomach

Pancreas

Duodenum

The intestinal wall has three layers:
— The smooth, outer peritoneal covering
— The muscle layer
— The inner layer, which consists of a folded mucous membrane

The intestine is suspended in the abdominal cavity by means of bands and folds of muscle leading from the peritoneum to the rear wall of the abdomen. The muscular motions (peristalsis) of the intestinal wall moves the food along.

The small intestine, 15 to 20 feet long, is the actual site of digestion; the intestinal villi on its inner surface absorb the nutrients. The large intestine withdraws water from the slurry of food remains. The undigested remains are passed on to the rectum, then eliminated through the anus.

IRRITABLE BOWEL SYNDROME

Complaints
Symptoms of irritable bowel syndrome include
— A vague belly ache whose nature and location aren't easy to describe
— An uncomfortably full feeling
— A hard, puffed-up belly, possibly with gurgling or passed gas
— Diarrhea alternating with constipation, or very frequent bowel movements

Causes
— If symptoms occur only occasionally, they are probably the body's normal reaction to certain types of food or psychosocial stress. If they recur repeatedly, you may be having difficulty coping with a stressful situation (see Health and Well-Being, p. 182).
— A food allergy may also be the cause.

Who's at Risk
In some families, digestive problems are considered a part of life.

Possible Aftereffects and Complications
Digestive problems may become chronic and determine the rhythm of daily life.

Prevention
Determine which foods give you abdominal pains. Onions, vegetables in the cabbage family, or legumes can subsequently be avoided, as can carbonated beverages if they are at fault.

When to Seek Medical Advice
Seek help if discomfort is stubborn.

Self-Help
Flatulence can be relieved by a hot water bottle, warm, moist compresses, baths, and teas. Don't hold the gas in; releasing it will relieve pain. If flatulence and abdominal pain occur between meals, eating a few bites usually calms them. Eating slowly and chewing thoroughly makes the work of digestion easier.

Be sure to eat fiber-rich, varied foods and keep to regular mealtimes (see Healthy Nutrition, p. 722). If you eat slowly, you will swallow less air.

Regularity is equally important. Don't repress bowel movements; go as soon as you need to, even if it means interrupting important work. You can train your bowels by spending a relaxed 10 minutes sitting on the toilet at the same time each day.

The most effective means of preventing an uncomfortably full feeling is to take on less: Less food, and less aggravation. Some herbal schnapps may help digestion, but be careful not to drink too much alcohol.

Regular exercise (walks, gymnastics, swimming, hiking, cycling) keeps the bowels in motion. Very important: drink 1½ to 2 quarts of liquid a day.

If symptoms appear as a regular result of conflicts or excitement, it may help to make a conscious effort to pause and take a rest, with breathing and relaxation exercises (see p. 693) or biofeedback (see p. 695). Various muscle relaxation techniques can support these behavioral changes.

Yoga (see p. 695) has its own exercises to support regular digestion. It is also helpful in reducing nervousness, even in the intestines.

Acupressure (see p. 680), learned from an experienced practitioner and applied by a partner, can also help.

Treatment

No medical treatment is necessary. If flatulence persists over time, a short course of treatment with antiflatulence medication can be tried (e.g., simethicone—Mylicon, Gas-X, Phazyme), although their effectiveness has been questioned by the U.S. Food and Drug Administration.

For antispasmodic medications to relieve cramps, see Acute Gastritis, p. 387.
Massages (see p. 686) can relieve symptoms.

Behavioral therapy (see p. 700) may be indicated if symptoms are accompanied by depression. Homeopathic treatments (see p. 684) have also been found to help.

GASTROENTERITIS

Complaints and Causes

The main symptom of all intestinal infections is diarrhea, sometimes coupled with vomiting.

Adults normally eliminate between 4 and 12 ounces of feces every day. Those who eat lots of vegetables, fruits, and whole-grain products produce significantly more.
Normal feces consist of 60 to 90 percent water; diarrhea contains more, which means the body is losing water. A single incident of loose feces is not unusual and no cause for alarm. Diarrhea is defined as a watery-liquid stool more than three times in a day.

The symptoms of gastroenteritis differ depending on the pathogen responsible for the infection.
Coliform bacteria: Which contaminate food through unsanitary practices or contact between food and/or drinking water and untreated sewage, cause slight diar-

---

Teas for Bloating and Cramps
Drink 2 to 4 cups of warm, freshly prepared tea in between meals.

Caraway Seed Tea
Pour 1 cup boiling water over 1 to 2 teaspoons mashed caraway seeds. Let steep for 15 minutes, then strain.

Fennel and Anise Seed Tea
Prepare as for caraway seed tee. For infants and small children use only 1 teaspoon. Milk or baby cereal can be mixed with this tea.

Chamomile Tea
Pour 1 cup boiling water over 1 tablespoon chamomile flowers. Let steep for 10 minutes, then strain.

Yarrow Tea
Prepare as for chamomile tea, except use 2 teaspoons of yarrow.

Stomach-Intestine Tea Blend
Pour 1 cup hot water over 1 tablespoon of blend. Let steep for 10 minutes, then strain. Prepare blend using: 1 ounce caraway seeds, 1 ounce peppermint leaves, 1 ounce chamomile flowers, and 1 ounce valerian root.

---

rhea, sometimes accompanied by vomiting and usually lasting a day or two. These infections often occur in summer and usually require no treatment.
Staphylococcal bacteria: Produce a heat-stable toxin that attacks the intestine. Symptoms of a staph infection are severe vomiting followed by intense diarrhea, and are typically preceded by salivation and stomachache. See a doctor if you have these symptoms.
Viral infections: Cause diarrhea with severe vomiting accompanied by headaches and muscle aches. A mild fever, sniffles, or sore throat may also be present. The illness may last up to a week; usually only bed rest is needed.
"Intestinal flu": Is often a combination of viral and bacterial infections. It can produce dizziness, vomiting, loud noises in the bowels, stomach cramps, and diarrhea in all varieties and degrees of severity. It often occurs in regular epidemics and usually subsides on its own after a few days.
Salmonella infections: Are transmitted by direct contact with infected persons or their feces, and by infected foods such as leftovers kept warm for a long time or

reheated several times, undercooked poultry, eggs, mayonnaise, salads, sweets, and milk products. Symptoms include a sudden feeling of illness and nausea followed by vomiting, stomachache and severe watery diarrhea which may last 2 to 5 days, often accompanied by fever.

Typhus and paratyphus: Are severe salmonella infections transmitted by contaminated drinking water and foods, especially eggs. They may begin with constipation, a gradually rising temperature, headache, loss of appetite, and bronchitis. In the second week, the fever can climb to 104°F. The body (with the usual exception of arms and legs) may become covered with small red spots. In the third week diarrhea begins, with pea soup consistency.

Helicobacter infections: Are acquired from contaminated foods or drinking water and cause fever, chills, stomach pains, watery diarrhea up to 20 times a day, vomiting, and flu-like symptoms.

Bacterial dysentery: Can be caused by a shigella infection from contaminated foods and drinking water. It begins with fever and severe stomach cramps, followed by frequent vomiting, bloody-slimy-watery diarrhea, and weakness.

Amoebic dysentery: Is caused by infection with amoebas from contaminated drinking water and foods. It begins with tiredness, stomachache, and nausea, but no fever. After a few days, the feces become glassy, bloody, and raspberry-red.

Cholera: Is caused by infection with cholera bacteria in contaminated drinking water and foods. Milky, watery feces ("rice water" stools) are accompanied by continuous vomiting and urine retention. There is no fever; in fact, body temperature may be below normal.

Even after these diseases have been treated successfully, patients may be infective for another 3 months. A test can reveal whether this is the case; if the patient works in the food industry, such testing is mandatory. Some carriers of infection never develop any symptoms.

Who's at Risk

The risk of "Montezuma's revenge" is increased by poor hygiene, epidemics, and travel. Bacterial and amoebic dysentery, typhus, and cholera are now practically nonexistent in developed countries; if they do occur, they are often imported by travelers.

Possible Aftereffects and Complications

Because the body loses vital potassium and magnesium (electrolytes) along with water, the circulation may collapse. This can happen very quickly in children, aged persons or those in fragile health, or those with severe diarrheal diseases like cholera. The resulting changes in the blood can stress the kidneys.

Prevention

Hygienic measures are important, especially when traveling in situations where you aren't certain that sewage is handled so as not to contaminate food or drinking water. Fecal matter dumped into the sea is often the source of seafood contamination (see Travel, p. 714).

People who work in the food industry are regularly tested to prevent salmonella outbreaks. For prevention in the home, see Bacterial Illnesses, p. 729.

Vaccinations exist for cholera (see p. 676) and typhus (see p. 677).

When to Seek Medical Advice

Seek help without fail if you see traces of blood, mucus, pus, or fat in your feces.

Self-Help

Don't eat anything. Drink large amounts of fluids: Sweetened tea, mineral water, diluted cola shaken to release the carbon dioxide, fruit juice. Fruits contain potassium, which is important to replace. Sugar promotes uptake of the mineral salts lost in severe diarrhea and vomiting. You should have a pinch of salt twice a day.

The ingredients for a fluid replacement beverage (see p. 406) are cheap and readily available in any pharmacy.

Electrolyte drinks are also available ready-made, but are more expensive (Pedialyte, etc.). Drink at least four times as much liquid as usual; this is the only way to make up for fluid loss. Take it easy and rest.

On the second and third day you can add grated apples and zwieback, or carrot soup to your diet.

Diarrhea and vomiting are the body's natural way of ridding itself of pathogens or toxins. Taking medicinal charcoal, Kaopectate, or apple pectin probably won't help, since they neither prevent water loss nor detoxify the pathogens or toxins. This is also true of any home remedies. Drinking liquids is the most important thing you can do.

If diarrhea lasts beyond 5 to 7 days, seek medical advice.

Fluid Replacement Beverage for Diarrhea
Dissolve 1 teaspoon table salt, $\frac{1}{2}$ teaspoon baking soda, $\frac{1}{4}$ teaspoon potassium chloride and 1 ounce sugar in 1 quart boiled water (World Health Organization oral rehydration solution).

Or, mix the juice of four oranges, seven teaspoons sugar, and one teaspoon salt. Fill to 1 quart mark with boiled water.

Treatment

If diarrhea is damaging to health, and its cause has been clearly determined, doctors may prescribe medications such as Imodium to reduce intestinal motility and limit loss of mineral salts.

The pathogens in bacterial infections should be identified, as some cannot be eliminated with antibiotics.

If the infection is known to be caused by a fungus, it should be treated with the appropriate antifungals.

Occasionally, extreme fluid and electrolyte loss necessitates a hospital stay for intravenous replacement therapy.

CONSTIPATION

Complaints

Symptoms include hard stool and difficult elimination, with the lingering feeling that the bowels aren't completely empty.

A bowel movement three times a week is considered normal; constipation is considered to be present only if there is no movement for more than 3 days.

Causes

Chronic constipation: Is often only a mistaken notion arising from the idea that bowels must be moved at least once a day, or that stools should be softer. Persons constantly preoccupied with expelling "unclean" waste from the body risk starting a vicious circle between expectation and a feeling of failure when the body refuses to comply.

If bowel movements are repeatedly repressed, the bowel becomes less active. After a time, its movement stops altogether.

Acute Constipation: If the bowels fail to move for a longer-than-usual period, anxiety or psychological factors may be at fault (see Health and Well-Being, p. 182). Constipation after traveling to a new location is considered part of the normal adaptation process.

Other causes of acute constipation include
— Various disorders of the intestines or nervous system.
— After-effect of surgery
— Side effect of medications such as those used for psychological disorders, aluminum-containing antacids, sleeping tablets, sedatives, and cough or pain remedies containing codeine.

Who's at Risk

A diet high in sugar and very low in fiber and fluid (see Drinks, above) promotes constipation.

Constipation is common during pregnancy.

Organic causes like hemorrhoids, tapeworm larvae (which may also be painful), or a tissue prolapse are rare.

Possible Aftereffects and Complications

Diverticula and diverticulitis (see p. 409) or possibly even bowel cancer (see p. 414) may result from chronic constipation, or from long-term consumption of certain laxatives, which may facilitate the development of cancer.

Prevention

The most important preventive is a fiber-rich diet including whole-grain bread, raw vegetables and fruit, and plenty of liquids. These foods fill the bowels and promote elimination. A glass of mineral water or fresh fruit juice every morning stimulates digestion, as do wheat bran or flax seeds. Regular exercise also keeps the bowels fit.

If you feel the need to go to the bathroom, don't put it off. It can be helpful to accustom yourself to going at the same time every day.

Relaxation exercises and yoga (see p. 695) may improve digestion.

If you are taking medications that promote constipation, consult your health-care provider.

Laxative Teas for Constipation

Take 1 cup of freshly prepared tea mornings and/or evenings. The effects are noticeable after 10 to 12 hours.

Senna Leaf Tea
Pour 1 cup of hot water over 1 teaspoon senna leaves. Let steep for 10 minutes, then strain.

Senna Fruit Tea
Prepare as for senna leaf tea, except use $^1/_2$ teaspoon of the senna fruit. The effect is somewhat milder.

Laxative Tea Blend
Pour 1 cup of hot water over 2 teaspoons of tea blend. Let steep for 10 minutes, then strain. Prepare blend using: 2 ounces senna leaves, $^1/_3$ ounce fennel, $^1/_3$ ounce chamomile flowers, and $^2/_3$ ounce peppermint leaves.

Important side effects of all laxative teas: Crampy abdominal pain, thin watery stools.
Warning: Not for prolonged use. Do not use during pregnancy or while breast feeding. The active ingredients pass into breast milk, and may cause diarrhea in infants.

When to Seek Medical Advice

Seek help for long-term constipation. If the frequency of bowel movements suddenly changes, the possibility of disease should be investigated.

Self-Help

At the first signs of constipation, eat more raw vegetables, fruit, and oils, and drink plenty of liquids. Sauerkraut, rhubarb, prunes, figs, and melons have laxative qualities.

Avoid laxatives if possible. All of them, even herbal laxatives, interfere with the body's water balance and, if taken regularly, damage the intestinal muscles, making them even less active. In addition, herbal remedies containing anthraquinones, including aloes, cascara bark, senna leaves and pods, and rhubarb root, are cathartics and are suspected of promoting cancer of the bowel with regular use. Laxative use is only justified to empty the bowels before surgery or X rays, or for painful conditions in the anal region. Laxatives should not be taken during pregnancy, by nursing mothers, or by children. If you need to help your bowels "get moving" once in a while, use glycerin suppositories and enemas. This must not become a habit because the bowel's own activity can be inhibited.

Treatment

People who have used laxatives for a long time need medical help to bring the bowel back to independent functioning.

Regularity can be established with the help of a mineral water cure with water containing large amounts of sodium sulfate or magnesium sulfate; breathing exercises; or massage. If constipation lasts more than a week, the hardened stool must sometimes be removed by a doctor. High colonic enema therapy is not suitable for chronic constipation.

INTESTINAL OBSTRUCTION AND ILEUS

In obstruction, the intestine may be partially or completely blocked, resulting in ileus.

Complaints

Symptoms of intestinal obstruction include constipation for more than five days, loss of appetite, and a full feeling. If this is not treated, ileus or complete blockage may result: Belching and painful abdominal cramps begin suddenly, and within a few hours, a serious illness has developed including vomiting of bile, inability to pass gas and stool, and a soft, distended abdomen. After hours of colic, if the intestine is unable to break through the blockage, it gives up. The abdominal noises stop and intestinal paralysis sets in. In most cases, circulatory collapse soon follows.

Causes

— A segment of the intestine gets stuck in a break in the abdominal wall (hernia)
— Gallstones (see p. 398)
— Inflammatory intestinal diseases (see Crohn's Disease, p. 412; Ulcerative Colitis, p. 411) and diverticulitis (see p. 409)
— Twisting of the intestine (volvulus)
— Intestinal cancer (see p. 414)
— Inflammation of the pancreas (see p. 400)
— Scarring after surgery, or tying off of a blood vessel
— Intake of bulk-creating nutritional supplements such as flax seed or bran without enough liquid

Who's at Risk
Complete intestinal obstruction is relatively rare.

Possible Aftereffects and Complications
Untreated intestinal obstruction leads to ileus, which is life-threatening if not treated.

Prevention
If there is an underlying illness, it should be treated. If an intestinal obstruction is present, high-fiber foods should be avoided.

When to Seek Medical Advice
Go immediately to a hospital if you have symptoms of intestinal obstruction.

Self-Help
Not possible.

Treatment
Complete intestinal obstruction requires immediate surgery. An X ray and/or endoscope is used to locate the constriction (see A Look Inside, p. 651). The lost fluid should be replaced and the underlying illness treated.

The abdomen is opened, and the part of the intestine pinched in the hernia or stuck to the abdominal wall is released. Some of the congested contents is pumped out through a tube inserted through the mouth or nose. If a piece of the intestine has already died, it must be removed.

APPENDICITIS

Complaints
In acute appendicitis, pain starts suddenly in the lower-right portion of the abdomen and is intensified by coughing, sneezing, or walking. Dizziness, vomiting, fever, constipation, flatulence, and bad breath are frequently present. The abdomen is hard and the pain may extend to the bladder and genitals.

Causes
The open end of the appendix is blocked either by feces, a crimped intestine, or, more rarely, a foreign body, a tumor, or worms. If it becomes infected, an abscess may develop.

Who's at Risk
Appendicitis is relatively common among children and young adults. Even children of preschool and school age often undergo appendectomies. However, a small percent of operations are based on an erroneous diagnosis. After the incision is made, it can be seen that the appendix was not inflamed.

Possible Aftereffects and Complications
Loops of the intestine may stick to the appendix and develop abscesses. If untreated, the infection can break into the peritoneal cavity within 24 hours; this usually occurs on the fourth day. In this case, the pain subsides temporarily, only to reappear with more intensity. The patient may vomit and develops a fever.

Prevention
Not possible.

When to Seek Medical Advice
A typical sign of appendicitis is pain felt when the extended right leg is gently rotated inward. Direct pressure on the area of the appendix also results in pain.

If abdominal pains persist for a number of hours and are not relieved (or are even made worse) by a hot water bottle, a doctor should be called. If symptoms are accompanied by greenish vomit and a pale, sweaty face, go to a hospital immediately.

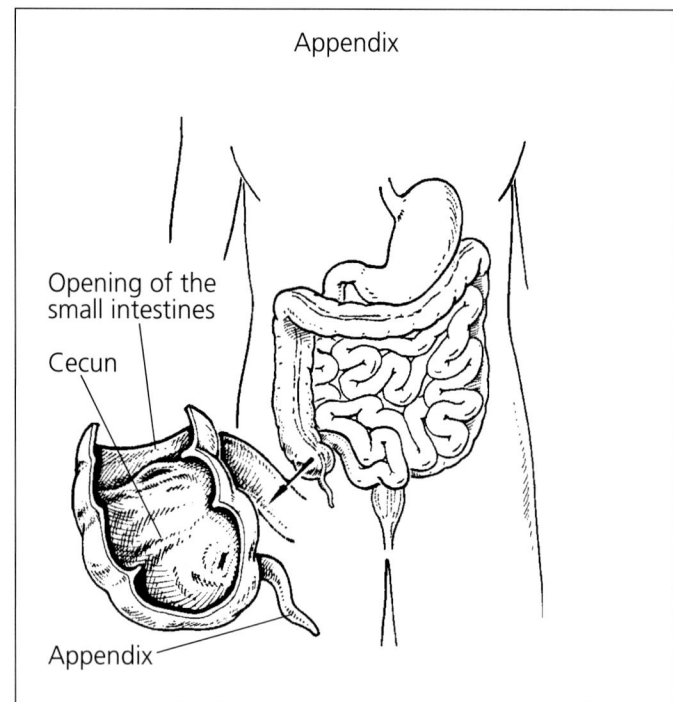

Appendix

Opening of the small intestines

Cecun

Appendix

Self-Help

Lie down and rest quietly. An ice pack may relieve pain. Because you may require surgery under general anesthesia, don't eat or drink anything. If you're thirsty, rinse your mouth with water. Don't take laxatives or pain medication.

Treatment

The physician must first confirm the diagnosis of acute appendicitis, which requires immediate surgery, since even if the current inflammation subsides, it will probably recur.

Patients should be encouraged to stand up soon after the operation. Only a few days' hospital stay is needed. Usually the patient can return to work after 3 weeks.

Laparoscopy is often used to remove appendices today (see p. 653).

If an abscess has formed, the pus must be drained out of the body through a tube, and the surgeon may wait a few weeks before removing the appendix.

PERITONITIS (INFLAMMATION OF THE PERITONEUM)

Complaints

The alarm signals for peritonitis are a hard, tense abdominal wall; inability to pass gas and stool; vomiting; violent abdominal pains; respiratory distress; rapid pulse; a cold forehead and hands; and pallor.

Causes

The peritoneum, the membrane enclosing and supporting the abdominal organs, becomes inflamed, and part of the abdominal cavity fills with pus.

Who's at Risk

— Appendicitis (see p. 408)
— Perforation of an ulcer of the small or large intestine
— Intestinal injury caused by laparoscopy
— Perforation of an inflamed gallbladder (see Gallbladder Inflammation, p.400)
— Perforation of an inflamed liver or abdominal wall abscess
— A tear in the uterus or a fallopian tube infection
— Tuberculosis (see p. 311)
— Lymph node infections; progressive inflammation of the pleural membranes and pericardium

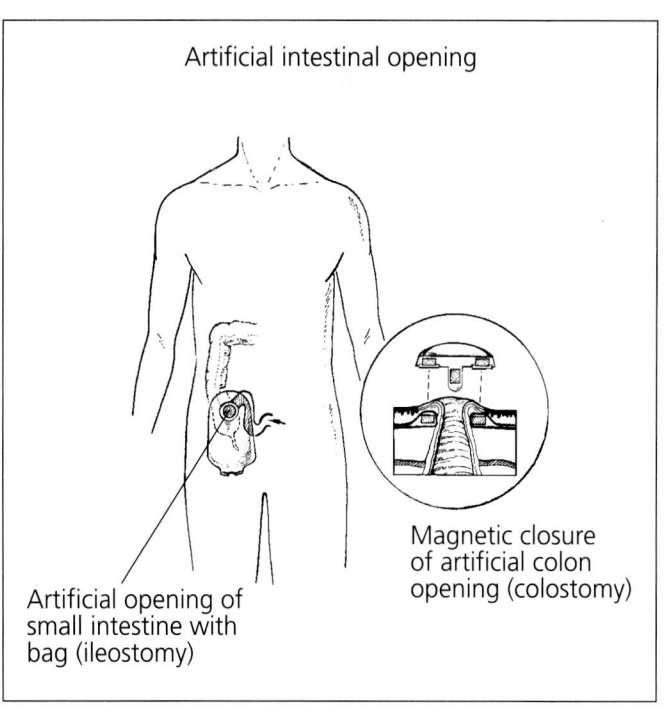

Artificial intestinal opening

Magnetic closure of artificial colon opening (colostomy)

Artificial opening of small intestine with bag (ileostomy)

— Infection after injury to the abdominal wall

Possible Aftereffects and Complications

Peritonitis is always life-threatening.

Prevention

Not possible.

When to Seek Medical Advice

Seek help immediately if symptoms are present.

Self-Help

Not possible.

Treatment

Depending on the cause, an immediate operation may be indicated, in conjunction with antibiotic treatment of the infection. If performed in time, surgery usually saves the patient's life.

DIVERTICULITIS

Complaints

Symptoms include a pronounced alternation between diarrhea and constipation accompanied by cramping, usually in the lower-left abdominal region. Sometimes there is blood in the stool.

Causes

Diverticulitis is diagnosed when diverticula become inflamed. *Diverticula* are areas of the intestine in which a segment of the inner lining protrudes through a crack in the muscular outer layer, forming a bulge that may grow as large as a cherry (this condition is known as diverticulosis). Diverticula are usually found in the part of the large intestine where the feces collect before being eliminated.

Who's at Risk

The more the large intestine contains, the better it can move. High-fiber diets fill the bowels and cause them to empty more effectively than low-fiber diets.

Persons who eat low-fiber diets are at greater risk of diverticulosis. The frequency of the disease increases with each decade of life until, at 70, one person in three in industrial countries has a diverticulum.

Possible Aftereffects and Complications

If the diverticula repeatedly become inflamed, there is danger of a perforation and peritonitis (see p. 409). Fistulas or pathways to neighboring organs, such as the bladder, may develop.

Prevention

People who exercise often and eat fiber-rich diets (see Healthy Nutrition, p. 722) have fewer inflammations.

When to Seek Medical Advice

Seek help if you have acute or chronic pains in the lower left part of the abdomen, or if there is blood in your stool.

Self-Help

Do not take laxatives; they cause constipation if taken for a long time. The bowels can be stimulated to more activity by eating a fiber-rich diet and getting plenty of exercise. This helps prevent congestion and inflammation. Bed rest and a day or two of fasting often cause the inflammation to subside rapidly.

Treatment

Because the symptoms may also indicate cancer of the bowel, a physician should examine the large intestine with an endoscope (see A Look Inside, p. 651).

Antibiotics will help clear up the inflammation.

If the diverticula bleed heavily and repeatedly, or if the disease leads to complications, the affected section of the bowel must be removed. If an artificial bowel outlet has to be inserted, it can usually be removed after four to six months in a second operation. Even in cases where it is possible to retain the natural bowel outlet, patients must occasionally live with an artificial outlet for a short time, to relieve the large intestine and promote healing.

In surgery for rectal cancer or operations on the large intestine for ulcerative colitis, a permanent artificial outlet must often be created. This is done by suturing the end of the remaining part of the large intestine to the abdominal wall (colostomy). In rare cases, the entire large intestine must be removed. In these cases, the end of the small intestine is pulled through and sutured to the abdominal wall and an outlet is created (ileostomy). Either type of opening is covered with a bag to collect the stool. Because the stool at the end of the small intestine is far more liquid than that produced by the large intestine, it is more difficult to care for an ileostomy than a colostomy.

In some cases, it is possible to create a stoma which allows the patient to empty the stool reservoir, using a tube. The opening is closed by a magnetic or balloon valve. The surgeon should inform the patient of all the details of the planned operation, options for the artificial outlet, and how to care for each type.

MALABSORPTION SYNDROMES

A number of disorders impair the intestine's ability to absorb nutrients, leading to deficiencies of minerals, vitamins, or proteins.

Complaints

A malabsorption disorder is always suspected if massive, foul-smelling diarrhea, loss of weight, and anemia occur together. Severe intolerance to lactose, gluten (see Celiac Disease, p. 411), or other substances also results in deficiency symptoms.

Treatment

It may take years to identify the cause of the disorder with the help of examinations and tests. Once the cause is identified, the patient is put on a special diet, including supplements of the substances the body isn't absorbing from foods.

CELIAC DISEASE

Complaints

This disease usually develops in childhood; in rare cases it appears in adults and goes under the name "sprue." Its symptoms may appear only sporadically, with long periods between episodes. Usually they first appear when a 6- to 12-month infant is introduced to cereal in addition to milk.

Children with celiac disease are usually sickly and pale and produce massive, yellowish, foul-smelling stools. Flatulence, a swollen belly, and anemia are present. If the disease lasts long enough, their growth can be stunted.

Adults with sprue have the following symptoms: Anemia, weight loss, reduced activity, bone pains, tingling sensations, edema, and skin disorders. They experience painful, foul-smelling diarrhea and bloating on a daily basis.

Fat in the stool is typical for the disease.

Causes

Celiac disease is caused by hypersensitivity to gluten, which is found in grains such as wheat, rye, and (in smaller amounts) barley, oats, spelt, and winter rye. The hypersensitivity promotes abnormal multiplication of a specific type of white blood cell, which damages the mucous lining of the small intestine (see Allergies, p. 360). This most important organ of resorption then atrophies, and nutrients can no longer be properly absorbed.

Who's at Risk

A predisposition to celiac disease is common in some families and in some countries.

Possible Aftereffects and Complications

In children, iron-deficiency anemia may result. In adults, iron-deficiency and folic acid-deficiency anemia may result. Depending on the course of the disease, the deficiency may also affect other organs, e.g., bones (see Osteoporosis, p. 430). The fact that the disease cannot be cured can be a great psychological burden, and depression is a common side effect. In women, menstruation may be affected, and potency may be affected in men.

Prevention

The later an infant is weaned from breast milk or a completely tolerated milk formula to a cereal diet (see Baby Foods, p. 738), the later the intestine is exposed to gluten, and the less severe any resulting illness will be.

When to Seek Medical Advice

Seek help if symptoms appear. Celiac disease can only be definitively diagnosed by a biopsy of the small intestine; this does not require hospitalization. If celiac disease is diagnosed, other family members should also be examined.

Self-Help

Switch to a diet completely free of gluten. Choose infant formula, baby cereals, and conventional flour-containing foods (bread, noodles, desserts, sauces, breaded fried foods) made with cornmeal, buckwheat, rice, millet flour, or potato flour. Fruit, vegetables, dairy products, eggs, meat, fish, etc. may be eaten.

Celiac patients must strictly observe their prescribed diets.

Treatment

Celiac disease cannot be treated with medications; only strict adherence to a gluten-free diet can help. After 6 to 9 months, the damage to the intestinal mucosa will heal, but the diet should be observed for the rest of your life to ensure continuing health.

Warning: If you start eating gluten again in spite of a nongluten diet and no symptoms appear, do not assume the disease is gone. Often no symptoms manifest for months or years, but suddenly reappear when the intestine is stressed, perhaps by a flu or pregnancy. The result may be a serious disorder that is difficult to treat.

Depending on the severity of nutritional deficiencies developed during acute celiac disease, vitamins, minerals, and iron may be prescribed as dietary supplements.

ULCERATIVE COLITIS

This chronic inflammation of the lining of the large intestine starts in the rectum and may spread upward through the entire large intestine, forming ulcers.

Complaints

Ulcerative colitis may progress intermittently, accompanied by abdominal pains and fever. It typically causes bloody, mucus-filled diarrhea; if the entire large intestine is affected, large amounts of blood may be lost. The results are lack of appetite, weight loss, and anemia, possibly accompanied by joint pain, skin disorders, and eye inflammations.

Causes

The causes of this chronic inflammatory intestinal disease are not yet known. There is probably a hereditary component, and there is evidence that bacteria and psychological factors also play a role (see Health and Well-Being, p. 182). Certain nonsteroidal anti-inflammatory medications, such as diclofenac and indomethacin, can also precipitate intestinal inflammation.

Who's at Risk

The annual incidence of ulcerative colitis is approximately 10 cases per 10,000 white adults, and is rising.

Possible Aftereffects and Complications

If the disease is treated promptly, 90 percent of patients have few aftereffects. However, stress may result from undergoing the required regular internal examinations, or from the knowledge that the risk of colon cancer increases after ten years of ulcerative colitis.

Prevention

Aside from consumption of a fiber-rich diet (see Healthy Nutrition, p. 722), no preventive measures are possible.

When to Seek Medical Advice

Seek help immediately if stool is bloody and contains mucus. The large intestine should be examined with an endoscope and biopsies should be taken (see A Look Inside, p. 651).

Self-Help

There is no effective special diet for ulcerative colitis. Patients may eat whatever agrees with them. A varied diet containing plenty of fiber is a good idea.

Treatment

The acute phase of the disease is treated with sulfasalazine (Azulfidine) and topical steroid enemas. Five-acetylsalicylic (5-ASA) derivatives—the mesalamine-group medications—may be substituted for sulfasalazine. These medications can prolong the remission phases of the disease, but do not cure it.

If the disease has caused dramatic losses of blood and weight, and if a large portion of the bowel is affected, a so-called toxic megacolon can develop. This is a serious condition which necessitates immediate hospitalization. The affected portion of the intestine must be surgically removed; thereafter, improvement is rapid.

Psychotherapy

As a chronic intestinal disease wears on, the psychological burden will grow. If colitis is running the patient's life, is getting distinctly worse, and is extremely stressful, therapy can help. Therapy also frequently reveals how the patient's self-image and attitudes contribute to the disease (see Counseling and Psychotherapy, p. 697).

CROHN'S DISEASE

Crohn's disease is a chronic inflammation of the intestinal mucosa and intestinal wall, which leaves scars that facilitate the formation of fistulas.

Usually the last loop of the small intestine is affected; segments of the small and large intestines and rectum are often also involved. However, the inflammation may appear in sections of the entire digestive tract, from the mouth to the anus.

Complaints

Symptoms include repeated episodes of violent abdominal cramps and a general feeling of illness, often accompanied by watery diarrhea which may contain blood.

Weight loss, recurrent fever, joint pains, skin lesions, disorders of the oral mucosa and eye inflammations may occur at the beginning of Crohn's disease, as may "appendicitis." Painful lesions and fistulas in the anus are typical. The disease develops slowly over a period of years, and progresses by episodes interspersed with remission periods of months or years.

Causes

The causes of Crohn's disease are not yet known, nor do we know why it appears with higher frequency in some families and has become more common in the last few decades. It is assumed that there is some connection with psychosocial stress (see Health and Well-Being, p. 182). The illness is more common in those with a predisposition toward allergies and a taste for sugar-containing foods. Whether bacteria are involved in its etiology is still unclear.

Who's at Risk

Crohn's disease usually begins in early adulthood. It is equally prevalent in women and men.

Possible Aftereffects and Complications

Anemia due to heavy bleeding.

In the advanced stages of Crohn's disease, fistulas may form and carry pus into healthy portions of the intestine or to the bladder, vagina, or anal area. There is a danger of intestinal obstruction (see p. 407) and perforation of affected segments of the intestine. The risk of intestinal cancer, however, is slight.

Two thirds of Crohn's disease patients are able to lead normal working lives. One third suffer persistent symptoms despite treatment.

Prevention

Aside from eating a healthy, varied diet, prevention is not possible (see Healthy Nutrition, p. 722).

When to Seek Medical Advice

Seek help if symptoms appear, especially changes in the anus, and bloody, mucus-filled diarrhea.

Self-Help

A fiber-rich diet, plenty of rest, and a stress-free lifestyle can positively influence the course of the disease.

Treatment

Crohn's disease is frequently discovered by chance during an appendectomy. The earlier it is discovered, the better the chances of treatment. To determine the extent of the disease and whether complications are present, the physician will need to examine the entire digestive tract from above and below, with the help of an endoscope and a biopsy (see A Look Inside, p. 651). Usually X rays of the small intestine are also needed.

Medications

Acute episodes can be eased, but not prevented, by medications. High doses of corticosteroids (see Corticosteroids, p. 665), possibly in combination with azathioprine (Imuran), are often prescribed to prolong the quiescent phase before the next flare-up.

If the large intestine is also affected, sulfasalazine (Azulfidine) or 5-ASA preparations (Asacol, Rowasa, Pentasa) can help.

Because the medications may need to be taken over a long period, considerable side effects may result.

There is no cure for Crohn's disease.

Surgery

Surgery usually becomes necessary in the course of Crohn's disease, e.g., to open a constricted intestine or close a fistula. Some patients need repeated surgery. Their quality of life may be seriously impaired by recurring symptoms and operations (see Artificial Intestinal Outlets, p. 410).

Diet

During the acute stage of Crohn's disease, a liquid diet—a nutritional solution completely absorbed by the small intestine—is often administered in the hospital, bringing about a reduction in diarrhea and abdominal pain, fever, and anemia. Due to the liquid's unappetizing taste, it is continuously pumped through a tube in the nose directly into the stomach. In rare cases, e.g. after removal of a large part of the intestine, the nutritional solution must be administered intravenously; patients are taught how to perform both procedures at home.

Psychotherapy

If the disease is a major stress factor, running a patient's life, or getting distinctly worse, psychotherapy (see p. 699) can help. It's also a good idea because in many cases, patients discover that their self-image and attitudes contribute to their condition (see Health and Well-Being, p. 182). Therapy cannot prevent relapses, but it can bring improvement, reduce symptoms, and above all, helps patients be more relaxed about the disease.

INTESTINAL POLYPS

Complaints
Intestinal polyps usually produce no symptoms. Occasionally, traces of blood and mucus are found in the stool.

Causes
There are many kinds of benign growths and tumors in the intestine that have no symptoms or known causes.

The large intestine especially may contain numerous polyps, either singly or in groups, which may bleed.

Who's at Risk
Intestinal polyps are found in 7 percent of the population. A rare hereditary form exists in which polyps are clustered in one region of the intestine.

Possible Aftereffects and Complications
The larger the polyps and other growths, the greater the risk of eventual malignancy. The risk of cancer is extremely high in people with hereditary polyps: By the age of 30, 50 percent have cancer; by age 40, 90 percent.

Some benign tumors can get so large that they close off the intestine.

Prevention
For early detection of polyps or colon cancer, an annual test for occult blood in the stool (hemoccult test) is a good idea after age 50.

When to Seek Medical Advice
Seek help immediately, if there are visible traces of blood and mucus in the stool.

Self-Help
Not possible.

Treatment
The physician will examine the bowel using an endoscope in order to exclude cancer (see A Look Inside, p. 651). Individual polyps are then removed and cauterized by an instrument introduced through the endoscope. This is possible without anesthesia, and the patient can return to work the next day.

Large tumors are completely removed because of danger of malignant transformation. This requires surgery under anesthesia, as the intestine must be opened from the outside. If polyps are clustered close together, it may be necessary to remove that entire intestinal section.

In the following year, the patient undergoes two endoscopic examinations, and any new tumors are surgically removed. Thereafter, the examinations are performed annually.

In the hereditary form of polyps, the polyps are so close together and the risk of cancer is so high, that the entire large intestine should be removed when the patient is 20 years old. An artificial intestinal outlet is then created (see p. 410).

COLON AND RECTAL CANCERS
(see also Cancer, p. 470).

Complaints
Early warning signals of colon cancer may be a sudden change in the type and frequency of bowel movements, resulting in either chronic constipation or diarrhea. The urge to eliminate increases, and small quantities of stool escape when gas is passed. The stool is formed like a thin rod and contains traces of mucus and dark red or black blood, though these are rarely noticed. Later symptoms include abdominal pain, loss of appetite, anemia, and weight loss.

Tumors in the anal region are externally palpable.

Causes
Colon cancer has several probable causes, including
— An imbalanced diet, low in fiber and rich in fats and carbohydrates; obesity.
— Carcinogens in food, including benzpyrenes in smoked or grilled foods, and nitrosomines in foods that are both fried and cured or smoked. Nitrosomines are also present in tobacco smoke, foods preserved with nitrites, and fruits and vegetables.
— Genetic factors are also assumed to be present, due to the high incidence of colon cancer in certain families.

Who's at Risk

Colon cancer is one of the most common forms of cancer. The risk is higher in people with polyps in the large intestine (see p. 411, 414), ulcerative colitis, or a family member with colon cancer.

Possible Aftereffects and Complications

As long as the cancer has not metastasized and is removed in time, surgery can save the lives of half of colon cancer patients. If other organs are affected, chances of survival are lower; if untreated, this condition is fatal within a year.

Prevention

A varied diet, rich in vitamins and including lots of fruits and vegetables, preferably organically grown, promotes a healthy large intestine (see Healthy Nutrition, p. 722).

After age 40, everyone should have an annual rectal exam by a physician. Rectal cancer can be detected early by examining the rectum with a finger. After age 50, all men and women should be tested annually for blood in the stool (hemoccult test) and have a colonoscopic examination every 3 to 5 years (see Colonoscopy, p. 653).

When to Seek Medical Advice

Seek help immediately if the first warning symptoms appear. People with hemorrhoids often disregard blood in their stool, at their peril.

Self-Help

Any attempts at self-help would only delay the necessary appointment with the doctor.

Treatment

If cancer of the bowel is suspected, an endoscopic examination will be performed (see Colonoscopy, p. 653) and the tumor surgically removed. Afterwards, if feasible, the two ends of the intestine will be stitched together. Occasionally, the cancer is so low in the rectum or anus that this part must be removed and an artificial outlet created (see p. 410).

If surgery is not an option, a course of radiation or cancer chemotherapy should be done. Tumor regrowth is not always prevented. The early detection of cancer recurrence after treatment does not guarantee a longer life expectancy.

Discuss all procedures with your treatment team, and develop a regime to relieve symptoms as much as possible. Anything that gives you pleasure and is good for you will improve your quality of life and strengthen your resistance to disease.

Psychotherapy and support groups can help patients cope with colon cancer. Alternative medicine may improve attitude, but has not been shown to inhibit tumor growth.

WORMS (PARASITES)

Worms live as internal parasites in human and animal bodies. In northern latitudes, the most common are pinworms, tapeworms, and roundworms (ascaris). There are many kinds of tropical worms, and their diagnosis and treatment may be difficult.

Complaints

Pinworms: Symptoms include anal itching and the urge to eliminate, caused by an inflamed rectum. In girls, the outer genitalia may be inflamed. Whitish, threadlike worms under half an inch long may be visible in stool, or around the anus.

Roundworms: Symptoms usually consist only of vague abdominal discomfort. Whitish worms, 6 to 8 inches long, may be visible in stool.

Tapeworms: Symptoms include inexplicable weight loss and vague abdominal discomfort. Fish tapeworms can also cause severe anemia. Pieces of the worm resembling flat egg noodles show up in the stool, or sometimes in the bed or underwear.

Dog tapeworms can cause irritable coughing.

Causes

Pinworm eggs are ingested in household dust or contaminated foods. The female worm leaves the anus at night to deposit thousands of eggs on the skin surrounding the anus, causing itching. When the itch is scratched, eggs lodge under fingernails and are transported back to the mouth.

Roundworm eggs are transmitted by contact with contaminated soil, or in salad or raw vegetables grown with human feces as fertilizer. The worms lodge in the small intestine.

Tapeworm larvae are ingested in raw or incompletely cooked meat or fish. In the intestine, they develop into worms up to 32 feet long consisting of flat segments.

Dog-tapeworm eggs are ingested in unwashed wild mushrooms and fruits growing close to the ground. The dog tapeworm forms fluid-filled cysts in the lungs.

Who's at Risk

Pinworms are common in children.

Tapeworms have become rare since almost all meat animals are now raised in feedlots. Dog tapeworms are relatively rare parasites of wild animals.

Possible Aftereffects and Complications

Pinworms: Weight loss; sometimes ulcers of the large intestine or "appendicitis," caused by immature eggs boring into the intestinal wall.

Roundworms: Inflammation of the lungs, gallbladder. and pancreas, where the larvae develop. Occasionally larvae may cause obstructions in the upper airways, nose-throat area, or small intestine.

Tapeworms: Lung cysts caused by the dog tapeworm usually encapsulate and cause no more symptoms.

Prevention

Pinworms: Wash hands thoroughly after every bowel movement.

Roundworms: Foods that might have been grown with human feces as fertilizer should be thoroughly washed and cooked before eating.

Tapeworms: Don't eat uncooked or undercooked meat or fish. Wash wild fruits and mushrooms carefully. Do not feed dogs meat that has been pronounced unfit for human consumption.

When to Seek Medical Advice

Seek help if symptoms appear.

Self-Help

For pinworms and roundworms:
After bowel movements,
— clean the anal region with a moist cotton cloth or under running water.
— wash hands with soap and use a nail brush.
— boil bed linens, underwear, nightclothes and washcloths to prevent reinfection.

Treatment

Physicians can prescribe medications for the various kinds of worms. Treatment for pinworms needs to be repeated more than once. In some cases, all members of the household must be treated simultaneously.

Dog tapeworm cysts can be removed surgically.

ANAL FISSURES

Complaints

Anal fissures are torn areas in the ring of tissue closing the anus, or the anal mucous membrane. They may bleed and cause pain, or tear open repeatedly.

Causes

Usually anal fissures are caused by hard stools, or sexual activities engaged in without sufficient lubrication.

Who's at Risk

The risk is increased by anal sex.

Possible Aftereffects and Complications

Sex without a condom increases the risk of sexually transmitted diseases, which may cause the mucous membrane lining the rectum to become inflamed (see Venereal Diseases, p. 545). The risk of AIDS (see p. 357) is also increased by unprotected anal sex.

Prevention

A high-fiber diet (see Constipation, p. 406), and use of a condom and sufficient lubricant during anal sex.

When to Seek Medical Advice

Seek help if pain and bleeding are present.

Self-Help

Eating fiber-rich foods and drinking plenty of liquids help keep stools soft. Avoid laxatives. Corticosteroid ointments and suppositories for relieving pain and reducing inflammation should be used for brief periods only, as they can facilitate fungal infections.

Medications Against Intestinal Parasites (Worms)

For pinworms: albendazole (Albenza), mebendazole (Vermox), pyrantel pamoate (Antiminth)
For roundworms (ascariasis): albendazole (Albenza), mebendazole (Vermox), pyrantel pamoate (Antiminth)
For tapeworms: paromycin sulfate (Humatin), praziquantel (Biltricide)

HEMORRHOIDS

The external anal swellings that are commonly called external hemorrhoids are characterized by painful bleeding due to burst blood vessels in the anal region.

Internal hemorrhoids, on the other hand, are dilations of the network of veins in the rectum.

Complaints

Symptoms include bright red bleeding, itching, and pain during bowel movements.

Causes

External hemorrhoids are a complication of skin folds in the anal region.
Internal hemorrhoids are caused by
— chronic constipation and increased pressure during bowel movements.
— laxatives, which not only do not prevent hemorrhoids, but force the bowel to empty when the anal sphincter is trying to stay closed. The resulting pressure strains the rectum.
— lack of exercise; excessive body weight.
— cirrhosis of the liver and increased pressure in the portal vein.

Who's at Risk

External hemorrhoids: The risk is higher among people whose jobs require them to sit for long periods of time.
Internal hemorrhoids: The risk is increased in people with hard stools or those who cough constantly.

Possible Aftereffects and Complications

Longstanding hemorrhoids can drop through the anus (prolapse); this condition is extremely painful and must be treated surgically.

Prevention

— A high-fiber diet will promote softer stools (see Constipation, p. 406; Healthy Nutrition, p. 722).
— Regular physical activity helps keep bowels fit.
— Sit on hard surfaces. Avoid long periods of standing or sitting, lifting heavy objects, and long sessions on the toilet.

When to Seek Medical Advice

Seek help if symptoms occur and self-help measures are ineffective.

Self-Help

Avoid straining at stool. Clean the anus with soapy water and a cotton cloth.

Treatment

Examination by palpation alone is not sufficient; sigmoidoscopy (theexamination of the rectum and sigmoid colon) can be used to detect internal hemorrhoids.

Medications cannot cure the disease, but can help ease symptoms.

Hemorrhoid preparations containing the following should not be used because they often cause allergies: formaldehyde, or local anesthetics such as benzocaine, procaine, and tetracaine. Corticosteroid products should also be avoided because they can cause skin damage, and because long-term use can facilitate fungal infections in the rectum and anus. Check product labels to determine whether these ingredients are present.

Internal hemorrhoids higher in the rectum should be cauterized or removed surgically.

If hemorrhoids drop through the anus, they should be removed surgically.

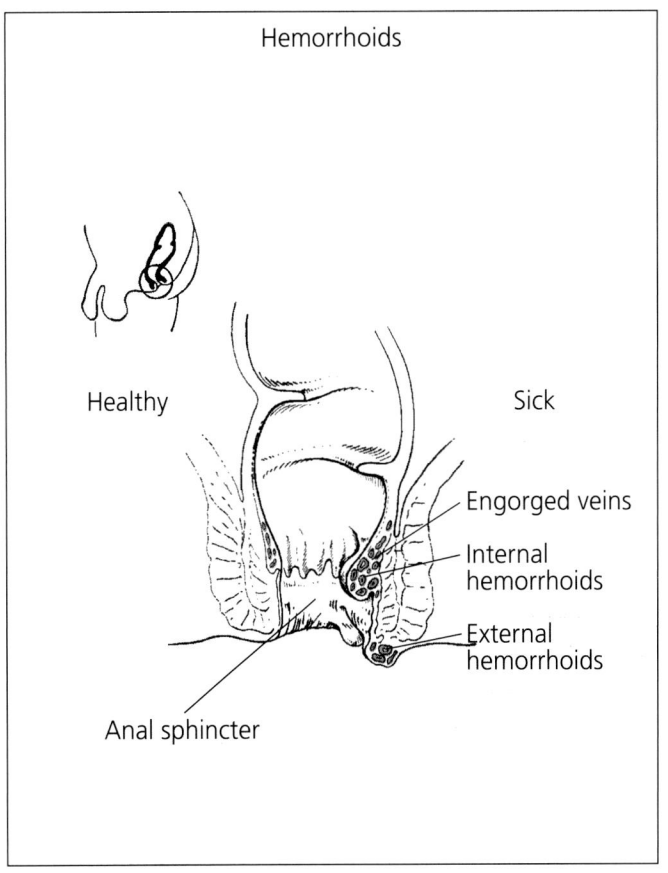

Hemorrhoids

Healthy

Sick

Engorged veins

Internal hemorrhoids

External hemorrhoids

Anal sphincter

KIDNEYS AND URINARY TRACT

When nutrients are taken in by the body and metabolized, by-products must be eliminated. Without the kidneys, toxins would accumulate to lethal levels in the body within a short time. Kidneys clear the blood of unusable substances and excrete them, along with excess water, as urine. In addition, the kidneys have the job of regulating salt and water levels.

They are involved in the production of vitamins and hormones, influence blood production, and play a role in the regulation of bone metabolism and blood pressure.

Everyone is born with two kidneys, each of which is composed of more than one million components, called nephrons; these consist of blood filters (glomeruli) and urine collectors (tubules).

Urine flows out of the tubules into a collection area called the renal pelvis; from there, it flows through a conduit (ureter) into the bladder. When the bladder has collected about ½ to 1 quart, it must be voided through the urethra.

The major illnesses of the urinary tract are infections caused by bacteria introduced through the bladder and ureter. In rare instances, the bacteria may be introduced from the bloodstream.

CYSTITIS (BLADDER INFECTION)

Complaints

Cystitis manifests as the constant need to urinate, accompanied by difficulty passing even small amounts of urine. Urination may be accompanied by burning or stinging. Occasionally, urine may contain blood or have a pungent odor.

Causes

Cystitis is caused by infection by microbes, mainly bacteria. In men,

these symptoms are usually due to an enlarged prostate gland (see p. 534).

Who's at Risk

Individuals with the following conditions are at increased risk for a bladder infection:
— Malformation of the urethra
— Kidney or bladder stones
— Psychological problems
— Use of a (permanent) catheter

Women have bladder infections fairly often. The urethra in women is only 1½ to 2 inches long, and bacteria that find their way into it can easily migrate to the bladder. In addition, any changes in the normal microbial inhabitants of the genital region can foster a

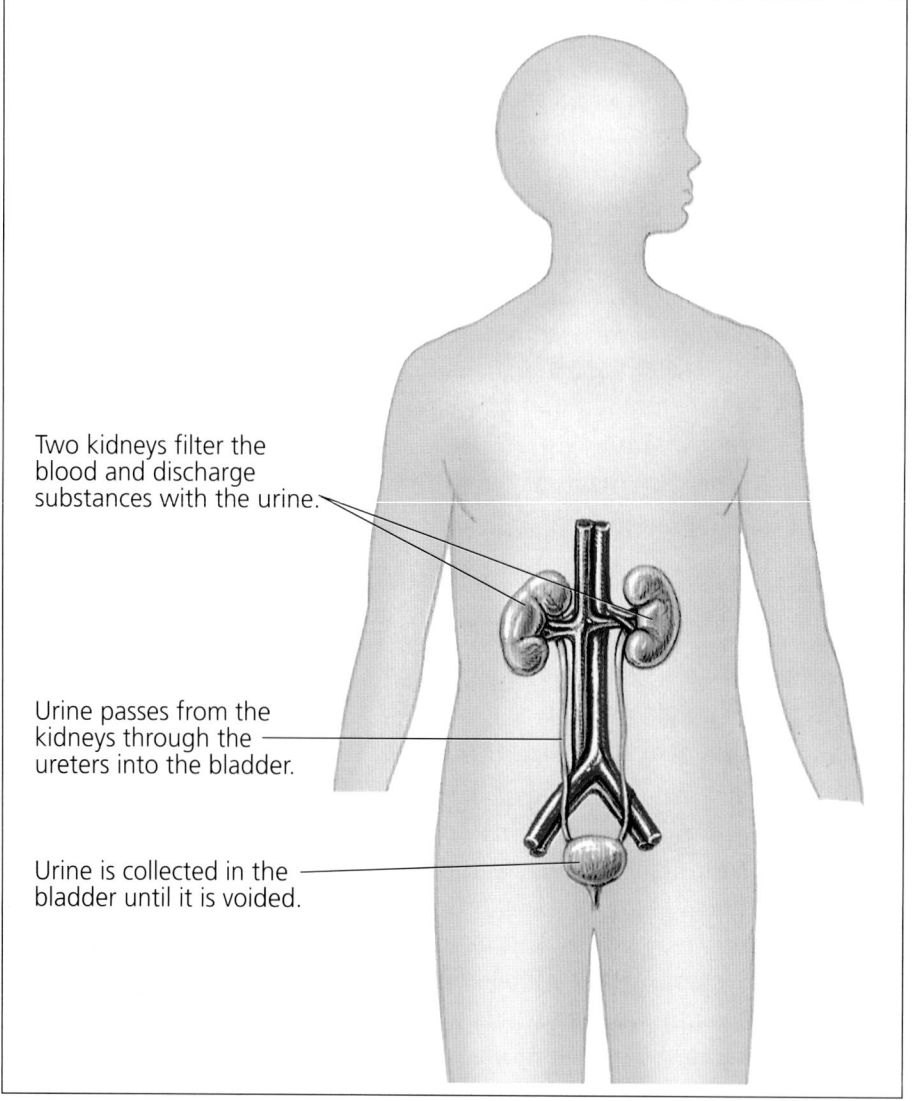

Two kidneys filter the blood and discharge substances with the urine.

Urine passes from the kidneys through the ureters into the bladder.

Urine is collected in the bladder until it is voided.

Bladder and Kidney Teas

Certain teas and infusions can help flush out the urinary system, but are of little use in infections. *Warning:* Avoid bladder teas if you suffer from water retention (edema) or congestive heart failure or kidney failure (see Heart Disease, p. 337; Chronic Glomerulonephritis, p. 423). In these cases excess liquid is a health hazard.

Birch Leaf Tea
Pour 1 cup hot water over 1 to 2 tablespoons birch leaves. Let steep for 15 minutes, then strain.

Horsetail Tea
Pour 1 cup boiling water over 1 to 2 teaspoons horsetail, and boil for 5 to 10 minutes. Let steep for 15 minutes, then strain.

Bladder and Kidney Tea Blend
Pour 1 cup hot water over 1 tablespoon tea blend. Let steep for 10 minutes, then strain. Prepare blend using: $2/3$ ounce birch leaves, $2/3$ ounce couchgrass root, $2/3$ ounce giant goldenrod, $2/3$ ounce spinosa root, and $2/3$ ounce licorice root.

This tea, freshly brewed, is recommended 3 or 4 times daily.

bladder infection.

These include
— Pregnancy (see p. 565)
— Vaginal inflammation (see p. 518)
— Intimate sprays, douches, and bubble baths
— Use of a diaphragm (see p. 554)
— Prolapse of the uterus or bladder (see p. 523)

In men, the risk is greater if the prostate is enlarged (see p. 534).

Possible Aftereffects and Complications

Bladder infections are always unpleasant. They can be dangerous if the bacteria spread into the kidneys and cause an inflammation of the renal pelvis (see Acute Pyelonephritis, p. 421).

Prevention in Women
— Use correct toilet hygiene (wipe from front to back).
— Avoid intimate deodorant sprays, bubble baths, soaps and disinfectant solutions. These change the surface environment in the genital region and provide a culture medium for bacteria.

— Chemical contraceptives change the vaginal environment and make the vagina more susceptible to infection.
— Drink plenty of liquid. Bacteria have more trouble infecting a well-flushed bladder.
— Do not retain urine too long: If the bladder is full, it is less resistant to bacteria.
— During sexual intercourse, bacteria are "rubbed" into the urethra. If the bladder is emptied soon afterward, they are rinsed out again.

When to Seek Medical Advice

Seek help as soon as you notice the symptoms. The doctor will examine your urine (see p. 644). If there is reason to suspect another illness, such as prostate trouble, kidney stones, etc., further tests will be necessary.

Self-Help

All forms of heat are helpful. Drink at least 2 quarts of liquid daily; bladder teas can help provide liquid. Increasing the amount of vitamin C in your diet will make your urine more acidic, causing bacteria in it to multiply less rapidly.

Treatment

For an uncomplicated bladder infection, prescription of a 1- or 3-day dose of antibiotics (amoxicillin, Bactrim, among others) is helpful (see Antibiotics, p. 661). If symptoms reappear after 2 to 3 days, not all the bacteria have been killed and it is advisable to take the antibiotic for 10 days.

Recurrent bladder infections may be due to anatomic problems, such as narrowing of the urethra. During urination, some of the urine may flow backward into the bladder from this narrowed segment. Surgical removal of this narrowed segment is the only long-term solution, so that the urine can flow out unhindered.

URINARY INCONTINENCE

Complaints

Symptoms include uncontrolled leakage of urine during the day or night; involuntary release of urine when coughing, straining at passing stool, sneezing, lifting weights, jumping, or engaging in other physical exertion.

Causes

Incontinence is caused by

— Weakness of the sphincter muscle closing the urethra (stress incontinence). The condition occurs in women because of weakness in the pelvic-floor muscles, caused either by the position of the muscles, by changes after childbirth, or by age-related sagging of tissues.

— Urinary tract infection (see Cystitis, p. 418)

— Congenital malformation of the urinary tract

— Psychosocial stress (see Health and Well-Being, p. 182)

— Diseases such as Parkinson's, Alzheimer's, or stroke; brain and spinal column injuries can also cause so-called neurogenic incontinence.

—Toxins that stress the nerves (Hazardous Substances, p. 729).

— Side effects of medications such as antihistamines (see p. 363), antidepressants (see p. 199) or pain killers like ibuprofen.

— In men, prostate diseases (see p. 534)

Who's at Risk

Eighty percent of those suffering from urinary incontinence are women. Stress incontinence accounts for more than 50 percent of urinary incontinence.

Possible Aftereffects and Complications

Most people are ashamed of admitting to this condition and attempt to deal with it on their own. The problem persists until the odor of urine can no longer be hidden, making the patient unwilling to appear in public. This may lead to social isolation.

Prevention

During childbirth, the pelvic floor muscles are subject to extreme stretching; they can be strengthened and toned by a suitable exercise regimen.

If the condition is due to an illness, proper treatment can usually prevent incontinence.

When to Seek Medical Advice

Seek help as soon as the symptoms appear. Urine tests, ultrasound and, in some cases, X-ray examination are used to determine the cause of the incontinence.

Self-Help

— Empty the bladder regularly, to prevent an involuntary release.

— Special underwear or incontinence pads may be worn to absorb urine and neutralize the smell.

— Men may wear a type of condom which conducts urine into a bag worn next to the body, under clothing.

Bladder Training

The bladder can be trained. For several days, empty the bladder completely every hour. If you feel the bladder still isn't empty, stand up, sit down again, lean back and try again. If underwear remains dry between trips to the toilet, lengthen the interval to 2 hours. A goal could be to use the toilet only every 3 to 4 hours.

Do not limit your intake of liquid during the day; toward evening, it may be limited.

Pelvic-Floor Exercises

Effective pelvic-floor exercises should be learned from an expert: physical therapists, midwives, and women's health centers can train women to use the right muscles. Although the advice is often given to tense muscles repeatedly as if interrupting a stream of urine, this usually only squeezes the urinary opening shut and does nothing to strengthen the pelvic floor.

Six months of daily pelvic-floor exercises, however, if done correctly and regularly, can greatly reduce stress incontinence, if not cure it altogether.

Treatment

Anatomical weaknesses of the bladder, such as congenital malformation, injuries, fistulas or prostate disease, are usually treated successfully with surgery.

In men, weak bladders are usually treated with muscle relaxants (anticholinergics), though these have unpleasant side effects like dryness of the mouth and visual impairment.

In women, weakness of the pelvic basin associated with hormonal changes during menopause is sometimes treated with estrogen ointments or suppositories (see p. 510).

Neurogenic bladder weakness is usually treated with medications, catheterization, or surgery, (to form a new passage for urine).

Surgery

If proper training of the pelvic-floor muscles does not help, a woman can have incontinence corrected surgically. The tilted bladder is straightened and attached within the abdominal cavity so that the urethra is stretched and the sphincter muscle can exert enough pressure on it. However, such operations are not always successful, and the correction often does not last long.

ACUTE PYELONEPHRITIS (KIDNEY INFECTION)

Complaints

Symptoms of this disorder include sudden outbreaks of chills, fever, sharp pain just above the hips, nausea and vomiting, frequent and difficult urination. The urine may be cloudy, or red if blood is present.

Causes

Usually this infection is caused by bacteria introduced through the ureters.

In children, a common cause is known as reflux: Because of a congenital defect in the ureter valves, urine in the bladder can flow back into the ureters.

In rare cases, kidney infections are caused by bacteria introduced through the bloodstream.

Who's at Risk

Individuals with frequent urinary-tract infections are at greater risk of kidney infections, as are those with reflux (see above), kidney and bladder stones, enlarged prostate glands or wearing a permanent catheter.

Possible Aftereffects and Complications

If the condition is treated early, complications are rare. In children, diabetics, or very frail people, the infection may enter the blood, causing blood poisoning (urosepsis).

Prevention in Women

— Use correct toilet hygiene (wipe from front to back).
— Avoid intimate deodorant sprays (douches), bubble baths, soaps, and disinfectant solutions. These change the surface environment in the genital region and provide a culture medium for bacteria.
— Chemical contraceptives change the vaginal environment and make the vagina more susceptible to infection.

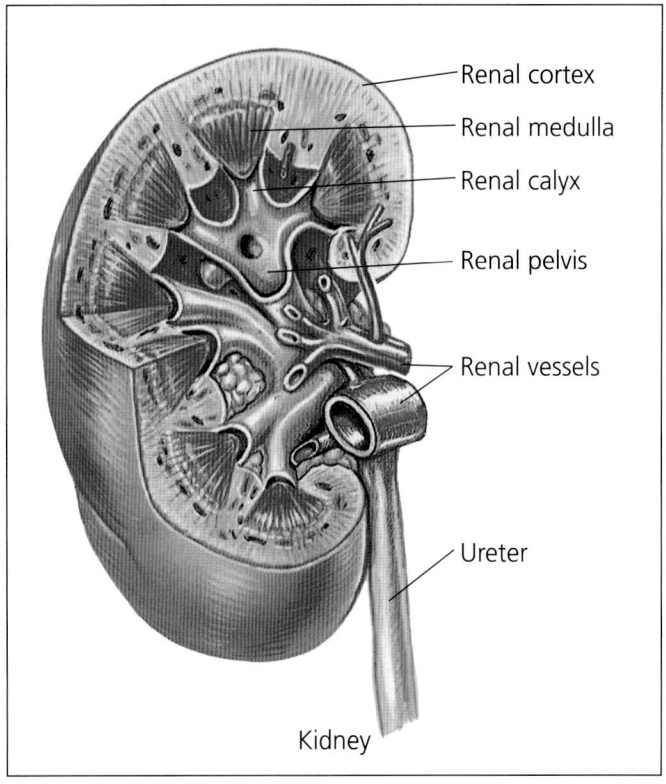

Renal cortex
Renal medulla
Renal calyx
Renal pelvis
Renal vessels
Ureter
Kidney

— Drink plenty of liquid. Bacteria have more trouble infecting a well-flushed bladder.
— Do not retain urine too long: if the bladder is full, it is less resistant to bacteria.
— During sexual intercourse, bacteria are "rubbed" into the urethra. If the bladder is emptied soon afterward, they are rinsed out again before they can cause an infection.

Prevention in Men

See Enlarged Prostate, p. 534.

When to Seek Medical Advice

Seek help immediately if symptoms are present.

Self-Help

Not possible. Bladder teas will not help with this condition.

Treatment

Treatment usually involves antibiotics. Although symptoms will lessen after a day or two, the antibiotics may need to be taken for 2 weeks or more.

In people who suffer from frequent kidney infections, tests may determine the cause of the disease. These are administered after recovery and include blood and urine tests, ultrasound, X-ray examination (see p. 635), checking for reflux, etc.

CHRONIC INTERSTITIAL NEPHRITIS

Complaints
This condition arises when a long-term kidney infection slowly and progressively damages the kidney. The patient becomes increasingly tired and lethargic; frequent urination, especially at night is common. If the disease progresses, nausea and itching skin may occur.

Causes
Chronic inflammations occur most often in patients who have suffered repeated infections of the urinary tract or kidneys, resulting in scarred and shriveled kidney tissues. Another cause is misuse of painkillers [nonsteroidal anti-inflammatory medications (NSAIDs)] over a period of many years (see p. 658) Kidney stones (see p. 424) may also lead to chronic interstitial nephritis.

Who's at Risk
The risk of disease increases:
— With repeated severe urinary tract infections
— With frequent recurrence of acute kidney infection
— With kidney stones
— After many years of painkiller (NSAIDs) use (see p. 661)

Possible Aftereffects and Complications
A damaged kidney can no longer carry out its function. As a result, blood pressure may rise (see p. 321) and toxins accumulate in the blood. During the final stage of the disease, known as uremia, the accumulation of toxins necessitates purification of the blood by dialysis or other medical technology (see Kidney Failure, p. 425).

Prevention
Avoid taking painkillers over an extended period of time.

For other preventive measures, see Acute Pyelonephritis, p. 421.

If you have frequent urinary-tract infections, you should have your urine and blood tested for early detection of chronic infections.

When to Seek Medical Advice
Seek help as soon as you suspect you have a chronic kidney inflammation.

Self-Help
— Immediately stop taking all painkillers (NSAIDs).
— Follow a diet prescribed by your doctor or a dietary counselor.

Treatment
Chronic interstitial nephritis should be treated by a kidney specialist.

The nature of the treatment depends on the stage of the disease.

If kidney stones or other obstructions are the cause of the inflammation, they must be treated.

Infections are treated with antibiotics. Often short-term use is sufficient, but in some cases, they are prescribed for longer periods at lower dosages.

In exceptional cases, the doctor may simply order regular examinations and not prescribe antibiotics.

Concurrent treatment may include medications to reduce blood pressure or stabilize the metabolism and vitamins B and D.

ACUTE GLOMERULONEPHRITIS

Complaints
Symptoms of this disorder include tiredness and feeling beaten down. Often the symptoms appear following a fever caused by viruses or bacteria (e.g., scarlet fever). After an interval of a few days, the fever reappears, urine production is reduced, and the urine is cloudy with protein or reddish brown with blood. The eyelids and knuckles may swell, and elevated blood pressure can lead to headaches.

Causes
The causes of this ailment are not precisely known. In some cases, it has been traced to an autoimmune reaction against the glomeruli, or filter cells, of the kidney.

The inflammation develops as protein components are caught in, or even attack, the filter cells, which become so inflamed that they can no longer prevent red blood cells and blood proteins from entering the urine. At the same time, metabolic waste products remain in the body and cause further damage to the kidney.

Who's at Risk

This disease is relatively rare.

Possible Aftereffects and Complications

Acute glomerulonephritis is always life-threatening. However, it can often be completely cured, although sometimes it can also lead to permanent loss of kidney function.

Prevention

Not possible.

When to Seek Medical Advice

Seek help as soon as symptoms appear. The sooner medical intervention begins, the greater the chances of a cure.

Self-Help

Attempts at self-help can be risky.

Treatment

A diagnosis of glomerulonephritis usually requires a biopsy of kidney tissue (see p. 655). This is done under local anesthesia, but it is risky and can be extremely painful. Other methods of examination include ultrasound, X rays, urine tests and blood tests (see Diagnostic Tests/Procedures, p. 635).

The treatment depends on the severity of the disease. The drugs of choice are antibiotics, corticosteroids, and immunosuppressants.

Blood plasma exchange or hemodialysis are also sometimes necessary (see Hemodialysis, p. 426).

CHRONIC GLOMERULONEPHRITIS

Complaints

The symptoms of this disorder are often the same as for other kidney problems (see Acute Glomerulonephritis, p. 422), with the urine containing protein and blood cells. The disease progresses gradually or in spurts; often it is only discovered by chance because of secondary symptoms such as high blood pressure.

One form of the disease (nephrotic syndrome) causes edema throughout the entire body, beginning in the face and lower legs. The urine is foamy and usually cloudy.

Causes

The causes of this ailment are not precisely known. In some cases, it has been traced to an autoimmune reaction against the glomeruli, or filter cells, of the kidney.

The inflammation develops as protein components are caught in, or even attack, the filter cells, which become so inflamed that they can no longer prevent red blood cells and blood proteins from entering the urine. At the same time, metabolic waste products remain in the body and cause further damage to the kidney.

Who's at Risk

About half of all patients requiring dialysis have had chronic glomerulonephritis.

Possible Aftereffects and Complications

The course of the disease varies greatly, but it often produces uremia and chronic kidney failure (see p. 425).

Prevention

Not possible.

When to Seek Medical Advice

Seek help if urine is cloudy, has a reddish tinge, or is very foamy.

Self-Help

Not possible.

Treatment

Urine and blood tests, ultrasound, and possibly X rays are needed for diagnosis. Sometimes a biopsy of the kidney is needed (see Biopsy, p. 655). This is carried out under local anesthesia. It is risky and can be painful.

Treatment of the underlying disease is often not possible, but elevated blood pressure must be reduced (see p. 321). It is also useful to follow a special low-protein diet under medical supervision, and to have regular checkups in a hospital nephrology unit.

In some cases, treatment with corticosteroids and/or immunosuppressants helps.

If treatment is not successful, hemodialysis (see p. 426) or a kidney transplant may be needed.

KIDNEY INJURIES

Complaints
A mild injury may cause fever, pains, and extreme sensitivity in the lower part of the back.

Sometimes traces of blood are found in the urine a day or two after the injury.

Severe pain and larger amounts of blood in the urine indicate a serious injury.

Causes
Blows, stab wounds, or crushing injuries in the kidney region.

Possible Aftereffects and Complications
Internal bleeding and infections.

When to Seek Medical Advice
Seek help if you are in pain and see blood in your urine. Ultrasound and X rays (see p. 646) are used to determine the extent of the injury.

Self-Help
The kidneys have a great capacity to heal themselves. Usually treatment consists of 7 to 10 days of bed rest.

Treatment
Severe injuries may require surgery, and need to be treated in the hospital.

If one kidney must be removed because of a severe injury, the other one takes over its work; even with only one kidney, a person can lead a normal life.

KIDNEY STONES

Complaints
If kidney stones are too large to pass from the kidney into the ureter, they usually cause no pain, or at most occasional mild pain in the kidney region.

If kidney stones are able to move, however, they become extremely painful. The best known symptoms are sudden, stabbing, dull pains in waves (so-called "renal colic"), caused by a stone moving toward the ureter. Usually pain begins in the back, below the ribs, and moves slowly downward over hours or days. It may be unbearable, necessitating emergency surgery, and may

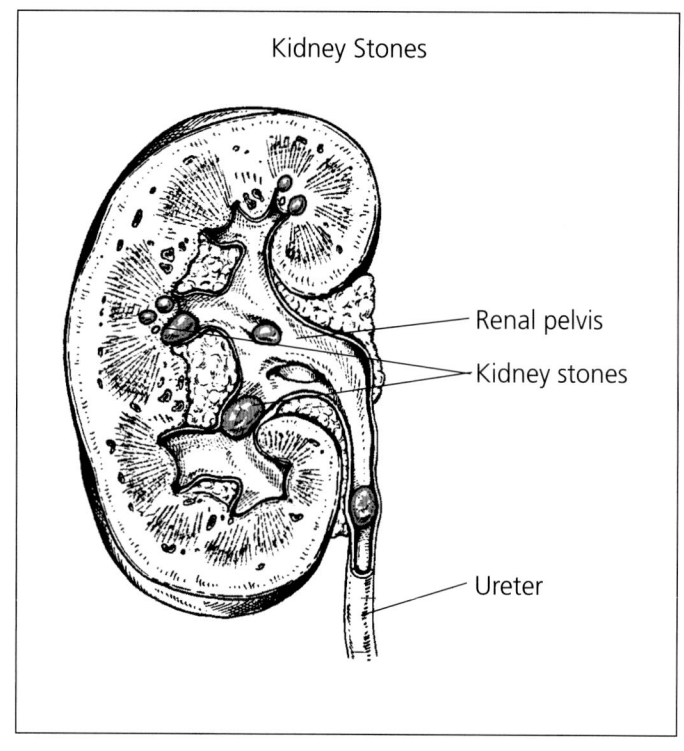

Kidney Stones

Renal pelvis
Kidney stones
Ureter

be accompanied by nausea. Sometimes traces of blood are found in the urine.

Once a stone reaches the bladder, it usually makes its way out through the urethra without causing much pain.

Causes
The following factors facilitate development of kidney stones:
— Chronic urinary-tract infections
— Parathyroid gland disease (see p. 500)
— Obstructions that cause urine to back up, e.g. scars, constrictions, or malformations
— A diet high in salts, which can crystallize into stones
— Insufficient intake of fluids
— Chronic intestinal diseases (see p. 402)
— Long-term use of painkillers (NSAIDs)

Who's at Risk
Men develop kidney stones more frequently than women, and they occur more frequently in older people.

The risk of disease increases in hot weather, when a larger quantity of liquid is excreted through the sweat glands, causing urine to become more concentrated. This can result in higher calcium levels in the urine, leading to easier formation of kidney stones.

Possible Aftereffects and Complications

Kidney stones increase the risk of

— Urinary tract infections (see Cystitis, p. 418)
— Scarring and constrictions, which increase the risk of subsequent stone formation
— Chronic interstitial nephritis (see p. 422).

Prevention

Drink plenty of fluids, especially in hot weather. People who have already had a kidney stone can sometimes prevent further formation of stones by changing their diets. This requires an analysis of the stone and consultation with a physician or dietary specialist.

Most kidney stones consist of calcium oxalate. Prevention includes limiting consumption of dairy products and salt, and avoiding spinach, rhubarb, and tomatoes.

When to Seek Medical Advice

Seek help if you have kidney pains. If you know you have a kidney stone, have regular checkups with a urologist or nephrologist.

Self-Help

Drink as much liquid as possible. Sometimes this floods out the stone and helps prevent formation of more stones.

A special diet may also prevent stone formation.

Treatment

An attempt is first made to flush out the stone by having the patient drink large quantities of liquid, take muscle relaxants, and apply a hot water bottle.

If the stone does not dislodge after a week or two, and if its position is favorable (in the lower third of the ureter or in the bladder), the physician may attempt to remove it by cystoscopy. This procedure is extremely unpleasant, however (See Cystoscopy, p. 654).

It is also possible to pulverize the stone (lithotripsy) using sound shock waves; this may be done under general anesthesia.

Surgery is needed under the following conditions:
— The renal colic does not respond to medication
— The kidney stone has caused a severe infection
— The stones are large
— The kidney is in acute danger from the stone
— Cystoscopy or lithotripsy have failed

After the stone has been removed, its chemical composition should be analyzed to determine which foods the patient should avoid to prevent formation of more stones. The diets for different kinds of stones vary considerably.

KIDNEY FAILURE (UREMIA)

Complaints

The symptoms of kidney failure are barely noticeable at first and often worsen slowly. The first indication is usually more frequent urination at night. The urine consists mainly of water, and more of the waste products remain in the body; as a result, tiredness and lethargy increase. Shortness of breath may appear. As the disease progresses, nausea, vomiting, loss of appetite and an unpleasant taste in the mouth are common. The skin acquires a yellowish-brown color and itches.

The last stages of uremia include pericarditis, pulmonary edema, paralysis, and finally, coma.

Causes

Repeated severe kidney inflammations, e.g., pyelonephritis or glomerulonephritis, can injure the kidney tissue and cause scarring, resulting in increasingly compromised kidney function.

Other causes include years of painkiller (NSAIDs) misuse (see p. 661), years of high blood pressure, and diabetes. In rare cases, inherited kidney diseases such as polycystic kidneys can lead to chronic kidney failure.

Who's at Risk

People of any age can develop kidney failure. Those who use painkillers (NSAIDs) for many years are especially at risk.

Possible Aftereffects and Complications

Chronic kidney failure can cause high blood pressure (see p. 321), reduced ability to concentrate, exhaustion, neurotic behavior, loss of weight, problems in the skeletal system, intense itchiness, loss of sexual drive, impotence, reduced resistance to infection, a tendency to bleed, anemia, heart damage, and other health problems. The final stage of the disease may be total kidney failure.

Prevention

Avoid misuse of painkillers (NSAIDs). Regular medical checkups can help identify problems early on.

When to Seek Medical Advice

Seek help if
—You need to urinate more frequently than usual
—You lose weight for no apparent reason
—You are chronically nauseous, especially in the morning
—You frequently vomit for no apparent reason
—You are always tired for no apparent reason.

Self-Help

Drink plenty of liquids. Do not take medications without consulting a physician.

Treatment

Only acute kidney failure can be reversed. A chronic, progressive failure will, sooner or later, require a replacement therapy: Hemodialysis, continuous ambulatory peritoneal dialysis (CAPD), or a kidney transplant.

Hemodialysis

If the kidneys are working at less than 5 percent of their normal capacity, the accumulated toxins must be removed from the blood by dialysis. As blood circulates through the filters of the dialysis machine, they remove most of the toxic substances. The blood is then circulated back into the body. Dialysis is usually performed 3 times a week, with each session lasting 4 to 5 hours.

The blood is usually tapped on the right or left lower arm through a small, permanent shunt surgically implanted into an artery and a vein, thus creating a short circuit. Alternatively, these two vessels are connected through a plastic prosthesis under the skin. Dialysis may take place either in the hospital or at home, if a family member is properly trained to perform it. Training at a dialysis center takes several weeks. Dialysis patients must adhere to a relatively strict diet low in protein and salt, and must limit their intake of fluids.

With the help of dialysis, many patients can continue working, and except for the dialysis itself, their daily routine is normal.

The kidneys are responsible not only for the excretion of liquid and metabolic products, but also for production of erythropoietin, which controls the production of red blood cells. The kidneys are also involved in the regulation of mineral levels in the body, and of blood pressure.

So, while a number of the symptoms of kidney failure are rapidly improved by dialysis, the functions of the kidneys are so varied that, even if the dialysis is done carefully, severe problems are unavoidable after a time. Therefore, a kidney transplant should be arranged as soon as possible.

The life expectancy of dialysis-dependent patients depends on the underlying illness. Many can now be dialysed for 10 years and longer.

Continuous Ambulatory Peritoneal Dialysis (CAPD)

In this procedure, the peritoneum, a membrane lining the inside of the abdomen, is used as a natural filter substitute for the kidneys.

First, under local anesthesia, a thin plastic tube is inserted into the abdomen of the patient. One end of the tube remains visible on the outside for as long as CAPD is administered, which may be for months or years. This end of the tube is then connected to a plastic bag filled with 2 to 3 quarts of a sterile, dialysate solution. The liquid flows by gravity into the abdominal cavity, over the course of 15 to 20 minutes. The tube and the empty bag remain attached, invisible under the patient's clothing.

The composition of the solution is such that it extracts water, and with it, toxins that would normally be excreted by the kidneys.

After about 4 to 8 hours, the empty bag is laid on the floor and the liquid containing the toxins flows back into the bag in about 15 to 20 minutes. A new bag of flushing liquid is then attached and the abdominal cavity filled again. In this way, toxic substances are continuously removed from the body, as they normally are by the kidneys.

Advantages: Patients are not dependent on others, as they would be with hemodialysis. Because the system is working continuously, patients' blood pressure is often better controlled than with hemodialysis, and their general condition and blood composition are usually better. In addition, a low-protein diet is not necessary.
Disadvantages: There is always the risk of a bacterial infection of the peritoneum, although it is lessened if bags are changed carefully, with attention to cleanli-

ness. Another disadvantage is that the patient must constantly carry an empty bag under the clothing. However, in the newer CAPD systems, this is no longer necessary.

Kidney Transplants

Kidney transplants are almost always the best solution for patients with chronic kidney failure, because they permit a complete cure—women can even maintain a pregnancy—and freedom from a hospital or dialysis center.

However, kidney transplants are often not possible for patients with severe additional diseases, such as chronic infections, circulatory disorders, etc., or elderly patients.

Preparation for the transplant requires a number of regular checkups. In the operation, performed only at special centers, the new kidney is set into the patient's lower abdomen, and the nonfunctional kidneys remain in the body.

There are long waiting lists for suitable kidneys. Availability depends on the patient's blood group and tissue type.

In some cases, a kidney can be taken from a living donor, a blood relative whose tissue matches that of the patient.

Transplants carry the following risks:
— Complications may arise during the operation, although they are rare.
— As long as the foreign kidney is in the body, immunosuppressant medications must be taken so that the kidney isn't rejected. These medications increase the risk of infection, and, over the long term, the risk of liver and kidney damage or cancer.

In spite of immunosuppressants, rejection of the kidney is still relatively common; either immediately or after some time. In this case, the patient must return to hemodialysis, CAPD, or another transplant.

TUMORS OF THE KIDNEY AND BLADDER

See also Cancer, p. 470.

Complaints

The first sign of kidney or bladder cancer is usually blood in the urine.

Causes

The causes are not known. Misuse of painkillers (NSAIDs) over many years (see p. 658) and smoking increase the risk of kidney or bladder cancer.

Who's at Risk

Tumors of the kidneys and bladder occur most frequently in people over the age of 50. Men are affected much more often than women. People who smoke or have taken painkillers (NSAIDs) regularly for years are at higher risk.

Possible Aftereffects and Complications

If not treated, the cancer cells may spread into other parts of the body.

Prevention

Stop smoking (see Smoking, p. 755). Take painkillers (NSAIDs) only for a short time (see Simple Analgesics, p. 660).

When to Seek Medical Advice

Seek help as soon as you notice the symptoms. Your health-care provider will perform a series of tests, including ultrasound and X ray examinations, if a tumor is suspected.

Self-Help

Not possible.

Treatment of Kidney Cancer

If recognized early, kidney cancers can often be completely cured by surgery and medications. However, because patients often seek help too late for surgery to be possible, the average survival rate is not high.

Treatment of Bladder Cancer

If recognized early, bladder cancer can be completely cured by surgery, radiation, and medications. In severe cases, removal of the entire bladder may be necessary. Patients are then supplied with an artificial urinary opening and a bag into which the urine empties.

BONES

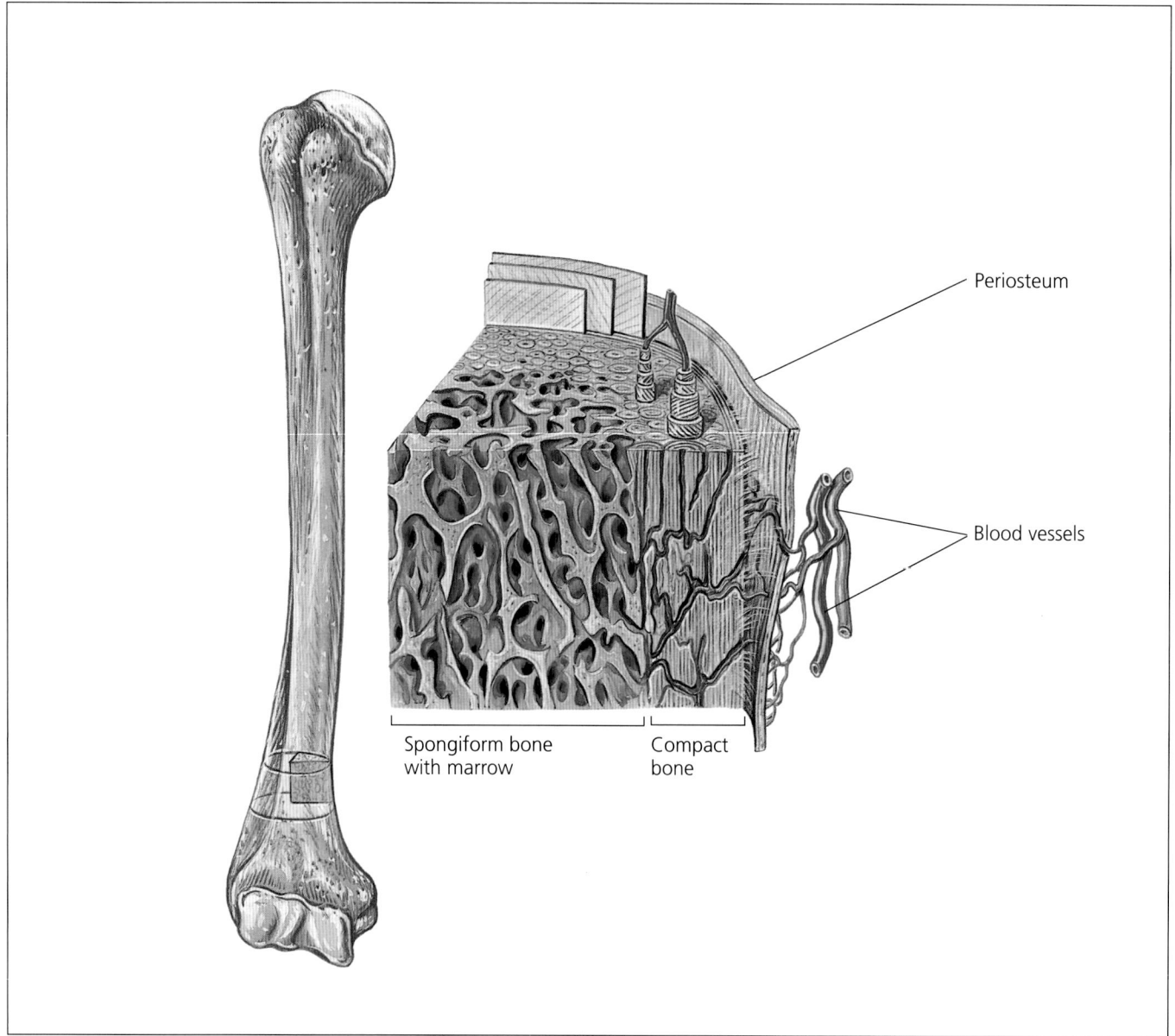

Periosteum

Blood vessels

Spongiform bone
with marrow

Compact
bone

The skeleton carries and supports the entire body; part of the functions of the internal organs and brain is to protect it. The bones are connected to the joints and tendons in such a way as to make movement possible. The bones are also storehouses of calcium and phosphates. Bone tissue is constantly increasing and decreasing, altering the skeleton in response to the various demands of the body.

Bones are surrounded by the periosteum, a tough, fibrous tissue containing blood vessels and nerves that enter the bones through tiny canals. The dense outer portion of the bone is called the compact bone. Long tubular bones, such as the thigh bones, consist almost entirely of compact bone. Inside the bone is the marrow cavity, filled in adults with fatty yellow marrow.

The spinal and pelvic bones are constructed differently, with tissue resembling a sponge: tiny inner walls form an extremely stable structure that gives the bones their firmness and ability to carry weight.

BONE STRUCTURE

A simultaneous bone-building and bone-destroying process constantly takes place within the bone. This is the work of the osteoblasts (the "building cells") and the osteoclasts (the "dismantling cells"). The process is controlled by hormones, by the calcium and phosphate content of the blood, and by the demands of bodily movement.

The building up of bone tissue is affected by:
— Parathyroid hormone (see Parathyroid Glands, p. 500).
— Calcitonin (see Thyroid, p. 493).
— Vitamin D, which the body needs to absorb calcium and store it in the bones.
— Sex hormones (estrogen and testosterone), which enhance calcitonin secretion.
— Exercise (strong muscles place heavy demands on bones, signaling the bones to become stronger to prevent breaking).
— Calcium, stored in the bones.

The breaking down of bone tissue is affected by:
— The parathyroid hormone/calcitonin balance (see Parathyroid Glands, p. 500; Thyroid, p. 493).
— Too much vitamin D.
— Too much phosphate in relation to calcium.
— Too little exercise.
— Corticosteroids taken in high doses and for a long time (see p. 665).

Children's Bones

Children have "soft" bones that are suitable for the normal requirements of childhood, but shouldn't carry heavy loads for long periods. The bone cells spend the first few years of life transforming children's bones to adult bones; this process requires a lot of calcium.

Children's long bones have areas of cartilage near the ends of the bones (growth plates) which enable their bodies to grow in length.

Mature Bones

After age 30, the human body undergoes a slow, unavoidable destruction of bone tissue. By age 70, about one-third of the bone mass has been lost. This does not automatically mean that older people suffer more bone fractures than younger people, however. In later years, stresses and strains on the body are usually less than in youth, and the weaker bones are often still adequate for these demands.

FRACTURES (BROKEN BONES)

Complaints

The area of the fracture is painful and swollen; the broken part may be in an unusual position and/or can be moved in unusual directions.

Causes

Any accident can cause a broken bone. If the bone mass is decreased, a fracture can result from a minor impact that would leave another person uninjured (see Osteoporosis, p. 430).

Who's at Risk

How easily bones break depends, among other things, on their strength; and this, in turn, depends upon age. The most frequent breaks are in the forearm and thumb. In later years, the hip bones break more easily.

Possible Aftereffects and Complications

Depending on the nature and severity of the accident, a fracture may involve damage to the soft tissues, blood vessels and nerves. This is less often the case if the fracture is the result of osteoporosis.

In open fractures where the bone pierces the skin, there is serious danger of infection. Poorly healed fractures can continue to be painful and limit mobility. This can cause abnormal strains on the joints, resulting in arthritic symptoms (see Arthritis, p. 452). In the worst-case scenario, problems during healing can even destroy the bone.

When recovering from a broken bone, elderly patients are especially at risk for blood clots, pneumonia, and bedsores during the time they must remain immobile.

A fracture of the spinal cord can result in paraplegia (see Spinal Injuries, p. 464).

Prevention

Accident prevention will help prevent broken bones.

When to Seek Medical Advice

A fracture should be suspected in the case of pain, inability to move a limb, or an abnormal position of the limb. See your health-care provider (see First Aid, p. 709).

Treatment

To heal a fracture, three conditions must be fulfilled: the broken bones must be joined; that part of the body must be immobilized; and there must be sufficient blood circulation.

If X rays reveal that the broken ends of the bone are out of alignment, the doctor will first attempt to reposition them so they can be joined as seamlessly as possible. Sedation and analgesics are usually required, both because the process is very painful and because it is easier when the patient's muscles are relaxed. Sometimes weights are used (traction) to separate dislocated bones.

If bones need to grow together, they can be immobilized by plaster casts and/or joined using metal pins, screws, plates, or wires.

In the rejoining of vertebrae as a result of osteoporosis, the spongy bone tissues hook together so as to support each other (see Osteoporosis, below). In these cases it is not possible, or necessary, to treat the fractures as such.

Casts

Patients in casts are usually taught isometric exercises; tensing the muscles inside the cast prevents muscles from atrophying and enhances circulation through the bones. Once the cast is removed, physical therapy may be required to restore muscle strength.

The doctor can also advise you how to walk correctly with a cane, and how much weight to put onto the broken limb.

Avoid bathing and showering with a cast, even though it may be protected by a plastic cover. If the skin under the cast gets wet, it will not dry easily and this could cause problems. (Cold air aimed under the cast by a hair dryer can help dry skin that does accidentally get wet.) Before leaving a hospital in a cast, you should discuss your home-care needs with the doctor or staff; for instance, will you need to hire a home health aide or other household help?

Surgery

Setting bones with the help of metal parts usually requires two operations: One to insert the part, one to remove it. Synthetic materials that the body can break down and absorb are still in the experimental stages. International studies have shown that fractures are operated on more frequently than necessary. Surgery is advisable if:

— The bones will probably not connect correctly except through surgery, as in fractures of the joints, spine, pelvis, or heel.
— The patient's health will be endangered by prolonged bed rest. Hip fractures in the elderly are always operated on, for instance.
— There is injury to the soft tissues, blood vessels or nerves, which requires surgical treatment.

Immediately following surgery, canes, braces, or plaster casts help take weight off the affected body part. Metal parts are only removed once the injured body part can support weight again on its own. Since the exact moment for this can be difficult to determine, it is preferable to wait a little longer than absolutely necessary. A thigh bone can take up to 2 years to be fully functional again.

Complications: In addition to the usual risks associated with surgery, working on broken bones brings the added danger of an incorrectly set bone or an infection from metal parts, which can damage soft tissue and bones.

FRACTURES IN CHILDREN

— The younger the child, the faster the healing process.
— Broken bones that grow together slightly shortened or out of alignment mostly will adapt in the course of the child's growth.
— Complications such as stiff joints, osteoporosis, stunting, or fluid retention due to lengthy bed rest are extremely rare.
— Fractures of the ends of the bones involving the joints, are rare, but usually require an operation.
— Fractures involving the growth plates of the bones can cause misalignments whose adverse effects increase with growth.

OSTEOPOROSIS

By age 35 or 40, the unavoidable, age-determined process of bone loss had already begun. By the age of 70, we lose about a third of our bone mass. As long as the bones still carry the body's weight plus occasional additional loads, the loss is fairly immaterial. Only if a fracture causes other complaints can osteoporosis be identified.

Debilitating spinal pains and a crooked spine

resulting from fractures, forming the so-called "widow's hump," were long ignored as women's problems. This attitude changed once the true costs of hip fractures due to osteoporosis were statistically calculated. Many women now benefit from the additional research engendered by this recognition of the economic significance of osteoporosis. They have thus been given the chance to practice prevention and benefit from a healthier old age.

Complaints

Osteoporosis usually begins as a slight backache, which can either subside or develop into unbearable pain. Some women notice that their height is decreasing; others seek treatment because of a bone broken by a very minor impact.

Causes

The factors listed on page 429, which hasten bone disintegration and prevent the building up of bone tissue, encourage the development of osteoporosis.
They include
— age-related decrease in sex hormones.
— too little exercise.
— insufficient calcium absorption, for instance, following a stomach operation (see Stomach and Duodenal Ulcers, p. 389) or inflammations of the lower digestive tract (see Ulcerative Colitis, p. 411; Crohn's Disease, p. 412).
— loss of kidney function (see Kidney Failure, p. 425).
— illnesses of the parathyroid glands (see p. 500).
— prolonged corticosteroid treatment (e.g., to treat rheumatism, asthma, or allergies; see p.665).

RISKS SPECIFIC TO WOMEN

Osteoporosis affects women in much greater numbers than men, because they produce much less of the protective hormone estrogen during menopause. But not all women get osteoporosis after menopause; only about one fourth are at special risk, losing so much bone mass so rapidly that they begin to suffer the results when they reach 65. In other women, it may be another 20 to 30 years before they experience the results of calcium depletion in their bones.

Women who meet the conditions listed under "Causes" and also have the following characteristics are particularly at risk:

— Female relatives who suffer from osteoporosis (heredity is a factor).
— Late onset of menstruation, and menopause beginning before age 40.
— Long periods without menstruation (e.g., in athletes or extreme dieters, see p. 509).
— Childlessness.
— Heavy smoking, which brings on earlier menopause.
— A very slender build. After menopause, the body makes estrogens out of other sex hormones and stores them in fatty tissue. Less fat means less estrogen.
— Frequent, heavy alcohol use. Alcohol reduces the absorption of calcium in the intestines and damages bone cells.

RISKS SPECIFIC TO MEN

Men are at risk of osteoporosis when the effects of their sex hormones are canceled out, e.g., by medications for prostate cancer (see p. 535).

Possible Aftereffects and Complications
Fractures of the vertebra:

This occurs in about 1 out of 500 women per year. The spinal cord always remains uninjured in these cases, so paraplegia does not result. The pain caused by the fracture is often misdiagnosed as lumbago and passes after a few weeks. When several vertebra collapse together in the area of the upper spinal column, a hump develops; the body's center of gravity shifts forward, increasing the danger of falls. Muscle pains and cramps often appear, as the muscles attempt to do the carrying work of the steadily weakening spine.

Hip fractures:

We know that approximately 15 percent of American women will suffer a broken hip during their lifetime. Their mortality risk from the complications is up to five times as great as that of uninjured women of the same age.

Bone fractures of any sort are often the cause of lack of mobility among the elderly, which, in turn, reduces their independence.

Prevention
— Do exercises daily; swim twice a week, or take a brisk half-hour walk every day.
— One and one-half grams of calcium every day is

recommended, either through a well-rounded diet, and/or with supplements in tablet form. This is relatively easy (see Calcium, p. 745): 2 ounces of hard cheese, or a quart of milk a day, will yield the right amount.

— Prevent falls: Avoid climbing ladders to clean windows or change light bulbs. Put nonslip pads under rugs. Wear sturdy shoes.

Prevention with Medications

Sex hormones have been proven to reduce the rate of fractures. Women taking estrogen after a hysterectomy are reducing their risk of osteoporosis; so are those women taking progesterone to lower the risk of estrogen-caused uterine cancer. Estrogen patches are also useful in preventing osteoporosis. But hormones should only be taken for about five years. After that time, the risk of uterine cancer outweighs the benefits. For more information on hormone treatment, see Menopause, p. 510.

When Women Should Seek Medical Advice

See a doctor if you are over 40 and have constant back pain. If you are approaching menopause and feel you belong to a high-risk group, request a bone density test.

When Men Should Seek Medical Advice

A decreasing interest in sex and/or impotence may indicate a lack of sex hormones. (see Men's Issues, p. 541). If you also have constant back pain, you should seek medical help.

Bone Density Measurement

These tests are usually conducted by X-raying the wrist twice at an interval of 3 months. To minimize radiation exposure for the patient see p. 646. If the two measurements indicate a bone loss of more than 3.5 percent per year, most gynecologists will recommend taking hormones. This baseline has been established by agreement among researchers. There is, as yet, no "normal curve" that unequivocally establishes the point for preventive hormone treatment to begin.

Bone density tests sometimes come under fire because too many doctors performing these tests are not sufficiently qualified, and because results may vary from one institution to another. You should always go to the same clinic for these tests.

Self-Help

— Bone density can only be maintained through regular exercise (see Physical Activity and Sports, p. 762). This also applies to people taking preventive medication.
— Get lots of calcium (see Calcium, p. 745).
— Prepared foods should be avoided because their high phosphate content can decrease the amount of calcium in the blood.

Alternative medicines, particularly herbal remedies used to alleviate menopausal complaints, are not effective against osteoporosis.

Treatment

Hormonal treatment is useful against osteoporosis, especially when started within 4 to 6 years after menopause. Together with exercise and calcium intake, they can prevent further loss of bone density.

Fluoride

Opinions on fluoride's effectiveness are divided. Its use is recommended only with clinical supervision, and with frequent checkups to determine that it is not doing more harm than good.

Side effects: Fluoride is ineffective in about one third of cases. In the remaining cases, fluoride is not likely to reduce further fractures because its strengthening effect is relatively minor. If unnecessarily high doses are given, ankles may swell and the digestive system may suffer.

Calcitonin

Women who cannot take estrogen might be able to use calcitonin as a preventive for osteoporosis. But if the disease is already present, calcitonin will not reduce the frequency of fractures. It can reduce pain, but may also cause nausea. It can be taken by injection or nasal spray.

Bisphosphonates

Lack of calcium in the bones is usually treated with etidronate and alendronate, which can also be used to treat osteoporosis. Bone density is markedly increased through these medications. It is not yet clear whether, over time, this treatment disturbs the storage of minerals in the bones.

Calcium

Calcium alone cannot strengthen bones after the onset of osteoporosis.

Vitamin D

It is doubtful that vitamin D can reduce bone loss.

OSTEOMALACIA (RICKETS, VITAMIN D DEFICIENCY)

If the basic substance of the bones does not harden sufficiently, the condition is known as rickets in children and osteomalacia in adults.

Complaints in Children

Symptoms include restless sleep, sweating, limited spontaneous movement, delayed crawling and walking, delayed teething, and distended abdomen.

Complaints in Adults

Symptoms include aching bones, particularly in the chest area, in the groin while walking, and in the spine.

Causes

It is caused by a lack of vitamin D, or insufficient exposure to sunlight.

In adults, additional causes are

— Lack of vitamin D, after a stomach operation or in connection with disorders of the small intestine or pancreas

— Kidney problems or cirrhosis of the liver

— Anticonvulsant medications

— Overuse of laxatives

Risks for Children

Rickets usually occurs between the ages of 3 months and 2 years. The risk is increased by a limited diet and insufficient exposure to sunlight.

Possible Aftereffects and Complications in Children

The long bones may bend as a result of the illness, causing bowlegs or knock-knees.

Possible Aftereffects and Complications in Adults

Since there is a tendency to avoid painful movements, muscle deterioration may set in. The skeleton may become deformed through unheeded vertebral collapse and frequent broken bones.

Prevention

Eat a balanced diet (see Vitamin D, p.743) and get lots of sunshine. Most infants are prescribed vitamin D in order to prevent rickets.

When to Seek Medical Advice

Seek help when symptoms appear.

Self-Help

Eat a diet rich in vitamin D (see p. 743) and calcium (see p. 742).

Treatment in Children

Children should receive five times the recommended daily allowance of vitamin D for 2 to 3 weeks. Sunlight or sunlamp treatment may also be effecive. After treatment, malformed bones usually correct themselves.

Treatment in Adults

Adults should likewise receive high doses of vitamin D. A back brace may be helpful to relieve pressure on the spinal column.

MUSCLES

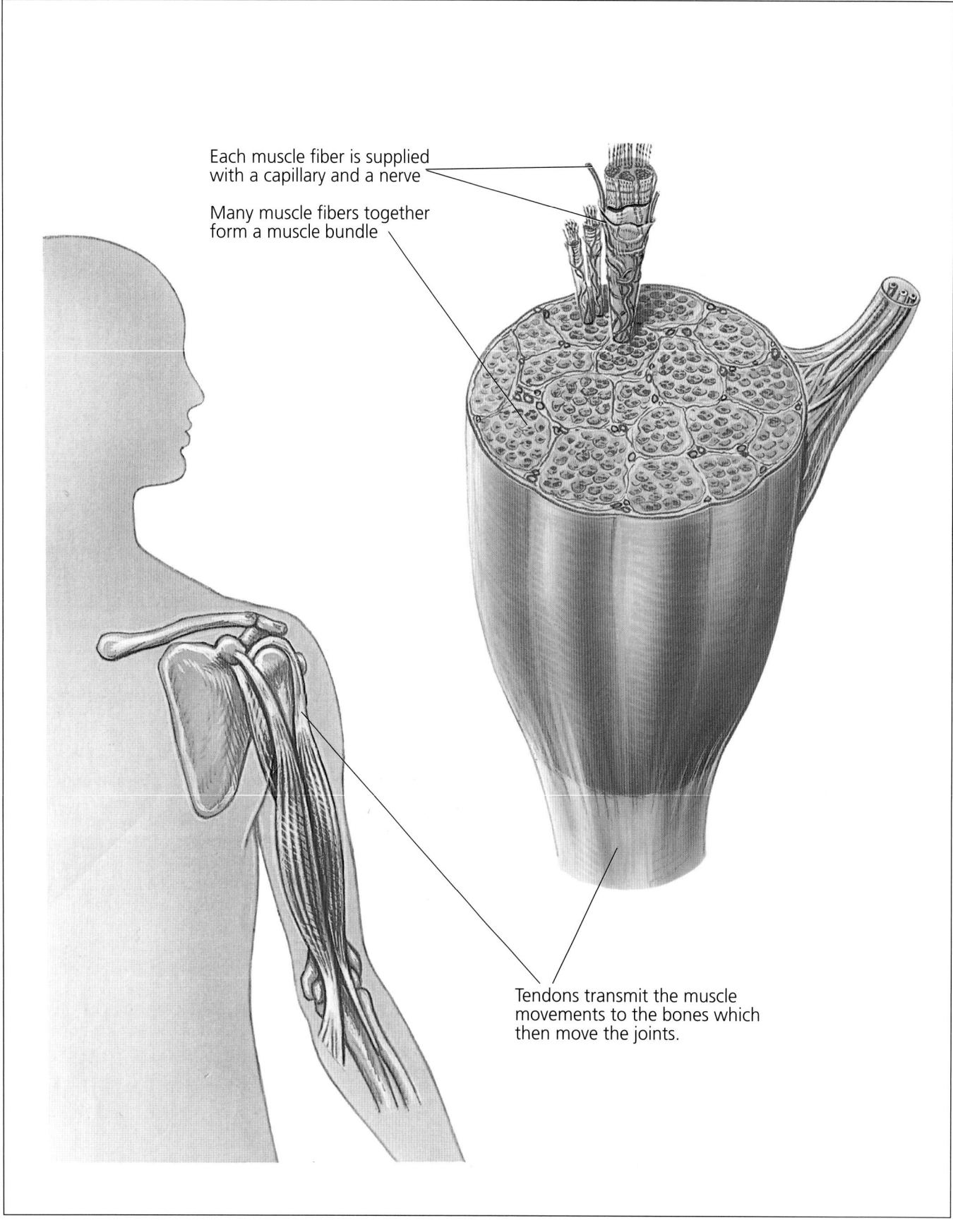

Each muscle fiber is supplied with a capillary and a nerve

Many muscle fibers together form a muscle bundle

Tendons transmit the muscle movements to the bones which then move the joints.

The skeletal muscles make body movements possible. Their fibers are capable of contracting and expanding in very quick succession; these actions are directed by nerve signals. Each muscle consists of a bundle of fibers held together by connective tissue. The individual fibers are between four thousandths and four ten-thousandths of an inch wide, and between 2 and 5 inches long. Muscles contain enough stored energy to allow them to work for a period of about 20 seconds; after that, they need to receive glucose and oxygen from the blood, which they metabolize into more energy. If a muscle is insufficiently supplied with oxygen, the products of its metabolic processes include undesirable substances such as lactic acid; these by-products are broken down by the muscle as soon as it is allowed to rest. Therefore, frequent short breaks are better than a few long ones when engaging in strenuous muscle activity.

MUSCLE SORENESS/STIFFNESS

Complaints
Aching, stiff, sore muscles ("charley horse") usually appear a day or two after engaging in unusually strenuous muscle activity.

Causes
Due to the unusual strain on muscles, lactic acid, and other metabolic by-products collect in the muscle fibers, resulting in tiny fissures.

Who's at Risk
You risk muscle soreness if you are unaccustomed to physical activity, or if you "overdo it" during sports.

Possible Aftereffects and Complications
The soreness and stiffness will subside on their own.

Prevention
Strengthen your muscles through regular physical activity (see Physical Activity and Sports, p.762).

When to Seek Medical Advice
Medical advice is not necessary.

Self-Help
—Warm water helps relax aching muscles.
— Exercise in the shower; the warm water will help loosen tight muscles.
—Take hot/cold baths: Immerse the aching limb in warm water for 3 minutes, then in cold water for 20 seconds. Repeat several times and follow with gymnastics to warm up the body.

Treatment
If pain is intolerable, take an analgesic (see Analgesics, p. 660).

MUSCLE CRAMPS

Complaints
The cramped muscles cause pain.

Causes
Muscle cramps are caused by insufficient circulation to the smallest muscles and metabolic changes in the muscle cells. Nerve damage may also increase muscle tension and cramping.

Who's at Risk
The risk of muscle cramps increases
— When the body's salt/water balance is disturbed, either because of faulty nutrition, diuretic or laxative use, or excessive perspiration
—During (and up to several hours after) unaccustomed exertion
— If you engage in strenuous activities in spite of physical exhaustion
— In the foot and lower leg, when wearing ill-fitting, uncomfortable shoes (see Feet, p. 443).

Possible Aftereffects and Complications
Muscle cramps usually have no lasting effect, but can cause real discomfort. After a muscle has cramped for a long time, it may be stiff and sore the next day.

Prevention
— Make sure you eat a balanced diet and drink plenty of fluids (see Drinks, p. 736). Don't bother taking calcium, magnesium, copper, or similar supplements unless a blood test shows a deficiency.
— Strengthen your muscles through regular exercise (see Physical Activity and Sports, p. 762).
— During heavy physical activity or profuse sweating, drink plenty of liquids, preferably mineral water

mixed with fruit juice.

— When taking medications, check labels or ask your health-care provider if cramps are a possible side effect.

Exercise for leg cramps
Face a wall at a distance of $1/2$ to 1 yard. Bend forward, keeping heels on the floor, without letting your forehead touch the wall. After 20 seconds, straighten up and shake your legs out. A slight pulling sensation in the calf is normal.

When to Seek Medical Advice
Seek help if you frequently have muscle cramps for no apparent reason, or if you suspect a medication is causing cramps.

Self-Help
Stimulating circulation will often loosen a cramp, e.g., gently shaking the affected area, massaging it, or applying warmth. Never apply cold. Cramps will often ameliorate when the affected muscles are stretched in the opposite direction.

Foot or Leg Cramps
— Try the related exercise (see box).
— Press your thumbs into the cramped area.
— Seated on the floor, hold onto your toes while stretching your leg out.
— Seated on the floor, bend your leg at the knee and have someone flex your foot back.

Cramps While Swimming
Turn over on your back; with your hand pull toes toward you while pressing heels in opposite direction.

Treatment
If a blood test shows a magnesium deficiency, it can be corrected by taking a dietary supplement.

Your physician may prescribe medication to calm you or relax your muscles. However, only a few products are available for this purpose, and their use is only advisable in selected instances.

Nightly leg cramps cannot be prevented by taking medication.

MUSCLE CONTUSIONS, BRUISES, ECCHYMOSIS

Complaints
A bruise may not appear until several days following an injury. The blue area (hematoma) indicates an effusion of blood under the skin. Mild pain is usually felt at the moment of injury and again when pressure is applied to the spot.

Causes
Any pressure, bump, or blow may cause bruising.

Who's at Risk
Bruising is risky in people with blood clotting disorders (e.g., low platelet levels, see p.345) or those taking medication that delays blood clotting.

Possible Aftereffects and Complications
The blue area is caused by bleeding of the broken blood vessels under the skin. If deeper blood vessels are injured, the bleeding shows as swelling. Extensive bleeding in the tissue may affect the functioning of joints and muscles.

After a major head injury or contusion, a hospital stay is necessary for purposes of observation. Sometimes several days pass before it becomes obvious that internal bleeding is putting pressure on the brain and endangering it (see Cerebral Contusions, p. 212). A computed tomography (CT) scan (see p. 649) may show tissue injuries of this type earlier. In emergencies, surgery may be necessary.

Prevention
Not possible.

When to Seek Medical Advice
Seek help if you have suffered a blow or severe contusion, especially to sensitive body parts such as the head and genitals.

Self-Help
— Limbs with extensive effusion (internal bleeding) should be elevated as high as possible.
— Cold packs applied around the clock for a 24 hour period (see p. 685) will keep effusions as small as possible.

—Warm compresses or baths can help the effusion subside after the swelling is gone.

Treatment

Ointments containing heparin are supposed to help the body absorb blood effusions more quickly, but their effectiveness is debatable. Heparin spray gels are more effective.

PULLED OR TORN MUSCLES

When muscle fibers are grossly overextended, tiny fissures form, resulting in a *"pulled" muscle*. A *"torn" muscle* is characterized by larger fissures in the muscle fibers. Only in very rare cases is the whole muscle literally torn through.

Complaints

Pulled muscle:
Stabbing pain, especially when applying pressure to affected spot.
Torn muscle:
Painful indentation at place of injury, sometimes with a bump above or below injury.

Causes

— Progressive, excessive strain on muscles
— Bump or blow to a very tense muscle
  Both types of injuries are especially frequent in sports.

Who's at Risk

The risk is increased in people with weak muscles.

Possible Aftereffects and Complications

Depending on the size of the injury and the quantity of torn fibers, the resulting effusion of blood will be smaller or larger. If the injury doesn't heal completely, scar tissue may bind some of the fibers together, causing a loss of muscle elasticity in those spots, and increasing the risk of further tearing of the muscle.

Hematomas may take about 4 to 6 days to subside. Pulled muscles heal in about four weeks, torn muscles in about 6 weeks. Three months may pass before the muscles fully regain their former strength.

Prevention

Warm up sufficiently and do conditioning exercises before engaging in strenuous physical activities. Don't overexert yourself. Wear support bandages or hose.

When to Seek Medical Advice

Seek help if you suspect a torn or pulled muscle; only a health-care professional can determine whether surgery may be necessary.

Self-Help

— Elevate injured limbs as high as possible.
— Round-the-clock cold packs for 24 hours (see p. 685) should keep the hematoma as small as possible.
—Warm compresses or baths can help the effusion subside after the swelling is gone.

External Treatment

A support bandage, tighter at the bottom and becoming looser toward the top, will relieve pain; it should be applied by a professional. Muscles should be moved regularly during treatment, e.g., with
— Nonstrenuous exercises in the tub or shower
— Physical therapy

Medications

Ointments containing heparin supposedly help the body absorb blood effusions more quickly, but their weffectiveness is debatable. Heparin spray gels are more effective.

Serious pain can be treated with analgesics (see Analgesics, p. 660).

Surgery

Extensively torn muscle fibers must be sutured to restore full functionality to the muscle.

MUSCLE ATROPHY

Muscle weakness or atrophy is a symptom of over a hundred different types of disorders of the skeletal muscles.

Neurogenic muscular atrophy results when the nerves governing the muscles are damaged or diseased and are no longer able to issue muscles "work orders." One indication of this ailment is that the arms and legs keep growing thinner and thinner.

Muscular dystrophy results when nerves are healthy, but muscles themselves are diseased and become progressively weaker. This ailment is not always externally visible, because connective tissues often replace the disintegrating muscle mass.

Both types of disorders are partially hereditary, and both are progressive. The later in life they appear, the slower their rate of advancement.

Muscle atrophy is treated by neurologists. Though complete remission is impossible, a targeted exercise regimen can considerably slow down the loss of muscle tone.

Having muscle atrophy means learning to live with the progressive loss of muscle tone and mobility. Over the course of years or decades, this usually leads to dependence on others and confinement to a wheelchair.

Support groups can help those affected by this disease and their families.

MYOSITIS (MUSCLE INFLAMMATION)

There are numerous types of muscle inflammations, all with similar symptoms.

Complaints

Symptoms begin with sore, stiff muscles, a slight temperature, weight loss, and an overall lack of energy.

Causes

Very occasionally, myositis is caused by an external pathogen. Usually, it is the result of an autoimmune disorder which causes the body to develop defenses against its own muscles (see Health and Well-Being, p. 182). Hereditary predisposition may also be a factor.

Who's at Risk

Women develop myositis more frequently than men.

Possible Aftereffects and Complications

Muscle weakness may progress slowly, or may come and go. In severe cases, respiratory and digestive muscles become paralyzed. The patient may lose the ability to walk. If the illness is not treated with medications, the by-products of muscle degeneration may trigger shock. Myositis is fatal in almost a fifth of cases.

Prevention
Not possible.

When to Seek Medical Advice
Seek help if muscles ache for more than a month.

Self-Help
Not possible.

Treatment
The affected muscles should be kept still as much as possible; bed rest is advisable. Later on, appropriate exercises should be introduced and carefully implemented. This is extremely important to keep the intact muscle fibers toned and strengthened.

Muscle inflammations caused by an autoimmune reaction should be treated with immunosuppressant medications, most commonly corticosteroids (see p. 665).

MYASTHENIA GRAVIS

Complaints

In this disease, the muscles tire easily and regain their strength very slowly. Voluntary movements of the eyes, gums, and pharynx are restricted to begin with, eventually followed by weakness in the arms, legs, neck, and torso.

Causes

Myasthenia gravis impairs the transmission of nerve impulses to the muscles. It is an autoimmune disease in which the body uses its defenses against itself (see Health and Well-Being, p. 182). The thymus gland, which is located behind the breastbone and shrinks following puberty, is extremely important for the functioning of the immune system (see p. 351), and is also thought to be connected to this disease.

Who's at Risk

Sixty percent of myasthenia gravis patients are women, 40 percent are men. This disease is not hereditary.

Possible Aftereffects and Complications

The disease may have an acute onset, appear and progress slowly, or come and go. Problems can arise if the respiratory muscles become paralyzed.

Prevention
Not possible.

When to Seek Medical Advice

Seek help at any sign of muscle weakness, especially if double vision or other visual disorders are present.

Self-Help

Not possible. Exercises or physical therapy are not helpful in this case.

Medications

Mild cases of the disease can be treated with neostigmine (Prostigmin and others) or pyridostigmine bromide (Mestinon, Regonol). More serious cases are treated with immunosuppressant medications like azathioprine (Imuran) and/or corticosteroids.

Surgery

The condition of about three fourths of myasthenia gravis patients improves significantly after removal of the thymus gland.

HERNIAS

Hernias are openings in the body tissues through which organs or tissues protrude.

Umbilical hernia: Parts of the peritoneum, the membrane lining the abdominal cavity, protrude through weak tissue surrounding the navel.

Epigastric hernia: Fatty tissue protrudes through weak connective tissue between navel and breastbone.

Inguinal hernia: Part(s) of the intestines protrude through a weak spot in the groin. In men this is a canal where the spermatic cord and blood vessels travel to the testicles; in women it is one of the uterine bands.

Femoral hernia: Parts of the peritoneum or intestines protrude low in the groin, at a point between trunk and legs where large blood vessels are present.

Hiatal hernia: Part of the stomach protrudes into the thoracic cavity through an opening in the diaphragm.

Complaints

Epigastric, umbilical, femoral and inguinal hernias: Usually swelling develops over the course of several weeks. The hernia may also appear suddenly after exertion, such as hoisting a heavy load.

Constricted (incarcerated) inguinal hernia: The hernial bulge enlarges and turns red, accompanied by severe pain. An incarcerated inguinal hernia is an acute emergency and must be treated immediately.

Hiatal hernia: Depending on the type, this hernia may produce no symptoms, or symptoms similar to those of angina pectoris: pressure in the stomach, heartburn, belching, vomiting, and pain in the upper-left portion of the abdomen, possibly extending to the back and heart area, especially when lying down.

Causes

Hernias result when connective tissues are unable to withstand the pressure of inner organs.

Who's at Risk

The risk of hernia is increased in
— Overweight individuals
— People with congenitally weakened connective tissues
— People who constantly or repeatedly strain the stomach muscles, either by heavy lifting or carrying; straining at passing stool; or coughing continuously
— Athletes and dancers

Possible Aftereffects and Complications

If the hernia can be pushed back into place, it is not a problem. If it cannot, or if it keeps recurring, the protruding tissues are at risk.

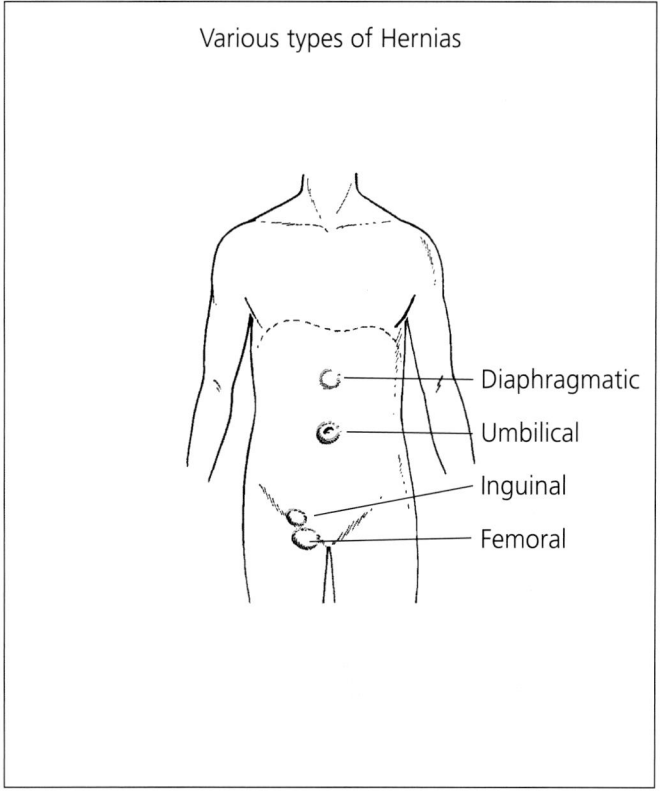

Various types of Hernias

Diaphragmatic
Umbilical
Inguinal
Femoral

Constricted (incarcerated) hernias (primarily inguinal and femoral): An intestinal loop may become lodged in the hernial opening and die off due to lack of circulation.

Hiatal Hernias: This type usually causes no problems. There is the danger, however, that a hiatal hernia may be needlessly operated on; or that a more serious disorder may be misdiagnosed as a hiatal hernia. Half of hiatal hernia patients are also suffering from a more serious disease, usually indicated by blood in the stool.

Prevention

— Lose excess weight (see p. 728).
— Make sure you have regular bowel movements (see Constipation, p. 406).
— Strengthen your connective tissues (see Physical Activity and Sports, p. 762).
— Carry heavy loads on shoulders, not in front of you.

When to Seek Medical Advice

Seek help if you notice swelling in the abdominal area, or if you frequently suffer from stomachache or heartburn.

Self-Help

Hernia supports are not helpful in the long term because their pressure may damage the underlying tissue, complicating future operations.

Inguinal hernias in children: A warm bath may soothe the child, after which the hernia may be able to be simply pushed back into place.

Umbilical hernias in children: Navel bands are not effective.

Treatment

Epigastric hernias: They may remain untreated as long as there are no problems. They have practically no life-threatening complications.

Hiatal hernias: An operation is very rarely necessary.

All other hernias: All other hernias should be sutured together surgically. A hospital stay of a few days may be required, followed by several weeks of taking it easy.

Endoscopic operations are also an option. These procedures require only two small slits in the abdomen, and are less taxing than a major abdominal operation.

Inguinal hernias in children: They may be treated on an outpatient basis.

Umbilical hernias in children: If the hernia has not closed by age 5, this should be done surgically.

Hernia Tip

An incarcerated hernia must be operated on immediately; so it is a good idea to have an operation before the hernia has a chance to become incarcerated.

TENDONS AND LIGAMENTS

Muscles are connected to the bones and joints by tendons, which transmit the muscles' movements to the bones. Tendons are extremely strong, but only slightly elastic. They slide in a track known as the tendon sheath. Mucus-filled sacs, the bursas, provide lubrication and distribute pressure evenly so skin, tendons, and muscles can glide smoothly over each other. The fluid in the sacs is similar to the fluid that lubricates the joints.

Ligaments are similar in structure to tendons. They, too, have great tensile strength but are inelastic; they do not stretch like rubber bands. Their function is to keep the joints together and in place. If the joint capsule is stretched too far during an injury, the ligaments are likely to tear; a sudden, severe stress may cause them to rupture or tear through.

If the ligaments are too loose, the joint becomes unstable, and the bones slip out of place and tend to wear down prematurely.

SPRAINS AND STRAINS

Complaints

Strains: Pain when the joint is moved.
Sprains: Sudden, sharp pain. The muscle connected to the tendon becomes immobile. Immediately after the injury, there is a depression above the site of the sprain, but this later disappears as the entire area swells.

Causes

If the tissue surrounding a tendon is poorly supplied with blood, or the tendon sheath is inflamed, the tendon cannot move freely. Such tendons are not able to withstand much stress, and if overloaded, may tear, although they rarely tear all the way through.
A tendon can be strained by an otherwise normal load if it hasn't moved in a while or hasn't been warmed up sufficiently, if it's wet, or if the weather is cold. Healthy tendons tear only when subjected to unusual stress, e.g.,
— Sudden interruption of a motion, as in a fall
— A blow to a tendon under tension

Who's at Risk

You are at higher risk for strains and sprains if you
— Run on an uneven surface, or on hard or sticky surfaces (especially in a gym)

— Play sports requiring quick, powerful movements, such as sprinting, broad jumping, hurdles, tennis or squash

Possible Aftereffects and Complications

A mild strain heals in 2 to 10 days, a more severe strain may require up to 6 weeks, and a sprain may take ten weeks. If the patient doesn't wait long enough before resuming regular activities, the injury will take still longer to heal. The joint connected to the ligament or tendon may be injured again. If the tendons and ligaments do not recover the ability to hold the joint tightly enough, it may be subject to arthritic changes as a late complication (see p. 462).

Prevention

— When training for a sport, start slowly and stay within your body's limits.
— If you have already had a number of strains, protect the joint with an elastic bandage.
— Warm up adequately before heavy exertion.
— Wear soft-soled shoes that fit correctly, especially when playing sports.

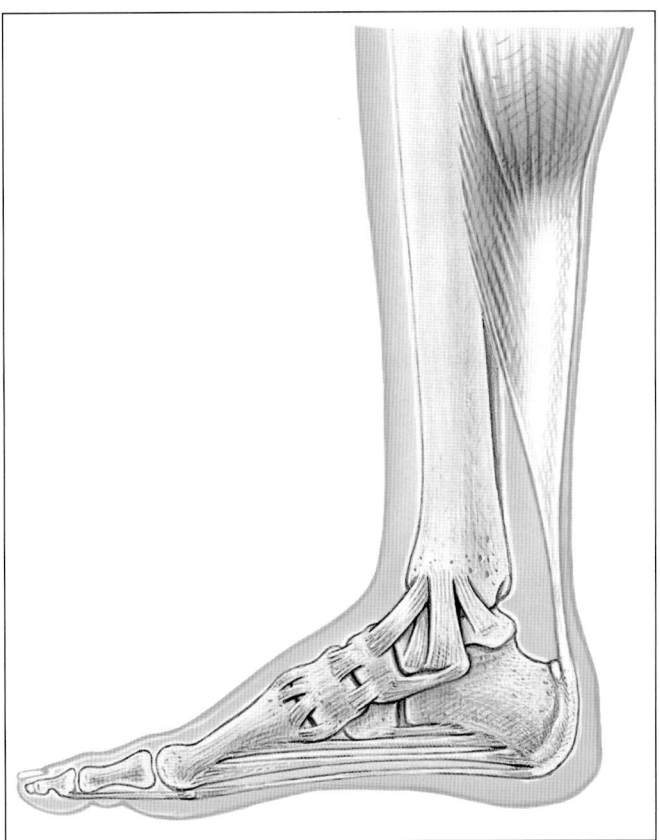

When to Seek Medical Advice

Seek help if you suspect you have a strain or a sprain.

Self-Help

— Keep the affected part of your body raised and don't move it.
— Apply cold packs (see p. 685).
— A strain can be treated with warmth the next day (see p. 691).

Apply compression packs or support bandages only if you have been taught how by a professional. Tension or pressure in the wrong places can compound the damage.

Treatment

Limbs with strained tendons or ligaments are immobilized with tape or functional bandages, which absorb some stress. Some cases require tendon bandages or even a plaster cast. A torn flexor or extensor tendon should be treated surgically as soon as possible.

When the doctor decides the time is right, he or she should prescribe physical therapy so you can learn how to increase stress on the joint gradually (see Physical Therapy, page 690).

TENDINITIS (TENOSYNOVITIS)

Complaints

Symptoms of this disorder include tendon pain during movement. If tendons of the lower arm are affected, it may not be possible to hold on to objects.

Causes

Tendinitis results when muscles, tendons and ligaments are subjected to more strain than is good for them. (For an explanation, see Fibromyalgia, p. 462.) The inside of the tendon sheath becomes rough, and motion of the tendon in this poorly lubricated channel is painful. Like the inner membranes of a joint affected by rheumatism (see p. 449), the inside of a tendon sheath can become inflamed. The swollen tissue then presses on the tendon.

Who's at Risk

The risk of tendinitis is increased by
— Constant overexertion and motions confined to one side of the body (e.g., typing or knitting)
— Playing sports on hard surfaces
— Increased muscle tension on inelastic tendons during sports training
— Improperly healed strains and sprains

Possible Aftereffects and Complications

Heavy loads or exertions may cause a tendon to tear.

The tendon may fuse with the tendon sheath, limiting its motility. This in turn causes the tendon to become shorter and still less mobile.

Prevention

— Don't continue repetitive motions for long periods of time. Vary your motions, and rest from time to time during repetitive work.
— In sports, build up your strength using exercises appropriate to your condition. Warm up well before heavy exertion; wear shoes with shock-absorbing soles.

When to Seek Medical Advice

Seek help if you are continuously in pain.

Doctors often forget that tendon sheath inflammations are one of the first symptoms of rheumatoid arthritis (see p. 455). If such an inflammation fails to heal even after lengthy treatment, ask for a referral to a specialist in rheumatic diseases.

Self-Help

— Immobilize the painful area.
— Apply cold packs (see p. 685).
— Apply warm packs (see p. 692).

Support bandages should only be applied by a professional, or someone who has learned from one. When symptoms ease, you can slowly and cautiously begin to use the joint again.

Treatment

Treatment first involves bandaging the affected area to immobilize it.

The following physical therapies are suitable: Ultrasound (see p. 651), electrical treatment, high-frequency treatment, and selected physical therapy exercises. Analgesics may be used if necessary (see p. 660). Corticosteroids are appropriate only in rare cases, when other measures have failed to reduce an inflammation (see p. 665).

BURSITIS

Complaints

Bursitis causes pain upon movement of the affected area. Mobility is reduced, and swelling appears above the affected joint.

Causes

Bursitis is caused by
— Bacteria, either from outside the body or introduced into the joint in the blood
— Overextending or overloading the affected area
— Deposits of uric acid in cases of gout (see p. 454)
— Inflammation in rheumatic diseases

The inner membrane of the sac is thickened and fluid collects in it.

Who's at Risk

The risk of bursitis is increased in people whose work causes pressure on one joint in particular, for example, jobs requiring frequent kneeling.

Possible Aftereffects and Complications

Bursitis can be the result of untreated ligament or tendon sprains.

When to Seek Medical Advice

Seek help if you feel pain in the bursa above a joint and are unable to relieve it, or if the area becomes red and swollen. Diseases such as gout or rheumatoid arthritis must be eliminated as possible causes.

Self-Help

— Rest the joint and prop it up.
— Apply cold packs as often as four times a day (see p. 685).
— Three days later, apply a warm compress (see p. 692) or rheumatism ointments (see Joints, p. 447).

Treatment

A bandage consisting of foam-rubber cushions can absorb the pressure on the inflamed bursa.

Cold packs (see p. 685), infrared or ultrasound treatments (see p. 651), or electrical therapy may be prescribed.

You should not use painkillers (see p. 660) unless it is absolutely necessary. Corticosteroids are appropriate only in rare instances when other measures have failed to reduce the inflammation (see p. 665).

Surgery

If a bursa is constantly inflamed and bacteria are not the cause, it can be surgically removed. If the inflammation is caused by bacteria, the pus is drained off and the disorder is treated with antibiotics.

Feet

Our feet are shaped so that we can stand in perfect balance. The arches distribute body weight so that two thirds is carried by the balls of the feet, one third by the heel. The interaction of ligaments and muscles keeps the arch from breaking. Footwear that maintains this equilibrium is good for the feet, but the best thing you can do for your feet is to walk barefoot on ground covered by grass or other vegetation. Since this is not an option for most of us, shoes and socks should meet these specifications:

— Socks or stockings should be roomy and end in a seam in front of the toes, rather than gathering to a point.
— Shoes should be wide and spacious enough for toes to move freely without constricting each other's movements.
— Soles should be flexible, to let the foot roll forward during the stride.
— The closest thing to going barefoot is wearing shoes without built-up heels. So-called "health shoes" come closest to this ideal, but are not considered especially attractive. It is unfortunate that women feel the need to wear "attractive" shoes and ruin their feet in the process. Men contribute to the situation by prizing slender legs visually lengthened by spindly high heels.
— Heels taller than an inch and a half throw most of the weight onto the balls of the feet and cram toes against the front of the shoe.
— Constantly wearing high heels shortens the achilles tendon and makes it practically impossible to wear flat shoes without pain.

If you must wear uncomfortable shoes during the day, do your feet a favor by wearing comfortable flat shoes whenever possible.

MOBILE FLAT FOOT

In this condition, the heel is bent outward to a considerable degree. In extreme cases, the sole's inner edge lies flat on the ground, and the person appears to be standing beside his or her own feet.

In children, this type of flat feet is normal and does not require treatment.

Complaints

Soles of the feet hurt in the evening, feet tire quickly, and calves cramp frequently (see Muscle Cramps, p. 435).

Causes

The foot's ligaments are too weak to keep the arch stable, and the muscles that lift the inner and outer parts of the foot are unequal in strength.

> **Foot exercises to do with bare feet**
> — Stand on tiptoes and straighten knees. Walk around in this position.
> — Stand on heels and bend knees. Walk around in this position.
> — Use your toes to lift objects (pencils, washcloths) off the floor and drop them.
> — Stand on tiptoes and move your heels in a circular motion, inward a few times, then outward. This exercise can also be done while sitting.
> — Stand on heels and make circles with your toes, inwards a few times, then outwards. This exercise can also be done while sitting.

Who's at Risk

People with weak ligaments and muscles are at increased risk of this disorder.

Possible Aftereffects and Complications

"Bent" ankles are usually associated with fallen arches.

Prevention

Do foot exercises (see above).

When to Seek Medical Advice

Seek help if you cannot relieve symptoms without help.

Self-Help

Arch supports often help.

Treatment

A physical therapist can teach you special exercises to counteract incorrect foot placement.

In severe cases, you could try raising the inner edge of the foot with a shoe insert that fits around the heels. Surgery is recommended only when the position of the foot is extremely abnormal.

RIGID FLAT FOOT

Complaints

Flat feet are a more extreme form of fallen arches than weak feet, and they cause pain.

Causes

Flat feet may be congenital or develop when weak feet cannot be corrected.

Who's at Risk

People with weak ligaments and muscles are at increased risk.

Possible Aftereffects and Complications

The tarsal joints may become prematurely arthritic.

Prevention

Do foot exercises (see above).

When to Seek Medical Advice

Seek help if you are unable to relieve the symptoms on your own.

Self-Help

Not possible.

Treatment

Arch supports cannot correct flat feet. It is better to gently support the feet, but finding good shoes for flat feet can be difficult; they may have to be custom-made. If the joints hurt, you should rest them for a long period and then, with professional help, slowly begin to use them again.

PARALYTIC DROP-FOOT (TALIPES EQUINUS)

In this condition, the toes point downward and the foot is nearly immobile. Only the ball of the foot rests on the ground; the heel does not touch it.

Complaints

Pain is caused by placing too much weight on the balls of the feet.

Causes

Paralytic drop-feet and talipes equinus are either congenital or caused by injuries. They are most common in cases of paralysis, for example, after a stroke. In the drop-foot position, the achilles tendon is shortened and the calf muscle contracted.

Who's at Risk

Drop-feet can develop in people whose feet are incorrectly placed during a long period of bed confinement. In bed, the foot automatically adopts a drop-foot position; the heavier the blankets, the greater the danger that a drop-foot will form. The drop-foot quickly becomes stiff and is nearly impossible to correct.

Possible Aftereffects and Complications

Limited mobility makes rehabilitation more difficult.

Prevention

If you are bedridden for a long time, make sure blankets aren't resting on your feet. In a hospital, physical therapy may help prevent this condition. In cases of paralysis, splints are applied.

When to Seek Medical Advice

Seek help if a drop-foot has developed.

Treatment

Sometimes physical therapy or a cast can correct a drop-foot, but only if used in the early stages. Usually surgery is needed to loosen the rigid soft tissues and to lengthen the achilles tendon.

CLAWFOOT (PES CAVUS)

The long arch of the foot is too high.

Complaints

Pressure spots appear on the highest part of the arch, on the ball and toes. The toes are curled under and rigid. Shoes wear most rapidly on the balls and outer edges of feet.

Causes

Nerve damage is thought to paralyze the small foot muscles, leading to clawfoot and finally to the curling of the toes.

Who's at Risk

Clawfoot is often the result of paralysis, or the first sign of a muscular weakness.

Possible Aftereffects and Complications

More frequent sprains.

Prevention

Not possible.

When to Seek Medical Advice

Seek help if you are unable to relieve the symptoms yourself.

Treatment

Shoe inserts can relieve pressure on the ball of the foot. Usually orthopedic shoes are needed, and in severe cases, surgery may be recommended.

BROAD FOOT (WIDENED FOREFOOT)

A broad foot widens out like a fan in front. The cross arch is flattened and broadened, and the arch by the ball of the foot protrudes.

Complaints

Pain in the ball of the foot. The toes hurt because the wide foot no longer fits into normal shoes. Pressure sites, calluses and corns form on the sole under the joints of the second, third and fourth toes. Finding appropriate shoes becomes a problem.

Causes

This condition is caused by overloading the front of the foot.

Who's at Risk

People with weak muscles and tendons are at increased risk of developing broad feet.

Possible After-effects and Complications

A bunion (or hallux valgus, see below) may form.

Prevention

Avoid letting muscles and tendons weaken.

When to Seek Medical Advice

Seek help if you are unable to relieve the symptoms on your own.

Self-Help

Broad-foot truss pads allow pressure to be distributed more evenly to the soles. They should be placed behind the ball of the foot, where the sole can easily be pressed in with a thumb.

Treatment

Calluses, pressure sites, and corns are best removed by a trained pedicurist.

A physical therapist can teach you exercises to strengthen the cross arch.

Orthopedic shoe inserts can be used to relieve the pressure on the foot.

BUNION (HALLUX VALGUS)

The foot is naturally widest at the base of the toes, with the big toe pointing straight ahead. *Hallux valgus* is a condition in which the big toe is bent in toward the other toes by more than 10 degrees.

Complaints

At first, nothing hurts, but the patient has trouble finding shoes that fit properly. Later, the pressure site on the side of the big toe may become very painful, and the bursa of this joint may also become inflamed (forming a bunion).

Causes

In a broad foot, shortened tendons may pull the big toe towards the others. The constant abnormal pressure can destroy the base joint of the big toe.

Who's at Risk

People with broad feet are at increased risk.

Possible Aftereffects and Complications

When the big toe pushes the other toes to the side, its base joint may wear down (see Arthritis, p. 452).

Prevention

Wear shoes that leave plenty of room for the toes to move. Do foot exercises (see p. 444).

When to Seek Medical Advice

Seek help if you cannot relieve the symptoms on your own.

Self-Help

Ring-shaped cushions can help relieve pressure. Shoemakers can widen shoes at the bunion point, or even cut out the leather. You could try to lessen the deformity by using truss pads for broad feet.

Treatment

A normal foot shape can be regained only through surgery, but because the results of the operation are not always satisfactory in the long run, surgery for purely cosmetic reasons is not recommended. In spite of this, the operation is frequently done because patients with bunions long to wear normal shoes again.

Deformities of the toes, rigidity, pain, and impaired gait are relatively frequent aftereffects of the surgery. If only the bunion is removed, the damage usually recurs after a while.

JOINTS

The bones in our bodies are connected to each other by joints, which make bodily movement possible.

Cartilage

The ends of the bones are tipped with rounded capsules of tough, elastic cartilage that can withstand pressure, allowing the bones to rub against one another without generating friction. Although cartilage contains no blood vessels, it is living tissue, containing building cells (chondrocytes) that allow the cartilage to grow and remain elastic. The cells receive a slow but steady supply of nutrients from the joint fluid that bathes them. If the flow of fluid is blocked, the cells die off; the dead cartilage is then slowly broken down, and the unprotected bone ends rub against each other, causing pain.

The Joint Capsule, Outside . . .

The exterior of a joint is a tight capsule of connective tissue, strengthened by groups of ligaments, which lead to tendons connected to muscles.

. . . and Inside

The joint capsule is lined with mucous membranes and contains blood vessels and the viscous joint fluid (synovial fluid). As long as the joint is in motion, the fluid acts as lubricant, shock absorber and protective coating, as well as transporting nutrients to the chondrocytes in the cartilage. Any changes in the blood, such as those caused by changes in diet or overall stress level, are also transmitted to the joint fluid. When the amount and viscosity of the fluid change, pain arises when the joint moves.

SPRAINS AND STRAINS

Complaints

Depending on the severity of the injury, symptoms can range from a brief period of pain during which the joint's weight-bearing capacity is only minimally affected, to long-lasting pain with visible swelling. In case of a serious injury, the joint can carry no weight.

Causes

If a joint is wrenched or overextended, the ligaments can become so stretched that they strain or even tear (see p. 441). Examples include twisting an ankle or falling on a knee while skiing.

Who's at Risk

The risk of strains and sprains is greater in people whose ligaments are weakened by frequent injuries, or who play sports, particularly those involving running.

Possible Aftereffects and Complications

Blood may enter the tissues or joints during an injury. If this happens frequently, the joint may develop arthritis (see Arthritis, p. 452).

Prevention

— If you often twist or turn a particular joint, you should protect the weakened area by wearing an elastic bandage.

—Wear soft-soled shoes that support your feet snugly, especially during exercise or sports.

—Wear flat-heeled shoes instead of high heels.

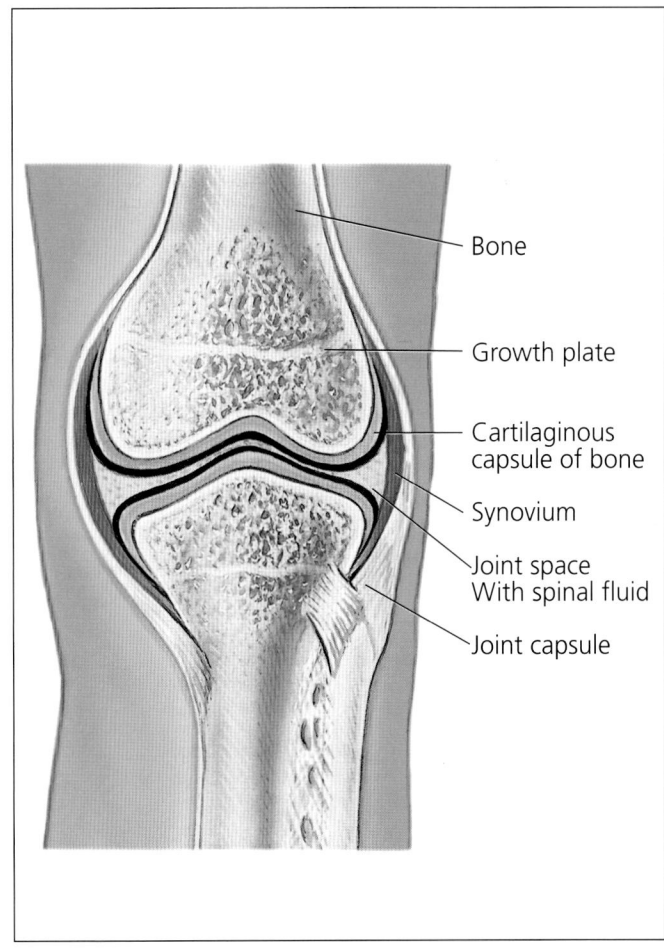

Bone

Growth plate

Cartilaginous capsule of bone

Synovium

Joint space
With spinal fluid

Joint capsule

When to Seek Medical Advice
Seek help if a joint is swollen and you have trouble moving it.

Self-Help
— Elevate and immobilize the injured body part.
— Apply cold compresses up to four times a day (see p. 692).
— After 12 to 24 hours of cold treatment, apply warm compresses to resolve blood effusion more quickly (see Heat Treatments, p. 691).

Treatment
Compression or support bandages should be applied by trained personnel; you can make matters worse by pushing or pulling the joint in the wrong direction. Don't start using the joint again until your health-care provider gives you the go-ahead. Then, with the help of physical therapy if necessary, gradually start moving the joint and applying pressure on it. Physical therapy strengthens the muscles, which in turn keep the joint stabilized while supporting the ligaments. Underwater exercises are also good for this purpose.

DISLOCATIONS
In a dislocation, the ends of the bones forming the joints are out of alignment. Sometimes they spring back into position almost immediately, sometimes they remain dislocated; in this case, they must be reset by a professional.

Complaints
Symptoms of a dislocation include
— Unbearable pain at the moment of injury
— Inability to move the joint; severe pain when it is attempted.
— Swelling

Causes
Dislocations often result when joints are made to move in directions they aren't meant to be moved in.

Who's at Risk
The risk of a dislocation is greater in people who
— Have weak ligaments due to repeated similar injuries
— Have relatively weak muscles
— Engage in sports or activities involving running, especially on uneven terrain

Possible After-Effects and Complications
The ligaments holding the joint and its connecting tendons may tear, and the bones may incur small tears or fractures.

If the joint has been the site of repeated blood effusions, arthritic symptoms may develop (see Arthritis, p. 452).

With each dislocation the joint becomes less stable, which in turn makes such injuries more frequent.

Prevention
— Support at-risk joints by bandaging or wrapping them as needed.
— Strengthen weak muscles by exercising.
— Warm up sufficiently before exercising (see p. 762).

When to Seek Medical Advice
Seek help if symptoms indicate a dislocated joint. An X ray will show whether there is also injury to the bone.

Self-Help
Elevate and immobilize the injured part.

Treatment
A dislocated joint should be reset by a professional as quickly as possible. The muscles may have been stretched so severely that this can only be done under anesthesia. Torn ligaments or tendons should be repaired. After such an operation, the joint will take at least 6 months to heal completely. Subsequent physical therapy will ensure pain-free movement in the future. For the treatment of injured bones, see Fractures, p. 429.

MENISCAL INJURY
The knee consists of three individual joints, held together by ligaments and tendons. Two movable cartilage disks shaped like half-moons (menisci) serve as buffers between the joints.

Complaints
Symptoms of injury to the meniscus include severe pain when the knee is stretched, when pressure is applied to it, or when the bent lower leg is turned. The joint feels wobbly, causing the patient to feel insecure on his or her feet.

Causes

When injured, the ligaments of the knee can strain or tear. One of the menisci may become wedged between the tibia and femur (the long bones of the upper and lower leg), or may even be torn off. Knee injuries are frequently a combination of injuries to the joint capsule, ligament, and menisci.

Who's at Risk

—The risk of meniscal injury is greater in people who engage in sports, especially soccer and skiing. If the body twists while the feet are stationary and the knees are slightly bent, the body's weight can pinch or crush a meniscus between the tibia and femur.

—The risk is also greater in people with jobs involving a lot of kneeling and crouching, for example, cleaning or gardening.

Possible Aftereffects and Complications

Knee injuries almost always involve bleeding into the joint. If the bleeding is not handled in a timely manner, the knee can lose its stability and develop arthritis (see p. 452).

After a menisal injury, risky sports such as tennis, skiing and soccer should be avoided for at least 6 months.

Prevention

Wear protective or support bandages when playing sports or exercising.

When to Seek Medical Advice

Seek help if you suspect the knee is seriously injured.

Self-Help

Immobilize the knee and immediately apply a cold compress (see p. 692).

Treatment

Damage to the meniscus can be verified by an arthroscopic examination (see p. 655), during which any loose pieces of cartilage can be removed. A pinched or torn meniscus requires an operation; this can often be performed arthroscopically.

Postoperative care varies according to the injury. Physical therapy or underwater therapy will help tone muscles and should be continued as long as possible.

RHEUMATISM (INFLAMMATION OR PAIN OF MUSCLES, JOINTS, OR FIBROUS TISSUE)

"Rheumatism" has become a catch-all term for joint or muscle aches, red, swollen or painful joints, a stiff knee, or a backache. These are all potential symptoms of disorders of the joints and connective tissue, which include more than a hundred different ailments, often with different causes and treatments.

These disorders can be grouped into the following categories:

— Inflammatory disorders: rheumatoid arthritis (see p. 455), ankylosing spondylitis (see p. 459), rheumatic fever (see p. 458) and systemic lupus erythematosus (see p. 460).

— Degenerative disorders (see Arthritis, p. 452).

— Fibromyalgia syndromes, affecting muscles, ligaments, tendons and mucous membranes (see p. 462).

— Gout (see p. 454).

Finding the Right Doctor

Patients suffering from muscle or joint pain usually consult their general practitioner, an internist, or an orthopedic surgeon. Unfortunately, their condition rarely improves as a result. Statistically, between 20 and 50 percent of all joint inflammations are misdiagnosed for at least 6 months. Needless to say, appropriate treatment can only start after the condition is correctly diagnosed.

It is usually a good idea to see a doctor in a rheumatology outpatient clinic or hospital department, especially if you have any doubts about the accuracy of another physician's diagnosis or prescribed treatment method (see Outpatient [Office] Medicine, p. 626).

Treatment Options

There is no general protocol for treatment of rheumatism. Together, you and your health-care provider should devise an individual treatment plan to alleviate your discomfort and keep you as mobile as possible. The treatment plan should of course be tailored to your overall physical condition, but it is also important that you feel comfortable committing yourself to it. You are unlikely to go through with a lifelong regimen of physical therapy if you aren't really willing to do so.

Diet
Strict fasting suppresses the activity of the immune system, so people with rheumatoid arthritis (an autoimmune disorder) can reap short-term benefits from fasting (see p. 683). Following a lacto-vegetarian diet is a good idea in the long run (see p. 723). Treatment for gout (see p. 454) always includes dietary recommendations.

Physical Therapy (see p. 690)
All treatments for rheumatism encourage movement. If moving is so painful for you that you're tempted to skip therapy, take a simple painkiller beforehand. Make sure you just take enough to make the pain tolerable, however, rather than completely erasing it. Physical therapy stimulates the body tissues with heat, cold, or electrical impulses. Massage is especially beneficial for this condition (see Massage, p. 686).

After a period of being under the care of others, your goal should be to become as independent and active as possible. Your physical therapist should design an individualized exercise program and practice it with you until you know it by heart; then, you need to continue practicing it faithfully and regularly on your own.

Occupational Therapy
An occupational therapist can teach you ways of performing daily tasks at home or at work more efficiently and ergonomically. These skills can make life easier and help you discover what you're capable of doing despite your illness.

Treatment with Medication
When prescribing medications, your physician must simultaneously consider the need to relieve immediate pain; the potential need to increase the dosage as time passes; and the need to limit any side effects or long-term damage the medications may cause.

Salves and Ointments
Arthritis ointments that purposely irritate the skin to generate heat deliver a specific form of heat therapy; they are indicated when the joints are chronically affected but not acutely inflamed.

Nonsteroidal Anti-Inflammatory Medications (NSAIDs)
These include medications that simultaneously relieve pain, inhibit inflammation and reduce swelling. They are indicated if you
— have severe pain, and physical therapy alone is not enough
— need medication to get through your physical therapy without severe pain
— have chronic rheumatoid arthritis, and are taking the basic medications for this disorder (see p. 455), but they still need to be supplemented

These medications don't work the same in all patients. You may have to try several kinds, under medical supervision, until you find the one that is best for you. In general, follow these guidelines:
— Use only established medications whose side effects have long been known.
— Use medications with short-term effectiveness. The danger of undesirable side effects is greatest with medications that have a long-lasting effect, particularly in people over 60.
— Take the medications for the shortest possible time.
— Don't mix different medications of this type; they don't work better in combination, and the danger of side effects is greater.
— By the same token, don't buy ready-made combination medications.

Pills, Suppositories, Injections, Creams
Nonsteroidal anti-inflammatory medications are usually taken orally. If this causes stomach problems, suppositories may be tried, though their effectiveness tends to be less. Some of these medications can be administered by injection.

NSAIDs also come as creams or salves whose effectiveness and side effects are both minimal. However, skin allergies often result (see Corticosteroids, p. 665).

Nonsteroidal Anti-Inflammatory Medications

Aspirin (Ecotrin, Empirin, Bayer, ASA)
Bromfenac (Duract)
Diclofenac (Voltaren, Cataflam)
Diflunisal (Dolobid)
Etodoloac (Lodine)
Flurbiprofen (Ansaid)
Ibuprofen (Motrin, Advil, Nuprin, Rufen)
Indomethacin (Indocin)
Ketoprofen (Orudis, Actron)
Ketorolac Tromethamine (Toradol)
Meclofenamate (Meclomen)
Mefenamic Acid (Ponstel)
Nabumetone (Relafen)
Naproxen (Naprosyn, Aleve)
Oxaprozin (Daypro)
Piroxicam (Feldene)
Salsalate (Salflex, Disalcid)
Sulindac (Clinoril)
Tolmentin Sodium (Tolectin)
Trilisate (Salicylate combination)

Principal side effects: Up to 40 percent of patients taking these medications complain of side effects which may be temporary but can also cause permanent damage: Stomach and intestinal disorders ranging from nausea to ulcers; kidney disorders ranging from infections to kidney failure; skin disorders ranging from eczema to permanent burnlike damage; liver damage; and neurological damage ranging from reduced sensitivity to seizures.

Joint Injections

You should only agree to corticosteroid injections in a joint if you thoroughly trust the doctor recommending them. Many doctors prescribe them more frequently than necessary. A joint injection may be indicated if a particular joint is unbearably painful while the rest of the body seems to be responding well to general treatment. Injections increase the risk of an infection in the joint to 1 in 10,000. Joint infections are fatal in 1 out of 13 cases, especially in older people. In addition, injections can destroy the bone, in which case the joint will become rigid. To lessen the risk of infection, the injection should be handled like a surgical operation, and the joint should be observed on a daily basis for at least 5 days following the injection.

Surgery

Two types of operations are common in the treatment of disorders of the joints and connective tissue: removal of the joint's mucous membrane lining (synovectomy) and replacement by an artificial joint.

Synovectomy

A synovectomy is useful during the early stages of the disease. The lining is removed to prevent the inflammation from further destroying the joint. The operation is performed under local anesthesia during arthroscopy (see p. 655).

Statistics show that approximately 20 percent of these operations must be repeated within the ensuing 10 years.

Artificial Joints

No synthetic material is as strong as natural cartilage and bone. Therefore, you and your doctor should carefully weigh the pros and cons of joint replacement. Before agreeing to a replacement, you should consider:
—Artificial joints have a limited life span (hips last about 10 to 15 years). Each time you move, a little of the synthetic material wears down, causing the joint to become progressively looser.
—Artificial joints can support less weight than natural joints.
—If the operation is not successful or the joint loosens over time, another replacement is not always possible.
—The operation carries a relatively high risk of infection—between 1 and 4 percent.

Hip Replacement

In this operation, the crown and socket of the hip are replaced by precious-metal, plastic, or ceramic prostheses. Costs may play a part in the choice of material. The replacement is either cemented or anchored into place.

Cementing the prosthesis to the bone has several advantages:
— The prosthesis takes a short time to cement into place, and can bear weight soon thereafter.
— Cemented prostheses have an almost 30-year history.

The disadvantage is that cemented prostheses only last 10 to 20 years.

Cemented prostheses are indicated if
—You are over 60

—You need to get back on your feet as quickly as possible
—You show signs of osteoporosis
—You don't need to go to work every day

In one study, 90 percent of cemented prostheses were still fully functional 10 years after the operation.

Noncemented prostheses, on the other hand, have a textured surface that stimulates the bones to grow into the device. These are indicated if
—You are under 60 years old
—You have healthy bones
—You know you'll never place undue stress on the joint at work or play

It was originally hoped that these prostheses would outlast the cemented kind, but this has not been shown to be the case. In addition, noncemented prostheses break significantly more often than cemented ones.

After the Operation

— Physical therapy is the most important part of recovery from a joint-replacement operation. Practice your exercises at home in between sessions.
— Appropriate sports include swimming (backstroke), bicycling, and walking.
— Inappropriate sports include all those involving sudden, jerky movements, such as tennis, squash, sprinting, jumping.
— Don't drive for at least 2 months. If your right hip was replaced, don't drive for 6 months or your right leg won't be strong enough to use the brake.

Knee Replacement

Artificial knees are significantly more complicated to construct and insert than artificial hips, and it has still not been established how long they can be expected to last.

Artificial Joints for the Shoulder, Arm, Hand, and Foot

These operations are complicated and so new that not enough is known about their long-term effectiveness. It is questionable whether they really improve the patient's mobility.

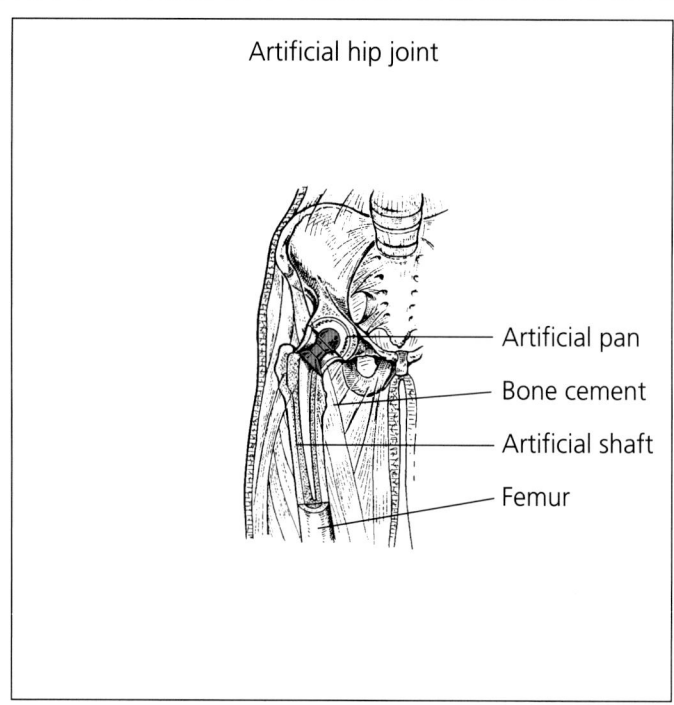

Artificial hip joint

— Artificial pan
— Bone cement
— Artificial shaft
— Femur

ARTHRITIS

Arthritis results when joints are worn down by years of bearing more stress than they should bear.

Complaints

The symptoms of arthritis include
— Joint pain that gradually diminishes while the joint is in use but eventually returns
— Swollen joints
— Nodules (hard lumps) on the middle or end joints of the fingers
— Pain when pressure is applied
— Increasing lack of mobility

Causes

Wearing down of the joints is the primary cause of arthritis. Although one could therefore expect arthritis to afflict all people who have done constant, hard physical work over the course of a long life, this is not necessarily the case. The development of the disease seems to be linked to anxiety over an anticipated loss of independence; long-term depression, grief, low spirits, and hopelessness also tend to worsen joint ailments (see Health and Well-Being, p. 182). The following conditions accelerate the wearing of joints:

— Skeletal malformations: knock-knees, bowlegs, developmental hip dislocations (see p. 433)
— Untreated meniscal injuries in the knee
— Poorly healed fractures
— Endurance sports
— Long-term obesity

Who's at Risk

Arthritic symptoms are found in half of all people over 50. Those engaged in certain professions are at greater risk than others. For instance, arthritis of the knees strikes roofers, miners (46 percent), and office workers (24 percent). Arthritis is recognized as an occupational hazard for tile installers and stonemasons, as is arthritis of the elbow in builders who constantly use pneumatic tools. It is unfortunately not recognized in the case of house cleaners and housewives. Arthritis of the hips afflicts 43 percent of miners, 28 percent of laborers who habitually carry heavy loads, but only 6 percent of office workers.

Possible Aftereffects and Complications

When there is continuous strain on a joint, the cartilage is undernourished and may become rough and stringy. Small fragments may break off and irritate the joint's mucous-membrane lining, causing it to become inflamed. The joint is no longer sufficiently lubricated, and the inflamed cells may release a substance that causes the cartilage to disintegrate.

Because of the pain, the patient may no longer move enough, causing muscles to deteriorate and cartilage to become further undernourished.

In arthritis of the knee, the legs may become deformed, resulting in knock-knees or bowlegs. The severe deformation associated with rheumatoid arthritis is not likely to occur, however.

Prevention

Get regular exercise that places equal strain on all the joints, such as swimming, cycling, or running (see Physical Activity and Sports, p. 762). Ten minutes of gymnastics a day will also help keep you fit and mobile (see Stretching, p. 765).

When to Seek Medical Advice

Seek help if your symptoms are significantly interfering with your life.

Self-Help

— Take time in the mornings to get going at your own pace.
— Schedule rest periods during the day.
— Avoid staying in one position too long, and avoid repetitive motions.
— Lose excess weight (see Body Weight, p. 727).
— Practice appropriate sports such as swimming and cycling.
— Wear soft-soled shoes to cushion the knees.
— If you have arthritis of the hip, walk with a cane holding it in the hand opposite the affected joint.

Treatment

Regular, moderate exercise can delay the progress of arthritis. Only when the body is exercised can the cartilage obtain the nutrients it needs from the circulating joint fluid.

Physical Therapy

Effective treatments include warmth (see p.691); high-frequency electric therapy; infrared; ultrasound (see p. 651); compresses (see p. 692); massage (see p. 686) and physical therapy (see p. 690).

Treatment with Medications

Ointments can reduce pain. Nonsteroidal anti-inflammatory medications (see p. 450) can make pain bearable, particularly before exercising. Corticosteroids (see p. 665) are almost never necessary in arthritis.

Surgery (see Surgery, p. 451)

An operation to correct a misalignment or deformation can often keep a joint functioning for a long time. If hip joints are causing continuous pain and inhibiting movement, they can be replaced, even in older people, with an artificial hip.

GOUT

Gout has historically been a disease of prosperous people, in whom a rich diet leads to uric acid crystals being deposited in the joints.

Complaints

In a gout attack, a joint (usually the big toe or knee) swells, reddens, and is extremely painful.

Causes

The tendency to develop this metabolic illness is genetic. The kidneys don't expel a sufficient amount of uric acid, a by-product of protein metabolism, and its concentration rises in the blood.

Who is at Risk

The risk of gout is greater in people with high levels of uric acid in the blood. About 2 percent of men between 18 and 20, and 8 percent of middle-aged men, show elevated uric acid levels; 3 percent of men will get gout by their 65th year. Women are less likely to develop this disease.

High uric acid levels are caused by
— A diet rich in meats and fats
— Alcohol
— Medications such as isoniazid (for tuberculosis), furosemide (Lasix) and ethacrynic acid (diuretics)

Possible Aftereffects and Complications

If the concentration of uric acid in the blood exceeds 9 mg/100 ml, uric acid crystallizes. If the crystallization occurs in the joints, an attack of gout will result which, if not treated, can last days or weeks.

Gout can become chronic, with no prior symptoms, in about 20 percent of cases. It attacks the cartilage and thus can destroy joints.

When the tissues encapsulate the uric acid crystals, gout nodules result. These are commonly found in cartilage, bones, tendons, skin, and kidneys. Over 70 percent of grout patients develop kidney damage.

Prevention

Maintain normal weight, and limit the fat in your diet to less than 30 percent.

When to Seek Medical Advice

Seek help at the first attack of gout.

Self-Help

— Eat a low-purine diet.
— Losing 15 to 20 pounds can reduce uric acid levels by 2 mg/100 ml.
— Drink lots of water that is low in minerals.

Gout sufferers should avoid:
Alcohol
Anchovies
Asparagus
Cauliflower
Egg yolks
Herring
Legumes
Mayonnaise
Meat
Mushrooms
Poultry
Sardines
Soups, sausage, etc. made from meat or poultry
Spinach
Strong spices

Treatment for Acute Gout Attack

Apply a cold compress or ice pack to the joint (see Cold Treatments, p. 685) and call your health-care provider. He or she will prescribe a medication to take in case the attack recurs.

Long–Term Treatment

Long-term gout medications either prevent the accumulation of uric acid (allopurinol) or accelerate its elimination. Gout should only be treated with medications if
— You are not overweight, and despite dietary changes, your blood uric acid level is still higher than 9 mg/100 ml
— In addition to high uric acid levels, you have high blood pressure
— In addition to high uric acid levels, you have kidney stones
— You have had several attacks of gout

RHEUMATOID ARTHRITIS

In this disorder, several joints are simultaneously inflamed; over time, they become deformed and immobile.

Complaints

Symptoms of rheumatoid arthritis include
— Fatigue, low endurance, fever.
— Painful finger joints, particularly the knuckles of the index and middle fingers; the end joints are rarely affected. Often, corresponding joints on both sides of the body hurt.
— Pain when shaking hands, if fingers are compressed.
— In the morning, stiffness in the fingers, lasting more than 30 minutes.
— In the morning, pain accompanying each movement.
— Pain or numbness in all the fingers except the little finger (see Carpal Tunnel Syndrome, p. 462).
— Swollen joints lasting more than 6 weeks.
— When hand is clenched in a fist, the knuckles are hardly distinguishable from the "valleys" between them.
— Pain in the cervical spine (neck area).
— Sudden, piercing pains in arm or leg.
— Palpable lumps or nodules under the skin near elbows, wrists, and fingers (except at the ends of fingers).

Causes

It is not clear why some people get rheumatoid arthritis. What is known is that it is a disorder of the immune system, possibly caused by an initial irritation, a subsequent reaction and then a continuation of the reaction, which apparently "jumps the tracks" of the body's self-regulating system. As with all immune disorders, the disease is affected by the patient's psychological state. Arthritis patients often find that when they feel "low," their arthritis worsens (see Health and Well-Being, p. 182).

The presence in the blood of certain antibodies to the body's proteins may be an indicator of rheumatoid arthritis, but this method of diagnosis is not foolproof. In chronic rheumatoid arthritis, the inflamed synovial membrane expels excessive quantities of modified fluid

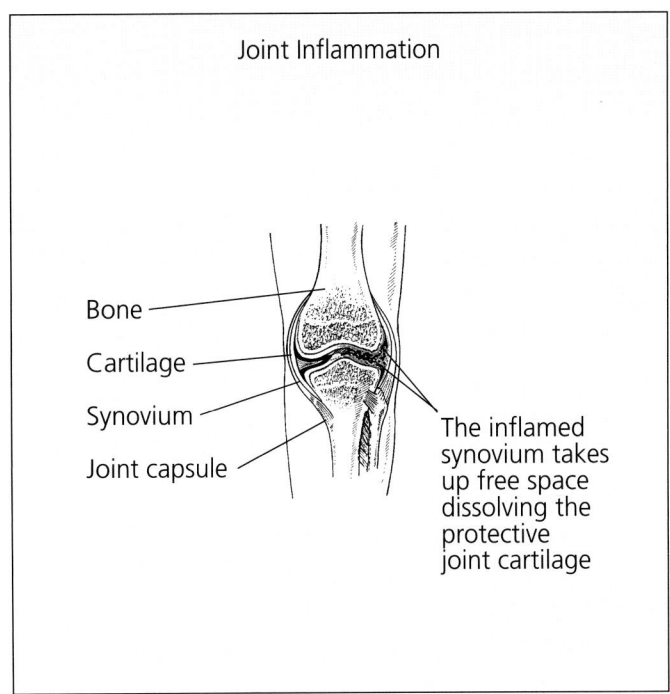

Joint Inflammation

Bone
Cartilage
Synovium
Joint capsule

The inflamed synovium takes up free space dissolving the protective joint cartilage

from the joint, causing the surrounding tissue to swell painfully. The membrane thickens and interferes with the smooth functioning of the joint. As a result, the cartilage becomes damaged, which in turn causes wear and tear on the bones. The joint gradually becomes deformed and rigid. The surrounding tendons and ligaments also suffer damage. Since it is now so painful to move, the patient avoids moving. As a result, the muscles finally atrophy.

Who's at Risk

It is not possible to predict which members of the population will develop rheumatoid arthritis, but we do know that women are twice as likely to get it as men, and that the incidence of the disease increases with age.

Possible Aftereffects and Complications

The prognosis of this disease is unpredictable. Some people remain symptom-free for months or years between attacks. In so-called "malignant" cases, the joints can suffer severe damage in only 1 or 2 years. In some forms of the disease, the heart, lungs, and eyes can become inflamed as well.

In about three quarters of afflicted children, only one joint is affected, the children recover from the disease, and their mobility is not seriously affected.

Living with Rheumatoid Arthritis

A diagnosis of rheumatoid arthritis can be difficult to face, both for the patient and family members. It conjures up images of a life dependent on doctors, medications, physical therapy, and other forms of assistance, not to mention the looming threat of becoming a total invalid. The burden of such a diagnosis is so heavy that it often becomes impossible to distinguish psychological factors that contributed to the development of the disease from psychological factors resulting from the disease. However, you might try accepting your diagnosis as a challenge to learn a new way of life, in which you practice going "with" instead of "against" your body. Try to develop a relationship to your body in which you learn to listen to its language and signals and grant it whatever will make it feel better.

Don't be afraid to accept help managing your life. Many arthritis patients have found life worth living again thanks to professional help. Support groups where information is shared with others suffering from the disease can also be very helpful (see Counseling and Psychotherapy, p. 697).

Daily Life
— Plan your day so that you can rest when pain is worst.
— Pause to let your joints recuperate, whenever necessary during the day.
— Avoid staying in one position or repeating a movement over a long period of time.
— Eat a balanced, nutritious diet to strengthen your resistance (see p. 722).
— Watch your weight: Every additional pound adds to the load on your joints.

At Work
Working gives us a sense of independence and accomplishment, and as an arthritis patient you should do your best to maintain an active working life. Start by discussing the prognosis of your illness with your physician. If appropriate, talk to a social worker as well.
— Find out from an occupational therapist whether and how your workspace could be adapted to place less stress on your body. Discuss this with those in charge of your facility.
— Find out whether other work is available in your company.

— Are any retraining possibilities open to you?
— Should you apply for disability?

The Right Way to Rest
During the one third of life that you spend in bed, it's easy to undo much of the progress you've painstakingly achieved during the day. This can be prevented if you
— Use a firm mattress on a wood-slat bedframe
— Use a small pillow or neck roll
— Lie as flat as possible
— Don't put a pillow under your knees during longer periods of bed rest; your hips or knees could stiffen in a bent position

Sexual Activity
Giving and receiving tenderness and love when your body is in pain or your joints are deformed can present difficulties. The fear of being undesirable and the burden of becoming dependent on others are enemies of sexual desire. And yet, you should do everything you can so as not to lose this important aspect of the joy of living.
— Lovemaking need not take place only at night. Arrange to meet your partner at a time of day when your pain is least noticeable (usually around midday).
— Take a warm, relaxing bath beforehand, or take a hot shower with your partner and see what happens.
— Ask your doctor if there's any pain medication you can take beforehand.
— The number of possible lovemaking positions is limited only by your imagination; discover together which are easiest for you.
— Have the courage to experiment: Hands, mouth, and skin can be used in lovemaking as well.

Prevention
Not possible.

When to Seek Medical Advice
If several symptoms appear at the same time, you should seek out a rheumatology specialist (see Choosing a Doctor, p. 626). General practitioners usually don't have sufficient experience to treat rheumatoid arthritis.

Children with this condition should be seen by an

ophthalmologist every 6 to 8 weeks. Only a thorough examination will detect the early signs of iritis, which develops in 20 percent of children with rheumatoid arthritis.

Self-Help

Switch to a balanced, nutritious diet (see p. 722).
If you have a child with rheumatoid arthritis, consider the following:

— If necessary, obtain written doctor's orders to enable your child to leave his or her books at school so as to avoid having to carry a heavy book bag.
— If your child has a writing handicap, arrange for easier assignments or a longer time to complete them.
— Discuss the issue of tutoring with your support group; perhaps several parents can get together and share costs.
— Learn the rules that will let you stay with your child when he or she is in the hospital (see Children in the Hospital, p. 633).

Nutritional Therapy

Fasting (see p. 683) often leads to marked improvement for many patients, although it is often preceded by a period of feeling worse. How soon symptoms reappear after the fast differs with each patient. Before starting a fast, consult your doctor. Among other things, fasting may affect dosages of medications you are taking.

Many patients benefit from a lacto-vegetarian, whole-grain diet; studies show that positive effects last over a year.

The gluten in grains and certain proteins in milk products can often trigger arthritic attacks. This sensitivity can be tested for, and the foods eliminated for a while. Long-term use of high doses of fish oils, evening primrose oil, and vitamin E can ease symptoms considerably and reduce the need for medication.

Physical Therapy

— Apply cold packs during periods of acute inflammation (see Cold Treatments, p. 685).
— At other times, warmth will help (see Heat Treatments, p. 692), as will baths (see p. 691) and mud packs.
— Do orthopedic exercises).
— Electrotherapy can be helpful.
— Occupational therapy can make life at home and work easier to manage.

Basic Medications as Therapy

Chronic rheumatoid arthritis should be treated early on with appropriate medications, despite possibly significant side effects. Immunosuppressants should be included in the picture because the immune system attacks bodily tissues in the course of the disease.

These medications slow down rapid joint destruction during the first 2 years of rheumatoid arthritis, as well as lessening related organ damage. Depending on the medication used, effects become evident after 2 to 6 months. Regular, careful monitoring is essential. Early treatment with medications is particularly important for children, since they respond most readily to its effect, and further joint destruction can be minimized.

Side effects: All medications used for rheumatoid arthritis have pronounced side effects. Have your health-care provider explain the risks involved.

Treatment with Nonsteroidal Anti-Inflammatory Medications

These are indicated if short-term pain relief is required during an acute attack, or if the other medications have not yet "kicked in" and aren't relieving pain and inflammation sufficiently (see Nonsteroid anti-inflammatory Medications, p. 450).

Corticosteroid Treatment

Corticosteroids can alleviate rheumatoid arthritis, but cannot cure it. If other efforts to reduce inflammation are insufficient, corticosteroids can help (see p. 665).

Surgery (see Surgery, p. 451)

A *synovectomy* (removal of the inflamed membrane in the joint) should be performed at an early point in the illness to delay destruction of the joint. This usually relieves symptoms, even if temporarily. Joints may also be replaced with artificial ones.

Medications used to treat rheumatoid arthritis

Auranofin (Ridaura)
Aurothioglucose (Solganal)
Azathioprine (Imuran)
Cyclosporine (Sandimmune, Neoral)
Hydroxychloroquine sulfate (Plaquenil)
Methotrexate (Rheumatrex)

PSORIATIC ARTHRITIS

Complaints

The symptoms of this disease combine psoriasis (see p. 278) with joint inflammation.

— Usually either all the joints of one finger or toe are inflamed, or corresponding joints on several fingers are inflamed.

— Ankle and knee joints may be affected.

— Sometimes no psoriatic symptoms develop. In children, the joints are often affected earlier than the skin.

— Pitting of fingernails in addition to the other complaints are diagnostic indicators of psoriatic arthritis.

Causes

The causes of this disease are unknown.

Who's at Risk

Psoriasis sufferers have a 20 percent chance of also developing inflamed joints.

Possible Aftereffects and Complications

Compared to rheumatoid arthritis, psoriatic arthritis is easier to live with (see also Living with Rheumatoid Arthritis, p.456).

Prevention

Prevention is not possible.

When to Seek Medical Advice

Seek medical advice if symptoms appear.

Self-Help

Follow procedures recommended in Self-Help for Rheumatoid Arthritis, p. 457.

Treatment

Joint pain can be managed with analgesics (see p. 660). The illness itself is treated with the basic anti-arthritic medications (see list on p. 457). Nonsteroid antiarthritic medications may exacerbate the skin condition.

RHEUMATIC FEVER, REACTIVE ARTHRITIS

Complaints

Symptoms include red, swollen, painful joints, usually in knees or ankles, possibly accompanied by fever, sore throat, scarlet fever, tendinitis, conjunctivitis or iritis, or kidney infections.

Causes

The joint inflammations typically are a delayed reaction to infections caused by

— Streptococci (throat infections or scarlet fever)

— Yersinia (various gastrointestinal ailments)

— Gonococci (sexually transmitted diseases)

— Chlamydia (bladder or genital infections)

— Lyme disease bacteria transmitted by tick bites

Who's at Risk

People who are HLA-B27 positive are at greater risk (see Ankylosing Spondylitis, p. 459). Rheumatic fever following a strep infection is found mostly in children and adolescents. Since the advent of antibiotics its incidence has declined in the industrialized nations.

Possible Aftereffects and Complications

The joint inflammations may take a long time to heal. Rheumatic fever caused by streptococci may result in heart valve damage. Even if the illness is successfully overcome, the resulting heart damage may lead to early death.

Prevention

The infectious illnesses should be treated promptly with antibiotics (see p. 661).

When to Seek Medical Advice

Seek help if your joints start to hurt during or after one of the illnesses listed under "Causes." Joint pain may take a while to appear: 2 to 3 weeks following strep throat or scarlet fever, several weeks to over a year following a tick bite.

Self-Help

Apply cold packs to joints (see Cold Treatments, p. 685).

Treatment
The infectious illness should be treated with antibiotics. Joint pain can be alleviated by nonsteroidal antiarthritis medications (see Rheumatism, p. 449). If the rheumatic fever is the result of a strep infection, a long-term course of penicillin is usually prescribed to prevent recurrence or reinfection.

ANKYLOSING SPONDYLITIS
This term refers to inflammations of the spine, though other joints may also be affected.

Complaints
Pain appears in the spine and lower back; it worsens when lying down and lessens when the patient is moving. The pain may at first be confused with sciatica, but tends to come on gradually rather than suddenly like sciatica. Picking something up off the floor becomes a major challenge.

Symptoms also include
— Recurring joint pains that come and go
— A feeling of tightness in the chest when inhaling, coughing or sneezing;
— Pains in the knees or heels—approximately one-third of the youngest patients experience these symptoms before the backache.

Causes
Ankylosing spondylitis is an autoimmune disorder (see Health and Well-Being, p. 182). The tendency to develop this illness is probably hereditary; one indication may be the HLA-B27 marker in the blood (see When to Seek Medical Advice, below).

Who's at Risk
Men are four times more likely to develop ankylosing spondylitis than women. Development usually occurs between the ages of 20 and 30. If a close relative has the disease, the risk is higher.

Possible Aftereffects and Complications
This disease progresses in stages, with possible long periods of remission between episodes. The vertebrae undergo a progressive stiffening from the lower to the upper back, resulting in the curvature of the spine typical of ankylosing spondylitis, which forces the head forward and down. The chest cavity becomes rigid, making breathing difficult. In only one fifth to one third of ankylosing spondylitis patients does the disease reach this stage, however; in most cases it stops earlier, even if the disease has been present for decades. Women usually have milder forms of the illness.

The role of heredity: The probability of the child of an ankylosing spondylitis patient developing the disease is uncertain. The probability is higher if both parents have the disease. Testing the children of ankylosing spondylitis patients for the HLA-B27 marker is pointless, however, since a positive result may simply engender severe anxiety and nothing can be done to prevent the disease.

Pregnancy: The symptoms of ankylosing spondylitis usually persist during pregnancy, but a caesarian section should only be necessary if the hips or pelvis are excessively rigid.

Prevention
There is no prevention for this disease.

When to Seek Medical Advice
Seek medical advice if symptoms are present. X rays may only show an inflamed sacro-iliac joint 4 to 12 months after symptoms appear. The most accurate diagnostic technology is a computed tomography (CT) scan (see p. 649).

Since the typical indicators of ankylosing spondylitis may not show up initially, patients are frequently misdiagnosed and treated for another disease, to the extent of undergoing an unnecessary disk operation.

Since about 75 percent of patients are HLA-B27 positive, initial testing for this marker in the white blood cells makes a correct diagnosis somewhat easier. However, about 10 percent of people without ankylosing spondylitis are also HLA-B27 positive.

Self-Help
— Lie on your stomach for at least an hour a day to prevent your spine from becoming bent to one side or the other. If you can't stand this position for long, break the hour up into shorter time periods, or try placing a pillow under your chest.
— Lie as flat, and on as hard a surface, as possible. If faced with a sagging bed when traveling, place the mattress on the floor.

— Avoid hard physical labor.
— Practice appropriate sports like swimming (back stroke or crawl), volleyball, cross-country skiing, or cycling.
—Take breaks during work and on car trips, and do exercises (including deep breathing exercises) to loosen you up. If possible, lie down, particularly on your stomach.
— If you work sitting down, get up and stretch your legs frequently.
— Singing and whistling are good breathing exercises.
—Wear soft-soled shoes to cushion the effects of walking on asphalt.

Treatment

The main goal of treatment is to keep the spine limber and flexible. Once it stiffens, the damage is done. You should incorporate therapeutic exercises (twice a day for 30 minutes) into your daily schedule so doing them becomes as automatic as brushing your teeth.

Physical Therapy

Therapies include orthopedic exercises, massage (see p. 686), and heat treatment to alleviate pain, but not during acute inflammations (see p. 692).

Medications (see Rheumatism, p. 449, 457)

Nonsteroidal antiarthritis drugs can reduce pain and make exercising an option. Corticosteroids should be used only in exceptionally severe cases.

Surgery (see Surgery, p. 451)

Replacing a rigid hip joint may be an option for younger patients.

Severe curvature of the spine forces the patient's head down. Surgical intervention can at least straighten the spine enough for the patient to be able to look directly in front of himself or herself.

SYSTEMIC LUPUS ERYTHEMATOSUS

Complaints

The symptoms of lupus include
—Long-term low-grade fever, accompanied by fatigue and weight loss
— Joint pain resembling rheumatoid arthritis (see p. 455)

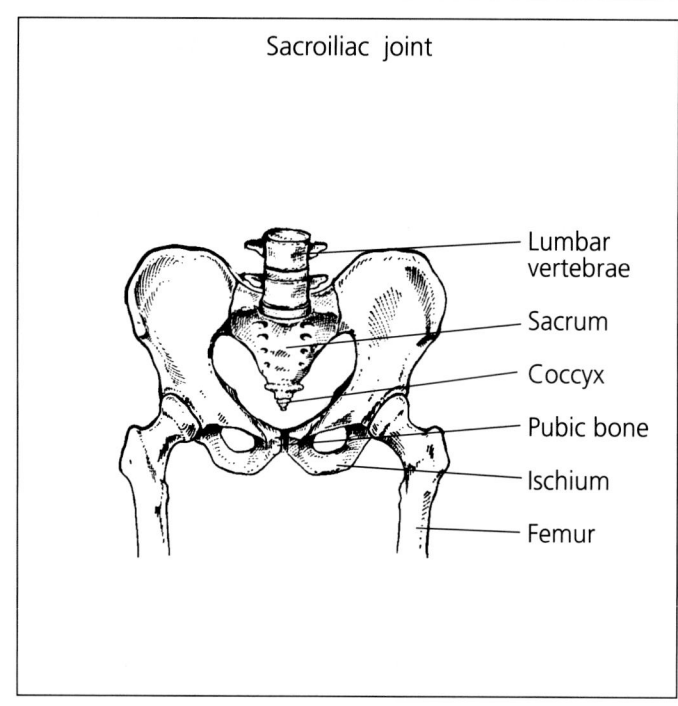

Sacroiliac joint

Lumbar vertebrae

Sacrum

Coccyx

Pubic bone

Ischium

Femur

— Skin rash, typically across the face in a butterfly shape
— Hair loss

Causes

The causes of lupus are not yet fully known. It is probably an autoimmune disorder (see Health and Well-Being, p. 182), possibly exacerbated by viruses, environmental factors, and/or medications.

Who's at Risk

Women develop lupus more often than men.

Possible Aftereffects and Complications

— Inflammations in various parts of the heart
— Kidney inflammations, potentially leading to kidney failure
— Diaphragm inflammation
— Increased susceptibility to other illnesses, due to a weakened immune system

Prevention

Prevention is not possible.

When to Seek Medical Advice

Seek help if symptoms are present.

Self-Help

Use sunscreen with a high SPF number. The skin rash tends to develop in response to sunlight.

Treatment

Like rheumatoid arthritis, less severe forms of lupus can be treated with nonsteroidal antiarthritic medications (see Rheumatoid Arthritis, p. 455).

If the organs are affected, the body's immune reactions need to be curbed using corticosteroids (see p. 665) and immunosuppressants. The skin condition may also be treated with corticosteroids.

SCLERODERMA

Complaints

Scleroderma is characterized by
— Painful whitish or bluish fingers and toes due to impaired circulation
— Sores on fingertips
— Joint pains
— Difficulty swallowing due to a constricted esophagus (see p. 384); loss of appetite and weight
— Tough, numb, rigid skin, gradually declining in flexibility and making it increasingly difficult to move the joints
— Dryness of the mouth and vagina; conjunctivitis
— Severe difficulty extending the tongue

Causes

The causes of scleroderma are not yet fully known. It is known to be an autoimmune disorder (see Health and Well-Being, p. 182) in which parts of the body's connective tissue become inflamed and thickened, causing damage to skin, membranes of the upper digestive tract, lungs, and kidneys.

Who's at Risk

Women develop scleroderma six times as often as men. People exposed to certain chemicals (e.g. the tuberculosis drug isoniazid, polyvinylchloride, or silicate dust) may be at greater risk. Women with silicone breast implants show a higher incidence of the illness.

Possible Aftereffects and Complications

— Blood vessels may become inflamed or constricted to the point of closure.
— The lungs may stop working efficiently; cough, shortness of breath, and oxygen insufficiency may ensue.
—The heart muscle may weaken due to the formation of scar tissue.
— Reduced blood flow to the kidneys may result in kidney failure.

The disease is usually more serious in men than in women.

Prevention

Not possible.

When to Seek Medical Advice

Seek help if several symptoms are present. A physician familiar with the condition can make an early diagnosis and try to tailor the treatment to match the estimated severity of the type of disease.

Self-Help

Avoid cold in any form, including food and drink.

Treatment

Physical therapy is essential.

No specific therapy is known. Many treatments, including corticosteroids, salicylates, chelating agents, chloroquine, penicillamine, and immunosuppressive medications have been tried. Severe forms of scleroderma may be treated with penicillamine, which may slow the progress of the disease although it has numerous side effects.

Various other therapies can bring symptoms under control.

POLYMYALGIA RHEUMATICA

This form of arthritis affects the connective tissue in the blood vessels of muscles.

Complaints

— Loss of appetite, weight loss, general weakness
— Severe pains in the neck, shoulder, and pelvis area, especially in the early morning
— Rapidly deteriorating vision

Causes

The causes of this disease are as yet unknown.

Who's at Risk

Polymyalgia rheumatica primarily affects people over 55. Women develop the disease about three times as often as men.

Possible Aftereffects and Complications

The inner walls of blood vessels, primarily the temporal artery, become inflamed, resulting in severely impaired vision and potential thromboses, vessel narrowing, and embolisms. The coronary vessels may also be affected.

When to Seek Medical Advice

Seek help if symptoms appear.

Self-Help

Not possible.

Treatment

If polymyalgia rheumatica is suspected, corticosteroids should be prescribed (see p. 665). If the eyes are already affected, the patient should be hospitalized.

FIBROMYALGIA SYNDROMES (SOFT-TISSUE PAIN AND STIFFNESS)

Fibromyalgia is a collective term for pain and discomfort in the soft connective tissues surrounding bones, muscles and joints. Fibromyalgia syndromes include the following disorders:

PAINFUL SHOULDERS, "TENNIS ELBOW," CARPAL TUNNEL SYNDROME

Complaints

The symptoms of these ailments can differ widely. In some patients, "everything hurts"; others can pinpoint the pain in certain body parts; still others experience an overall burning sensation combined with weakness and exhaustion. The pain may begin gradually or appear suddenly; it may pass quickly and recur, worsen or stay the same.

Painful shoulders: Repeated movements cause the shoulder to ache.

Tennis elbow: Pain in the exterior elbow joint extends down the forearm; it hurts to make a fist.

Carpal tunnel syndrome: The palms of the hands hurt, especially at night. Pain may extend up through the arm, shoulder, and neck. In the morning the fingers are stiff and weak, with numbness in the thumb, index and middle finger. The muscles in the ball of the thumb may atrophy.

Causes

When a few muscles are used repeatedly, or are constantly tense due to psychological factors, they require increased quantities of oxygen. When no additional oxygen is supplied, muscle cells die off and harden, affecting the surrounding tendons, ligaments, and other tissues.

Carpal tunnel syndrome occurs when a nerve in the wrist becomes pinched due to chronic tendinitis.

Who's at Risk

Fibromyalgia syndromes account for more than half of all movement-related complaints. The incidence of fibromyalgia syndromes is greatest in

— People who habitually overcompensate or "overdo" things in daily life
— People whose jobs require repetitive movements (e.g., typing, operating a machine or tool, working a cash register)
— People who play sports with an incorrect grip, stroke or throwing technique
— People whose muscles are compensating for a physical misalignment, e.g., one leg shorter than the other

Possible Aftereffects and Complications

Any incorrect position or movement places strain on the muscles, whose oxygen requirement rises as a result. Poorly oxygenated tissues cause pain, which causes the patient to exaggerate the incorrect placement that started the whole vicious circle. If this process lasts long enough, it will result in irreversible atrophy.

In some people these symptoms become so severe that after repeated episodes, they finally become unable to hold a job. In such cases the mind-body connection is often a crucial factor in the disease, but unless this is recognized in time and appropriate action is taken, a constantly ill "career patient" may well result (see Health and Well-Being, p. 182).

Prevention

— Alternate hands when working.
— In sports, learn to throw or hit the right way. If you play tennis, make sure your racquet handle is the right size for your hand.

How to choose the right handle size for your tennis racquet:
The circumference of the handle should be equal to the distance from the tip of the middle finger to the midline of the palm.

When to Seek Medical Advice

Seek help if pain is unbearable despite relaxation and limbering exercises.

Fibromyalgia syndromes often take a long time to diagnose correctly, because several factors must simultaneously be present: a doctor experienced both in arthritis and psychosomatic illnesses, and a patient who understands that his or her behavior and attitude play a role in the disease.

Self-Help

Anything that you find relaxing will lessen your symptoms. Relaxation exercises, refreshing sleep, and resting the painful limb will all help. During the acute stage, cold compresses should be applied three or four times a day (see p. 692); later, switch to warm compresses (see p. 692).

Treatment with Physical Therapy (see p. 690).

— Physical therapy (see p. 690); massage (see p. 686).
— Heat applications: infrared lamp, diathermy (see p.693).
— If your illness is caused by conditions at your place of work, an occupational therapist can help improve them.

Treatment with Medications

— Analgesics (see p. 660)
— Prescription Muscle relaxants
— Sedatives (see p. 189)

For counseling and psychotherapy options, see p. 697.

Operations

For carpal tunnel syndrome: If other treatments, e.g., a one-time corticosteroid injection, are not effective, surgery should be chosen before matters get worse. The ligament crossing the wrist is cut so that it no longer compresses the nerve.

SPINAL COLUMN

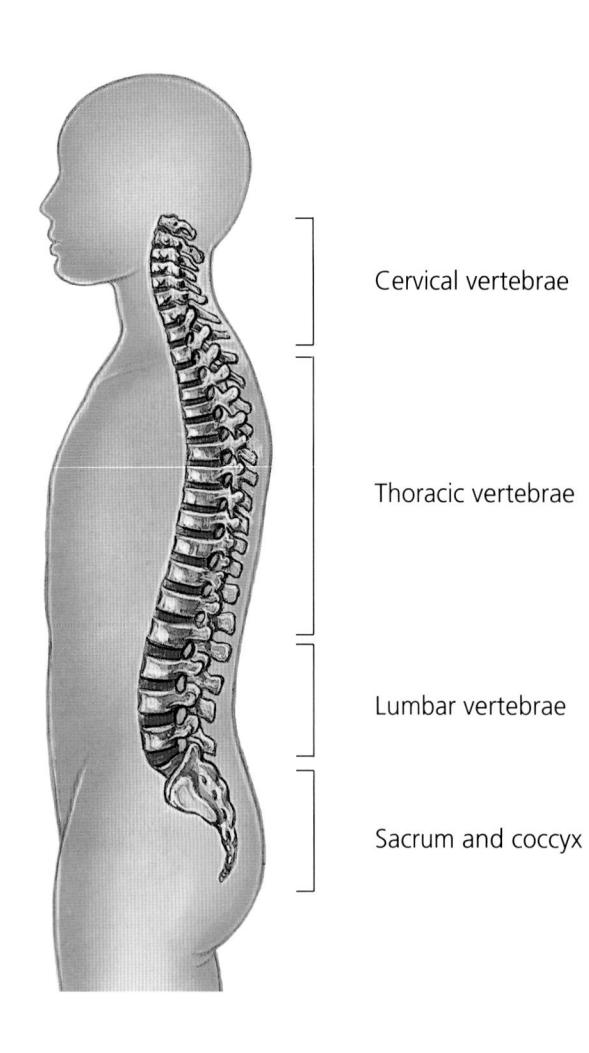

Cervical vertebrae

Thoracic vertebrae

Lumbar vertebrae

Sacrum and coccyx

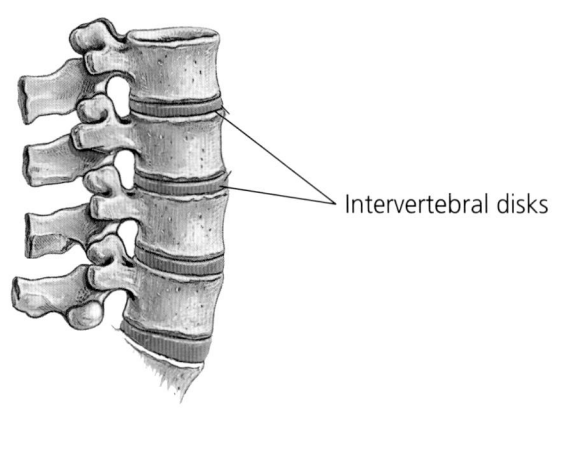

Intervertebral disks

Human beings achieve upright posture thanks to the spinal column and its connections to complex muscular systems. All the muscles of the trunk and limbs are connected, directly or indirectly, to the spine. The ring-shaped vertebrae, one above the other, enclose and protect the spinal cord while leaving room for the nerves to enter and exit. Small joints connect the vertebrae, allowing for some flexibility.

The Spine's Three Segments

The uppermost segment, the neck, consists of seven cervical vertebrae which support the head. The cervical vertebrae with their intercalated cartilage discs are very mobile.

What we call the "back" consists of the 12 thoracic vertebrae, which are relatively immobile because they are connected to the ribs. This segment provides bony protection for the sensitive heart and lungs.

The "lower back," or lumbar region, consists of five vertebrae, and is extremely flexible. Most of the body's weight is supported by the lowest lumbar vertebra and the sacrum just below it. The sacrum, and its lower extension, the coccyx, consist of fused vertebrae.

The spinal column curves slightly outward in the thoracic area (behind the chest), which, when exaggerated, forms a humpback (kyphosis). In the lumbar region, the spine is curved slightly inward; if the curve is extremely pronounced, it is called *lordosis*.

Intervertebral Discs as Buffers

The cartilaginous discs between the vertebrae serve as shock absorbers and account for about one fourth of the length of the spine. They consist of a fibrous outer ring and a gelatinous core that is not supplied with blood. The normal stresses of a day compress the soft cores of the discs, so that in the evening you may be almost an inch shorter than in the morning.

Lying down relieves the spinal column of its duties and lets the discs expand again by absorbing liquids out of the surrounding tissues. The more relaxed the spine is, the more completely the discs recover their shape; this capacity decreases with age, however.

BACK AND LOWER BACK PAIN

Causes

Backaches are the result of a vicious circle. When back muscles are tense, they are inadequately supplied with oxygen because circulation is impaired. The lack of oxygen causes pain, which in turn causes the muscles to tense further. The spinal discs are unable to recover sufficiently, causing the interactions between the vertebrae to be disturbed. The muscles try in vain to rectify the situation, intensifying their tension.

Muscle spasms are usually an expression of an imbalance elsewhere in life (see Health and Well-Being, p. 182). Just as the word "posture" can refer to both one's inner and outer bearing, our emotional state and body position influence each other reciprocally.

Who's at Risk

The very mobile segments and the load-bearing segments of the spinal column are most subject to wear and tear. All aging spines show wear, but are not necessarily painful.

People who are under great physical or emotional stress over a long period of time tend to experience greater muscle tension (see Health and Well-Being, p. 182).

Possible Aftereffects and Complications

Damaged intervertebral discs may press on nerves (see Ruptured Disc Damage, p. 466). Incorrect weight distribution or overloading the small joints between the vertebrae causes them to wear out more quickly (see Arthritis, p. 452; in the spine, this is called spondylarthrosis). The tendons, nerves, and blood vessels connected to the vertebrae can conduct pain and tension into other parts of the body, causing, for example, aching in the head, forearm, and lower leg, or impaired vision, hearing, or balance. Many applications for early retirement due to disability are based on back trouble.

Prevention

Strong back and stomach muscles keep the spine upright and encourage good posture. Physically active people are much better able to deal with back problems than those who are sedentary. The rule of thumb for preventing back problems is "get plenty of exercise." Balancing exercises, such as the following are also helpful:

— While standing on one leg, wave one arm vigorously. Or use the other foot to write a name in the air, the faster the better. There are many balance exercises in yoga.
— Walk or climb stairs holding a small sandbag (or this book) on your head. To exercise the spine thoroughly, carry a weight on your head for 20 minutes, twice a day.
— Walk in shoulder-deep water; swim, doing the crawl.
— Stand and do balancing exercises on a seesaw.
— Alternate between activities that are as different as possible from one another.

Day-to-day back-protection tips:

— Change positions repeatedly over the course of the day, to relieve your joints of weight and give them a rest.
— Adjust the height of your chair and work surface correctly for all jobs, so that knees, hips, and elbows are all bent at right angles.
— If necessary, rearrange your workplace, with the help of an ergonomics expert or occupational therapist if possible.
— Lie on your stomach as often as possible, for example, while reading or watching television.
— Never carry anything that you could roll or push instead.
— Let both arms share the weight when carrying things.
— When you need to lift a heavy object, squat to pick it up so your legs carry much of the weight, instead of bending over and lifting it with straight arms and legs, which strains the back.
— Back pain clinics often offer classes on strengthening the back and avoiding injuries.

Any kind of relaxation will help prevent backache and, in conjunction with a more balanced outlook on life, can help balance and reenergize the rest of the body.

When to Seek Medical Advice

Seek help if back pain is present for an extended period of time and you are unable to relieve it with relaxation exercises and self-help methods.

Self-Help

The following can often relieve back pain:

— Bed rest, or positions described under Sciatica (see p. 692).
— Warm packs (see p. 682) or rheumatism ointments (see p. 450).
— If pain is in the neck region: A neck support, to immobilize and support the cervical vertebrae.
— Rubber soles, to cushion the impact of walking on hard surfaces.
— Swimming, balancing exercises.
— Relaxation exercises (see p. 693).

Treatment with Physical Therapy

— Therapeutic exercises (see p. 690) are extremely important. At first they should relax the tense muscles, and later strengthen them.
— Massage (see p. 686).
— Acupuncture is often successful (see p. 679).

Treatment with Medications

Painkillers (see Analgesics, p. 660) relax tense muscles; if they are insufficient, a doctor may additionally prescribe a short-term course of diazepam (Valium) (see Sedatives, p. 189).

LUMBAGO, SCIATICA, HERNIATED OR RUPTURED DISC DAMAGE

Complaints

Lumbago: Sudden, sharp pain in the lower back, often when bending over, straightening up, twisting or lifting, which intensifies when coughing, sneezing or pressing with the abdominal muscles. The muscles around the spine are contracted in a spasm. It's almost impossible to move, or to find a comfortable position lying down.

Sciatica: The same symptoms, but lower down in the back. The pain radiates into the buttock area, along the outside or back of the thighs, and often extends to the calves, ankles, and feet. Paralysis is possible.

Causes

A disc may be protruding or may have "slipped" or shifted out of its normal position, causing its cartilaginous core to press on the nerves leading out of the spinal canal at that site. This leads to: muscle spasms, numbness and paralysis, and/or impaired posture.

Who's at Risk

In people with congenital disorders of the connective tissue, the intervertebral discs may become prematurely weakened. Persons burdened with long-term physical or psychological stresses subject their discs to tensions which may result in damage.

Possible Aftereffects and Complications

To avoid pain, lumbago or sciatica sufferers may adopt a posture that actually puts additional strain on the muscles.

If a disc presses on a nerve long enough, it may cause permanent damage.

Prevention

— Find the right mix of stimulation and relaxation for you, and adjust your lifestyle accordingly.
— Insist on working conditions that spare your back; exercise to counteract unsatisfactory conditions.
— Strengthen your stomach and back muscles.

When to Seek Medical Advice

— Seek help immediately if paralysis sets in.
— Make an appointment to see a doctor if pain becomes unbearable in spite of self-help measures, or if pain doesn't lessen appreciably in a month's time, or recurs repeatedly.

Self-Help

Any type of relaxation should help: Bed rest, moist warm compresses(see p. 692), baths, and relaxation exercises (see p. 693).

Treatment

Lumbago and sciatica are signals from your body that you need to balance tension and relaxation more effectively. If you often can't find the time to relax, it would be worth your while to discuss things with a professional (see Counseling and Psychotherapy, p. 697).

Physical therapy

— Massage (see p. 686)
— Mud treatments or warm packs (see p. 692)
    After acute symptoms have receded:
— Back-strengthening exercises
— Acupuncture (see p. 679)

Medications

Painkillers will relieve acute pain (see Analgesics, p. 660). For muscle relaxants, see "Back and Lower Back Pain: Treatment with Medication," p. 466.

An injection of a local anesthetic such as procaine is sometimes used, but it should be given only to break the vicious circle of pain and muscle tension.

Surgery

If a disc is causing paralysis by pressing on nerves in the spinal column, it should be removed as soon as possible. In all other cases, surgery should be postponed until several weeks of treatment have brought no improvement and pain is recurring repeatedly. Disc problems require surgery in only about 10 percent of patients.

Before an operation, it must be established that a slipped disc is actually causing the problem; this can be shown by a CT scan, magnetic resonance imaging (MRI), or myelogram. Two thirds of patients who undergo this type of surgery are symptom-free thereafter; the rest continue to experience pain. In a few cases, the patient's condition actually worsens.

SCHEUERMANN'S DISEASE

This disease of the spine causes a pronounced "humpback" in youths.

Complaints

In rare cases, the tense back muscles hurt.

Causes

For unknown reasons, a portion of the patient's vertebral bone dies. The vertebrae then become wedge-shaped, and the discs sink into the vertebrae.

Who is at Risk

The progress of this disease stops at puberty. It mainly affects youths around the age of 14. The later it appears, the more slowly it will progress and the less curvature of the spine results.

Possible Aftereffects and Complications

The back may become rigid in its curvature. Pain may result.

Prevention

—Allow your children freedom to grow; don't repress them with words or actions.
— Swim often to strengthen back muscles.
— Lie on your stomach as much as possible.
— Make sure chairs and tables are the right height.
— If possible, do closeup work at an inclined table.

When to Seek Medical Advice

Seek help if your child constantly has bad posture, especially if combined with backache.

Many children that don't stand up straight don't have Scheuermann's disease, however, and the diagnosis is often made incorrectly, causing the child needless anxiety together with unnecessary physical therapy.

Self-Help

—Warm compresses (see p. 692) or rheumatism ointments (see p. 450).
— Don't carry heavy objects.
— Don't sit hunched over for long periods; don't work slumped over your desk.

Treatment

Much as parents may wish their children to stand up straight and make a good impression, a bent back often expresses in body language some psychological burden the child is carrying. If matters are straightened out, the spine will often straighten as well (see Counseling and Psychotherapy, p. 697). Time-consuming physical therapy or uncomfortable support corsets can add to a child's emotional burden; achieving a straight spine at all costs makes little sense in such cases.

In general, this condition lasts about 2 years. During this time, patients should receive special care; afterward, they can and should lead normal lives.

Physical Therapy

Any type of physical therapy will require responsible cooperation, and therefore a certain degree of maturity, on the child's part.

Medications

Painkillers should be used only in case of severe pain (see Analgesics, p. 660).

SCOLIOSIS

Scoliosis is a condition characterized by a laterally curved and twisted spine.

Complaints

The curved spine characteristic of scoliosis is usually noticed by someone other than the patient, perhaps while fitting clothing. By the time the curve is visible, the disease has progressed, with the following symptoms:

— One hip leads the other.
— One shoulder (usually the right one) is higher than the other, and the shoulder blade protrudes.
— When the patient bends forward, it is apparent from behind that the spine is twisted, and that part of half of the back is higher (protrudes).

Causes

The causes of most scolioses are unknown. Only occasionally is scoliosis caused by paralysis or birth defects.

Who is at Risk

Two to 4 percent of the population have a lateral curve to their spines, but only 2 to 4 percent of this group need to be treated for scoliosis. Usually scoliosis appears in 13- or 14-year-olds. Girls are four times more likely to be affected than boys. The gradual curving of the spine slows down after the child stops growing, and sometimes stops altogether.

Children with scoliosis in the family are at greater risk of developing this disorder.

Possible After-effects and Complications

— Pain.
— The ribcage may be distorted, interfering with heart or lung function.
— Scoliosis patients often find their lives negatively affected by the disease. Nearly half of female patients and a third of male patients never marry, and patients of both sexes are much more likely to be unemployed or invalids than healthy individuals.

Prevention

The best prevention is early detection. Children with mild scoliosis should be checked every six months by an orthopedic physician.

When to Seek Medical Advice

Seek help if symptoms are present.

If a child isn't standing completely still during an X ray, the resulting image will show an apparent curve in the spine, which may be mistaken for scoliosis by an inexperienced physician. Scoliosis can be ruled out by the absence of twisting along the vertical axis, however.

Self-Help

Not possible.

Treatment

If the scoliosis is mild (under 20 degrees) but appears to be worsening, the patient should be fitted for a support brace (orthesis). If a child with over 30 degrees of curvature is experiencing a growth spurt, a brace should be fitted immediately to prevent the condition from becoming more pronounced. Braces push and pull the spine in the desired direction. Treatment is supplemented by physical therapy.

How long the brace is needed depends on the severity of the disease and the age of the patient. It is usually worn between 14 and 23 hours a day. Treatment continues until the patient has stopped growing, which is usually about age 15 for girls, and about 2 years later for boys.

The downside: Braces are confining, uncomfortable, and hard to hide under fashionable clothes. It may be hard to force an active young person into such a shell; after all, he or she is not in pain, and may have trouble imagining the consequences of leaving his or her condition untreated.

The upside: In many cases, wearing a brace makes it possible to avoid further deterioration, and thus surgery.

Surgery

If the scoliosis curvature is greater than 50 degrees, it can be expected to worsen and should be corrected surgically. Surgery will also prevent pain and the negative psychological effect of a serious deformity.

A scoliosis operation is major surgery. Two rods are inserted into the spine, which is fused at one site so that it becomes immobile there. After the operation, the patient wears a cast or plastic brace for about a year to let the site of the surgery "set." Recent developments in surgery can in some cases avoid the need for the brace or cast.

Results: The curvature of the spine is reduced by half, on average.

Risks: In addition to the usual risks of surgery (anesthesia, blood transfusion, infection), there is a 0.3 to 0.8 percent risk of nerve damage, which in the most severe cases results in paraplegia.

If the twisting occurs in the small of the back, it may be possible to operate from the front, through the abdominal cavity. This method gives better results and carries a lower risk of paraplegia, although the operation itself is more complicated.

During treatment with braces and following surgery, the patient can usually claim disability status.

CANCER

Until now, cancer has thwarted all efforts to fully understand the secrets of its origin. Advances in effective treatment, too, take place one small step at a time. In the industrialized countries, one in three people will get some sort of cancer at some point in life; one in five will die of it.

These figures have improved only slightly over the past 20 years; the longer one lives, the longer one's exposure to environmental factors that contribute to cancer. On the bright side, rare and unusual forms of cancer, particularly in children, can frequently be cured today.

A diagnosis of cancer gives rise to shock and anxiety, both in patients and their families; as a result, cancer patients often feel abandoned by others at a time when they need them the most. This worsens the odds, since the more supported patients are by a community of family and friends, the more positive their experiences, and the better their prognosis.

WHAT IS CANCER?

The catch-all term *cancer* refers to different kinds of malignant tumors. Cancer can occur in all organs and areas of the body.

The cells of the body perform different, specialized functions. Their function, properties, and growth are all determined by genetic programming. If this programming is disrupted, the cells become abnormal and grow uncontrollably.

It can take years for a "normal" cell to become cancerous; the process actually takes place constantly, throughout the body. Cancer cells are more aggressive and robust than other cells. In all instances, the body's system of defenses recognizes the cancer cells and attempts to render them harmless (see Immune System Disorders, p 351). If this is unsuccessful, the cells grow uncontrollably, and a tumor develops.

Whether a tumor is benign or malignant is determined by what kind of cells gave rise to it, and what kind of defect has arisen in the cells' control system.
Benign tumors: Are those which remain isolated from the adjacent tissue and do not invade surrounding organs.
Malignant tumors: These tumors invade and ravage the surrounding area. They spread cancer cells through the blood and/or lymphatic system and can give rise to tumors in other organs (metastasis).

In general:
— The smaller the tumor, the better the prognosis or chance of a cure.
— Once a tumor exceeds about half an inch in diameter, numerous metastases have most likely already occurred.
— Some tumors metastasize very quickly, others more slowly.
— Depending on where tumors develop, metastases can be expected in certain organs.
— In 7 percent of cancer patients, metastases are in evidence, but not the original tumor. In these cases, chances of a cure are slim.
— Some metastases grow very slowly and have no negative effects on the patients' general well-being for years.
Basically:
— A cancerous tumor, if operable, should be surgically removed as soon as possible.
— If indicated by a biopsy, some malignant tumors should be treated with chemotherapy or radiation therapy instead.

HOW DOES CANCER DEVELOP?

Cancer develops slowly, generally taking years or decades. There is no single cause for the more than a hundred different types of cancer, and not all the contributing factors are known. In all cases, several contributing factors must be present, resulting in a command to the cell that launches the abnormal development. For the most part, these involve a combination of external and internal factors: Diet, smoking and alcohol, carcinogens in the workplace and in the environment, sunlight and radiation can all promote cancer. Genetic mutations can also increase the risk. Viruses and bacteria may play a role. Chronic inflammations, disruptions in normal cell activity, or immune disorders can all lead to cancer.

It's likely that psychological factors such as emotional overload, unresolved conflicts, and traumatic experiences such as the loss of a loved one can increase the risk as well; however, these cannot be considered causes of the disease. Recent studies show that there is no such thing as a cancer-prone personality.

Cancer can happen to anyone; however, a tumor develops only when the equilibrium of the organism as a whole is disturbed.

Lifestyle Risk Factors
Food
Experts believe that 30 to 40 percent of all cancers can be traced to poor diet. Excessive consumption of animal fats increases the chance of intestinal cancer and possibly breast cancer as well. Food can be a source of a range of carcinogens, including nitrosamines in cured and smoked meats, fish, and cheeses. The nitrate content in vegetables (see Hazardous Substances in Food, p.729) and drinking water (see Drinks, p. 736) also contributes. However, nitrosamines also occur naturally in the body.

Carcinogens (benzyprenes) are produced when fat drips onto the coals while grilling meat or by overheating fat to the smoking point; they are also found in the dark rind of smoked meats.

Aflatoxins, a mold by-product found principally in nuts, smoked ham, bread, and marmalade, contributes to cancer of the liver and stomach. Therefore, even if food has only one moldy portion, the entire piece or batch should be thrown away. The molds used in the production of cheeses do not contain aflatoxins.

Cancer-causing heavy metals, such as cadmium, chromium, nickel, and arsenic, are found increasingly in farm produce, grains, fruit, in mushrooms, egg yolks, meat, and fish (see Hazardous Substances in Food, p. 729).

Smoking
Smoking (see p. 754) causes one third of all cancer deaths and nearly 90 percent of all lung cancer cases. The risk of lung cancer increases with every cigarette: Smoking 10 cigarettes a day makes one 5 times as likely to develop lung cancer; more than 35 cigarettes, 40 times as likely. Breathing second-hand smoke in the home or workplace also increases the risk of cancer.

Alcohol
Alcohol, too, is suspected of causing cancer. Excessive alcohol consumption intensifies the effects of cigarette smoking and increases the risk of cancer between 20 and 40 times.

Medications
Estrogen therapy, prescribed for menopause or osteoporosis, increases the risk of uterine cancer; however, it reduces the risk of ovarian cancer (see Hormone Therapy, p. 477).

Risk reduction
Diet: A balanced, nutritious diet high in vegetables (organically grown, if possible) is the best precaution one can take in the area of food (see Preventing Cancer through Diet, p. 472).
Smoking: Quit smoking (see How to Quit Smoking, p. 755). If this isn't possible, cut back drastically, and avoid inhaling deeply.
Alcohol: Cut back on alcohol consumption (see Alcoholism, p.205).
Sun: Avoid excessive sun exposure (see Sunburn, p. 263).
Personal hygiene: In men, good personal hygiene helps prevent cancer of the penis and also helps protect female sex partners against cervical cancer.
Chronic inflammations: These should be cleared up wherever possible.
Hobbies: Avoid working with asbestos (see Asbestos, p.776, 784); handle paints, varnishes and adhesives with care, or switch to nontoxic alternatives.
Gardening and housework: Always wear gloves. When working with compost, wear a mask to avoid breathing in airborne molds. Where possible, don't use pesticides and herbicides; switch to natural pest- and weed-control products and methods.

ENVIRONMENTAL RISK FACTORS
Environmental factors cannot cause cancer on their own, but they play an important role in the complex interplay of factors that results in cancer.

The quantities and concentrations of chemical compounds in the environment and workplace are steadily rising. A considerable number of cancers can be traced to environmental factors. Embryos and small children are at especially high risk from chemicals.

Cancer-causing agents include all of the ubiquitous aromatic hydrocarbons, amines, alkalis, tobacco, nickel, asbestos, chromates, thorium dioxide, aflatoxin, and oxymetholone. These substances directly cause the transformation of normal cells into cancer cells.

See The Most Common Pollutants, p. 773.

See Cancer in the Workplace, p. 793.

Exposure to ionizing radiation greatly increases the

risk of leukemia. For example, following the 1986 Chernobyl nuclear reactor disaster, the incidence of cancer in the region more than doubled.

The biggest source of exposure to radiation is from diagnostic tests and therapeutic interventions (see X rays, p. 646). About one fourth of overall exposure comes from radon in building materials and poorly ventilated structures (see Radioactiviy, p. 777). Smoking also exposes oneself significantly to radioactivity: The intensely radioactive polonium 210, found in tobacco smoke, reaches into the farthest corners of the lungs. Finally, airline crews are constantly exposed to high levels of radiation from the atmosphere.

PREVENTION

Preventing Cancer Through Diet

A diet high in fiber and low in fat is an important tool in the fight against cancer (see Nutrition, p. 722).

Certain types of vegetables and fruit have been shown to help prevent the development of stomach and intestinal cancer, and possibly lung cancer as well. The most important of these is broccoli, followed by soy, cabbage, cauliflower, Brussels sprouts, and sauerkraut. Carrots, onions, white cabbage and beets protect against cancer of the intestines, uterus, and tongue. The cabbage family, root vegetables, lettuce, and cucumber protect against breast cancer. Tomatoes, strawberries, pineapple, and hot pepper can slow the formation of nitrosamines. Garlic also works to prevent cancer. It is thought that certain compounds found in berries, citrus, grapes, walnuts, and caraway can detoxify the body in cancer's initial stages. It has been established that certain compounds in soy and broccoli have cancer-fighting properties.

The immune system is weakened by deficiencies in trace elements such as magnesium, iron, copper, zinc, and selenium, among others. Because trace elements are present in unprocessed foods, a healthy, well-balanced diet rich in these foods can ensure sufficient quantities of these substances.

The role of vitamins in the fight against cancer appears smaller than previously thought. Vitamin C inhibits the formation of nitrosamines in the stomach; whether vitamins A and E prevent tumors is still a matter of debate. Under no circumstances should one self-medicate with megadoses of vitamins; too much of a good thing can be dangerous (see Vitamins, p. 740).

Preventing Cancer Through Exercise

Today it is accepted that regular exercise (see Physical Activity and Sports, p. 762) keeps one healthy and can guard against the development of cancer.

EARLY DETECTION

The patient is in the best position to detect slight changes in or on the body. You are, after all, most familiar with your own body. Having your partner examine you—and examining your partner—can also be helpful. Ask a trusted doctor how often to examine breasts, skin, and testicles, as well as what you should be looking out for (see Breast Self-Exam, p. 473; Testicle Self-Exam, p. 473).

Do not pass up an opportunity for early detection screening. When cancer is diagnosed in someone at an early age, the chance of cancer developing in immediate family members increases significantly, and they should categorically avail themselves of any and all screening methods.

Warning Signals

Many people don't go for routine checkups because they dread a diagnosis of cancer; or they report any suspicious symptoms or observations incompletely, if at all. Keep in mind that your health-care provider can help you only once he or she has all the relevant information.

Any unusual changes should be reported without hesitation to your health-care provider; most of them will turn out to be insignificant, but even if you are not so lucky, at least your cancer will be detected as early as possible. The earlier the diagnosis, the better the prognosis. About 40 percent of cancer cases can be cured through conventional methods.

Recommended exams for early cancer detection for both men and women
Skin self-exam—monthly after age 20
Skin exam by doctor—annually after age 30
Digital rectal exam—annually after age 40
Fecal occult blood test—annually after age 50
Sigmoidoscopy—every 3 to 5 years after age 50

Men

Testicular self–exam—two monthly between ages of 20 and 40

Prostate exam—annually after age 50

Women

Breast self-exam—monthly after age 18

Clinical breast exam—every 3 years between ages 18 and 40, then annually; semiannually for women taking hormones

Mammography—baseline exam between ages 35 and 40; every 1 to 2 years between ages 40 and 49, annually after age 50

Pelvic exam—every 1 to 3 years between ages 18 and 40, then annually

Pap smear—annually between ages 18 and 65; after 3 or more consecutive normal exams it may be done less frequently at the health-care provider's discretion

DIAGNOSIS: CANCER

The period between the voicing of a suspicion and a definitive diagnosis of cancer can be stressful for family and friends. Everyone should have someone to talk to during this time, be it the doctor or somebody from one of the numerous cancer support groups available. The patient would do well to contact a support group as early as possible. Such groups can often be a good source of information when difficult decisions on treatment must be made (support groups are listed by disease in your local telephone directory). If the anxiety becomes unbearable, seek crisis intervention at a clinic.

Some people are plagued by the fear that the doctor is withholding the true diagnosis from them. Physicians are, however, required to give truthful and complete information to all patients who make it unmistakably clear that they want to know what is going on with their bodies.

When going to the doctor for a definitive diagnosis, the patient should be accompanied by someone he or she trusts who can help retain what has been said and process the new information. Often, unanswered questions arise only while discussing the events after the fact with the other person present.

The doctor may outline the treatment plan or procedure. Patients can choose the extent to which they want to participate in their treatment. They must be advised and informed comprehensively and make sure they understand the primary and secondary effects of the proposed treatment. This is critically important. Even if a recognized cancer needs to be surgically removed as quickly as possible, the patient can decide in his or her own good time which treatment to choose. It's always a good idea to sleep on an important decision; this certainly applies here. Often, many conversations take place between doctor and patient after diagnosis and before treatment.

Feel free also to ask your doctor for information on alternative forms of treatment.

Regarding the odds of surviving cancer, the doctor can only extrapolate from statistical data. However, this says nothing about how the disease will actually progress in your case. Each individual's chances depend not simply on medicine and pharmaceuticals; they are also fundamentally bound with the patient's desire to live, the available support network of friends and family, and the patient's positive outlook on the future, including the expectation of a meaningful life after treatment.

Warning signals of cancer

The following symptoms are common to several illnesses, but they can also be signs of cancer. If you notice any of these and cannot determine their source, see your doctor.
— Fatigue, low energy levels of recent origin
— Weight loss
— Digestive problems that persist for more than 6 weeks: alternating diarrhea and constipation, poorly formed stool
— Aversion to certain foods (e.g., meat)
— Vomiting blood
— Mucus or blood in stool
— Blood in urine
— Coughing up blood
— Persistent pain
— Cough that persists more than 6 weeks; lasting hoarseness
— Changes to warts, moles, or spots on the skin
— Any new growths on the skin, particularly in areas exposed to the sun
— Wounds or sores that heal slowly, if at all, even with treatment
— Bloody vaginal discharge between periods, after intercourse, or following menopause
— Lumps in breast
— Lumps in testicles
— Swelling in the throat, armpit, or groin
— Unexplained pains in bones

TREATMENT OPTIONS

The goals of cancer treatments differ depending on the prospects of a cure. They should be clearly formulated within the framework of the treatment and monitored in the day-to-day course of the illness.

Ideally, the goal is a full cure, and doctors operate in "full cure mode." A cure is possible if the tumor continues to respond well to treatment appropriate to its type and the stage of disease. The goal is full remission: i.e., the tumor disappears and is no longer evident even after careful testing. When full remission persists, one can speak of a complete cure. Cancer patients are considered cured after five years following treatment without relapse.

In the case of many cancers involving tumors, a cure is not possible, and the goal is then a positive impact on the progress of the disease, or palliative care. If the tumor can be shrunk, this usually means a prolonged life span and/or an improvement in the symptoms caused by the tumor. About a third of all cancer patients live with the disease for years in this way. Radiation therapy for cancer that has metastasized to the bones, even if it doesn't cure the disease, can considerably improve the patient's quality of life by drastically reducing pain and preventing broken bones.

Doctors need to explain the sense and purpose of palliative care as thoroughly as possible to patients with inoperable cancer. The metastasis of a tumor alone is not sufficient cause for treatment, but the amelioration of tumor-related symptoms certainly warrants consideration. On the other hand, it would be senseless to subject a patient with inoperable cancer and no symptoms to extended treatment. In such cases, preserving a better quality of life means sparing the patient the burden of radical therapy.

Competent doctors aim for realistic, achievable treatment goals and line up diagnostic and therapeutic preventive measures to support these goals. They are more likely to prescribe intensive diagnostic procedures and onerous therapies for patients with a good prognosis and a strong desire to live than for those who can only receive palliative care.

It is vitally important that doctor and patient discuss the treatment plan thoroughly. Informed patients, fully aware of what's going on, do not feel powerless in the face of their disease. Feeling in control of one's destiny contributes to good health.

Many patients fear that the treatment will make them sicker than they already are. They must have faith that their treatment is designed so that the cure is not worse than the disease.

An international standard of care exists for every type of cancer and each of its stages. Sometimes one form of treatment is considered sufficient; sometimes several types of treatment together have been most successful.

Surgery

The oldest and surest way to treat cancer is surgery. A large margin of healthy tissue around the cancerous mass is also removed to ensure that no microscopic tendrils remain, which could mean a return of the cancer. Most cancer patients owe their lives to such radical surgery. If the cancer has spread to the lymph nodes, the affected areas, and if possible the compromised lymph vessels, must be completely removed ("en bloc" surgery). However, in cases where the cancer has spread throughout the body, such radical surgery usually makes little sense. Its costs can be prohibitive, and, except in the case of ovarian cancer, it is usually considered "overkill"; just because something is technically feasible doesn't mean it is the best option.

Radiation Therapy

Radiation can cure cancer. Ionizing rays are directed at the tumor to check its rapid cell division. The dose of radiation, its precise delivery, and the simultaneous protecting of surrounding healthy tissue make it possible for radiation therapy to shrink tumors significantly. These days it is possible to deliver a targeted dose of radiation directly to any part of the body.

Recent advances in radiation therapy have made it less onerous today than it was in the past.

Chances of Recovery

The prognosis depends on how well the tumor mass responds to radiation. This is determined by the type of tissue and how well it is supplied with blood: Oxygen-rich tissue is most responsive to radiation. However, because every tumor contains oxygen-poor cells, the tumor may grow back in time after radiation therapy even though it may have shrunk immediately following the therapy. Some tumors do not respond at all to radiation.

Radiation therapy plays an important role in the treatment of carcinomas of the prostate and the early stages of breast cancer, among other forms. It is also used to supplement chemotherapy in the treatment of rectal cancer, and cancer of the uterus, cervix, and vulva.

Radiation therapy is also frequently prescribed in palliative care.

Side Effects

The side effects of radiation therapy depend on the targeted region and the responsiveness of the surrounding healthy tissue. The bigger the irradiated area, the more compromised the patient's condition can become. For the most part, symptoms consist of sleepiness, general exhaustion, and loss of appetite. In the head and throat regions, mucous membranes may become inflamed, causing difficulty in swallowing. Radiation in the abdominal area can give rise to gastritis and intestinal inflammations accompanied by diarrhea, vomiting, flatulence, and cramps. These symptoms often continue after the treatment ends.

Out of fear of overtaxing their gastrointestinal tract, many radiation patients eat very little and end up losing weight. In general, symptoms can be controlled with medication and diet. Metoclopramide (Reglan), as well as dexamethasone (Decadron), are prescribed for vomiting. Medication taken before meals to help settle the stomach, and antidiarrhea medication, can help the body absorb as many nutrients as possible from food.

The skin reacts to radiation as it would to sunburn: It gets red and itchy. Sometimes little blisters or freckles develop. Irradiated areas of the skin may lose hair after 3 weeks; it usually grows back within a few months. The effectiveness of radiation treatment, and some of its side effects as well, may only become evident after weeks or months. Discuss your observations and any related concerns with your caregivers, even if the radiation therapy has concluded.

Tips for cancer patients

— A diagnosis of cancer can be a shock to you and those around you. From now on, you will be bombarded with recommendations; before you follow any of them, speak with your doctor.

— Set up a consultation with a doctor you trust. Demand the doctor take time to answer all your questions to the best of his or her abilities. Prepare a list of questions in advance so you don't forget to have any of them answered.

— If you are at all uncertain, seek the advice of a specialist. The better informed you are regarding the different chances, risks, and side effects of each procedure, the better you and your team of care givers can select the approach that will work best for you.

— Having someone you trust accompany you to the hospital can help you cope with strenuous treatments.

— Clarify with the doctor what you can do personally to further your recovery. You can't change your genes, but you can change your life to avoid unhealthy circumstances: Quit a high-stress job, rid your home of sources of toxic materials, or change your diet. It might also be time to rearrange your daily routine or to analyze or rethink your relationships with family members, partners, or other important people in your life.

— Relatives and friends often feel insecure and unsure of how to act with the cancer patient; speaking openly about your feelings with them can reduce stress.

— If you would rather speak with an uninvolved third party, contact the Cancer Information and Counseling Line Center (see p. 479). People at the center are there to answer all your questions, medical and psychological. You can also get counseling (see Counseling and Psychotherapy, p. 697).

— Recruit help in taking your life in hand. It could be a friend who will listen to your problems and respect your decisions. It could be a self-help group where people with similar issues can share with and gain strength from each other. It could be a psychologist or counselor who can help you get on your feet and accompany you on your way. Even if the disease wins out in the end, you can spend the time you have left the way you want to, and live consciously.

Self-help for side effects of radiation treatment

— For fatigue, try to rest as often as possible. Do not take sleeping pills without first consulting your doctor.

— Eat smaller meals frequently throughout the day. For snacks, keep on hand fresh, easy-to-digest fruit, fruit juice, milk, cottage cheese, etc.

— Get some exercise about an hour and a half before eating, to stimulate your appetite. Prepare your favorite foods, and make them especially appetizing. Eating in good spirits and good company helps digestion.

— Protect the part of the skin that's been irradiated from any contact with soap, cosmetics, perfume, ointments, heat lamps, or hot water bottles; these irritate the skin. Clean the area only with lukewarm water. Avoid sunlight or extreme cold.

Chemotherapy and Other Remedies

Certain cancers can be treated with medication, either exclusively or in tandem with surgery and/or radiation therapy. Cytotoxic agents check the growth of all fast-dividing cells, which include not only cancer cells but blood-cell production, mucous membranes, germ cells, and hair cells.

Today more than a hundred different cancer medications are prescribed clinically, including:
— Cytotoxic agents
— Alkylating agents
— Platinum compounds
— Antimetabolites
— Herbal cytotoxins
— Cytotoxic antibiotics
— Hormone treatments
— Biological response modifiers (e.g., Interferon)

Treatment can be administered intravenously, by injection, by mouth or in ointment form (for skin cancer). Many are given in combination to boost effectiveness and cut back on side effects. The length of treatment is tailored to each individual case.

Prognoses

Chemotherapy brings real prospects for a cure in about 10 percent of all tumors. Cytotoxic agents can cure or help cure the following diseases: Testicular cancer, Hodgkin's disease, one form of non-Hodgkin's lymphoma, acute leukemia, Wilms' tumor, choriocarcinoma,

ovarian cancer; to prevent recurrence of metastasis in certain types of breast cancer, where it is given directly after surgery; colon cancer; and as partial medication for Ewing's sarcoma.

Diseases for which cytotoxins can be prescribed as palliative or life-prolonging medication: Breast cancer that has already metastasized; chronic leukemia type CML and CLL; one form of non-Hodgkin's lymphoma; small-cell lung carcinoma; metastasized colon cancer; tumors of the ear, nose, and throat area and esophagus. It is worth noting that, in order for a cure to be possible, you may have to endure severe side effects as part of chemotherapy. A common mistake is under-medication, which will certainly produce fewer side effects, but may also be largely ineffective against the cancer.

In the case of palliative care, the treating physician should critically analyze—and patients should ask—whether chemotherapy will really prolong life in this case; which tumor-related symptoms should be treated; and what side effects and difficulties the therapy may entail. The weighing of needs against risks is especially important here.

It is your right as a patient to have your desires known with regard to treatment.

Side Effects

The various side effects of cancer medications may be moderate or intense, and may manifest early or late in treatment.

Nausea and vomiting
Effective drugs (e.g., Zofran) for these common, sometimes very severe symptoms can be given in tandem with cytotoxins.

Smoking marijuana is effective against nausea. Although it is illegal in this country, a drug containing the active ingredient in marijuana is legally available in England.

Some cancer medications cause considerable discomfort, especially in young patients. Fear of vomiting often results in loss of appetite during chemotherapy, and the patient may even become ill before chemotherapy sessions. Behavior therapy can help (see p.476).

Hair loss
Many people lose some or all of their hair during

chemotherapy and suffer profoundly as a result. With some cytotoxins, and if the chemotherapy is restricted to only a few treatments, hair loss can be minimal or nonexistent. In any case, hair growth will resume after treatment is completed.

Inflammation of the mucous membranes

Some cancer medications affect the oral and vaginal mucosa, first by drying it out, then through lesions and inflammations. For this reason, particular attention must be paid to hygiene in these areas while the chemotherapy is in course.

Infections

Most cancer medications cause the white-blood-cell count to drop within 10 days. This is temporary, but it can be months before levels return to normal. If levels are especially low, there is a mounting risk of infection. Good oral hygiene, including gargling, and regular checkups are essential. Avoid exposing yourself to sources of infection, and at the first sign of an infection, see your doctor.

Bleeding

The production of platelets, the blood cells involved in coagulation, is also temporarily disrupted. Therefore, cuts and bleeding wounds may be risky; exercise caution.

Hormone Therapy

Hormone treatment or hormone deprivation can slow growth and prevent metastasis in tumors in which growth is hormone-dependent—primarily cancers of the breast and prostate.

Hormone deprivation can be performed either through surgery or medication. In the case of breast cancer, the ovaries are removed. With prostate cancer, it means either removal of the testes, or radiation therapy to destroy their hormone-producing tissues. Since this effectively amounts to castration with all its implications, such treatment can have serious psychological impact.

When hormone receptors are found in the tumor cells, matching antihormones can slow growth and prevent metastasis, resulting in a gradual "chemical castration" over time. Compared to chemotherapy, hormone therapy causes fewer side effects in the rest of the body.

Combined Treatment

In the case of certain cancers, combining treatments makes sense. The combination of surgery, radiation therapy, and cytotoxins can significantly increase children's chances of surviving Wilms' tumor. Cancer medication can increase life expectancy following surgery for breast or stomach cancer. Radiation can be helpful prior to surgery for bladder cancer. Combined radiation and drug therapy is effective with cancer of the rectum, throat, nose, and ear; in certain circumstances, contained small-cell lung cancers can also be cured by these methods.

Immunotherapy

Because the body's own system of defenses plays such an important role in preventing cancer, research has been going on for years to find ways to strengthen the immune defense.

What seems logical in theory, however, doesn't necessarily work in practice. The fact that the immune system responds to treatment doesn't mean the tumor will shrink. Perhaps the immune system doesn't recognize every cancer cell, so its defensive reaction doesn't kick in; or perhaps the number of cancer cells multiplies so quickly that the defense system is overwhelmed.

Initial success with turberculosis (TB) immunization Bacille Calmette-Guerin (BCG), with *Cornybacterium parvum*, levamisole, thymus gland hormones, and other drugs has ended in disappointment: BCG is relatively effective only in bladder cancer. The initial euphoria over interferon, a drug developed at colossal expense, has also disappeared, except when it comes to treating certain forms of leukemia.

Attempts to influence the body's cancer defenses using genetic engineering is still in research stages.

LIVING WITH CANCER

Because social and psychological factors contribute significantly to how cancer runs its course, friends and family play an important supporting role. Solid relationships strengthen the immune response, and patients who establish a good relationship with their doctor beforehand can play an active role in, and take responsibility for, their treatment. They handle suffering better, develop self-confidence, and cope better in general. Nevertheless, many cancer patients experience

Self-help for side effects of cancer treatment

— Eat frequent, small snacks as opposed to large meals; eat slowly, sip your drinks; avoid sweets and fatty foods, citrus fruit, and strong spices. Toast and crackers can settle your stomach.

— Eat something light (soup or crackers) before taking medication.

— If you develop an aversion to meat, preparing it with soy sauce, fruit juice, or wine may make it more palatable.

— Good oral hygiene is important. Use a soft-bristle toothbrush and avoid mouthwash that contains alcohol or salt. Choose a mild, fluoride toothpaste.

— Keep your lips moist with lip balm.

— Avoid large gatherings, people with contagious diseases, and travel, all of which expose you to potential infection. Should you experience fever, diarrhea, pain when urinating, or any other signs of infection, contact your health-care provider immediately.

— Due to the risk of hemorrhage, be especially careful with knives and tools; wear gloves while gardening. Avoid contact sports.

anxiety and depression that leaves them withdrawn and alienated; this can be greatly relieved simply by talking about it. But unfortunately, medical treatment teams often don't allow patients anywhere near the time they need for talking through their doubts and fears, whether before, during, or after treatment.

Patients who regularly practice relaxation techniques (see p. 694) handle the difficulties of treatment better; meditation and regular yoga routines (see p. 695) can also provide relief. The healing process can be helped along by good diet (such as one adapted from the Preventing Cancer Through Diet section, p. 472) and an exercise routine including walking, hiking, swimming and nonstrenuous aerobic exercise, including underwater aerobics.

Psychological Support

The concept of an illness is very different from the actual experience of being ill. An illness affects not only the diseased organ, but the whole person and his or her various relationships. Therefore, a holistic or comprehensive approach will take into account the patient's childhood, family, work situation, and personal relationships; the fear of pain will be taken seriously, as will the

fear of death.

If you have received a diagnosis of cancer and feel shattered, depressed, and hopeless, and are unable to cope with this on your own, by all means talk to your doctor; this is often the first big step toward recovery. If you can't talk to your doctor or don't find it helps, then seek psychological help. Experts say that one in three cancer patients needs counseling.

Counseling can improve the quality of life and in some cases even prolong life expectancy. There are therapists (psychooncologists) who specialize in treating cancer patients. Behavioral modification (see p. 700) can be helpful in controlling anxiety, coping with despair, handling treatment better, and getting back in control of one's life and experience.

The Simonton program is designed to get cancer patients in touch with their disease through role-playing and creative visualization of the disease and treatment. Ultimately, recovery is visualized, as well as drawn or painted. You can learn Simonton techniques from your therapist and use them daily at home. They can improve your quality of life, and may also increase life expectancy.

Group therapy can achieve similar results, along with giving you the courage to speak openly about your fears and reassess your life this far.

Occupational therapy and art therapies using creative expressions such as painting, dance, or music can help the recovery process. For information on psychological counseling and support, see Counseling and Psychotherapy, p. 697.

FOLLOW-UP TREATMENT

The type and length of treatment will determine the extent of stress on cancer patient and family alike. Most surgery involves 2 to 4 weeks in the hospital. Radiation treatment is generally done on an outpatient basis and lasts between 6 to 8 weeks. Chemotherapy, given mostly on an outpatient basis, takes the longest and lasts 4 to 12 months or longer, including rest periods between courses of treatment.

Following treatment, all cancer patients are advised to go for regular checkups to monitor progress. If the tumor returns or another develops (such as in the previously unaffected breast), it must be caught as quickly as possible. Such relapses usually occur within two years, but they can also appear 5 or more years following treatment; they can usually be overcome with renewed therapy.

If the cancer has spread, a different follow-up procedure is used. With breast cancer, for example, regular monitoring for recurrences is recommended, but the metastases are not exhaustively hunted down. If the cancer has metastasized to the bones, lungs, or liver, treatment will not prolong life expectancy; in these cases it's preferable not to treat until symptoms appear.

The doctor should always discuss the recommended follow-up care with the patient and clarify the goal of any exams.

Career and Earning Capacity

Cancer patients suffer especially intensely from isolation, loss of the sense of self-worth, and the decreased capacity for work. Therefore it's important to maintain a regular relationship with the "outside world" and keep a foot in the professional door. Ideally, doctor and patient together develop a regimen in which this is taken into consideration. Losing a job usually means losing an entire community.

If this can't be avoided, doctors should also be supportive during this difficult time and help enroll the patient in benefit programs. Cancer can cause financial hardships for many patients.
The Cancer Information Service is a good resource for information on support programs, benefit eligibility, rebates and lists of organizations that offer help.

Cancer Information and Counseling Line
800-525-3777

ALTERNATIVE TREATMENTS

The majority of cancer patients supplement conventional treatment with alternative or unconventional remedies, often without informing their doctor or health-care team.

The reasons for this are many. Many cancer patients want to participate more actively in their treatment; others are dissatisfied with medical care or afraid of its side effects. The desire to be cured also drives many patients to doctors, healers, and laypersons offering alternative therapies touted variously as being gentler on the body, having no side effects, embracing the holistic view of illness, or resulting in "victory" over cancer.

Unconventional theories appeal to the popular imagination, playing up the connection between cancer and psychological causes and recommending life changes and the strengthening of immunity and powers.

Unfortunately, their promises are rarely fulfilled. There is no evidence that unconventional diagnoses are reliable. Alternative treatments frequently have side effects, and their effectiveness is usually questionable. To date, no alternative approach has a documented, incontrovertible success rate to match that achieved by conventional medicine in the treatment of childhood and testicular cancer, for example. For all these reasons, there is increasing pressure on alternative practitioners to provide replicable, repeatable evidence of the success of their methods.

Alternative treatments, therefore, cannot replace conventional cancer treatment such as targeted tumor therapy; but as supplements to this therapy, they can in certain cases alleviate symptoms and help recovery.

This is why many health-care providers recommend nontraditional methods for follow-up cancer care. While the cancer patient cannot gauge the objective effectiveness of such treatment, the patient can tell if he or she is feeling better and coping more easily with the disease.

Miracle Cures and Miracle Workers

Promises of miraculous cures and pseudoscientific discoveries make it next to impossible to distinguish dubious claims from valid ones. Stories of alleged cancer cures, spread by word of mouth, and stubbornly persistent, prove that faith can move mountains, and self-anointed "wonder doctors" seem to take advantage of such stories on a regular basis to help them hawk their services in the popular press. So-called "miracle" cures do happen occasionally because patients want to believe in them, and because spontaneous cures do exist. There are documented—albeit very rare—cases of cancer being healed through religious rites or shamanistic rituals.

A spiritual hope for release from suffering may give a cancer patient strength, but if such hopes are dashed, pain and suffering may be even harder to bear than before. As a rule of thumb when attempting to decide whether a claim is serious or frivolous, use your common sense. Adopt a healthy skepticism

— If there is talk of "miracles"

— If, at the other end of the spectrum, a diagnosis of cancer is made to sound like a sure sentence to agony and death

— If somebody claims to have all the answers

A cancer treatment is worthwhile if it can
— cure the cancer
— prolong life expectancy
— improve quality of life

It may not be sufficient to avoid a relapse.
Regarding alternative treatments:

— Don't take too many at once. More isn't necessarily better, and side effects can become impossible to track.

— Watch for side effects; even herbal remedies may have them. Stop treatment if necessary.

— Beware of a remedy that simply purports to help against "cancer": the word refers not to one single condition but rather to many distinct diseases, with distinct causes and prognoses. Anyone who makes such an oversimplified claim is revealing a fundamental ignorance of the facts.

— Remember that people who promote alternative therapies also have financial interests at stake. Many patients would give everything they own for a cure, but a high price tag doesn't guarantee a treatment's success.

— Find out whether your insurance covers alternative medicine.

— Ask your doctor or the Cancer Information and Counseling Line (see p. 479) about approaches to alleviate symptoms and support the healing process.

MANAGING CANCER PAIN

Pain appears early in about half of all cancers; a third of inoperable cancers are accompanied by severe chronic pain. Some pain is stronger than pain medication.

At what point pain occurs and how severe it is does not depend entirely on the medical team. If you can lower your perception of pain or focus your attention elsewhere, your pain sensitivity can be reduced. Behavioral therapy (see p. 700) or hypnosis (p. 701) can help. The World Health Organization (WHO) has issued the following guidelines for cancer pain management:

— Initially, simple pain medication is given, such as aspirin and acetaminophen (Tylenol) (see Analge-sics, p. 660), or nonsteroidal anti-inflammatory pain medication.

— When these are no longer effective, supplemental opioids are prescribed. The weakest of these is codeine, followed by tramadol. Either may be combined with nonsteroidal anti-inflammatory drugs for maximum effectiveness.

— If this approach doesn't bring freedom from pain, morphine compounds are prescribed. They may be taken as drops, tablets, lozenges, suppositories, injections, or may be administered intravenously.

A significant advantage of self-dosing is that the patient is independent and, if circumstances permit, can take care of him- or herself at home.

All pain medications, particularly opioids, should be prescribed according to a fixed schedule. The doses should be sufficient to kill pain, and timed so that pain will not return before the next dose is taken.

The WHO has determined that doctors worldwide tend to prescribe insufficient amounts of morphine for cancer patients. This may be due in part to the complexities of prescribing a controlled substance, or to widespread fear of causing a morphine addiction. This fear is unfounded.

These days, cancer clinics are setting up panels of experts to offer advice on the best possible care for each individual patient and to take a proactive approach toward pain, seeking to manage it before its onset. Pain management specialists tend to recommend such a comprehensive approach of treatment.

Supplemental Pain Management

Physiotherapy and massage can alleviate pain, but should be done only with the doctor's approval to avoid any possible risk. Transcutaneous electrical nerve stimulation (TENS) is a technique that stimulates nerves via electrical impulses. Its effectiveness is limited in the case of chronic cancer pain. Pain management can be enhanced by antidepressants, neuroleptics and other neuropharmaceutical drugs (not to mention alcohol), which alleviate pain and relieve related symptoms such as sleep disturbances.

Cannabis products such as hashish and marijuana not only relieve pain, but can also minimize the side effects of cancer treatment. They prevent nausea, induce euphoria, and restore appetite. Although cannabis products are illegal, medications containing synthetic cannabis are available in the United States. and Canada.

In rare cases, extreme pain can necessitate neurosurgical intervention. Surgeons may sever nerve centers in the spinal cord, or block individual nerves by injecting alcohol or a local anesthetic.

GUIDELINES FOR FRIENDS AND FAMILY

Few people feel prepared or equipped to care for a cancer-stricken relative. Yet while being a cancer caregiver is stressful, it can also be psychologically rewarding. The Cancer Information and Counseling Line can offer information on relief programs. The hospice movement offers courses for nonprofessional caregivers.

What you should know:

— Uncertainty in this situation is normal—cancer causes anxiety in the caregiver as it does in the patient. Don't give in: Cancer patients have an uncanny sense of when someone is not speaking openly. Be honest with the patient when you're feeling bewildered or sad. It may give him or her the courage to talk about his or her own feelings.

— Hang in there when the patient expresses grief, doubt, or despair, or is tormented by shame, guilt, or self-hatred. This is when he or she really needs you to be there. Assistance may be available from friends, experts, the Cancer Information and Counseling Line, support groups, social workers, psychologists, members of the clergy, or the treating physician.

— Honesty should be the bottom line in your life together. The patient will let you know how much he or she wants to know about his or her condition; usually only small amounts of information can be processed at a time. Commonly, the initial reaction to a diagnosis of cancer is denial, followed by rage, attempts to negotiate, depression, and finally, hope. Try to stay with the patient through these stages. Fight the urge to flee. If you can't take reality and resort to acting overly comforting or reassuring, the patient will only feel more alone.

— Touch the patient a lot. Physical contact is extremely important. If the patient feels you are avoiding him or her, he or she will be overwhelmed with a sense of worthlessness.

Unconventional and unproven cancer treatments

Diets—Cancer cannot be "starved" out. No diet is effective against tumors. These diets, including the macrobiotic diet, all put additional stress on the body.

Heat therapy (hyperthermia)—The Ardenne method combines overheating and oxygen therapy with equivocal success; the Weisenburg method combines hyperthermia with megadoses of vitamins and is still in the experimental stages.

Anthroposophical medicine—The tumor-inhibiting effect of mistletoe-compound injections has not been definitively proven in spite of large-scale studies; they may minimize the side effects of conventional cancer treatments.

Homeopathy—Won't stop the tumor, but may improve the patient's overall condition.

Herbal medicines—The effect of herbal remedies on tumors is dubious; injections of echinacea are risky.

Ozone therapy—May cause blood clots.

Organ-extract preparations—Treatments with preparations made from the thymus gland are risky; those made from stem cells can be life-threatening.

Microorganisms—Fermented drinks such as kampucha are of dubious value.

Bioenergetic procedures—Bioresonance therapy, for example, has unknown effects; acupuncture can raise the risk of wounds and infections.

Immune strengthening—The effectiveness of techniques such as the Wiedemann, Theuer, or Schleicher method is as yet unknown.

Preparations from bodily fluids and tissue—These include preparations from tumor mass, cytokines, and lymphocyte vaccines. Effectiveness: Highly questionable; attendant risks: Unknown.

Folk remedies—Beet juice does not cure tumors; drinking petroleum is extremely dangerous.

Unconventional diagnostic tools (not recommended)

The following methods can produce a false diagnosis of cancer:

Iridology—diagnosis based on irregularities in the iris

Electroacupuncture—Voll technique, based on imprecise measurements

Blood tests—diagnosis based on the shape of drying blood drops

Fringe medical practitioners also claim the existence of cancer-causing factors in the blood, or use dowsing rods to locate supposed cancer-causing earth emanations. No evidence exists for the effectiveness of either phenomenon.

— Do nothing behind the patient's back. Try to make all decisions together.

— Try to keep a dialogue open with the patient's employer: Cancer patients are often let go because of irrational fears or mistaken conclusions on an employer's part.

— Find out about possible financial help from a social services center. The Cancer Information and Counseling Line is also a good source of information.

— Respond to the patient's questions about the future with answers that hold out hope, but don't make empty promises.

— Find out what services are offered in your community—visiting nurses, home health aides, respite services.

— Try not to do everything yourself in this chronically stressful situation; you need breaks, too. Set limits. It may be helpful to keep in mind an image of the patient separate from the disease. What this person needs most from you is your compassion, not your suffering.

— If you start to feel overwhelmed, don't push yourself any further. Investigate having the patient cared for in a hospital or hospice setting, so you can save up your strength for all-important visits.

HORMONAL DISORDERS

Most people know that hormones have something to do with love and sex; they may have heard of the sex hormones estrogen and testosterone. Fewer have heard of insulin, the hormone that regulates blood-sugar levels; fewer still are familiar with thyroid stimulating hormone (TSH). Yet these are only a fraction of all the hormones in the body's arsenal.

Together with other regulatory mechanisms, the hormone-secreting glands work to harmonize the functions of all the organs. Via the bloodstream, hormones carry signals from the glands to the particular organs that contain the receptors for them. Specific hormones and specific organs fit together like lock and key.

All the hormone-secreting glands work in close cooperation. They are connected via a complex system of regulation and control that generally works in three phases: (1) The hypothalamus and pituitary (hypophysis), regulatory glands located in the brain, signal particular glands throughout the body such as the thyroid, pancreas, and adrenals, to produce hormones. (2) This takes place, for example, the pancreas secretes insulin. (3) The hypothalamus and pituitary then review the body glands' performance by checking concentrations of that hormone in the blood.

Pancreas

The pancreas produces digestive enzymes as well as hormones. In the beta cells of the islets of Langerhans in the pancreas, insulin is produced; in the alpha cells, glucagon, an insulin antagonist, is produced.

Insulin

Insulin has several functions in the metabolism. Among other things it maintains the blood-sugar level within a specific range: it should not drop below 60 mg%, or exceed 140 mg% after eating. If blood sugar levels are too high, insulin causes the sugar to be stored in liver, muscle, and fat cells.

A small amount of insulin should always be in circulation in the bloodstream, even when no food has been ingested.

Glucagon

If the pancreas registers insufficient sugar in the blood, the insulin antagonists are activated. For example, the hormone glucagon signals the liver to release its sugar stores.

DIABETES

Symptoms

Common signs of diabetes are
— Excessive thirst and urination, at night as well as during the day
— Weight loss
  Other signs can include
— Fatigue, exhaustion
— Itching all over the body, especially the vagina
— Deteriorating eyesight
— Soreness in folds of the skin (between the buttocks or thighs, under the breasts)
— Slow healing of sores
— Frequent sores in the mouth or vagina, or on penis

Hypothalamus
Pituitary gland

Thyroid

Adrenals
Pancreas

— Leg cramps at night

— Pins and needles in hands or feet ("going to sleep")

On the other hand, adult diabetics may remain symptom-free. Children may experience sudden, drastic drops in insulin levels without showing any symptoms; their condition quickly becomes life-threatening (diabetic coma). Signs include

— Nausea, vomiting

— Abdominal aches or cramps

— Dry skin and mucosa

— Breath smelling like acetone

— Rapid, heavy breathing

— Impaired consciousness to total loss of consciousness

Someone in diabetic coma should be taken to the hospital immediately.

Causes

Type I (insulin-dependent diabetes mellitus, or juvenile-onset diabetes): Is in part hereditary. Its causes and triggering factors are still mostly unknown. In Type I diabetes, the body's immune system destroys more than 80 percent of the pancreas' insulin-producing cells (see Health and Well-Being, p.182).

Type II (noninsulin-dependent diabetes mellitus, or adult-onset diabetes): Is hereditary, the insulin-producing cells cannot handle various stresses.

Obesity is a primary stressor. In obese people, fat cells may become largely unresponsive to insulin, and the pancreas must produce substantially more insulin than in people of normal weight in order for blood sugar to be stored in the fat cells. This demand strains the pancreas until it is exhausted. In addition, adequate insulin is no longer produced following food intake.

Who's at Risk

The following stress factors increase the chances of developing diabetes:

— Surgery

— Accidents

— Pregnancy

— Medications

Possible Aftereffects and Complications

It is possible to live to old age if diabetes is stabilized. However, living for years with fair or poor sugar levels can lead to secondary disease or eventual damage.

Medications that can trigger type II diabetes

— Corticosteroid medications (e.g., for rheumatism, allergies, asthma, immune system disorders, or following organ transplants). Even short-term corticosteroid treatment may trigger diabetes.

— Diuretics (e.g., to reduce fluid buildup in the tissue and to lower blood pressure).

— Birth-control pills.

Generally, blood sugar levels return to normal when medication is stopped.

Damage to Small Vessels (Microangiopathy)

Sugar levels in the body's proteins rise, causing the tissues' condition and functional capacity to be compromised. Blood vessels are particularly affected, disrupting circulation. At worst, vascular damage affects the kidneys, eyes, and nerves.

Kidney Damage (Nephropathy)

Changes to the small vessels in the kidneys lead ultimately to kidney failure (see p.425). Metabolic waste that the kidneys can no longer process poisons the body. After years of poor blood-sugar levels, about a third of diabetics develop kidney damage, many eventually requiring dialysis. Many die from the cardiovascular diseases that often result from kidney damage.

Eye Damage (Retinopathy)

Capillaries in the eye weaken and bleed into the retina. New blood vessels may proliferate in the transparent vitreous body, compromising eyesight. If unchecked, this may lead to blindness. Ninety percent of all Type I diabetics experience changes in eyesight due to poor control of blood-sugar levels.

Cataracts (see p. 243)

Glaucoma (see p. 244)

Damage to Larger Blood Vessels (Macroangiopathy)

All diabetics are in danger of vascular damage, but especially older Type II diabetics, in whom many risk factors are combined.

Various organs are affected. Nerve damage combined with constriction of the coronary arteries can be especially dangerous: Diabetics are less likely to notice the warning signs of a heart attack. Seventy percent of diabetics die from cardiovascular diseases.

Circulation in the legs can also be compromised (see Poor Circulation, p. 326).

Nerve Damage (Neuropathy)

The nerves become less responsive to stimuli. Early signs of this include
— Tingling or pins and needles in feet and legs.
— Burning sensation in soles of feet.
— Leg cramps at night.
— Aching legs: For example, the weight of bedcovers may seem unbearable.

Later a dangerous lack of sensation develops. The patient can no longer feel surface wounds. Small, superficial cuts can develop unnoticed into an ulcer, destroying tissue and bones. The feet are especially at risk. When neuropathy develops, the gait gradually changes until the ball of the foot supports one third more body weight than before.

If parts of the foot darken, gangrene has set in. If a diabetic has severe circulatory disorders in conjunction with gangrene, amputation may be unavoidable to prevent the infection from poisoning the rest of the body. However, too many diabetics today undergo amputations unnecessarily; they could live on intact with antibiotic treatments, correct and periodic cleaning of the infection, and appropriate resting of the foot. Never allow a foot or leg to be amputated without consulting a diabetes specialist.

Neuropathy may also affect the nerves of inner organs, causing
— Accelerated heartbeat
— Unregulated emptying of the stomach
— Constipation and diarrhea
— Incomplete emptying of the bladder; and pathogens can multiply in the retained urine
— Impotence in men, because of weakening of the reflex that causes the penis to engorge with blood

Prevention

Type I: Self-help measures will not prevent the disease. Experiments using drugs to prevent the immune system from destroying insulin-producing cells have not been successful. Treatment may lead to kidney damage or cancer, especially since the medication must be taken for the rest of one's life.

Type II: Contracting this disease can be postponed through measures that protect the pancreas, including
— Maintaining normal weight
— Getting regular exercise
— Avoiding medications that might trigger diabetes (see p. 484)

Preventing Aftereffects

Diabetics usually don't notice the gradual development of complications, which can be prevented only by keeping blood-sugar levels as close to normal as possible. Regular doctor visits are extremely important for early detection of the signs of diabetic damage. The following measures may keep damage to a minimum:
— Don't smoke. The risk of retinal damage is almost doubled in diabetics who smoke. Kidney damage also occurs more than twice as often as in non-smoking diabetics.
— Maintain normal weight (see Body Weight, p. 727).
— Maintain normal blood pressure, by medication if necessary (see High Blood Pressure, p. 321).
— Maintain good cholesterol levels through diet, taking medication if necessary (see Atherosclerosis, p. 318).
— Get regular physical exercise. If this is no longer possible, maintain vascular fitness by doing exercises prescribed for circulatory disorders (see p. 327).
— If possible, use birth control methods other than the pill (see p. 493).
— Avoid substances that cause kidney damage, including painkillers (see Analgesics, p. 660), and dyes such as those administered by the doctor prior to X ray analysis of kidney function.
— Older diabetics and people with incipient neuropathy should pay close attention to the condition of their feet.

When to Seek Medical Advice

If you experience the aforementioned symptoms, and you are overweight and diabetes runs in the family, see a doctor.

If there is a suspicion that you are diabetic, your blood-sugar levels should be measured before breakfast and about two hours after breakfast. You may have diabetes if
— Your fasting blood-sugar level exceeds 120 mg%
— Your blood-sugar level after eating exceeds 180 mg%.

Fasting blood-sugar levels between 80 and 120 mg%, or levels between 120 and 180 mg% after eating, are considered borderline. In these cases, your doctor can administer an exact amount of sugar and monitor how your body reacts. This oral glucose tolerance test is extremely important for pregnant women, who should try to maintain levels within normal range (see p. 493).

Self-Help
Natural remedies can supplement, but not replace, medical treatment.

Treatment for Diabetes
— A diabetes-appropriate diet rich in fiber
— Adequate physical activity
— Monitoring of sugar content in urine or blood
— Blood-sugar-reducing tablets, in some cases
— Insulin, in some cases

Diabetes Education
All diabetics should inform themselves fully about their disease, regardless of whether they need to inject insulin or not. Most diabetics have to change their eating habits. In addition, they need to familiarize themselves with tablets or insulin, and learn how to do the necessary tests. Special educational programs exist for both types of diabetes.

Treating Diabetes Through Exercise
There is a clear connection between diabetes and exercise: Lots of exercise, little medication; little exercise, lots of medication. Exercise in this case means a minimum of 30 minutes of physical exertion sufficient to work up a sweat, at least three times a week. Endurance sports are best, such as running, cycling, swimming, cross-country skiing, or even vigorous gardening.

Treating Diabetes through Diet
Nutritional principles for diabetics depend on what type of diabetes you have; whether you are an overweight Type II diabetic; and whether you inject insulin.

If you are an overweight Type II diabetic, you probably have sufficient insulin, but because of your weight it is unable to function optimally. Once you lose weight, the situation will probably correct itself. A diabetic diet for you simply means eating frequent, small, fiber-rich meals, with the goal of losing weight.

Foot care for diabetics with neuropathy
— Wash feet daily with lukewarm water and mild soap; dry with a soft towel.
— Check the feet and between the toes carefully for fissures, redness, rash, and blisters.
— Put a mirror on the floor and use it to check the soles of your feet.
— Use lanolin to moisturize feet after washing.
— Don't alternate hot and cold baths; your decreased sensitivity to temperature places you at risk of scalding.
— Don't use a hot water bottle or heating pad to keep feet warm.
— Protect feet from sunburn.
— Never go barefoot or wear shoes without socks. In summer, avoid hot stones and sand.
— Wear socks and shoes that give your feet plenty of room. Nothing should rub; toes should lie comfortably side by side, not squeezed together.
— If you're no longer certain of the fit of your shoes, draw an outline of your feet on paper at home, cut it out, take it with you to the store and insert it into shoes. It should slip into the correct size without forcing.
— Choose shoes made of soft leather, with flexible soles.
— Opt for wide, flat heels.
— Change shoes often, if possible.
— File, do not cut, toenails to avoid the risk of cutting yourself.
— When you can no longer care for your feet as directed, ask friends or family to help.
— Otherwise, go regularly to the foot doctor. Advise beforehand that you are diabetic and need special care.

Nonoverweight Type II diabetics can adjust their diets in order to get by on the little insulin their bodies produce. They can avoid large fluctuations in blood sugar levels by
— eating high-fiber foods (see p. 726)
— avoiding refined sugar and carbohydrates that make blood-sugar levels soar (see p. 726)
— eating smaller meals more often during the day, rather than a few big meals

Insulin-injecting diabetics need to coordinate their diets with their insulin requirements. Because only foods high in carbohydrates raise the blood-sugar level, they must be eaten with great care. Food is divided into "free" and "restricted" carbohydrates according to the insulin necessary for its metabolism.

How fast the blood-sugar level rises depends not only on the type of carbohydrate ingested, but mainly on how quickly food is metabolized and how long it takes to pass from intestine to bloodstream. Fat, for example, takes longer to be processed.

Free carbohydrates
All vegetables and nuts with the exception of potatoes and corn.

Restricted carbohydrates
Depending on carbohydrate content, different foods cause the blood sugar level to rise at different rates.

Malt sugar, mashed potatoes, baked potatoes, honey, rice, corn flakes and cola drinks effect a rapid rise.

Bread, cake, muesli (granola), pudding, beer, oatmeal, bananas, corn, potatoes, table sugar and fruit juices cause a moderate rise.

Milk, yogurt, fruit, pasta and ice cream effect a slow rise.

Food Exchange
A food-exchange list is very helpful in coordinating insulin dose with carbohydrate intake. One carbohydrate unit contains about 10 grams or one third ounce of carbohydrate, equivalent to half a hard roll, half a slice of rye bread, half a banana, or a small pear. (This list is not intended as a strict indication of weight, but rather as a general guide for blood-sugar control purposes.)

The concept of food exchange makes it easier for insulin-injecting diabetics to eat a more varied diet. Any 10-gram serving of carbohydrates can be substituted for another portion of the same value.

How many carbohydrate units insulin-injecting diabetics should eat per day depends on their body size and how many calories they expend.

People who take blood-sugar-reducing tablets usually also have strict carbohydrate-unit guidelines in order to avoid hypoglycemia.

Alcohol
Alcohol can cause hypoglycemia in diabetics (see p. 490). However, two glasses of the following drinks should not cause damage: Distilled spirits (clear schnapps, aquavit, fruit brandy, cognac, whiskey), dry wine, dry champagne, or one glass of beer. It's best to drink alcohol together with food.

— Some wines contain less than 9 grams of sugar per liter. When it contains less than 4 grams of sugar, wine can be labeled "Suitable for diabetic consumption."

— "Sparkling wine for diabetics" must contain no more than two grams of sugar or 40 grams of sugar substitute per liter.

Sugar-containing drinks such as large quantities of beer, liqueurs, fortified wines, sweet or fruity wines (especially late-vintage wine, or wine from specially selected grapes), and most American sparkling wines are not advisable. "Dry" or "brut" wines can contain lots of sugar. Use caution when drinking "diabetic beer": Some kinds contain high amounts of alcohol.

For sugar substitutes, see p. 733; for diabetic foods, see p. 735.

Treatment with Pills
Blood-sugar-reducing pills are effective only if the pancreas is still producing insulin, and under no circumstances can they compensate for poor diet. Taking pills makes sense when the diabetes is causing symptoms and the patient

— Is of normal weight or has lost a significant amount of weight (depending on basal weight, between 6.5 and 11 pounds.), *and*

— Gets regular exercise, *and*

— The pills cause a definitive drop in blood-sugar levels within 2 weeks.

According to these guidelines, less than a third of diabetics should be treated with pills; unfortunately, these guidelines are not always adhered to.

The pills prescribed to reduce blood-sugar levels are mostly sulfonylureas. Their biggest drawback is that overweight diabetics taking them may gain even more weight. The pills can also cause hypoglycemia (see p. 490).

Pills containing biguanides should be prescribed only in rare cases due to potential severe side effects.

Acarbose prevents the absorption of carbohydrates in the upper portions of the intestine, thus leveling the blood-sugar profile. However, many diabetics find it hard to put up with the associated side effects, which include flatulence, abdominal pains, and diarrhea.

Sulfonylurea Sugar Pills

First generation:
Chlorpropamide (Diabinese)
Tolazamide (Tolinase)
Tofbutamide (Orinase)
Second generation:
Glimepiride (Amaryl)
Glipizide (Glucotrol)
Glyburide (Micronase, DiaBeta)
Undesirable effects: gradual, unnoticed onset of hypoglycemia (see p. 490); usually, weight gain.
Monitoring (see also p.489)*:* To begin with, test urine daily two hours after breakfast; later, do this two or three times a week. If sugar level is high three days in a row, see your doctor.
If you get sick during this period (e.g., cold, vomiting, fever), test for ketones. If ketones are high, see your doctor.

Treatment with Insulin

Diabetics must categorically take insulin if
— their body no longer produces insulin
— they have had a previous metabolic disorder with high ketone levels in the urine
They should inject insulin if they have high blood-sugar levels despite average weight, sufficient physical activity, and an appropriate diet, *and*
— they are under 60 years old
— their blood sugar levels don't drop appreciably after 2 weeks of taking sugar pills
— the liver and kidneys no longer function satisfactorily;
— they are pregnant
Combining insulin and sugar pill use is not advisable in the long term.

Two Approaches

Fixed Insulin Therapy: The doctor determines how much insulin is injected and how often, as well as which, how much, and how often food is taken. The patient checks urine or blood sugar and regularly goes in for checkups. In this approach the patient is dependent on the doctor.

Intensive Insulin Therapy: Diabetics are trained to determine insulin dosage on their own, depending on what they want to eat, how much exercise they're getting, and whether or not they're ill. They inject two different kinds of insulin between three and five times daily, either separately or mixed together, and test their blood-sugar level four times daily. This approach allows diabetics to be substantially independent.

Insulin pens

Syringes have largely been replaced by insulin "pens," so named because they resemble a pen, containing insulin instead of ink and a needle in place of a nib. The injections are usually given in the belly or thigh. A fold of skin is pinched between thumb and forefinger of one hand while the shot is administered at a 45 degree angle with the other.

There is little danger of infection, so disinfecting the skin may not be necessary. (Exception: When using an insulin pump.)
Disadvantages
— Because of the "low-tech" nature of this approach, bits of lint or debris can get in the way of the injection.
— If air enters the pen, pressure is lost and no insulin, or too little, will come out.
— Each manufacturer makes a different type of insulin cartridge. In an emergency the patient may have trouble obtaining the correct cartridge.
— Patients accustomed to mixing regular and time-release insulin on their own have to use the pen more frequently, since the cartridges come pre-mixed.

Insulin Pumps

An insulin pump is smaller than a cigarette box and is worn on the body. A thin feed-line takes insulin from the reservoir to the needle, which is inserted in the fatty tissue of the belly and secured with an adhesive bandage strip. The pump releases constant small doses of insulin on its own in accordance with the body's basal metabolic rate. Patients must adjust insulin delivery at mealtimes, however.

The effectiveness of insulin delivery by pump is the same as that of other insulin delivery methods.
Advantages
— Especially good for people with irregular daily routines (such as shift workers) and for pregnant women.
Disadvantages
— The tube can kink or clog.
— The feed-line can get clogged or fall out.

— Keeping a needle in the belly may hurt or cause an inflammation.

—The needle's entry point may redden, swell, or harden.

— The patient is dependent on the pump's manufacturer for insulin.

— The pump becomes like a prosthesis.

— Insulin pumps are very expensive.

Different Kinds of Insulin

There is quick and short-acting (normal) insulin and slow and long-acting (time-release) insulin. The slower-acting type provides the body with a constant low dose; the quick-acting type prevents blood sugar spikes after eating. Both are available singly in tubes, or premixed together. Insulin for pens and pumps comes in higher concentration.

Handling Insulin

Keep insulin in the refrigerator if you won't be using it immediately; do not freeze. Don't use insulin that has expired.

Monitoring Levels

Sugar levels in the blood or urine must be monitored several times daily. How often and at what time of day these measurements should be taken differ for each individual and should be discussed with the doctor. If you happen to have an acute illness (e.g., cold, flu), you should also test for acetone.

Transplants

Transplants of the pancreas or cells from the islets of Langerhans are in experimental stages; results are not yet conclusive.

Self-Monitoring

Sugar-monitoring kits are standard-issue equipment for all diabetics.

Sugar in the Urine

One to 2 hours after eating, a test strip is held in the urine stream. The patient can determine the sugar content of the urine by matching the color to a chart on the package.

If the sugar level exceeds 2 percent over 3 consecutive days, try to determine the cause: Weight gain? Not enough exercise? Illness? Medication? If you can't figure it out, see your doctor.

Ketones in the Urine

Elevated blood- or urine-sugar levels and simultaneous detection of ketones in the urine is always an alarm signal. Contact your doctor as soon as possible.

Sugar in the Blood

For this you need a drop of blood from the fingertip or earlobe, obtained by pricking yourself. Consult the instruction manual on how to apply the blood to the test strip and read the results. The coloring on the tester corresponds to the chart on the package.

Blood-Sugar-Measuring Kits

Some devices don't use color matching but give measurements in numbers; be advised, however, that very low or very high measurements often come out inexact with this method.

Monitoring by a Doctor

Every 3 months, your doctor should measure your glycosylated hemoglobin, which gives an indication of how well your blood-sugar levels have been controlled over the previous quarter. Ask for all test results and measurements in numbers, and know what the "normal" values are. Different test methods yield different results. Stabilized diabetics have glycosylated hemoglobin readings of between 6.5 to 7.5 percent.

Blood pressure and weight should be measured at every visit.

Once a year, the doctor should perform the following tests:

— Kidney function (including testing for protein in the urine, see p. 645).

— Blood analysis (including creatinine level, see p. 641; cholesterol, see p. 640).

— Electrocardiogram (EKG), see p. 646.

— Reflex testing of the feet to determine nerve function.

—Taking pulse in the feet.

— Eye exams to measure pressure in the eyeball, examine the retina, and to check eyesight.

If changes are noted, more frequent exams may be necessary.

Money-saving tips for diabetics

Blood-sugar-self-test strips can be cut in half length-wise so they last twice as long and require less blood for testing. Cutting them will not hinder their effectiveness.

For insulin pump users: Pumps and related equipment from lesser-known manufacturers are a better value for your money and just as effective.

Possible Side Effects: Hypoglycemia

Hypoglycemia (too little sugar in the blood) is a warning sign. It can arise if blood-insulin levels are too high, either because of injections or blood-sugar-reducing tablets. Mild hypoglycemia has no repercussions if it is rectified immediately; severe hypoglycemia can cause brain damage. Signs of hypoglycemia include

— Sweating
— Trembling and agitation, especially trembling hands, weak knees, pounding heart
— Nervousness
— Headaches
— Hunger
— Difficulty concentrating
— Tiredness
— Speech disturbances
— Vision disturbances
— Aggressiveness

If treatment is not immediate, seizures and loss of consciousness can result.

How to Counteract Hypoglycemia

At the first sign of hypoglycemia, take 10 to 20 grams of glucose or 6 ounces of fruit juice. Always have glucose tablets on hand. Afterwards, eat two carbohydrate units of bread, fruit, chocolate, or similar food. Then look for the cause of the hypoglycemia. Possible causes include:

— Overdose of insulin, incorrect dose of pills
— Not eating enough
— Unexpectedly high physical-stress level
— Excessive alcohol consumption
— Vomiting or diarrhea
— Dieting
— Drug interactions that cause blood-sugar levels to drop

In an emergency:

Diabetics should carry an emergency kit at all times. Inform your relatives, colleagues and sports partners that you are diabetic, that you inject insulin, and that they can inject you with glucagon if you lose consciousness during a hypoglycemic episode. Explain

— The signs of hypoglycemia.
— Where you keep sugar and glucagon (see p. 483).
— That they should give you sugar if you start acting strangely or attract excessive attention, even if you resist (hypoglycemia makes some people aggressive).
— That if you lose consciousness, it's likely due to too little rather than too much sugar in your blood.

With Inadequate Treatment: Hyperglycemia

Hyperglycemia (too much sugar in the blood) arises if blood-insulin levels are too low. It can be avoided by regularly checking blood- and urine-sugar levels and taking appropriate action. Hyperglycemia damages all the organs, which can lead to complications.

The signs of hyperglycemia are the same as those listed as symptoms of diabetes on p. 483.

How to Counteract Hyperglycemia

Test urine for sugar and ketones. If levels are extremely high, follow instructions below. Once you've stabilized, talk to your doctor about possible causes.

If you don't inject insulin, or have no quick-acting insulin on hand:

— If urine sugar level exceeds 2 percent, test three times daily.
— If urine-sugar level exceeds 3 percent for three consecutive days, *or*
— If sugar and ketone levels in urine are very high, see your doctor immediately.
— Drink lots of water until you can get to the doctor.

If you have quick-acting insulin on hand:

If you have a high blood-sugar level or your urine-sugar level exceeds two percent, and you have a high ketone level:

— Inject 20 percent of your daily insulin dose as quick-acting insulin. Drink lots of water.
— After two hours, test blood sugar and ketone levels.

If both are still too high, inject the same amount of insulin again.

— After two hours, test again. If blood sugar measures less than 240 mg% but ketones are still high, inject half of the original dose of insulin

— If blood sugar is below 180 mg%, drink lots of water and eat two carbohydrate units.

Treating Complications

The most important treatment for complications caught in their early stages is to maintain a daily average blood-sugar level of less than 150 mg%.

Damage to Large Blood Vessels

First and most important: Quit smoking (see p.755). For the treatment of circulatory diseases, see p. 316.

Nerve Damage

There is no medical treatment for nerve damage.

Kidney Damage

At the first sign of kidney damage, blood pressure should be stabilized at 120/80. This can prevent kidney function from worsening.

In diabetics under age 45 with kidney failure, a kidney transplant may be performed (see Kidney Failure, p. 425). In patients over 65, weekly dialysis is often performed (see Kidney Failure, p. 425). For people between 45 and 65, treatment depends primarily on the condition of the large blood vessels and on other diabetes-related damage.

Eye Damage

Laser treatment can remove damaged areas of the retina (see Retinal Detachment, p. 247). This prevents further damage but makes vision nearly impossible in the affected area. About half of patients prefer such treatment to blindness.

In the case of bleeding into the vitreous humor, the entire vitreous and all affected tissue is surgically removed. The patient should not expect to be able to see again immediately, but blindness can at least be avoided. Unfortunately, bleeding often recurs some time after such an operation.

A cataract can be surgically removed (see Cataracts, p. 243).

For treatment of glaucoma, see p. 244.

Impotence

For treatment of impotence, see Men's Issues, p. 541.

Wound Treatment

Any wounds or sores that don't start to heal after a week, are red in color, and secrete yellow or greenish fluid, require professional treatment. An inflamed foot should be kept completely still, propped up on pillows to ensure that there's no pressure on the foot. The wound should be flushed with antiseptic solution; sometimes antibiotics, either oral or intravenous, are prescribed as well.

Counteracting Hypoglycemia
Appropriate to take for hypoglycemia:
3 to 4 glucose tablets (corresponding to 1 to 2 carbo-hydrate units).
Fruit juice, lemonade, cola drinks.
Sugar cubes, raisins, crackers.
Not recommended: Chocolate and other fatty sweets.

Emergency kit for diabetics who take blood-sugar-reducing pills: several glucose tablets.

Emergency kit for diabetics who inject insulin: Blood-sugar test kit; several glucose tablets; a packet of glucagon (check occasionally to make sure it hasn't expired); at least two carbohydrate units to tide you over, such as raisins, chocolate, a bottle of juice.

If a diabetic loses consciousness:
Clear the airways (remove any food and dental devices from mouth). Lay patient on his or her side.

If possible, measure blood-sugar level.

Inject glucagon.

If no glucagon is on hand, call a doctor.

Never give an unconscious person something to drink.

If consciousness is not regained ten minutes after an injection of glucagon, call a doctor.

When the patient wakes up, give two carbohydrate units.

Glucagon, the first-aid fallback:
Glucagon signals the liver to release all its sugar reserves. A glucagon kit contains a syringe and needle, a vial of water, and a vial of powder.
— Remove safety cap from the needle.
— Poke the needle through the protective seal of the water vial and draw water into the syringe.
— Poke the needle through the protective seal of the second vial and empty the water into the powder.
— Shake the vial till the powder is dissolved.
— Draw the solution into the barrel of the syringe. The needle must be completely submerged in the fluid, otherwise air will enter the barrel.
— Stick the needle in the skin of the thigh, buttocks, or belly and slowly press the plunger. In an emergency, you can safely inject directly through clothes.

Living as a Diabetic
Diabetics and parents of diabetic children can become overwhelmed. Support groups, available almost everywhere, can help remove the impression that you are alone in dealing with your difficulties.

Patients who have been sick for years often need professional help to keep their spirits up. For information on how to get help, see Counseling and Psychotherapy, p. 697.

Professional Life
Because of the risk of hypoglycemic episodes, diabetics should avoid professions in which they might pose a danger to themselves or others, such as work that involves moving parts, presses, stamping machines, rollers, blast furnaces, monitoring electrical controls, or high tension installations. They should not work as roofers, chimney sweeps, scaffolders, police officers, soldiers, border guards, long-distance truck drivers, taxi drivers, bus drivers, pilots, or navigators.

Diabetics have more trouble reconciling treatment and calling in some professions than in others, although this needn't mean that these professions are off limits. Piecework can cause problems because one can't always take lunch hours punctually; shift or night work may make it difficult to adjust insulin doses because conditions or schedules may change constantly. In such cases an insulin pump can be useful (see p. 488). The appropriateness of a profession depends on your particular type of diabetes; diabetes alone is usually insufficient ground to be turned down for a job.

Unemployment
In principle, diabetics with no complications are capable of normal work levels. Nevertheless, many employers hesitate to employ diabetics on the grounds that they are sick more frequently than their colleagues. This false assumption is the legacy of a former age, when many diabetics were poorly educated about their condition and therefore insufficiently stabilized. However, studies have shown that, on average, diabetics actually miss fewer days of work annually than others, and that properly trained diabetics are neither hospitalized more often nor for longer periods than nondiabetics.

If You're Traveling
— Take along everything you need to manage your diabetes.
— When going overseas: Definitely take along papers that identify you as a diabetic. This makes it easier to explain to border officials why you are carrying syringes and needles.
— When flying: Pack diabetes gear in your carry-on luggage.
— When taking road trips in summer: During the ride, keep your insulin in the shade under your seat. If you have to leave it in a parked car, keep it in a cooler.

When Driving
The general rules for driving apply equally to Type I and Type II diabetics. All diabetics are responsible for ensuring that they do not have a hypoglycemic episode while behind the wheel. In practice, this means you should do a blood test before setting out.
— Don't set out on an empty stomach.
— Don't set out if you feel sick in any way.
— Keep your emergency kit (see p. 491) within arm's reach.
— At the slightest sign of hypoglycemia, pull over to the side of the road immediately.
— Do not smoke or drink alcohol during the ride.
— Have your eyesight tested every 6 months.
Do not drive if:
— Your diabetes is difficult to stabilize and your levels are frequently out of kilter.
— Your diabetes has affected your heart.

—Your doctor has established that you have advanced cerebral blood-vessel hardening.

You should also not drive:

— During the first 3 months of treatment, since this is the time you're most likely to experience vision disturbances and/or hypoglycemic attacks.

When applying for a driver's license, you'll need a form filled out by your doctor attesting that you are capable of driving. It may help to demonstrate that you have your diabetes under control.

Birth Control

Diabetics should try to avoid birth-control pills, if this doesn't have an adverse effect on their love life, and use a mechanical (rather than chemical) means of birth control instead (see p. 551). Intrauterine devices (IUD) are also appropriate. The pill can cause vascular damage, and in diabetics the vascular system is especially susceptible. Do not use the pill if you

— Are older than 35
— Have vascular damage
— Have high blood pressure
— Have high cholesterol levels
— Are overweight
— Smoke

For those who can't warm to the idea of an IUD, the appropriate choice may be the socalled "minipill." If these are unavailable, use only pills with low hormone content. The estrogen content should definitely be less than 30 mcg, the progesterone content less than 1 mg (see p. 556).

Pregnancy

A diabetic should plan her pregnancy. Before getting pregnant, if possible, you should

— Switch from blood-sugar-reducing drugs to insulin
— Switch to purified insulin or human insulin
— Get used to paying even closer attention to your insulin/sugar balance

During pregnancy, your health and the health of your baby depend on keeping sugar levels as close to normal as possible. To this end, you should count on at least three insulin injections and five blood-sugar tests a day.

The pregnancy of a diabetic is always high-risk, so have frequent obstetrics and gynecology (OB/GYN) checkups.

You won't have to spend the last 4 to 8 weeks before childbirth hospitalized if

—You are certain you have your diabetes firmly under control
— Your OB/GYN confirms through a checkup two to three times a week that you and the baby are doing fine
— The hospital is close to your home

Women who are routinely admitted to the hospital early for childbirth just because they are diabetic should be aware that, statistically, about half of these pregnancies end in an early cesarean section. On the other hand, in cases where only extremely high-risk pregnancies are admitted early, only about a quarter of the pregnancies end in a cesarean, with no ill effects to the babies. It goes without saying that diabetic mothers may and should breast feed their children.

Predicting Diabetes in Children

The following conclusions may be drawn from analyzing the occurrence of diabetes in families:

— If one parent has Type I diabetes, there is a smaller than 5 percent chance that an offspring will develop diabetes over the course of his or her life.
— If both parents have Type I diabetes, the risk to the child is between 10 and 25 percent. Siblings of Type I diabetics have a risk of 6 to 7 percent of developing Type I diabetes themselves.

With Type II diabetes the risk is considerably greater if there are diabetic relatives. Following the measures listed on p. 485 under "Prevention" can help prevent onset of the disease.

Thyroid

The thyroid gland is located below the larynx. Under normal conditions it is not noticeable, but if it becomes abnormally enlarged, a goiter appears.

The thyroid regulates the basal metabolism—the rate at which the body produces and uses energy to maintain its processes.

High levels of thyroid hormone mean high energy usage; low levels mean less energy usage. The thyroid hormones triiodothyronine (T3) and thyroxine accelerate (T4) the metabolism; iodine is required for their production.

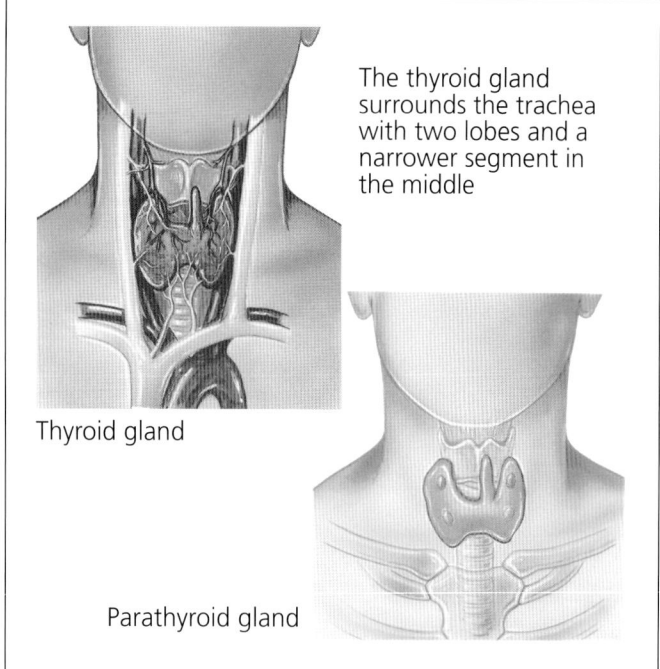

The thyroid gland surrounds the trachea with two lobes and a narrower segment in the middle

Thyroid gland

Parathyroid gland

If thyroid hormone levels are too low, the glands in the brain kick in: The hypothalamus (see p. 501) signals the pituitary to release thyroid-stimulating hormone (TSH), which in turn stimulates the thyroid to produce more hormones. The hypothalamus checks to see that this has taken place. The cycle can be disrupted in several ways:

— The pituitary and/or hypothalamus produce insufficient thyroid stimulating hormones.
— The thyroid is unable to respond to the brain's command to send more hormones into the blood stream.
— There is insufficient available iodine.

In all three cases the body will be deficient in thyroid hormones. Overproduction of thyroid hormones, however, always originates with the thyroid gland.

The thyroid also produces the hormone calcitonin, which is involved in the metabolism of calcium and phosphate.

GOITER

A goiter is an enlarged thyroid. Most goiters don't affect normal thyroid function; they are usually caused by iodine deficiency.

A goiter is also a clear indication that the regulation of thyroid production and function is disturbed. This can be caused by either hypothyroidism (see p. 495) or hyperthyroidism (see p. 496).

Symptoms

An enlarging thyroid generally has no symptoms. Once it starts to take up room in the throat, the enlargement may become visible and lumps may be felt; hoarseness and difficulty breathing may result.

Causes

Goiter due to iodine deficiency: A lack of iodine causes the thyroid to grow, because more thyroid tissue will result in the production of more hormones. The body is usually successful in rectifying its deficiency in this way.

Goiter due to nitrate overload: An excess of nitrates, e.g., in the water supply (see p. 731), prevents the thyroid from absorbing iodine.

Goiter due to thyroid underfunction: The pituitary and hypothalamus continuously register insufficient thyroid hormone levels, so the pituitary produces TSH, but the thyroid is already working overtime to supply the body with hormones, albeit inadequately. For more on hypothyroidism, see p. 495.

Who is at Risk

The risk of goiter is greater in people
— Who eat iodine-poor diets and whose water supply contains too little iodide (see Trace Elements, p. 747)
— Whose water supply contains high nitrate levels
— Who smoke
— Who are on medication

Possible Aftereffects and Complications

In an enlarged thyroid, parts of the tissue may cease producing hormones. Such "cold nodules" can in rare cases become cancerous (see Thyroid Cancer, p. 499).

Other areas of the tissue can turn into "hot nodules": these no longer respond to the pituitary's instructions or produce the correct level of hormones.

Iodine insufficiency during pregnancy poses a danger to the baby: Miscarriages are more common; the baby may develop a goiter. If the thyroid hormones are deficient, the baby's intellectual development may be affected (see Congenital Hypothyroidism, p. 496).

Prevention

Iodine deficiency can be prevented through an iodine-rich diet (see Iodized Salt, p. 736 and Trace Elements, p. 747); iodine-containing toothpaste, mineral water, or tonics can also help. Dried kelp also contains iodine.

Keeping nitrate levels low (see Hazardous Substances in Food, p. 729, and Drinks, p. 736) will help the thyroid use available iodine.

Undesirable Side Effects

Although they may be unaware of it, about 65 percent of people over 45 with goiters (diagnosed or not) have hormone-producing tissue in their thyroids that no longer responds to the pituitary's commands. In these people, increased iodine intake can lead to hyperthyroidism; in the worst case this can lead to so-called thyroid storm, which, even today, is fatal in 50 percent of cases. Such a thyrotoxic episode is particularly life-threatening for the elderly.

For people with hyperthyroidism (see p. 496) even the smallest amount of iodine is harmful, stimulating the production of yet more hormones.

In some people, however, for unknown reasons, iodine has the opposite effect, leading to a goiter or even hypothyroidism.

When to Seek Medical Advice

Seek help if you notice your throat has thickened or you feel lumps there. The following exams will determine why a goiter has developed:
— Ultrasound, to ascertain thyroid size (see Ultrasound, p. 651)
— Blood test to check TSH level

If the ultrasound confirms that the thyroid has undergone changes, a scintiscan is necessary (see Scintigraphy, p. 650).

Self-Help

Not possible.

Treatment with Medications

Today, goiters are treated with iodide. They gradually shrink as a result of treatment, and stay small after medication is discontinued. A year-long treatment with thyroid pills is sometimes prescribed before starting the iodine therapy, to stimulate the pituitary to stop producing the hormones that overwork the thyroid. In these cases, however, the resulting thyroid shrinkage is not permanent: Within four months it tends to return to its previous size.

Surgical Removal of Goiter

A goiter can be treated with radioactive iodine therapy (see Graves' Disease, Radiation Treatment, p. 496), or surgically removed. This is necessary if
— The airways are constricted by more than half, or blood supply to the throat area is severely restricted. People under 25 should try to control the situation with medication for a minimum of 2 years before opting for surgery.
— A single "cold nodule" develops. This is especially likely in people over 40 who have had a goiter for some time.
— Thyroid cancer is suspected.

Most goiters are preventively removed to ensure that no malignancy develops, although the risk is low (see Thyroid Cancer, p. 499).

Possible Complications Following Surgery
— One to 3 percent of thyroid operations incur irreparable nerve damage to the muscles of the larynx. In the case of such laryngeal paralysis, the voice changes and speech (and occasionally breathing) is compromised. If the operation has to be repeated, 10 to 20 percent of patients suffer laryngeal paralysis.
— The parathyroid glands can be inadvertently removed as well, causing painful muscle cramps in up to 2 percent of patients (see Hypoparathyroidism, p. 500).
— Only patients whose residual thyroid is extremely small must take thyroid hormone supplements for the rest of their lives; for all other patients, iodide supplementation is sufficient.

HYPOTHYROIDISM (UNDERACTIVE THYROID)

Hypothyroidism may be congenital or develop over the course of life. Symptoms differ depending whether the thyroid functions insufficiently or ceases to function completely. Hypothyroidism causes cretinism and myxedema.

CONGENITAL HYPOTHYROIDISM (CRETINISM)

Hypothyroidism left uncorrected during pregnancy can lead to skeletal deformities and nervous disorders in the child.

If thyroid hormones are completely absent, the child may be born with severe intellectual and physical defects. Treatment can address only the hormonal situation: The developmental damage is irreparable. In the first week of life, one of the battery of screening tests performed on every newborn checks for the presence of TSH.

MYXEDEMA

Symptoms

The symptoms of myxedema include reduced endurance, poor concentration, fatigue, and sensitivity to cold. Both internal and external rhythms slow; the patient becomes apathetic, lethargic, and depressive. These signs are often misdiagnosed as nonspecific symptoms of aging. A goiter may or may or not be present.

In the case of marked hormone deficiency, the skin becomes remarkably pale and dry, hair becomes bristly and the voice turns hoarse. Affected babies are excessively quiet, feed poorly, and suffer from constipation. Older children grow slowly and reach puberty late; their intelligence may be affected.

Causes
— All factors that cause goiter (see p. 494) can also signal hypothyroidism.
— Insufficient thyroid hormone can result from drug treatment, surgery, radiation, or inflammation of the thyroid.
— The immune system may attack the thyroid.
— In rare cases, the glands in the brain don't produce enough regulating hormones, so the thyroid receives no stimulus for hormone production.

Who is at Risk
About one in a hundred people suffers from hypothyroidism. Women are five times as likely as men to be affected. The condition is usually discovered between ages 40 and 60.

Possible Aftereffects and Complications
These include circulatory disorders, changes in the heart and lungs, edema (e.g., around the eyes), and anemia. In women the menstrual cycle may be irregular; men may lose their sex drive.

If the illness is detected late in a child and the deficient hormones aren't supplied on a regular basis, intellectual and physical development may be compromised. In extremely rare cases, hypothyroidism can cause obesity.

Prevention
See Goiter, p. 494.
Newborns are tested for hypothyroidism through early-detection newborn screening.

When to Seek Medical Advice
— Seek help if you notice the listed symptoms in yourself or your child.
— If there are cases of goiter in your family or neighborhood, special vigilance is advisable.

Self-Help
Not possible.

Treatment
Thyroxin pills will supply the missing hormones. These must initially be given at extremely low doses and increased only gradually, lest the accelerated metabolism exhaust the organs.

HYPERTHYROIDISM (OVERACTIVE THYROID)

Several factors can cause excessive levels of thyroid hormone in the bloodstream. The resulting symptoms are the same, but treatments differ.

GRAVES' DISEASE

Symptoms
Excessive amounts of thyroid hormone cause the patient to "live in the fast lane," both internally and externally. Symptoms include
— Nervousness, pounding heart, trembling fingers
— Always feeling too hot, sweating profusely
— Weight loss despite large appetite

— Rapid speech, hurried movements, unconcentrated behavior
— Goiter (may or may not be present)
— In people over 60, reduced functioning, apathy

In at least a third of patients with hyperthyroidism the eyeballs protrude (exophthalmus) and the following symptoms are present:
— Burning, runny eyes; sensitivity to light
— Seeing double or blurred vision

Causes

Graves' disease is an autoimmune disorder in which the thyroid produces excessive, unregulated amounts of hormones.

Who is at Risk

Women are five times more likely to be affected than men. The disease usually appears during puberty, pregnancy, or menopause.

Possible Aftereffects and Complications

The heart may become overtaxed by constantly working under pressure; bones may become brittle.

Eyelids may no longer close completely over the protruding eyeballs; corneal problems and conjunctivitis can develop. In the worst cases, blindness results.

Prevention

Not possible.

When to Seek Medical Advice

Seek help if symptoms are present. Graves' disease is often misdiagnosed as a nervous disorder, vegetative dystonia (see Health and Well-Being, p. 182), or old age. Testing for pituitary thyroid-regulating hormones will permit a correct diagnosis. An ultrasound exam can detect any lumpy areas in the thyroid.

Self-Help

Take reasonable precautions; try to take life easy.
— Alternate between work and rest throughout the day.
— Eat a nutritious, vitamin-rich diet (see Healthy Nutrition, p. 722).
— Drink plenty of liquids, but avoid alcohol and caffeine.
— Don't smoke.

— Avoid excessive exposure to sun.
— Avoid saunas.
— Avoid iodine (e.g. in seafood or iodine-containing medications like antiseptic solutions).
— Avoid swimming in water with high iodine content.

If your eyes are affected:
— Wear tinted glasses
— Sleep with head elevated
— Use artificial tear eye drops (see Eye Strain, p. 228)

Treatment

An autoimmune disease like Graves' disease needs to be dealt with both physically and psychologically. Help is necessary (see Counseling and Psychotherapy, p. 697).

Medications

Medications can prevent the thyroid from producing excessive amounts of hormones. Methimazole (Tapazole) is commonly prescribed. Propylthiouracil (PTU) is usually prescribed as second line treatment. Generally, thyroid hormone is prescribed simultaneously with the hormone-suppressing medication, to suppress production of thyroid-stimulating hormone. If this fails, a goiter develops.

Disadvantages: Treatment lasts at least a year. Medication must be taken regularly, and frequently checkups are required. In about 40 percent of patients undergoing this type of treatment, the thyroid resumes overproduction of hormones after the medication is stopped. At this point, lifelong treatment becomes inevitable.

Radiotherapy

Patients are given radioactive iodine, administered orally. It is stored in the thyroid and gradually destroys the thyroid tissue. Radiation exposure to the other organs is equivalent to that of an X ray. This method is successful in treating about half of all cases of overactive thyroid, if
— The patient is over 40
— Treatment with medications was unsuccessful or is not possible

Radioactive iodine treatment has been used for 50 years; it is more user-friendly and poses fewer hazards than surgery, and has a higher success rate than treatment with medications. There is no evidence that it increases the risk of cancer.

Disadvantages: Patients continue to emit radioactivity for a while, and the thyroid is "hot" for a time. They may be confined to a special wing of the hospital until radioactivity is no longer detectable. Depending on the patient's situation, a hospital stay may last from 2 to 10 days, or outpatient treatment may even be an option, as long as special precautions are taken.

After about 6 months, the radiation has usually destroyed so much thyroid tissue that treatment can be stopped. In some cases, however, the thyroid is now unable to produce hormones at all. The risk of reversing the situation (substituting underfunction for overfunction) through radiation therapy is between 3 and 20 percent.

Surgery

The quickest way to treat an overfunctioning thyroid is surgery. But because of the risk of serious complications, doctors choose this option only in special cases. Possible complications include:
— Those listed under Goiter Surgery, p. 495.
— Up to a third of thyroid-surgery patients have to take thyroid pills after the operation because hormone production is no longer sufficient.

Treatment for the Eyes

Depending on how much the eyes protrude, the following approaches can be useful:
— Painkillers
— Iodine-free eye drops or ointments
— Radiation of the area behind the eyeball
— Immunosuppressant medications such as corticosteroids (see p. 665).
Treatment should be handled by both an eye doctor and an endocrinologist.

HASHIMOTO'S THYROIDITIS (AUTOIMMUNE THYROIDITIS)

This involves the development of a free-standing mass in the thyroid, which no longer responds to signals from the pituitary gland, and produces unregulated hormone levels.

Symptoms

The symptoms of these adenomas resemble those of Graves' disease (see p. 496), except that in this case the eyes do not protrude.

Causes

When the thyroid enlarges due to iodine deficiency, a free-standing mass or adenoma may develop (see Goiter, p. 494) and remain undetected until the body receives a large dose of iodine (often contained in the contrast media used in diagnostic X rays), which suddenly promotes the production of excessive amounts of hormones.

Who is at Risk

Ten to 50 percent of all hyperthyroid cases result in such adenomas. The risk of contracting the disease increases with iodine deficiency.

Possible Aftereffects and Complications

The healthy part of the thyroid may stop functioning, with the adenoma's hormone production leading to hyperthyroidism.

Prevention

Prevent iodine deficiency (see Goiter, p. 494).

When to Seek Medical Advice

Seek help if symptoms listed under Graves' Disease (p. 496) are present.

Self-Help

Not possible.

Treatment

If the adenoma is smaller than about an inch and a half, and the patient's metabolism is stable, the lump should simply be checked regularly. In addition, iodine should be avoided. General recommendations often include either surgically removing the adenoma or destroying it with radiotherapy (see Hyperthyroidism Treatment, p. 497).

THYROIDITIS (INFLAMMATION OF THE THYROID GLAND)

The various forms of thyroiditis are distinguished according to their symptoms: Sudden and severe (acute thyroiditis), moderate (subacute thyroiditis), or low-level and continuous (chronic thyroiditis).

Symptoms of Acute Thyroiditis
— Throat pain
— Sensitivity to pressure in throat; swelling
— Difficulty swallowing
— Hoarseness
— High fever

Symptoms of Subacute Thyroiditis
Same as above, except fever is only rarely present.

Symptoms of Chronic Thyroiditis
This condition may be present for long periods without any symptoms. It is generally identified by its result, an underactive thyroid (see Hypothyroidism, p. 495).

Causes of Acute Thyroiditis
Causes may include a bacterial infection or an aftereffect of treating another thyroid disorder with radioactive iodine.

Causes of Subacute Thyroiditis
Viral infection.

Causes of Chronic Thyroiditis
Autoimmune disease.

Who's at Risk for Acute Thyroiditis
This disease is extremely rare.

Who's at Risk for Subacute Thyroiditis
This condition usually appears following a cold or viral infection of the upper respiratory tract. Women are four times as likely as men to be affected.

Who's at Risk for Chronic Thyroiditis
This is the most common of all thyroid inflammations. Women are 20 times as likely as men to be affected.

Possible Aftereffects and Complications
Each inflammation destroys thyroid tissue; depending on the extent of the damage, thyroid hormone production is reduced to some degree. The result is hypothyroidism (see p. 495).

Prevention
Not possible.

When to Seek Medical Advice
Seek help if symptoms are present.

Self-Help
— Get bed rest.
— Keep throat cool with an ice pack (see p. 685).

Treatment for Acute Thyroiditis
Antibiotics (see p. 661) are prescribed to fight the disease-causing bacteria. Anti-inflammatories, such as those used for collagen vascular diseases, can also ease symptoms. If the inflammation causes an abscess, it should be lanced and drained by a health-care professional.

Treatment for Subacute Thyroiditis
In mild cases, anti-inflammatory medications like those used for collagen vascular diseases are sufficient. In more severe cases, corticosteroids (see p. 665) are used to reduce the inflammation. Antibiotics won't help against this viral disease.

Treatment for Chronic Thyroiditis
Chronic thyroiditis is almost always recognized only after it has caused hypothyroidism. Taking thyroid hormones will rectify this deficiency and also provide relief and rest for the struggling thyroid. In severe cases, corticosteroids can diminish the body's autoimmune reaction (see p. 186, 353).

THYROID CANCER
See also Cancer, p. 470.
Thyroid cancer is rare. Ten to 30 people in a million contract the disease annually; it is fatal in five of the cases.

Thyroid cancer requires an immediate operation. Where necessary, this is followed by treatment with radioactive iodine (see Hyperthyroidism, p. 496).

There is no connection between thyroid cancer and iodine deficiency or hypo- or hyperthyroidism; and in adults, radiation therapy does not increase the chances of thyroid cancer.

For any changes in the throat area, doctors will examine the thyroid for nodules. Every "cold nodule" that turns up in scintigraphy (see Goiter, p. 494) is considered potentially cancerous until proved otherwise. A "cold nodule" is always a compelling reason to undergo radioactive iodine therapy to shrink the thyroid.

Parathyroid Glands

The four peppercorn-sized parathyroid glands are located right next to the thyroid. They produce parathormone, which maintains blood-calcium levels within strict limits. If the parathyroid glands register a drop in blood calcium levels, they release parathormone into the bloodstream. This stimulates the bones (see Bones, p. 428) to release calcium and directs the kidneys not to eliminate any more calcium. Parathormone also enables vitamin D to release calcium contained in the intestines into the bloodstream.

HYPERPARATHYROIDISM

Symptoms
Slightly elevated blood-calcium levels produce no symptoms. If there is a great excess of calcium in the blood, the following symptoms may appear:
— Loss of appetite and weight
—Constipation and flatulence
— Increased thirst and frequent urination
— Psychological disorders
— Osteoporosis (see p. 430)
    If blood-calcium levels remain high over a period of years, kidney stones may develop, resulting in frequent urinary tract infections and renal colic.

Causes
Not yet known.

Who is at Risk
Not known.

Possible Aftereffects and Complications
Usually the parathyroid glands become enlarged due to tissue overgrowth and produce too much parathormone, causing the bones to leach calcium. More calcium is now circulating in the blood than the kidneys can process, and kidney stones develop. In addition, duodenal ulcers, pancreatic inflammations or gout may develop.

When to Seek Medical Advice
Seek help if symptoms are present.

Treatment
Extensive growths on the parathyroid glands should always be surgically removed. One percent of these operations may result in laryngeal paralysis (see Goiter, p. 494).

HYPOPARATHYROIDISM

Symptoms
The symptoms of hypoparathyroidism resemble those of hyperventilation (inhaling too fast and exhaling too little):
— Tingling in the hands, feet, and around the mouth
— Idiosyncratic cramping in the fingers and toes
—Acute shortness of breath caused by laryngeospasms and/or cramped respiratory muscles
— Abdominal cramping and diarrhea
    Sometimes a seizure is the sole sign of underfunctioning parathyroid glands.

Causes
Hypoparathyroidism generally develops following a thyroid operation; it may be congenital in rare cases.

Who is at Risk
The risk of developing this disorder increases with every thyroid operation.

Possible Aftereffects and Complications
— Cataracts (see p.243)
— Dry, cracked skin; deformed fingernails
In children:
— Defective dental enamel
— Delayed intellectual and physical development

Prevention
Not possible.

When to Seek Medical Advice
Tetanic fits must be treated immediately by a professional. Cramping of the muscles involved in breathing can be life-threatening.

Self-Help
Not possible.

Treatment
Calcium injections are used to treat tetany. Long-term treatment includes megadoses of vitamin D and calcium.

Hypothalamus

The hypothalamus is located in the brain and functions as the master control for most of the hormone glands. It produces at least nine hormones, known as "releasing hormones," which it sends to the pituitary (see below), stimulating it to regulate many body functions. In this indirect way, the hypothalamus influences the thyroid, the adrenal glands, the gonads, milk production during lactation, and growth.

The hypothalamus can sense "calls for action" coming from other regions of the brain; it translates these nerve impulses into hormonal messages. It also monitors hormone levels in the blood, and uses a feedback mechanism to regulate its own functioning.

Pituitary Gland

The pituitary gland, or hypophysis, lies just below the hypothalamus, connected to it by a stalk. It is divided into anterior and posterior lobes.

The anterior lobe of the pituitary responds to a command of "release hormones" with the following six hormones:
— Adrenocorticotropic hormone (ACTH), which stimulates the adrenal glands to produce hormones
— Somatotropin or growth hormone (STH or GH), which stimulates the liver and is involved in sugar metabolism
— Thyroid-stimulating hormone (TSH), which stimulates the thyroid to secrete hormones
— Leutinizing hormone (LH), which stimulates ovulation and the hormones required following conception in women, and signals the gonads to produce hormones in men
— Follicle-stimulating hormone (FSH), which stimulates follicle development in the ovaries in women, and regulates sperm maturation in men
— Prolactin, which stimulates the development of milk-producing glands at the end of pregnancy

The posterior lobe of the pituitary produces two hormones:
— Vasopressin or antidiuretic hormone (ADH), which regulates water balance
— Oxytocin, which stimulates labor during childbirth

ACROMEGALY (GIANTISM)
The symptoms of acromegaly differ in children and adults; its causes and aftereffects are the same in both groups.

Symptoms
In children: Children grow abnormally fast and keep growing after their peers have stopped; many grow over 6 and a half feet tall.
In adults: The extremities enlarge and elongate. Shoes and rings no longer fit, lips and tongue thicken, the growing jaw lengthens the face. The voice becomes hoarse and deep. Acromegaly patients sweat profusely and suffer from joint pain.

Causes
Acromegaly is caused by excessive production of growth hormone due to an abnormal growth in the pituitary gland. In children, all the organs may be affected proportionally as the body grows excessively tall. In adults the bones, cartilage, and connective tissue thicken and broaden. The internal organs can also become enlarged.

Who is at Risk
Both sexes are affected equally. Adults are usually affected between the ages of 30 and 40.

Possible Aftereffects and Complications
Changes in the bones can lead to arthritis (see p. 452) and brittle bones (see Osteoporosis, p. 430). Eighty to 90 percent of patients develop a goiter, about a quarter become diabetic (see Diabetes, p. 483); 10 to 15 percent develop high blood pressure.

Many patients die in their sixties from heart disease. Children mostly die early from one of the many infectious diseases they contract.

Prevention
Not possible.

When to Seek Medical Advice

In children: Seek help if early detection screening suggests that growth is abnormal (see Weight and Height, p. 592).

In adults: Seek help if symptoms are present. An abnormal growth causing the pituitary to malfunction can be diagnosed by testing blood-hormone levels. In addition, an X ray and computed tomography (CT) scan of the entire skull region should be taken.

Self-Help

Not possible.

Treatment

Pituitary tumors are surgically removed where possible. How the surgery is performed depends upon which lobe the tumor is on, and how big it is. Following surgery, pituitary function must be carefully monitored for life. Pituitary hormones must usually be supplemented or substituted with specific medications.

HYPOPITUITARISM

Symptoms

At about age 2, the smaller size and slower growth of a child with hypopituitarism will become apparent.

Causes

Hypopituitarism is caused by growth-hormone deficiency.

Who is at Risk

Boys are almost three times as likely to be affected as girls. The risk is increased if the child's delivery was complicated.

Possible Aftereffects and Complications

If the disease is untreated, the child's height will remain below 4 feet 8 inches. The child's intelligence will be normal. Puberty is usually delayed, but it may also never arrive.

Prevention

Not possible.

When to Seek Medical Advice

Seek help if the child's growth curve shows he or she is growing markedly less, and more slowly, than other children the same age (see Growth Charts, p. 592). Many factors can cause a child to grow slowly; if hypopituitarism is suspected, low-growth-hormone levels will confirm the diagnosis.

Self-Help

Not possible.

Treatment

Injections of human growth hormone are prescribed for this disease. Because this involves years of treatment several times a week, it makes sense for the child or someone in the family to learn to give the injections. In the first year of treatment the child may grow 3 to 5 inches; thereafter, growth will be slower. As an adult, the child will be short.

Almost always, sexual development must be managed with hormones; these should be administered as late as possible (around age 20) because they cause growth to cease.

Adrenal Glands

On top of each kidney sits an adrenal gland, with two hormone-secreting parts: The adrenal cortex on the outside, and the adrenal medulla on the inside. The most important function of the adrenal hormones is to enable the body to adapt readily to external conditions; for example, to go from "normal" to "fight or flight" in a split second. The adrenal hormones also determine long-term stress endurance levels.

The Adrenal Cortex

The adrenal cortex secretes glucocorticoids and aldosterone, hormones with distinctly different functions. Aldosterone regulates electrolytic balance; it affects the kidneys and the circulatory system.

Glucocorticoids regulate the liver's metabolizing of blood fats and proteins into sugar; prevent inflammation by slowing the proliferation of certain white blood cells; and retard the production of antibodies. Corticosteroid medications make use of these properties.

Excessive amounts of glucocorticoids weaken the immune system.

Glucocorticoids also play a role in the body's reaction to stress (see p. 182).

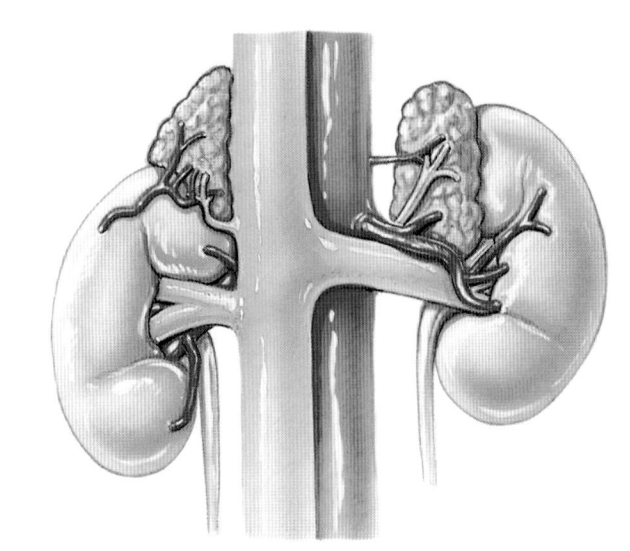

The adrenals sit on top of the kidneys like a hat. They are especially well supplied with blood vessels

The Chain of Command

The actions of the adrenal glands are regulated by the hormone-producing glands in the brain. The hypothalamus signals to the pituitary that there are insufficient glucocorticoids in the blood. The pituitary reacts by sending ACTH to the adrenal glands. Meanwhile, the hypothalamus checks to make sure both other glands are reacting properly. These glands have different activity levels throughout the day. The day's biggest dose of glucocorticoid is released by the adrenal glands at about 5 a.m., at a signal from the pituitary. Smaller amounts are delivered as needed during the day, either when the hypothalamus's blood glucocorticoid sensors register low levels, or when the nerves are in a state of alarm (see Stress, p. 182).

The Adrenal Medulla

The adrenal medulla secretes the "alarm hormones" epinephrine and norepinephrine. When a child runs in front of your moving car, the adrenal medulla floods your system with these hormones, producing the following effects, among others:

— Lung capacity increases, allowing more oxygenation of the blood.
— The heart beats faster and stronger, causing increased blood supply to all the organs.
— The liver and muscles release their energy reserves: for a brief period, you are capable of great strength and speed.

— The nerves are on high alert; reactions are quicker and concentration is better.
— Blood pressure rises.

If no emergency exists, epinephrine and norepinephrine perform these functions at normal levels.

CUSHING'S SYNDROME

Symptoms

The symptoms of Cushing's syndrome include the following:

— Fat deposits develop in the face and on the neck ("moon facies" and "buffalo hump"), not necessarily with overall weight gain.
— Skin becomes thin and stretch marks appear.
— Acne develops; body hair increases. (These symptoms are not present if the disease is caused by medications.)
— The menstrual cycle is disrupted.
— The patient's psychological condition deteriorates.

Causes

An abnormal growth in the pituitary causes it to produce too much ACTH (see Pituitary Gland, p. 501), which stimulates the adrenal glands to release too much glucocorticoid. Glucocorticoid overproduction can also be caused by an abnormal growth in the adrenal cortex itself.

Who's at Risk

One person in 10,000 will develop this disease as a result of overactive glands in the brain. In all other cases, Cushing's syndrome is caused by long-term corticosteroid treatment (see p. 665).

Possible Aftereffects and Complications

— Diabetes can develop or worsen.
— High blood pressure may develop.
— Calcium can leach from the bones (see Osteoporosis, p. 430).

These three aftereffects are more common and more intense if the condition is caused by medications.

— Children may stop growing.
— Following treatment with medications, cataracts can develop (see p. 243).

If left untreated, Cushing's syndrome is usually terminal.

Prevention

It is impossible to prevent Cushing's syndrome caused by abnormalities in the hormone glands. For prevention of Cushing's syndrome due to medication, see Corticosteroids, p. 665.

When to Seek Medical Advice

Seek help if symptoms appear and/or you are taking corticosteroids.

Self-Help

Not possible.

Treatment

Growths on the pituitary or adrenal glands must be surgically removed. To treat side effects of long-term medication, see Corticosteroids, p. 665.

ADDISON'S DISEASE

In this rare disorder, the cortex of both adrenal glands is seriously damaged by the body's immune system. Addison's disease sometimes develops as a complication of tuberculosis or cancer of another organ, such as the lung. The resulting deficiency in glucocorticoids and aldosterone must be rectified by medication.

WOMEN'S ILLNESSES

The external female sex organs are the breasts, mons, labia, clitoris, and vaginal opening; the internal organs are the vagina, cervix, uterus, fallopian tubes, and ovaries. The hormones affect all aspects of these organs, changing and synchronizing the position, size, sensitivity and function of each respective organ depending on the stage of the individual's life. This is manifest during the monthly menstrual cycle, and especially during pregnancy, breastfeeding, and menopause (see p. 510). All these factors also affect the sex drive.

A woman's health, fertility and sexual desire depend first and foremost on her psychological condition (see p. 537); the interactions of hormones are extremely sensitive to psychological factors. This is especially clear in the case of menstrual disturbances and menopause (see p. 508). Therefore, to consider sex organs strictly in terms of their function is to comprehend them incompletely.

THE GYNECOLOGICAL EXAM

Gynecological checkups can't replace the most important part of preventive care: Awareness of ones own body and the self-exam. The more familiar you are with your own rhythms, hormonal fluctuations, variations in discharges, changes in breasts and appearance of the vulva, the more informative your gynecological exam will be.

What to Look Out For

— If your gynecologist's office has an unfriendly atmosphere or an overworked staff, or you feel like a number, chances are good that not much time will be dedicated to you, the patient. If you are considering switching doctors, consult your local women's health center for help.

— Every gynecological exam should start with a detailed conversation, since any gynecological dysfunctions may be linked to other factors such as birth-control issues and sexual or relationship problems. This consult should not be subject to time pressure.

— Your doctor, not an assistant, should be the one to ask important questions regarding your first and/or last period, the length of your cycle, how many births you've had, any medication you're taking, and your general health.

— For most women, having to get undressed before the beginning of the consultation can feel like a violation. Standing naked and exposed in front of

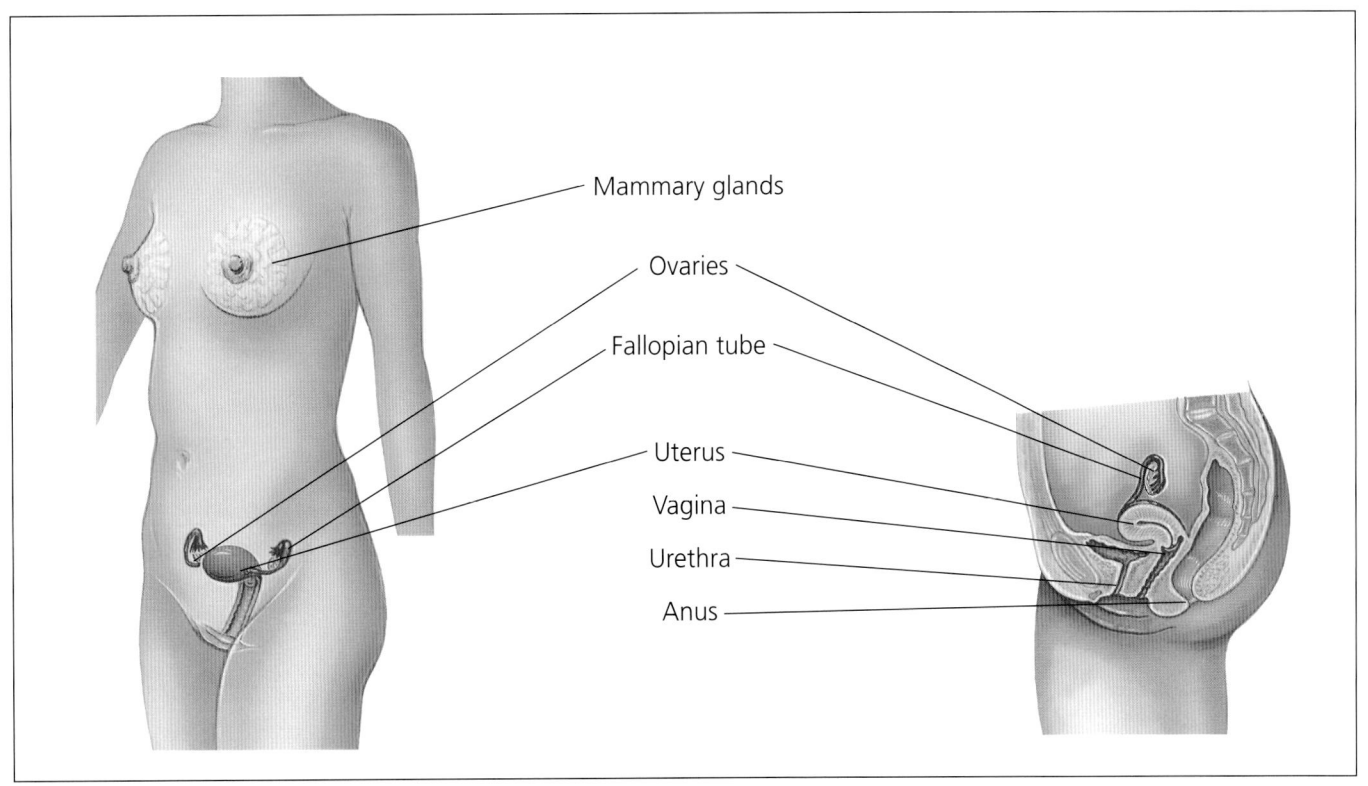

Mammary glands

Ovaries

Fallopian tube

Uterus

Vagina

Urethra

Anus

someone fully clothed does not make for an atmosphere of trust.
— The vaginal exam always involves a speculum and manual exam (palpation). The doctor uses the speculum to check the vaginal walls, any discharge, and the cervix.
— Swabs of the cervix and vagina are taken for a Pap test. This early screening test for cancer can also catch viral infections that could lead to cervical cancer (see p. 524).
— After age 20, all women should have annual check ups with Pap smears. Women taking birth control pills or hormone replacement therapy for menopause should be checked every six months.
— During the speculum exam the doctor can inspect the cervix directly using a special lens called a colposcope. The magnification reveals conspicuous changes in the mucosa; and a tissue sample (biopsy) may be taken.
— The manual exam determines the position and size of the uterus and ovaries.
— Regular breast exams from age 30 on are part of early detection for cancer. Make sure your gynecological exam includes palpating your breasts for hardening or lumps.

MENSTRUATION

From the first day of one menstrual period until the first day of the next, a constant rhythm is repeated in the female body. No two cycles are the same: Stress hormones, released by the body during times of crisis and positive events alike, influence overall hormone levels and can cause changes in individual cycles.

Follicular Phase (Proliferative Phase)

An ovum (egg) takes from the first day of the menstrual cycle until ovulation to ripen. In each ovary, a mass of cells (the follicle) surrounds an unripe ovum. The follicle-stimulating hormone (FSH) regulates the production of more follicles after, or even during, the cycle. Usually one ovum ripens at a time; in exceptional cases, more than one ripens. Estrogen production increases during follicle growth, resulting in the creation of a new uterine lining to replace the one expelled during the last menstruation.

Ovulation

The leutinizing hormone (LH) from the pituitary, influenced by estrogen, gives the command to ovulate. The ripened follicle breaks, the egg is expelled, and the second half of the menstrual cycle begins.

Luteal Phase (Secretory Phase)

The time between ovulation and onset of the next menstrual bleeding is the most fertile phase of the cycle. It is followed by the regression, "breakdown" phase.
The funnel-shaped fallopian tube catches the egg; the egg moves along the tube toward the uterus, which it reaches after 4 to 5 days. For the 12 to 24 hours following its release, the egg is ready to be fertilized. Meanwhile, in the ovaries, the ruptured follicle has developed into the corpus luteum, which produces the hormone progesterone. Progesterone causes a thickening of the uterine lining in anticipation of possible pregnancy.

If no fertilization occurs, the egg decomposes. A few days after ovulation, the corpus luteum begins to wither; the process is complete after about 2 weeks. Hormone levels (estrogen and progesterone) drop; the uterine lining detaches from the walls of the uterus and is expelled during menstruation, as a new cycle begins.

Length of the Cycle

A cycle is calculated from the first day of one period of bleeding until the first day of the next bleeding. In almost all standard medical references this time is given as 28 days, but it merely represents an average: a "normal" cycle can be anywhere from 21 to 35 days.

To learn your individual rhythm, keep accurate records and learn to measure your own basal temperature (see Natural Contraception, p. 551). It's advisable to keep as accurate a record as possible of your periods, recording the first day every time.

Possible Premenstrual Symptoms

As women vary in shape, weight, and personal comfort levels, so do their premenstrual symptoms. The many symptoms possible before the onset of menstrual bleeding are known collectively as premenstrual syndrome (PMS).

Changes in Weight

In the second half of the menstrual cycle—after ovulation—water may be retained in the tissues, giving rise to tenderness in the breasts but also in the legs or arms. The water is expelled in the urine when bleeding begins. In some women, the difference in weight before and after their period can be considerable.

Breast Tenderness

Following ovulation, the breasts may enlarge. The connective tissue thickens, circulation to the breast intensifies, and water is retained. The breasts become sensitive to pressure and pain. These sensations disappear with the onset of bleeding.

Emotional Changes

Prior to their period some women feel not only under physical pressure, but under emotional pressure as well. Whether hormonal changes are responsible for this is still a matter of debate. Feelings of increased vulnerability usually appear a few days before the onset and almost always disappear by the second day of bleeding. In some women, physical symptoms and premenstrual tension intensify after age 30.

Pain in the Back and Lower Back

These may be caused by tipped or prolapsed sex organs, chronic inflammations, reactions to an intrauterine contraceptive device (IUD), problems with posture, or overwork. However, the most common cause of back pain is psychosocial stress, which affects the autonomic nervous system (see Health and Well-Being, p. 182).

DYSMENORRHEA (MENSTRUAL PAIN)

Symptoms

Dysmenorrhea ("cramps") manifests as an ache or pulling sensation, either sharp or dull, which may extend to the thighs, upper abdomen, or back. It may start shortly before the onset of bleeding and usually disappears by the second or third day.

Causes

The individual's physical and emotional condition play a major role in the presence or absence of menstrual pain. There is a close relationship between pain-free menstrual cycles and emotional stability and self-confidence (see Health and Well-Being, p. 182).

Possible organic causes, often at the root of intense or prolonged bleeding (see Menstrual Disorders, p. 508), can be checked during a gynecological exam (see p. 505).

Who's at Risk

Organic causes aside, the risk of psycho-physical disorders during the menstrual cycle can be very high (see Health and Well-Being, p. 182). Many women live with conflicting demands in their professional lives, families, and relationships. Long-standing conflicts and constant stress overload can have painful physical manifestations.

Possible Aftereffects and Complications

Extremely painful menstruation can lead to a vicious circle of anxiety, tension, and other symptoms. If the quality of life is continuously undermined in this way, there are usually negative consequences for a woman's relationship with her body.

Prevention

The best preventive medicine is whatever will bring your physical, emotional, and social well-being into harmony (see p. 184). Basic prevention of menstrual difficulties, however, begins even earlier. Young girls should be nurtured in their self-esteem, encouraged to feel comfortable with their bodies and enjoy physical exercise, and supported in withstanding peer pressure. They should also be given the freedom to explore their bodies and sexuality undisturbed. Mothers and older sisters are important role models, too, in determining whether or not menstruation is treated as a "curse" or a normal part of a woman's life.

When to Seek Medical Advice

Seek help if
— You have been symptom-free and suddenly suffer from menstrual pain
— Cramps become unusually intense
— The pain feels different this time
— Pain and bleeding last unusually long
— You have unusually heavy bleeding

Self-Help

Exercise: Physical exercise can release tension, if you

avoid excessive strain. Try taking a walk, swimming, dancing, or doing gymnastics. See Relaxation, p. 693.

Rest: Get enough sleep, avoid especially stressful or demanding tasks during your period, and pamper yourself. Don't work as hard.

Warmth: Moist warmth is good for cramps. Take a bath, or use a hot water bottle or heating pad on your belly or back.

Herbal remedies: Try calming, cramp-relaxing teas like chamomile or lemon balm.

Medication: Take a simple painkiller such as aspirin or ibuprofen. Excessive cramping can often be avoided by taking these drugs up to 3 days before the beginning of the period. They hinder the body's production of prostaglandins, which can produce symptoms similar to labor pains. See Analgesics, p. 660.

Sexuality: Orgasm, achieved through sex or masturbation, can ease menstrual cramps.

Smoking: Nicotine narrows the blood vessels and makes circulation difficult, which can cause symptoms to intensify. Don't smoke if you have menstrual pain (see Smoking, p. 754).

Treatment

For disorders with organic causes, the underlying causes should be treated professionally.

For symptoms with nonorganic causes, see
— Analgesics, p. 660
— Reflexology, p. 684
— Acupuncture, p. 679
— Acupressure, p. 680

MENSTRUAL DISORDERS

Menstrual disorders are grouped into three categories:
—Very light bleeding
—Very heavy bleeding
— Prolonged bleeding (menorrhagia)

Light bleeding is only very rarely a sign of illness. It can be an early sign of pregnancy, lack of ovulation, or taking birth-control pills. Very heavy or prolonged bleeding, on the other hand, almost always signals disease. Bleeding is classified as "heavy" if 6 or more pads or tampons a day (or 20 or more per period) are not sufficient to handle the menstrual flow. A period is considered excessively long if it lasts over 7 days and/or requires more than 20 pads or tampons.

Symptoms

Heavy blood loss can lead to weakness, dizziness, and circulatory problems.

Causes

Very heavy or lengthy bleeding usually has an organic cause, such as
— Intolerance of an IUD (see p. 555)
— Uterine inflammation (see p. 520)
— Benign muscle-tissue tumors in the uterine wall (see Myoma, p. 521)
— Benign growths in the uterus (see Polyps, p. 521);
— Endometriosis (see p. 52)
— Loss of muscle tone in the uterus, which happens occasionally after many births
— Anticoagulant medications
— Malignant uterine tumors (see Uterine Cancer, p. 525).

Who's at Risk

Refer to risks of the underlying disease or organic cause.

Possible Aftereffects and Complications

Very heavy or prolonged bleeding can lead to anemia (see Anemia: Iron Deficiency, p. 345).

Prevention

Prevention depends on the underlying disease or organic cause.

When to Seek Medical Advice

Seek help if symptoms are present.

Self-Help

If no organic cause can be determined
— Relax, rest, and rid your life of as many stresses as possible
— Seek help and support from others, particularly women.

Treatment

Treatment depends on the underlying disease or organic cause.

What to do for irregular bleeding

Spotting after your period: Spotty, dark bleeding that continues for days after normal bleeding stops may be caused by a uterine inflammation. See your health-care provider.

Spotting before your period: Spotty, dark bleeding some days prior to menstruation is a sign that the corpus luteum is producing too little progesterone; no cause for alarm unless you're trying to become pregnant (see p.565).

Constant bleeding: If bleeding continues regardless of cycle and menstrual phase, commonly in conjunction with taking birth-control pills, consult your health-care provider.

OLIGOMENORRHEA (EXCESSIVELY LONG CYCLES)

In oligomenorrhea, the time between periods is more than 35 days but less than three months, and bleeding is usually light and lasts a relatively short time. Organic causes are occasionally to blame (see Cysts, p. 527), but overload, worry, or stress are more likely to be affecting the cycle.

These psychological factors result in changes in hormone levels, and ovulation may be absent or delayed. You can determine when or whether ovulation is taking place by measuring your body temperature first thing in the morning (see Natural Contraception, p. 551).

If organic causes are ruled out, no action need be taken unless:

— You want to become pregnant and the extra-long cycle suggests you are not ovulating (see Infertility, p. 559).

— You want a shorter period between ovulations to facilitate contraception.

If you feel fine and your overall health is good, there is no need to treat oligomenorrhea. For Self-Help, the same rules apply as for amenorrhea (see p. 510).

POLYMENORRHEA (EXCESSIVELY SHORT CYCLES)

In polymenorrhea, menstrual periods are fewer than 21 days apart. The principal causes are

— An abbreviated luteal phase: The buildup phase of the uterine lining is shorter, and it regresses and detaches sooner.

— Earlier ovulation.

— Lack of ovulation.

As with overly long periods, the causes are largely psychological in nature. You need take no action unless:

— You wish to get pregnant. If the luteal phase is too short, the fertilized egg may not have enough time to attach to the uterine wall.

— The short cycles are accompanied by heavy bleeding. Increased blood loss can lead to anemia.

If you feel fine and your overall health is good, there is no need to treat polymenorrhea. For Self-Help, the same rules apply as for amenorrhea (p. 510).

AMENORRHEA (ABSENCE OF PERIOD)

Symptoms

After more or less regular periods, menstruation is absent for intervals of longer than 3 months.

Causes

In women of childbearing age, the most common cause of amenorrhea is pregnancy. If there is no pregnancy, 80 percent of cases are attributable to psychological difficulties. A change in lifestyle, adjusting to a new situation, extremely tense or stressful situations, or severe emotional conflicts can bring on amenorrhea. There is a close connection between emotional overload and the possibility of hormonal changes.

Anorexia and excessive overeating are similarly manifestations of psychological emergency (see Eating Disorders, p. 202). Anorexia usually leads to absence of menstruation, but extreme weight gain can also cause it.

Occasionally disease, injuries, or accidents can result in amenorrhea, for example:

— General illnesses such as thyroid disorders, diabetes or tuberculosis, or inflammations of the sex organs.

— Faulty or deficient development of ovaries or uterus.

— Benign or malignant growths on ovaries or adrenals.

— Too much of the hormone prolactin in the blood.

— Insufficient hormone production in the anterior lobe of the pituitary gland, or growths on the pituitary.

— After a severe head injury or very complicated, prolonged childbirth involving loss of blood, this important gland sometimes stops functioning.

— Disrupted hormone production by the adrenal gland (see p. 502).

— Faulty surgery, such as an incompetently performed curettage.

Who's at Risk

The risk of complete absence of menstruation is increased in women under long-term emotional and/or physical strain. For example, high-performance athletes are at higher risk of amenorrhea. However, environmental toxins or medications can also interfere with the hormone cycle (see Causes of Infertility, p. 559).

— The pill (see p. 556): About 1 to 2 percent of women who take birth control pills suffer from postpill amenorrhea after discontinuing.

— Other hormone-containing medications can have similar effects, as can antipsychotic medications containing phenothiazines, and anticancer medication containing chlorambucil or cyclophosphamide.

Read the inserts that come with your prescription drugs and ask your health-care provider about side effects if you think your amenorrhea is the result of medication.

Possible Aftereffects and Complications

Lack of ovulation means that you can't get pregnant at this time.

Prevention

Avoid toxins in the workplace and environment, and medications that impair infertility.

When to Seek Medical Advice

Seek help if you stop getting your period.

Self-Help

Diet: A poorly balanced, one-sided, or insufficient diet can disrupt the cycle (see Nutrition, p. 722).
Exercise: Dance, gymnastics, or swimming can bring the hormones back into rhythm. However, avoid excessive high-performance sports and excessive physical exertion.

Some naturopathic remedies can bring the hormones into balance and can also be taken during early pregnancy. However, most other menstruation-inducing herbs have an abortive effect. Therefore, make sure you're not pregnant before using such preparations, and always consult your doctor beforehand.
Massage: One can stimulate menstruation by vigorous massage in the direction of the heart. This should be performed only by qualified practitioners.
Sexuality: A satisfying sex life helps promote emotional and physical balance and stimulates hormones as well.

Treatment

If your general health is good, you're not planning to get pregnant, and you have no problem with not menstruating, there is no need for treatment. However, women under 40 who don't menstruate for over 6 months due to hormonal insufficiency should consider hormone replacement therapy in order to avoid osteoporosis (see p. 430) later on. Treatment options for amenorrhea include

— Exercising, getting enough rest and fresh air, massage, tonics, and cleansing or "detox" diets can offer the body additional support.

— Hormones. Hormone therapy is based on the (disputed) belief that suddenly stopping hormone therapy will "jump-start" the body's production of regulating hormones. This treatment is justified if it can be established without a doubt that the body is not producing sufficient sex hormones and a pregnancy is desired, or in very young women with hormone deficiencies. In all such cases, however, the emotional causes of the hormone deficiency should also be explored (see Infertility, p.559).

— Counseling and psychotherapy. Investigating the patient's past suppressed or repressed conflicts (see Conflict-Centered Techniques, p. 699) is the best method for uncovering the causes of amenorrhea.

MENOPAUSE

Menopause occurs more or less between ages 45 and 55. It is a time during which ovarian activity slows and hormone levels slowly drop. Toward the end of this time, menstruation becomes irregular, lighter in flow or shorter in duration; the final cycles occur without ovulation. The final menstruation is defined as menopause; it can be identified only in retrospect, after menstruation has been absent for a full year.

How a woman experiences and copes with menopause depends directly on her contentment with herself and her life as a woman. It also depends on how her body reacts, and how she experiences her body. The transition phase may be accompanied by difficult symptoms, completely symptom-free, or somewhere in between.

Symptoms of Menopause

Because of fluctuating hormone levels, women undergoing the transition to menopause may experience hot flashes and sweating, often followed by chills. Other symptoms may include changes in blood pressure, dizzy spells, a pounding heart, tingling fingers or toes, numb or "asleep" extremities, or swollen joints.

The vagina becomes less moist and elastic; skin and mucosa may become drier. Bladder problems and difficulties with bladder control sometimes develop as well. Menopausal symptoms vary greatly from woman to woman: Some have no problems at all, and only relatively few experience strong and uncomfortable symptoms. Many women find the physical symptoms bearable and get used to them.

Risks

— The risk of cardiovascular disease is increased because of hormonal changes that affect cholesterol levels.
— There is a risk of osteoporosis (see p. 430).

Emotional Changes

Psychological symptoms may accompany the physical changes of menopause. Many women experience occasional sleeplessness, tiredness, anxiety, headaches, dejectedness, or irritability (see Health and Well-Being, p. 182). Menopause may be accompanied by other life changes that make it harder to stay serene and poised.

Physical Changes

The body starts to look different. While wrinkles are still acceptable on men, many women take it hard when skin grows less elastic, hair grows thinner (see p. 290) and they put on a few pounds (see Aging, p. 606).

Social Changes

Menopause is often marked by losses of various kinds. Women not only have to let go of their children: Personal dreams and hopes, too, may be given up because they no longer seem attainable. Returning to the work force can be hard; finding a new professional direction involves great personal effort. Often there are crises in the relationship with a partner.

Self-Help

Professional help is only necessary if symptoms are taking over your life and your general well-being is compromised. Menopausal symptoms are not a disease.

— Exercise and sports will help maintain physical fitness (see p. 762); a balanced diet will keep body weight steadier (see p. 723). Regular exercise and a calcium-rich diet are important in preventing osteoporosis (see p. 430).
— Be aware of your needs and be good to yourself. Try to adapt your lifestyle to your new physical condition (see Health and Well-Being, p. 182; Relaxation, p.693).
— Take advantage of natural healing with herbal baths, body brushing, heat packs, mud packs, or movement therapies (see Natural Healing and Alternative Medicine, p. 679; Physical Therapy, p. 690).
— If you are experiencing psychological problems, depression, or periods of sadness, turn to friends. Keeping a sketchbook or journal can help you take an active part in processing and working through your feelings.
— Professional counseling can help through difficult periods (see Counseling and Psychotherapy, p. 697). Treating menopause with sedatives (see p. 189) or antidepressants (see p. 199) is not advisable.
— Some herbal remedies can ease symptoms. St. John's wort extract can help against depression; valerian and hops can help with sleep disturbances (see p. 688).

Early menopause

— Menopause can occur up to 6 years earlier in heavy smokers than in nonsmokers (see Smoking, p. 754).
— "Early" menopause is defined by symptoms of hormonal deficiency and menopause prior to age 45. Hormone-replacement therapy is frequently prescribed in these cases to minimize the danger of osteoporosis and arteriosclerosis.

Hormone Therapy

For some women, the symptoms of menopause are a heavy burden. Hormone supplementation can make life easier and render the symptoms bearable. In such cases, combined estrogen and progesterone must be prescribed: Estrogen alone is justified only in rare cases, for example following a hysterectomy (see Risks from Hormones section, p. 512).

Women who tolerate hormones well are usually advised to take them for 2 to 5 years, especially if there is a high risk of osteoporosis (see p. 430). The side effects and risks of hormone therapy can be considerable. Their prescription is especially controversial for certain symptoms which could be treated in other, less risky ways (see Self-Help section, p. 511).

Prior to any hormone treatment, the doctor should establish the patient's hormonal status by a Pap smear and blood test. The ratio of estrogen to progesterone is usually more important than the exact amounts of these hormones. Regular checkups are necessary during the course of hormone therapy.

When to Take Hormones

Hormone therapy should be considered only if
— You suffer excessively from hot flashes or sleep disturbances and want short-term, fast relief.
— You want immediate help because your job or family situation will not allow you to adjust to slower-acting measures or alternative procedures.
— You are at relatively high risk for osteoporosis (see p. 430).
— You suffer excessively from hormonal changes and consequent symptoms in the bladder and vaginal areas, such as dryness, irritable bladder, or vaginal atrophy or constriction.
(You suffer recurring, heavy spotting, or constant bleeding, for which organic causes have been ruled out (see Menstrual Disorders, p. 508). If the bleeding does

Avoid hormone therapy in the event of:
— Liver disease
— A history of blood clots
— Problematic metabolism of fats
— Endometriosis
— Breast cancer, or a history of breast cancer in female relatives
— Uterine cancer

Discontinue hormone therapy, with a doctor's approval, in the event of
— Acute thrombosis, heart attack, stroke
— Intensified migraines, or the onset thereof
— Jaundice, pancreatic inflammation, gallbladder disease
— Allergic reactions
— The onset of high blood pressure

not respond to hormone therapy, the cause should be determined by an endometrial curettage.

Estrogens

Different kinds of estrogen function differently. Estriol can treat uncomfortable skin symptoms, including those in the vagina, and have a beneficial effect on fat metabolism.

Estrogens slow the aging process up to a certain point: the skin and mucosa stay moister, bones stay more stable, and blood vessels are less susceptible to arteriosclerosis. This effect, however, can be duplicated by regular physical training, which stimulates the metabolism and benefits the skin, bones and psyche.

Estrogens and Progesterone

The high risk of uterine cancer from estrogens is mitigated somewhat by simultaneous doses of progesterone, so many medications combine the two. Progesterone therapy is omitted only in women who no longer have their uterus. In all other cases, the prescription of estrogen without progesterone constitutes medical malpractice.

Risks of Hormone Therapy

The risk of developing breast cancer from estrogen therapy over the course of years is still not definitively established, but women with an increased risk of breast cancer (see p. 515) should avoid long-term estrogen therapy. Combined estrogen-progesterone injections given at monthly intervals are prescribed in exceptional cases only since the hormone levels are impossible to regulate.

BREAST

The female breast consists for the most part of fatty tissue, in which the lactiferous (milk) glands are embedded like a many-branched bunches of grapes. The lobes of the glands connect to about two dozen mammary gland ducts which lead to the nipple. The breast is also covered and permeated by a fine network of lymph vessels. In the middle of the areola is the sensitive nipple, which may contract and harden when sexually stimulated. Sebaceous glands in the nipple look like little lumps; during breastfeeding, these glands secrete a fatty fluid that protects the nipples.

The size and shape of both breasts is almost always

different. The structure of the fat tissue, usually inherited, determines the size of the breast. Breast size also varies throughout the menstrual cycle. Following menopause (see p. 510) the glandular tissue shrinks and the surrounding skin becomes flaccid.

MASTITIS (BREAST INFECTION)

Symptoms
In mastitis, the nipples or glandular tissue becomes inflamed.

The nipples may be sensitive to pressure and pain and secrete fluid. Usually one breast starts to hurt considerably and become swollen, red, warm or even hot. A high fever may accompany these symptoms, especially in mastitis after childbirth (see Nursing, p. 584).

Causes
Mastitis is almost always connected to breastfeeding (see Nursing, p. 584). The newborn's suckling can damage the nipples (through scabs, fissures, tears). Bacterial infections may spread through the lymph ducts, especially if a milk duct is blocked.

In nonbreastfeeding women, mastitis may appear in connection with certain breast disorders (see Breast Lumps and Cysts, p. 514) or increased levels of milk-producing hormone (prolactin). In these cases, too, the milk glands swell and milk blocks the ducts. Possible causes include stress, thyroid disturbances, or high-blood-pressure medication.

Who's at Risk
Mastitis occurs most frequently in women who
— Practice poor hygiene after childbirth and have even slightly injured nipples
— Are below age 30, whether or not they've given birth (the reason for this is unknown)
— Have breast disorders

Possible Aftereffects and Complications
Fever and chills may intensify, and the lymph nodes in the armpits become increasingly painful and inflamed.

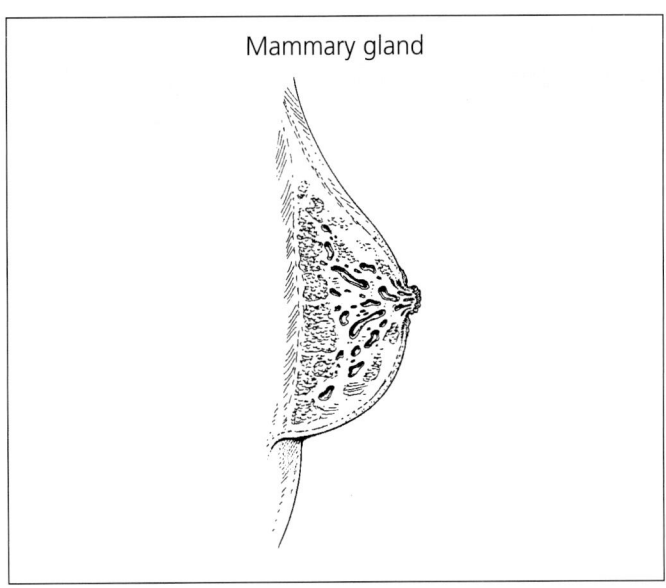

Mammary gland

The infection may come to a head in a suppurating abscess. Mastitis, especially if not caused by childbirth, can become chronic.

Prevention
Practice proper hygiene after childbirth and while breastfeeding.

When to Seek Medical Advice
Seek help at the first sign of pain, redness or swelling. It must be determined whether the mastitis is masking another disease (such as breast disorders; see Breast Lumps and Cysts, p. 514). Occasionally, breast cancer (see p. 515) can cause these symptoms.

Self-Help
In early stages, compresses can help; in later stages, home remedies are ineffective.
— If you are nursing, free the blocked glands by expressing milk or using a breast pump.

Treatment
Antibiotics are used to treat mastitis (see p. 661). In the advanced stages, warm packs or tar-based ointment may be used to induce the formation of an abscess, which is then surgically lanced to release the pus.

BREAST LUMPS AND CYSTS (MASTOPATHY)

The term mastopathy refers to all benign changes of the milk ducts and/or connective tissue of the breast. The most common of these is fibrocystic breast disease. Through excessive cell production the tiny cavities of the gland tissue fill up with fluid, resulting in cysts. Less common are fibroadenomas, caused by overdeveloped connective tissue; these individual lumps contain no fluid.

Symptoms

Often the lumps or cysts are not noticed until, depending on their stage of development about a week before menstruation, the breast becomes painful, sensitive, and swollen; there may be discharge from the nipple.

The breast tissue feels fibrous, and the lumps, which can feel as small as a cherry pit or as large as a hazelnut, move freely under the skin when palpated.

Breast Self-Exam

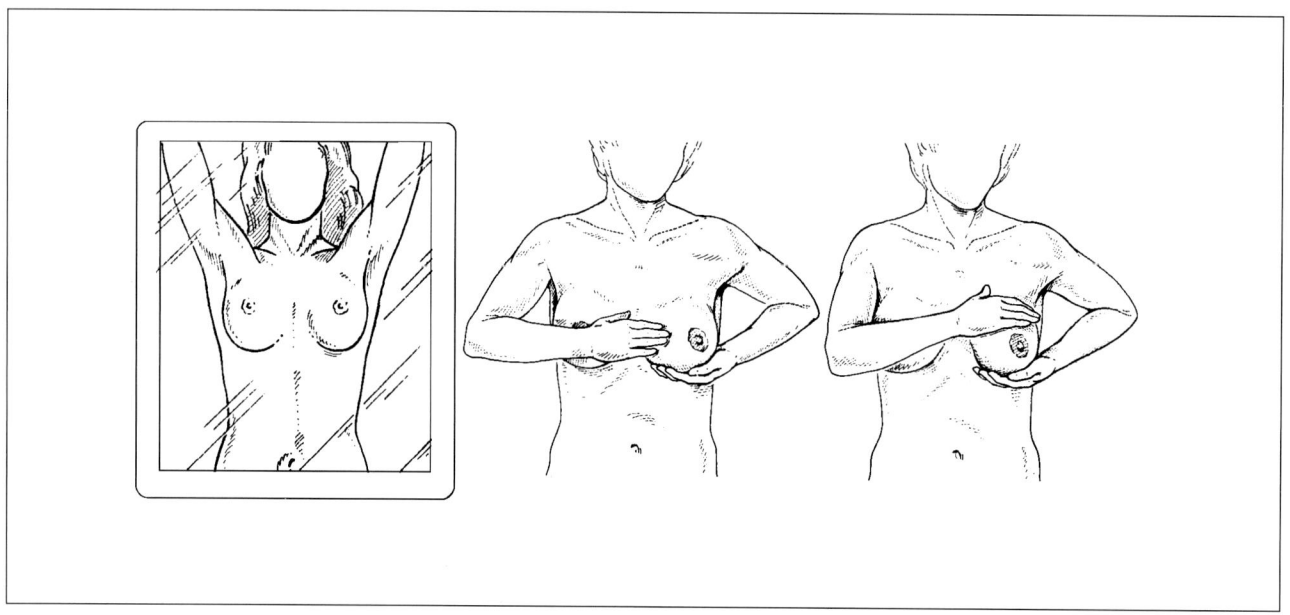

It's best to examine your breasts on the second or third day after the onset of menstruation, when the tissue is especially loose and easily palpated.
1. Stand naked before a mirror, letting your arms hang loosely: Are there any unusual changes to the shape, size, or silhouette of the breasts, or bulges or puckers in the skin?

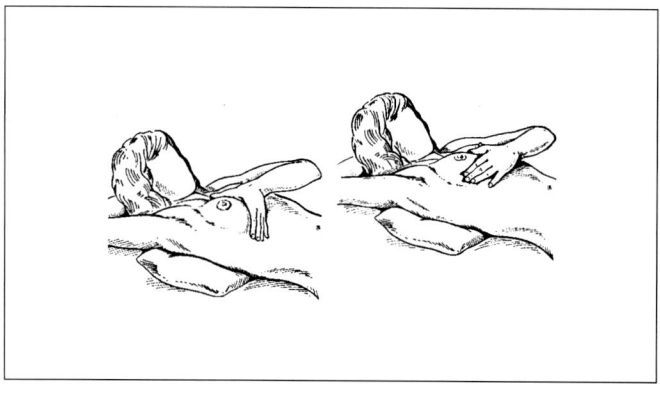

2. Raise your arms over your head and check again, from different angles, for shape and size.
3. Lie relaxed on your back. Tuck your left arm under your head and examine your left breast with your right hand: Is the tissue soft and does it move easily? Do you feel any lumps? Manipulate the whole breast slowly and thoroughly. Examine the entire breast from the outside to under the armpit. Do you feel any nodelike formations?
4. Carefully push the nipple aside: How does the flesh below feel? Does anything hurt?
5. Either sitting or standing, support the breast from below; with the other hand, stroke carefully but firmly from outside to inside, from top to bottom, from back to front. Also press carefully toward the nipple: Is there any discharge? Is it bloody, milky or watery? Repeat the whole procedure with the other breast.
6. If you detect any changes, hardening, lumps, or discharge, consult your doctor.

Causes

Mastopathy is caused by too much estrogen in relation to progesterone. Male hormones, prolactin, and thyroid hormones also play a role, but their exact connection is not yet understood. An indication of such a hormonal situation is considerable breast pain immediately prior to menstruation, when estrogen and progesterone levels are at their highest.

If a discharge from the nipple is present, it is usually caused by fluid buildup in enlarged lobes of the milk glands, or by increased levels of the milk-producing hormone prolactin. Sometimes a discharge can be indicative of growths in the milk ducts.

Who's at Risk

About half of all women between ages 30 and 50 experience a benign breast disorder. Fibrocystic changes account for 70 to 80 percent of all cases. It appears during puberty and is at its riskiest around age 40. After menopause the symptoms diminish in intensity.

Possible Aftereffects and Complications

Simple cystic or fibrocystic disease is seldom associated with complications. It sometimes increases the risk of breast inflammation (see Mastitis, p. 513).

A mastopathy with significant growths in the connective tissue of the milk glands and ducts may lead to abnormal cell development and destruction of the gland; this may further develop into a malignant tumor (see Breast Cancer, p. 515).

Prevention

Do regular breast self-examination (see p. 514) and have regular gynecological exams (see p. 505).

When to Seek Medical Advice

Seek help at the first sign of unusual lumps or swelling, or if you have unusual breast pain prior to menstruation.

Fibrocystic disease can be identified by ultrasound (see p 516). A mammogram (see p. 516) can further help identify a fibrous mastopathy. It should be determined whether or not the growth has developed into a malignancy; a needle biopsy may be additionally necessary for this.

Self-Help

Not possible.

Treatment

Once it is determined that the growth or mastopathy in question is benign, alternative treatments can be tried. Acupuncture can ease pain and tightness (see Acupuncture and Moxibustion, p. 679). Herbal remedies, some of which help stabilize the hormone balance, can be tried.

If there is no improvement, the next treatment option is hormone therapy (progesterone ointment, prolactin antagonists, or danazol, which impedes hormone production of the ovaries).

A mastopathy cannot be cured, but the sometimes intense pains and tenderness can be eased. The breast should be checked regularly by a doctor on an ongoing basis.

BREAST CANCER

See also Cancer, p. 470.

Symptoms

Breast cancer can develop in the nipples, the glands or the milk ducts. It usually manifests as hard lumps that rarely hurt. They can appear not only in the breast itself but also around its edge or even in the armpit. A bloody or mucous discharge from the nipple, or eczema-like inflammation, may also be present. A puckered, painful or itchy nipple can also indicate cancer. Changes to the skin can manifest as orange-peel skin, in which pits appear in a hardened surface.

Causes

Breast cancer is caused partly by hormones. Estrogens encourage the growth of existing tumors; whether they causes them is a matter of debate. For this reason, it is especially important that women who take birth control pills (see p. 556) regularly do breast self-exams or have them performed by a doctor.

Genetic factors and as-yet unknown causes—possibly viruses or environmental toxins as well—also play a distinct role in the development of cancer.

Who's at Risk

About one in 10 women will develop breast cancer. It is the most common form of cancer in women. Two thirds of breast cancers develop in women over 50. Women who are at greater risk of developing a tumor include

— Those with close relatives (mother or sister) who have the disease, since genetics plays a role; those who have not given birth or have done so later in life; who don't breast feed or do so only briefly; those with early menstruation and/or late m e n o - pause (breast tissue is subjected to prolonged exposure to estrogen);

— Those with complicated and/or fibrocystic breast disease.

Possible Aftereffects and Complications

Stage I: The cancer is limited to the glandular tissue. The tumor measures less than an inch across (T1). There is a 60 percent chance of complete recovery—defined as ten years without a relapse.

Stage II: The tumor measures between 1 and 2 inches across (T2), and/or the lymph nodes in the armpit are affected. There is a 40 percent chance of complete recovery. About two thirds of all breast cancers are diagnosed at this stage.

Stage III: The lymph nodes are more extensively involved and/or the tumor is larger than 2 inches across (T3). There is a 10 percent chance of complete recovery.

Stage IV: The cancer has reached beyond the chest and metastasized to more distant organs.

The maturity of the cancer cells and their sensitivity to hormones must also be taken into account when calculating the patient's prospects of recovery.

Prevention

In eight out of ten cases, a woman discovers her own breast cancer. Regular breast self-exams (see p. 514) and gynecological early-detection exams (see p. 505) are extremely important in helping to detect cancers at Stage I.

In addition there are genetic tests that check for the so-called breast cancer gene, which has been found in women whose mothers or sisters have breast cancer. However, the dependability of such tests has still not

MAMMOGRAMS AND ULTRASOUND SCREENING

Mammograms

Before you decide on regular mammograms, you and a doctor you trust should weigh the pros and cons. A mammogram involves X rays, or exposure to radiation. In addition, it has not yet been proven that in women under 50 who undergo routine mammography, breast cancer is usually detected early enough to improve their chances of survival significantly. The following points may help you decide:

— Women under 50 generally have very dense breasts that undergo considerable changes with every menstrual cycle. The dense tissue makes it hard to spot changes, so mammograms only rarely show a clear image and evidence is often inconclusive. If a lump can already be felt or other abnormalities have appeared, a mammogram should be used as a supplement to an ultrasound examination (see below).

— Women over 50 who take hormones have relatively dense breasts, similar to those under 50, because of the hormone therapy; therefore the above applies to them as well.

— In women over 50 who are not taking hormones, the breast's glandular tissue decreases in size; as a result of menopause, the tissue is barely responsive to hormones. Therefore, mammograms show a clearer

image in women of this age group, and studies show that women over 50 who go for regular mammograms die of breast cancer significantly less often than those who don't. Regular mammograms are therefore strongly recommended for this group.

— Most doctors recommend annual mammograms for women at high risk of breast cancer (those whose mammograms reveal sufficient data).

Ultrasound

Ultrasound involves no radiation (see Ultrasound Breast Examination, p. 651) and gives a clear image of the breast tissue. In order to interpret ultrasound images correctly, however, personnel must be specially trained and experienced in the field. Each woman's breast tissue is individual in appearance, and undergoes its own monthly changes according to where she is in her cycle. An ultrasound exam can determine whether a palpable lump is a cyst or another type of tissue change (see Breast Lumps and Cysts, p. 514).

Experienced ultrasound specialists using high-quality images can also distinguish between benign and malignant tumors; high-quality images can depict even the milk ducts very precisely. However, state-of-the-art ultrasound equipment may not be available in every medical setting, so ultrasound is not recommended as the only routine method for early detection of breast cancer.

been proved. It is also questionable how worthwhile they are, since genetic predisposition alone says nothing about when and to what extent cancer might actually develop (see Cancer, p. 470).

When to Seek Medical Advice

Seek help at the first sign of an unusual lump, swelling, skin change or discharge from the breast. If the results of a mammogram are inconclusive (see Mammography, p. 649), a biopsy must be done to determine whether the cancer is benign or malignant.

Magnetic resonance imaging (see MRI, p. 650), a relatively new diagnostic tool, produces images that are often inconclusive. Time and again, MRI examination shows suspicious areas that are not found during surgery, or conversely, fails to show lumps in the breast that are palpable.

Self-Help

Not possible.

Treatment

Following the biopsy, the results of the cell analysis (histology) determine what happens next.

— If tests reveal a carcinoma (malignant tumor), doctors will probably want to operate. They first need to obtain your consent as the patient, however. Experts caution against panicking after a diagnosis of cancer. If a week or two goes by between the diagnosis and the treatment, nothing serious will happen, and you will gain valuable time to think.

— Increasing numbers of patients are keeping their breasts and having lumpectomies. This may be an option if: Only one tumor is evident, it is no larger than ⁴/₅ of an inch, it can be easily located, the underarm lymph nodes are not affected, the tumor is not located directly under the nipple, and the breast is not too large to permit the necessary follow-up radiation.

— In a lumpectomy, the tumor, part of the surrounding healthy tissue, and the underarm lymph nodes are all removed. This results in a loss of between one eighth to one quarter of the breast. During the operation the surgeons fashion a slightly smaller breast. The size difference can be corrected surgically later on.

— If a lumpectomy is not an option, the breast tissue and underarm lymph nodes are removed. The chest musculature and skin may remain intact.

Breast Reconstruction Surgery— What You Should Know

Whether you opt for breast reconstruction surgery, and if so what kind, depends on your physical and emotional state, the surgical possibilities, and the previous shape of your breasts.

— When you get a silicon implant, a silicon sac is implanted under the breast muscle. In 5 to 10% of women with implants, the connective tissue overreacts by trying to encapsulate the implants, growing uncontrollably and deforming the breast.

— Silicon may leach from the implants, which may tear, resulting in possible health risks.

— The "new" breast remains scarred and often looks markedly different from the other breast. It also feels different and is less sensitive.

— Apart from appearance, an honest emotional relationship with your partner is the most important aspect of this whole question. You should discuss what the operation means to you, well before undergoing it.

— A reconstructed breast is no guarantee that you'll be freed from fears and uncertainties. Whether or not you are lovable and desirable depends on the quality of your relationship, not your breasts.

— Your personality and presence needn't be affected by surgery. Involve your partner in respecting and caring for your body. Don't hide: You have a whole body to stroke and embrace.

— Surgical removal of a breast can affect your self-image and sense of identity as a woman. Remember that you are not alone; many support groups and sources of information are readily available.

VULVA AND VAGINA

Vulva

"Vulva" is the term for the area including the major and minor labia, the clitoris, the urethra and the vaginal opening. Also visible from the outside are the mons veneris and, beneath the vaginal opening, the perineum, ending at the anus.

The labia have a primarily protective function. Embedded between the labia majora are the Bartholin's glands, whose two exit ducts lie directly at the vaginal opening. These secrete a viscous fluid that keeps the area moist.

Vagina

The vagina curves backward in a slight arch extending from the vaginal opening to behind the cervical opening. Just before the top of the vaginal canal, the smooth, round, firm cervix can be felt, which opens into the uterus.

Only the outer portion of the vagina has sensitive nerve endings; the innermost part contains very few nerves, which is why a woman can wear a tampon without feeling it. This muscular canal's tremendous elasticity and relative insensitivity to pain make childbirth possible. Its sides consist of numerous folds that feel like horizontal ridges.

The vagina is lined with skin that feels either dry or damp depending on age and phase of the menstrual cycle. The vaginal lining can change in reaction to emotional burdens or problems, usually secreting increased amounts of discharge.

VAGINITIS (VAGINAL INFLAMMATION)

Infections of the vulva and vagina have various causes. For example, disease-causing agents may be transmitted through poor hygiene, or sexual intercourse (see Sexually Transmitted Diseases, p. 545).

Symptoms

Symptoms of vaginitis include an unusual or increased discharge which may be yellowish to greenish in color and smell unpleasant. The vulva may itch. The symptoms may be so minor, however, that they go unnoticed.

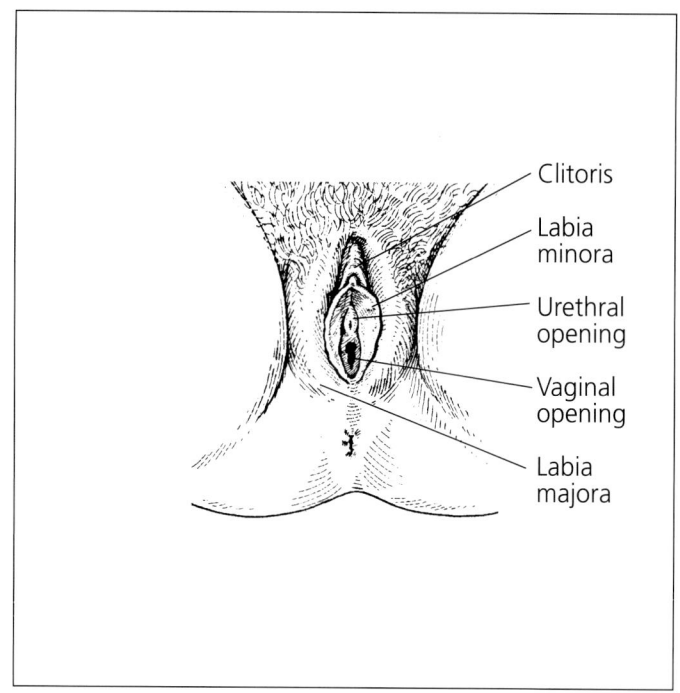

Clitoris

Labia minora

Urethral opening

Vaginal opening

Labia majora

Causes

A variety of germs may be responsible for vaginitis:
— Coliforms that are carried to the vulvovaginal area in stool
— Bacteria of the skin, such as staphylococcus or streptococcus, that can proliferate in an immuno-compromised vaginal area
— Gardnerella bacteria, which may settle in the vaginal environment following intercourse
— Viruses, fungi, or chlamydia (see Sexually Transmitted Diseases, p. 545)

Who's at Risk

The risk of developing vaginitis is increased in women who
— Practice poor hygiene, particularly poor genital and anal care (see Prevention section, p. 519)
— Change sexual partners and/or have partners with poor hygiene (see Penile Cancer, p. 531)
— Are older, because of hormonal changes which often hinder the vagina's infection-fighting abilities (see Menopause, p. 510);
— Wear an IUD (see p. 555)
— Have undergone surgical or medical intervention in the uterus area, e.g., a curettage or abortion

Possible Aftereffects and Complications

If untreated, a vaginal infection may lead to an inflammation of the uterus, and eventually of the fallopian tubes and ovaries. The end result can be infertility (see p. 559).

Prevention

The most important method of prevention is thorough cleanliness following bowel movements. Always wipe yourself from front to back. Also:

— Don't use douches, intimate sprays or similar products. They alter the vaginal environment and make it more susceptible to germs.
— Clean your genital area daily, preferably just with water. Change underwear and towels regularly. Wear underpants made of natural fibers (cotton or silk).
— If you notice an increased discharge, your vaginal environment may be out of balance; yogurt containing live lactobacillus can help stabilize it (see Vaginal Candidiasis, p. 545).
— Use condoms to guard against sexually transmitted diseases (STDs) and passing diseases back and forth. As long as the vaginal lining is irritated, avoid intercourse.

When to Seek Medical Advice

— Seek help if you have unusual-looking, strong-smelling or increased discharge.
— Seek help immediately if you have unexplained pain in the lower abdomen, especially if accompanied by fever.

Self-Help

Not possible if infection is already present.

Treatment

— A laboratory test may determine which microbe is responsible for the infection, and a bacteria-appropriate antibiotic will usually be prescribed.
— Antibiotic vaginal creams/suppositories can be used with only minor side effects.
— After antibiotic treatment, build up the vaginal lactobacillus colonies with yogurt (see Prevention, above).

INFLAMMATION OF THE BARTHOLIN'S GLANDS

Symptoms

Very uncomfortable, painful swelling and redness on one side of the labia, possibly accompanied by general signs of inflammation such as fever.

Causes

Infections of the Bartholin's gland and ducts can be caused by pathogens on the skin or bacteria from the colon that have been transferred to the labia from the anal area. This infection is also an aftereffect of gonorrhea (see p. 549).

Who's at Risk

Infected Bartholin's glands are rare and occur mostly in younger women. Having multiple sex partners increases the risk, as do recurring or long-term vaginal infections that are bacterial in nature.

Possible Aftereffects and Complications

If not treated, the infection can become chronic or lead to an abscess.

Prevention

Follow the steps outlined for vaginitis (see above).

When to Seek Medical Advice

Seek help if symptoms are present.

Self-Help

In early stages, the inflammation can be stopped with sitz baths with a solution of potassium permanganate, or a concentrate of chamomile or witch hazel.

Treatment

A combination of disinfectant sitz baths with potassium permanganate and ointments can draw the pus to a head. The resulting abscess can be lanced surgically by your doctor. At the same time the opening of the duct can be surgically widened; in some cases the entire gland is removed. In rare instances the abscess disappears following the sitz bath treatment.

VULVA AND VAGINAL CANCER

See also Cancer, p. 470

Symptoms

Symptoms usually include small, weeping, sometimes painful sores or swellings of the skin that don't heal. Because the vulvovaginal area is usually moist, early signs often go unnoticed.

Causes

Largely unknown. The human papilloma virus (HPV) may be involved (see Genital Warts, p. 547).

Who's at Risk

Cancer of the vulva and vaginal area is extremely rare. The risk increases after age 70.

Possible Aftereffects and Complications

Pain and bleeding. If the tumor spreads outward, sitting and walking can become difficult. Vulval carcinomas grow slowly. Prospects are relatively good if they are detected early. In contrast, vaginal carcinomas grow fast and metastasize relatively aggressively (see Cancer, p. 470).

Prevention

Regular checkups (see p. 505).

When to Seek Medical Advice

Seek help immediately at the appearance of skin changes such as inflammation, unexplained sores, or abrasions.

Self Help

Not possible.

Treatment

Radiation or surgery, depending on the stage and type of tumor. In the case of vulvar carcinoma, the tumor and some of the surrounding healthy tissue is removed. If possible, the clitoris and vaginal opening are preserved. With vaginal carcinoma the vagina is removed, after which vaginal intercourse is no longer possible. Hardened lymph nodes in the groin must also be removed.

CERVIX AND UTERUS

Cervix

The cervix—the opening to the uterus—is shaped like a cherry and can be felt at the back of the vaginal vault. Its front part is sensation-free, with an opening about the width of a needle; nothing that enters the vagina can thus "get lost" in the uterus. However, the cervix is flexible enough to allow a baby to pass through during childbirth. Both uterus and cervix are lined with mucous membrane that changes with the rhythms of the menstrual cycle (see Menstruation, p. 506).

Uterus

The uterus is shaped like a pear, 2½ to 3½ inches long. Its thick walls are heavily muscled. Normally it lies folded in on itself between bladder and intestine. The widely held image of a hollow womb is erroneous. Only in the event of pregnancy or a growth are the uterine walls pushed apart.

UTERINE INFLAMMATION

Symptoms

Discharge as with vaginitis (see p. 518).
Pain and pressure in the abdomen, if abscess cannot drain.

Causes

Infections of the cervix and uterus can be caused by a vaginal infection or during insertion of an IUD. Later, bacteria can also be transferred from the vagina into the uterus via the IUD cord (see Intrauterine Devices, p. 555).

Who's at Risk

Abscesses occur more frequently in older women with a narrowed cervix.

Possible Aftereffects and Complications

If pus collects in the uterus, the risk of general blood infection (septicemia) increases.

Uterine infections can spread to the fallopian tubes and ovaries later, potentially resulting in infertility.

Prevention

Follow steps outlined for vaginitis (see p. 519).

When to Seek Medical Advice

Seek help
— If you have unusual or increased discharge
— Immediately if you have unexplained abdominal pains, especially when accompanied by fever

Self-Help

Not possible.

Treatment

A short-term estrogen treatment that induces light bleeding can heal minor surface inflammations of the mucous membrane.

As a rule, this infection is treated with antibiotics. If pus has collected in the uterus, the cervical opening must be dilated to release it. After the course of antibiotics, a curettage should be done to determine whether the tissue has undergone malignant changes.

POLYPS

Polyps are benign growths that appear either in patches or on stalks on the cervical opening and in the cervix or uterus.

Symptoms

Polyps don't necessarily produce symptoms. Sometimes a heavy discharge containing blood may result, or spotting, mainly after intercourse. Polyps may cause painful cramping in the uterus as it tries to expel what it perceives to be foreign bodies.

Causes

Polyps are often the result of excessive tissue production. A high estrogen level is also presumed to cause polyps.

Who's at Risk

Polyps can occur at all stages of life. During menopause there is a slightly increased risk of uterine polyps. However, these occur far more rarely than cervical polyps.

Possible Aftereffects and Complications

Thick discharge or spotting, especially after intercourse, that can turn into constant bleeding. Excessive blood loss calls for professional intervention. Occasionally a carcinoma can develop behind a polyp.

Prevention

Not possible.

When to Seek Medical Advice

Seek help if you have a significantly bloody discharge or spotting.

Self-Help

Not possible.

Treatment

Uterine polyps that cause no side effects do not require treatment except in post-menopausal women, where they pose an increased risk of cancer. Any unexplained bleeding must be stopped with a dilation and curettage (D&C) and the polyps should be surgically removed from the uterus. The tissue of the uterine lining removed during the D&C is analyzed for malignancies. The lining will repair itself.

Large polyps growing in patches on the cervix are "burned off" with a laser or electrical current under local anesthesia. This is usually done on an outpatient basis.

Polyps on stalks are usually removed in a hospital so extensive bleeding can be prevented. The stalk is gripped and severed with a cautery instrument. No further treatment is needed once the lesion has healed.

FIBROIDS

Fibroids are benign tumors in the muscles of the uterus. Twenty percent of women over 30 develop them. They can either be bunched on the outside or grow into the uterus.

Symptoms

About 20 percent of all women with fibroids have no symptoms whatsoever. Others experience menstrual pain (see p. 507), menstrual disorders (see p. 508), spotting or constant bleeding, depending on the position and size of the tumor. Pressure on surrounding organs can manifest as bladder problems, lower back pain, or constipation.

Causes

Not known.

Who's at Risk

Fibroids occur more frequently after age 30. Their growth slows during menopause due to a drop in estrogen production. After this they tend to redevelop.

Possible Aftereffects and Complications

— Spotting and constant bleeding can lead to anemia (see Anemia: Iron Deficiency, p. 345).
— Fibroids can intensify menstrual symptoms and/or crowd a developing embryo or pose an obstacle to child birth.
— Fibroids develop into malignancies in fewer than 1 percent of all cases.

Prevention

Not possible.

When to Seek Medical Advice

Seek help if spotting or constant bleeding or painful or heavy menstruation are present. A manual and ultrasound examination will reveal the presence of any fibroids.

Self Help

Not possible.

Treatment

If pain and bleeding are intense, or a gynecological exam reveals the presence of a fibroid, the following measures can be taken:

— A fibroid extending into the uterus can be surgically removed through the vagina. After cervical dilation, the fibroid is removed from the muscles with the uterus remaining intact.
— A fibroid that has intruded into the abdominal cavity is removed through an abdominal incision. In this procedure, too, the uterus is retained. The uterine wall is opened, the fibroid removed, and the uterus is sewn shut.
— If several fibroids are growing in the uterus, the entire uterus may need to be removed (hysterectomy). The fallopian tubes and ovaries are preserved. Depending on its size, the uterus may be removed through the vagina with no abdominal incision.

— It is sometimes possible to keep a uterus even if it is heavily overgrown with fibroids. This involves preoperative injections of hypothalamus hormones known as gonadotropin-releasing hormone (Gn-RH) analogs, which stop the ovaries from producing estrogen, thereby depriving the fibroids of nourishment. This causes a menopausal state with associated side effects.

Hormone treatment causes the fibroids to shrink, facilitating surgical removal. The uterus is preserved. After the medication is discontinued, the hormonal balance will right itself within a few weeks.

ENDOMETRIOSIS

Endometriosis is defined as small islets or implants of uterine lining that have settled outside the uterus. They can occur on the fallopian tubes, ovaries, cervix or vagina, but also in the abdominal cavity, bladder or intestine. In rare instances they can settle in the lungs, extremities or groin.

Symptoms

The endometrial implants, like the uterine lining they come from, respond to the hormonal changes of the menstrual cycle. The growths swell and cause cramps. Unexplained abdominal pains usually appear before, and during the first few days of menstruation. Heavier menstrual flow can also result (see p. 508).

Causes

The implanted cells are transferred from the uterine lining by a process that is not fully known. The uterine lining may invade the muscles of the uterine wall following surgical intervention such as diagnostic or therapeutic D&Cs, cesarean sections, operations on the uterus, or biopsies. Endometrial cells may be transferred to the abdominal cavity via the fallopian tubes and carried to distant organs through the lymph and bloodstream. Endometriosis may occur in organs connected to the uterus during the development of an embryo.

Who's at Risk

Endometriosis is diagnosed more commonly in the industrialized world today than it was 50 years ago. A possible reason for this is the increasing frequency of surgical and diagnostic intervention.

Possible Aftereffects and Complications

During the menstrual cycle the implants bleed slightly and, because blood collects, develop into small cysts. Depending on their size, the cysts can cause pressure and abdominal pain outside the regular menstrual cycle. Infertility is the most common result of endometriosis of the fallopian tubes, ovaries, or abdominal organs.

Prevention

Physicians should exercise appropriate care particularly when performing cesarean sections and surgery for fibroids. Patients should always get detailed reasons as to why an operation is necessary. If possible, get second or third opinions.

When to Seek Medical Advice

Seek help
— If menstrual symptoms intensify over time and unexplained, diffuse abdominal pains develop.
— If periodic pains occur elsewhere in your body.

Self Help

Not possible.

Treatment

Treatment is necessary only if daily life is adversely affected.
— Laparoscopy (see p. 653): In this procedure, implants in the abdomen can be detected and immediately cauterized.
— Hormones: Some endometrial implants respond to hormones. Hormone treatment can significantly cut back the body's production of estrogen and progesterone, preventing menstruation and stimulation of the implants. This eases symptoms considerably. After discontinuing medication, the ovaries will resume their function.

Oral contraceptives (see p. 556), synthetic gonadotropin-releasing hormones (Gn-RH analogs), progestins or danazol are used to treat endometriosis. Except for birth-control pills, no treatment should exceed 1 year at most. An estrogen deficit increases the risk of osteoporosis (see p. 430). Side effects of hormone therapy may include weight gain, acne, increased body hair, fatigue, migraines, sweating, and a reduced interest in sex. You should opt for hormone treatment only if you are in constant pain or are infertile as a result of endometriosis.

Large, painful endometrial implants almost always require surgical removal.

Questions to ask before having a uterine operation

No organ—particularly one like the uterus—is superfluous or unnecessary. For most women the uterus is a sign of womanhood. Therefore, get all the information you can about the need for, and risks of, any operation on the uterus.
— Why is this surgery unavoidable? Are there really no alternatives?
— What are the chances of success?
— Will it be performed vaginally or abdominally, and why?
— Will the ovaries be removed? If so, why? Postmenopausal women, or those about to undergo menopause, are often advised to have the ovaries removed during a hysterectomy to avoid possible cancer, but a hypothetical future event does not necessarily justify such invasive surgery.
— Confirm before surgery that your vagina will not be so scarred as to affect sexual intercourse after the operation. Many doctors simply assume that older women are not sexually active.

PROLAPSED UTERUS

A prolapsed uterus usually occurs in conjunction with a prolapse of the bladder and surrounding tissue. You can determine this for yourself by feeling the cervix and uterus with your finger: If the uterus protrudes into the vaginal canal and the cervix is near the vaginal opening, it has prolapsed. In rare cases, the uterus may slide so far down that it appears at the vaginal opening (uterovaginal prolapse).

Symptoms

Pressure, a pulling (downward) sensation, frequent and possibly uncontrollable urination with little urine.

Causes

Prolapse is caused by weakening of the connective tissue and tendons that hold the abdominal organs in place. Along with an enlarging of the vagina and loss of muscle tone of the pelvic floor, the organs begin to droop.

Who's at Risk

The risk of a prolapsed uterus is increased after multiple births or years of physically stressful and/or constant labor. It also increases when hormone production is reduced (e.g., during menopause), and in the presence of obesity and weak muscles from insufficient physical activity.

Possible Aftereffects and Complications

Constant pressure and a pulling sensation can be extremely uncomfortable and adversely affect daily life, particularly if coughing or exertion causes you to urinate involuntarily (see Urinary Incontinence, p. 419).

Prevention

An exercise regimen specifically designed to strengthen the pelvic floor should be followed regularly after each delivery and for the next 4 to 6 months.

When to Seek Medical Advice

Seek help if symptoms are present.

Self Help

Regular and intensive pelvic-floor muscle exercises can often strengthen the supporting tissue sufficiently (see Urinary Incontinence, p. 419).

Treatment

Initially, an intensive regimen of pelvic-floor muscle-strengthening exercise is recommended. It may be supplemented with estrogen therapy (vaginal suppositories or tablets).

If exercise proves unsuccessful, surgery may be advisable to tighten the supporting muscles of the bladder and intestine. The prolapsed uterus is usually removed—except in younger women who want to have children—to increase chances of long-term success and prospects for a physically active life. The ovaries are retained.

CERVICAL CANCER

See also Cancer, p. 470.

Symptoms

In the early stages, cervical cancer produces no symptoms. Later, bleeding may occur, for example following intercourse. Pain usually develops only if the surrounding organs are affected.

Causes

The principal cause is believed to be human papilloma virus (HPV), which also causes genital warts (see p.547). It also seems that the sebaceous secretions (smegma) of glands in the male foreskin can have a cancer-stimulating effect on the cervix and cervical opening.

Who's at Risk

Cervical cancer is the most common cancer of the female reproductive organs. The risk of HPV infection increases with multiple sex partners. Your partner's hygiene also plays an important role. Heterosexual women contract cervical cancer far less frequently in cultures where men are circumcised .

Possible Aftereffects and Complications

Cervical cancer may metastasize to the uterus and other organs such as bones, liver, bladder, intestine, and lymph nodes.

Prevention

The earlier the cancer is detected, the better the prospects (see Gynecological Exams, p. 505). Use condoms to prevent infection with HPV. Your partner can also do his part in prevention by thoroughly washing his penis daily.

When to Seek Medical Advice

Seek help if unexplained bleeding occurs outside the menstrual cycle. All women should have regular gynecological exams.

Self-Help

Not possible.

Treatment

If the cancer cells are confined to the surface of the uterine lining, they can be treated with laser surgery. A cone biopsy, in which a section of the cervical tissue is removed, is simultaneously diagnostic and therapeutic: The tissue sample can be used to determine how advanced the cancer is. If it has already spread to the underlying tissue; the uterus, cervix, and lymph nodes of the groin are removed.

UTERINE CANCER

See also Cancer, p. 470
Uterine carcinoma is primarily a cancer of the uterine lining, since malignancies rarely develop in the muscles of the uterus.

Symptoms

Symptoms include unusual, heavy or prolonged bleeding, or light bleeding outside menstruation.

Causes

Not known.

Who's at Risk

The risk of uterine cancer increases slowly after age 40 and peaks between 55 and 60. Uterine cancer is the second most frequent cancer of the female reproductive organs.

It occurs more often in women who have never given birth. Women who are obese or diabetic or who have high blood pressure are also thought to be at higher risk.

Possible Aftereffects and Complications

Uterine cancer grows slowly and signals its onset early with bleeding. Early detection and intervention can help prevent life-threatening aftereffects. If left untreated, the uterus enlarges, pressure and pain may develop, and the cancer may spread to the cervix, the pelvic cavity, and beyond.

Prevention

Not possible.

When to Seek Medical Advice

Seek help if you experience unexplained, unusual, increased, or prolonged bleeding, or any bleeding at all after menopause.

Self-Help

Not possible.

Treatment

The uterus is removed, along with the fallopian tubes. Because the growth of uterine cancer depends on hormones, the ovaries are often removed as well. If this happens early, the chances of surviving through the 5 year observation period are 70 to 80 percent. If the tumor was confined to the uterine lining, radiation therapy is not required; otherwise it may be prescribed following surgery.

After a hysterectomy, you will no longer menstruate, nor will you be able to bear children. Your sex life, however, need not be affected.

FALLOPIAN TUBES AND OVARIES

Fallopian Tubes

The fallopian tubes are between 3 and 5 inches long. They are flexible transport ducts for the egg (ovum). At the ovary end, fingerlike projections form a kind of funnel. The projections and tubes are in a state of constant slight undulation, which enables them to catch the egg expelled into the abdominal cavity by the ovary at ovulation. The wavelike movement then helps the fallopian tube propel the ovum toward the uterus, helped along by fine cilia or hairlike cells lining the tube.

Ovaries

The ovaries are the size and shape of small plums. They are situated in the pelvic cavity on either side of the uterus, next to the peritoneum or abdominal wall, and connected to the uterus by the utero-ovarian ligament. Each ovary consists of an inner core (medulla) and a 1- to 2-mm-thick outer cortex. In the cortex are the liquid-filled follicles, like small blisters, which contain the eggs. The total number of eggs in the ovaries at puberty is about 400,000. When a follicle is ripe, it grows on the surface of the ovary. Ovulation occurs when it ruptures, releasing the egg into the abdominal cavity in the middle of the menstrual cycle. The follicle then turns into the corpus luteum and starts producing progesterone (see Menstruation, p. 506).

SALPINGITIS (INFLAMMATION OF THE FALLOPIAN TUBES, PELVIC INFLAMMATORY DISEASE)

What is commonly referred to as an inflamed ovary is usually actually an inflammation of the fallopian tubes, or salpingitis.

Symptoms

Pain usually appears on both sides of the abdomen, but it is frequently stronger on one side than the other and may extend to the groin. Pulling pains may also be present, extending into the thighs, knees or back, possibly accompanied by high fever.

Causes

Salpingitis can be a complication of a vaginal or uterine infection (see Vaginitis, p. 518). It is often also caused by gonococcal bacterial and chlamydia (see p. 546). If the ovaries are also inflamed, salpingitis may affect the tissue surrounding the ovary.

Who's at Risk

Women with infections of the reproductive organs are at higher risk for salpingitis.

Possible Aftereffects and Complications

— Salpingitis can affect the flexibility of the projections of the fallopian tube, making catching the egg difficult.
— Fallopian tubes that are stuck together can obstruct the egg's passage considerably and may result in ectopic pregnancy (see p. 526).
— If salpingitis is not treated in time, peritonitis or an tubo-ovarian abscess may develop, which then may need to be surgically removed along with the affected organs.

Ultimately, chronic inflammation can cause scarring of the fallopian tubes, potentially resulting in infertility (see p. 559).

Prevention

Treat vaginal infections appropriately (see p. 519).

When to Seek Medical Advice

Seek help
— If you experience unusual or increased discharge
— Immediately if you experience unexplained abdominal pain, especially in conjunction with fever

Self-Help

Not possible.

Treatment

Salpingitis is treated with antibiotics (see p. 661).

Inflammations of the fallopian tubes or ovaries can be treated at home only if you have no fever; if that is the case, stay in bed, take it easy and keep warm.

If fever is present, you are almost always admitted to the hospital and given antibiotics intravenously. The hospital stay lasts between 7 to 10 days. Warmth and bed rest are very important: Both may help prevent complications.

After the worst of the inflammation is over, localized warmth (heating pads, hotwater bottles) are beneficial. During the acute inflammation, however, an ice pack should be applied.

ECTOPIC PREGNANCY

A fertilized egg can attach itself to any blood-rich tissue, and the embryo can start to grow outside the uterus. A pregnancy in the abdominal cavity is relatively rare. Tubal pregnancies are more common. These occur when a fertilized egg lodges in the fallopian tube on its way to the utcrus.

Symptoms

The initial symptoms of an ectopic pregnancy resemble those of a normal pregnancy: Menstrual bleeding is absent, or lighter than usual. A pregnancy test is positive. After about 6 weeks, pains in the lower abdomen appear, usually only on one side; light bleeding is often present as well.

If an ectopic pregnancy is not terminated, the egg may continue to develop, bursting the fallopian tube. The pain moves from the abdomen to the upper belly and shoulders. Shoulder pain is diagnostic for a ruptured ectopic pregnancy.

Pallor and loss of consciousness may result. They are signs of life-threatening shock.

Causes

Usually, an ectopic pregnancy is the result of narrowed, obstructed fallopian tubes following salpingitis. Poor flexibility and stiffened muscles in the tubes can prevent the fertilized egg from reaching the uterus.

Who's at Risk

The risk of ectopic pregnancy is increased in women who have had salpingitis and in women who wear an intrauterme device (IUD). It is unclear whether copper ions absorbed from the IUD can impair the flexibility of the tubes. The risk is also increased in women with previous ectopic pregnancies or terminations, and early infertility. Ectopic pregnancies occur more often with in vitro fertilization.

Possible Aftereffects and Complications

The fallopian tubes may rupture, causing bleeding into the abdominal cavity. Hemorrhagic shock is always life-threatening and calls for immediate medical intervention (see Shock, p. 712).

Prevention

Not possible.

When to Seek Medical Advice

Seek help immediately if you have abdominal pain and your period is absent or very light.

Self-Help

Not possible.

Treatment

An ectopic pregnancy requires surgery, usually a laparoscopy through the navel—an abdominal incision is rarely necessary. If the tubes are not damaged or bleeding, the surgeon will attempt to squeeze the implanted egg out of the upper end of the tube. If this is not possible, it is removed by microsurgery. The fallopian tube is retained, if at all possible.

In the event of large, bleeding tears in the fallopian tube, this relatively gentle procedure is no longer possible. The tubes are completely removed, since this is the only way to stanch the bleeding.

CYSTS

Cysts are the most commonly occurring benign tumors. They can appear throughout the body and are not exclusive to women. A cyst is nothing more than a fluid-filled sac. If a cyst is involved with the function of the ovaries, such as a follicular or luteal cyst, it is called a "functional cyst."

Cysts are rare on the fallopian tubes, but not on the ovaries, where cysts commonly occur either on the ovarian cortex itself or on a stalk, showing up in ultrasound images as an appendage on the ovary.

A cyst that comprises tissue (*cystadenoma*) is rarer

and can be problematic; it will usually not disappear on its own, and may develop into ovarian cancer.

Symptoms

Depending on the size of the cyst and phase of the cycle, a vague, pulling ache may appear on one side of the abdomen. In the early stages, cysts usually cause no symptoms.

Causes

Cysts arise when a ripe follicle does not rupture, either because it contains no egg or because the egg has died. This can be caused by hormonal disturbances. In the absence of ovulation, the follicle may continue to grow; fluid collects inside it, and a cyst develops.

Who's at Risk

Cysts develop more easily in younger women. They occur only as long as the ovaries are active. It is believed that psychological stress contributes to their development.

Possible Aftereffects and Complications

If multiple cysts develop, the ovarian cortex can get crowded, with insufficient room for viable follicles to ripen. This can be a cause of infertility (see p. 559).

In extreme cases, large cysts can rupture and bleed into the abdominal cavity. In rare instances the cyst can cause abnormal twisting. This calls for emergent surgical removal, otherwise it can lead to blocked circulation and the death of the ovary.

Cystadenomas (tissue-containing cysts) can become cancerous. Large cystadenomas can press on nearby healthy organs, crowding them.

Prevention

In younger women prone to recurring cysts and needing birth control, taking oral contraceptives can have a calming effect on the ovaries.

When to Seek Medical Advice

Seek help if you have unexplained lower abdominal pain.

Self-Help

Warm compresses may help.

Treatment

Functional cysts do not require treatment as long as they neither hurt nor exert considerable pressure. They often disappear on their own after a month or two, or rupture without major complications. However, many doctors treat cysts anyway. A common bad practice is aspiration—puncturing the cyst and drawing off the fluid—even though the cyst will only refill with fluid. Cysts that continue to grow, becoming increasingly sensitive and causing noticeable symptoms, should be surgically removed, as should those that are suspected to be complex, cystadenomas, or even cancerous.

During surgery, only the cyst is removed. The ovary is retained, if at all possible. However, the entire ovary may need to be removed if multiple cysts have formed.

OVARIAN CANCER
See also Cancer, p. 470

Symptoms

The ovaries can enlarge over time without causing any symptoms. Pain usually arises only when some boundary is reached and another organ affected, for instance, peritoneal irritation, or pressure on the bladder or intestine.

Causes

Not known.

Who's at Risk

The risk of ovarian cancer increases after age 40.

Possible Aftereffects and Complications

Malignant tumors on the ovary are insidious. They are often discovered purely by chance. They grow very quickly and metastasize in the abdominal cavity, accompanied by accumulations of fluid.

Prevention

Ultrasound can help detect ovarian cancer early.

When to Seek Medical Advice

Seek help if you experience unexplained swelling or expansion in the abdomen, accompanied by a vague ache and possibly nausea and general weakness.

Self-Help

Not possible.

Treatment

Surgery is always required with ovarian cancer. Usually, both ovaries are diseased, but even if only one is compromised, both are removed to prevent the cancer from spreading to the healthy one. The operation is almost always followed up with chemotherapy. Radiation is rarely recommended.

After removal of the ovaries, hormone-replacement therapy (see p. 477) is usually prescribed to restore those hormones the body no longer produces. Your sex life need not be affected.

MEN'S ILLNESSES

The male sex organs consist of penis, testicles, epididymis, seminal vesicles, seminal duct, and prostate gland. The erectile tissue, which is permeated by blood vessels, is important to the penis' function as a sex organ. The glans is at the tip of the penis, surrounded by the foreskin. If the organ is stimulated mechanically or otherwise, blood congestion causes the erectile tissue to thicken and the penis becomes erect; further stimulation results in ejaculation.

The male gonads or testicles lie in a protective sac, the scrotum. They produce male sex hormones (in the interstitial cells) and sperm (in the canals). Sperm is transferred to the epididymis, situated behind the testes, which accumulates sperm for the next ejaculation. The sperm are then pressed into the seminal duct and transported to the prostate.

The prostate is the size of a chestnut and surrounds the section of the urethra leading out of the bladder. Before the two seminal ducts empty into the prostate, they take up the fluid secreted by the seminal vesicles as well as the prostate. The seminal fluid is important in that it enables the sperm discharged during ejaculation to be mobile. The seminal fluid and the sperm are discharged together into the urinary tract. A special mechanism prevents urine and semen from being released at the same time. The male sex organs are so interconnected with the urinary tract that disease in one system can result in disease in the other.

ACCIDENTS AND INJURIES OF THE GENITAL ORGANS

Urethra

After accidents, instruments used by doctors during exams cause the most frequent injuries to the urethra (see Cystoscopy, p. 654). Blood in the urine is usually the result. Often no treatment is necessary for mild urinary-tract injuries, or a urinary catheter may be installed for a few days. For severe injuries, surgery is necessary. A potential consequence is narrowing of the urethra.

Penis

Penile injuries are usually the result of sexual practices in which the penis is inserted into various foreign objects. They also result from self-gratification or from inserting the penis into a partner's mouth. Though it is rare, a rigid penis can be snapped forcibly, leading to a penile fracture or tear in the sheath of erectile tissue.

Forestry and farm workers are at risk of penile injuries caused when clothing gets caught in running machinery.

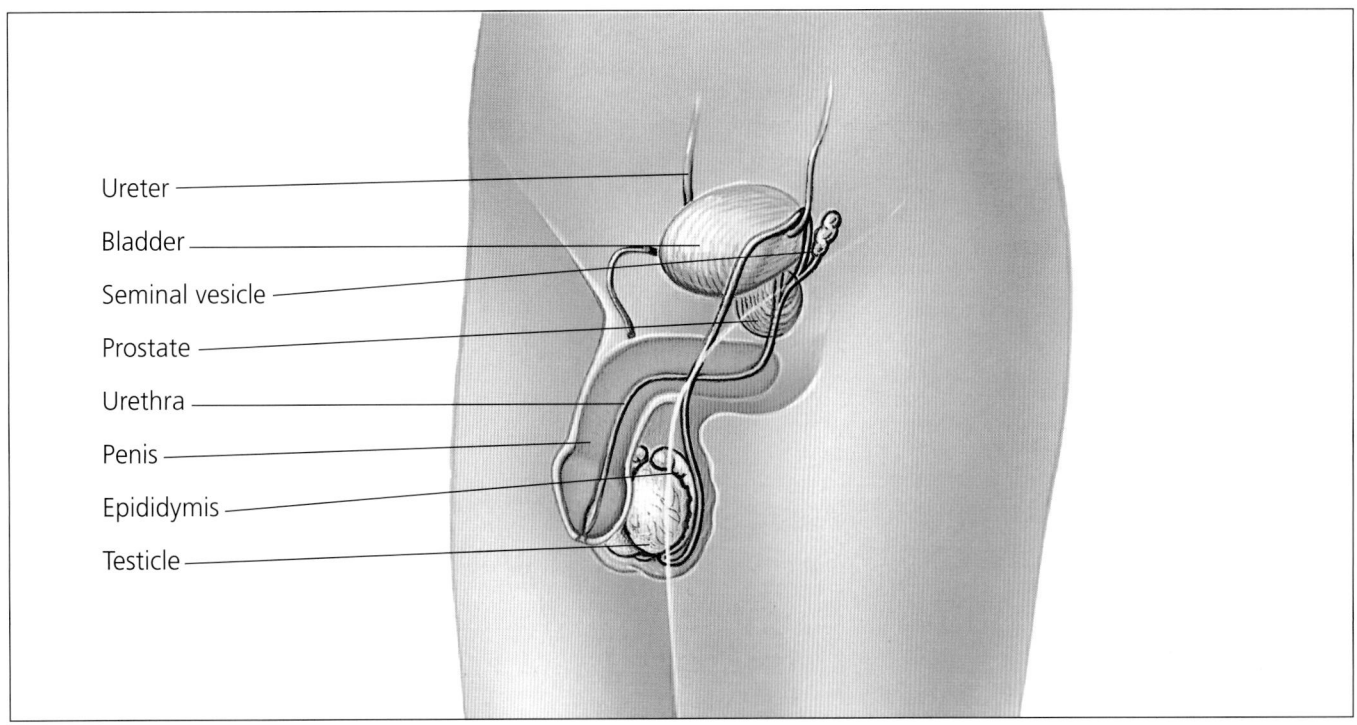

Ureter
Bladder
Seminal vesicle
Prostate
Urethra
Penis
Epididymis
Testicle

External injuries require immediate medical attention. Torn-off parts of skin or tissue should be placed back on the wound as quickly as possible or into a cooler for transport to the site where clinical repair will be performed.

Testes
Bruises
Injuries to the testicles are often caused by kicks or impact. They are very painful. A bruise where pain subsides within an hour is harmless. However, if the pain lasts longer, or the testicle swells up and an effusion of blood develops, contact your health-care provider. In such cases, surgery can prevent long-term damage. An open wound always requires immediate intervention to avoid losing the testicle.

Testicular Torsion
The twisting of the vascular stem of the testicles occurs almost exclusively in boys and youths. It is often caused by sudden movement while playing or during sports, but can also happen during sleep. The arterial flow is cut, causing severe, piercing pain in one testicle, which swells up quickly. No fever or nausea are present. The testicle can best be saved if it is operated on within six hours.

Warning: Testicular torsion is often confused with testicular inflammation, epididymitis, which hardly ever occurs in children.

URETHRITIS
(INFECTION OF THE URETHRA)

Symptoms
The symptoms of urethritis include a burning sensation during urination, a discharge that may be whitish or yellowish, pus-filled, or clear, and the strong urge to urinate.

Causes
— Bacterial or viral infections
— Trichomoniasis (see p. 546), gonorrhea (see p. 549)
— Allergies
— Sexual practices
— Narrowing of the urethra

Who's at Risk
You are at increased risk of urethritis if you have

— Unprotected sex with multiple partners whose habits you don't know
— Poor hygienic habits
— An injury to the urethra
— An infection

Possible Aftereffects and Complications
— Chronic urinary tract inflammation can cause narrowing because of resulting scars, resulting in a thinner urine stream, recurring bladder infections, and urinary retention.
— Abscesses can form in the urinary tract. They require treatment with antibiotics. In certain cases surgery is necessary.

Prevention
Using a condom (protected sex); daily cleaning of the penis, particularly under the foreskin.

When to Seek Medical Advice
Seek help if symptoms are present.

Self-Help
Not possible.

Treatment
Medical treatment of urethritis depends on its cause.

Special tubes can be inserted to help release urine, but work only temporarily. The narrowed tract should be widened surgically; the success rate for this procedure is between 60 and 80 percent. Scars from the intervention, however, may lead to further constriction of the urethra.

BALANITIS AND POSTHITIS
(INFLAMMATION OF THE GLANS
AND FORESKIN)

Symptoms
In this condition, the glans and foreskin are inflamed and are red, swollen and painful. On the reddened areas there may be
— Whitish, removable spots
— Skin abrasions, red with white borders
— Painful blisters
Warning: Reddish, firm lumps that weep or bleed can be signs of cancer. Seek professional care immediately.

Causes

— Bacterial infection, phimosis (see p. 594), mechanical damage, use of disinfectant or antiseptic solutions, early sign of diabetes.
— Fungal infections (see p. 545). These commonly affect diabetics and can be spread by sexual contact.
— Ulcerated lesions can be spread by sexual contact. They can also be signs of syphilis (see p. 548).
— Infection with herpes virus: This can be spread by sexual contact (see Genital Herpes, p. 547).

Who's at Risk

The risk of balanitis and posthitis is higher in those who practice poor hygiene or, alternatively, are excessive about cleaning and disinfecting themselves; and in those who practice unprotected sex.

Possible Aftereffects and Complications

You run the risk of infecting your sex partner or partners. Chronic inflammations of the foreskin and glans increase the risk of cancer.

Prevention

The best prevention is thorough daily cleaning of the foreskin and glans, with the foreskin pulled back, preferably using soap and water. Use a condom to prevent cross-infection of partner(s).

When to Seek Medical Advice

See your doctor immediately if you see signs of inflammation of the foreskin or glans.

Self-Help

Not possible.

Treatment

The underlying disease must be treated professionally.

PENILE CANCER

See also Cancer, p. 470

Symptoms

Small, firm, reddish lumps that appear on the glans or foreskin and weep or bleed easily may be a sign of syphilis or of cancer. Other signs of cancer include inflammations on the shaft of the penis that don't heal, or an unpleasant-smelling, pus-filled discharge possibly accompanied by phimosis.

Causes

One contributing factor to penile cancer is smegma, the secretion that collects under the foreskin. The additional factors necessary for cancer to develop, however, are not known.

Who's at Risk

Penile cancer accounts for 2 percent of malignancies in men. The risk increases in individuals with poor hygiene. Penile cancer is extremely rare in circumcised men.

Prevention

This is the only form of cancer in which prevention is possible and even simple: Daily washing with soap and water of the foreskin and glans, with the foreskin pulled back. Phimosis or narrowing of the foreskin (see p. 594) should be treated by circumcision performed by healthcare professionals. Examine the glans regularly.

When to Seek Medical Advice

Seek help if symptoms are present.

Self-Help

Not possible.

Treatment

If penile cancer is detected in its early stages, laser treatment or partial removal of the penis is sufficient. Loss of the glans can result in loss of sexual desire. Early surgery results in recovery in nine out of ten cases. If the lymph nodes are already involved, chemotherapy is necessary following surgery (see p. 476).

There is no evidence that herbal or alternative medicine can slow the cancer. Psychotherapy, however, can bring psychological release. Anything that will bring you joy and do you good will improve your quality of life.

ORCHITIS (TESTICULAR INFLAMMATION/INFECTION)

Symptoms

In orchitis, one or both testicles swell(s) painfully; the scrotum turns red; the pain worsens and is accompanied by fever.

Causes

Orchitis is usually caused by pathogens in the blood or by an injury to the testicles. An inflammation in the epididymis can also reach the testicles, in which case only one testicle becomes painfully swollen. Orchitis is most often found in youths who have mumps.

Possible Aftereffects and Complications

Orchitis can result in infertility.

Prevention

Not possible.

When to Seek Medical Advice

Seek help if symptoms are present. Testicular torsion may result in similar symptoms (see p. 530).

Self-Help

Bed rest and ice packs can help lessen pain. Wear looser pants.

Treatment

Orchitis is customarily treated with antibiotics. If an abscess forms and antibiotics don't help, as happens almost exclusively with older, weaker patients, surgical removal of the testicle(s) may be necessary.

EPIDIDYMITIS (INFECTION OF THE EPIDIDYMIS)

Symptoms

In this condition, the epididymis swells painfully and the scrotum becomes red and hard.

Causes

Epididymitis is usually caused by a urethral infection that spreads to the epididymis (see p. 530). It may also be caused by gonorrhea (see p. 549), an infection of the prostate (see p. 534), or long-term use of a catheter.

Who's at Risk

The risk of epididymitis is increased in individuals with the diseases listed above.

Possible Aftereffects and Complications

The infection usually progresses rapidly to the testicles.

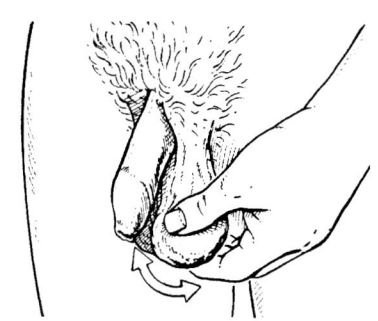

Self-exam of the testicles

It's best to examine yourself while in the shower. Heat makes the scrotal skin slack, while cold causes a muscle to pull the testes up toward the warmth of the body.

Grasp the right testicle with the right hand, without stretching the skin; with the fingers of your left hand, gently palpate the testicle, from top to bottom and back to front. Repeat with the left testicle. Once you become familiar with the way your testicles feel, you'll notice any changes right away.

Prevention

Not possible.

Self-Help

Bed rest and an ice pack may ease the pain.

When to Seek Medical Advice

Seek help if symptoms are present.

Treatment

Like orchitis, epididymitis is treated with antibiotics.

HYDROCELE, HEMATOCELE, VARICOCELE

Symptoms

Hydrocele: The scrotum enlarges, with no associated pain. A smooth, tight, colorless swelling is present, sometimes separate from the testes.

Hematocele: The testicles swell painfully, with internal bleeding.

Varicocele: In 90 percent of cases these occur on the left side. Particularly when the affected individual is standing, the scrotum is filled with varicose veins, with their distinctive wormlike appearance.

Causes

Hydrocele: Usually injuries or inflammations cause the pooling of fluid.

Hematocele: Usually this is the acute aftereffect of an injury or contusion of the testicle. In older men it can follow a genital inflammation.

Varicocele: Various causes are possible, including weak bloodvessel walls, or failure or absence of the venous valves.

Who's at Risk

Men exposed to contusions and injury are at increased risk for these conditions.

Possible Aftereffects and Complications

Varicocele can negatively affect fertility in young men.

Prevention

Not possible.

When to Seek Medical Advice

Seek help if the scrotum becomes enlarged.

Self-Help

Not possible.

Treatment

Hydrocele: A hydrocele rarely disappears spontaneously and must be surgically removed. Aspirating is usually unsuccessful.

Hematocele: This may disappear on its own after a few weeks. If the body does not reabsorb the blood, the hematocele must be surgically removed through a simple procedure performed under general anesthesia.

Varicocele: Depending on the circumstances, the varicose veins may need to be tied off.

TESTICULAR CANCER

See also Cancer, p. 470

Symptoms

The symptoms of testicular cancer include
— Enlargement of a testicle, without pain; lumps may also develop and harden
— In rare cases, additional pain or pulling sensation in the groin

Causes

Most testicular tumors arise from germ cells (seminomas). The causes are not known, but environmental toxins that affect the hormones may be implicated.

Who's at Risk

Testicular cancer occurs predominantly between the ages of 20 and 40 and accounts for 1 to 2 percent of all cancers. It is the most common cancer in men between the ages of 20 and 32.

Possible Aftereffects and Complications

If treated in time, testicular cancer can be cured. Left untreated, it leads to death in 1 to 2 years.

Prevention

After age 20, inspect your testicles every month and go for a medical checkup every year.

When to Seek Medical Advice

If you find any changes during your self-exam, contact your health-care provider immediately. An ultrasound exam can help establish whether or not you have testicular cancer.

Self-Help

Not possible.

Treatment

If your doctor suspects testicular cancer, under no circumstances should you consent to an aspiration as this procedure may increase the risk of metastasis.

Testicular cancer calls for swift surgical intervention. The testicle, epididymis and a part of the seminal ducts are removed. In certain circumstances the lymph nodes in the rear wall of the abdominal cavity are removed as well. For physical and emotional well-being, a testicular prosthesis (like a prosthetic breast after mastectomy) can be implanted after the scrotum heals. The remaining healthy testicle then regulates all sexual functions on its own. Potency and fertility are retained.

After surgery, a course of chemotherapy is often necessary and helpful (see p. 476).

The effectiveness of herbal remedies and alternative medicine has not been established. Psychotherapy or counseling can make living with the disease easier. Anything that you enjoy and that is good for you will improve your quality of life.

PROSTATITIS (INFLAMMATION/INFECTION OF THE PROSTATE GLAND)

Symptoms

Symptoms include frequent urination, pain and problems while urinating, and also during bowel movements; bloody, sometimes pus-filled urine; fever often is present.

Causes

Causes include agents such as colon bacteria or streptococci, transferred through the urinary tract or bloodstream.

Who's at Risk

One out of every 2,000 men will have a prostate inflammation at some point in his life.

Possible Aftereffects and Complications

An incompletely treated prostatitis can become chronic and lead to impaired fertility and potency.
Abscesses or fistulas may develop.

Prevention

Not possible.

When to Seek Medical Advice

Seek help if symptoms appear and intensify.

Self-Help

Not possible.

Treatment

The infection is treated with antibiotics for a minimum of 10 days. If abscesses or fistulas develop, surgery is necessary.

PROSTATE ENLARGEMENT (BENIGN PROSTATIC HYPERTROPHY)

Symptoms

Some men with enlarged prostates experience no symptoms. Usually the disease develops in three stages:
— Urination (including at night) increases in frequency.
— Next, the strength of the urine stream diminishes; the bladder can no longer be emptied completely.

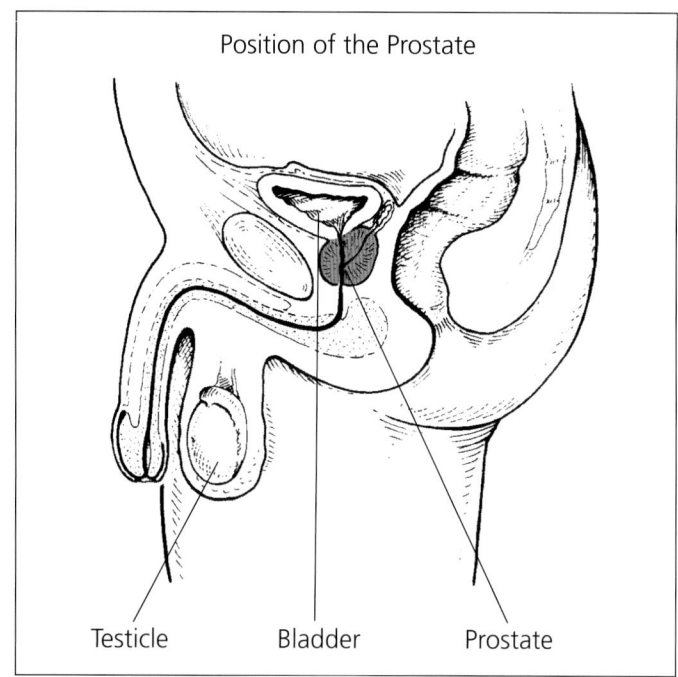

Position of the Prostate

Testicle   Bladder   Prostate

— Finally, complete inability to empty the bladder may result, accompanied by constant dribbling. Nightly bedwetting or enuresis (loss of bladder control) results. Signs of kidney failure follow, including thirst, weight loss, vomiting, diarrhea, and dizziness.

Causes

The male body produces both male and female hormones. The female hormones affect the inner glands of the prostate, the male hormones the outer glands. In older age the production of male hormones drops. Because the hormone balance favors the female hormones, the inner glands enlarge. The outer glands atrophy and become compressed over the years. The swelling eventually obstructs the urinary tract.

Who's at Risk

Prostate changes begin around age 50. A third of men in their seventies are affected by prostate enlargement; by age 90, all men are affected. How long an individual will remain symptom-free depends on the location of the enlargement.

Possible Aftereffects and Complications

Urine retained in the bladder fosters infections that don't heal because the irrigating effect of passing urine is lacking. This may result in inflammations of the renal pelvis, renal degeneration, renal failure, and septicemia (blood poisoning).

At any stage of prostate enlargement, it can suddenly become impossible to urinate. Drinking alcohol often triggers this development.

Prevention
Prostate enlargement caused by old age cannot be prevented.

When to Seek Medical Advice
Seek help if symptoms are present.

Self-Help
— Avoid sitting for long periods. Make sure you get plenty of exercise.
— Drink small amounts throughout the day; give up alcohol.
— Don't suppress the urge to urinate, so as to avoid the bladder becoming overfull.
— Make sure you have regular bowel movements.
— Take warm sitz baths, and take foot baths in increasingly hot water.
— Learn relaxation techniques (see p. 693).

Treatment
Herbal medications containing sitosterols can temporarily reduce swelling in the prostate, easing symptoms. A varied, high-quality diet will also provide sufficient sitosterols.

Although extracts of pumpkin seed, nettle root, and saw palmetto are purported to have a beneficial effect, the Food and Drug Administration (FDA) has not approved their use.

In 40 to 80 percent of cases, placebos—or discussions with a doctor—are effective in treating prostate enlargement.

Symptoms may be lessened by 5-Alpha-reductase inhibitors, such as finasteride (Proscar), but these have the disadvantage that they must be taken for the rest of the patient's life. If the prostate enlargement has reached the second or third stage, the inner gland must be surgically removed. The choice of surgery depends on the size of the prostate.

In 75 percent of cases, the swelling can be treated electrically with an instrument inserted through the urethra. The advantage of this method is a hospital stay of only five to seven days, relatively little pain, and swift recovery. Larger swellings require an incision, prolonging the hospital stay to 8 to 10 days.

Laser therapy and heat therapy are promising techniques, but don't allow for histological diagnosis, and are not widely available.

Postoperative Effects
The obligatory use of a catheter can lead to urinary-tract infections, which require treatment with antibiotics.

Most men are rendered infertile after prostate surgery because the seminal ducts now empty into the bladder, and semen is released along with urine.

In most, however, erectile capacity remains. If you're worried about whether and how your sex life will be affected after surgery, consult your doctor.

PROSTATE CANCER
See also Cancer, p. 470

Symptoms
In the early stages, prostate cancer usually produces no symptoms. In advanced stages the symptoms are similar to those of prostatic hypertrophy: Urge to urinate, thin urine stream, dribbling, and decreasing volume of urine passed. Later the urine or semen may contain blood. Back pain usually appears only after metastasis has occurred.

Causes
The causes are as yet unknown. Environmental toxins with hormone-mimicking effects may play a role.

Who's at Risk
Prostate cancer is the most common form of cancer in men over 50.

Possible Aftereffects and Complications
As the urinary tract is increasingly obstructed, consequences resembling those of benign prostate enlargement occur. Advanced prostate cancer may metastasize to the lymph nodes and especially to the bones of the spinal column and pelvis.

Prevention
Prevention is not possible. A rectal exam and a blood test for a prostate tumor marker can lead to fairly early detection of prostate cancer. Every man over 45 should

undergo these evaluations annually as part of a general checkup.

When to Seek Medical Advice
Seek help if symptoms appear.

Self-Help
Not possible.

Treatment
Rectal and ultrasound exams cannot establish for certain whether cancer is present. This can be confirmed only by microscopic analysis of sampled cells.

Surgical removal of the prostate and seminal vesicles can cure prostate cancer that is still contained. This is the case in 80 to 90 percent of patients.

If the tumor is large and has breached the border of the prostate but not affected the lymph nodes, radiation therapy is administered either externally, or by implanting radioactive material (radionuclide implantation) into the tumor.

If prostate cancer has already metastasized, hormone therapy may be necessary. This completely removes all effects of the male hormones. In 80 percent of patients this treatment can delay tumor growth for many years. The cancer and metastases may even disappear. Occasionally this approach is supplemented by removing the hormone-producing tissue of the testicles. The incontrovertible side effect of chemical and/or surgical castration is loss of sexual desire.

If hormone therapy fails, chemotherapy is possible. Radiation therapy will reduce the pains associated with metastases to the bones.

Counseling can make living with the disease easier. Anything that is enjoyable for the patient and is good for him will improve his quality of life.

DESIRE AND LOVE

Sexual desire is one of the most powerful human drives. Over the course of a lifetime it is possible to experience untold variations in sexuality, ranging from the open expression of desire, sensuality and warmth to feelings of anxiety, repression and shame, and everything in between. During times of heightened stress, sexuality may almost seem to disappear, only to reappear stronger and more urgent than ever afterward. Throughout life, our level of desire fluctuates; times of heightened sexual activity alternate with periods of abstinence, and no definition exists of when or how often it is "normal" or "healthy" to express sexuality. When lovemaking will take place, how intense it will be, and how it will be expressed, all depend on you and your partner. The only limits are those determined by your combined comfort level: Living out your sexuality is fine as long as it doesn't make you or your partner uncomfortable or cause suffering.

Sensuality seems to come especially easily to people who were allowed to experience pleasure through their bodies in childhood, by being hugged and stroked, feeling the joy of movement, and learning to receive and give tenderness, to themselves as well as others. This capacity for exhilaration in one's own body—rather than the degree to which one conforms to some norm of physical attractiveness—is the main ingredient of a positive sensual and sexual outlook.

HOMOSEXUALITY

The wide variety of possible human sexual activities and needs are always subject to prevailing societal norms; what is condemned as "sick" at one time may be considered perfectly healthy at another. For centuries, homosexual love was strictly taboo and harshly punished; the only permissible expression of human sexuality was narrowly defined by religious and political authorities as heterosexual intercourse between married partners, with the intent to procreate. Today, this narrow viewpoint has broadened in many societies; still, the ability to live freely and openly in a same-sex partnership without discrimination is often the hard-won result of a struggle against social, political, and religious prejudice.

SEXUAL DYSFUNCTIONS

The skyrocketing number of sexual dysfunctions has

nothing to do with the sex organs per se; these disorders are psychological in origin (see Men's Issues, p. 541; Women's Issues, p. 537).

Counseling is readily available from physicians trained in psychosexual issues, sex therapists, and sex counselors.

PROBLEMATIC SEX

Couples who enjoy long-term sexual relationships have generally reached consensus in their sexual preferences. Wildly differing preferences, in contrast, can rapidly lead to the end of a relationship. You owe it to yourself not to hide, or even simply endure, lasting feelings of resistance, aversion or revulsion at a partner's sexual wishes; you should honor those feelings and act accordingly. Merely going through the motions of sex can make life miserable, or even lead to illness.

Women's Issues

Sexual problems are some of the most common psychosomatic disorders encountered in gynecological practice. Of these, 25 percent involve lack of desire or inability to achieve orgasm, and about 10 percent involve pain during intercourse. In many classical medical texts these symptoms are classified as diseases—frigidity, anorgasmy, and vaginismus—but in actuality their causes are almost always psychological. The suggested treatments and self-help recommendations for all these disorders are very similar; only the symptoms differ. The term *frigidity* is heard less and less nowadays; *libido disorder* is often used instead.

LACK OF DESIRE, PAINFUL INTERCOURSE, DIFFICULTIES WITH ORGASM

Symptoms

Low or nonexistent sexual desire can manifest as complete disinterest in sexual contact, usually combined with feelings of unhappiness about this situation. In some women this symptom has been present since early childhood; they have simply never experienced sexual desire. This is known as a primary inhibition. Others have experienced desire at other times, but lack it in their current life situation or with their current partner (secondary inhibition).

A woman who has difficulty achieving orgasm, on the other hand, usually experiences sexual desire but does not reach its climax, the orgasm. She may never have achieved orgasm (primary inhibition) or simply be unable to achieve it in her current situation (secondary inhibition).

Vaginismus is a functional disorder that manifests as pain in the vaginal area during intercourse. If no organic cause can be determined, it is considered a psychosomatic reaction to deep, unconscious conflicts. As with all other sexual problems, it may date from childhood or puberty (primary) or have developed only recently (secondary; see Psychosomatic Disorders, p. 185).

The physiological distinctions between these disorders show up during sexual intercourse in general or the orgasm phase in particular (see box opposite).

Lack of desire (libido disorder): The arousal phase is slight or nonexistent; all physical and psychological changes associated with the following phases are absent:

Difficulty achieving orgasm (anorgasmy): Sexual arousal is experienced intensely and passionately until the plateau phase, but is directly followed by the afterglow phase, with no release of sexual tension. The tension may cause discomfort and take a long time to subside.

Pain or cramping: If penetration causes great pain or is impossible, vaginismus is usually diagnosed. In this disorder, the vaginal muscles involuntarily become strongly contracted, and the front third of the vagina cramps up. Such a reaction can be caused by the autonomic nervous system, which is not controlled by the conscious will.

Causes

Just about no other aspect of life is so sensitive to crises and problems as sexuality (see Sexual Dysfunctions, p. 537).

Primary inhibition of desire or orgasm, or pain during intercourse: These often arise as a result of psychological conflicts in early childhood, of which the individual is usually unconscious as an adult, and traumatic childhood or teenage experiences. A home life that was characterized by any of the following: Extreme rigidity or strictness, emotional coldness, repressed or puritanical atti-

The Road to Orgasm

THE AROUSAL PHASE
— The vagina becomes moist and its uppermost part enlarges; the labia and clitoris engorge with blood; the vulva secretes increased mucus.
— The breasts increase somewhat in size and sensitivity.
— The uterus enlarges upward.
— Breathing and heart rate quicken.
— Muscle tension increases, especially in the genital area.

THE PLATEAU PHASE
— The upper part of the vagina continues to widen; its front third narrows.
— The entire genital area continues to engorge; sensations are focused onto this area.
— The uterus contracts still farther upwards; breathing becomes faster; muscle tension increases.
— The clitoris contracts under its hood.

THE CLIMAX PHASE
— Orgasm begins with muscular contractions lasting 2 to 4 seconds, usually followed by further rhythmic contractions in the front third of the vagina.
— A feeling of relaxation and tenderness usually floods the entire body.
— Depending on desire and stimulation, multiple orgasms are possible.

THE INVOLUTION PHASE (AFTERGLOW)
— The engorged areas return to their normal size within half an hour; the muscles relax.
— The clitoris, vagina, and uterus return to their usual size and position.

tudes; domestic violence, rape, physical or sexual abuse; alcohol or drug abuse; divorce or abandonment; constant rejection or belittling as a female—can distort the development of a young girl's sense of self. Her capacity for adventure, self-confidence and trust in others can fail to develop. As a result, her sexuality may be profoundly inhibited (see Psychosomatic Disorders, p. 185).

Secondary inhibition of desire, or of orgasm: These appear in adult life, following periods of successful sexual expression. The three critical issues to be addressed are

— Relationship: How well do you get along with your partner? Has anything in your relationship changed? Do you understand and trust your partner? Do you share intimate experiences, fantasies, desires, discusions? Do you know how to play together?

— Environment: How are you doing in your family

and professional environments? Are you overworked, overburdened, stressed, overextended, exhausted, restless, nervous, generally run down?
— Body image: How do you feel about your body? Do you like yourself even though you may consider yourself too pudgy/skinny, or have breasts you consider too large/small, legs you consider too long/short, etc.?

Relationship

Conflicts with your partner, constant arguments, a lack of respect or emotional warmth, humiliation, lovelessness, mistrust and/or violence (see Alcoholism, p. 205) are the most common causes of loss of libido. Many women live in dependent relationships that continuously undermine their self-worth, self-confidence and self-esteem.

However, your partner may also be sexually inept, not patient enough, and poorly informed. The art of lovemaking includes taking the time to learn what makes a partner feel good. This is not always, or not only, communicated verbally, but requires attention to visual, tactile, and auditory clues, and their correct interpretation.

Men are notoriously less adept than women at the art of "feeling" what another person wants, which leads to countless misunderstandings and disappointments.

Environment

Feeling overburdened, overworked and constantly exhausted is especially common after childbirth and while children are young, and can dampen sexual enthusiasm to a considerable extent. Interpersonal conflicts often intensify at such times, and feeling unappreciated at home or work can contribute to feelings of resentment or frustration, which can inhibit your sex life.

Seemingly inconsequential things can also have a negative impact, such as cramped living quarters in which you share a room with small children or sleep next door to parents or inlaws. Light and noise in the bedroom can be disturbing; keeping the television on constantly can strip you of any motivation.

Body Image

A woman's physical well-being is profoundly influenced by prevalent ideals of beauty, even though she will never look as perfect as the retouched photographs of models in magazines. She may consistently conceal or camouflage certain body parts or odors, resulting in an excessive concern with cleanliness. She may renounce whole areas of life's pleasures in the process: The simple joy of bodily movement, the multiplicity of sensory perceptions and feelings, the sensuality of being naked.

The whole issue of contraception is also an important one: If birth control pills or an intrauterine device are poorly tolerated, or if there is fear of pregnancy or possible complications, sexual desire can be compromised (see Contraception, p. 551).

Organic Causes

Sexual problems are rarely caused by organic factors. At your routine checkup, your doctor can determine whether sexual problems might be traceable to
— Changes, inflammations, tumors, scar tissue, or abnormalities in or around the genitals, which can interfere with sexual activity or cause pain
— Neurologic disorders resulting from traumatic injury or inflammations in the lower spinal cord or changes in the hypothalamus (see p. 501), which can affect sexual desire
— Specific chronic or long-term illnesses, which can diminish sexual desire considerably
— Hormonal changes, which can influence lovemaking during menopause and in old age. Because of lowered estrogen production, the vagina loses its elasticity and becomes drier. This can be remedied with lubricants (see Menopause, p. 510; Aging, p. 606).

Who's at Risk

Because sexuality is one of the most sensitive barometers of emotion, women are at high risk of experiencing sexual difficulties. Research suggests that women with a lack of desire or problems achieving orgasm have more to overcome than men with similar difficulties—not because of basic biological differences between the sexes, but rather because of the different ways in which women relate to the world: Even today, young girls and women are more prone to self-denial and geared to accommodate others than young men. Therefore, women have greater difficulty revealing and gratifying their selves and their desires—not least in the area of sex.

Possible Aftereffects and Complications

Going for years with no sexual desire, or experiencing constant pain during intercourse, can eventually affect general physical, mental and social well-being. Long-lasting attachments to men, or to women, may be rendered more difficult or even impossible. Those considering divorce or separation on grounds of sexual incompatibility, however, should be clear that relational problems are usually the cause of sexual problems, rather than the result.

Prevention

To be able to experience your sexuality fully, you need to be content with yourself; this is absolutely vital for a trusting, intimate sharing of yourself with another person. Feeling good about yourself includes taking pleasure in your own body and being comfortable with your own sensations, feelings, and fantasies.

A woman's sexual fantasies may be soft and tender, or violent and pornographic. They don't necessarily fit the stereotyped image of women as passive. They may change over the course of her life, and with different partners. The more a woman can free herself from societal ideals, norms, and prohibitions, the better she can know herself. It is also possible, of course, to go off the deep end in the opposite direction: Breaking down taboos should not be confused with becoming indiscriminate in your choice of partners, or having too many partners. Just because you can do something is no reason to do it; you should only do what will contribute to your happiness and self-esteem.

Maintaining a balance between periods of closeness and time spent apart, expressions of independence and requests for intimacy, and dominant and submissive roles can help keep sexual interest alive for partners in a satisfying relationship.

When to Seek Medical Advice

If your sexual problems become a real burden which isn't lessened by talking to your partner, and the self-help suggestions below don't work, make an appointment with a doctor you trust.

Self-Help

— Get in touch with your body and discover what makes you feel good. See the suggested self-help measures for psychosomatic disorders (p. 185) for additional support.

— Explore your fantasies, perhaps with the help of erotic literature, pictures, or videos. Many women are ashamed of having erotic thoughts and suppress or deny them, perhaps afraid that describing a fantasy might be mistaken for the desire to live it out. There is no obligation to reveal your fantasies, however— they can fuel the flames of sexual passion even when unspoken.

— Discover your tendencies. Maybe you're more attracted to women than to men and don't dare admit it. Seek support from women's self-help groups or counseling centers; find like-minded people in lesbian locales (see Homosexuality, p. 537).

— Explore your sensuality. Your skin is the largest and most important sense organ. Every inch of it can be touched in a sensual, arousing, calming, or irritating way. Explore smells, tastes, sounds, or words that you find erotic.

— Discover self-gratification. The clitoris is one of the most important erogenous zones; depending on your body, the breasts, labia, vulva, or anus may react more or less sensitively to stimulation. For many women, masturbation is one of the most important sources of, and pathways to discovery of, sexual desire. It can also be integrated into lovemaking with your partner.

— Explore your relationship. It is a myth that aging partners in a long-term relationship must renounce sexuality. On the contrary, for many couples the quality of the sexual relationship increases with the length of their partnership. Factors that may inhibit sexuality include boredom, indifference, and emotional distance—which are not unique to long-term relationships.

— Discover communication. Maybe you like certain games, caresses, erogenous zones or positions your partner doesn't know about. Talk about your desires and needs if you want them gratified. Exploring new, different forms of sexuality can help lessen vaginal cramping accompanying intercourse.

— Pay attention to your rhythms. There are times when you're extremely active sexually, and others when your head, heart, and imagination are occupied with other things—a newborn baby, for example. You might simply be going through a less sexual phase; discuss this with your partner.

Treatment

Professional support is available at women's counseling centers and family therapy centers. For primary sexual inhibitions that you've been carrying around since childhood, comprehensive psychotherapy can be worthwhile (see Conflict-Centered Techniques, p. 699).

Couples therapy can offer significant help for secondary inhibitions (see Couples and Family Therapy, p. 698).

Men's Issues

The penis has deep symbolic significance: It's a sign of strength and potency, a wonderful toy with a will of its own. Lovers may treat it like a third partner. Male identity is closely identified with the penis: If it doesn't work, a man doesn't feel like a man. Male prowess can't be measured in terms of penis length, however; neither can a woman's likelihood of achieving orgasm. No penis is too big or too small for mutual enjoyment. In the throes of pressure to "perform," many men forget that a wide variety of sexual activities exists in addition to intercourse.

Factors affecting sexual intercourse include not only the "tool" but psychological and cultural factors as well: your expectations, degree of desire, vascular circulation, and quality of orgasm. After ejaculation, tension is released, muscles relax and a feeling of well-being pervades the body. After some time has passed, another erection and orgasm become possible. The entire sexual cycle consists of reflexes regulated by the carefully balanced interplay of the autonomic nervous systems; any of the reflexes can be inhibited or interrupted at any point by thoughts and feelings, hormones, the nervous system or the effects of medications and illness. Interpersonal factors, such as the need to adhere to socially acceptable male-female behavior, can also interfere with sexual potency.

SEX IN MIDDLE AND OLD AGE

A man's peak sexual performance is achieved at about age 20; erection and ejaculation happen quickly and can be repeated after a few minutes. By the time he's 50, sexual potency has diminished noticeably. A full erection may take longer to achieve and require longer, more vigorous stimulation. The ejaculation is usually not as strong and can be delayed.

All of this need not be a disadvantage. Many women enjoy more pleasurable play and tenderness as their partner becomes less single-minded, and they usually enjoy oral or manual stimulation.

Even if the penis is less hard than it used to be and sex results only infrequently in orgasm, desire and fantasy need not be affected. A fulfilled sex life is possible in later years, even if the need for sex is absent for periods at a time.

MID-LIFE CRISIS

The so-called middle years of life can bring increased professional pressures and problems with wife and children, as well as the added realization that it's time to let go of youth; the sex hormones also undergo changes. One sixth of all men suffer from this "male menopause."

Chronic diseases may appear during this period. Though sex can provide a welcome respite from life's problems and improve your overall health and equilibrium, the libido may become problematic or repressed. Talk honestly to your partner about this, and seek help from a trusted doctor or a sex therapist. Rest assured that this isn't the end: It's only a change.

LACK OF DESIRE, IMPOTENCE, DISORDERS OF ERECTION AND EJACULATION

Lack of desire: Although you are capable of being aroused, you have no sustained interest in sex.
Impotence and erection disorders: The penis is not hard enough for sexual intercourse. Impotence may or may not be a factor.

In priapism (constant erection), the penis remains hard for extended periods, causing considerable pain. Intercourse can be painful if the penis is unnaturally bent or the foreskin is too tight.
Ejaculation disorders: Most men need to learn to delay ejaculation in order to avoid the urge to come soon after penetration: For most women, a short period of penetration is not satisfactory, and neither partner has enough time to really enjoy sex to the fullest. Ejaculation in the absence of mechanical stimulation is considered a disorder.

Causes

The occasional inability to achieve an erection is every man's lot at some point in life. In 30 percent of cases, long-term disturbances of libido and potency have a mental/emotional cause.

Emotional Causes

An inhibited sex life usually stems from onerous sexual experiences in childhood or youth, or an upbringing that powerfully repressed sexual fantasy and desire.

Libido disorders: These may be the expression of problems—even unconscious ones—in your relationship with your partner. Perhaps you've chosen the wrong partner, and the penis is expressing what you can't—namely "no." Perhaps you are unmoved or even repulsed by your partner's sexual practices. This may show up only when you've been living together for a while, helped along by waning desire and growing boredom. In addition, overwork, exhaustion, stress, agitation, nervousness, depression, cramped living quarters, excessive noise levels, or constant background interference from the television set can be alienating and distracting, as can an unconscious fear of women or one woman in particular, fear of fathering a child, or fear of failure.

If you don't feel attracted to women or fantasize about men, you may have homosexual tendencies. Many men have such fantasies without necessarily wanting to live them out. At least 5 percent of men are homosexually inclined; 15 percent are bisexual.

Ejaculation disorders: Some men learn only gradually to control ejaculation and accommodate their partner's different arousal phases and wishes. Various anxieties can hasten ejaculation; unresolved performance anxiety can make premature ejaculation chronic.

Organic Causes

Lack of sexual desire can be due in rare cases to congenital underdevelopment of the gonads, or insufficient production of testosterone. Sexual desire naturally diminishes gradually with age.

The main causes of potency disorders are usually vascular diseases (occasionally congenital ones), followed by chronic diseases such as diabetes, liver damage, hypothyroidism, asthma and high blood pressure.

Infrequently, hormone deficiencies can cause sexual problems, as can the following: Damage to the erectile tissue; central nervous system disorders including paralysis, multiple sclerosis (see p. 220), shingles (see p. 284), or tumors; disorders of nerve conduction between the erection nerve center in the lower spine and the sex organs, e.g., after certain types of pelvic surgery.

These organic disorders invariably lead to psychological problems over time, and can cause a vicious circle of anxiety and failure.

Other Causes

These disorders can also be caused by medication, excessive alcohol consumption, obesity, and nicotine abuse.

Who's at Risk

Men with any of the listed root causes are at risk; if the causes are not discovered and addressed, problems can proliferate.

Possible Aftereffects and Complications

Failure to perform can heighten performance anxiety and lead to renewed failure, establishing a vicious circle. Feelings of frustration and disappointment can endanger a relationship; fear of failure can cause a man to avoid intimacy with women altogether.

Sex therapy and counseling

You don't necessarily need a sex therapist for counseling in matters of sex: A general practitioner can also help if he or she knows you well and is familiar with your life situation and the people you live with. Your general practitioner can gauge whether disease, behavior or medication may be causing your problems, and will probably refer you to a urologist for a medical assessment, and/or to a specialist in psychosomatic illnesses. Your doctor may also recommend psychotherapy (see Counseling and Psychotherapy, p. 697). Be sure to talk your decision over with your partner beforehand.

Medications with libido-affecting side effects:

— First among these are high-blood-pressure medication, especially beta blockers (see Hypertension, p. 321)
— Antidepressants and antipsychotic medication
— Medication for ulcers, the so-called H2-antagonists
— Amphetamines
— Female hormones
— Cancer medication

Prevention

For parents

An open attitude toward sex can help avoid many of these problems. Protect your child against sexual abuse by talking about what constitutes sexual violation. Don't hesitate to intercede if the child reports advances or improprieties by relatives, friends, or trusted people.

For the patient

Avoid excessive alcohol and nicotine, excessive weight, stress, overwork, and insufficient sleep.

Listen to your intuition when choosing a sexual partner and dealing with your relationship. Little things or situations that annoy you or cause you to get defensive right from the start aren't going to go anywhere.

When possible, avoid contraceptive methods that can inhibit desire, even if only temporarily. For possible alternatives, see Contraception, p. 551.

Communicating openly with your partner about what you're going through will relieve a lot of the emotional pressure.

When to Seek Medical Advice

Seek help if you're unhappy because you don't want to have sex, or can't, or can't do it the way you'd like to.

Self-Help

If you have a compassionate partner, sexual difficulties need not develop into a problem requiring treatment, although you can't expect your partner to cure you. However, if your partner is lacking in compassion or sensitivity toward your difficulties, you might want to rethink the relationship.

If you're already in the vicious circle of performance anxiety and fear of failure, and your partner is feeling frustrated, disappointed, or rejected, forgo intercourse for a while and try what many women enjoy: Gentle, tender, sensual play involving the whole body, using hands and tongue. You may discover new forms of togetherness and find that your partner wants things you hadn't known about.

— Be honest and open in mutual communication with your partner about what arouses or alienates both of you. This will help prevent misunderstandings and overstepped boundaries.

— Create—alone or together—erotic situations. Play-act new situations; try new positions. Explorations accompanied by tenderness and imagination can disrupt the tedium of routine.

— There are positions that make penetration possible even with a slight erection, such as when the woman, lying on her side, raises her upper thigh and presents her bottom.

— A predetermined period of time spent apart from your partner can kindle renewed interest or help you determine whether it's time to move on.

— If you have homosexual interests, make contact with a gay support group; speaking openly in the group, you may be able to clarify your desires and decide which ones to act on.

Sexual Aids

Folk medicine claims aphrodisiacal powers for a variety of common herbs and plants; most owe their effectiveness to magical beliefs or wishful thinking. Asparagus, for instance, supposedly gives men sexual endurance, and celery, garlic, and nettleseed can improve erections. If you believe this, go ahead and try them. The effects of other folk remedies throughout history have been dubious and even dangerous, but some techniques have proven effective.

For ejaculation disorders:

— After a premature ejaculation, try, try again; you may be more successful the second time around.

— Prolong foreplay. An impending ejaculation can be delayed by tightly gripping the shaft of the penis under the glans.

— Changing positions during intercourse will delay ejaculation; in the dominant position the woman can stimulate her clitoris especially strongly.

— You can "win time" by disengaging mentally and thinking of other things.

Treatment

Any organic causes should be identified and treated.

If you are on any of the medications listed on p. 542, discuss your situation with your doctor; don't simply stop taking them.

Doctors often prescribe testosterone for sexual dysfunctions; this is helpful only if an actual hormone deficiency exists. If you are undergoing hormone treatment, a urologist should check you regularly for possible side effects, which could include prostate cancer.

Disadvantages of aphrodisiacs

Ginseng: improves sexual endurance, but not potency in men. In women, ginseng can increase sexual receptiveness and cause the nipples to swell. Its side effects are significant: High blood pressure, diarrhea, skin rashes, edema, nervousness, sleeplessness, euphoria and depression. In high doses, ginseng causes confusion. Many ginseng preparations contain additional synthetic or inert ingredients.

Spanish fly: Is derived from an insect, which is crushed into a powder (containing cantharides) and rubbed on the genitals, irritating the skin and mucosa. Ingestion causes uterine bleeding in women and painful erections without increased sexual desire in men. In higher doses, cantharides have the same effect as mustard gas on the central nervous system. Ingesting 10 to 50 mg leads to death within twelve hours from liver poisoning, circulatory breakdown, and kidney and heart failure.

Yohimbine: Causes the vascular system of the erectile tissue to dilate. It should not be taken by people with kidney or liver problems.

Strychnine: Affects the whole central nervous system. It leads to convulsions and muscle cramps causing stiffness in the face and neck.

Treatment of Psychologically Caused Libido Disorders

Professional help can be useful in sexual disorders of psychological origin. Counseling shouldn't be a source of shame; to the contrary, it takes courage to resolve to clear out emotional garbage and take on the hard work of getting to the bottom of things. Make sure, however, that you select a counselor experienced in sex therapy. You can get referrals from an outpatient urology clinic (see Counseling and Psychotherapy, p. 697).

One widely used approach to breaking the vicious circle is to agree to a "no sex" period lasting a predetermined amount of time. During this period, follow these steps:

Step 1: Three evenings a week, create a relaxed atmosphere with your partner: Enjoy peace and quiet, have a light meal by candlelight, listen to music together. Make sure the house is warm and you won't be interrupted. Get undressed and stroke each other all over. Explore every area of your partner's body—except for the breasts, genitals, and anal area. Give yourself at least half an hour for this. Enjoyment can be intensified by using aromatic skin lotion. Give yourself over to your feelings and take pleasure in feeling another body with your fingers. After three or four evenings, proceed to step two.

Step 2: In the same setting, luxuriate in the sensual and erotic pleasures you learned in step 1, but take things a step further by stroking and massaging each other's breasts, genitals, and anal area.

Step 3: Usually, the compelling desire for complete physical union appears after a few days of step 2; once you break the "no sex" rule, the program can be considered a success.

Treatment for Erection Disorders

There is a range of medical options for treating organically-caused erection disorders; however, they don't always satisfactorily solve the problem.

Medications

Circulation-boosting medications such as papaverine are injected directly into the erectile tissue. Only two out of three men actually achieve erection if the shot is given in the doctor's office; the method is usually more successful if administered by you or your partner in a private atmosphere.

These medications cause blood to rush into the erectile tissue and constrict the veins so blood can't flow out again. The shot should be given about a quarter hour prior to planned intercourse. With a correct dose, the penis relaxes again after erection; if the dose is too high, dangerous priapism (abnormal erection of the penis, usually without sexual desire, accompanied by tenderness and pain) can result.

Side effects: Tension to the point of pain in the penis; also orgasm disorders. Two to 5 percent of patients experience painful priapism that must be treated with medication or by drawing blood off the erectile tissue with a syringe.

Injuries to the nerves or urethra can result from injecting medication into the penis.

Surgical Options

— If a blocked pelvic artery prevents successful engorging of the penis with blood, a bypass operation can create a detour through a vein or artery.

— An artificial penile implant can stiffen a penis sufficiently for vaginal penetration. These prostheses usually fall short of expectations, nevertheless.

— If you are producing too little testosterone, your doctor can prescribe the hormone as medication. With hormone treatment, a urologist should check you regularly for possible side effects, including prostate cancer.

Treatment for Ejaculation Disorders

Delay training: The partner manually brings the penis to the point of ejaculation, then grips the shaft of the penis under the glans until the erection subsides. After a short time, the partner stimulates the penis again. This is repeated several times before gratification.

Sexually Transmitted Diseases

Sexually transmitted diseases (STDs) are the world's most prevalent infectious diseases; the number of cases continues to rise. Reasons for this include increased mobility of the population and a more permissive attitude toward sex in general and various sexual practices in particular, as well as widespread ignorance and embarrassment at discussing sexual matters. Advanced diagnostic and treatment protocols can quickly return most infected patients to health.

The classic genital diseases—syphilis, gonorrhea, chancroid, lymphogranuloma venereum, and granuloma inguinale—must be reported to local health authorities, but only details of the disease are registered: Confidentiality is preserved.

Today, the classic diseases are less common than other STDs such as trichomoniasis, chlamydia, and herpes simplex. Two to 5 percent of all gynecological patients have genital herpes; extrapolated to the adult population, this means that 0.2 percent are infected with trichomonas and 4 to 10 percent with chlamydia.

Condom use is the most effective tool in preventing the spread of STDs.

CANDIDIASIS

Fungal or yeast infections of the genitalia (candidiasis) can be transmitted through sexual contact, but in women they usually develop independently of sexual contact.

Symptoms

In women: Symptoms usually include a severe vaginal inflammation with light to very heavy discharge. The labia are red, swollen and itchy and become covered with a crumbly discharge resembling cottage cheese. Burning pain and a sensation of heat and weight in the pelvis may be present as well.

In men: The glans and foreskin are inflamed and red, often with weeping lesions, occasionally with whitish deposits.

Causes

Fungi normally inhabit the skin and mucosa of healthy people. If disease results, it's usually due to a failure of the immune system. This can be facilitated by
— Constant moistness of the skin
— Diabetes
— Changes in hormone levels (e.g., taking birth control pills, pregnancy, old age, cortisone intake)
— Antibiotics or immunosuppressants
— Severe anemia

Who's at Risk

Yeast infections are increasingly common. The causes for this may include excessive sugar consumption and the effect on the skin's acid mantle of excessive showers and baths, swimming, or saunas. Yeast infections are also fostered by overly tight underwear. Many women take birth control pills, and more and more antibiotics are prescribed; both the hormones in the pill and antibiotics can reduce the lactobacillus population in the vagina that usually holds the pathogens in check, resulting in unhampered proliferation of the fungus.

Possible Aftereffects and Complications

Your sex partner may become infected; stubborn recurrent infections may occur.

Prevention

Wear loose cotton underwear and eat a low-sugar diet. Women who tend to get vaginal and yeast infections can stabilize the acid balance of the vagina by taking weekly lactobacillus.

During menstruation, use sanitary pads rather than tampons so as not to irritate the vagina. Condoms can prevent infection of partners (see p. 553).

When to Seek Medical Advice

Seek help if symptoms are present.

Self-Help

Self-help with lactobacillus treatment rarely helps once the infection has already set in.

Treatment

All factors that can encourage yeast infections should be avoided. Stop taking birth-control pills for 1 month. Avoid sexual contact so as to avoid reinfection. In case of recurrent infections, your partner must also be treated.

In women: Antifungal medications such as clotrimazole, miconazol enitrate, terconazole vaginal tablets and/or cream are inserted into the vagina daily for up to 6 days. Alternative options include a single oral dose of fluconazole (Diflucan).

In men: Anitfungal creams applied for 7 to 10 days usually clear up the inflammation. Relapses are common if the treatment is not carried through conscientiously and thoroughly.

TRICHOMONIASIS

Symptoms

In women: Burning sensation in the vagina, inflammation with greenish-yellow discharge, pain in the vulva, pain while urinating.

In men: A trichomonad infection is usually not noticed. Some have milky discharge in their first urination of the day; a sensation of burning, pulling, or tickling in the urethra; oozing.

Causes

Infection with a parasite.

Who's at Risk

Trichomonad infections have dropped in the past few years. The pathogens are spread almost exclusively through sexual intercourse, and only rarely by toilet seats, towels, or saunas. Infection can occur in small children as well, most likely through manual cross-infection from adults.

Trichomoniasis occurs more often in women than in men.

Possible Aftereffects and Complications

In women: Chronic vaginal inflammations; Bartholin's gland inflammations; bladder infections.

In men: Inflammation of glans and prostate.

Prevention

Protected sex through condom use (see p. 553); proper hygiene.

When to Seek Medical Advice

Seek help if symptoms are present.

Self-Help

Not possible.

Treatment

Treating with metronidazole-containing medications such as Flagyl is usually successful.

Warning: Even if your partner is completely symptom-free, he or she should absolutely be treated simultaneously to avoid reinfection.

Important: The medication listed above should not be taken during the first trimester of pregnancy or while breastfeeding.

CHLAMYDIAL AND UREAPLASMAL INFECTIONS

Symptoms

In women: Symptoms may include the frequent urge to urinate, difficult urination, pains in the lower abdomen and during intercourse, mild discharge, and mild inflammations of the urethra and cervix. Most women, however, don't even notice the infection.

In men: One to 2 weeks after exposure, symptoms include difficulty urinating, strong urge to urinate, a pulling sensation in the urethra, and mucous or pus-filled discharge. Often the opening of the urethra is stuck together first thing in the morning.

In rare instances, inflammation of the mouth and throat can result from oral sex, and inflammations of the rectum from anal sex.

Causes

The majority of common diseases formerly termed "nonspecific urethral and genital inflammations" are caused by chlamydia organisms, the remainder by ureaplasma and mycoplasma.

Who's at Risk

This STD is the most common in the West, about 10 times more common than gonorrhea.

Possible Aftereffects and Complications

In women: The most common complication is pelvic inflammation. Infertility, resulting from an infection of the fallopian tubes, is also possible. Possible growths on the fallopian tubes may predispose for tubal pregnancies. Further complications can include inflammations of the liver capsule or Bartholin's glands, and arthritis. In 40 percent of cases, babies are born infected. This is why pregnant women who present for prenatal care are routinely tested for chlamydia. In newborns, the disease manifests as conjunctivitis or, more rarely, pneumonia.

In men: This infection is the most common cause of epididymitis and prostatitis in men under age 35.

Warning: Even without treatment, symptoms usually clear up after a month in two out of three cases.

However, the disease can also become chronic. In women it can lead to painful pelvic inflammations, infertility, and ectopic pregnancies.

Prevention

Protected sex through condom use (see p. 553).

When to Seek Medical Advice

Seek help if symptoms are present.

Self-Help

Not possible.

Treatment

A 10-day course of doxycycline, or single dose of azithromycin (see Antibiotics, p. 661) is recommended. During pregnancy, erythromycin or azithromycin is recommended. Infected people should avoid intercourse until symptoms have disappeared and treatment is complete. Your sex partner should also be checked and treated, and checked again after 3 months. It may be wise for former sex partners to get checked as well.

GENITAL WARTS

Symptoms

In women: Warts may appear on the labia, anus, cervix, vagina, or rectum.

In men: Warts may appear on the foreskin, urethral opening, shaft of the penis, anus, or rectum. The warts are small and pale pink and grow quickly, often in a group.

During pregnancy and in the presence of a chronic discharge they can grow more quickly. They usually cause no pain but may itch.

Causes

Infection with the human papilloma virus (HPV), usually through sexual contact.

Who's at Risk

Genital warts can be spread very quickly to others.

Possible Aftereffects and Complications

Genital warts may be a precursor to cervical cancer and may be associated with the development of other forms of cancer.

During childbirth, HPV can be transmitted to the child, who may subsequently develop growths.

Prevention

Protected sex through condom use (see p. 553).

When to Seek Medical Advice

If you notice wartlike growths, you and your sex partner(s) should see a doctor. Examinations of the affected areas can rule out syphilis or cancer.

Self-Help

Not possible.

Treatment

Recovery after direct application of podophyllin to small warts is possible.

Wart tissue can also be destroyed with applications of liquid nitrogen/cryosurgery, surgery, or laser therapy.

Wait to have intercourse until you are completely recovered. You and your partner(s) should be checked after three months.

Important: After successful treatment, women should get a Pap smear at least once a year for early detection of any possible cancer.

GENITAL HERPES

Symptoms

A red swelling appears on the genital mucosa and possibly also the anus; many flat blisters appear in groups and sometimes run together. After the blisters burst, they develop into painful sores. Often the lymph nodes in the groin are swollen, sometimes accompanied by general malaise, a slight fever, and difficulty urinating. After a few days the open sores disappear; occasionally, larger sores may develop.

Causes

The pathogens are the herpes simplex virus, type I or II. After initial infection they lie dormant in the body. If the immune system is disturbed or taxed (e.g., due to sunburn, fever, injuries, digestive-tract disorders, menstruation, or corticosteroid treatment), the pathogens are reactivated.

Who's at Risk

Herpes is one of the most common STDs, with up to 50 percent of adults in Europe (70 percent in Africa) having been exposed to this virus and having developed antibodies. In most people the immune system is able to hold the virus in check without symptoms. In only about 1 percent of infected people do the characteristic blisters recur.

Possible Aftereffects and Complications

In men, these may include inability to urinate, constipation, and erection disorders.

Like herpes labialis, genital herpes can spread to other parts of the body and affect the eyes; with resulting scar tissue on the conjunctiva or cornea. In rare cases, if the immune system is severely compromised (e.g., by leukemia), genital herpes can be accompanied by encephalitis. This can manifest as fever, headaches, stiff neck, vomiting, and sensitivity to light.

During acute outbreaks of herpes, newborns can be infected in the birth canal. Because this can have life-threatening consequences, cesarean sections are often performed protectively.

Prevention

Protected sex through condom use (see p. 553). If you are having an outbreak, avoid sexual contact.

When to Seek Medical Advice

Seek help if symptoms are present.

Self-Help

Not possible.

Treatment

Acyclovir taken in pill form or given intravenously can ease the symptoms, restrict the spread of blisters, speed healing, help prevent outbreaks, and minimize the severity of relapses, but it cannot do away with the latent infection.

SYPHILIS

Syphilis is a bacterial disease that can affect the whole body. If untreated it can last for decades and may lead to death. However, only one third of untreated syphilitics manifest the symptoms of the final phase.

Symptoms

Initial phase: Two to 4 weeks after infection a hard "primary" ulcer appears—a painless, firm, red-brown sore on the skin or mucosa directly at the site of infection, which may go unnoticed. Without treatment, the ulcer heals after about 6 weeks. Lymph nodes in the area of the source-point of infection swell after about a month and remain enlarged.

Second phase: About 9 to 10 weeks following infection, a characteristic light- to red-brown spotted rash develops on the skin and mucosa in various parts of the body; it may be raised or bumpy. Hair loss and liver inflammation may accompany this phase, and the central nervous system may be affected. Exhaustion, joint pain, slightly elevated temperature, and mild headaches may occur. After a few months the symptoms may disappear, as the pathogens become dormant again.

Third phase: After 3 to 5 years, every organ of the body may come under attack by the disease. Rubbery lumps can develop on the skin and in liver, testicles, and brain. Vascular disease, especially of the cerebral vessels, is a particularly dangerous complication.

Fourth phase: After 20 to 30 years, progressive paralysis may ensue.

Causes

Syphilis is caused by *Treponema pallidum* bacteria, usually spread through sexual contact.

Bacteria can enter the skin through microscopic fissures in the skin and mucosa. They can—rarely—also be spread by kissing, but not through sharing utensils, cups, or towels. Outside the body, the bacteria die quickly.

Who's at Risk

Individuals who have unprotected sex with multiple partners are at increased risk for syphilis.

Possible Aftereffects and Complications

About 10 percent of untreated patients die from late complications of the disease.

Beginning in the fifth month of pregnancy, syphilis can be transmitted from mother to baby. Depending on the stage of the mother's infection, the child may be stillborn or born with birth defects. Penicillin given before the fourth month can prevent this, which is why prenatal screening includes a blood test for syphilis. There is no immunity to syphilis.

Prevention

Protected sex through condom use (see p. 553).

When to Seek Medical Advice

Syphilis is insidious: Its earliest symptoms are easy to miss, it remains dormant for long periods, and the skin eruptions of the second phase are harmless, yet contagious. If you suspect you have syphilis and notice sores and eruptions, see a dermatologist as soon as possible. This disease should not be spread.

There are two ways to test for syphilis: Either by proof of the pathogens in initial stages, or through evidence of antibodies in the blood.

Self-Help

Not possible.

Treatment

The treatment of choice is penicillin. If you can't tolerate it, the doctor can prescribe tetracycline, or erythromycin for pregnant women. These medications can stop syphilis as late as the third stage.

After healing, blood tests should be done after 1, 3, 6, and 12 months. After 2 years of clear tests, the patient is considered cured. Only after treatment is completed is intercourse possible without danger of infection.

Patients whose syphilis is detected early enough should contact any sexual partners from the previous 3 months to inform them that they may also be infected and should avoid sexual intercourse until they have been checked and possibly treated. Patients diagnosed in the second phase should inform sexual partners from the previous 12 months.

Syphilis must be reported to health authorities.

GONORRHEA

Symptoms

In women: Two to 4 days after infection, many women may experience pus-filled discharge from the urethra after markedly frequent urination. This may be misdiagnosed as natural mucous discharge from the vagina. Chronic gonorrhea affecting the cervix, fallopian tubes, and ovaries may go undetected even by the woman herself, because there may be no symptoms. Often the infection is first noticed when the male partner is infected, since his symptoms generally are unmistakable. *In men:* About 3 days after infection, burning pains accompany urination; shortly afterward, there is a yellowish, creamy pus-filled discharge from the urethra.

Causes

The bacteria *Neisseria gonorrhea* cause the disease, which is spread through sexual intercourse. The bacteria can invade undamaged mucosa.

Who's at Risk

The risk of contracting gonorrhea through unprotected sex is great, since many women and some men don't exhibit signs of infection. It is possible to be repeatedly reinfected.

Possible Aftereffects and Complications

In women: If a pregnant woman doesn't know she is infected, the pathogens may pass to the newborn in the birth canal. In the past, a solution of silver nitrate was routinely dropped in the eyes of newborns as a preventive measure. Currently, erythromycin ointment applied to the newborns' eyes is used.

In about 20 percent of women an abscess can result from an infection of one of the Bartholin's glands. Common consequences include inflammations of the uterine lining, ovaries, fallopian tubes, and peritoneum; liver-capsule inflammations are less frequent.

In men: Possible complications include prostatitis or epididymitis.

In both women and men: About half of all women develop anal gonorrhea through local contact. It is also widespread among homosexual men. There may be no symptoms, or mucous and pus may appear in the stool. Rectal gonorrhea should be treated in all cases. Gonorrhea can also be spread to the oral cavity through oral sex.

Chronic gonorrhea can lead to infertility through occlusion of seminal ducts in men and fallopian tubes in women. It is common for individuals with gonorrhea to experience simultaneous infection with other pathogens, e.g., chlamydia or HPV (see Genital Warts, p. 547), or in rare cases, syphilis. For this reason, when gonorrhea is diagnosed, tests should also be made for other infections.

Prevention
The risk of cross-infection can be reduced by protected sex through condom use (see Condoms, p. 553) and by immediately seeking medical advice at the first suspicion of infection.

When to Seek Medical Advice
In women: If you notice unusual vaginal discharge, contact your gynecologist. If gonorrhea is suspected and the culture test is negative, another test should be done during your next menstrual cycle. Often the organism is first detected this way.

In men: If you notice burning during urination or discharge from the urethra, contact a specialist in STDs. Personal responsibility dictates that you inform your sex partner of your status. If you have (or have had) sex with a gonorrhea-infected person, see your health-care provider immediately, even if no symptoms have appeared.

Self-Help
Not possible.

Treatment
Special culture tests for gonorrhea take about 3 days to process.

Antibiotics in the cephalosporin group, such as ceftriaxone, cefixime, or cefpodoxime are given or prescribed in single-dose form.

To ensure that the risk of cross-infection is past, samples of the affected areas should be analyzed a week after treatment. These will determine whether the infection is gone and sex can once more be engaged in without danger of infection.

Gonorrhea must be reported to health authorities.

CHANCROID

Symptoms
Within 3 to 5 days after infection, flat, white, painful, lentil-sized sores with overhanging bright-red edges appear, in men on the glans and foreskin, in women on the labia. Some days later the nearby lymph nodes swell up with slight pain. Abscesses may develop.

Causes
Bacterial infection. A concurrent infection with syphilis is also possible, as it is with all STDs.

Who's at Risk
Chancroid is very rare. Men are five times as likely to be affected as women. Chancroid may facilitate HIV transmission.

Possible Aftereffects and Complications
Phimosis, constriction or fistulas in the groin area after an abscess bursts, and serious tissue destruction are possible complications.

Prevention
Protected sex through condom use (see p. 553).

When to Seek Medical Advice
Seek help if symptoms are present. A dermatologist should rule out other STDs, whose symptoms may resemble those of chancroid.

Self-Help
Not possible.

Treatment
Chancroid is treated with a single dose of ceftriaxone or azithromycin.

Chancroid should be reported to health authorities.

CONTRACEPTION

The ideal contraceptive is one that is reliable, safe, cheap, available on demand, and easy to use, and won't interrupt lovemaking. Such a contraceptive does not yet exist. Even existing contraceptive methods, however, are not used to best advantage, often because of insufficient information or lack of support from the partner.

Contraception continues to be primarily a women's issue; this allows men to deny that the birth of an unplanned child has consequences for them, too.

In choosing a contraceptive method, various factors should be taken into account:
— Success rate (this is determined by the Pearl index— or failure rate—of the method: The total number of pregnancies per 100 women using the method for 1 year)
— Possible health risks
— Cost per month
— Your attitude toward daily ingestion of a pill
— Your attitude toward the possible pregnancy or abortion, in case of failure
— Stability or instability of your life circumstances at the moment
— Whether you're forgetful or well-disciplined
— How actively your partner is involved
— Frequency of sexual intercourse
— How much time and attention you can or want to devote to contraception
— Chances of conceiving and bringing to term healthy babies after discontinuing the method

NATURAL CONTRACEPTION

The Rhythm Method
The failure rate of the rhythm method is notorious. According to the Pearl index (see above), between 15 and 35 unplanned pregnancies per hundred women result from this method.

The rhythm method supposedly allows one to calculate when one is ovulating, and therefore at peak fertility, by counting the days of the menstrual cycle and relying on information from previous cycles. However, environmental and emotional factors can alter even the most regular of cycles unpredictably, making this method very undependable.

Coitus Interruptus
Coitus interruptus is one of the oldest and most fallible contraceptive methods, with a Pearl index rating of between 10 and 20 pregnancies per hundred. In this method, the man withdraws his penis from the vagina shortly before ejaculation. Even if the man has learned to hold back his ejaculation, drops of semen often enter the vagina in the preejaculatory fluid, causing a pregnancy. Besides, many women can't reach orgasm with this method, so both partners lose out on the moment of release.

Self-Observation (Natural Family Planning)
This method, if used correctly and conscientiously, has a high success rate: Only 0.8 to 3 pregnancies per hundred. There are negligible side effects and it costs nothing, but it's not for everyone.

Women can conceive during only about 60 hours of each cycle. Natural contraception requires getting in touch with your body, observing it carefully, learning to identify your fertile times with certainty, and avoiding sexual intercourse during these days. (You can also use this method to become pregnant.) For contraception, self-observation can be combined with other methods such as using a condom or diaphragm during days of peak fertility.

The natural method involves constant monitoring of the body's basal temperature and changes in the cervical mucus. Absolute prerequisites are a good knowledge of your own body, a relatively stable life and regular menstrual cycle, experience with the method over the long term, and sufficient self-discipline.

This method is not as effective in sporadic or irregular sexual relationships. Even in a stable relationship, it requires the full cooperation of both partners: During days of peak fertility, sexual intercourse must be avoided or a condom or diaphragm used. This method is not suitable for nursing mothers.

Measuring Basal Temperature
Due to increased progesterone levels, body temperature at ovulation rises from about 97.7°F to about 98.6°F and remains elevated until the onset of menstruation, when it returns to normal.

The exact day of ovulation cannot be determined through temperature measurement alone; for this reason, taking your temperature must always be combined with observing the cervical mucus. It can only be determined after the fact that ovulation has occurred.

Things to pay attention to:

— Your body's *basal temperature* is its temperature on waking. You must take your temperature at the same time every morning when you get up. The most exact reading is rectal.

— Leave the thermometer in for at least 5 minutes after you have slept at least 6 hours. Always record the reading on a chart.

— If you've slept less than 6 hours or spent a restless night, your basal temperature will be affected. Record on your chart anything that might affect the temperature, whether you danced till dawn or worked a night shift; note any psychological stress as well. Over time, you'll learn to interpret your temperature fluctuations.

— Other factors that affect temperature include an illness accompanied by fever; alcohol consumption the night before (raises temperature); certain pain medications like aspirin or acetaminophen (lower temperature).

— If, under normal circumstances, you get three consecutive readings that are at least 0.36°F higher than those of the previous 6 days, you can conclude that ovulation has taken place (see p. 506).

— Always use the same thermometer; clean it only with lukewarm water, and shake it down the evening before.

Observing Cervical Mucus

Estrogen levels rise before ovulation, causing increased mucus production in the cervix. The normal vaginal discharge increases, signaling that ovulation is now possible. Every woman can learn to detect changes in the volume and consistency of cervical mucus throughout her cycle, and thus to predict the ovulation phase.

It is important not to use vaginal douches, sprays, or similar products. These disturb the chemical balance of the vagina, promote infections and change the composition of the mucus. Also be aware that if you use vaginal suppositories or creams for contraception, these also change the mucus. The method of analyzing cervical mucus is only practicable with a healthy vaginal environment. Therefore, if you have a vaginal inflammation, choose some other method of birth control: A condom is doubly useful because it also protects against cross-infection.

You can generally detect the cervical mucus at the vaginal opening. Don't try to detect it by placing a finger into the vagina: Since the vagina is usually moist, this makes a "reading" difficult. Record all your observations, along with basal temperature, on your chart.

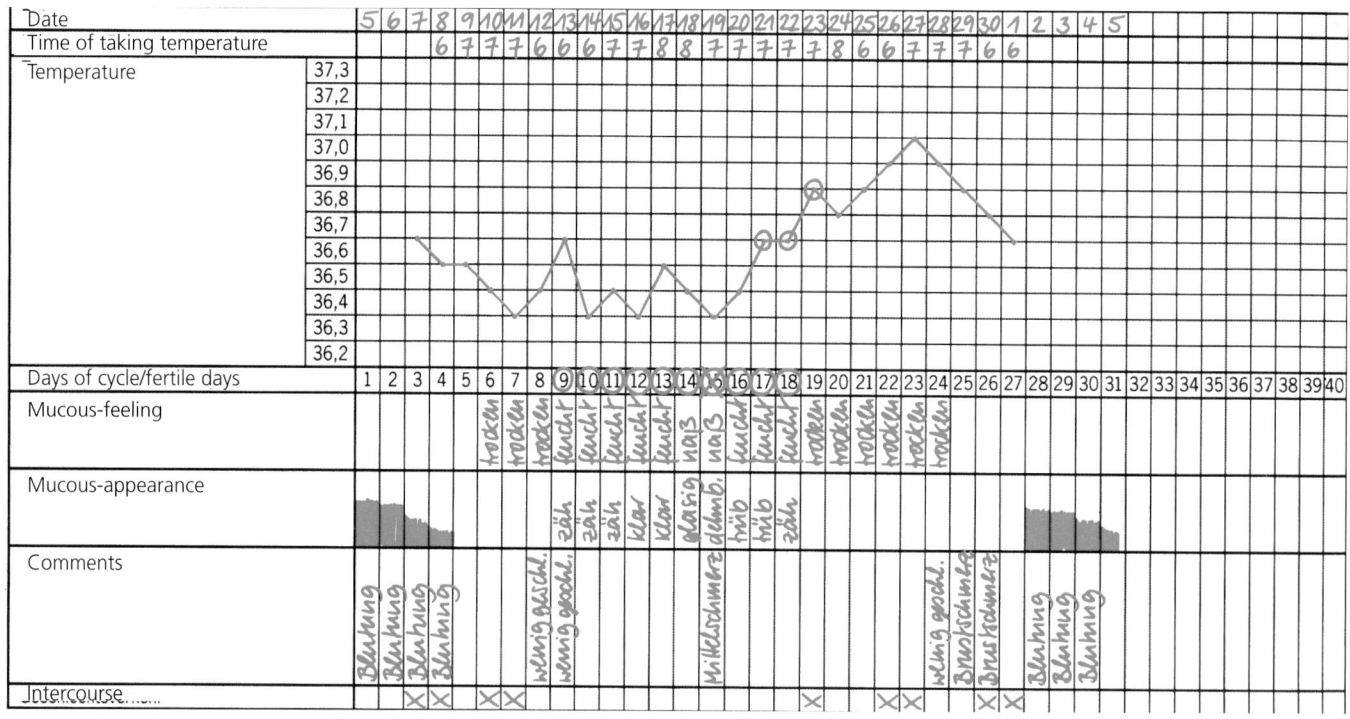

Things to pay attention to:

— A cycle begins on the first day of your period. Menstrual fluid hides mucus discharge, so for women with particularly long bleeding and very early ovulation, menstruation is not a safe time for unprotected sexual intercourse.

— After the end of menstruation there is a sensation of dryness around the vaginal opening; no discharge is evident. These are the days of lowest fertility. Sperm cannot survive the acidic vaginal environment in the absence of mucus.

— During ovulation, the cervix in most women creates so much mucus that it flows out and the vagina is covered with a thin, fluid film. In this environment, sperm can survive up to 72 hours, waiting for ovulation.

— The mucus is initially whitish or yellowish, sticky, lumpy or creamy; immediately before ovulation it usually becomes clearer and more liquid. Check its consistency by taking a bit between thumb and forefinger; if it's stringy, this indicates ovulation. On the day they ovulate, some women feel a pulling sensation in the abdomen.

— The fertile period begins with the cycle's first sign of moistness or mucus, and ends the evening of the fourth day after mucus production reaches its peak.

— The infertile phase begins at that point and lasts until the onset of menstruation. A few days after ovulation, most women experience the vagina as drier and/or the discharge as thicker. Menstruation begins at the latest 12 to 16 days after peak mucus production.

Only by combining basal-temperature measurements with observation of the amount and consistency of cervical mucus is reliable natural contraception possible. Its failure rate can be as low as that of the intrauterine device (IUD), if you leave a "safety interval" of seven days prior to your ovulation phase, determined over the course of several months.

CONDOMS

A condom is a sheath made of thin rubber or latex about 7 inches long, which is fitted onto the erect penis prior to sexual intercourse. Condoms are one of the few contraceptive devices that place responsibility on the male as well as the female partner. Some men resist condom use because they fear it will inhibit sexual

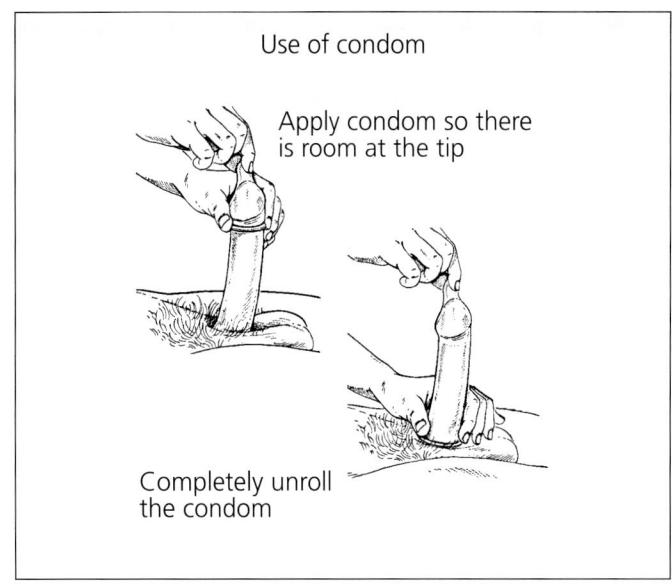

Use of condom

Apply condom so there is room at the tip

Completely unroll the condom

arousal; this will only occur, however, if applying the condom is thought of as an unwelcome interruption. As with so many other sexual issues, it's all in how you think about it. If you learn to include condom application in foreplay, it usually causes no difficulties whatsoever. Moreover, when combined with the natural family-planning method, condoms need not be used every time sexual intercourse takes place. Condoms are to date the sole effective protection against HIV and most other sexually transmitted diseases (STDs). Condoms are available in ready-to-use packs, and are cheap, easy to use, and almost completely free of side effects. Some are coated with lubricants that contain a spermicide, augmenting protection. Latex allergies or intolerance of the spermicide are very rare.

If used correctly, condoms are 96 to 97 percent reliable (Pearl index rating 3.3). The most common causes of accidents are putting the condom on too early, too late, or incompletely. The statistical (and needlessly high) failure rate, taking user error into account, is between 10 and 15 pregnancies per hundred users per year. To increase protection, condoms may be used in conjunction with contraceptive foams (see p. 555).

Things to pay attention to:

— The condom should be applied onto a fully erect penis, before the penis is inserted into the vagina, well before (not immediately preceding) ejaculation.

— The condom should be completely unrolled over the shaft of the penis. Leave some room at the tip to contain the semen, if the condom isn't already designed with a reservoir at the tip.

— When removing the penis from the vagina, hold the condom's rim to keep it on the penis and prevent semen from entering the vagina.
— After ejaculation and removal of the condom, the still-moist penis should not be placed anywhere near the vaginal opening.
— Use a new condom each time sexual intercourse occurs. Never reuse a condom.
— After use, it's advisable to check the condom for any damage. If a rip or hole is found, a "morning-after" pill can be used up to 72 hours after intercourse.
— Condoms are made of rubber and have a shelf life. After long or inappropriate storage (i.e. in heat or sunlight) they can become brittle and tear easily. Condoms packed in aluminum foil last longer. Buy only brand-name condoms, and check expiration dates.
— For lubrication, use only water-based creams. Oil-based products may affect the rubber and compromise its integrity, as may other contraceptives used simultaneously (e.g., foams), or medications against infections.

DIAPHRAGMS

A diaphragm consists of a rubber dome with a flexible rim, which is inserted so as to cover the cervix and prevent sperm in the vagina from entering the uterus. Before deciding to use a diaphragm, have a comprehensive professional consultation. The diaphragm must be individually fitted by an experienced gynecologist who should also instruct you on proper insertion and positioning. You can also get fitted for a diaphragm and receive information on its proper use at women's health centers and clinics.

Diaphragms are effective only when used in conjunction with spermicidal jelly or cream. They work well in conjunction with natural contraceptive methods; like them, diaphragm use requires a good knowledge of your own body.

When used properly, diaphragms very rarely cause side effects. If they are left in place for too long (over 12 hours), foul-smelling discharge or vaginal inflammations can develop. In some women, diaphragm use increases the incidence of bladder inflammations. Skin irritations or allergic reactions to certain creams or jellies are rare; if they occur, stop using the product and consult your doctor.

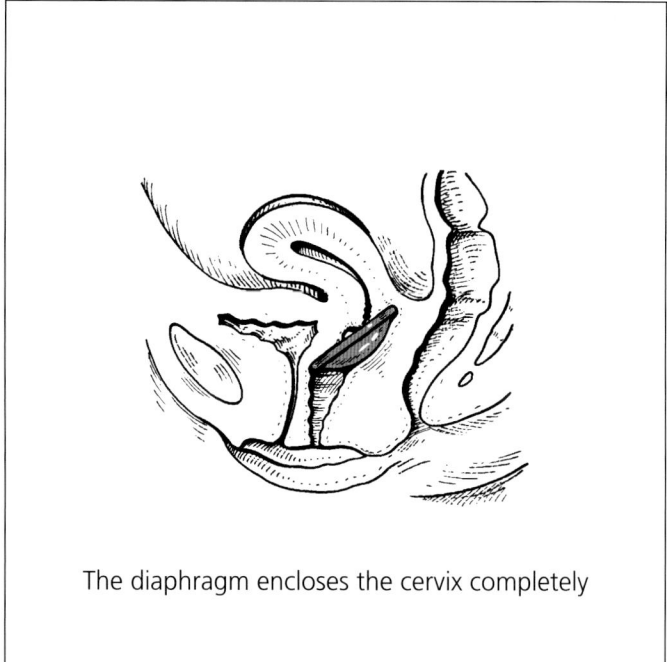

The diaphragm encloses the cervix completely

After childbirth or a gain or drop in body weight of more than seven to ten pounds, have your diaphragm checked; you may need to be fitted for a new one. Young girls whose sex organs are still growing and changing should have their diaphragms checked at least every 6 months. The diaphragm is endorsed by many women's groups because it does not interfere with hormonal balance, it promotes familiarity with one's own body, and with proper use it offers a relatively high success rate (in conjunction with contraceptive jelly, it has a Pearl index rating of 2 to 4).

Inserting a diaphragm is like inserting a tampon: Both get easier with practice. First, learn to locate and feel your cervix. Before you insert the diaphragm, apply about a teaspoonful of contraceptive jelly on the inside of the dome; then pinch the diaphragm between thumb and middle finger and insert it deep into the vagina along the vaginal walls, as far as possible. With your finger, push the leading edge of the diaphragm upwards so it's tucked behind your pubic bone. Check to make sure the cervix is completely covered.

Things to pay attention to:
— The diaphragm should not be inserted more than 6 hours before intercourse, lest spermicidal jellies and creams start to lose their effectiveness. The shorter the interval prior to intercourse, the better.
— You can insert your diaphragm prior to intercourse, or integrate it into lovemaking. Your partner can

also learn how to insert it properly.
— If intercourse is repeated, insert more jelly deep into the vagina using an applicator. Do not remove the diaphragm.
— The diaphragm should be removed no less than 8 and no more than 12 hours following intercourse.

SUPPOSITORIES, CREAMS, AND GELS

The most commonly used contraceptives are chemicals like foam suppositories. They must be inserted in the vagina at least 10 minutes prior to sexual intercourse. They release a sticky foam that blocks off the cervix, hinders sperm's ability to move, and also contains a spermicide.

Side effects consist primarily of skin irritations, allergies, and discomfort including burning or the sensation of heat. Women prone to vaginal infections should not use these products.

The reliability of foam suppositories is subject to interpretation; accordingly, their Pearl index rating ranges from 8 to 36. To be on the safe side, they should therefore be used only in combination with a diaphragm. The thin rubber of a condom can be compromised by the chemicals in foams or jellies (see Condoms, p. 553).

IUDS (INTRAUTERINE DEVICES)

The IUD is a very reliable method of birth control, although it interferes with physiological processes; its Pearl rating is 1 to 2.

Modern IUDs have little in common with the prototypes of the early 1960s. IUDs today are made of flexible synthetics wrapped in thin copper wire. They are inserted by a doctor into the uterus. A thread attached to the lower end reaches down into the vagina so the woman can check for herself that the IUD is still in place.

It is recommended that the position of the IUD be checked, using ultrasound, 2 weeks and then 3 months after insertion. Afterwards, checkups should be done semiannually. When the effectiveness of the copper starts to diminish, after 2 to 3 years, a new IUD must be inserted.

How Do IUDs Work?

How the IUD works is still not understood completely; it seems that the presence of copper in the uterine environment restricts the movement of sperm.

If an IUD wearer gets pregnant
— If a woman gets pregnant with an IUD in place, the risk of ectopic pregnancy increases 10 to 15 times. For this reason, and because of the possibility of inflammations and subsequent infertility, it is recommended that young women who have not borne children use some other form of contraception.
— If a normal pregnancy develops with an IUD in place, the IUD should be removed to avoid the danger of severe inflammation leading to miscarriage. Although removing the IUD can also cause miscarriage, if it remains in place the risk of miscarriage increases by a factor of 4.
— If the pregnancy proceeds normally in spite of the presence of an IUD, no fetal abnormalities need be expected .

In about 8 percent of women fitted with an IUD, the body quickly expels the device or it must be removed because of severe pain or other symptoms.

Signals of the body rejecting or poorly tolerating an IUD include painful, prolonged, or intensive bleeding, spotting, and inflammations in or around the uterus and fallopian tubes, possibly resulting in fertility problems.

Insertion of the IUD

A comprehensive gynecological exam should always precede insertion of an IUD. Most doctors will insert the IUD during the menstrual period, because at this

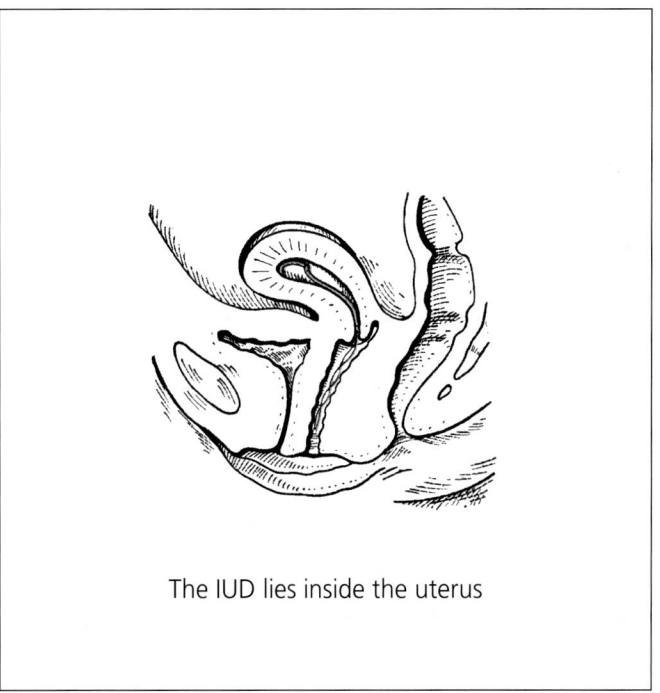

The IUD lies inside the uterus

time the uterine canal is wider, and it can be determined with certainty that the woman is not pregnant. Insertion may prove painful as the sensitive inside of the cervix becomes irritated and the muscles cramp in an effort to expel the foreign object. In rare instances, this can lead to injury or perforation of the uterus, in which case surgical intervention may be necessary. A local anesthetic during insertion is an option; having a friend or your partner present can help relax you.

ORAL CONTRACEPTIVES (BIRTH CONTROL PILLS)

Many women develop fatigue after long-term use of oral contraceptives, despite official doubts that a steady stream of hormones might have negative side effects.

In theory, the failure rate of the pill is nil; it prevents ovulation, making it the most dependable form of contraception. If a pregnancy does occur, it is attributed exclusively to human error.

Monophasic Pills

These pills consist of a predetermined combination of estrogen and progesterone, taken over the course of 21 days. The high estrogen level simulates a pregnancy and prevents the maturation of eggs in the ovaries, so that ovulation does not occur. In addition, the progesterone transforms the mucous plugs that block the cervix into a sticky fluid impenetrable to sperm.

Today, the estrogen levels in many single-phase pills are very low: They contain 0.02 to 0.035 mg of ethinyl estradiol. These micropills are as reliable as pills with higher doses, but generally cause fewer side effects.

After 21 days the pill is discontinued for one week; the sudden drop in estrogen and progesterone levels causes the uterine lining to be expelled, and bleeding begins.

Although most people are unaware of the fact, this pill-induced bleeding is not the natural menstrual cycle kicking in; rather, it is artificially caused by hormone withdrawal. The 28-day cycle was adopted for purely psychological reasons, to make it seem as natural as possible. If pill use were to continue uninterrupted, irregular, severe, and/or prolonged bleeding might occur as the expanded uterine lining breaks down because the hormones are unable to keep it sufficiently supplied with nutrients.

There may be a risk of blood clots (thrombosis) associated with certain monophasic pills.

Biphasic Pills

These pills are designed to simulate a natural 28-day cycle. They function similarly to monophasic pills but contain only estrogen in the first phase, and a combination of estrogen and progesterone in the second. To ensure effectiveness, they contain relatively high levels of estrogen. They must be taken in the prescribed order and are available in 21- and 28-day packages.

Triphasic Pills

Usually these consist of usually three phases, with estrogen levels about equivalent to that of monophasic pills. Progesterone and estrogen are taken simultaneously, but their ratio varies from phase to phase.

Triphasic pills try to emulate the natural 28-day cycle. They are as reliable as monophasic pills (Pearl index rating: 0.1 to 0.9); however, following the prescribed sequence is critical. Spotting is occasionally present.

Progestin-only Tablets (Minipill)

The minipill contains only progesterone, which renders the mucus in the cervical canal impenetrable to sperm.

The minipill usually doesn't suppress ovulation. At first, the cycle proceeds as usual. After long-term use, however, the cycle may change, with bleeding lessening or stopping altogether. Long-term spotting may also occur.

It is essential that the minipill be taken regularly at the same time each day; there is only a three-hour maximum grace period. The pills are identical and come in packages of 35. Minipills must be taken without interruption starting the first day of the period.

Even with optimal use, the minipill has a failure rate of 0.5 to 4. Because it contains no estrogen, it is appropriate for nursing mothers (the estrogen in other kinds of birth control pills may hinder lactation).

Aside from possible bleeding irregularities, minipills have far fewer side effects than other birth control pills, particularly those that affect the blood vessels (see Risks Associated with The Pill, p. 557). This is why they are also appropriate for diabetics (see Diabetes, p. 483).

Medroxyprogesterone (Depo-Provera), The 3-Month Injection

This method of birth control involves an injection of large amounts of time-release progestin every 3 months. It can cause menstrual disorders that last even after the injections are discontinued. The suspicion that it can cause cancer has not been proved. However, bleeding disorders are a relatively common consequence.

"The Morning-After Pill"

These pills contain relatively high doses of estrogen and progesterone and are indicated in emergencies only, following unprotected sex during a woman's fertile period. They must be taken within 72 hours of intercourse.

The large dose of hormones usually leads to nausea, vomiting, breast tenderness, and irregular bleeding.

Risks Associated with the Pill

Women with high blood pressure or heart disease who take oral contraceptives are at greater risk of blood clots, heart attack, and stroke. If they are also smokers, the risk of heart disease and vascular disorders rises significantly; the increase is due to the effects of nicotine.

Further side effects include liver damage, especially in women who have already had jaundice, as well as changes in skin color, migraines, nausea, nervousness, depression, breast pain, weight gain, changes in sexuality, spotting, and vaginal fungal infections.

Contradictory studies show higher risks of breast and cervical cancer on the one hand, and suggest on the other that higher doses and long-term pill therapy may protect against ovarian and uterine cancer.

Under no circumstances should you take the pill
— If you are pregnant
— If you have a vascular disorder
— After a heart attack
— After a stroke
— If you have high blood pressure (defined as higher than 160/95)
— If you have diabetes
— If you are a smoker over 35
— If you have severe liver or gallbladder disease
— If you have a hormone-dependent tumor (such as breast cancer)

You should take the pill only with caution and under careful supervision
— If you smoke
— If you have pronounced varicose veins,
— If you are epileptic
— If you suffer from migraines
— If you have mildly elevated blood pressure
— If you have high cholesterol
— If immediate family members under age 40 develop thrombosis, lung embolism, or heart attack
— If you are prone to vaginal infections (e.g., fungi),
— If you are immobilized over the long term (e.g., in you are wheelchair-bound)

Discontinue pill use immediately
— If blood clots appear (swelling, leg pains)
— If blood pressure rises sharply
— If visual disturbances occur
— If you become pregnant
— Prior to major surgery or leg operations
— In the presence of jaundice
— In the presence of severe circulatory disorders (e.g., angina pectoris, infarction)
— In the presence of severe migraine

Basically, every woman who takes oral contraceptives should undergo regular checkups of liver and kidney function, blood pressure, blood-sugar level as well as half-year gynecological checkups and early screening with Pap smears.

Severe side effects are rare with the widely prescribed "minipills"—except for the possible elevated risk of thrombosis carried by certain products (see Monophasic Pills, p. 556). The health risks posed by pregnancy and childbirth, or abortion, are greater than those posed by the pill. If there are no risks or contraindications, the pill can be taken up to menopause.

Advantages of the Pill
— Lighter menstrual bleeding, less menstrual discomfort, and a regular cycle
— Reduced frequency of ovarian cysts
— Lessening of premenstrual syndrome
— Positive effects on acne, hair loss, and endometriosis

Frequently Asked Questions

What If I Miss a Day?

Take the pill as soon as you realize you missed a day, and take the next pill at the usual time, even if it means taking two pills in one day. If the interval between two pills is greater than 36 hours, you can no longer count on complete protection. In order to be certain of full protection, use an additional form of birth control till your next menstrual period.

Important: When taking the minipill, the grace period must not exceed 3 hours.

When Am I Protected?

If you start taking the pill on the first day of your period, you can count on complete protection. If you start after that, it's a good idea to use an additional method of contraception.

You should also use an additional method if you
— Have diarrhea
— Vomit up to four hours after taking the pill
— Take certain medications (e.g., certain antibiotics, medications for epilepsy or tuberculosis)

What If I Want to Get Pregnant?

Even after long-term use of the pill, fertility is normally not affected. If you want to get pregnant, stop taking the pill at least 3 months before your target conception date; use other forms of contraception in the interim. This way, your body has enough time to return to its natural hormone balance.

STERILIZATION

Sterilization is a definitive method of contraception, appropriate for both men and women. It is nonreversible, or only possibly reversible by means of a complex operation. The statistical failure rate of sterilization is between one and two cases per thousand procedures.

Tubal Ligation

The most common form of sterilization is endoscopic sterilization: With laparoscopy (see p. 653), the fallopian tubes are cauterized and often removed. This is usually done under general anesthesia in the hospital or on an outpatient basis.

In the past, an incision was made in the abdomen, the fallopian tubes were removed and both ends tied off and tucked into the surrounding tissue. These days, this procedure is usually done only in conjunction with a cesarean section, when the abdomen is already opened.

Complications

Unlike a vasectomy, sterilization in a woman is a more involved operation.

Possible complications include
— Fallopian pregnancies (rare)
— Heavier (10 to 40 percent) and more irregular menstrual bleeding than before, as well as intensified menstrual symptoms (20 to 30 percent)

The cause of the increased bleeding is a matter of debate. Occasionally, isolating the ovaries affects circulation to that area, rendering hormone production weaker and more irregular. If the woman has difficulties coming to terms with her infertility after surgery, this can also affect menstruation.

Vasectomy

The removal of the vas deferens is called vasectomy and is usually performed in the doctor's office in a brief, half-hour operation on an outpatient basis and under local anesthesia. The doctor makes 2-inch-long incisions in the back of the scrotum, clips two small pieces out of each vas and ties off the severed ends with stitches. The patient can go home after a couple of hours.

After several weeks, the patient is tested to ensure his semen is not potent.

Complications

Minor pain, localized bleeding, or mild inflammations may occur.

Side Effects

The functional capacity of the sex organs is unchanged. The testes produce the same amount of male sex hormones and sperm as before; the sperm reach the epididymis, where they ripen; but instead of going into the ejaculate, the mature sperm cells go into the dead ends of the vas deferens, where they are reabsorbed into the tissue.

The volume of ejaculate diminishes by about 10 percent—the amount formerly comprised of the sperm. The smell, taste and appearance of the ejaculate remain unchanged.

Virility is not affected by the physical results of vasectomy. Infrequently, however, sadness over the loss of reproductive capacity may cause temporary psychological problems.

Infertility

Nowadays, it's no longer possible simply to decide to have children—or leave the decision to chance—and be reasonably sure of conceiving. In the past 35 years, the number of people unable to have children has more than doubled. At the start of the 1960s only 8 percent of young couples wanting children were childless; today, this applies to 17 percent.

A diagnosis of infertility can set off a profound life crisis—even in women and men whose lifestyle and identities haven't necessarily been geared toward parenthood. A couple is defined as infertile if they have not conceived after 1 to 2 years of regular, unprotected sexual intercourse.

CAUSES OF INFERTILITY

Research has to date not yet found an explanation for the increasing infertility rate. It is, however, known that toxins, increasing environmental hazards, and psychosocial problems affect reproductive capacity, including conception and development of the embryo. A third of infertility cases are due to the fact that more people are planning children later, after achieving career goals. Infertility increases with age.

Workplace Factors

Environmental toxins may have a detrimental effect on fertility. One indication of this is the number of cases in certain professions. Men and women who work in the following fields are more frequently infertile than others (see Health in the Workplace, p. 789) and women in these fields are at increased risk of miscarriage:

— Agricultural and vineyard laborers, forest industry workers, and florists who work with herbicides and insecticides
— Laboratory and chemical industry workers
— Anesthesiologists and palliative care workers
— Health-care and medical personnel in oncology wards who handle cancer treatments without sufficient protection
— Dental employees
— Textile and leather-industry workers
— Artists and house painters
— People who handle lead or copper

Environmental Factors

Chlorinated hydrocarbons, which are found everywhere in the human environment (see p. 774), can definitely kill sperm. Heavy metals such as mercury (possibly also from amalgam dental fillings), cadmium, and lead, as well as insecticides and herbicides all increase the risk. Ionizing radiation can damage the gonads of both sexes (see X Rays, p. 646).

Environmental toxins are also toxic to the fetus. Scientists believe they cause 20 to 30 percent of all miscarriages. Studies of premature deliveries have revealed the presence of lindane, dichlorodipheryltrichloroethane (DDT) and polychlorinatedbiphenyls (PCB)—all chlorinated hydrocarbons—in the blood of both mother and fetus (see Substances that Compromise Fertility, p. 560).

Stress Factors

In one out of every six couples seeking professional treatment for infertility, the cause is diagnosed as psychological factors, and the condition is usually temporary. Not infrequently, sex is hindered by such disorders as premature ejaculation or difficulties with arousal or orgasm. Sexual disorders may also be the end result of unaddressed, repeatedly unsatisfying sexual relations; breaking the cycle of noncommunication and resentment will often clear up the disorder.

Stress can have a direct or indirect impact on the delicate balance of hormones regulating sexual function. Career pressures, excessive physical stress, medication, consumption of caffeine, nicotine, and alcohol—even the unfulfilled desire for a child—can all create stress. Exhaustion or the pressure to succeed with fertility treatment can dispel sexual desire; relationship conflicts or unconscious rejection of the idea of pregnancy can have contraceptive effects.

The negative effects of a rigid desire to have a child at any price cannot be underestimated. Follow-up studies have shown that many women end up becoming pregnant without medical help when, after failed attempts at artificial fertilization, they finally give up trying to get pregnant and come to terms with being childless. The decision to adopt can have a similar effect. Lifting the pressure to conceive often bears more fruit than medical intervention.

Some Substances that may Compromise Fertility in Men (M) and Women (W)

Ethyl alcohol	M
Cadmium	M
Sulfur dioxide	M/W
DDT	W
Ethylene bromide	M/W
Ethylene oxide	M/W
Lead	M/W
Mercury	M/W
Bromated biphenyls	W
Polychlorinated biphenyls (PCB)	W
Toluene	W
Vinyl chloride	M/W

THE INFERTILE COUPLE

Infertility is present in equal proportions in both sexes. In one out of three infertile couples, no medical cause can be found. While a couple's fertility depends on the potential of both partners, and decreased fertility in one might be compensated for by high fertility in the other, fertility cannot be predicted in individual cases. Depending on the circumstances, both partners might well be fertile with another partner; women also occasionally develop antibodies to their partner's sperm.

If a couple is unable to conceive, both partners should be tested, preferably at a clinic specializing in fertility issues. This can shorten testing and treatment time and cut down on stress, both physical and psychological.

Fertility treatment involves 3 to 6 months of daily temperature checks for the woman and a large proportion of time spent on tests, examinations, and procedures. Having sex on command—at a specific time on specific days—can put a damper on the experience, and living with the constant hope and expectation of conceiving can lead to problems between partners.

MALE INFERTILITY

Infertility in men may be congenital or acquired, permanent or temporary. Because sperm take 3 months to develop, disorders usually take that long to manifest, as does the process of reversing the disorder.

The most important criterion for fertility is the number of healthy and sufficiently motile sperm in the ejaculate. If the sperm count is low, this diminishes the odds of one or more sperm overcoming the obstacles nature places in its way: the mucous cervical plug, the uterine environment, and the outer layer of the egg.

Causes

The medical cause of infertility remains unknown in about 30 percent of men seeking medical help. There can be multiple reasons for infertility.

Relationship problems can play a major role, though these often remain unconscious. Not infrequently, an unacknowledged rejection of pregnancy, children, or fatherhood underlie reproductive problems.

Congenital Disorders

These are rare. They include

— Undescended testicle, if not treated successfully: In about 5 percent of newborn boys, the testes have

What to Do If Nothing Seems to Work

For both partners:

— Avoid medications that may impair fertility (see above); limit cigarette and alcohol consumption.

— Have sex every 3 days, if possible, especially during the period of peak fertility (see Contraception, p. 551). Shorter intervals reduce the chances of success because of lowered concentration of sperm in the ejaculate. After intercourse, the woman should stay on her back for 10 minutes (optimally, with a cushion under her pelvis).

— Take time for yourself and for each other; try to make your lives less hectic and stressed.

— Better yet, take a vacation. Get away by yourselves for a while, cut loose and just enjoy each other.

— Learn relaxation techniques (see p. 693).

— Massages (see p. 686) and hot compresses (see p. 692) are relaxing; think of them as giving yourself a treat, not as "going for treatment."

— Keep physically fit with a balanced, nonstrenuous exercise regimen (see p. 765).

— Perhaps a change in eating habits is long overdue: A balanced diet with lots of fresh vegetables and fruit can make a big difference in your overall energy level (see p. 723).

For the woman:

— If you're always dieting or trying to starve yourself into a perfect figure, stop now. Dieting can disrupt the hormone cycle. Eat moderate amounts of a variety of nutritious foods.

For the man:

— Wear loose, roomy pants and undershorts, made of natural fibers. Don't sleep under a down quilt and avoid trips to the sauna and spa: Excessive heat causes a drop in sperm quality that can take 3 to 6 months to reverse.

not descended into the scrotum (see Undescended Testis, p. 593).

— Klinefelter's syndrome: in addition to the X and Y chromosome which determine male gender, an extra X chromosome is present in the genes.

Acquired Disorders

These comprise disorders caused by developmental or infectious factors, and include:

— Loss of sex hormone function prior to or during puberty.
— Orchitis due to mumps, syphilis or injury, which can impair sperm production even after recovery (see p. 531).
— Epididymitis (see p. 532).
— Prostatitis (see p. 534).
— Urethritis (see p. 530) can block the seminal ducts, causing problems with urination and aberrations of the immune system: If semen appears outside the normal channels, antigens to the body's own sperm are produced. Antibodies are found in one in three infertile men.
— Chlamydial and ureaplasmal infections (see p. 546). The connection with diminished sperm quality is not precisely known, but such infections are common among infertile men. STDs can damage the seminal ducts through adhesions or scar tissue.
— Varicoceles and insufficient emptying of the blood vessel of the scrotum, which keeps the testicles warmer than they should be for optimal sperm function.
— Chronic anemia (see p. 345).
— Diabetes.
— Male hormone deficiency (extremely rare).

External Causes

External causes account for 10 percent of infertility problems (usually, inhibited sperm production). These include
— Anxiety, work-related pressures, relationship problems, psychological stress from worrying about infertility
— Excessively tight pants, which create an overly warm, damp environment; saunas and very warm bedding should be avoided for the same reason
— Excessive alcohol consumption
— Heavy smoking

Medications that May Inhibit Sperm Production

— Ulcer medications with cimetidine (Tagamet) and ranitidine (Zantac).
— Sulfasalazine, used in treating ulcerative colitis and rheumatoid arthritis.
— Medications for urinary tract infections containing nitrofurantoin and trimethoprim.
— Cancer medications (methotrexate, cyclophosphamide) taken for longer than 6 months.
— Antipsychotic medication (see box on Neuroleptics, p. 202).
— The epilepsy drugs phenytoin (Dilantin) and carbamazepine (Tegretol).
— Beta-blockers (especially propanolol) taken for highblood pressure, migraines, circulatory and heart rhythm disorders, and as a sedative.
— Nontopical (ingested) corticosteroids.
— All anabolic steroids that promote physical endurance, strength and performance, especially those used in bodybuilding. Other hormones such as estrogen, progesterone, androgen, and antiandrogens also affect sperm production.

— Hair growth treatments containing cadmium or estradiol
— Medications that partly or completely inhibit sperm production (see box)
— Damage from X rays (see p. 646)
— Shock or trauma
— Undernourishment
— Extremes of altitude or depth (pilots, mountain climbers, deep-sea divers)

Necessary Tests

— Discussion of your sex life with your partner, medical history (infectious diseases, surgery, diabetes, nervous disorders), cigarette smoking, alcohol, and drug abuse
— Examination of sex organs
— Sperm count, taken 4 to 6 days after the last ejaculation; this must be performed twice, since results can vary considerably
— Hormone testing, if sperm count is below five million
— Biopsy of testicle tissue, if sperm-duct blockage is suspected
— Microscopic analysis of hair follicles or cells from the oral mucosa, if chromosomal anomalies are suspected

Treatment
— Surgery for varicocele (see p. 532)
— Antibiotics for acute or chronic infection
— Hormone-replacement therapy for a demonstrable deficiency
— Corticosteroids or immunosuppressants if antibodies are present; but often these techniques are not successful
— Microsurgery to open blocked seminal ducts

Sperm Stimulation
In mild to moderate cases of low sperm count or poor sperm motility, acupuncture may prove effective in stimulating the sperm: After 10 half-hour sessions, sperm quality usually improves.
 Other, less successful efforts at stimulation include:
— Hormones (antiestrogens, gonadotropins, androgens)
— Tissue hormones and enzymes to stimulate semen production in the gonad
— Pentoxifylline to stimulate circulation

FEMALE INFERTILITY
Statistically, the principal causes of infertility in women break down more or less as follows:
— In 45 percent of cases, the complex hormonal regulation of the ovaries is disturbed (see Menstrual Disorders, p. 508). This can result in the egg not ripening, not being released, or not attaching to the uterine lining after fertilization
— In 35 percent, blocked or insufficiently flexible fallopian tubes are responsible
— 5 percent of cases are due to cervical problems
— 15 percent are due to other causes

Causes
Hormonal disturbances because of
— Under- or overproduction of hormones other than sex hormones, such as hypo- or hyperthyroidism, liver or kidney disease, diseases of the adrenal cortex, tuberculosis; overproduction of male sex hormones or of prolactin, the hormone that regulates milk production
— Obesity
— Underweight, weight loss diets, poor nutrition
— Medications, especially antipsychotics and all hormone therapy. (After discontinuing use of birth control pills, the hormone cycle needs to stabilize.)
— Alcohol or tobacco abuse
— Stress or agitation

Blocked Fallopian Tubes
— Fallopian tubes may be blocked by adhesions as a result of past inflammations, STDs (see Chlamydial and Ureaplasmal Infections, p. 546), endometriosis (see p. 522), or surgery (e.g., an appendectomy or ovarian cyst operation).
— The fallopian tube may rupture after an ectopic pregnancy, or after surgery to restore fertility.
— Adhesions of the abdominal tissue can result in the fallopian tubes' inability to "catch" the ripened ovum.

Cervical Problems
— The cervix may be too narrow or produce too little mucus.
— The cervical mucus may be infected.
— The vaginal mucosa may be too acidic.
— The cervical mucus may contain antibodies to sperm.

Necessary Tests
— As with men, an initial examination should include discussion of sex life and relationship, medical history, evidence of fertility problems in the family, general or childhood illnesses.
— The gynecological exam should include smears of vaginal secretions, to determine if any infections are present.
— In the event of irregular menstruation, blood serum hormone levels should be checked for abnormalities. Usually several blood tests are necessary.
— Basal temperature measurements (see Natural Contraception, p. 551) should be taken for three complete cycles. A comparison of the temperature curve with results of hormone tests will determine further courses of treatment.
— At this point, a sperm motility test is usually performed to determine whether enough viable sperm are making it into the cervical mucus. If no (or too few) normal sperm are found, this may indicate either low sperm quality, or low penetrability of the cervical mucus. This test must be performed several hours after intercourse. Your physician will advise you when during your cycle to have sex, and you must not have intercourse for 5 days prior to the test.

— If there is reason to suspect that the cervical mucus and semen are incompatible, a laboratory test is performed exposing the mucus to sperm from another donor.

— Using laparoscopy (see p. 653) and dye, the fallopian tubes can be checked for blockages. An additional scope can check the uterus for fibroids or polyps. Small adhesions or cysts or mild endometriosis can be removed during this process. The surgery is performed under general anesthesia on an outpatient or inpatient basis.

— The viability of fallopian tubes can also be checked by ultrasound, using a special contrast medium. No anesthesia is necessary for this procedure.

— These tests should be performed before the tenth day of the menstrual cycle, since they may be sufficient to dislodge adhesions and thus promote pregnancy without further treatment.

Treatment

— Infections are treated with antibiotics.

— In the rare cases of incompatibility between sperm and cervical mucus, there are no effective treatment options. Impenetrable cervical mucus plugs can be bypassed by artificial insemination.

— In the case of hormonal imbalance, different approaches can help eggs ripen or correct the hormone balance. In many cases, hormone or drug therapy can set the stage for natural conception. Diagnosis and treatment may take months, however, and can be very stressful for this reason. In some cases, adhering to a strict schedule may require taking time off from work.

— Blocked fallopian tubes can be corrected through microsurgery in about 50 to 60 percent of cases. The risk of a resultant tubal pregnancy is about 10 percent. A procedure involving pumping carbon dioxide through the tubes to unblock them is only rarely successful.

— In the case of severe adhesions, surgery should not be considered. The danger of a tubal pregnancy following such an operation, necessitating complete removal of the fallopian tubes, is too great. Attempts to transplant fallopian tubes or implant artificial tubes have not been very successful to date.

— If the fallopian tubes cannot be made passable, there is only one option for conception: Egg and sperm

must be obtained separately, at which point one of the following procedures can take place:

— Gamete transfer, in which egg and sperm are inserted into the fallopian tubes together. This method is usually more successful than in vitro fertilization (IVF) but it carries a high risk of tubal pregnancy

— IVF, in which the egg is fertilized in a test tube and the embryo implanted in the uterus (see In Vitro Fertilization and Embryo Transfer, below).

ARTIFICIAL FERTILIZATION

If the abovementioned individual treatments for men and women prove fruitless, the last resort is artificial fertilization or IVF. Taking this step should be carefully considered in light of the associated psychological and physical stresses and potential legal issues.

Insemination

For artificial insemination, the male partner produces semen by masturbating. If necessary, the sperm are "activated" (see Sperm Stimulation, p. 562).

The semen is then injected into a cap which is placed on the cervix at peak fertility. In case of cervical problems, or if the sperm is of low quality, injecting the semen directly into the cervix is more successful. One to 2 out of every 4 couples routinely conceives by way of this procedure.

Fertilization with the partner's semen is known as homologous insemination. If the partner is infertile, heterological insemination, using donor sperm, is an option. Donor semen is routinely tested for infectious diseases (human immunodeficiency virus [HIV], hepatitis); but some risk remains. The semen is deep-frozen and collected in sperm banks. After thawing, the sperm are completely viable but 30 to 50 percent less motile than nonfrozen sperm, lowering their success rate.

In Vitro (Test Tube) Fertilization (IVF) and Embryo Transfer

This technology is considerably less successful and far riskier than generally believed. Its advent has given rise to profound ethical dilemmas involving issues like human genetic engineering. Despite the fact that trafficking in eggs and embryos is illegal, and despite protestations from the medical community, the technology is abused for such industries as egg harvesting and surrogate mothering. The social repercussions of

IVF and its psychological effect on parents, surrogates and children are not yet fully known.

Medical Indications

These procedures are prescribed in instances of irreparable damage to both fallopian tubes, immunologically caused infertility, and fallopian tube disorders due to endometriosis.

If the female partner is over 40 or the male partner's sperm count and motility are very low, IVF is not recommended because of the low chances of success.

The conception rate per treatment cycle is about 19.5 precent if more attempts are made, the rate rises. However, since about a third of IVF pregnancies end prematurely in miscarriage, only about 12 percent of such pregnancies actually result in successful births.

Preparation and Egg Extraction

In a normal cycle, only one egg follicle is produced, but the ovaries can be overstimulated with a combination of different hormones, causing several follicles to produce eggs to be harvested for test-tube fertilization.

Depending on the position of the ovaries, the eggs are extracted either through the vagina or through the abdominal wall using laparoscopy (see p. 653).

Sperm Extraction

Only half of the males in couples participating in test-tube fertilization have normal sperm quality. In cases of extremely poor sperm quality, a technique known as intracytoplasmatic sperm injection is used: Using a microscopic glass pipette, a single sperm is injected directly into an egg. The pregnancy rate with this procedure is 13 percent, with a miscarriage rate of 37 percent. If the ejaculate contains no sperm whatsoever, fertilization may be attempted through extracting sperm cells directly from the epididymis.

Fertilization and Embryo Transfer

Egg and sperm are combined in a petri dish. Normally, fertilization occurs within 18 hours. The egg undergoes its first cell division about 20 to 30 hours after fertilization; after about 48 hours, it is implanted into the uterus through the cervix, via a soft plastic tube.

A test-tube embryo has a 1 in 10 chance of developing into a normal fetus. If the IVF is successful, multiple pregnancies are common. With this technique, the risk of an extrauterine pregnancy is about 5 percent.

Legal Issues

IVF technology has made it possible for a child to have up to six theoretical parents: One "mother" who donates the egg, another who carries it to term, and a third who raises the child; one "father" who donates sperm; a fifth parent who helps raise the child, and a sixth parent—the doctor—who helped the child into existence. (And, in certain cases, not one of the fathers pays child support.)

In separating sex from procreation, artificial fertilization has given rise to unforeseen and dubious possibilities: A woman can now bear a genetically alien child, and a grandmother can give birth to her own grandchild.

The legal questions raised by this technology are so difficult to answer that despite existing laws and guidelines, they are far from resolved. The objective of the legal considerations thus far has been to determine "ownership": to whom does the child "belong"? Who is responsible for his or her support? Whose heir is he or she? To whom do excess semen, eggs, or embryos belong?

Psychological Consequences for Parents and Child

The few existing long-term studies on artificial fertilization suggest that emotional stress is consistently present prior to such treatment, that it intensifies during the treatment, and that it continues to be present thereafter.

A huge time commitment for diagnosis and therapy with dubious chances of success; possible depression due to failure or the side effects of drugs; mounting fears of complications if a pregnancy does take place—these are only a few of the most common stress factors. Half of all couples remain childless despite all attempts to conceive; 85 to 90 percent of those attempting test-tube fertilization remain childless. All must cope with the psychological fallout.

PREGNANCY AND BIRTH

As a woman, your body is perfectly suited for pregnancy and birth, and these are natural experiences in your life. This fact, however, is often ignored by modern obstetrics, which prefers to see pregnancy as a "disease" and delivery as a "risk" to be dealt with using the full arsenal of modern technology. And although the World Health Organization (WHO) has long issued recommendations contradicting procedures common in most modern hospitals, the majority of births in industrialized countries continue to be electronically monitored and involve anesthesia and surgery—most of it medically superfluous, since more than 80 percent of all deliveries do not require intervention.

A normal pregnancy lasts 10 lunar months, or 280 days, or 40 weeks—give or take a couple. During this time, you will gradually get used to the new presence in your life; usually, the experience is accompanied by emotional highs and lows alternating between joy and misgivings, serenity and anxiety. This is also a time of receiving well-intentioned advice from family and friends, which may actually cause more harm than good: Nearly all preconceptions surrounding pregnancy are false. Contrary to popular belief, you won't have a miscarriage if you take a hot bath, nor will the umbilical cord become twisted if you do a lot of stretching, nor will a shock during pregnancy lead to a baby with deformities, nor will a passionate love life harm your baby. To the contrary, "relaxed mother = relaxed baby" is the equation for the well-being of your unborn child. Trust your body and feelings, and try to follow their requirements as much as possible; you'll stand the best chance of a pleasant pregnancy.

FIRST TRIMESTER (WEEK 1–12)

A pregnancy can be confirmed as early as 1 week after conception with a urine test that checks for traces of the hormone human chorionic gonadotropin (HGC). It takes a week until the ovum has implanted in the uterine wall. You can also simply wait for your period not to come. If you discover you are pregnant and have recently drunk alcohol or taken medication, there is no cause for concern. Damaged egg cells have little chance of survival and usually won't even succeed in implanting in the uterus. If you lose the baby within the first 3 months, you can simply conclude that it wasn't viable; excessive caution isn't necessary during this time unless your body is sending alarm signals. In any case, however, once you know you're pregnant, you should quit smoking and stop drinking alcohol. If you take medication, ask your doctor whether it poses a risk to the fetus.

Physical and Emotional Changes

The first trimester of pregnancy is a period of intensive changes. The ovaries, and later the placenta, produce hormones that affect your entire organism. Blood flow to the skin increases; breasts become larger; internal organs operate more efficiently. This process of transformation can tire you out; you may experience nausea and vomiting, especially in the morning. Although your belly probably doesn't look pregnant yet, your overall weight may increase by up to 5 pounds, because you are retaining water or are craving and eating high-calorie foods.

The awareness of another life growing inside you may make you more alert and sensitive, and irritable at times. If the pregnancy is unplanned, you need to establish whether or not you want to bring it to term. Even if the pregnancy is the realization of a long-held dream, life might get a little overwhelming for a time—between the realization that there's no going back, the dawning of new responsibility, and any financial and/or career concerns.

Development of the Baby

During the first week, the fertilized egg divides repeatedly, travels down the fallopian tube to the uterus, and lodges as a clump of cells in the uterine mucous mem-

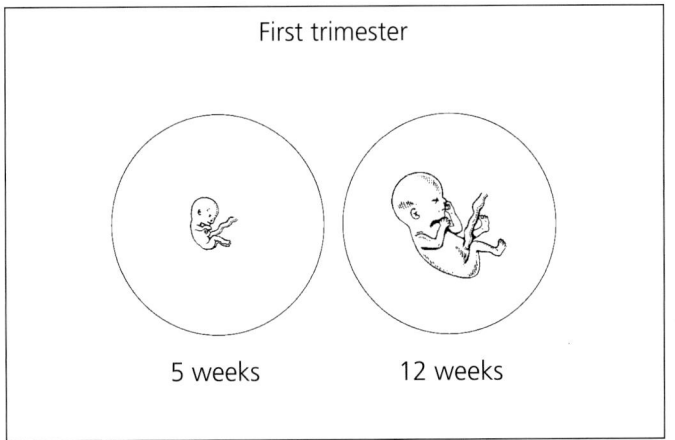

First trimester

5 weeks   12 weeks

brane; the embryo, placenta and umbilical cord all develop out of it. Enclosed in the fetal membrane, the embryo and umbilical cord float in amniotic fluid. After the third week, the organs begin to develop. In the fifth week the central nervous system (brain and spine) starts to develop, as does the head with eyes and mouth, and the digestive system. The heart begins to beat, the arm buds appear followed by the leg buds, and the skeleton develops. In the eighth week, arms with distinct hands, facial contours, ears, and airways develop. In the ninth to tenth week, testes or ovaries start to develop; the flexible skeleton begins to ossify. At the end of the third month the embryo is about 3 to 4 inches in length.

Examinations and Tests

At your first visit, the doctor can determine how advanced the pregnancy is by the size of the uterus. If the evidence doesn't correspond to your calculations of the date of your last period or of conception, an ultrasound exam is recommended (see Ultrasound, p. 516, 570, 651). A precise medical history is taken and a gynecological exam performed, including an internal exam, a Pap smear, and a microscopic analysis of vaginal secretions. The pelvis is measured to establish whether a vaginal birth is feasible.

Laboratory analysis determines your blood type, Rh factor, and blood count. Your blood is also screened for antibodies against rubella, syphilis, human immuno-deficiency virus and hepatitis, and toxoplasmosis if risk is determined (see Blood Tests, p. 636). Your general practitioner should also check your overall condition.

SECOND TRIMESTER (WEEK 13–26)

For many women, the second trimester is the easiest part of pregnancy. The upheaval of the first few months is over, you've settled in, and the pregnancy isn't cramping your style yet. If you're feeling fine, there's no need to make major adjustments; but remember to take seriously any body signals such as exhaustion, sluggishness, aches or pains, and respond to them as soon as possible.

Physical and Emotional Changes

The baby feels more and more "real." Between the 16th and 23rd week you'll notice its first movements. Morning sickness is usually past, and your body is noticeably rounder. It doesn't matter whether you've gained 7

pounds or 12: As long as you feel well and your weight gain isn't unhealthy (see Preeclampsia, p. 574), you shouldn't let the weight charts terrorize you. The latest WHO guidelines recommend that doctors not monitor the weight of expectant mothers since this often leads to undue distress. Light swelling in the hands, lower legs and feet from water retention is normal. If you tend toward vascular weakness, blood may collect in the lower part of your body, causing varicose veins and hemorrhoids. The intestine may also become sluggish (see Complaints During Pregnancy, p. 570).

In midpregnancy, many women feel fine, with only this or that minor complaint. However, you may also find your swelling belly and voluptuous shape hard to accept, since they don't match today's narrow standards of beauty. Talk this over with your partner or other pregnant women. Many support groups and courses offer relaxation techniques specially tailored for expectant mothers.

Development of the Baby

Your baby is now developing its muscles—kicking its legs, flexing its toes, opening and closing its hands, moving its head. By the fourth month the principal reflexes are present. During this period, the senses of taste and touch begin to develop and, from the fifth month on, the sense of hearing and balance (the vestibular system). The sense of sight is already so developed that the baby can distinguish between light and dark. It practices breathing and swallowing, and can already react to its environment, changing position if it's uncomfortable. At the end of 5 months you may feel the baby move for the first time: A slight tapping, followed days or weeks later by quite definite kicking and acrobatics. In the sixth month, the baby starts to par-

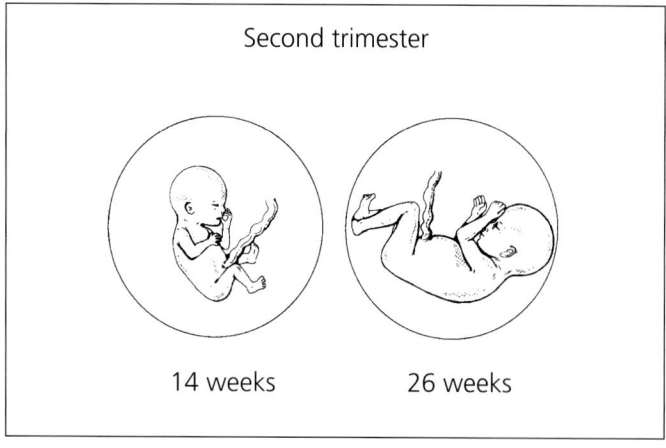

Second trimester

14 weeks   26 weeks

ticipate increasingly in your physical and psychological life: For instance, it will turn away from a disturbing sound and react differently to loud and soft music. It can sense irritation, stress, and anxiety on your part, as well as feelings of security and contentment. At the end of the sixth month the baby is about 1 foot long and weighs 1 to 2 pounds. If born now, it has a slight chance of survival.

Examinations and Tests

You should now be going for prenatal checkups every 4 to 6 weeks. Each exam should include a fetal heartbeat check, urine tests for protein and sugar, blood pressure measurement, external (noninvasive) measurement of the uterus, and monitoring of edema (swelling) and varicose veins. Your weight shouldn't need to be checked unless there is a risk of preeclampsia.

If your health-care provider wants to do an ultrasound exam (see p. 516, 570, 651), ask why.

FINAL TRIMESTER

During the final trimester of pregnancy the fetus keeps growing, and your impatience level may be right up there, too. How you experience this time depends on your life circumstances and attitude. You may be able to enjoy "the calm before the storm," or your fast-growing belly may simply get on your nerves.

As before, anything goes if it makes you feel good. Remember to pay attention to your body's signals, though, and don't wear yourself out. It can mean the difference between your child coming into the world at the right time or a few weeks early.

Physical and Emotional Changes

The baby is starting to outgrow its cramped quarters: It communicates this by pushing and kicking. Because of its rapidly increasing weight, your spinal column is overburdened and blood flow to the pelvis is increasingly obstructed. Lower back pain, varicose veins, hemorrhoids, and swelling and heaviness in the legs can get worse. The increasing pressure on your bladder leads to more frequent urination; getting up at night to urinate is common. The uterus presses upward onto the stomach, making it necessary to eat smaller portions at a time. The intestines become sluggish and the tendency to constipation increases. The joint cartilage and skin grow soft and elastic, in preparation for the delivery.

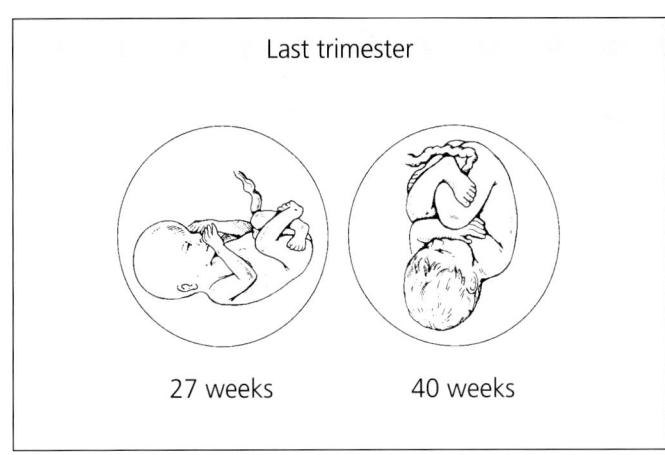

Last trimester

27 weeks   40 weeks

Along with the physical symptoms, you may be feeling fearful about a painful delivery, or worried about the baby's health. Widely fluctuating moods ranging from "Will this never end?" to "I'm not ready for this yet!" are completely normal.

Now is a good time to join a childbirth class where you can prepare yourself optimally for the delivery. It would also be ideal to get to know the midwife and/or doctor who will be attending at your delivery. Many midwives are affiliated with a hospital, and have a doctor as "backup."

Development of the Baby

The baby is fast readying itself for life on the outside. In the last months it usually gains the most weight, seemingly aiming for its highest possible birthweight. The nervous system is developing, and with it, consciousness and memory. During the eighth month the baby is usually already in its birth position: 95 percent of babies are positioned with their heads down.

After 40 weeks, the fetus is between 19 and 22 inches in length and weighs about 6 to 10 pounds.

Examinations and Tests

Until week 37, monthly checkups are sufficient; after that, you should be examined every ten days. In addition to the regular tests, a blood count may be indicated, because anemia often develops in the final trimester.

Ultrasound is necessary only in certain cases (see p. 516, 570, 651). If you're planning a home birth, you should definitely get an ultrasound to determine the exact position of both placenta and baby.

UNWANTED PREGNANCY

Only 25 to 40 percent of all pregnancies are planned. If you find yourself unexpectedly pregnant, you have until week 12 to figure out how you want to deal with the situation. During this period, an abortion is still a less complicated procedure.

If you have no partner to help you with this difficult decision, seek input from friends or a professional counselor. Even for a couple, the decision to have the baby or not has repercussions. It could mean the end of the relationship either way. It is essential that you discuss this in total honesty. All too often, relationships break up years later when it comes out that partners either stayed together only for the sake of the child, or secretly blame themselves or each other for an abortion.

Methods

An abortion can usually be performed relatively safely 7 to 9 weeks after the last period. Complications are rare. Despite this fact, it is not uncommon for a woman facing an abortion to be afraid of the finality of this decision, afraid of sustaining an injury, and afraid of risking infertility.

Dilation and Curettage (D&C)

D&C is the most "user-friendly" method of terminating a pregnancy. Under local or general anesthesia, the cervix is carefully dilated and a thin tube inserted into the uterus. The placental tissue is suctioned from the uterus; usually a curettage (scraping of the uterine lining) is necessary to remove all tissue.

The procedure lasts a few minutes; blood loss is minimal. Immediately afterwards, the patient is given an injection that causes the cervix to contract; this slows bleeding and prevents infection. An hour after surgery, the patient can go home.

Prostaglandins

This method is usually used if the pregnancy is terminated after week 12. The most common reason for this is that tests have detected deformities of the embryo.

Prostaglandins are hormones that cause the cervix to soften and the uterus to contract, resulting in a miscarriage. The procedure is performed on an inpatient basis in the hospital. The hormone is given intravenously or applied to the cervix in gel or other topical form. This induces labor, and the placental tissue is aborted. Because prostaglandin works slowly, this can take up to 2 days. Often another labor-inducing drug, such as oxytocin in dilute form, must be administered additionally. Painkillers are given to counteract the usually considerable pain. To avoid infection, a D&C is usually performed to remove the uterine lining and what remains of the placental tissue.

The patient can return home a day after the operation if there are no complications, such as fever or bleeding.

Scraping

This method is obsolete and best avoided.

RU-486

RU-486 is an antihormone that terminates pregnancy and is legal in some countries. It makes abortion considerably less rigorous for women and may soon be available on a wider basis, since the manufacturer has released its claim on the patent.

Recovering

Following an abortion, you will probably feel sad, and perhaps guilty as well. You may feel freed from an unbearable burden, yet still mourn the loss of the child. Be gentle with yourself. Take the time to process recent events. Turn to your partner, friends, or professional counselors for help.

The physical wounds will heal more quickly. Bleeding usually stops after 8 to 10 days. Don't use tampons or have sex until your doctor has done the necessary follow-up checkup.

Menstruation will usually reappear after 4 to 6 weeks.

NUTRITION DURING PREGNANCY

If you "eat for two" while pregnant, you'll gain unnecessary weight. As long as you eat a balanced diet high in fresh, healthy foods (see Nutrition, p. 722), your baby will take all that he or she needs. In the first 4 months, you don't need to increase calorie intake; later, you can meet your body's slightly elevated calorie requirement by eating fruit, vegetables, and dairy products. If you have food cravings, go ahead and satisfy them; they may be your body's way of telling you you're not getting enough of a certain food group.

SEX DURING PREGNANCY

Forget anything you may have heard about the dangers of sex during pregnancy. Your baby is well cushioned in a fluid-filled sac and won't be harmed by an active love life. On the contrary: If you feel good, your baby will feel good. During pregnancy, the physical conditions for sex are optimal: The body produces more sex hormones, making the vagina moister and increasing blood flow to the area; and fears of an unwanted pregnancy are no longer an issue. You and your partner may especially enjoy your new voluptuousness (bigger breasts and rounder hips).

However, it may also be the case that your partner feels threatened by all this womanliness, or that in his image of femininity, voluptuous means unattractive. Don't sweep these issues under the rug; open communication can bring about understanding and change.

Similarly, you yourself may have no desire for sex. If this is the case, don't feel pressured; maybe your corpulent body is inhibiting you, or you feel that the baby is literally coming between you and your partner. Verbalize your feelings. Unexpressed emotional stress can affect your baby.

Avoid sex if
— you have no desire for it. Stress can lead to miscarriage
— you have lower abdominal pains
— you notice bleeding
— there is any danger of miscarriage or premature birth
— the amniotic sac (bag of water) has broken.

TESTING

Genetic Counseling

Genetic counseling can determine your personal chances of producing an unhealthy or disabled child. It makes sense only if you already have a child with disabilities, or if there is a history of profound hereditary disorders in your or your partner's family, or if you're related to your partner.

From a detailed medical history of both partners' families, the statistical likelihood of a child inheriting the disease or condition can be calculated (see Disabilities, p. 618).

Genetic counseling centers exist in almost all major cities. Your gynecologist can help you find the nearest one.

Prenatal Testing

Certain disabilities can be detected during pregnancy (e.g., Down's syndrome; see p. 619). Critics of such testing argue that the baby may be damaged during the test, or that the test may induce a miscarriage.

You should not agree to prenatal testing unless you are certain that terminating the pregnancy is an option you would consider.

Amniocentesis (Amniotic Fluid Exam)

This time-tested method involves sampling fetal cells taken from the amniotic fluid and analyzing them for chromosomal abnormalities and defects of the central nervous system (neural tube defects).

A hypodermic needle is inserted through the abdomen into the amniotic sac and some fluid is aspirated. Local anesthesia is usually not necessary at the entry point, which is determined by ultrasound.

The test is performed between week 15 and week 18 of pregnancy. It takes two to three weeks to obtain the results. The pregnancy is that much farther along if you need to consider terminating. Amniocentesis should be performed only by well-trained specialists. In about 1 percent of cases, it may result in miscarriage.

Chorionic Villus Sampling (CVS)

With this procedure, congenital defects can be detected as early as week 7 to 10. The chorionic villi are parts of the placenta that have the same genetic pattern as the fetus.

Chorionic villi samples are suctioned from the uterus through a thin, flexible tube inserted in the vagina. Results are available the following day.

The advantage of this procedure over amniocentesis is the early date at which chromosomal abnormalities can be determined. The disadvantage is increased risk: CVS is twice as likely to cause miscarriage as amniocentesis. Moreover, studies have determined that children born following this procedure are more likely to have deformities of the fingers and toes.

Either CVS or amniocentesis is advisable if
— you are over 35, or the combined ages of you and your partner exceed 75
— there is a family history of congenital disorders
— you already have a child with a congenital disorder.

Ultrasound

Ultrasound is used freely by many doctors and mid-wives despite the fact it remains controversial. The WHO rejects this procedure as "standard of care" because there is as yet no definitive proof that it is advisable for mother and child. Moreover, sonograms are often misinterpreted, leading to needless anxiety and hasty surgical intervention.

The WHO recommends this test only in cases where

— the date of the last period, or of conception, is unknown
— the size of the uterus cannot be determined through physical exam
— there is bleeding or pain
— the fetal heartbeat cannot be detected
— the fetus has not moved for some time
— the birth position cannot be determined with certainty
— there are indications of twins
— there is some fear of developmental disorder
— the baby is more than 10 days overdue
— a birth defect is suspected, in which case testing should be performed in a center specializing in birth defects
— amniocentesis is planned.

Doppler Ultrasound

This type of ultrasonic device is useful in cases where defective development is suspected, for instance if the mother's abdomen is smaller than it should be. Blood flow in certain blood vessels, such as the umbilical cord or the aorta, is measured using this procedure.

As with ultrasound, routine use of this technique is not advisable.

Blood Tests

All expectant mothers undergo blood tests, and the results often deviate widely from "the norm" (see Diagnostic Tests/Procedures, p. 635). However, this is rarely cause for alarm. Talk to your doctor.

Blood Count

Red blood cells (erythrocytes): During pregnancy, blood volume increases 40 percent and the number of red blood cells drops, often to lower than normal levels. This doesn't necessarily mean you are anemic. The overall hemoglobin level is more important than the red-blood-cell count.

Hemoglobin: Critical threshold is about 10 gm/dl.

White blood cells (leukocytes): Increased levels of white blood cells are normal. During childbirth, levels can soar to 15,000 (normal is between 4,800 and 10,000/mm).

Iron in Blood Serum

Throughout pregnancy, the blood-iron content is usually at the low edge of the normal range.

Erythrocyte Sedimentation Rate (ESR)

The ESR is always increased.

Antibody Testing

Antibodies are defense substances produced in the bloodstream when foreign bodies, such as pathogens or alien blood, are encountered.

All pregnant women are tested for antibodies to measles, syphilis, HIV and hepatitis, and in many cases toxoplasmosis.

If you are Rh-negative, you'll also be tested for Rh antibodies. This test is repeated in the final trimester, or in case bleeding appears.

COMPLAINTS DURING PREGNANCY

Pregnancy makes demands on the body that it isn't accustomed to. The resulting symptoms are usually harmless, but if you don't feel well, contact your doctor.

Shortness of Breath

In the final trimester, the growing uterus pushes against the diaphragm. Breathing can become difficult, particularly during exertion like climbing stairs. Don't worry: The baby is getting enough oxygen. Around 3 weeks prior to delivery, the belly drops, making breathing easier.

Self-Help

Try not to gain excessive amounts of weight. Sleep on your left side, if possible.

Discharge

As the vaginal environment undergoes changes, a light, odorless discharge is normal. If you have heavy discharge or additional symptoms, see Vaginitis, p. 518.

Self-Help

Sitz baths can help, as can yogurt containing live acidophilus cultures.

Incontinence/Weak Bladder

In the final months of pregnancy, the baby's head may press down on the bladder. It's normal to need to urinate more frequently, or uncontrollably to release the occasional few drops of urine. If other symptoms arise, such as pain while urinating or pain in the kidney area, see p. 418.

Self-Help

Wear panty liners if you feel insecure. Don't drink less: Your body needs fluids.

Flatulence

Flatulence can often be extremely painful. If it occurs in conjunction with other symptoms, see Intestines, p. 402.

Self-Help

Avoid foods that cause flatulence; drink antiflatulence tea (see Irritable Bowel Syndrome, p. 403).

High Blood Pressure

High blood pressure that first manifests during pregnancy can be a warning sign of preeclampsia (see p. 574). Contact your health-care provider.

Low Blood Pressure

Low blood pressure in pregnancy can lead to circulatory disorders.

Self-Help

Regular exercise and alternating hot and cold showers usually help.

Bleeding

Vaginal bleeding must always be taken seriously. Only a health professional can determine whether it is harmless or indicates a serious condition (see Miscarriage, p. 574; Premature Delivery, p. 574).

Skin Pigmentation

Brown spots in the face, darkened nipples, and a brown line down the middle of the belly are normal signs of pregnancy. They result from changes in the body's pigment (see Pigmentation Disorders, p. 280).

Self-Help

Not possible. The spots usually disappear gradually after delivery.

Hemorrhoids

Hemorrhoids develop more easily during pregnancy, as veins in the pelvis become distended by the weight of the uterus (see p. 417).

Self-Help

Wash your anal area regularly with cold water. Push any painful lumps back into the anus and apply a topical ointment. Keep bowel movements regular and loose by eating lots of fiber (see p. 726).

Food Cravings

Craving certain foods is completely normal; indulge your cravings when possible. Sometimes they are your body's way of telling you that you have certain nutritional deficits.

Varicose Veins

Pregnancy can worsen an existing predisposition to vascular weakness. The pressure of the uterus also hinders the blood flow returning to the heart (see Varicose Veins, p. 328).

Self-Help

Get lots of exercise (swimming, biking). Wear support hose. Sit while working; standing can cause the blood to pool in the leg veins. Keep your legs elevated. Try hot and cold alternating baths (see Foot Baths, p. 692).

Muscle Cramps

Muscle cramps are usually harmless and often affect the lower legs. Persistent cramps may indicate calcium, magnesium, or vitamin B-complex deficiencies.

Self-Help

Try putting all your weight onto the cramping leg or flexing the toes to stretch the calf muscle (see p. 436).

Fatigue

Fatigue is normal particularly during the first months

of pregnancy, as your body adjusts to changes. However, if you constantly feel exhausted, you may be overtaxing your body.

Self-Help

If you're tired, get lots of rest. Tiredness may also be a sign of insufficient physical activity; try to get regular exercise, or play your favorite sport, where you can breathe lots of fresh air.

Back Pain

Backache, especially toward the end of pregnancy, may be caused by the baby's head pressing down on the sacrum, the general strain of carrying more weight around, overweight, or preexisting poor posture exacerbated by the pregnancy (see Back and Lower Back Pain, p. 465).

Self-Help

Relieve your spine as often as possible by lying on your side, with your back curved. Swim or do pregnancy exercises and relaxation exercises (see Relaxation, p. 693).

Sleep Disturbances

In the final trimester, your big belly or the baby's "gymnastics" can disturb your sleep. You may also be feeling worried or anxious.

Self-Help

Take a relaxing bath or go for a walk. Avoid hard-to-digest food at dinner; drink soothing herbal tea (see Sleep Disorders, p. 588).

Swollen Hands and Feet

Swelling in the extremities is usually harmless. During pregnancy, the body retains more water than usual. Nevertheless, contact your health-care provider if your hands or feet are swollen. In rare cases, swelling can be the first sign of dangerous preeclampsia (see p. 574), which requires professional treatment.

Self-Help

Keep your legs elevated as much as possible. Massage your legs daily in the direction of your heart. Cold showers can help, as can warm baths for at least an hour (see Baths, p. 691).

Heartburn

Heartburn can begin at the start of pregnancy, as the lower esophageal sphincter at the entrance to the stomach relaxes and stomach acid enters the esophagus. Also, in advanced stages of pregnancy, the uterus can press against the stomach, causing the same symptoms.

Self-Help

Avoid spicy or hard-to-digest foods. Eat smaller meals, but eat more frequently. Chew nuts or dry bread to neutralize stomach acid (see Acid Reflux, p. 383).

Nausea and Vomiting

It may take a while to adjust to your changed circumstances, both physically and psychologically. This is why nausea and vomiting may occur early in pregnancy. If you lose weight, or the symptoms don't stop, contact your health-care provider.

Self-Help

Have breakfast in bed and lie down for a while afterward, if possible. Drink small amounts of mineral water or herbal tea throughout the day. Avoid heavy meals.

Constipation

Due to relaxed intestinal muscles, food is processed more slowly, which can lead to constipation.

You may also have a misguided idea of what constitutes "normal" elimination: as long as you move your bowels three times a week, there's no need to worry (see Constipation, p. 406).

Self-Help

Under no circumstances should you take a laxative without your doctor's consent; it could damage the baby. High-fiber foods and dried fruit almost always clear up the problem (see Constipation, p. 406).

DANGERS DURING PREGNANCY

Coffee

There's no reason to avoid your customary cup of morning coffee during pregnancy, but large amounts can cause damage. More than 600 mg of caffeine daily (two to four cups, depending on how it's prepared) can lead to premature birth or miscarriage (see Caffeine, p. 758).

Although tea contains caffeine, its potential danger during pregnancy has not been proved.

Tobacco
Every cigarette you smoke, your baby smokes, too. Nicotine constricts the blood vessels and inhibits the transport of oxygen, causing your baby to get less "air." Babies born to heavy smokers weigh 6 to 14 ounces less and have a higher mortality rate than those born to nonsmokers. If the father smokes heavily prior to conception, this can also cause fetal damage (see Smoking, p. 754).

Alcohol
Regular alcohol consumption doubles the risk of miscarriage. Alcohol slows fetal development and can cause premature birth. A third to half of all children of alcoholic mothers are born damaged (see Alcohol, p. 756). Fetal alcohol syndrome is a serious and completely preventable problem.

Drugs of Abuse
All drugs cross the placenta and affect the fetus. Drugs taken immediately before delivery can cause respiratory and circulatory disorders in the newborn. Addicted mothers bear addicted babies, whose symptoms (breathing disorders, trembling, anxiety, screaming, etc.) require treatment (see Addiction to Illegal Drugs, p. 208).

Medication
Almost all medications cross the placenta to the baby; ask your health-care provider whether any medications you are taking can cause damage to the fetus.

Infectious Disease
Certain infectious diseases in the mother, particularly during the first trimester, can severely damage the fetus.

Rubella
Before planning a pregnancy, have your rubella titer—the level of antibodies in your blood—checked. If you've never been exposed or were never immunized and have no antibodies against German measles in your blood, you should get immunized (see Immunizations, p. 667).

As a precaution, you should avoid getting pregnant for 3 months after the vaccination. The rate of defor-mities and damage in children exposed to rubella in utero is extremely high: More than 50 percent of children born to mothers who get rubella during the first month of pregnancy experience disorders; during the second month, about 25 percent, and in the third month about 15 percent. New studies show that children whose mothers were exposed to rubella in the fourth month of pregnancy run little or no risk of damage; at most, temporary developmental or growth delays may result. If you have been exposed to rubella and don't know whether you've been infected, have your rubella titer checked immediately. If your antibody level is low, you should receive an injection of rubella immunoglobulin within 4 days of your exposure to the disease.

If you were definately exposed during the first trimester, serious consideration should be given to terminating the pregnancy.

Measles, mumps, chicken pox
Nearly all women are immune to these childhood diseases. If you have not developed any antibodies and come into contact with an infected person while pregnant, your doctor should give you an injection of the requisite immunoglobulin (see Immunizations, p. 667).

Toxoplasmosis
Toxoplasmosis is a rare infection that is primarily transmitted through raw meat. It can also be transmitted if handling infected cats, i.e., cat feces. Studies have shown that the danger of fetal damage is less than previously believed.

X Rays
Fetal damage from X rays depends on phase of pregnancy, type and dose of radiation, and the mother's general condition. If exposed between the first and twentieth day, the fetus will die if it is damaged. If you are exposed to radiation within the first four months of pregnancy, see an experienced specialist for an assessment of any possible damage to the baby (see X Rays, p. 646).

Toxins
All substances that compromise fertility (see p. 560) can also affect fetal development. The effects are similar to that of smoking during pregnancy (see above). It is known that even small levels of poly-chlorinated

biphenyls (PCB) and lead can impair fetal brain development, resulting in lower intelligence, short attention span, and hyperactivity. Heavy metals and halogenated hydrocarbons are believed to have similar effects.

Preeclampsia

The causes of preeclampsia are still not known. It is known only that women expecting their first child are more frequently affected, and that women from lower socioeconomic levels are at greater risk. High blood pressure during pregnancy must be treated immediately, because it can damage the baby: Reduced blood flow to the placenta may result in the baby not getting enough oxygen.

The principal signs of preeclampsia are
— High blood pressure (greater than 135/85)
— Swollen legs, feet, hands, and face (edema), when in conjunction with high blood pressure
— Protein in urine (dangerous only in conjunction with above symptoms)
— Sudden significant weight gain

Treatment

If the disease is recognized in time, sufficient rest and relaxation are often enough. The strict bed rest that is often prescribed is controversial; enforced rest during the day often leads to insomnia at night.

Preeclampsia that persists despite increased rest and relaxation should be treated in a hospital. Sodium-restricted diets are often prescribed as part of treatment, but their efficacy is debatable.

In severe cases, the pregnancy may need to be ended prematurely in a cesarean to save the baby. After childbirth, the symptoms usually disappear on their own.

Miscarriage

If you lose your baby in the first three months, this often means that it wasn't healthy.

Spontaneous abortion or miscarriage refers to a pregnancy that terminates before week 20 (calculated from the first day of your last period). An impending miscarriage is marked by contractions and bleeding; sometimes it can be staved off through bed rest.

Hormone treatment early in pregnancy appears to be worthless. Numerous studies have shown that the successful pregnancy rate with and without treatment is about equal.

The most common causes of miscarriage are infectious (e.g., viral) diseases, damage from environmental toxins (e.g. heavy metals), and various systemic diseases (e.g., immune disorders, kidney diseases, diabetes). Only very few spontaneous abortions can be traced back to hormonal imbalance in the mother. During the second half of pregnancy, emotional problems can cause a miscarriage as well.

If miscarriage is inevitable, heavy bleeding and abdominal cramping develop. In many cases a curettage (scraping of the uterine lining) must be performed.

Sexual intercourse is possible after a miscarriage as soon as your sexual desire returns. Medically speaking, a new pregnancy can be planned as soon as the menstrual cycle stabilizes, but it's better to give yourself time. One child should not be used to replace another.

Premature Delivery

A child weighing less than 5 pounds and born prior to week 37 is considered premature. Possible causes of premature delivery include heavy smoking, alcohol, environmental toxins, heavy physical exertion, stress, conscious or unconscious rejection of the baby, or overwhelming circumstances at home (problems with your partner, financial troubles, a major move, etc.). Women who are well prepared for the arrival of the baby have fewer premature deliveries than women who are abandoned to cope on their own.

If you pay attention to your body's alarm signals, you may be able to prevent a premature delivery. At the first sign of the following, contact your doctor.
— If you need to urinate often (more than twice) during the night and don't have a bladder infection, you may be suffering from a nervous disorder.
— If you can't fall asleep in the evening, even if you're tired, or if you wake frequently during the night, you are probably suffering from exhaustion.
— Uterine contractions several times a day lasting more than 30 to 60 seconds, and occurring more frequently than three times in an hour, constitute an alarm signal. These contractions are rarely painful and are often noticeable only by a hardening of the abdomen.

Medical Options

Medication: Although the use of labor-inhibiting drugs is controversial, doctors often give them. An Irish study of more than 104,000 premature deliveries showed that the total number did not rise if these drugs were avoided. Moreover, they can damage the fetal heart muscle and lead to unpleasant side effects for the mother, such as a rapid drop in blood pressure, a racing heart, sweating, trembling, and anxiety.

In critical situations, however, such as to buy time during a delivery, labor-inhibitors are appropriate. *Cerclage:* Cerclage is the surgical closure of the cervix. This surgery is necessary only in the event of a known weakness in the uterus (such as after multiple miscarriages), in the presence of disease-related abnormalities (see Fibroids, p. 521) or following an operation.

The closing of the uterus after labor has already begun is an operation that runs counter to all scientific knowledge.

High-Risk Pregnancy

The term "high-risk pregnancy" is used far too freely. Doctors are trained to attend to complications; reading the medical textbooks, one might expect "normal" pregnancies to be the exception rather than the rule. If a pregnant woman is defined as a high-risk case, she will feel herself to be at higher risk and undergo needless anxiety. Typical examples include the "elderly *prima gravida,*" the very young (less than 17 years of age), twins, breech births, and Rh-negative cases. Very few pregnancies are actually high-risk; those that are include the following:

— Previous stillbirth or premature delivery
— Threatened premature delivery
— Suspected deficient fetal growth
— Systemic diseases (diabetes, kidney diseases)
— Psychological problems (excessive anxiety, stress or trauma)

PREPARATION FOR LABOR AND DELIVERY

Start preparing for labor and delivery by taking a childbirth class as early as the seventh month of pregnancy: It's worth the effort. Numerous studies show that well-prepared expectant mothers experience premature deliveries and preeclampsia less frequently, labor is shorter, and painkillers and surgical intervention are required less frequently.

Which type of class you attend is entirely up to you; the main thing is that you feel well supported and that the class meets your needs.

The childbirth class curriculum should offer the following:

— Discussions of questions, anxieties, worries, possible surgical interventions, changed life circumstances, healthy diet, etc.
— Exercises to tone your body so that you're well conditioned for the stresses of childbirth
— Relaxation and breathing techniques. It is less important that you learn a specific technique than that you find one that works for you.

LABOR AND DELIVERY

The birth of your child is an experience that, as far as possible, should be the way you—the mother—want it to be. Should your partner be present or not? Should it be high-tech, lower-tech, "natural" or medically assisted? There are a lot of factors to decide. Fortunately, various options are usually available, no matter where you live. The important thing is to learn as much as you can ahead of time, and make an informed decision before your first contractions appear!

Choosing a Place

The best place to have your baby is wherever you feel safest and most comfortable. Whether that's in the hospital, birthing center, or at home—only you can decide, possibly with a partner's help. Very few conditions limit your options (see High-Risk Pregnancy, above).

Hospital Delivery

Most babies are born in a hospital. Because the quality of obstetrics/maternity wards differs widely, however, it's worth your while to visit different hospitals in your area for the sake of comparison.

Don't hesitate to ask direct, detailed questions. You're preparing for a very important experience in your life: The birth of your baby.

Outpatient

If you want to go home with your baby as soon as possible, you may be able to find a hospital or birthing center geared to discharging mother and baby a few hours after delivery. (Some hospitals even allow you to provide your own midwife.) If this is not an option where you live, you can always check yourself out of the hospital when you want to, provided both you and the baby are doing fine. Either way, you should be under a midwife's or health-care provider's care once you return home.

Home Birth

A well-planned home birth can be just as safe as a hospital birth, as long as you bear in mind the following vital points:

— A home birth is appropriate only if you are in excellent health and can reasonably expect a delivery with no complications (see High-Risk Pregnancy p. 575).
— You need to feel completely comfortable with the idea of a home birth.
— Make sure you prepare yourself with a thorough childbirth-education class beforehand.
— Your midwife will be calling the shots as your labor coach and right-hand person during and after delivery. Find someone you trust, who will be able to take care of you for 10 days after the birth.
— The nearest hospital should not be more than 20 minutes away.

Support During Delivery

Choose with care the person(s) you want to be present to support you during this profound experience. Most women want their partners to be there for them in their "hour of need"—but you may have no partner, or your partner may not be up to it. In this case, it's especially important for you to decide on a labor coach. Don't choose somebody simply to do them a favor: You won't be doing yourself or your baby any favors. Ideally, you should get to know the attending physician(s) and midwife before delivery, but this is usually difficult in large hospitals with rotating staff.

Stages of Labor

Early (First) Stage

The onset of labor is usually characterized by back pain. These initial signals may start and stop, or occur at irregular intervals over a period of hours or days.

As labor progresses, contractions begin: The muscles at the top and sides of the uterus push down with increasing regularity, gradually moving the baby toward the cervix. As long as your contractions occur at 10- to 20-minute intervals, and you feel fine, you can stay at home. Relaxing in familiar surroundings can shorten this first stage. How long your baby will need to make

its way into birth position is hard to predict. It may take as little as 6 hours. With your first child, it may take 16 hours for the cervix to be fully dilated.

If this is your first child, don't worry about getting to the hospital too late; experience has shown that you have at least 3 to 4 hours to go.

Get to the hospital or inform your doctor and/or midwife if

— Contractions occur regularly every 5 minutes.
— The amniotic sac (bag of water) has broken. Lie down immediately (don't take a shower or bath, and don't stop to pack your hospital bag) and, unless you're planning a home birth, have yourself transported to the hospital as soon as possible, lying down. When the amniotic sac ruptures, the umbilical cord may get into a position where it can hamper the baby's breathing. Once the doctor has determined that this isn't the case and that the baby's head is sealing off the vagina, you can stand up again.
— You have unexplained pains not like regular contractions, which come at regular intervals and then subside.
— You experience bleeding that is not the "bloody show" caused by the dislodging of the mucus plug that seals the uterus till birth.

Second (Transition) Stage

The cervix is now completely dilated; contractions come at short, often irregular intervals and are usually extremely painful. You may already be feeling a powerful urge to push: Don't give in yet. This usually short transitional phase of labor is uncomfortable for almost everybody.

Final Stage: Advanced Active Labor

Now is the time to start pushing to help your baby into the world. For decades, women were instructed to breathe deeply and squeeze the child out with great effort. It's usually better to find your own rhythm. Most women who aren't made to follow a prescribed method push for shorter periods, and take longer breaks than usually advised by hospital personnel. During the pauses you can recover a bit, and your baby gets more oxygen. The practice of keeping the mother lying on her back, still common in many hospitals, actually makes labor more difficult. Birth positions that use the weight of the baby's head to help dilate the cervix (see p. 577) are simpler and make more sense.

Some time after delivery, the placenta (afterbirth) is delivered with the final contractions. Whether this takes place 15 minutes or an hour later makes no difference as long as there is no uterine bleeding.

Cutting the Umbilical Cord

It is still common practice in many hospitals to cut the umbilical cords of healthy babies immediately following delivery. There are no medical grounds for this. In fact, a baby can adjust more easily to the shock of life outside the womb if it doesn't have to deal simultaneously with the shock of the umbilical cord being cut. Especially gentle treatment is important for newborns in acute circumstances (e.g., premature babies), yet such a procedure goes against hospital routine. As it is, sickly or weak newborns usually have their cords cut immediately and are transported to the appropriate area for resuscitation. It would be preferable to bring the apparatus to the baby while it is still attached to the mother, if at all possible. It is vital that the newborn be kept lower than the placenta, so that blood will continue to flow to the child.

Immediate cutting of the umbilical cord is necessary only in rare cases in which the mother has a serious blood disease or mother and child are Rh–incompatible.

The First Hours After Birth

Give yourself time to experience this miracle fully. Your baby has arrived; now it needs peace and quiet and protection. In the hospital, however, this isn't always possible. Often the baby is removed from the mother right after birth to be measured, weighed, and examined. In a healthy baby, all neonatal testing, including Apgar scores which provide information on breathing, appearance, heartbeat, reflex, and muscle tone, can be performed while the baby is lying on the mother's belly or in the crook of her arm. All other tests can wait a couple of hours.

Object if hospital staff want to wash and dress the baby immediately: It may get too cold. You are the best source of warmth for your baby; all you need is a blanket. Now is the time to put your child to your breast: He or she will learn to suckle right away. The first milk, or colostrum, is especially full of nutrients. Perhaps your partner can bathe the baby while you rest.

Choose a hospital that respects your first moments together as a family.

Questions to ask hospitals

— Do you offer a childbirth-education class in which I can meet the staff?

— Whom can I bring along as my support person/labor coach? Can they stay with me through all stages of the delivery?

— How many midwives do you have on staff? (One per mother is ideal.)

— Can I bring my own midwife?

— Can I design my own childbirth: Walk around freely, take a warm bath, choose my own birth position, etc.? (See Natural Childbirth Aids, p. 579; Birthing Positions, p. 577).

— Is it hospital policy to monitor all labor patients electronically?

— Can I have a portable monitor? (See p. 578.)

— What are your standard procedures for childbirth, such as shaving the pubic area, labor-inducing IV, rupturing the amniotic sac, episiotomy, etc? (See Routine/Standard Procedures, p. 578; Natural Childbirth Aids, p. 579; Medical Intervention, p. 581.)

— Is it hospital policy to give pain medication routinely?

— What percent of births at this hospital are cesarean, vacuum extraction, or forceps deliveries?

— How many episiotomies are performed?

— What are the grounds for a routine cesarean? (See p. 581.)

— Can the baby stay with me (and my partner) right after birth?

— How soon after birth is the umbilical cord cut? Can I start nursing the baby immediately? (See The Post-Delivery Period, p. 584.)

— How long can mother, father, and baby stay together undisturbed after the birth?

— Do you have rooming-in, and if so, what kind? (See Rooming-in, p. 584.)

— Is there a neonatal intensive care unit (NICU)? In case of emergency, would the baby be transferred to a children's hospital? Which one? Would I be transferred there as well?

BIRTH POSITIONS (PRESENTATIONS)

In the early months the fetus moves around freely in the womb; its quarters gradually become increasingly cramped. By week 32, 90% of babies have adopted their final birth position. The remaining 10% continue to try out positions till week 37, and some change at the last minute, or can be helped to do so through different techniques.

Vertex Presentation

About 94 percent of babies are born head first. This is optimal for both mother and child, since the head widens the birth canal and stretches the vagina gently.

Breech Presentation

The fear many women (and doctors) have of a breech birth is unfounded: The risk for both mother and baby is only slightly increased. Because the baby's narrow body needs to lead the way in widening the birth canal, labor usually lasts longer. The common practice of performing a cesarean as a precautionary measure may be misguided. It minimizes the risk to the child only in very specific cases (see Cesarean Section, p. 581).

Sometimes it may be possible to change the baby's position. On no account should you try to do this without guidance from your midwife or doctor.

"Indian Bridge"

Twice a day, lie on your back for ten minutes with your belly and pelvis elevated 10 to 12 inches above the rest of your body. Your head and legs should hang down and be as relaxed as possible. This way, the abdominal wall is stretched taut—an uncomfortable position for mother and child alike, which is presumably why some babies change their position as a result.

Gentle Turning

This new method for turning the baby is based on the theory that physical and emotional tension can lead to muscles so tight that the baby can't move itself into position. A combination of dialogue, massage, and specific exercises can loosen the tissues sufficiently so the baby can turn.

External Turning

In this method, the doctor tries to turn the baby by manipulating it with both hands on the mother's belly. This can be risky (if the umbilical cord is too short, for example) and should be performed with care only by experienced practitioners.

Transverse Position

Only 0.5 percent of babies are in the transverse position prior to delivery; a cesarean delivery is the only option. As with breech birth, the doctor or midwife may attempt to turn the child beforehand.

If your baby doesn't want to change position, you and your obstetrics team should respect this.

MONITORED DELIVERY

The word monitoring says it all: Any procedure considered "dangerous" requires watching over. Many of the interventions that women undergo during childbirth result directly from monitoring, which frequently leads to measures that are misguided or at best unnecessary.

Fetal Heartbeat Monitor

Many hospitals subject all labor patients to electronic monitoring of the fetal heartbeat, although the procedure is useless. There is no evidence that it has a positive influence on birth outcome. Because the monitor often detects "suspicious" heartbeats, this procedure contributes to the rising number of cesarean, forceps, and vacuum-extraction deliveries. Fetal heartbeat monitors should be employed only in carefully selected high-risk cases.

Doppler Device

In noninvasive settings, in which the expectant mother is allowed maximal freedom of movement and top-quality care takes the place of constant electronic monitoring, doctors and midwives frequently use this portable ultrasound fetal heartbeat monitor.

Stethoscope

The traditional stethoscope is coming back into vogue. The World Health Organization recommends its use, instead of electronic monitoring, during normal births. In a study of 13,000 births, half the women were monitored with a stethoscope and the other half electronically. There was no qualitative difference in the outcome. The stethoscope has the advantage of not using ultrasound, unlike Doppler devices.

ROUTINE/STANDARD PROCEDURES

Standard procedures aren't necessarily determined by what's best for mother and child. Some are traditional, others are designed to provide comfort and have no medical justification.

Shaving the Pubic Area

Some hospitals still shave expectant mothers' pubic hair,

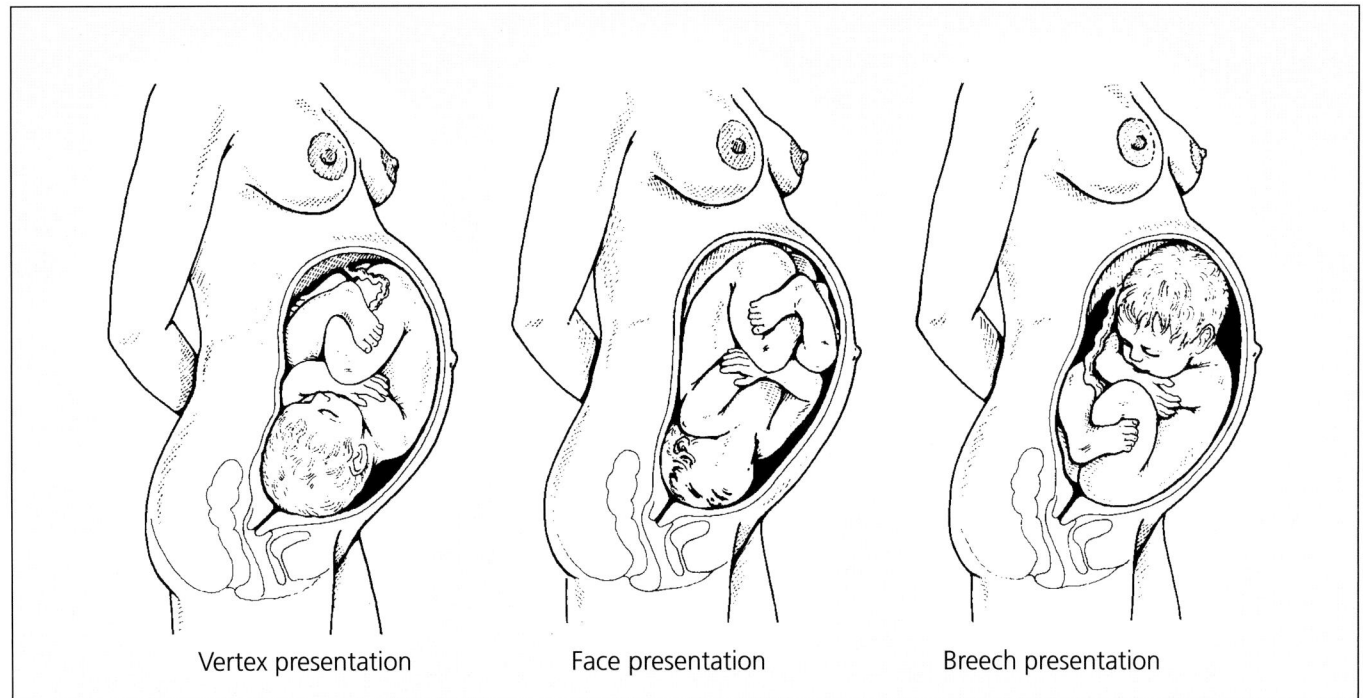

Vertex presentation   Face presentation   Breech presentation

though it is medically unnecessary.

The argument that hair might contaminate an episiotomy while suturing and cause infection has long been disproved.

Enema

Even though it's not necessary, many women are prepped for delivery with an enema or anal suppository. Any stool passed during labor and delivery may pose an aesthetic problem for personnel, but certainly not a medical or hygienic one.

Food and Drink

The mother is usually not allowed to eat or drink once labor has begun, the rationale being that this is a precautionary measure in case anesthesia becomes necessary later on. If you consider that at least 90 percent of all women need no surgical intervention, the explanation holds no water.

Easily digestible foods such as broth or white bread are recommended to keep your strength up if labor takes a long time.

As an alternative, some hospitals have a policy of hooking mothers-to-be to a glucose intravenous (IV) drip to compensate for the calorie deficit incurred by not eating. There is no reason for this during a normal birth. In fact, the drip restricts movement and contributes to the sense of being sick and dependent.

Natural Childbirth Aids

There are many things you can do to help make the birth of your child as pain-free and pleasant as possible.

Exercise

Women who are able to move about freely usually need less pain medication and have fewer surgical interventions during childbirth. If you feel like walking around, by all means do so; it will help your baby press down on the cervix, speeding delivery.

Changing Position

Alternating positions between sitting, standing, crouching, squatting, and lying works for many women. It lessens contractions but doubles their effectiveness and ultimately may shorten the first stage of labor.

Warm Baths

Pain sensitivity is substantially reduced by warm water. Despite this, many doctors discourage this tested relaxation technique for fear that the baby might be born underwater. Their concern is unnecessary, however. If a baby is unexpectedly delivered underwater, it will not begin breathing until it is lifted into the air. Likewise, supposed higher rates of infection in the mother due to baths have not been proven. Once the water has broken, bathing is not recommended. A warm shower may be helpful.

In some hospitals and birthing centers, in fact, underwater births are encouraged or routinely planned, with very positive results.

Massage

Massage from your partner or labor coach can help ease labor pain; there are several simple, easy-to-learn techniques.

Sacral Massage

There are two dimples above the tailbone, a few inches to either side of the spine; vigorous pressure using thumbs or knuckles in this area can bring relief, especially during the second stage of labor.

Reflex-Zone Massage

Directly under the ribcage, four finger-widths to either side of the spine, the skin should be vigorously massaged with broad circular movements until it turns red.

Belly Massage

Many women enjoy having their belly massaged, upward in the middle (on the top of the belly) and down on the sides.

Thigh Massage

This massage is especially helpful if the vagina is tense. The insides of the thighs are stroked toward the knees, preferably in time with your breathing.

There may be times you don't want to be touched. Some women find massage in the last stage of pregnancy unpleasant. Don't hesitate to let your partner know.

Acupuncture, Autogenic Training, Yoga, Hypnosis

These are gentle methods of facilitating childbirth that should only be used and taught by trained specialists (see Relaxation, p. 693).

PHARMACEUTICAL INTERVENTION

Almost all medical methods for easing childbirth have disadvantages for the baby; however, they should not be rejected out of hand. If you are extremely apprehensive about childbirth or find the pain unbearable, you should select one of these options with a clear conscience.

Medications

All medication taken during childbirth reaches the baby through the placenta. A commonly dispensed painkiller and muscle relaxant, Demerol, can lead to uterine inertia and breathing problems in newborns. Ideally, you should not be given Demerol right before delivery because the baby needs 4 hours to process just half the dose.

Pain Relief

There are various methods for numbing or killing pain associated with childbirth. They are practical if required in individual cases, such as when the stress caused by labor is greater than the stress caused by the medication.

As a rule, however, they make little sense. The stage when the child is passing through the vagina and perineum is perceived by most women as painful, but also as not very stressful because it doesn't last long, and because they're actively participating by pushing.

Pudendal Block

A local anesthetic is injected into the ischial tuberosity, lessening pain by blocking nerve communication to the external genitalia.

This block is not advisable for an episiotomy, or for vacuum extraction or forceps delivery: A perineal anesthetic is just as effective.

Perineal Anesthesia

A local anesthetic is injected into the perineum, where the episiotomy will be performed. This procedure is necessary only in case of an early episiotomy (see p. 581), otherwise the incision is made without anesthesia during labor. This procedure is also appropriate for suturing the episiotomy. It has no negative effects, and side effects are rare.

Caudal Block

Avoid any hospital that still uses this method, which poses potential risk to the child.

Nitrous Oxide

Laughing gas creates a condition similar to general anesthesia. You won't feel much pain, but you also won't be an active participant in delivery. This method is outdated and should no longer be offered.

Epidural Anesthesia

This method is used widely although it may have severe repercussions for both mother and baby. An anesthetic is injected into the mother's spine, rendering the lower part of the body insensitive. The consequences may be serious:

— The delivery must be monitored closely, since blood pressure may drop (see Fetal Heartbeat Monitor, p. 578).
— An IV drip of oxytocin is often necessary (see p. 583).
— You feel no urge to push, so the work of labor is left to the baby, significantly prolonging delivery.
— Vacuum extraction and forceps delivery are considerably more frequent.
— Headaches lasting for days or temporary paralysis in the legs are not uncommon.

An epidural is advisable only if you are extremely apprehensive about labor or if it is replacing sedatives during a cesarean section.

MEDICAL INTERVENTION

Artifical Rupture of Membranes (Amniotomy)

The longer the placenta remains intact, the less stressful the birth. The membranes will usually rupture on their own at the end of the first stage of labor.

In spite of this, many obstetricians rupture the amniotic sac membranes artificially when the cervix is just 5 cm dilated. This causes contractions to intensify. Lacerations of the cervix and trauma to the baby's head can result. A surgical opening of the sac is justified only if labor has been very long and you are exhausted. An artificial rupture to induce labor is not routinely recommended.

Episiotomy

Although episiotomy is, surgically speaking, a minor procedure, it can be a source of discomfort after childbirth. Its consequences may last weeks and even months: Pain while sitting, urinating, or having sex. Despite this, many hospitals still routinely perform episiotomies without medical justification. Contrary to long-held belief, a surgical cut does not heal better than a tear, and tears extending deep into the tissue are rare.

If during your pregnancy you massage your perineum, vulva, and labia with wheat-germ oil, your tissues will be able to stretch more easily during childbirth. Your midwife should be able to tell you how best to care for your perineum.

An episiotomy is justified if
— The baby is short of oxygen just before crowning
— The baby is premature and therefore less viable
— It's a breech delivery
— The perineum is not stretching properly
— A forceps or vacuum delivery is necessary
— The mother cannot push for medical reasons (e.g., heart or eye problems)

Techniques for Episiotomy

A medial episiotomy is much less unpleasant than a lateral episiotomy: The incision is made on the less sensitive perineum, it is smaller, and it heals faster. In spite of this, some doctors prefer the lateral because the anus is not as easily injured. However, this technique is justifiable only in cases of breech birth, forceps or vacuum extraction delivery, or if the perineum is too narrow to allow for a sufficient medial cut.

Forceps and Vacuum Extraction Delivery

Sometimes childbirth must be concluded swiftly because the fetal heartbeat is slowing down, the mother is too exhausted to push, or the baby is in a problematic position.

Whether your obstetrician chooses forceps or vacuum extraction depends in part on which procedure he or she is more experienced. It has not been proven that one is preferable to the other. Forceps may prompt premature intervention, because the head can be grasped before it's at the pelvic outlet.

Cesarean Section

Far more cesareans are performed today than are medically necessary. Doctors almost always cite the baby's safety as justification, but they may be more concerned with protecting themselves against litigation. Hospitals in which doctors and midwives take the time to monitor each patient carefully usually have no more than 5 to 10 percent cesarean deliveries.

A cesarean is justified in the following situations:
— The fetal heart rate drops suddenly, and the cervix is still not completely dilated.
— The child is positioned in such a way (e.g., transverse) that normal vaginal birth is not possible.

— The child is in breech position in a first-time mother, and ultrasound data estimates its weight at 8 pounds or more.
— The mother's pelvis is unusually small (less than 8 inches in diameter). Experience has shown, however, that this is often measured incorrectly: Before opting for a cesarean, have a second doctor remeasure you.
— The child's head is too large in relation to the mother's pelvis.
— Contractions are weak and don't improve after administration of labor-inducing drugs.
— The placenta is at or near the opening of the cervix, so that it tends to precede the child at birth.
— The placenta prematurely detaches from the wall of the uterus.
— The umbilical cord is twisted around the baby's head.
— There is a risk of uterine lacerations due to heavy contractions or previous surgery.
— Despite strong contractions, the cervix is still not open (effaced).

Techniques for cesarean section

In a cesarean section, the abdomen is cut open with a longitudinal or transverse incision.

A transverse incision is less troublesome for the mother because it's made at the top of the pubic hairline and the scar is hardly visible later. Doctors sometimes justify a lengthwise incision in emergencies in terms of safety, but this is questionable since it shortens the procedure by no more than 30 to 60 seconds. A lengthwise incision should be performed only if a previous birth was performed with a lengthwise cesarean, or in the event of previous abdominal surgery, or obesity.

Epidurals during cesarean section

This procedure presents a favorable alternative to general anesthesia during a cesarean, since it renders only the lower part of the body pain-insensitive for a limited time (see p. 581). It has the following advantages:
— Mother and child aren't subjected to general anesthesia
— The mother doesn't sleep through her first contact with her child
— The sense of "childbirth as illness" is limited, and there are fewer complications (fever, exhaustion, constipation) and less postoperative pain.

High-Risk Delivery

This term is used far too frequently. Anyone whose pregnancy is labeled "high-risk" or "problematic" and who faces a "high-risk" birth will naturally be much more apprehensive and fearful than someone without these labels. The resulting anxiety and stress, in turn, can make childbirth truly risky, requiring medical intervention. This self-fulfilling prophecy can be broken only by not classifying pregnancies into predetermined categories. Each and every childbirth should be attentively cared for and monitored so the obstetrics team can intervene immediately in case of emergency.

Having said this, some mothers and babies definitely require special attention.

Premature Delivery

Premature babies require an especially careful delivery. Where possible, medication should be avoided, since it stresses the baby.

An episiotomy may be necessary. A pediatrician and neonatal intensive care unit (NICU) should be the standard of care.

Multiple Births

Twins and multiple births require special attention, because the babies are usually small and frail, and monitoring the fetal heartbeat may be more difficult.

Rh Factor

If the mother is Rh-negative, this need only be significant if she has not received RHO immune globulin (RhoGAM), and has Rh antibodies in her blood, in which case the child must be closely monitored and, in an emergency, given an immediate blood transfusion.

Maternal Diseases

Mothers with serious conditions such as diabetes and heart disease require special attention, since childbirth may be a profound ordeal for them.

Birth Defects

If ultrasound or amniocentesis show evidence of a fetal deformity, delivery should take place if possible in a center that can provide the requisite special care. In any case, rapid transportation to a NICU should be organized.

Breech Delivery

Breech deliveries continue to be defined as "high risk," even though numerous studies show that they are only slightly riskier as long as certain critical ground rules are observed (see Breech Presentation, p. 578).

DELIVERY AFTER DUE DATE

Only a few babies are born on their calculated due date; however, the fault usually lies with the calculations. A normal pregnancy lasts 280 days, give or take 14. The World Health Organization defines a prolonged gestation as one lasting more than 293 days.

In case of a bona fide prolonged gestation there is a danger that the baby is no longer receiving sufficient nutrients and oxygen. If you are already 10 days past your calculated due date, your doctor may determine whether to induce labor using some of the following tests.

Amniotic Fluid Sampling

A metal tube is inserted through the vagina and into the cervix, through which the obstetrician draws a sample of amniotic fluid. This procedure can be performed only if the cervix is already open. The baby's health can be determined by the color of the amniotic fluid. The exam is repeated every two days. The procedure often induces labor.

Heartbeat Monitoring

The fetal heartbeat is carefully monitored during a half-hour exam every other day. If results are inconclusive, an oxytocin challenge test may be given.

INDUCED LABOR

Natural Methods of Inducing Labor

If you are past your due date, there are a few things you can do on your own to induce labor.

Hunger and Thirst

One midwife's trick is to fast for 48 hours. This works for many women. The baby won't suffer as long as you eat something as soon as labor starts to keep your strength up.

Stimulating the Nipples

If you or your partner stimulate your nipples manually or orally several times a day, this can induce labor. Have patience and keep trying if it doesn't work right away.

Sexual Intercourse

If you still feel like having sex, it's a good method of stimulating labor. Semen contains prostaglandins that can induce labor.

Enemas

Nerve irritation caused by an enema can induce labor. Complement the effect with a warm bath.

Medically Induced Labor

Inducing labor artificially is a massive intervention in the natural process, and should be done only on good medical grounds.

Oxytocin

The hormone oxytocin, which the body naturally produces during childbirth, is injected into the veins, stimulating labor. This causes considerable stress to both mother and child because the uterus is under significantly more strain and the cervix is not yet softened. Moreover, postpartum bleeding can result because the uterus does not contract properly.

Prostaglandin

Prostaglandins are hormones present in semen as well as other sources, which induce labor naturally. The advantage to using prostaglandins is that they simultaneously soften the cervix. The disadvantage is that because the hormone is inserted into the vagina in gel or tablet form, an exact dose is not possible. This can result in rare cases of uterine tetany, which must then be treated with labor inhibitors.

Rupturing the Amniotic Sac

Rupturing the amniotic sac to induce labor is not recommended.

"Programmed Childbirth"

The natural process of labor and delivery should not be interfered with without good medical cause. If you set a date for labor to be induced, you take away the uncertainty, but you may have to deal with increased complications.

Inducing labor medically is justified in the following circumstances:

— In the event of a bona fide prolonged gestation (see p. 583).
— if you are suffering from pre-eclampsia (see p. 574).
— If the placenta is no longer providing the baby with enough nourishment or oxygen (placental insufficiency). The child's condition can be determined through a stress test or oxytocin challenge, in which a labor inducer is injected intravenously and the child's heart function is monitored simultaneously. An ultrasound image alone will correctly gauge the status of the placenta in only one out of two cases.
— If you are physically and emotionally exhausted. An exhausted, weakened mother is a greater risk to the child than an induced birth.

THE POST-DELIVERY PERIOD

After the first few hours of joy, excitement, relief, and exhaustion, life will return to "normal"—except that things will be very different. Suddenly there's someone new in your life who needs your attention around the clock. Don't try to act like some stereotype of the happy new mother if you don't feel like one. Let your true feelings show. It's okay to feel anxious, overwhelmed, or let down. Your breasts may hurt, your episiotomy suture may hurt, and when your hormone levels drop you may feel depressed. This is when you need other people's help. Arrange to get support, and relieve yourself of some household duties. It's okay to stay in your pyjamas till afternoon; your baby is monopolizing your day.

Rooming-In

This is the modern term for the most natural event in the world: For a newborn to stay with mother. The advantages of this are obvious: Everything a baby urgently needs—warmth, tenderness, attention—is constantly available; the milk bar is always open if he or she is hungry; mother is always there to hear if he or she cries.

This doesn't mean you should ignore your own needs. If you need a little peace and quiet, by all means leave your baby in the care of a nurse (while in the hospital) or other helper (at home) without misgivings. Rooming-in is offered by birthing centers almost everywhere, and also by many hospitals, although you can't always be sure exactly what is meant by the term in a hospital. In some maternity wards, for example, it's still customary for babies to sleep separate from their mothers at night. When choosing a hospital, find out beforehand whether you'll be able to care for the baby according to your own needs, without intervention.

NURSING/BREASTFEEDING

Mother's milk is the best nourishment for the baby during the first few months. However, many women don't breastfeed at all or only for a short time, because they have "too little" milk. If breastfeeding doesn't work, it's usually due to poor instruction at the hospital, a misunderstanding of how milk is produced, or supplemental feeding.

How the Breast Works

Anxiety and tension pose the biggest threat to a peaceful mother/child nursing relationship. Worrying about not having enough milk affects not only the baby but also your lactation reflex.

As long as you follow these tips, not much can go wrong:

— Nursing takes time and patience. Arrange not to be interrupted; make sure you and your baby are comfortable. Some children drink faster than others; relax and don't worry about following "the rules."
— Milk production is a dynamic of supply and demand. The earlier and more frequently you give your baby the breast during the first days, the better your milk production.
— Try to ensure that the entire areola, and not only the nipple, is in the baby's mouth, to lessen the likelihood of nipple soreness. If necessary, use your index finger to keep the breast from obstructing air flow to and from the baby's nose.
— If the breast is taut, massage some milk out to begin with so that it's easier for the baby to suckle.
— Alternate breasts when feeding so that milk production is the same from both breasts.
— If your milk doesn't start to flow for two or three days, don't let hospital staff feed your baby; water will tide a healthy newborn over until the mother's milk comes in. What you're trying to avoid is having your baby arrive at your breast already half-full and accustomed to sweet food. Your milk just won't taste quite right after that.

Difficulties Nursing

You should decide freely whether or not to breastfeed, without worrying about matching some "ideal" image of motherhood. Nursing a baby even though you don't really want to is worse for the baby than bottle-feeding. On the other hand, if you do want to breastfeed, there are a few things that could go wrong.

Not Enough Milk

Not having "enough" milk may simply be due to a lack of correct information. Sometimes, however, you may be inhibited by unspoken family anxieties or semiconscious worries (like, "My mother and her mother couldn't produce enough milk, so I probably can't either"). Consult your health-care provider or the La Leche League.

Breast Pain

If you have pain when nursing or your nipples are inverted, contact a lactation consultant. Breast infection is usually no cause to stop nursing as long as no yellowish or greenish pus appears.

Toxins in Mother's Milk

Although levels have been decreasing in recent years, mother's milk may still contain more toxins than cow's milk. This is no reason not to breastfeed, however: The special composition of mother's milk and the intimate mother/child contact it provides outweigh any negative impact from the potential toxins. You should take care not to lose weight while you are nursing. Many toxins are stored in the body's fatty tissue, and when fat deposits are metabolized, the toxins may pass into the mother's milk. If you live in a highly polluted area, you may be able to have your milk examined at the toxicology unit of the nearest university.

If you drink large amounts of coffee, your child may have difficulties sleeping, since caffeine is passed on through mother's milk.

Diseases

There are few diseases that preclude breastfeeding: in both developed and (especially) developing countries, two of these are tuberculosis and human immuneo-deficiency virus (HIV). However, if you are weakened following a severe infection or due to cancer, you should not breastfeed.

Medication

When you take your medication, so does your baby. Find out from your doctor whether your medication can hurt the baby.

Nursing Problems in the Baby

If your child is unable to drink because of extreme weakness or a deformity of the mouth or cheeks, it is especially important that he or she get your milk. Milk expressed with the help of a breast pump can be fed to your baby by bottle or via tube feeding.

Weaning

How long you breastfeed depends on you and your baby's well-being: One or the other of you will determine when it's time to wean.

Children who are breastfed for longer than 9 months usually won't wean without a struggle. Substitute a bottle or cup for the breast more and more at feeding time, so your baby can adjust gradually.

Bottle Baby

Contrary to what you might hear, bottle-feeding will not have lasting repercussions in your child's life. The most important benefits of breastfeeding—intimacy and security—can be given equally well when bottle-feeding. Hold and snuggle with your baby often; carry him or her close to your body. Bottle-feeding may also come in handy at times when breastfeeding is inconvenient.

Don't bottle-feed according to a strict schedule; feed on demand, and use a nipple with a smaller hole (see Baby Foods, Infant Formula, p. 738).

CHILDREN

Children are not little adults; a child's body acts and reacts differently from that of a teenager or adult. Illnesses are often important milestones in a child's development, as the immune system practices distinguishing between "self" and "other."

The adage "everything in its own time" holds just as true in childhood as in other phases of life. Although a child's development is considered "normal" when his or her behavior conforms to that of most other children with undisturbed development during a specified time period, this doesn't mean deviations are necessarily "abnormal." Of course, they might also indicate a disorder.

Your child's physical development is monitored by the pediatrician during "well baby" exams and regular childhood checkups (see p. 591). Emotional development is harder to measure. Some behaviors are closely linked to certain stages of development; if they outlast the appropriate stage significantly, they should be discussed with a specialist.

DEVELOPMENTAL MILESTONES

During the first year of life, a baby gains its primary experiences of the surrounding world. It learns to touch the environment, feel it, see it, hear it, move around in it. It reacts, and expresses these reactions. There is no precise road map for this stage of development; various skills can develop at different times and rates, in various sequences. You should observe your child carefully, and consult a pediatrician at the first sign of delayed (or missing) development. The earlier a developmental delay is detected, the more easily it can often be rectified. The following developmental abilities can help you determine what your child should be able to do at what stage.

By 3 Months

The baby should be able to kick vigorously, raise its head 90 degrees while lying on its stomach, play with its own fingers, hold an object for a short time, track with its eyes, move its head toward the source of a sound, notice when you speak to it and, possibly, smile.

By 6 Months

The baby should be able to turn over from its stomach onto its back and vice versa, grasp and play with its toes, play with blocks or other toys, shake a rattle. The baby should be able to make four different kinds of sounds, react when called, and stretch out its arms to be picked up when it sees someone coming.

By 9 Months

The baby should be able to crawl forward, pull itself up on a piece of furniture, stand holding onto something, spend long periods of time sitting on the floor playing, throw objects, pick things up using thumb and forefinger, shake a little box containing rattling objects, knock two blocks together when you demonstrate, and distinguish between familiar people and strangers.

By 12 Months

The baby should be able to walk with assistance, climb low steps, take paper wrappings off something or find a toy hidden from its sight, scrawl something on a piece of paper using a pencil, know his or her own name, speak three words clearly and follow simple commands. If a child hasn't developed certain skills by a certain time, this doesn't necessarily indicate a developmental delay; discuss it with your pediatrician.

SEXUAL DEVELOPMENT

Sexuality does not begin with puberty; people are born as sexual beings. Babies enjoy the sensual experiences of breastfeeding and stroking, the delights of being bathed, cuddled, and rocked. The freedom to discover one's own body and explore one's genitalia are necessary steps toward sexual maturity, and predispose a person to enjoy a healthy, fulfilling sexuality from childhood through old age.

Small children want to explore their bodies and know no taboos. Such behavior may be shocking to adults who are the products of repressed upbringing. Girls, in particular, tend to be discouraged from sexual play; nevertheless, anyone who overtly or covertly prevents a child from such natural behavior is interfering with the child's sexual health.

Adult-imposed strictures regarding toileting and personal hygiene are often based on the idea that bodily functions are "dirty"; this can also affect the child's developing sexuality.

Around kindergarten age, children discover that boys and girls are different. Role-playing, including playing doctor and playing house, helps them experiment with gender roles. During this time they also begin to see their parents as sexual beings. How they experience father's masculinity and mother's femininity has a significant impact on their own sexuality.

Locked bathroom doors, "prudishness" on the part of the child, and the keeping of bodily functions secret often appear around the age of 10. This behavior is the child's natural protection against a sexuality that is not yet appropriate. If this boundary is not respected, the child will be psychologically damaged.

Many children masturbate before puberty, which often disturbs adults, who may overreact or forbid such activity. However, together with curiosity about—and perhaps touching—children of the other or same sex, this is a natural stage of sexual maturation. Repressing a child's sexual needs during this period will only lead to insecurity. On the other hand, talking openly to older children about sexuality will help them to feel better about themselves and realize they are normal, thus paving the way for healthy sexual development.

Sexual Abuse

Sexual abuse is found in about 6 percent of confirmed reports of maltreatment. However, it may occur much more often. The perpetrator is almost always somebody in a position to care for, nurture, protect, or act as a role model for the child.

In almost half of cases, the child knows the abuser, who may be a caregiver, teacher, clergyperson or athleteic coach. The incidence among stepfathers is about five times higher than among natural fathers.

The consequences of such abused trust are devastating. External injuries to the sex organs will heal, but the lasting damage to the child's psyche will be felt throughout the child's life and in all his or her subsequent relationships, intimate or not (see Counseling and Psychotherapy, p. 697).

BED-WETTING

Symptoms
The term "bed-wetting" should only be used if a child over the age of 5 repeatedly and unconsciously wets the bed while sleeping. If younger children are wetting the bed, parents may simply need to let go of their agenda and put the child back in diapers at night until he or she is developmentally ready to stay dry.

Causes
Emotional problems are frequently the catalyst for bed-wetting: family, a new sibling, problems at school, or the desire to "be a baby" again.

Bed-wetting also frequently indicates a urinary tract infection (see Cystitis, p. 418) or previously undetected diabetes (see p. 483).

Who's at Risk
Rigorous toilet training can turn the child's bodily functions into a major issue.

Orders, threats, and punishment only create anxiety. You can't force a child to defecate or urinate. You may just cause the child to regress.

Possible After-effects and Complications
A child who wets the bed is usually pretty unhappy about it; lecturing or punishing the child will cause his or her self-esteem to sink even lower. This can transform relatively benign bed-wetting into a vicious circle.

Prevention
Patience and care are the prerequisites for not turning toilet-training into a battle between parents and child. Have faith: The child will eventually decide on his or her own that he or she has had enough of bulky diapers. If you can regard a full potty as a gift instead of the spoils of war, you will save yourself a lot of trouble during toilet training. Also, children naturally want to imitate adults, so seeing their parents or older siblings going to the bathroom helps them to want to do the same.

When to Seek Medical Advice
Seek help if:
— A previously toilet-trained child regresses
— A child still wets himself regularly after the age of 4
— You suspect a bladder infection or other disease

Self-Help
Small rewards for "dry" nights, and a calendar highlighting them, can boost the child's self-esteem. Allow for accidents; avoid making much of them.

Alarm devices and similar transitional measures should be avoided because they reinforce the idea that there is still a problem.

Withholding drinks in the evening or waking the child in the middle of the night do not work.

Treatment
If the bed-wetting mushrooms into a problem involving the whole family, counseling is advisable (see Couples and Family Therapy, p. 697). Bed-wetting is a classic theme in child therapy.

Treatment with Medications
The prescription of medication—usually an antidepressant—for bed-wetting is considered by pediatricians and child psychologists as a last (and usually unsuccessful) resort. In about a third of cases the drug works temporarily, but many children are wetting their beds again within 3 months. Relatively common side effects are a dry mouth and circulatory and vision disorders.

Desmopressin (DDAVP) works very reliably, but only while being used.

SLEEP DISORDERS

Symptoms
Every child needs to establish his or her own sleep patterns. Some babies sleep for 10 hours straight by the age of 6 weeks; others still aren't sleeping through the night at 9 months. This is a problem only for the person who needs to get up and calm the baby; for the baby, waking at night is completely normal.

Older children sometimes lie awake for long periods, tossing and turning restlessly.

Actual sleep disorders are rare in children, however. It's pretty normal for children, even very young ones, not to want to go to bed or fall asleep.

It should also cause no great concern if children sometimes wake during the night, as happens often with 3- to 8-year-olds. Some 5- to 12-year-olds are even occasional sleepwalkers: They wander around, disoriented and clumsy, yet cause themselves no harm.

Causes
Breastfeeding infants wake at night mainly from hunger; prolongued, heartbreaking wails can also mean "I'm all alone—come pick me up!"

Bona fide sleep disorders, like chronic nightmares, are almost always the result of traumatic experiences which are causing the child unexpressed anguish.

Who's at Risk
Children suffering from separation anxiety or insecurity because of new, unfamiliar surroundings or other circumstances may have a variety of sleep problems.

Possible Aftereffects and Complications
A child's sleep problems can profoundly affect family life and the relationship between parents or adult partners.

Prevention
Small children in particular suffer from separation anxiety. Children need security and the sense that they can count on their guardians.

When to Seek Medical Advice
Seek help if sleep disturbances are frequent and you are unable to determine their cause or do anything about them. If possible, consult with a doctor who knows your child and family well.

Self-Help
As long as your partner has no objection, let the child sleep in bed with you. Don't worry that you'll crush or suffocate an infant: Adults quickly learn to be alert to a child's slightest signal, even during deep sleep. Your baby will let you know by kicking if he's uncomfortable.

If this is not possible, the job of night watchman needs to be shared by both partners. Otherwise the household will soon be out of kilter, with someone (usually the mother) perpetually overtired and exhausted.

Treatment

Locating the source of the child's anxiety and resolving the problem sometimes calls for family therapy (see Counseling and Psychotherapy, p. 697). Giving medication is justifiable only in extreme cases. Unfortunately, although doctors are aware that psychopharmaceuticals, including sedatives and tranquilizers, can be addictive, they are often reluctant to disappoint parents who are just longing for a good night's sleep.

LEARNING DISORDERS

Symptoms

Disturbances that can lead to learning disorders are often first detected at school age. A child may have difficulty perceiving an image or sound correctly, retaining or remembering information, or recognizing relationships. Undiagnosed problems in the sense organs themselves may be at fault: It may become apparent that the child hasn't been seeing or hearing properly for a long time.

Some so-called learning disorders may actually be behavioral disorders such as difficulty concentrating (see Hyperactivity, below), communicating, or setting personal boundaries.

Dyslexia: This is a congenital condition in which, despite normal vision, a child cannot read or understand words or sentences. Particularly when confronted with unfamiliar words, the child transposes letters, leaves some out, or creates a whole new word. Dyslexics often lag several years behind their peers in reading skills, although they usually perform well in most other subjects and most are of normal or above average intelligence. This is why the disorder is often detected only when the child is in the second or third grade.

Causes

Any physical or psychological disorder can lead to a learning disability.

Dyslexia is probably a brain function disorder that hampers the decoding of graphic symbols.

Who's at Risk

Dyslexia often runs in families with speech disabilities.

Boys are affected more often than girls.

Possible Aftereffects and Complications

An unrecognized learning disability can present constant problems for a child in school. As a result, going to school may be fraught with anxiety, and behavioral problems may develop.

Prevention

Carefully monitor the progress of the growing child. Take advantage of early screening and diagnostic tests (see p. 591).

When to Seek Medical Advice

Seek help if a learning disorder is suspected. If possible, consult a doctor that knows the child and family well.

Treatment

Finding the source of a learning disability requires careful physiological and psychological examinations. First of all, hearing and vision problems should be ruled out. The child's strengths should be emphasized, and help should be offered for overcoming his or her weaknesses. This might include special learning programs or behavioral therapy (see p. 700).

Dyslexia: A special program (phonics) teaches reading by emphasizing hearing skills. Until around age 10 this is often successful in helping children overcome dyslexia.

Treatment with Medications

Drugs that allegedly boost concentration or learning capacity are mostly worthless and dangerous, as well as potentially addictive. Children medicated for learning disabilities learn that taking a pill, rather than developing a useful problem-solving strategy, is an acceptable response to adversity. More than one drug addict has started out this way.

HYPERACTIVITY

Symptoms

Hyperactivity is usually already noticeable by age 2 or 3. Hyperactive children are extremely lively and incapable of occupying themselves for long periods with a toy. If they don't get their way, they quickly get angry. They don't get along well with other children.

School-age hyperactive children are unable to concentrate and exhibit unruly behavior.

Causes

Theories on the causes of hyperactivity abound, but none has yet been proved.

Who's at Risk

Boys are at higher risk of hyperactivity than girls.

Possible Aftereffects and Complications

Hyperactive children often have serious difficulty getting along with playmates. This may be why they are prone to both aggressiveness and depression. Relations with their families are also often difficult, causing behavioral problems to intensify.

Uncontrolled behavior often puts these children into dangerous situations, such as playing on a busy street, climbing too high, etc.

Prevention

Not possible.

When to Seek Medical Advice

Seek help if the hyperactivity becomes a burden for the child, the class, and/or the family.

Self-Help

A low-phosphate diet has been touted as a cure for hyperactivity, but its benefits are unproven. The most important thing parents and teachers can do is to realize, and reinforce, that hyperactive children aren't being "bad": They simply can't help their behavior.

Treatment

Family therapy is advisable, to teach parents how to deal appropriately with a "problem" child, and teach the child how to cope better with his environment.

The psychostimulant drug Ritalin is often prescribed to combat attention-deficit syndromes, but its use is controversial.

Special diets or megadoses of vitamins are useless and can often be dangerous.

AUTISM

Symptoms

Autism becomes evident in a baby's first year of life. The child makes no contact with his or her environment: The child makes no eye contact, shows no need for physical contact, and his or her speech development is disturbed or absent entirely. Idiosyncratic behavior may develop: Adherence to strict rituals, repetitive behaviors, constant playing with the same objects.

Causes

It is presumed that brain damage, either congenital or damage sustained in the early stages of life may be the cause, resulting in the child's inability to distinguish between people and inanimate objects.

Who's at Risk

Boys are at higher risk of autism than girls.

Possible Aftereffects and Complications

Autism can develop to varying degrees: Some children are of below average intelligence and need special care throughout their lives. Autistic children of average or above-average intelligence can grow up to be functioning, independent adults provided they receive the right help.

In rare cases, aging adults suffering from autism can develop psychoses (see p. 200).

Prevention

Not possible.

When to Seek Medical Advice

Seek help if autism is suspected.

Self-Help

Not possible.

Treatment

Both parents and children should enter behavioral therapy. Speech therapy should begin as early as possible.

Preventive Measures

ACCIDENTS AND INJURY PREVENTION

Children are especially accident-prone. They're active and like to explore; and their environments are becoming increasingly hazardous. Infants and toddlers are frequently injured in falls; toddlers are often attracted to kitchens and bathrooms, where they are the most common victims of burns from hot water, hot plates, irons, etc.

Despite all the warning labels required by industry codes, increasing numbers of children are poisoned in the home, especially by medications and cleaning products (see Poisoning, p. 708).

As soon as children reach school age, their proneness toward outdoor accidents rises, especially those connected with automobiles.

Accidents to infants can be prevented by taking necessary precautions and protective measures. For older children, the best precaution is developing the child's own capacity to evaluate danger. General pronouncements and prohibitions are meaningless to children if you don't bother to explain them. In the long run, children are much more likely to obey your wishes if they can understand them. Understanding the presence of risks will lead to the child learning to gauge risks for himself. Nevertheless, your home and play areas should be childproofed as completely as possible, with obvious hazards removed. Remember that children are children and should not be expected to act or reason like adults.

Early Detection/ Screening

Many developmental disorders or diseases can be prevented if detected in time and treated properly. This is the idea behind the standard newborn screening exams done on all newborns prior to discharge from the hospital.

"WELL BABY" EXAMS

The most important monitoring of your baby is performed by you—the parent—as you observe your child closely. If you suspect a developmental delay or anomaly, don't hesitate to discuss it with your pediatrician. Time may heal all ills in some cases, but if you wait too long you may be passing up the opportunity for early treatment, thus inadvertently hurting your child.

What's Being Checked

The first "well baby" exam takes place right after birth and determines how the baby has come through child-

Preventing accidents
Infants
— Never leave an infant unsupervised on a changing table, bed, or sofa.
— Keep small objects and anything that could be swallowed well out of reach.
Toddlers and small children
— Childproof stairs and windows with gates and window guards.
— Keep anything that can be climbed on away from windows.
— Don't leave heavy objects or containers with hot contents on tables within a child's reach. Be careful with tablecloths: Children often use them to pull themselves up.
— Childproof all electrical outlets.
— Never leave detergents, cleansers, paints, lacquer, alcohol (including liqueur-filled chocolates or sweets) or medication unlocked, and especially not stored on a low shelf.
— Never leave cigarettes, ashtrays, and matches or lighters on coffee tables or low surfaces. Keep all smoking paraphernalia out of reach of children.
— Don't plant anything toxic (laburnum, yew, deadly nightshade, oleander) in your garden.
Kindergarten and school-aged kids
— Start teaching traffic rules early and set a good example. Follow up at home by playing "stop, look and listen."
— Never leave children unsupervised near swimming or wading pools, ponds, or brooks, unless they are excellent swimmers. Children should wear water wings or life preservers; inflatable rings won't do the trick.

birth and whether any birth defects are evident. Weight, length, and head circumference are measured. Newborn screening blood tests will check for certain latent metabolic diseases, such as phenylketonuria (PKU), which affects one out of every 6,000 to 10,000 children. Untreated, PKU can lead to mental retardation. This can be avoided by following a strict diet for 8 to 10 years which omits foods known to cause the disease. After age 10, brain development is mostly complete, and the diet need not be followed as strictly.

The second exam is performed 3 to 10 days after birth. Again, the doctor looks for any injuries resulting from the birth process, searches for anomalies and checks on the child's physical development. The function of the nervous system is checked by testing the child's relexes.

The third exam takes place from 3 to 4 weeks after birth. Thereafter, during the first year the baby is examined every 2 to 3 months, then semiannually, and after age 3 annually if there are no discovered problems. On these occasions the pediatrician assesses the child's overall physiological and psychological development. It's best if the same pediatrician performs all the exams, so that he or she can better gauge overall development.

Weight and Height

As part of these early diagnostic tests, the child is measured and weighed. Although children are growing constantly, exceptional growth spurts usually take place in the first year, then between ages 5 and 7, and finally during puberty.

The doctor records the child's weight and height and checks it against a general growth curve. If a growth disorder is suspected, a hand X ray can show the developmental stage of the bones.

DEVELOPMENTAL DISLOCATION OF THE HIP

Normally, the head of the femur, or hip bone, lies comfortably in the hip socket.

In hip dysplasia, or developmental dislocation of the hip, the bone and socket don't fit together well. In extreme cases, the hip is functionally dislocated: The head of the femur continually slips out of the socket.

Symptoms

Hip dysplasia is often detected only by early screening. One sign of this may be abduction difficulty: If a healthy infant lies on its back, the legs fall to either side; in an anomaly of the hip, the legs are held more closely to the body.

Hip subluxation/dislocation: The leg on the side of the malformed hip may appear shorter, and the creases between and under the buttocks may not be symmetrical.

All these signs can easily go unnoticed in an infant, especially if both hip joints are simultaneously affected.

Causes

The causes of developmental hip dislocation are not known.

Who's at Risk

Two to 4 percent of all children are born with hip dysplasia. Hip anomalies are especially common
— In breech deliveries

Growth Charts

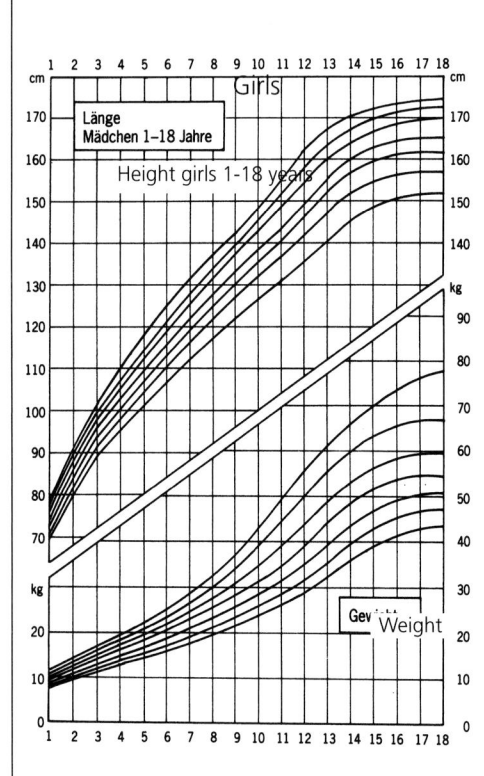

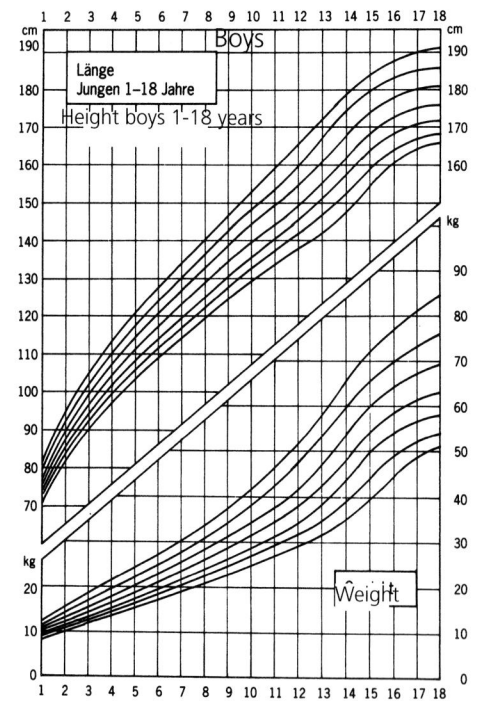

The lines give information about average growth: half the children will be larger at any point in time, and half will be smaller. It is only abnormal if your child's growth is more than 2 lines from the middle one. It should then be investigated by your health care provider. It is also meaningful to note if there is a change in curves, that is if your child was always tall, but now is only of average height. This may indicate a growth problem. By comparing the height and weight curves it is possible to determine whether a child is under-or-overweight.

— If the condition runs in the family
— In children with malformations or anomalies of the spine, legs or feet
Girls are six times as likely to be affected as boys.

Possible After-effects and Complications
If left untreated, hip dysplasia can lead to difficulties with walking. Even a mild hip anomaly can affect walking so significantly that arthritis soon develops.

Prevention
Early treatment is essential.

When to Seek Medical Advice
Seek help if a hip dislocation is suspected, at which point the child should be referred to an orthopedist. Ultrasound can diagnose dysplasia in a newborn; There is no scientific evidence that ultrasound hurts the baby. Because such a diagnosis can be tricky, this should be performed only by a specialist.

If this condition is diagnosed early, treatment can be shortened considerably. In children who have undergone long-term hip treatment, follow-up X rays will determine the success of the treatment.

Self-Help
Not possible.

Treatment
During treatment, the child's legs are placed in a specific harness so they splay apart. The head of the femur is pressed into the socket and secured, ensuring that ball and socket develop normally. This treatment must continue until the joint is completely formed. The devices are adapted to allow the child to learn to crawl, and must be worn around the clock. In some cases, casts need to be applied, usually in the hospital.

If none of these interventions is successful, or if they are begun too late, the hip joint must be corrected through surgery.

UNDESCENDED TESTES

Symptoms
During the final weeks of pregnancy, the testes in a male baby descend from the abdomen into the scrotum. In a normally developed newborn, both testes can be felt in the scrotum. In case of an undescended testis, one or both gonads can't be felt, or can be felt only at the entrance of the inguinal canal.

Causes
A narrow inguinal canal may prevent the testes from descending to the scrotum. In other cases, the testes don't respond to the hormonal command to move into the scrotum, or the hormones are insufficient.

Evidently, hormonelike toxins can also impair the development of the gonads in the placenta (see Causes of Infertility, p. 559).

Who's at Risk
This condition is found in around 5 percent of newborn boys. In some, it corrects itself on its own during the first few months of life.

Over the past 40 years, the incidence of newborns with congenital defects of the urogenital tract has tripled. It is suspected that environmental toxins are the cause.

Possible Aftereffects and Complications
If the testes have not descended after two to three years, the higher ambient temperature of the abdomen can damage the sperm, resulting in possible infertility.

Moreover, men born with this condition have 20 times the normal chance of developing testicular cancer (see p. 533). The risk diminishes if the testes are surgically brought into the scrotum early on.

Prevention
Not possible.

When to Seek Medical Advice
Seek help if one or both testes cannot be felt, or if they can be felt only in the inguinal canal and it hurts to have them pulled downward.

Self-Help
Not possible.

Treatment
Treatment should occur after the child is a year old.

The testes are surgically brought down into the scrotum. There is some risk that the seminal tissue may be crushed during the procedure.

PHIMOSIS

Symptoms
In phimosis, the foreskin of the uncircumcised penis is pulled so tightly over the head that it cannot retract properly over the glans. This may cause fluid to build up between glans and foreskin, occasionally causing pain when urinating.

Causes
The condition can be congenital or develop as a result of inflammation or scarring.

Who's at Risk
In newborns and infants it's fairly normal for part of the foreskin to be attached to the glans. By age 2 or 3 at the latest, however, the foreskin can usually be pulled back easily.

Possible Aftereffects and Complications
Phimosis in adults can cause pain, impeding erection. It also increases the risk of penile cancer, since proper hygiene is difficult due to the tight foreskin, and secretions can collect under it.

Prevention
Never try to pull back the foreskin forcibly in newborns or infants. Though this is often done in an attempt to stretch the foreskin gently, it can actually cause small fissures that lead to scarring, and ultimately to phimosis.

When to Seek Medical Advice
Seek help if
— A male infant has trouble urinating
— You suspect an inflammation (redness, swelling, pain—especially when urinating)
— By age 3 the foreskin doesn't retract over the glans

Self-Help
Not possible.

Treatment
If phimosis is caused by scarring, it is occasionally possible to correct the condition surgically. However, generally circumcision is recommended.

Early Childhood Diseases

NEWBORN JAUNDICE

Symptoms
Many newborns have yellowish skin during the first few days of life; this "newborn jaundice" slowly disappears after 5 to 7 days. In nursing infants it may last a bit longer, but this is no reason for the mother to stop breastfeeding.

Causes
During the first few days of life, the infant's body breaks down red blood cells. The liver can't yet quickly process the bile pigment (bilirubin) that's produced, resulting in jaundice.

Who's at Risk
All newborns have mild jaundice. Severe cases can be caused by incompatibility of the blood group of mother and child, or an infection contracted after birth.

Possible Aftereffects and Complications
Mild newborn jaundice in newborns is not dangerous. However, if blood levels of bilirubin exceed a certain limit, brain damage can result.

Prevention
If the incompatibility between mother's and baby's blood groups is detected prenatally, it can be treated.

When to Seek Medical Advice
Seek help if the child develops a yellowish skin color. The doctor can determine whether this results from blood group incompatibility or infection. The doctor checks the newborn's bilirubin level. In severe cases of newborn jaundice, additional daily blood tests are necessary.

Self-Help
Self-help is not necessary in mild cases, and not possible in severe cases.

Treatment

In severe cases the child is placed under an ultraviolet light (phototherapy). Ultraviolet rays transform the yellow bilirubin pigment into a water-soluble substance, which is then processed and excreted by the kidneys.

Sometimes giving the child glucose intravenously is enough to hasten the processing of the pigment.

COLIC

Symptoms

Symptoms of colic often appear during the first 3 months of life. Especially after a meal, but also at night, the infant may cry loudly and appear inconsolable. Often the child's belly is distended.

Causes

The causes of colic are not known for certain, but probably bubbles of air become trapped in the infant's gastrointestinal tract when he or she gulps milk or formula very quickly. Additives in infant formula (see p. 738) may also be responsible.

Who's at Risk

Not known.

Possible Aftereffects and Complications

While screaming with colic, the child may swallow yet more air, worsening the colic.

Colic is not fun, both for infant and family, but it is also not dangerous and usually clears up by the third or fourth month. It can be dangerous only if rare, serious gastrointestinal conditions (such as twisted bowel) are misdiagnosed as colic, and thus go undetected and untreated.

Prevention

Not possible.

When to Seek Medical Advice

Seek help if additional symptoms appear, such as fever, problems in drinking, vomiting, constipation, stool that is bloody or contains mucus, or if the child is seriously ill and has a greyish cast to the skin.

Self-Help

— Burp the baby after mealtimes.

— Feed the child smaller quantities, more frequently.
— If bottle-feeding, use a nipple with slightly larger hole.
— Gently massage the baby's belly.

Treatment

No reliable treatment for colic has yet been discovered.

THRUSH, YEAST (CANDIDAL) DIAPER RASH

Symptoms

Thrush is seen as white patches on the mucous membrane of the mouth which, unlike milk residue, can't be wiped away. Severe cases can interfere with feeding. Oral thrush often clears up after a few days. As diaper rash, yeast is seen as fine blisters that grow and eventually slough off, leaving the skin reddened and sore.

Causes

Yeast fungi.

Who's at Risk

The risk of these infections is increased in babies
—Who are undergoing antibiotic treatment
—Whose mothers have vaginal yeast infections at the time of birth
—Whose pacifiers and bottle nipples aren't disinfected properly

Possible Aftereffects and Complications

Oral thrush is dangerous only in children with congenital immune weakness.

Prevention

Thoroughly wash a newborn's pacifier and bottle nipples, and sterilize them once a day.

When to Seek Medical Advice

Seek help if yeast infection is suspected.

Self-Help

While the child is being treated for thrush, sterilize pacifier and nipples several times a day. Thrush is no reason to stop breastfeeding; the mother can use the same medication on her nipples that she's swabbing into the baby's mouth. Anything that prevents a moist environment in the diaper area will help heal diaper rash: Keep the baby's bottom naked as much as possible, and use cloth diapers without rubber pants instead of disposables.

Treatment

After feeding, the child's mouth is swabbed with an antifungal medication, such as nystatin. There's no need to worry if the baby happens to swallow some. For diaper rash, nystatin, or another antifungal, is prescribed in cream form.

CRADLE CAP

Symptoms

Cradle cap usually appears in babies during the first 3 months of age. The skin on the scalp and in the creases of the body becomes flaky, oily and itchy.

Causes

The causes of cradle cap are not yet known.

Who's at Risk

Not known.

Possible Aftereffects and Complications

Areas that the baby scratches can become infected. Itching can disturb the child's sleep (and therefore the sleep of at least one parent, as well). Cradle cap can be a precursor of eczema (see p. 272).

Prevention

Not possible.

When to Seek Medical Advice

Seek help if itching and rash are severe.

Self-Help

Dress baby in cotton clothing; relieve itching by applying cool, damp compresses, and adding moisturizers to baby's bath. Oil may also be applied to baby's scalp and hair.

Treatment

Usually, no treatment is necessary; cradle cap disappears on its own.

CROUP

Symptoms

One form of croup is a sign of diphtheria, the other is a viral disease. It's the latter form that children develop either after coming down with a mild cold, or without warning out of the blue. The illness usually starts at night with a barking cough and hoarseness. Because the airway is constricted, breathing becomes more and more difficult, and the sensation of suffocation causes panic.

The child looks anxious and acts restless, and has a pounding heart. By morning the symptoms have usually subsided, to be followed the next day by a pronounced cold with cough and fever.

Causes

This type of croup is usually caused by viruses. Air pollution contributes to croup, as does breathing secondhand smoke in confined spaces.

Who's at Risk

The risk of croup is increased in children who
— Are exposed to secondhand smoke
— Live in heavily polluted areas, especially in the winter (see Smog, p. 787)

Possible Aftereffects and Complications

Severe cases of croup can cause respiratory distress and exhaustion, necessitating hospital treatment.

Prevention

To reduce the chance of croup in your baby
— Spend as much time as possible in areas with clean air (mountains, seaside, away from major roadways and industrial smokestacks).
— Don't smoke at home.

When to Seek Medical Advice

Seek help if the child has had an attack of croup.
Get help immediately if
— The child's voice sounds muffled
— The child has severe throat pain or difficulty swallowing
— A high fever develops
— Respiratory distress does not improve within an hour, despite treatment
— The child turns blue

Self-Help
— Sit with baby near an open window: Cool, damp air will often alleviate symptoms. If you have doubts about outside air quality, hang damp towels around the room, or sit in the bathroom with the shower running.
— Soothe your baby by speaking calmly and handling him or her gently, to give a sense of safety, security, and comfort. Keep the baby with you so he or she won't feel alone. Anxiety and crying only increase the need for air.

Treatment
Corticosteroid products shrink swelling in the mucous membranes and are highly effective, but long-term use can cause serious side effects (see Corticosteroids, p. 665). They are available in oral form for use at home.

In severe cases the child should be treated in the hospital with nebulizers and corticosteroids to reduce the swelling.

EPIGLOTTITIS

Symptoms
Epiglottitis is an inflammation and swelling of the epiglottis that occurs almost exclusively in early childhood. The epiglottis and surrounding area swell quickly and can completely block the airways. Epiglottitis usually starts with a high fever and sore throat. Symptoms include muffled voice, difficulty swallowing, and drooling. It can quickly lead to respiratory failure.

Causes
Epiglottitis is caused by bacteria, especially *Haemophilus influenza* type B (HIB).

Who's at Risk
Children aged 3 to 6 contract epiglottitis most frequently.

Possible Aftereffects and Complications
Epiglottitis can quickly become life-threatening because of the danger of suffocation.

Prevention
Immunizing for HIB protects against the pathogens that usually cause epiglottitis (see p. 674).

When to Seek Medical Advice
Immediately: Take the child to the hospital if the child has high fever, muffled speech, difficulty swallowing, and gasps loudly when breathing in.

Self-Help
Not possible.

Treatment
Epiglottitis must be treated as soon as possible with intravenous antibiotics. Fluids should also be given intravenously if swallowing difficulties have caused dehydration. In extreme cases the child is intubated—a tube is inserted in the windpipe—and kept for a few days on an artificial respirator.

BRONCHIOLITIS

Symptoms
Bronchiolitis usually starts with a mild cold. After a day or two, coughing starts, often in fits. The baby breathes rapidly and wheezes, with a whistling sound. Breathing can be so constricted that respiratory distress results and the skin starts to turn blue.

Causes
Swelling in the bronchi is usually caused by viruses. Because a baby's bronchi are much smaller than an adult's, this leads very swiftly to respiratory distress. As with asthma (see p. 307), it is extremely likely that airborne irritants and allergens can trigger this condition.

Who's at Risk
Children are most frequently affected between the ages of 6 months and 3 years.

Possible Aftereffects and Complications
Some children with chronic bronchiolitis eventually develop asthma.

Because breathing is so difficult for babies with bronchiolitis, they tire easily and often get insufficient fluids. Dehydration worsens the symptoms. In certain cases, hospital treatment is necessary.

Prevention

In children who suffer recurring bronchiolitis it is especially important to keep the house free of tobacco smoke and other toxins (see Healthy Living, p. 772). At the first sign of a cold, you can give a nebulizer treatment to a child prone to getting bronchiolitis.

When to Seek Medical Advice

Seek help if:

— The child wheezes during a coughing fit.

— The coughing is accompanied by fever.

An X ray and blood tests may need to be taken to determine whether pneumonia has developed. *Get the child to a hospital (preferably a children's hospital) immediately if*

— The child has respiratory distress, or his or her skin turns blue, or the child won't drink enough

— The child seems to be seriously ill

Self-Help

Keep the child as calm as possible. Crying can cause stress and worsen breathing difficulties.

Using a room humidifier can benefit children with recurring bronchiolitis.

The child should always drink as much as possible.

Treatment

In cases of severe respiratory distress, humidified, oxygenated air should be administered, and the child should be rehydrated by means of intravenous fluids. Nebulizer treatments with bronchodilating medication, such as abluterol can help.

CYSTIC FIBROSIS

Symptoms

The first sign of cystic fibrosis (CF) is often constant, heavy perspiration, with the sweat or skin tasting especially salty.

Respiratory Tract Symptoms

Children with CF often had severe bronchitis as infants and develop chronic bronchitis over the years, with cough, heavy mucus production, and constant shortness of breath. Frequently recurring pneumonia often develops as well.

Digestive Tract Symptoms

Children with CF eat and drink sufficiently, yet their growth and development is poor. Their stool is frequently thin, light in color, shiny, and especially foul-smelling. As a result of protein imbalance, they may retain water in the body.

Causes

Cystic fibrosis is hereditary.

Who's at Risk

Cystic fibrosis is a metabolic disorder and is fairly common.

Possible Aftereffects and Complications

Although years of regular daily treatment can make the child's condition bearable, it may place tremendous strain on both child and family.

Possible Respiratory Aftereffects and Complications

If the child has trouble coughing up phlegm from the bronchi, respiratory distress may develop. Phlegm enables the growth of pathogens that can cause pneumonia.

Over the course of years the child's lungs change: Blebs may develop and the alveoli may shrink (see Emphysema, p. 309). Changes in the lungs can repeatedly lead to pneumothorax (see p. 314) and compromise the heart.

Possible Digestive Aftereffects and Complications

The secretions of the pancreas are unusually thick in children with CF, impairing digestion, which can lead to undernourishment and stunted growth. In some children, the meconium (the first bowel movement after delivery) is so thick that it causes an intestinal blockage that may require surgery.

Prevention

Cystic fibrosis cannot yet be prevented. Early detection—by means of a sweat test to analyze the child's salt content— and prompt treatment can, however, make the patient's life easier. If a family member is known to have CF, parents should have their newborn checked for the disease.

When to Seek Medical Advice

Seek help if:
— A family member has CF
— Symptoms are present

Self-Help

Self-help is not possible without instruction from a health-care professional.

Treatment

Cystic fibrosis is a disease that lasts for life. Symptoms can be alleviated only with close cooperation between child, parents, and doctors. Children need constant professional treatment and care, preferably at a center that specializes in this disease.

Treatment of Respiratory Symptoms

Thumping the chest several times a day, and inhaling humidified air (aerosol therapy), can help loosen mucus so it can be coughed up. Older children can help themselves using postural drainage and other special techniques.
Important: See a doctor any time general health deteriorates, breathing becomes difficult, or an infection arises.

Treatment of Digestive Symptoms

Eat a diet high in protein and calories. Infants sometimes need a special formula. Cystic fibrosis patients must also take digestive enzymes with every meal, usually in the form of many tablets to swallow at once.

Cystic fibrosis is one of the few diseases that requires constant intake of vitamin supplements. These provide sufficient doses of the fat-soluble vitamins the child's CF-ridden body can't absorb adequately on its own.

LACTOSE INTOLERANCE

See also Allergies, p. 353, 360.

Symptoms

Children with lactose intolerance digest poorly and vomit frequently. The stool occasionally contains blood.

Causes

Lactose intolerance results when the mucous lining of the digestive tract will not tolerate the protein in cow's milk. This condition may be congenital, or may develop following an intestinal infection.

Who's at Risk

The risk of lactose intolerance is increased in
— Children who have had a severe gastrointestinal infection with diarrhea and vomiting.
— Children from families with a history of lactose intolerance, who are fed lactose-containing infant formula very early in life. The risk is not elevated in children who do not receive lactose-containing formula until later in life.

Possible Aftereffects and Complications

In rare instances, prolonged diarrhea can dehydrate the child and lead to digestive disorders and malnutrition, necessitating intravenous feeding in a hospital.

Prevention

Breastfeed for as long as possible. If the mother can't produce enough milk at first, supplement the baby's diet with hypoallergenic formula. If mother's milk isn't an option, hypoallergenic formula (Alimentum, Nutramigen) may reduce the risk of allergy.

When to Seek Medical Advice

Seek help if symptoms are present.

Self-Help

The child should completely avoid cow's milk. About a third of children who can't tolerate cow's milk protein are also unable to tolerate soy milk. A custom-developed diet needs to be instituted in these cases.

Treatment

Treatment of lactose intolerance consists of the restricted diet mentioned above.

GASTROINTESTINAL INFECTIONS/ GASTROENTERITIS

Symptoms

As in adults, infections of the gastrointestinal tract in children cause diarrhea and vomiting, and occasionally fever. However, infants and young children often get far sicker than adults because they suffer dehydration much more quickly. They often react to the fluid loss caused by diarrhea and vomiting by rejecting any and all fluids.

Causes

Gastrointestinal infections are caused mostly by viruses transmitted through contact with feces or saliva.

Who's at Risk

Children are at increased risk for a gastrointestinal tract infection if someone in the community (family, kindergarten, or day care) has one.

Possible Aftereffects and Complications

Dehydration in young children, especially infants, can have serious ramifications, sometimes ending in death.

Prevention

If someone in the baby's environment has a gastrointestinal tract infection, hygiene is very important. Wash hands thoroughly before and after changing the baby. Keep pacifiers and bottle nipples separate from those of other children.

When to Seek Medical Advice

Seek help if:
— A child with diarrhea isn't drinking enough liquids
— Diarrhea persists for longer than 3 days
— The child vomits constantly over a period of 12 hours
— The child vomits after every effort to get him or her to drink
— An infant does not urinate for longer than 4 to 6 hours
— The child's skin is slack and does not return to its original position after being pinched lightly between thumb and forefinger
— The child's eyes appear sunken
— The child appears seriously ill

Self-Help

Water and electrolytes lost through diarrhea and vomiting must be replaced. Have the child drink as much as possible, as often as possible. Follow the recipe in the box above for an electrolyte solution. Commercial products, such as Pedialyte, are also available, though costly.

If the child has an appetite, feed a normal diet. Rice, applesauce, banana, saltines, dry toast, or broth are all easily digested, restorative foods. Expensive prepared foods and formulas are not necessary.

> **Rehydration Electrolyte Solution**
> Dissolve in 1 liter of boiled water:
> 2.5 gram baking soda
> 3.5 gram table salt
> 1.5 gram potassium chloride
> 20 gram dextrose

Treatment

Severely dehydrated and weakened children must be rehydrated intravenously in a hospital setting. Medications to stop the vomiting and/or diarrhea are unnecessary.

Antibiotics should be prescribed only for seriously ill children whose gastrointestinal illness is caused by bacteria.

MEASLES

Symptoms

The incubation period of measles—from exposure to the manifestations of the disease—takes 8 to 14 days. Usually, measles starts with cold symptoms, a cough, conjunctivitis, and a fever of about 102°F. Three to 4 days later the characteristic rash appears and the fever rises to 104°F. A measles rash begins with bright red spots behind the ears and spreads over the head and torso all the way down to the legs. Usually there is no itching. After 3 days the spots get darker and fade; occasionally brown patches remain visible for a week or two. Inflamed eyes and light sensitivity, dry cough and sore throat are generally the most bothersome symptoms.

Causes

Measles is caused by a virus. It is spread by direct contact; less commonly, the virus is airborne.

Who's at Risk

Children who come in contact with other children with measles are at high risk of developing the disease.

Possible Aftereffects and Complications

Measles may be accompanied by bacterial infections that can lead to middle-ear infections or pneumonia. Its most serious complication is encephalitis (see p. 213).

Prevention

Measles is one of the highly infectious children's diseases. Newborns are generally protected from infection during the first 4 months of life by antibodies acquired from the mother.

The most infectious period starts 4 days prior to, and ends 4 days following, the appearance of the rash. To prevent the spread of disease, the child should be separated from other children for a week following the appearance of the rash.

See Immunizations: Measles, p. 672.

When to Seek Medical Advice

Seek help if measles is suspected. A thorough examination may help the doctor determine whether the measles is accompanied by a bacterial infection, in which case antibiotics should be prescribed.

Warning: To reduce the risk of contagion, advise your pediatrician that you suspect measles before bringing your child to the office.

Take your child to a pediatrician or children's clinic immediately if

— The child's neck is stiff (the chin can't be lowered to touch the chest)
— Seizures develop
— The child is lethargic and barely responsive
— Unusual bleeding (e.g., of the mucous membranes) develops, and dark red patches appear under the skin (possible signs of blood clotting disorder)

Self-Help

Keep the child in bed. Because of fluid loss due to elevated temperature and sweating, encourage the child to drink as much as possible.

Don't overdress a child with a fever. Cotton clothing or a light bedcover should be sufficient, together with a relatively cool room temperature (about 68°F).

Cool compresses on the calves will help cool the body (see Compresses, p. 692)—but apply them only if the child's hands and feet are warm.

Cool drinks and cool, humidified rooms will make a sore throat feel better. Avoid giving fruit juices, whose acid content can irritate the mouth and throat. If the child is having trouble swallowing, soft or pureed food will go down more easily. A darkened room is more comfortable for the child's light-sensitive eyes.

Treatment

As with most viral diseases, only the symptoms of measles can be treated.

Fever-reducing medication should be used for fever or if the general condition of the child is severely affected.

Use products containing acetaminophen or ibuprofen (see Analgesics, p. 660).

GERMAN MEASLES/RUBELLA

Symptoms

German measles or rubella usually manifests as a rash, 11 to 21 days after infection. The pea-sized, bright red spots appear first on the face and then spread over the whole body. It's common for the lymph nodes in the throat and at the back of the neck to swell. They can be felt as little lumps. The child has no fever or other signs of illness; in fact, in a quarter to a third of all children with rubella, there is no sign whatsoever of the disease.

Causes

Rubella is caused by a virus and transmitted through direct contact.

Who's at Risk

Children old enough to go to school are most likely to be exposed to rubella and are therefore at highest risk.

Possible Aftereffects and Complications

In extremely rare cases, rubella may be accompanied by a bacterial infection or encephalitis.

Prevention

Warning: Pregnant women must be not be brought in contact with a rubella-infected child. If you are pregnant and have been exposed, contact your doctor immediately.

Rubella is contagious 7 days prior to, and 5 days following, the appearance of the rash. Having the infection during childhood offers better protection than immunization.

See Immunizations: Rubella, p. 673.

When to Seek Medical Advice

Seek help if other symptoms, such as cough or earaches, accompany rubella.

To prevent contagion, advise your pediatrician of suspected rubella by phone before an office visit.

Take the child to a pediatrician or children's clinic immediately if

— The child has seizures

— The child acts apathetic or unresponsive

Self-Help

Because the disease produces few (if any) symptoms in children, no special measures are necessary.

Treatment

Treatment is usually not necessary.

SCARLET FEVER

Symptoms

Two to 3 days after infection, the child's temperature suddenly spikes. The child may develop a headache, severe sore throat, and trouble swallowing; he or she may vomit once or twice.

Two to 3 days later the fever rises again, and the typical scarlet fever rash appears: A dense field of tiny, pinpricklike, rough, red spots, almost like sandpaper, which lighten in color for a moment when pressed with a finger.

The rash starts on the chest and groin area and spreads over the entire body, although the face is usually unaffected. After a week or two the topmost layer of skin becomes flaky; on the hands and feet it may peel off in patches.

Further classic signs of scarlet fever include red cheeks; a red-dotted, swollen "strawberry tongue"; painful, swollen lymph nodes of the neck and jaw.

Causes

Scarlet fever is caused by a bacterial (streptococcal) infection.

Who's at Risk

Children are at higher risk of contracting scarlet fever if others nearby have it, and during the colder seasons.

Possible Aftereffects and Complications

Before scarlet fever was treated with antibiotics, it was feared because of its severity and capacity to affect certain organs especially acutely. Complications include rheumatic fever (see Rheumatic Fever, p. 458).

Prevention

One day after starting antibiotics, a child with scarlet fever is no longer contagious. Without antibiotic treatment, the disease remains contagious for weeks. The child should stay home until the infectious period ends.

When to Seek Medical Advice

Seek help if scarlet fever is suspected. To avoid spreading the disease, advise your pediatrician by phone before you go for an office visit.

Take the child to a pediatrician or children's clinic immediately if

— The child's temperature does not go below 104°F even with fever-reducing medication

— The child develops seizures

— The child seems beside himself or herself and very restless

— The child has severe vomiting and diarrhea

Self-Help

See Throat Disorders, p. 157; Fever, p. 29; Headaches, p. 193. Cool the child's throat with an ice pack (see Cold Packs, p. 685).

Treatment

Call your pediatrician if you suspect your child has scarlet fever. The child should be treated with antibiotics and may need to undergo further tests (urinalysis, throat culture).

PERTUSSIS (WHOOPING COUGH)

Symptoms

Whooping cough is highly infectious and runs a long course. According to popular wisdom, it takes 3 weeks to come, stays three weeks, and then takes at least three weeks to leave.

The incubation period actually lasts a week or two, but because whooping cough symptoms mimic a cold for the first 2 weeks, it often goes undetected. Over the course of the next 3 to 6 weeks, the classic symptoms develop: Coughing fits with sharp breath intake, and short hacking coughs with the final "whoop" that gives the disease its name. In the final phase the child's face may be red, the eyes glassy, and the child is usually exhausted. It's common for children to have no fever and seem healthy apart from the coughing fits, which may number at least 15 to 20 a day. Infants with whooping cough often don't "whoop." After about 6 to 9 weeks, the fits finally become less frequent.

Causes

Whooping cough is caused by a bacterial infection; the brain's "cough center" is affected by the toxins released by the bacteria.

Who's at Risk

In contrast to most other childhood diseases, even newborns can get whooping cough. There is a greater risk to children who have contact with a carrier before the carrier has been diagnosed with the disease. Children not immunized are at increased risk.

Possible Aftereffects and Complications

Whooping cough can be especially dangerous for young infants. Infants with whooping cough must be monitored constantly, because they can stop breathing during coughing or sneezing fits. If this happens, immediately pick up the child and resuscitate him or her.

Prevention

Whooping cough is at its most infectious during the first 2 weeks, before it is likely to have been diagnosed. Because the disease can be significantly more dangerous for infants than older children, keep infants carefully separated. If infants are exposed, give them preventive antibiotics (erythromycin). All household contacts should receive prophylactic antibiotics.

If not treated with antibiotics, the disease is contagious for about 3 weeks after the first typical coughing fit. With appropriate treatment, this period is reduced to about a week.

See Immunization, p. 671.

When to Seek Medical Advice

Seek help if
— Whooping cough is suspected
— The child develops a fever
— The child develops an earache

To prevent the spread of disease, advise your pediatrician by phone before an office visit.

Take the child to a pediatrician or children's clinic immediately if
— The child's face takes on a light bluish cast and the nostrils tremble when breathing.
— The child develops seizures, paralysis, or loses consciousness.

Self-Help

The sick child does not need to be confined to bed, but should stay in a well-ventilated, warm environment (about 70°F), with an ambient humidity of at least 40 percent.

Because children with whooping cough frequently vomit after a coughing fit, they should eat light meals frequently during the day.

If the child is vomiting, it's important that he or she drink a lot, to compensate for fluid loss and ease coughing somewhat.

Treatment

Cough suppressants are hardly capable of suppressing the fits of whooping cough.

Antibiotics (erythromycin) should be prescribed for whooping cough during the early phase to ameliorate the illness; and are also recommended during the coughing phase primarily to limit the spread of the organisms to others.

Infants younger than 6 months and other patients with severe disease often require hospitalization for supportive care.

MUMPS

Symptoms

Eighteen to 21 days after infection with mumps, swelling starts in front of the ears by the angle of the jaw, first on one side, then a day or two later on the other, causing "chipmunk cheeks" which feel spongy to the touch and are very painful. The child may complain of earaches and pain when chewing or turning the head. A high fever is not uncommon, but the child may also remain fever-free. The illness generally clears up after about a week, usually with no lasting effect.

Causes

Mumps is caused by a virus that especially affects the parotid glands.

Who's at Risk

Children are most likely to be affected between the ages of 4 and 10. An adult can catch mumps too, however, if the effect of an immunization has worn off, or if he or she did not have mumps as a child, or was not immunized.

Possible Aftereffects and Complications

In rare cases, mumps can lead to complications such as pancreatitis or meningitis. In boys, mumps can lead to orchitis, which may cause sterility.

Prevention

Mumps is contagious from 4 days prior until 7 days after the first signs of illness.
See Immunizations: Mumps, p. 673.

When to Seek Medical Advice

Seek help if
— Symptoms grow worse with the application of heat.
— The child complains of a severe earache, or a severe earache ends suddenly and the ear begins to ooze.
— The child's temperature won't go below 104°F despite use of fever-reducing medication.

Take the child to a pediatrician or children's clinic immediately if
— Headaches develop, the neck is stiff (the chin can't be touched to the chest), or the child is unresponsive.
— Vomiting or severe stomachache develop.
— Post-pubescent boys complain of pain in the gonads.

Self-Help

Applying warmth to the parotid glands can help alleviate symptoms.

Treatment

Antibiotics have no effect on mumps. Keep ears and cheeks warm and, if necessary, try to bring down the fever.

CHICKENPOX

Symptoms

Chickenpox (varicella) generally starts with headache and fever. Usually about 2 to 3 weeks after infection, a rash appears on the torso and quickly spreads.

Within a few hours, the bright red bumps turn into small, easily burst blisters that may or may not ooze clear liquid. Fresh blisters appear in waves and keep crusting over. They may also appear on the scalp or mucous membranes (mouth, genitals).

Body temperature is usually only mildly elevated; signs of illness other than the blisters are rare. The rash itches severely.

Causes

Chickenpox is a highly infectious viral disease which can be transmitted by direct contact and occasionally may be spread by airborne means up to a distance of 30 feet from the source.

Who's at Risk

Children between ages 2 and 7 are most likely to contract chickenpox.

Possible Aftereffects and Complications

Normally, one gets chickenpox only once and is immune thereafter. People who had chickenpox as a child may develop shingles as an adult, if the latent virus is triggered (see Shingles, p. 284).

Occasionally, the brain is affected. This may cause balance disorders, which almost always clear up again within a few weeks.

Prevention

It is almost impossible to prevent infection in a child.

In exceptional cases, chickenpox immunoglobulin (varicella-zoster immune globulin [VZIG]) can be injected in newborns if the mother developed chickenpox 5 days or less before delivery, or in children who are being treated with cytostatic drugs, corticosteroids, or other immunosuppressants for conditions like cancer or severe rheumatism.

Immunization to prevent disease is currently recommended for most children.

When to Seek Medical Advice

Call your pediatrician if
— The itching cannot be relieved (see Self-Help, p. 605).
— The rash has become inflamed: The blisters are red and ooze a yellow, purulent liquid.

Take the child to a pediatrician or children's clinic immediately if

— The child has a headache, the neck is stiff (the chin can no longer touch the chest), or vomiting is severe.
— The child is apathetic and unresponsive.
— The child staggers or his or her speech is unintelligible.

Self-Help

Fingernails: Cut nails as short as possible so the child can't scratch open the pustules. Frequent handwashing and nailbrushing also reduce the chance of infection. Sometimes it is necessary for the child to wear cotton gloves to prevent scratching.

Clothing: Loose cotton clothing is the least irritating to the rash.

Rinses: If mouth or eyes are affected by the rash, gargling and eyewashes with saline solution (1 teaspoon table salt dissolved in a glass of sterilized water) can reduce the itching.

Baths: Frequent showers or rinsing with lukewarm water can ease the itching and prevent inflammation of the pustules. A daily bath of lukewarm water with a cup of baking powder, or oatmeal in a sock, added can also help. Always use a fresh washcloth.

Infants: Careful hygiene and frequent changing of bedclothes and diapers is especially important to try to avoid a bacterial infection of the blisters.

Treatment

Powders or lotions that claim to stop the itching caused by chickenpox are probably actually substituting a sensation of cold or warmth for that of irritation.

You can purchase calamine lotion, among others from the pharmacy. Children often feel better after a solution is swabbed onto their blisters.

ROSEOLA

Symptoms

Roseola almost always begins with a high fever lasting 3 or 4 days, with no further signs of disease such as a cold or cough. In rare cases, the child vomits or has diarrhea.

After 3 to 4 days the fever quickly drops. A rash of tiny red spots appears, especially on the belly and back, and clears up in a week or two.

The disease is not very infectious.

Causes

The cause of roseola is a virus.

Who's at Risk

Children usually contract roseola between the ages of 3 months and 4 years.

Possible Aftereffects and Complications

Roseola has no lasting ill effects. However, because of the associated high temperatures at a time when the child's brain reacts sensitively to fever, febrile seizures can occur.

Prevention

Not possible.

When to Seek Medical Advice

Seek help if

— Body temperature does not drop despite fever-reducing medication (see Compresses, p. 692).
— The fever remains constantly elevated for more than 2 days.
— The child continues to have a fever, especially at night.
— Other signs of illness appear (such as pain when urinating).

Self-Help

Bed rest will help the body conserve energy and devote all its reserves to the immune system. Because the child is losing fluids due to his or her elevated temperature, he or she should be encouraged to drink as much as possible.

Often children with a fever are dressed too warmly. Cotton clothing or a light coverlet are best. Keep the ambient temperature on the cool side (around 68°F).

Cool compresses can help cool the body down (see Compresses, p. 692).

Treatment

If necessary, take steps to reduce the child's fever.

AGING

The population of the industrialized world is aging. In 1994, average life expectancy was 72 years for men and 79 for women, so the "golden years" portion of the average lifespan keeps increasing. It is a time that can be filled with all sorts of purposeful activity and new perspectives on life. If your attitude toward aging is one of curiosity and you don't lose interest in the world or in yourself, you'll probably cope just fine with the inevitable physical changes aging entails. The limits that old age gradually sets need not signify the end of anything: On the contrary, they can challenge you intellectually to stay flexible, adapt continually to new conditions, and make the most of remaining possibilities.

CAREFREE AGING?

How the aging process runs its course depends ultimately on your specific situation and how you choose to experience it. Your physical condition will usually reflect how you've lived your life, revealing whether you labored for years at strenuous physical work, got no physical exercise at all, or suffered from major psychological problems, excessive worries, or chronic overwork. Current life circumstances can also play a major role in your experience of aging: Living on a fixed income at or near the poverty line will affect both body and soul. Depending on the individual's physical health, emotional condition and mental attitudes, life's various stress factors may or may not contribute to premature aging or chronic illness.

Planning Ahead

If, like many people, you plan to retire from active professional life around age 65, the best way to prevent a major shock is to start cultivating other interests well ahead of time.

For example, if you start planning for a secure, fulfilling old age when you're 50, you have excellent chances of making your dream a reality. It's a safe bet that in retirement you'll continue to build on the foundations you've developed over the course of your lifetime. Research shows that older people are very unlikely to make radical relationship and lifestyle changes.

Life offers a infinite of options for the older person:

— Do something just for yourself. What have you always wanted to do, experience, know, learn? The range of possibilities is limitless: travel, take up a new sport or language, cultivate roses, make short films, learn acupressure, work on cars, and so on and on.
— Get involved and make your voice heard. Maybe you've always been frustrated by social injustice, but never had the time to devote serious attention to the issues. Active participants—including many older people—are the lifeblood of civic and environmental organizations, political parties, and interest groups.
— Do something for others. Especially in the social service arena, helping hands are needed almost everywhere. Become a volunteer at your local hospital or community hotline; share your professional skills and life experience with college students through a mentorship program or senior executives service; join Literacy Volunteers of America; help children of recent immigrants with their homework; provide home daycare.

HOW WE AGE

The aging process actually begins with the first breath we take, as older cells begin to die off and are replaced by younger ones. While we're young, the process happens quickly and efficiently, but the older we get, the less smoothly it runs: The individual phases of cell division take longer, and errors in cell and nuclear division increase. The organism's capacity to compensate for such errors diminishes, and it generally loses flexibility. The following signs of aging are all part of the body's natural process:

— The water content of the cells lessens. A young person's body tissues contain about 62 percent water; over the years this figure drops to 54 percent, causing organs to shrink and their functionality to be reduced. For this reason, older people should drink plenty of liquids (see Drinks, p. 736).
— Heart function diminishes. Hardening of the arteries may set in, constricting the blood vessels.
— Lung capacity decreases. The rib joints stiffen and the chest loses elasticity, making breathing more difficult.
— The muscles and mucous membranes of the

gastrointestinal tract change; food takes longer to digest, and medications are absorbed more slowly.

— The cholesterol level in the liver rises. Toxins are broken down more slowly. Because the liver requires good circulation to function optimally, it is especially affected by reduced heart function and circulation.

— Blood flow to the kidneys diminishes, causing them to shrink, and causing residues, toxins, and medications to be broken down and excreted more slowly.

— In the tissues of the musculoskeletal system, lost water is partially replaced by fat deposits. Bone tissue is broken down faster than it is replaced; muscle mass is reduced. Joints, vertebrae, and disks show signs of wear.

— After age 40, the eyes gradually lose their capacity to focus on near objects (see Presbyopia, p. 232). Light sensitivity is also reduced, which is why older people require better-lighted environments than younger folks.

— Hearing deteriorates: Parts of the ears ossify, the ear canal narrows, the total number of auditory cells drops (see Hearing Loss, p. 250).

— The circulation to the skin decreases, and the skin loses its ability to bind water. It is no longer as elastic, becomes drier, and wrinkled.

Senility (Failing Memory)

With advancing age, the blood vessels narrow and circulation becomes more sluggish. If organs are insufficiently supplied with blood, the brain in particular is affected (see Arteriosclerosis, p. 318). This may result in

— Loss of memory and concentration
— Loss of orientation
— Rapid mood swings

Such changes can be prevented. Mental skills decline less the more they're used. You can compensate for deteriorating alertness and reaction times by increasing the care, time, and foresight with which you approach daily tasks. Some skills actually improve with age: these include judgment, grasp of intellectual connections and relationships, independence, forethought, sense of responsibility, and reliability.

The cliché that older people are forgetful is something of an overstatement. Granted, short-term memory does tend to fade to varying degrees in different people, but long-term memory usually works flawlessly. If your

How to Live Longer

Although there's no surefire, all-purpose recipe for living to a ripe and healthy old age, the following ingredients will certainly increase your chances:
— Get appropriate physical activity (see Physical Activity and Sports, p. 762).
— Eat a balanced diet (see p. 723).
— Limit your use of mood-altering substances (see Smoking, Alcohol, p. 754).
— Work on maintaining intellectual stimulation and an active interest in political, social, and cultural events.
— Work on maintaining your psychic well-being. Lively relationships with friends and family will help keep you "forever young." Happiness and a positive outlook promote health, whereas loneliness and bitterness damage it.
— Sexual activity can make your spirits soar.

memory isn't so dependable anymore, use crib sheets and notes.

The capacity to grasp the finer details of a situation as well as retaining a sense for the whole remains fully functional—until you decide that something is no longer of interest to you. Indeed, not having to be interested in every little thing any more is a privilege of old age. Even though it may look like stubbornness to others, it is a liberating experience to pay attention only to those things in life that are important to you.

Changes in Sleep Patterns

Sleep patterns start to change around age 50: Nightly deep-sleep periods become less frequent, and sleep becomes less restful.

The daily ratio of sleeping to waking changes, too. It's harder to stay awake through a long day and then sleep soundly all night. A 60-year-old is more rested after a shorter period of sleep than a 20-year-old, but will need a nap sooner.

If possible, adjust your daily schedule to these new rhythms: Determine what your sleep requirements are, and plan activities and commitments for times when you know you'll have more energy.

Relaxation techniques (see p. 693) can boost your energy and help you make it through the day, and can also help you fall asleep on restless nights. Lost sleep due to age-related symptoms can usually be satisfactorily supplemented by a siesta, or a catnap or two, over the course of the day.

Sexuality

The concept of older people, especially women, as sexual beings is largely taboo in our society, although the capacity for sexual experience and responsiveness actually endures until the very end of life. From the traditional male perspective, procreation and sexuality are closely linked; therefore, women past childbearing age are considered "desexualized" or sexually neutral. This misconception is furthered by the media, which seldom represent older women as experienced, mature, knowing, sensual beings. Many aging women suffer more from this devaluation of their sexuality and eroticism than from an actual disease or changing family circumstances.

In Women

Hormonal changes during menopause (see p. 510) don't substantially influence the libido. Some women only really bloom sexually during this stage: Older women usually have more sexual experience and know their own bodies better than younger women.

The effects of physiological changes such as vaginal dryness can be counteracted by using lubricants, or experimenting with new sexual techniques such as prolonged, uninhibited foreplay.

You can unlock your ability to live your sexuality fully if you are able to let go of preconceptions about what's "allowed" and what isn't. Physical love need not be narrowly defined as permissible only between males and females of a particular age: It can also encompass self-gratification and erotic contact with other women, or with younger men.

In Men

Like women, men retain their capacity for orgasm well into advanced old age. If you are prepared for the usual physiological changes, it will be easier to adapt to them: Erections take a bit longer than they used to, sometimes requiring longer periods of stimulation, and ejaculation is more fleeting, but the experience of orgasm itself remains unchanged. There's no general rule for how long men remain potent; depending on your personal life circumstances and whether or not you established an active sensuality in your youth, you might start cutting back on sex, or give it up altogether, at 60 or at 90.

A problematic erection need not be a hindrance to physical love: Keep in mind that many women profoundly enjoy sexuality that doesn't involve intercourse but offers lots of warmth and tenderness (see Desire and Love, p. 537).

DISEASES OF THE ELDERLY

In later years, health disorders often manifest in various combinations. Their impact on quality of life depends on the individual; no matter what your circumstances, you can always make a conscious effort to use and strengthen the capacities that remain to you.

Look up resources for prevention, self-help, and treatment under the respective headings in this book.

Medications for the Elderly

More than half the pharmaceuticals dispensed today go to people over sixty, mainly for conditions such as cardiovascular disease, musculoskeletal, or metabolic problems, diseases of the lungs and airways, and psychological problems such as depression.

Older people often habitually take several medications at a time; the resulting risk of side effects is 3 to 7 times higher than in younger people, because of age-related changes in the organism and metabolism. For this reason, it's generally a good idea to keep medications to a minimum. Always ask your doctor whether all your medications are absolutely necessary (see Medication Summary, p. 657).

Geriatric Drugs

The pharmaceutical industry markets a multiplicity of geriatric drugs, many of which claim to stop or slow aging. However, a healthy, balanced diet, physical exercise, and intellectual stimulation can help postpone aging much better than any drug.

In addition to their frequently exaggerated promises, geriatric drugs have the added disadvantages of undesirable side effects and (usually) considerable expense.

The following herbs, used for centuries in many countries, have beneficial effects in treating symptoms of aging: Gingko, ginseng, garlic, rosemary, and hawthorn berry.

Beware of miracle cures

— Many commercially available geriatric supplements contain useful ingredients, but in concentrations too low to have any effect. A fresh bulb of garlic from the greengrocer's will usually be more effective than the infinitesimal amounts of garlic in many products. Likewise, if you're interested in the salutary effects of hawthorn extract, buy it straight instead of diluted with other ingredients.

— The reason many geriatric products have a stimulant effect is that they contain alcohol.

— The iron, vitamins, and minerals contained in many antiaging elixirs and geriatric supplements are unnecessary. If you have an actual vitamin or mineral deficiency, your health-care professional should determine this and treat it accordingly.

LIVING SITUATIONS FOR THE ELDERLY

Most people want to stay independent for as long as possible and move into an assisted-living situation only when it's unavoidable; however, they usually misjudge the most appropriate moment to make the transition.

If you're still mentally and physically agile, you're much more likely to adapt well to new living quarters than if you're sick and need care. You're also more likely to form strong new friendships, creating a circle of support that will be there for you until the end. That's why it's so important to select, well in advance, the living situation in which you'd like to pass your final years.

Living at Home

The ideal home for an older person would be

— Not too big
— Close to shopping and services
— Close to a medical center
— Easily accessible to transportation
— Within walking distance of entertainment (movies, restaurants, senior center, etc.)
— Single-level or equipped with an elevator
— Close to a park or garden, or provided with a terrace or balcony

Basic Requirements

— The house or apartment should be simple and easy to heat; coal or kerosene stoves should be avoided.
— In the kitchen, everything should be within easy reach without climbing or bending. Work surfaces should be appropriate for your height: Ideally, they

should be about 4 inches below your forearms when you bend your arms at right angles. Electrical appliances that switch off automatically after a certain period of time are also a good idea.

— The shower should have a low rim, so getting in isn't a problem. Non-skid floors and handrails in the shower and by the toilet are important safety features.
— Furniture should be stable and/or secured in place, so you can lean on it safely. The ideal height for seating is about 18" off the floor. Sofas and beds that are too low, deep or soft can make getting up difficult.
— Easy-care, no-wax floors are best to prevent slipping. Arrange rugs and carpets so you won't slip on or trip over them. If possible, remove door sills to minimize the risk of stumbling.
— Have your electric wiring checked if you live in an old house; old wires are often a fire hazard. Make sure light switches are conveniently located so you don't have to grope in the dark.
— Older people require better light than younger people, so don't skimp on lighting. If necessary, demand that your landlord provide better lighting in entry halls and stairwells.
— Telephone cords should be short to prevent tripping over them; instead of dragging a long cord through the house, install a second phone in the bedroom or get a cordless model.
— A First Alert device worn (or another such device) on the body can be very useful in case you fall or need to call for help and are not near a telephone.

Social Services

Many services are available to the elderly, depending on the community. These include Meals On Wheels, bookmobiles, and mobile health-care units of various types. Inquire at your local senior center or community services office.

Retirement Communities

Today, more and more apartments are available for purchase or rental in retirement communities, with the advantage that many services are available right on the premises, just a phone call away. You pay only for the services you use. If you feel like cooking for yourself, you can; if you choose, meals can be delivered to your apartment. The same may go for housekeeping and personal assistance. Nursing and medical services are available around the clock, so the chances are good of being able to convalesce in the privacy of your own home, should it become necessary.

Group Living

Group homes for the elderly are becoming more common, too. These are especially valuable for partnerless people who could use a regular source of social interaction. There are many advantages:

— You have your own room and independence, and are responsible for yourself.
— When you want to, you can enjoy the benefits of community in your small group.
— If you feel like it, you can stay in your room.
— Communal housekeeping is cheaper than living alone.
— You can choose the people you want to live with. There are also potential disadvantages:
— Living with other people on a daily basis can be a source of conflict. It's often hard for older people to adapt their living customs and habits to other people's requirements.
— You can't avoid anybody for long periods, the way you can in a large apartment building. Therefore, it's important to communicate honestly and state your requirements and expectations in advance. Conflicts in a group living situation should always be addressed promptly so they don't mushroom out of control.
— Live-in nurses or homecare assistants are often permitted only on a limited basis, so a good source of outpatient care or affiliation with a nursing home is important.

Assisted-living Communities

These are for older people who are fully capable of caring for themselves and their living quarters, usually small furnished units with kitchen or kitchenette and bath. The advantage of an assisted living community is that meals and care are available if you need them. Usually activity programs and social gatherings are part of the daily and weekly schedule.

Nursing Homes

Nursing homes are for people who can no longer live completely on their own and require varying degrees of assistance. You can sometimes bring your own furniture. Housekeeping and all other services are provided.

Finding a Good Nursing Home

Ideally, finding a home in your own neighborhood would be best; staying in familiar surroundings will make the transition easier.

Send a list of questions to different homes in your chosen area; Be suspicious if they're not forthcoming with answers.

Ask about

— Surrounding infrastructure (shopping, parks, etc.)
— Accessibility to transportation
— Total number of inhabitants, size and layout of units, how the rooms are outfitted
— An exact breakdown of costs (meals, laundry, housekeeping, etc.)
— Availability of medical care
— Availability of psychological care
— How long you can stay in the home if you are temporarily bedridden and need in-home care, and available alternatives in case on-site convalescing is not available
— How the place is organized (obligatory meals, individual house key, phone use, scheduled visiting hours, payment plans, etc.)
— Communal facilities (sauna, library, snack bar) and available activities

Take a tour of those homes that interest you, and speak to as many residents as possible.

Home Care

Millions of disabled children, chronically ill, and bedridden people, and aging parents and relatives are cared for at home. Even with periodic help from visiting nurses, community or welfare organizations, private institutions or churches, experts warn caregivers in these situations against overestimating their own abilities. To be able to provide home care for chronically ill and older loved ones, goodwill isn't enough: The external circumstances need to be favorable, too. These include financial and social provisions for the caregivers, adequate living space, the opportunity for respite and rest and relaxation (R&R), and the availability of support from friends and neighbors (see Times of Crisis, p. 611).

Caring for the Caregiver

Eighty percent of the time, home care is provided by women—daughters, daughters-in-law, sisters, wives, and life partners. For many of them, the cost of this care is the neglect of their own children, careers, and earning power.

Respite programs (see Social Services, p. 609) can provide relief services to caregivers; information is available from your town's social services department.

Relationships

Conflicts inevitably arise within families caring for sick or elderly members. Relationships that may already have been stressed are suddenly put to the test and may come to a boil very quickly. Feelings of disgust, frustration, resentment, anger, and guilt can create a situation of constant friction. It's crucial to be able to talk about these feelings (see Counseling, p. 697); contact with other caregivers in similar situations, such as in support groups, can be extremely helpful.

Times of Crisis

Even in a basically problem-free situation, crises can arise; the disease or condition may worsen, pain may increase, communication problems may arise, or the caregiver may be dealing with additional issues of her own and feel unable to cope with everything. The situation will be especially difficult if antipathy and resentment are allowed to blossom between patient and caregiver.

Be familiar with the warning signs: The patient may reject certain treatments, pull away or withdraw, or act

Dependent and Helpless?

A chronic illness and/or the need for constant care can change a patient's life profoundly, often overnight. Someone who can no longer wash himself, or needs help getting dressed or going shopping, usually feels helpless, dependent, and defeated. Add to this the actual pain or weakness generated by the disease, not to mention existential fears of the future, of death, of being a burden to others or leaving them alone in the world, the overwhelming sensation of not being needed any more, or not being able to bear it any longer, can all pave the way for severe depression and thoughts of suicide (see p. 197, 199).

To counteract this sort of assault on your outlook on life, you'll need a lot of patience. Relief often comes gradually, in small steps, for patient and family alike. Given time, however, it is altogether possible to develop a new perspective on life despite any disability or disease (see Counseling and Psychotherapy, p. 697).

defeated or aggressive; the caregiver may act irritable, impatient or rough; at times she may seem to be the sick one, or she may obviously be neglecting her own care.

As a caregiver, you need to be aware of your own needs:

— Make sure you get enough time off to be able to maintain some perspective on the situation. Look into counseling; join a support group for caregivers.

— If the situation becomes unbearable, consider a short- or long-term respite program, or other arrangements (see Older People in the Hospital, p. 634).

THE HOME

If you are providing live-in care, your household's daily routine will necessarily undergo some changes. Be sure to discuss all changes in advance with all members of the household. You may need to consider issues such as the setup of the sickroom, rearrangments in the kitchen, or structural changes (e.g. wheelchair access) in the bathroom (see Disabilities, p. 618).

The Sickroom

To ensure the patient's comfort, as many as possible of the following requirements should be met:

—The patient needs his or her own room, located near the rest of the family—even if this just means he or she can hear familiar voices through the open door—while at the same time providing a quiet refuge. Proximity to a bathroom is also important.

—The patient's favorite furniture, knickknacks, books, pictures, and plants should be in the room, in addition to a radio and/or television if desired.

— The room should have lots of sunlight and good artificial lighting; it should also be possible to darken the room as necessary.

—The heating system should be individually controlled: Bedridden patients usually like room temperatures around 68°F. The room should not be too cold, however, since older people are more sensitive to cold than younger individuals.

Encouraging Exercise

Anytime we are prevented from moving normally, our attitude towards life takes a distinct downturn. If you are a homebound patient, you should exercise on a regular basis and practice your remaining skills. Perform as

Changing sheets for the bedridden

1. Loosen old sheet at all four corners and position patient on side.

2. Holding patient's shoulder and hip, roll patient toward you to edge of bed. Place lower leg backwards, pull upper leg at an angle forward. Roll old sheet up to the back of patient. Place new sheet on exposed bed area lengthwise with fold in the middle

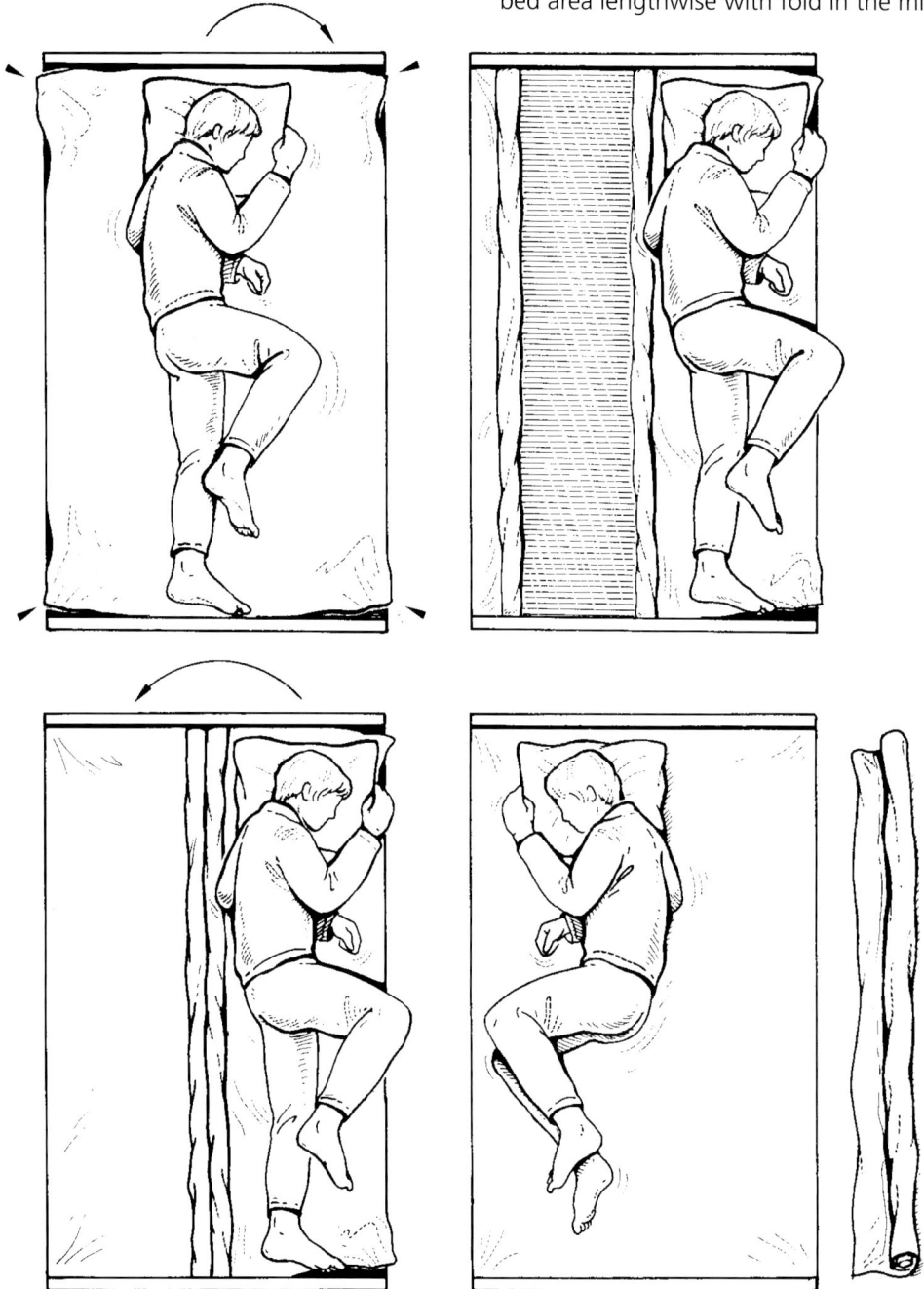

3. Roll upper part of new sheet toward middle of bed, and fasten lower part of new sheet under mattress. Then roll patient on his back, and then onto his/her other side. Holding shoulder and hip, pull patient to other side of bed.

4. Now you can remove the old sheet, and roll out the new one, fastening it under the mattress.

many daily tasks for yourself as possible; the more you can achieve, the better your psychological condition will be.

Even in bed some exercise is possible, depending on your circumstances and physical condition. Skilled help is available from a physical therapist acting on the recommendations of your doctor. If you are bedridden, you should sit up at regular intervals to keep your breathing as deep as possible.

If you are not confined to bed, you can regain lost ground with a walker. Regular short walks will help you keep up your coordination.

Preventing Falls

If you are in bed a lot, you gradually lose your reaction and coordination skills, which increases your risk of falling. Older people break bones and joints more easily than younger people. After a fall, they may be afraid of falling again and exercise even less as a result.

— Bend and stretch your legs a few times when you stand up after sitting or lying down for a long time. This helps joint flexibility and improves circulation.
— Wear sturdy shoes with closed backs and flat, slip-proof soles for extra security.
— Longer distances, such as corridors, are easier to master if you have a conveniently placed chair to rest on, or if railings or handholds are available.
— There should be nothing for you to stumble over such as rugs, door sills, or telephone cords.
— Watch for medication-induced side effects such as unsteady gait, fainting, or confusion. Some sedatives and tranquilizers can remain in the body for a long time (see Aging, p. 606).
— If you have a tendency to fall, have a doctor examine you. Muscle weakness, sensory disorders, or disorders of the vestibular system (sense of balance) can be treated.

Stimulating the Senses

The senses of hearing, vision, and taste fade with advancing age (see Food and Drink, p. 616). Prescription eyeglasses, a magnifying glass for reading, and an appropriate hearing aid can help you maintain contact with the world. Sensory stimulants like flowers, colors, and music can touch the soul and enliven your spirits.

The Bed

For many chronically ill or frail older people, the bed is where they live. Accordingly, its quality and position are important.
—The mattress should distribute body weight well and be neither too hard nor too soft. Choose a mattress that has good support properties. A slip-proof, washable mattress pad will prevent damage due to incontinence.
— Adjustable head and foot sections can facilitate sitting upright or keeping legs elevated.
— The patient's individual preferences, such as a favorite cushion, extra covers for the legs, neckrolls/ bolsters or patterned sheets, should always be accommodated.
— A hospital bed that can be raised and lowered can make getting in and out easier, and is easier on the patient's back.
—The bed should be easily accessible from both sides and the floor underneath it should be of the non-skid, easy-care variety.
—The bedroom door and a window should be within full view of the bed.
Important: The bed should be within easy reach of a sturdy surface large enough to hold a drink, a radio, books, a telephone, a good reading lamp, and a bell or buzzer to call for help.

Care of the Sickbed

The bed should be made twice a day, morning and evening, preferably after the patient washes and changes clothes. When changing bedlinen, take care that the patient doesn't fall off the other side of the bed: Move a heavy object such as an armchair to the unprotected side, or, better yet, get someone to help you.

Personal Hygiene

For most people it's extraordinarily embarrassing not to be able to wash or care for themselves any more. For as long as possible, therefore, the patient should be helped only as much as he or she absolutely needs it (see Encouraging Exercise, p. 611): Even the smallest skill should be encouraged and incorporated into the daily routine.

For example, patients may still be able to wash hands and face, comb their hair or apply cream to their hands. A change in routine can also act as a stimulant: For example, alternating between various grooming aids, brushes, sponges, bath scents, or bath times.

Full-Body Wash

— If the condition of the sick or frail patient allows it, a daily head-to-foot washing and change of underwear should be standard procedure. Aside from fulfilling basic hygienic needs, washing, drying, and moisturizing feel good. Set aside enough time for this ritual: Being touched will help the patient inhabit the body more fully, and is also essential to psychic well-being.

— Don't use excessively soft towels and washcloths: Slightly rougher fabrics will massage the skin and stimulate circulation.

— If you're using a wash bowl or pan, make sure the water doesn't get cold. If necessary, use bath gel or liquid soap, which is easier to handle than bar soap. The best option is clear water with no additives: It won't dry out the skin.

—The order in which the body is washed should follow the patient's preference. If none is forthcoming, experience has shown that the following sequence is most comfortable for most people:

First wash hands and arms, and dry them quickly; then face and neck. Then come chest, belly, legs, and genitals. After each area is washed, it should be carefully dried. Moisture in the folds of the skin can cause sores and yeast infections of the skin and genitals. Afterward, turn the patient on his or her side and wash back and buttocks. Following the final drying, rub with skin lotion and massage lightly.

Breathing and Pulse

Older people, especially those confined to bed, usually breathe too weakly and shallowly. This results in insufficient oxygen in circulation, which can lead to sleepiness and sleep disorders as well as a deterioration of lung function. The worst complication is pneumonia (see p. 310), one of the most common causes of death in old age.

To improve breathing, it is crucial to get lots of fresh air, drink plenty of liquids, and exercise regularly. Daily breathing exercises can also help:

— Encourage the patient to stretch regularly, and consciously breathe in deeply. Give him or her a balloon to inflate, or try to keep a puff of cotton in the air between you by blowing out together.

— To ensure that air gets deep into the lungs, the patient should practice abdominal breathing, lying relaxed on the back and resting hands on the belly. Ask the patient to breathe in through the nose rather than the mouth, then to breathe out in slow puffs on a "P" or "F" sound.

— Deep breathing can be encouraged in bedridden patients by laying them on their sides and placing their upper arm over the head. This stretches the upper part of the lung.

Heart Rate and Body Temperature

In frail, bedridden, and/or chronically ill patients, body temperature and pulse should be taken regularly, preferably once in the morning and once while resting before supper. A rate over 80 beats per minute is deemed rapid; under 60, slow. If the numbers increase or decrease significantly, contact the doctor.

Bodily Fluids

Some caregivers react to the unexpected release of urine or feces with disgust and unwillingness to deal with this new development. Patients, too, need to come to terms with it; the first "accidents" on the bedpan or sheets usually trigger incalculably deep feelings of shame and guilt. Long-term incontinence (see Urinary Incontinence, p. 419) can be a great strain on patient and caregiver alike.

Loss of Self-Control

Incontinence can have psychological causes as well as being associated with nervous disorders, diabetes, or stroke (see Urinary Incontinence, p. 419). Loss of bladder or bowel control may indicate withdrawal or a reaction to stress, such as when an older person loses an especially important support person or resists changes in home or family. Also, if a caregiver gives "too much care" and doesn't require the patient to do as much as possible, this may have the unintended effect of encouraging the patient to relinquish self-control.

Combating Incontinence

If a patient's control skills are actively encouraged and practiced, they will be retained longer and may even improve. Regular exercises can help strengthen the pelvic floor muscles and bladder (see Urinary Incontinence, p. 419).

Incontinent patients should always wear underpants to keep them warm; colder temperatures promote the urge to urinate. In addition, without the familiar contact of underwear against the pelvic area, the patient can easily lose awareness of that part of the body.

Bedsores

Bedridden people are at risk of developing bedsores. Their skin should be kept dry, cared for thoroughly and checked regularly. Places to watch especially are the heels, tailbone, hips, spine, shoulder blades, and any other place that's subjected to pressure for long periods.

Any patch of red that doesn't disappear may indicate a developing bedsore and requires immediate professional attention (see Bedsores, p. 288).

Changing Position

The best prevention against bedsores is to change position regularly. Alternating sides and back is effective. With the help of two cushions or other devices (e.g. a foam wedge) the patient is moved into a diagonal position, from which he or she is rolled onto the right side, back, left side, back, etc.—every 2 hours. Before moving someone, always state your intentions clearly; being handled without warning can easily cause the patient to feel anxious, defensive, and insecure.

Antibedsore Mattresses

These special mattresses help prevent bedsores and may be reimbursed by your insurance company. Over the long term, however, supersoft mattresses are not an optimal solution, for they reinforce bedridden patients' waning body awareness, caused by their lack of exercise and movement. Many such patients, unsure of exactly where they and the bed begin and end, constantly worry about falling out of bed. Therefore, one advantage of using regular bedding is that the patient's position must be changed regularly, providing him or her with periodic contact and movement.

SPEAKING AND COMMUNICATING

Communicating with a home-care patient can become extraordinarily difficult if a stroke or brain tumor has interfered significantly with the patient's ability to form words, hear distinctly, or think clearly.

If speech alone is affected, keeping paper and pen-

Cleanliness and hygiene for the caregiver

— Wear easily washable clothing without jewelry; tie long hair back; take your own hygiene seriously.
— Empty dustbin or remove waste from the sickroom every day, and don't leave soiled clothing lying around.
— Urine can and will thoroughly soak bedding, rugs, clothes, and diapers. Options for men include urine bottles and condom catheters.
— After every use, thoroughly clean bedpans, urine bottle, washbowls, and grooming aids. A hospital-like sterile environment is not necessary, with the exception of a catheter, which must be sterile.
— Catheters are hollow, sterile tubes that are inserted into the bladder via the urethra or abdomen and collect urine into a bag outside the body. Catheter use and care must be taught by a skilled professional and performed scrupulously.
— Costly devices such as toilet chairs can be rented; if your doctor prescribes them, your insurance may pick up the cost, as it may cover the cost of diapers/overpants, rugs, special mattresses or bed pads, urine bottles, or bedpans.
— For more information on hygiene, contact your health-care provider, local clinic or health maintenance organization (HMO).

cils on hand can help. In the event of severe disabilities, a speech board featuring simple symbols from daily life, or an electronic keyboard, can facilitate communication.

Physical Contact

The loving touch of a fellow human being is not just an elemental form of interpersonal communication; it can also be particularly helpful in aiding confused or paralyzed patients to regain body awareness and sense of orientation. Bedridden patients especially should be touched as often and gently as possible, since they are in greatest danger of losing body awareness (see Encouraging Exercise, p. 611). A constantly moving pressure, such as that of a body brush, is especially effective. All touch should start from the trunk, for example the shoulder: Being touched unexpectedly on the hands or

Bedsore Prevention Aids

In addition to special mattresses, body weight-distribution aids include gel cushions, foam wedges or sheepskin pads. More information is available from your local visiting nurse service or medical supplier.

fingers may cause the patient to react defensively.

In a Few Words

— Practice speaking with the patient. The goal is functional communication, not error-free speech. If necessary, supplement verbalization with simple gestures or body language.

— Speak distinctly, in simple, short, precise sentences. Ask questions that can be answered yes or no by the patient's nodding or shaking his or her head, squeezing your hand (one squeeze for yes, two for no), or blinking.

— Keep in mind that factors such as dry mouth, pain, or fatigue can be additional hindrances to communication.

— Avoid speaking for the patient. He or she should always make as much of an effort as possible to be intelligible.

— Always inform the patient regularly of the date and time, where he or she is, and what's going on around him or her. Prepare the patient in advance for any visits and changes.

— Offer praise and encouragement often.

Disorientation

Caring for a confused patient in a home setting is extremely stressful and usually places strain on the whole family structure. Make sure you get time off regularly as caregiver, whether it's free weekends or longer vacations. If the patient's disorientation and confusion accelerate quickly, have the doctor determine what changes may be going on in the brain (see Alzheimer's Disease, p. 219).

For confused older people and their family members as well, it is important to establish solid routines and rules. The daily routine should be as consistent as possible, with regular times for meals, exercise, and rest. Familiar, long-established routines are significant reference points in a potentially chaotic day; they should be observed to the minute as much as possible. An Alzheimer's disease patient can handle anything familiar better than something that's apparently unfamiliar. By sticking to a routine, the patient may be able to improve or maintain existing skills.

— Personal hygiene and getting dressed are often overwhelming for a disoriented person. You can help by dividing procedures into smaller steps, such as laying clothes out in the sequence in which they should be put on, or serving a meal one dish at a time instead of bringing everything to the table at once.

— Contact with friends and family is very important: Keep the patient as involved as possible in family life.

— Calendars, large clocks, labels, and signs on cupboards and doors can all help the patient stay oriented in the immediate environment. Favorite objects such as photographs or mementos are also helpful.

— When they're feeling overwhelmed, confused patients may act anxious, agitated, or even violent, so their environment should be kept as tranquil and unchanging as possible.

— Restless pacing around the house often relaxes older people and should be allowed (see Preventing a Fall, p. 613).

FOOD AND DRINK

Regular meals help structure the day into manageable portions and have an energizing effect on the chronically ill or disabled patient. The patient should feed himself or herself as long as he or she is able, even if the hands tremble or are weak, or the patient is uncoordinated. Useful aids include foam-covered knobs and handles, plates with high rims, and cups with spouts or long, curved straws. Combination utensils are also helpful, if a meal calls for several utensils at once. For more ideas, contact a visiting nurse service or medical supply store.

Potential Eating Problems

Bedridden or chronically ill older people usually have little appetite and are almost never thirsty; most don't drink enough liquids. Sometimes it helps simply to serve drinks in larger cups or glasses; they will often keep sipping until the cup is empty. Increase fluid intake by offering fruit juice or tea, stewed or pureed fruit, soup, and the like. At least 1½ to 2 quarts of water should be drunk daily.

A confused person may also forget to eat and drink if not regularly reminded. Problems chewing and swallowing, missing teeth, or ill-fitting dentures may further interfere with eating (see Dental Care, p. 364); unfortunately, this often results in patients being served foods that have been "cooked to death," until they are quite soft, but also practically devoid of nutritional value. To prevent malnutrition, the main thing is to help the patient maintain pleasure in eating:

— Set aside enough time for the patient's mealtime. If you act impatient and pressured, you'll reduce his or her appetite.

— The patient should be sitting as upright as possible, either at a table or securely propped up against the raised head of the bed.

— Eating will be more fun if the patient is with other people and/or in a pleasant dining atmosphere, for example with soft music in the background.

— Many small meals—five or six times a day—can relieve the stress of having to cope with one or two larger meals.

— One's favorite foods always taste best. To keep the patient's appetite stimulated, try to serve his or her favorite dishes as often as possible.

Eating Aids

— Allow enough time and establish an unhurried mood, especially if the patient has problems chewing and swallowing.

— Give the patient gum or a crust of bread to activate chewing; give him or her a lemon to sniff, to stimulate the flow of saliva.

— Always start meals with small amounts of solid food: Drinking is usually harder for the patient and can easily lead to choking.

— Place the patient's hand on the hand you are feeding him or her with. This will heighten the patient's sense of involvement in the process and usually cause him or her to open his or her mouth (lightly stroking the lower lip has the same effect).

— When giving the patient liquids through a straw, make sure no air gets swallowed.

— The patient's mouth and teeth should be rinsed or brushed following every meal.

DISABILITIES

Most of us don't know how to act with disabled people: Our behavior ranges from pity to embarrassment. Blind and deaf persons, paraplegics, and the intellectually disabled are at a distinct disadvantage in a society that places a big premium on youth, competitiveness, and high achievement. This list also encompasses people disabled from diseases such as polio and multiple sclerosis, and those who suffer disabilities due to accidents, war injuries, etc. Despite legal, social, and medical advances over the last two decades, the marginalization of people with severe disabilities continues. They are effectively kept out of the mainstream, especially in times of economic crisis.

WHAT CONSTITUTES A DISABILITY?

In medical terms, a disability is a disorder that permanently impairs a person physically, intellectually, or emotionally. In the strict sense, therefore, the approximately 25 percent of the population suffering from allergies, arthritis, or other chronic ailments qualifies as disabled, although the people involved certainly would not want to be labeled in that way. For the purposes of everyday language, disabled people are identified as those on crutches, in a wheelchair, psychologically disturbed, and so on. The percentage of disability is calculated according to the patient's level of productivity and autonomy.

Physical Disability

A physical disability is defined as a condition in which elements of the musculoskeletal system are damaged, or their functions disturbed.

Intellectual Disability

Intellectual disability is defined by the World Health Organization (WHO) primarily as significantly impaired intellectual faculties that first became evident in early childhood. Intellectually disabled people have problems forming social bonds with others. Their capacity to adapt and general aptitude are impaired, but not their capacity to experience joy or contentment.

The varying degrees of mental impairment are defined by the WHO as severe, moderate, and mild. Basically, intellectually disabled people develop the same way all people do; however, they require more time for each developmental stage, and in some areas never reach the advanced stages. They are thus unable to acquire the capacities and skills one generally expects of adults. Despite this, many intellectually disabled people, especially the mildly disabled, can lead relatively independent lives. The severely intellectually disabled can be somewhat independent as well, although they require the input of others to a greater degree. Most intellectually disabled people would not need to be institutionalized if alternatives were available; because many are limited only in their ability to establish ties with other people, they could live normal human lives with appropriate help and support.

Multiple Disabilities

Multiple disabilities can develop from a single disability that isn't detected and treated early enough. For example, a child's hearing problem, if not corrected in time, can lead to speech and learning disabilities, since hearing, speaking, and thinking are inextricably linked. The same goes for dyslexia (see p. 589).

Multiple disabilities can also indicate damage or dysfunction of several organs or systems of the body.

CAUSES

Physical or intellectual disabilities are caused by a variety of factors; parental chromosomes are by no means the principal cause. Most disabilities arise during fetal development and after birth; a large proportion are the result of work-, traffic-, and recreation-related accidents over the course of life.

Heredity

The exact causes of about 60 percent of all severe malformations remain unknown; in about 20 percent, a combination of congenital defects and acquired factors has been identified (e.g., spina bifida, cleft palate). A scant 7.5 percent of malformations are traceable to mutations in a particular gene (e.g. cystic fibrosis, Huntington's disease, Marfan's syndrome, neurofibromatosis). In the case of intellectual disabilities, 30 to 40 percent have unknown causes. It is often difficult to distinguish between genetic and acquired factors.

Acquired Factors

Nonhereditary factors present before birth cause

disabling conditions far more frequently than congenital factors. The following can cause developmental disorders in the fetus: maternal infections such as rubella early in pregnancy; chronic diseases in the mother (diabetes, epilepsy, high blood pressure, thyroid diseases, asthma, kidney disease); medications; alcohol, drug and tobacco use (see Dangers During Pregnancy, p. 572).

During or after birth, lack of oxygen can cause a disability; in later life, other causes include accidents, diseases, wars, and natural disasters. Under specific circumstances, existing disabilities can give rise to additional disabilities (see Multiple Disabilities, p. 618).

EARLY SCREENING

Thanks to genetic counseling, a couple concerned with the possibility of hereditary diseases can get help with decisions before conceiving and during the first few weeks of pregnancy (see Testing, p. 569). Some conditions such as Down's syndrome, spina bifida, or cystic fibrosis can be detected between the seventh and tenth weeks of pregnancy.

A range of tests administered during well-baby exams are designed to detect otherwise inconspicuous changes in babies. Early detection and treatment can also limit developmental disorders or diseases later in life (see Early Detection Screening, p. 591).

DISEASES AND DISABILITIES

Down's Syndrome

Characteristic signs of this disease include the epicanthal fold of the eyelid, a short skull, and small fingers. Children with Down's syndrome learn much more slowly than others and reach typical developmental stages much later. Often there are associated diseases or disorders. About a third of these children have heart defects, many have gastrointestinal problems, eyesight, and hearing are often impaired, and susceptibility to infections is greater.

Causes

Chromosome 21 has 3 components rather than the customary 2: hence the name trisomy 21.

Incidence

Down's syndrome is the most common human chromosomal disorder; 11 to 12 people in 10,000 are affected. One child in 700 is born with Down's syndrome, and the older the mother, the greater the risk: A 35-year-old has a 0.25 percent chance of bearing a child with trisomy 21, a 44-year-old has a 2.5 percent chance—ten times higher.

Treatment

Early intervention in children with Down's syndrome is critical and can significantly improve their chances for development. Therapies are comparable to those for other developmentally and intellectually disabled children. Practice and repetition are essential, since learning takes time and effort and is often achieved only after years of training. Even parents who play an active role in their Down's syndrome child's development should always take advantage of available medical and therapeutic resources, including home-based components. The experiences and input of other parents can also be helpful.

A primary goal of the child's journey to adulthood should be the attainment of independent living.

Huntington's Disease

This hereditary disease usually becomes apparent between age 35 and 50. It causes physical and mental changes that can appear sequentially, simultaneously or in an alternating fashion. Physical changes include uncontrollable, jerky movements, difficulties speaking and swallowing, and restlessness. Personality changes include irritability, indifference, depression, deteriorating intellectual skills, and social withdrawal. The disease leads to death within 15 to 20 years.

Causes

Huntington's disease (Huntington's chorea) is a degenerative disease of the central nervous system and is caused by an abnormal gene on chromosome 4. It was identified in 1983 and isolated and analyzed in 1993. The gene is inherited by both men and women. The offspring of people with the disease have a 50 percent chance of inheriting it: If they inherit the mutated gene, they can pass it on to their children, but if they don't inherit the gene, the disease will not be passed on.

Incidence

One person in 10,000 is affected.

Treatment

Although predicting the disease genetically before its

onset is now possible, there is as yet no definitive treatment. The goal of existing therapies is to enhance the patient's well-being, prolong life expectancy and ease symptoms.

Cleft Palate

Cleft palate is a common, visible congenital deformity. With early intervention, children with cleft palate can be successfully treated for this disability.

Causes

Most cases of cleft palate have genetic causes. The cleft develops through the interaction of several genes in conjunction with external factors such as a viral infection in the mother (rubella) or medications such as vitamin A derivatives (such as Accutane) prescribed for skin conditions like acne. Environmental factors (e.g., dioxin) are also thought to be associated with the incidence of cleft palate.

Incidence

One child out of every 500 to 1,000 is born with lip and/or cleft palate. Isolated cleft palate occurs in one out of every 2,500 births.

Treatment

Early intervention is crucial. Because parents and pediatricians can be ill-informed, they may miss the optimal moment for surgery, orthopedic intervention, and speech therapy, leading to a malformation that can be only partially corrected later in life.

In any case, intervention is also important to guarantee the child's normal psychosocial development. Parents can obtain information and help from the appropriate support group.

Dwarfism

Women with dwarfism stop growing once they reach a height of 36 to 56 inches; men's height is between 36 and 60 inches. Children with dwarfism are 20 to 30 percent below average height for their age. There are about 100 known types of dwarfism. Depending on the type, it may involve additional disorders such as intellectual disabilities, obesity, or muscle weakness. People with dwarfism have to cope with major psychosocial issues such as prejudice, lack of respect, and lack of societal acceptance.

Causes

Many factors cause growth disorders. Only 5 to 8 percent of those affected are missing human growth hormone, which can be replaced through injections (see Hypopituitarism, p. 502). In most cases a genetic connection is suspected or proven.

Incidence

One out of every 800 to 1,000 people is born with dwarfism.

Treatment

Medical diagnosis and monitoring are critical in preventing complications, as are early intervention and physiotherapy. In some cases, surgical extension of the leg and arm bones is possible, but risk-intensive.

Psychological support for people with dwarfism is essential, to prevent anxiety and the tendency to withdraw from society.

Spina Bifida

In the second to fourth week of pregnancy, the vertebrae develop into a bony column surrounding the spinal cord. If development is incomplete, it leaves a gap through which the spinal cord can protrude. In the most extreme cases, the spinal cord and nerve tissue are exposed. The baby is born with severe paralysis and associated conditions. This disability may include paralysis of the musculature, bladder, and intestine, as well as disorders of skin sensitivity. Eighty percent of children with spina bifida also develop hydrocephalus, a disturbance of fluid circulation in the brain, which in turn leads to further disorders.

Causes

The causes of spina bifida are not known for certain. It has been determined that it can result from an interplay of genetic and environmental factors, such as a folic-acid deficiency.

Incidence

Spina bifida is one of the most common birth defects. One in ten newborns has a mild spinal defect that does not affect the spinal cord (spina bifida occulta). If a couple has a child with this anomaly, their subsequent children are ten times as likely to have this anomaly as children born to other parents.

Treatment

In 9 cases out of 10, amniocentesis and ultrasound can detect fetal spina bifida and hydrocephalus.

For almost 40 years now, hydrocephalus has been successfully treated with surgery; and complications of spina bifida can be limited by simultaneous treatment on different fronts. Despite the complexity of this condition, prospects for rehabilitation are good if the child receives skilled care and support from the community.

Neurofibromatosis

Symptoms of this condition are light-brown patches on the skin and neurofibromas, or benign tumors of selected nerve and connective tissues. In severe cases, the tumors can appear by the thousands on the face and the whole body. Other forms of the disease are recurring tumors in the brain and spine as well as on the nerves of the eyes and ears. The severe consequences include paraplegia, blindness, and deafness. In children, the condition can cause problems with psychomotor skills, learning disabilities, and achievement and behavioral problems.

Because the condition can take many different forms, the disease is often diagnosed fairly late. This often leads to multiple doctor visits and hospital stays; in addition, symptoms may worsen because of incorrect treatment.

Causes

Neurofibromatosis is inherited from one parent in about half of all cases; in the other half, it is triggered by genetic mutations whose causes are unknown.

Incidence

Neurofibromatosis is a relatively common genetic disorder: One person in 2,000 is affected.

Treatment

This chronic disease affects the patient (and the patient's family) for his or her entire life.

Psychological help is as important as medical care. Intensive early intervention can compensate for children's psychomotor developmental problems and learning, performance and behavioral disabilities. In addition, blind or deaf patients can develop more of a social life thanks to new technologies (see Help from Computers, p. 623).

A therapy based on genetic engineering is in the research phase (see p. 753).

LIVING WITH DISABILITIES

With the passage of the Americans with Disabilities Act (ADA) in 1990, discrimination against people with disabilities was made illegal in this country. This has not been entirely effective to date: Disability continues to be measured exclusively in terms of one's capacity to work, given as percentages of "normal" activity.

This bias toward "normality" complicates the life of the disabled person and his or her interaction with nondisabled people. It undervalues and discriminates against the disabled person. It erects walls that prevent the disabled from living normally.

But what is "normal" and what isn't? In the complex arena of human life, even "normal" people may well be "different" in some areas, downright "disabled" in others. A child who learns things more slowly due to a disability still feels and experiences things like a "normal" child.

The 1975 United Nations Declaration on the Rights of the Disabled recognizes the needs of disabled people and addresses the barriers that prevent a person with congenital or acquired challenges from leading a substantially independent professional and private life. Despite some advances in certain areas—which are always at risk during times of economic crisis—the public mindset is only slowly coming to reflect the idea that people with disabilities have the right to the same living conditions we all do. In concrete terms, this means that the scope of their independence and responsibility should extend as far as the disability will allow. Disabled people should be able to grow up, learn, live, work, and play as much as possible within society.

Sexuality in the Intellectually Disabled

With few exceptions, sexual development in the intellectually disabled is substantially the same as in other people. They seek sexual contact and intimacy and are capable of developing an erotic relationship as a couple; sexuality is as much a part of their personality as it is in others. In spite of the right to sexuality of intellectually disabled persons, however, the issue is controversial and tends to make both the experts and the parents of intellectually disabled people uncomfortable. Some object to any form of sexual activity between the intellectually disabled; some advocate supervised sex. It is a matter of debate whether such individuals have sufficient capacities for empathy and mutual caring to maintain a mature relationship.

The arguments against self-determined sexuality completely ignore the fact that many things seen as peculiar to the disabled are actually the products of limited education, deficient sexual education, and abnormal living conditions, such as the lack of intimacy in group homes.

The desire to have a child is often included in a retarded person's desire for sexuality and partnership. In these cases, parents or guardians need to evaluate the situation and provide counsel to help the individuals in question realistically gauge their capacity for the responsibility that parenthood requires.

Sexuality in the Physically Disabled

Sexual problems in physically disabled persons are usually because of the fact that their bodies are "different"; many people have trouble associating deformed body parts with giving and getting love. Especially for this reason, parents of disabled children should encourage as normal and healthy an affective development as possible.

Contraception

Like everybody else, disabled people who are heterosexually active need to be able to prevent unwanted pregnancies. In principle, all methods are appropriate (see Contraception, p. 551).

Sterilization

Sterilization should only be considered for the intellectually disabled if the use of other forms of birth control can't guarantee against unwanted pregnancy. If the patient can comprehend the consequences of sterilization, he or she can decide in favor of the operation, with a guardian's consent and legal sanction. Forced sterilization is illegal. If the patient expresses any reaction that could be construed as a lack of consent, sterilization is prohibited. Sterilization of minors is expressly forbidden (see Sterilization, p. 558).

Living at Home or Away?

For a person with disabilities, living in a group home is the closest alternative to staying with the family of origin. In group homes, small groups of people live together with a supervisor; they hold jobs or attend school; they enjoy skilled supervision, care, and help at home; and they are in daily contact with peers, with whom they can interact, teaching and learning important life skills such as feeding and dressing themselves and handling emotions.

Institutions

Disabled people are often housed in institutions because of a shortage of supervised group homes. Institutions combine more or less restricted living and working spaces with facilities for recreation, occupational training, and therapy. Adequate psychospiritual support and stimulation are usually lacking. As if in compensation, institutionalized patients often have many daily physical tasks performed for them which they could benefit greatly from having to perform themselves.

Institutionalized patients live isolated from society. Sleeping and living areas are usually communal; they have little or no privacy or space to call their own. Treatment is geared more toward maintenance than development and eventual mainstreaming.

Troubling images of children warehoused in such institutions touch the heart, while perpetuating a false image of what disabled people could actually achieve with appropriate care.

Nursing Homes

Nursing homes are designed mainly to care for older patients. Younger residents don't get anywhere near the help they need. Rather than emphasizing potential, these institutions, too, focus on maintenance

Lifesharing Communities

These village settings include living, working, occupational, recreational, and therapeutic facilities for both disabled and nondisabled people. The ratio and setup vary from one type of community to the other. The Rudolf Steiner Camp Hill villages, for example, have a familylike structure.

Living and working together enriches the lives of disabled and nondisabled persons alike, but as in institutions, the disabled person is still isolated from the rest of society. Living quarters and lifestyles in the various villages also tend to be rather uniform, though this is not a serious offense.

Disabled-living Centers

These centers provide a place for disabled people who are able to function in a supervised workplace and either can't, or don't want to, live with their families. To be accepted into such a center, the person must be in a position to care for herself in large measure without help. Contact with housemates is abundantly available; free time can be spent in a variety of ways. Disadvantages are isolation and lack of contact with nondisabled people.

Group Homes

In this arrangement, three to eight disabled people share a house or apartment in a regular residential area, which is owned or rented by the sponsoring organization. The sponsor provides supervision and help. Members go to school or work during the day; care and supervision are provided at specific times. This approach requires that the housemates demonstrate a certain measure of independence.

These homes offer members the possibility for contact with neighbors. Everyday activities like shopping, going to the doctor, taking walks, etc., take place within the context of a nondisabled environment; daily experiences resemble those of the nondisabled. Close contact with housemates helps the individual get a sense of his or her own potential and limitations. Members experience life's ups and downs in the company of a close, supportive community.

The problems that develop are the same as any encountered when a number of people live together under one roof; the atmosphere can get tense. Since the groups are smaller than those in institutions, however, problems are usually easier to resolve.

Communities

In communities for the disabled, people live together voluntarily and organize their own assistance programs. Some communities are composed exclusively of disabled people, others are mixed. There are independent communities as well as those organized and supported by various societies.

Independent Living

Living solo works as long as the disabled person has access to good outpatient care. Such arrangements may be organized by the state, a support group, or a sponsor. Independent and autonomous living is possible in this situation. If support services are insufficient, however, the individual may feel isolated and easily overwhelmed, for example, by the prospect of having to organize cultural or recreational activities during free time.

Respite Homes

Disabled people can be temporarily accommodated in respite homes or hostels when the family needs a break, be it for a vacation or during a crisis. At some facilities, patients may have access to occupational training and programs to prepare them for alternative living situations, mainstreaming, and/or halfway houses.

HELP FROM COMPUTERS

New technologies incorporating microchips and computers can significantly improve daily life for the disabled. Microchips can replace an ear or an eye to a certain extent; modern communication techniques can enable even severely disabled persons to work on a computer. Some technologies are already a reality, others are in experimental phases.

Microchips Replace Body Parts

Artificial ears: An electronic prosthesis (cochlear implant) is inserted under the skin. A microphone picks up vibrations, which are transmitted as electrical impulses to the implant and then to the brain. While conventional hearing aids can only intensify vibrations, a cochlear implant can, in certain cases, actually help a child born deaf to hear (see Deafness, p. 251).

Artificial eyes: Devices similar to the artificial ear will one day help people with retinitis pigmentosa (see p. 248) to see. Scientists are working on a microchip that converts light into electrical impulses that stimulate the remaining intact nerve cells.

Artificial limbs: Prostheses controlled by microchips are already being used in animal experiments. In the future, prostheses such as artificial hands will be moved by the body's own nerves via microchips embedded in neural pathways: The chips will interpret brain commands that control movements of hands or legs and transmit them to the prosthesis.

IRIS for the Blind

The IRIS system being developed in Austria can help a blind pedestrian navigate street traffic with more confidence. It works by way of infrared signals transmitted from a traffic light to a receiver held by the pedestrian, which then translates the data into synthetic speech. Much information can be transmitted this way.

Computerized Workstations

Body signals can be picked up, digitized and processed by means of a bioelectrical interface. This makes it possible for severely disabled people to use a computer by eye or head movements, which are transmitted to the computer via an optical motion detector in the mouse.

Speech-Activated Manipulation

This device makes it possible to perform a multiplicity of tasks through voice activation. The spoken word is translated into signals that are transmitted via cable or infrared technology to operate a specially adapted wheelchair, window, door, radio, television, or stereo.

Examination and Treatment

THE PATIENT-DOCTOR RELATIONSHIP

Although we entrust our health-care providers with the health of our bodies and psyches, many of us spend a lot longer looking for a good car than a good doctor. Yet, in order not to be treated like a faceless "case" when we require medical care, we should be willing to put time and energy into finding a health-care provider who will get to know us, our families and our circumstances, and to whom we can always turn first in time of need.

During a hospital stay, it can seem overwhelmingly tempting simply to give up responsibility for our health along with our clothes and personal belongings. Questioning or challenging authority can be intimidating even when we're healthy; for an ill person, it is often that much harder. It's easier just to hope "the system" will take care of everything—yet this hope is often accompanied by a nagging sense of being at the complete mercy of an institution. A lot of anxiety could be prevented if we took the time while still healthy to familiarize ourselves with local hospitals and staff.

Outpatient (Office) Medicine

CHOOSING A DOCTOR

Choose your health-care providers while you are still healthy: A general practitioner, a gynecologist, a specialist for any chronic conditions. Your sense of judgment will be better, and so will your flexibility in switching doctors if necessary. Doctors vary both as individuals and as practitioners, so it is important to have clear expectations and be as well-informed as possible.
— Do you favor certain types of therapeutic approaches, for example, anthroposophic medicine, naturopathy, homeopathy, or acupuncture?
— Whom do you feel you would trust more: a young doctor who (you assume) is more knowledgeable about the latest advances in medicine, or an older one with more years of experience?
— Would you be more comfortable confiding your health problems or intimate details to a male or female practitioner?
— Would you feel more secure or more anxious in an office stocked with the latest technology?

— Would you feel more relaxed in an informal atmosphere?

Location, Scheduling, Services
Where a medical practice is located, how it's organized, and how it operates can help you decide if it's right for you.
— Is it near public transportation, or is parking available?
— Is it handicapped-accessible?
— Are office hours flexible? Are evening or Saturday hours available?
— Are appointments necessary, or are patients seen on a first-come, first-served basis?
— Can you get an appointment on short notice, or do you have to sign up weeks in advance? A long wait doesn't always indicate a good doctor—it might just indicate a badly managed office.
— Do multiple consulting rooms make you feel part of an assembly line—the sooner you're in and out, the better—or do you feel you can take your time dressing and undressing without gumming up the works?
— Is the phone constantly busy?
— Does the doctor make house calls in emergencies?
— Is he or she associated with a hospital or clinic?
— Is he or she associated with a home health-care agency or visiting nurse service?
— Does the practice offer special services: Nutritional counseling for diabetics or people on low-cholesterol diets; stress management counseling; etc.?

When asking friends, family members, or colleagues to recommend a physician, the above questions may come in handy. Keep in mind that, especially in cities, competing medical practices often try to outdo each other by offering special services. While this should work to the patient's advantage, all services may not be administered by qualified personnel. To avoid disappointment, periodically ask yourself: Is this service something I need? Did it really help me? Do I feel comfortable?

Office Organization
How a medical practice is organized can tell you a lot about it. Depending on what is important to you, the following details may be worth noting:

— How does the doctor interact with the staff? This will probably give you a good idea of how he or she will deal with you.
— Do the doctors and staff wear name tags? These can make communicating with them easier.
— Are patients in the waiting room kept informed of unexpected delays in the appointment schedule, or are they left waiting without explanation?
— Are magazines the only reading material in the waiting room, or is there informational literature as well? The latter may indicate that the doctor welcomes well-informed patients.
— Is patients' privacy respected? Are files lying around for all to read? Are you asked for personal information or read test results in a crowded waiting room?
— Are you given informative literature to take home in anticipation of particular tests or procedures so you will be better prepared? Are you given a written record of upcoming appointments to prevent misunderstandings?
— Is anybody smoking in the office? If so, how seriously will you be able to take health advice from this source?
— If you are obviously disabled in any way, are you offered help dressing and undressing?

BEFORE THE DOCTOR VISIT

Before seeing a doctor, know what you want and expect from the appointment. Are you seeking immediate help for an acute condition, treatment for a chronic illness, or a better understanding of how your lifestyle may be contributing to ill health, and assistance in changing it?

It doesn't make sense to come away with a prescription for antibiotics, for example, if you don't plan to take them. On the other hand, some adjustments in your lifestyle may be necessary for a proposed treatment to be effective.

Preparing at Home

Preparing for a doctor appointment should be no different from preparing for a business meeting. Writing down beforehand what you wish to discuss will help you organize your thoughts.
— What are the symptoms? How long have you had them? When do they appear, and under what circumstances? Exactly where does it hurt? Also note any past symptoms, even if they seem unrelated.
— How have you treated the ailment so far?
— What medications are you taking? Include all prescription medications and any over-the-counter analgesics, vitamins, tonics, etc.
— Record the results of home tests such as urinalysis or temperature readings.
— Keep a home file of your medical history, containing pertinent information on vaccinations, illnesses, examinations, operations, etc.
— Keep documentation on allergies and vaccinations, and prescriptions for medications or treatments, with you at all times.
— If symptoms vary over the course of the day or are more pronounced at certain times, schedule your medical appointment for the time when they are most evident.

COMMUNICATING WITH THE DOCTOR

As an adult, you are basically responsible for your own health. You can freely decide whether or not to undergo treatment and may choose whatever treatment modality you prefer, even though others might consider your decisions misguided. Physicians are required to discuss with you, the patient, all information necessary for you to make an informed decision, including risk factors, possible side effects and consequences of treatment, chances of recovery, and alternative treatment options.

Some examinations or treatments may require serious pondering before you can come to a decision. You can ask to be given time for this, and you'll know you are in good hands if your doctor understands and agrees. Only you can judge whether you have enough information and understand the situation clearly enough to arrive at a decision. Most doctors will only take the time to talk things through if you ask, so do ask if necessary. It might be wise to make another appointment for this purpose, since physicians are often on tight schedules and other patients may be waiting.

Of course, all patients have the "right to not know," if that's what they prefer. However, experience with chronically and acutely ill patients has shown that people are usually better off with a thorough comprehension of their situation, and answers to questions like: What will affect the course of this illness? What are its causes? What is the prognosis? How does the treatment work?

Communication Hangups

Patients sometimes come away from a doctor's appointment upset because they still have unanswered questions or an incomplete understanding of something that was discussed. This may be partly the doctor's fault, but remember, doctors can't read minds. The more common reason is that communicating with a health professional can be a source of anxiety. How many of the following sentiments feel familiar to you?

"If I ask to have too many things explained, I might sound stupid."

"If I ask the doctor how he or she arrived at the diagnosis, he or she might think I don't trust him or her."

"If I tell the doctor he or she is hurting me during the checkup, he or she might feel criticized and get angry."

"If I talk about my drinking or sexual problems, he or she might disapprove of me or even refuse me treatment."

"My problems are probably unimportant compared to other people's. I shouldn't take up too much of the doctor's time."

Though such worries are common, you should do your best to ignore them. If your physician is worth his or her salt, they will prove to be unfounded. It is in your best interest to make sure you understand things completely. You can only follow instructions that you understand. It's a good idea to write things down as you hear them in the doctor's office, and ask right away about anything that isn't clear.

The Medical History

A definitive diagnosis and customized treatment program are only possible if the doctor knows your complete medical history. This includes information on your lifestyle, job, and past illnesses as well as current symptoms. A complete physical exam is also essential, and at least a half hour will be required for this aspect alone.

Make sure to tell the doctor if you have already received treatment for your current complaint from another source, be it conventional or alternative.

Getting the Diagnosis

The doctor should share test results with you in person. The following points should be covered:
— The name of the illness.
— Is the diagnosis definitive, or is it simply the most likely one? How was it arrived at?

— What is the normal course of the illness, and what complications are possible?
— Is the illness contagious?
— Is it hereditary?

The doctor may recommend additional tests, such as endoscopy, X rays, or radioactive isotope tests (see Diagnostic Tests/Procedures, p. 635). You should find out why they are necessary, what the risks are, and exactly what the results are expected to reveal. Modern diagnostic techniques can produce large quantities of detailed information, which doesn't necessarily translate into useful treatment options. Ask yourself whether you are willing to go through with extensive testing procedures just to find out something nobody can do anything about anyway.

Guidelines for Treatment

In general, provided the patient gives permission, a physician is free to treat the illness as he or she thinks best. Certain guidelines for patient protection exist, including the following:
— The chosen treatment method must be effective and appropriate.
— A method whose risks might outweigh its benefits should not be used, even if the doctor disagrees with this risk assessment.
— A doctor may not do anything that general medical practice considers pointless. For example, he or she may not pull healthy teeth under the assumption that they are a breeding ground for some disease.
— If an unconventional method of treatment is to be used, the patient needs to be especially well informed about it beforehand. Even treatment of a common cold requires some explanation from the doctor.
— How should the illness be treated?
— What are the risks of treatment?
— Can a change in lifestyle or working conditions replace treatment, or lower its risks?
— What is likely to happen if the illness is left untreated?
— What is likely to happen if the treatment isn't followed through to its conclusion?
— What do I do if my symptoms get worse?
— How do I know whether the illness is getting worse?
— Can the treatment be increased or intensified?
— Are there other forms of treatment, and why was this one chosen?

Prescription Medications

Don't feel you automatically need to come away with a prescription after a visit to the doctor; many successful treatments involve no medication. Instead, you should always ask the doctor whether any prescribed medication is absolutely necessary.

If you do receive a prescription, be sure to get clear, complete instructions from the doctor before leaving the office. Medication labels can be so confusing that some people end up not taking the medicine at all (see Medication Summary, p. 657). The instructions should include anything you should or shouldn't do while taking the medication, as well as what to do if you can't tolerate it.

Again, taking notes is a good idea to remind yourself of all the details.

Living Wills

If you want to be sure not to receive specific medical treatments even after you are no longer capable of making a decision, a "living will" may be the answer. A living will is a document in which you state your wishes regarding medical procedures; for example, you may not wish to be put on a life-support system, should the time come.

You should understand, however, that doctors don't necessarily have to abide by the living will if they feel its directives contradict their better judgment. If the document is notarized, it may carry more weight.

Checkups and Early Detection

It is well established that regular checkups can detect illnesses in their early stages, which are the easiest to treat effectively. For example, use of a hearing aid early in life can do much to ensure healthy psychological development in a hearing-impaired child. In adults, lowering elevated pressure in the eyeball before it causes problems can prevent cataracts which could eventually ruin eyesight.

Cholesterol and liver function tests, on the other hand, are important because the potential illnesses they may reveal can be prevented simply by making changes in lifestyle or diet. Of course, if you are unwilling to make such changes, treatment may eventually be the only remaining course of action.

PATIENTS' RIGHTS

Patients have the right to receive thorough information on diagnoses and treatments (see Communicating with the Doctor, p. 627). Doctors must obtain patient consent before taking action. If the patient is underage, parents must be informed; for example, children may not be given routine immunizations at school unless parents are informed of the reasons, risks, and possible consequences. Patients must give written informed consent before receiving certain injections or undergoing certain tests, procedures, and/or treatments. A doctor who tests someone for human immunodeficiency virus (HIV) without their consent can be sued.

Patients have additional rights, including

— Medical records must be made available to all health-care personnel involved in the patient's care.
— Patients may obtain copies of their medical records.
— Patients may see the results of all their lab tests, X rays, and diagnostic procedures, and may obtain copies.
— Patients have the right to be informed of the contents of a sealed letter they are taking from one doctor to another, but may not open it.
— Your doctor is under no obligation to inform your employer or anybody else about your health condition, unless not doing so would increase health risks to others.

Getting a Second Opinion

You may feel justified in seeking out another doctor beside your own if

— Your doctor cannot provide a service which has been deemed necessary in your case (e.g., psychotherapy).
— You feel your doctor is not correctly diagnosing your condition.
— Treatment has not been effective within an allotted time period.
— You want a second opinion before undergoing surgery.

In an emergency, all doctors are required to be of service. In nonemergency situations, however, they have the right not to treat a patient, or to terminate treatment.

When You Disagree with the Doctor

If you feel you were incorrectly treated by a doctor, it is a good idea to follow the steps outlined below. The goal of the process is usually financial compensation from the doctor's malpractice insurance company. Settling out of court is much less costly and time-consuming than taking the case to court. Statistically, about half the medical cases that make it to civil court are thrown out; in about 40 percent a settlement is arrived at.

— First of all, talk to the doctor. This can make the next steps unnecessary.
— Get expert advice on patients' rights and possible avenues of recourse. Many support groups can supply this.
— Make a written record of all the pertinent events as they occurred: Dates, names, fellow patients who could serve as potential witnesses.
— Obtain copies of all relevant medical records.
— You are responsible for the fees of lawyers or medical experts from whom you request reports or evidence.
— Find a competent lawyer who will help you decide which course to follow: reaching an agreement with the doctor's and/or institution's insurance company; or filing suit in court.

Inpatient (Hospital) Medicine

In general, hospital stays are becoming shorter, with patients released earlier than they used to be. This development is not always in the best interest of the patient, unfortunately. Many procedures that used to require a day or two in the hospital are now handled on an outpatient basis, and policies are constantly changing.

CHOOSING A HOSPITAL

It is not always possible to choose a hospital, especially in emergencies. However, if you have the opportunity to choose, it is to your advantage to do so.

General Hospitals

General, nonspecialized hospitals are often a better choice for common ailments than specialized medical centers. You will probably not be subjected to unnecessary tests or operations, especially for a simple procedure such as an appendectomy. Because of a possible lack of experience on the part of the staff, however, you may choose not to have less common types of surgery performed at such a hospital (e.g., plastic surgery or heart operations).

Specialized Hospitals

If you can find an institution that specializes in your particular condition, it is probably a good idea to go there. A surgeon who performs three ureter operations a day is likely to be more familiar with the procedure than one who does one a month. A possible disadvantage of such an institution, however, might be a tendency to perform surgery simply because it is the norm at that hospital or because the hospital possesses the latest in medical technology—even if this approach or procedure is not necessarily indicated in your case. When in doubt, get a second opinion.

Teaching/University Hospitals

Teaching hospitals often have the most advanced techniques and equipment, but you may find yourself in the following situations: You may be surrounded by medical students while being examined or operated on; an inexperienced doctor may perform procedures on you under the close guidance of an experienced teacher; or (with your prior consent) you may be treated as the "case of the day" and operated on with an entire class watching.

Day Hospitals/Outpatient Clinics

Outpatient clinics do not provide overnight care. Patients requiring follow-up treatment return to the clinic if and when necessary. If you are slated for outpatient surgery, make arrangements beforehand for supplementary help or care at home, in case you are very weak after the operation or experience complications.

When a doctor decides to assign you to a certain hospital, what is the basis for the decision?
— Does the hospital specialize in treating your particular condition?
— "It's the best hospital in town" is not a satisfactory answer; it's extremely rare for every department in a hospital to be "the best." How does the department you'll be in rate?

Guidelines for Choosing a Hospital

The most important aspect to consider when choosing a hospital is the quality of its medical care. Since hospitals are not required to publicize their statistics regarding successes and failures, you will probably need to depend on recommendations from friends, colleagues, or health-care providers.

Also important when choosing a hospital, however, is the quality of life it offers. This checklist may serve as a guide:
— Are the rooms quiet and well-lit?
— Are they pleasant and well-organized? Is there room for personal belongings?
— How many patients share a room?
— How close together are the beds?
— Does the room contain a place to wash, separated by a curtain or wall?
— Are there enough showers and toilets in the ward?
— Is there a pleasant waiting room?
— Are patients lying in beds outside rooms? Is there an odor of food or excrement in rooms or hallways?

Rules and regulations
— Do visiting hours suit your needs?
— Are children allowed to visit?
— Can family members stay overnight with a child or critically ill person?
— Can a patient leave the hospital for a few hours, health permitting?

— Can patients sleep whenever they want, or are there strict rules?

Staff
Some aspects of hospital life only become evident once one is actually a patient. However, even a casual visit will give an impression of the general atmosphere:
— Do staff members appear friendly and courteous, or harried and overworked?
— Are their interactions with patients respectful and appropriate?
— If you ask to speak to someone in charge, how is your request received?
— Are your questions considered an intrusive nuisance, or are you accepted as someone who simply wishes to be well-informed?

Food
Healthy, tasty meals can significantly speed the healing process. Daily menus are usually posted in hospitals; is a varied vegetarian option included, or does "vegetarian" mean wilted salad and hard-boiled eggs day after day? Don't be afraid to ask questions, such as:
— Is the food prepared fresh daily, or is it frozen?
— Is there a choice of menus?
— Is food served warm? How long is it kept warm before being served?

— Does the doctor have other patients in this hospital, making it more convenient for him or her to keep tabs on you? This is not the best reason for choosing a particular hospital.
— Does the doctor have friends on the aftercare staff? This is only an advantage if the hospital has high standards of medical care.

COMMUNICATING WITH DOCTORS AND HOSPITAL STAFF

Partly for their own protection, people who are around illness and suffering on a daily basis tend to become somewhat desensitized to these phenomena, and may come across as unsympathetic or emotionally uninvolved.

As a patient, you are nevertheless entitled to be treated with respect and dignity, and to receive understandable answers to your questions. Be sure to ask immediately about anything that is unclear to you.

Daily Rounds

The doctor's daily rounds are designed to update doctors and patient on the patient's condition, but they are also often the patient's only opportunity of the day for one-on-one dialogue with the doctor. If you feel rushed, ignored, bewildered by jargon, or if the only remark addressed to you is a formulaic "How are we doing today?" you need to take responsibility for the situation.
— Ask medical personnel to speak clearly in terminology you can understand.
— If a new treatment or test is prescribed during rounds, ask your questions now. The person who will actually be administering the procedure later won't have the complete picture.
— If you have questions regarding your current treatment, ask them now.
— If time runs out and all your concerns aren't put to rest, make an appointment to see the doctor later, at a more convenient time.

Medical Records

Everything that happens to you in the hospital is recorded: All your tests, treatments, therapies, medications, surgery, and so on. Often patient files are kept in a central location or on a computer. The advantages of such centralized data storage are accessibility and organization; the disadvantage is the increasing erosion of patient privacy.

As a patient, you have the right to inspect your files and receive copies of your records. Your doctor will usually personally share information regarding your case with you, your family members, and any other doctors involved in your care. If you are opposed to this practice you need to make your wishes known.

Decoding Records

If you need help making sense of your medical records, you could either consult a medical dictionary or (the simpler solution) ask your doctor to explain them, translating any unfamiliar words, cryptic codes, or abbreviations into laypersons' language. Ask about anything you don't understand. Some hospitals have their own code symbols for certain confidential procedures, such as tests for HIV.

Your Right to Know

Physicians are required by law to personally inform you about all procedures, treatments, and typical risks involved in your situation; merely handing you preprinted literature is not sufficient.

In an emergency situation, however, it is understood that doctors may not have the time to explain everything fully.

Medical personnel must answer all your questions truthfully, but only you can decide how much you want to know. Some people feel better knowing every detail, others don't want to be burdened by all that information. In any case, you are within your rights asking the following questions:

— What are the risks of this procedure?

— What complications may arise?

— What are my other treatment options and their risks? (For example: Could I have laser treatment instead of surgery, or epidural or spinal anesthesia (see p. 581) instead of general anesthesia?)

— Is the recommended treatment relatively new or controversial?

— What are the effects and side effects of the recommended medications?

— Is the doctor proposing an experimental treatment? (You have the right to refuse guinea pig status.)

It's All in the Timing

When you're lying there sedated and prepared for surgery, it's too late to change your mind—so make sure you are informed in advance of the possible risks and consequences of all procedures. You need time to think things over with a clear head, get a second opinion, or check out other alternatives if you wish to do so.

ARE HOSPITALS DANGEROUS?

If you believe the media, hospitals are fraught with lurking dangers: Patients routinely undergo operations meant for someone else, scalpels are sewn up in patients' bodies, infections run rampant. Most of this is hype, with the possible exception of the fact that you stand about a 4 percent risk of contracting an infection in a hospital.

The Risk of Infection

It's impossible to avoid some exposure to infections in a hospital. Wherever microorganisms and antibiotics are concentrated in such close quarters, resistant strains develop much more quickly, so new varieties are constantly being hatched. Among the most common infections are those of the urinary tract, followed by wound infections and respiratory infections.

Seventy to 80 percent are transmitted by doctors and other hospital personnel.

The following guidelines can help you lower the risk of infection:

— Avoid hospital stays if outpatient treatment is an option, especially if your immune defenses are low. This may be the case in older people, who contract hospital infections at an above-average rate.

— Don't routinely take antibiotics if not strictly necessary. They are neither cure-alls nor some sort of internal disinfectant, and they hasten the development of resistant microorganisms.

— Make sure catheters are removed as soon as possible. Catheters are often left in longer than necessary, and the risk of infection rises with each passing day. After 10 days, 50 percent of patients with urinary catheters develop a bladder infection.

— Avoid invasive examination methods. Choose noninvasive options whenever possible.

The Risk of Mistakes

Every year, a certain percentage of mistakes are made in hospitals. You can do your part to reduce the chances of this happening to you:

— If you have doubts about your treatment or your diagnosis, don't hesitate to get a second opinion.

— In larger hospitals, "assembly-line" operations are common, with pre-surgical exams and actual surgery performed by different doctors. Ask to meet your surgery team in order to reduce your chances of being mistaken for another patient.

The Risk of Complications from Anesthesia

If you are in generally good shape, the risk of complications from anesthesia is extremely low. Even if you have heart disease, diabetes, hypertension, asthma, or cirrhosis of the liver, you can lower your risk of complications considerably by taking appropriate measures in preparation for anesthesia. However, if you require emergency surgery, e.g., as an accident victim, neither the doctor nor the anesthesiologist is likely to know your general state of health and, therefore, your particular level of risk. Similarly, they are unlikely to know whether your stomach is full or how extensive your loss of blood was. Both these factors can influence your reaction to anesthesia.

If you require surgery, there is usually no way around anesthesia, but you can improve your chances by asking the following questions in advance:

— Is your anesthesiologist also working on other patients? Mistakes are often the result of fatigue or overwork due to understaffing.

— Can you meet your anesthetist beforehand? This will help you feel more comfortable.

— Are local or regional anesthesia viable alternatives to general anesthesia, which is not always necessary?

Malpractice

If you feel hospital malpractice has caused you pain and suffering, the path ahead promises to be strewn with obstacles. Like members of any other profession, medical personnel are reluctant to speak ill of each other. Malpractice cases often take years to settle. Your best recourse is to get a lawyer and try to settle out of court.

Going to trial only makes sense if you have the money, time, and stamina for a long legal battle, and/or are trying to focus public attention on a particular cause.

Preparing for Legal Action

— Make sure you have a paper trail of reliable evidence. Even if you aren't out for blood and hope to come to an agreement, it is still advisable to secure copies of all relevant records before revealing that you're considering legal action. It is not uncommon to find information altered or omitted from records if you wait until the legal process has begun. If you encounter problems dealing directly with the hospital, try to get the necessary information through a doctor you trust who is not personally involved in the case. If this is not possible, a patients' rights organization may be able to help you.

— Secure the services of a reputable attorney. Some lawyers are known to specialize in malpractice. Support groups or patients' rights organizations can supply you with names. Malpractice attorneys will almost always aim for a financial settlement with hospitals, doctors, and insurance companies.

— Keep detailed records. Clearly document everything related to your illness as soon as you suspect malpractice. It may be harder to remember the details at a later date. Some patients' organizations have forms to fill out for this purpose. Make sure you include:

— What damage or injury you suffered, and what caused it.

— A detailed description of events leading up to the alleged malpractice.

— Names and addresses of fellow patients and relevant medical personnel.

CHILDREN IN THE HOSPITAL

To feel sick in a strange place, surrounded by strangers, can be a very stressful situation for children, who especially need a parent's loving presence at such a time. Bedwetting, eating disorders, fear of the dark, depression, aggressive behavior, and communication problems are only a few of the symptoms that may result from a traumatic hospital experience. To reduce this risk, most children's hospitals and wards have extended visiting hours and permit overnight stays for parents or guardians.

Hospital Trauma

Children experience traumatic events in three distinct phases: protest, hopelessness, and denial.

Protest

The child throws tantrums or weeps inconsolably, either clinging to the nurses or angrily fighting them off. He or she misses her parents desperately and can't understand why she has suddenly been separated from them. This phase may last several hours or even days.

Hopelessness

The child realizes his or her parents will not return. He or she stops crying or showing emotion, lapses into apathy, and stops interacting with her surroundings. This phase is repeatedly misunderstood. Often caregivers believe the child is finally being "good" and has gotten used to the new situation.

Denial

The child has given up inside, but acts outwardly "reasonable," showing interest in his or her surroundings again. When family members come to visit, he or she doesn't pay attention, or may even reject them. This phase is often misinterpreted as successful adjustment.

What You Can Do for Your Child

— Before a hospital stay, prepare your child at home. Play doctor; listen to each other's heart and lungs, give pretend injections, etc. Even after the hospital stay, role-playing can help the child process traumatic experiences. Pay attention to your child's play: Whatever the dolls or stuffed animals are preoccupied with will offer a clue to what the child is trying to cope with but not expressing.

— If your child can be treated as an outpatient, choose that option—as long as someone will be able to care for him or her at home.

— If hospitalization is required, make sure its duration is as brief as possible.

— Visit your child as often as possible and arrange to have other family members visit.

— Don't forget that babies can feel and suffer even though they can't talk. They need the same amount of care and loving reassurance as older children.

— Ask to stay with your child around the clock; you may have the legal right to do so.

— If you stay in the hospital with your child, make sure you trade off with another family member or someone close to the child. Spending day in, day out in a hospital can be extremely stressful for a healthy person.

— Ask to be present during difficult or painful examinations or procedures. Your presence will contribute to their success.

— If your child will be undergoing surgery, try to stay with him until he or she is anesthetized. Be there without fail when he wakes up.

OLDER PEOPLE IN THE HOSPITAL

Hospitals are often filled with elderly patients that don't really belong there. Older patients may be relegated to understaffed wards where their needs are not sufficiently met and opportunities for rehabilitation or counseling are scarce. The patient may feel abandoned and afraid he or she will never leave the hospital, which in turn worsens his or her condition.

If you have an older relative in the hospital who can no longer take care of his or her affairs, step in.

— Find out whether hospitalization is really required: Can the person be treated on an outpatient basis?

— Try to determine whether all the procedures the person is undergoing are actually necessary. Procedures unnecessary for health but convenient for the caregiver (e.g., installing a catheter in the bladder) are common in older patients.

— Try to arrange for rehabilitation services for the patient, such as physical therapy.

— Time your visits to coincide with the greatest opportunity to help the patient, e.g., mealtimes to help him or her eat, or bedtime to help him or her wash. Very few hospitals have enough staff to give individual attention to all patients.

— Don't do things for the patient unless absolutely necessary. Encourage him or her to be as independent as possible. This will stimulate a sense of capability and well-being, and hasten healing.

— The sooner the older person can get back to familiar surroundings, the sooner he or she will get better. Try to shorten the hospital stay as much as possible.

If the patient becomes an invalid, insurance will usually no longer cover hospitalization costs, and finding a nursing home may be necessary.

DIAGNOSTIC TESTS/PROCEDURES

Everyone makes mistakes. We know this is true of people, yet we mistakenly assume that, on the contrary, machines and technologies can't be wrong. Many patients feel more secure if they can take home charts full of numbers or X ray results. Physicians, too, tend to place more confidence in a technological diagnosis than in the evidence of their own senses when examining a patient. Yet a recent long-term study showed that despite their increasing reliance on technology, doctors' rate of misdiagnoses remained constant at 10 percent.

The more physicians and patients depend on technology, the less intimacy is required of the relationship. This spares both sides from having to deal with often unpleasant feelings and problems. However, the trend toward mechanization also tends to obscure the psychological components of illness, for example the connection between a disease and the patient's situation at home or at work (see Health and Well-Being, p. 182).

The desire for perfection is costly. In the United States, approximately a billion laboratory tests are ordered annually, at a cost of billions of dollars. According to the American Medical Association, at least millions are spent annually on unnecessary tests.

Because the lifetime of fancy medical equipment—and the time manufacturers will service it—keeps on getting shorter, it is becoming more and more difficult for individual doctors to purchase the equipment, and for laboratories to amortize the high initial cost. In order to make the device pay for itself, physicians and laboratories need to use it as much as possible to run patient tests—keeping medical costs spiraling upward.

Another reason test costs are constantly on the increase is that the medical technology industry keeps developing more complex and expensive methods, which are erroneously assumed to be automatically superior to older methods. In reality, it has only occasionally been proven that "newer" means "better" when it comes to medical testing technology.

Many diagnostic tests also contribute to environmental problems. Disposable instruments pile up in landfills; reagent solutions flow down the drain to ... somewhere; radioactive substances are transported to the medical facility, used, and then disposed of ... some-where. Questions also remain as to the cumulative health effects on medical personnel who work with these substances every day of their working lives.

TESTS AS ENDS IN THEMSELVES

So-called "screening tests" examine as many people as possible, repeatedly, for one characteristic. For example, the general population is encouraged to have blood cholesterol levels checked regularly. This test is appropriate for people who are at especially high risk of dying of coronary heart disease and who are willing to change their lives to reduce the risk (see Atherosclerosis, p. 318)—but it is useless if the test subject is simply left on his or her own with a poor test result. By itself, such a diagnostic test not followed by treatment serves no useful purpose

Large numbers of unnecessary tests cost health insurance carriers (and therefore their subscribers) huge amounts of money. They may also be hazardous to the health of the patient, sometimes significantly so. One study, for example, showed how casually doctors order routine chest X rays for no obvious reason. In over 25 percent of referrals to one X ray specialist, it was unclear why the X ray was ordered. Over 25 percent of the patients did in fact show something unexpected in their results, and in some cases, this led to more tests—but did not in any way alter the diagnosis.

The same goes for the array of tests often routinely administered during the course of admission to a hospital: They are only rarely essential for diagnosis or treatment. All these ills can be avoided if you, together with your doctor, determine your goals and the procedure to be followed to achieve them.

Determining Goals and Procedures

Even though lots of things can be tested, that doesn't mean they need to be.

From your description of the symptoms and a general examination, your doctor should determine as precisely as possible which disease he or she suspects, and which he or she wishes to rule out. Before you undergo any tests, both you and your doctor should be clear about the purpose to be served by each procedure. Does it

— Provide, confirm, or rule out a diagnosis

— Determine the severity of the disease
— Show how the disease is progressing
— help in determining the right treatment
— Show what results a treatment has had
— Determine the level of a drug in your body
— Check whether you have been following your doctor's orders

How reliable are the test results? Before you make a decision with serious consequences

— Have the results checked again.
— Find out whether the results can be obtained by a less problematic test.
— Find out what conclusions should be drawn from the results.
— Be sure to tell your doctor, before every test, which drugs you are taking. Some deviations from the norm can be caused by medications and are not indications of disease.

Routine Tests

When a patient is admitted to a hospital, some tests are routinely administered. These may include

— Sodium (Na), potassium (K), and sometimes chloride (Cl) or magnesium (Mg). The levels of these ions in the blood help determine whether certain heart and kidney conditions are present, possibly caused by dehydration, or if the composition of the body fluids has changed.
— Phosphate (PO^4) is an indicator of kidney function.
— Calcium (Ca) gives information on parathyroid gland function. Calcium and phosphate together indicate whether nutrients are being properly absorbed from the stomach and intestines.
— Blood urea nitrogen (BUN) and creatinine can indicate kidney function.
— Alkaline phosphate (AP) can indicate bone disease and whether the bile tract is blocked.
— Protein. An abnormally low value can impart information about diseases that consume body mass, and possible disorders of resorption. An abnormally high value can be an indicator of a type of malignant disease.
— Blood sugar. The level indicates whether carbohydrate metabolism and insulin production are in balance.
— Glutamic oxalacetic transaminase (GOT) (see p. 643),

glutamic-pyruvic transpeptidase (GPT) (see p. 642), gamma-glutamyl transpeptidase (see p. 643), lactic dehydrogenase(LDH) (see p. 643). These tests are indicators of liver function.

When comparing numerical values from your tests with those on the following pages, you may run into differences caused by the use of different units in expressing the results. While internationally standardized (Système international d'unités or SI) units for these tests have existed for a long time, not all medical facilities use them.

The type of assay used, the temperature at which it was carried out, and many other variables can yield abnormal numerical results, which still do not indicate the presence of disease. If you are in doubt, ask the laboratory what range it considers normal.

What follows is an overview of the most common diagnostic testing methods. The test results you are given by your doctor may, however, include other terms and numbers; always ask for clarification if you need it.

BLOOD TESTS

Applications

These tests are used when doctors want a general idea of the body's condition, or to learn more about certain blood components. Many changes in organs and immune-system processes are reflected in the blood.

Purpose and Reliability

Changes in blood values confirm the suspicion that something is wrong. In order to determine exactly what this is, more tests are needed.

Procedure

Depending on what is to be determined, blood may be taken either by pricking a fingertip and collecting the blood drops (capillary blood), or by inserting a needle into a vein, usually in the arm, and withdrawing blood through it. Today this is done with disposable vacuum tubes with which the person drawing the blood cannot be injured; this method also protects you from infection.

Blood drawn in this way is used for plasma or serum tests.

Blood Cell Counts

About 45 percent of the blood consists of solid particles: red cells, white cells, and platelets. Blood cell counts reveal the numbers of individual cell types, and sometimes, sub-types.

Red Blood Cell Count

The red blood cells (erythrocytes) are formed in the bone marrow. They consist mainly of hemoglobin, the protein which transports oxygen in the blood.

Normal Range

Adult women: 3.5 to 5.5 millions/mm^3
Adult men: 4.3 to 5.9 millions/mm^3
The values for children are somewhat lower than those for adults, and vary with age.

Applications

In common illnesses; when anemia is suspected; and in blood diseases.

Purpose and Reliability

Values below the normal range indicate anemia (see Anemia, p. 345). Values above the normal range (polycythemia) are found in disorders of blood cell formation, chronic lung diseases and tumors. It is normal for the number of red blood cells to increase in individuals who engage in physically demanding work or sports, or who are acclimated to high altitude.

Hematocrit

The hematocrit value is the percentage of blood volume occupied by solids (cells).

Normal Range

Adult women: 37 to 47 percent
Adult men: 42 to 52 percent

Applications

In general illnesses; when anemia is suspected; and in disorders of blood formation.

Purpose and Reliability

See Red Blood Cell Count, above.

Hemoglobin

Application

To determine how much hemoglobin is present in the red blood cells.

Normal Range

Adult women: 12 to 16 g/dl
Adult men: 14 to 18 g/dl

Purpose and Reliability

The type of anemia present can be deduced by comparing the hemoglobin content to the red blood cell count or the hematocrit value. This is necessary in order to treat the anemia properly.

Iron Level

Iron is one component of hemoglobin. It is also found in the protein transferrin, which transports iron in the blood, and in ferritin, which is a storage protein for iron. If the blood is lacking in iron, the body normally attempts to compensate by synthesizing more transferrin than normal.

Normal Range for Iron

Adult women: 40 to 150 mcg/dl
Adult men: 50 to 160 mcg/dl

Normal Range for Transferrin

Adults: 200 to 400 mg/dl

Normal Range for Ferritin

Adult women: 13 to 125 ng/ml
Adult men: 27 to 220 ng/ml

Applications

To determine whether anemia is due to an iron deficiency; if it is suspected that there is too much iron in the blood.

Purpose and Reliability

Iron values are low
— After severe bleeding, e.g. after an operation, but also when there has been unnoticed loss of blood through the gastrointestinal tract, or due to inflammation or tumors. Nursing mothers also have low iron values.

—When iron intake is not sufficient to meet the body's need.

— If gastrointestinal disease prevents uptake of iron out of food.

Iron values are high:

— In diseases in which liver cells degenerate;

— In disorders of hemoglobin formation (see Hemolytic Anemia, p. 347).

A single blood-iron test is meaningful only if it shows values far below or far above the normal range. Blood's "normal" iron content may differ from person to person. It is almost always lower in older people than in younger ones. In everyone, it is higher in the morning than in the afternoon. Only a combined test of iron, transferrin and, if possible, ferritin, can give reliable information about an iron deficiency. If both iron and ferritin values are low but the transferrin value is high, the diet may have contained too little iron for a long period. If all three values are low, this suggests a chronic inflammation or a tumor.

White Blood Cell Count

The white blood cells (leukocytes) are part of the body's immune system. There are three large groups of white blood cells: Granulocytes, monocytes, and lymphocytes. There are also further subdivisions of these large groups.

Normal Range

Adults: 4.5 to 10 thousand/mm³

Newborns have up to 30,000 white blood cells/mm³. The number drops gradually until the 15th year of life, when adult values are attained.

Applications

In cases with general symptoms, such as fever without an obvious cause, or fatigue; also, to confirm suspicions of a particular disease.

Purpose and Reliability

Either an elevated or a depressed number of white blood cells can indicate that the immune system is challenged, for example by infection, tissue necrosis after a burn, heart infarct or cancer.

Some medications can reduce the leukocyte count.

A slightly elevated leukocyte count is normal during pregnancy, after physical exertion, or in cases of psy-

chological stress. The leukocyte count drops in old age.

White Blood Cell Count Differential

The several different types of white blood cells are counted in a blood smear, and their proportions are reported as percentages.

Normal Range (adults)

Immature granulocytes: < 3 percent
Polymorphonuclear granulocytes: 60 to 70 percent
Eosinophils: 1 to 5 percent
Basophils: < 1 percent
Lymphocytes: 20 to 30 percent
Monocytes: 2 to 6 percent

Application

A differential count shows which types of leukocytes are present in larger or smaller numbers than normal. This knowledge improves the odds of a correct diagnosis, because other possible diseases can be ruled out more easily.

Purpose and Reliability

Changes in the granulocytes can indicate a bone marrow disorder. Granulocytes go through a process of maturation, and their appearance depends on their level of maturity. If the distribution of the cells at various levels of maturity deviates from normal, this is another indication of disease.

The entire lymphatic system, especially the spleen and lymph nodes, forms lymphocytes. If the lymphatic system is diseased, for example by cancer, the lymphocyte count is reduced. Treatment with cancer medications also reduces the lymphocyte count. The count is increased during infectious diseases and diseases of the blood-forming organs.

Erythrocyte Sedimentation Rate (ESR)

Freshly drawn blood is prevented from clotting by an additive; it is then placed in a measuring tube. The blood cells gradually sink to the bottom. After an hour, the distance they have settled is measured.

Application

The ESR is a common laboratory test. Its purpose is to reveal a "poor general condition" if it exists. It is a marker of tissue inflammation.

Normal Range

Neonates and children: 3 to 13 mm/hr

Post-adolescent women (< 40 years): 1 to 20 mm/hr

Post-adolescent men (< 40 years): 1 to 15 mm/hr

Women > 40 years: (age in years + 10)/2

Men > 40 years: age in years/2

Purpose and Reliability

The ESR is accelerated by inflammations, cancer and severe anemia. It is slowed by diseases in which red blood cell counts are elevated. An ESR in the normal range is neither an indication of good health nor of disease. If the value is moderately elevated, the reason should be sought, if there are important accompanying symptoms. An ESR from 80 to 100 is always a reason for further testing. In older people who have been ill for a long time and whose ESR rate has become worse, it is prudent to test for an unnoticed cancer. However, the ESR is not suitable as a general "cancer test." When the ESR is evaluated, it is often forgotten that the values tend to rise with age.

Causes of Error

The ESR is extremely sensitive to errors.

Oral contraceptives, vitamin A, and phenothiazine accelerate the ESR, while corticosteroids, acetylsalicylic acid (aspirin,) and indomethacin (all used against rheumatism) retard the ESR.

Coagulation Profile

The process of blood coagulation (clotting) involves three components: The injured tissue, the platelets (thrombocytes), and the clotting factors in the blood. Clotting is a multistep process.

Applications

— When a blood-clotting disorder is suspected. Its presence is first confirmed with broad-spectrum tests, and then the precise site at which the clotting process is interrupted is located by more specific tests.

— To monitor the patient's blood when anticlotting drugs are administered; for example, in order to prevent thromboses or after a heart attack.

Platelet Count

Platelets develop from cells in the bone marrow and are involved in blood clotting.

Application

— To determine whether a clotting disorder is due to a defect in the platelets.

Purpose and Reliability

The number of thrombocytes is elevated (thrombocytosis) in diseases of the bone marrow, during severe general illness, following removal of the spleen, and following severe blood loss. Their number is depleted (thrombocytopenia) if the bone marrow is producing too few platelets or their lifespan is unusually short. This can happen, for example, if antibodies are attacking the platelets.

Normal Range

Adults: 150,000 to 400,000/mm^3

In children it varies with age.

Prothrombin Time Test

The prothrombin time compares clotting time against normal values and measures a selection of specific clotting factors.

Applications

— To determine whether a clotting disorder is due to specific clotting factors.

— To test the effectiveness of medications intended to increase clotting time, e.g., those administered after a heart attack (Coumadin).

Purpose and Reliability

The prothrombin time test gives low values when

— A vitamin K deficiency is present

— Clotting factors are absent

— There is liver damage

— Certain medications have been ingested

Normal Range

10 t 13 seconds.

Blood Lipid (Fat) Levels

The fats we take in with food consist, chemically speaking, of a variety of individual substances, including cholesterol. After absorption from the intestine, these fats are found in the blood. An excess of fats can damage the body in a variety of ways (see Atherosclerosis, p.318).

Applications

Elevated blood fat levels are considered risk factors for hardening of the arteries, and thus for coronary heart disease. Patients who are aware of their risks can reduce them by changing their lifestyle. Therefore, it is reasonable to test for blood cholesterol and high-density lipoproteins (HDL) (see Lipoproteins, below) levels about every 5 years after one's 20th birthday. Some diseases and a variety of medications affect the amount and composition of blood fats, so in these cases it is also wise to check for the associated risk of atherosclerosis.

Purpose and Reliability

The ratio of blood cholesterol to HDL is the most reliable method for determining one's personal risk of atherosclerosis.

Triglycerides

Application

Provides a general indication of blood-fat content.

Normal Range

Age 0 to 19:   10 to 140 mg/dl
Age 20 to 29: 10 to 140 mg/dl
Age 20 to 39: 10 to 150 mg/dl
Age 40 to 49: 10 to 160 mg/dl
Age 50 to 59: 10 to 190 mg/dl

Purpose and Reliability

Elevated triglyceride values are usually related to nutrition (see Atherosclerosis, p. 318), but they also occur in disorders of fat metabolism, gout, inflammation of the liver, kidneys or pancreas, and in diabetes.

After a fatty meal, the triglyceride content of the blood is high. In addition, it is quite variable for any individual, and depends on age and gender as well.

Cholesterol

Cholesterol is taken in with foods containing animal fats. However, the body synthesizes considerable amounts of cholesterol on its own.

Applications

— To confirm the suspicion of a disorder of fat metabolism.
— To obtain a better estimate of the risk of coronary heart disease.

Values for Selecting Men and Women at Risk for Treatment

Age	Moderate Risk (mg/dl)	High Risk (mg/dl)
20 to 29 years:	>200	>220
30 to 39 years:	>220	>240
40 and over:`	>240	>260

Purpose and Reliability

Coronary heart disease is practically unknown in people with cholesterol values below 200 mg/dl, and this is a value which adults should attempt to maintain. The risk increases significantly between 200 and 240 mg/dl. Above 250 mg/dl, the risk is high (see Atherosclerosis, p. 318). However, age should always be taken into account in such evaluations.

Causes of Error

Corticosteroids (see p. 665) and oral contraceptives can cause cholesterol levels to rise.

Lipoproteins

Fats are linked to proteins in order to be transported by the blood. The combination of fat and protein is called a *lipoprotein*. There are three main types:
Very low-density lipoproteins (VLDL)—contain large amounts of triglycerides and little cholesterol.
Low-density lipoproteins (LDL)—contain small amounts of triglycerides and large amounts of cholesterol (these are the "bad" lipoproteins).
High-density lipoproteins (HDL)—contain little triglyceride or cholesterol, and are able to absorb deposits of cholesterol (these are the "good" lipoproteins).

The designations "good" and "bad" refer to the influence of these lipoproteins on atherosclerosis (see Atherosclerosis, p. 318).

Application

Determination of the risk of atherosclerosis is based on the fat content of the blood.

Purpose and Reliability

An assessment of lipoprotein levels can help in identifying the right treatment for a fat metabolism disorder. The ratio of cholesterol to HDL in the blood may be used by physicians as part of an examination for early warning of atherosclerosis risk. The numerical ratio should be lower than seven.

Causes of Error

When interpreting the results, the physician should take into account that many diseases affect the lipoprotein composition, as do oral hormones and pregnancy.

Normal Distributions for Lipoproteins

Age	VLDL (mg/dl)	LDL	HDL (mg/dl) Men	(mg/dl) Women
0–19	5–25	50–170	30–65	30–70
20–29	5–25	60–170	35–70	35–75
30–39	5–35	70–190	30–65	35–80
40–49	5–35	80–190	30–65	40–95
50–59	10–40	80–210	30–65	35–85

Sugar

The blood carries sugar as an energy source for cells. The body regulates the concentration of sugar in the blood by means of the hormonal system, and keeps it within narrow limits (see Diabetes, p. 483).

Application

Every routine blood examination should include a glucose test. Especially in older people, diabetes can remain undiagnosed for a long time (see Diabetes, p. 483).

Purpose and Reliability

Significantly elevated blood sugar, or high values obtained repeatedly, indicate diabetes (see p. 483).

Procedure

Blood is drawn for the test when the patient has fasted overnight. Then, on the same day, it is drawn again 1 or 2 hours after a meal.

Causes of Error

Some medications elevate blood-sugar levels, including diuretics, corticosteroids, oral contraceptives, thyroid hormones, and medications for mental illness, rheumatism, epilepsy and circulatory disorders. Alcohol reduces the blood-sugar level.

Other Methods

Sugar can be measured in urine, but only when levels are higher than normal.

Normal Range

— Fasting blood sugar: < 100 mg percent
— One hour after eating: < 180 mg percent

Uric Acid

The kidneys normally excrete as much uric acid as the body produces, but excessive production or insufficient excretion can upset the balance.

Application

— To confirm suspicion of gout or monitor its treatment.
— To check for excessive uric acid in the body during a fast or treatment of a serious illness.

Normal Range

Women: 2.5 to 6.2 mg/dl
Men: 3.5 to 8.0 mg/dl

Purpose and Reliability

Above normal uric acid values are found in connection with:
— Gout
— Kidney function disorders
— Fasting
— Diseases in which cells degenerate (some muscle diseases, psoriasis, leukemia, and cancer)
  Below-normal uric acid values may indicate several extremely rare diseases.

Sources of Error

Diuretics (thiazides) increase blood uric acid levels.

Creatinine

Creatinine is a metabolic end-product formed when muscles contract. It is excreted by the kidneys.

Application

Test of kidney function.

Normal Range

Adults: 0.7 to 1.5 mg/dl

Purpose and Reliability

Creatinine values increase slightly in cases of cardiac arrest, liver coma, and lack of fluids. Values over 2 mg/dl clearly indicate that the filtration capacity of the kidneys is limited (see Kidney Failure, p. 425). In cases of severe injury, burns, or muscular dystrophy, the muscles may contribute to elevated creatinine values. In the borderline region between the upper end of the normal range, the test gives little reliable information about kidney function. However, even values below 1.1 mg/dl do not guarantee that the kidneys are functioning perfectly.

Bilirubin

Bilirubin is formed when red blood cells break down. It links to a protein and is then transported to the liver by the blood. After further changes in the liver, the bilirubin becomes part of the bile and is excreted.

Application

— To test liver function, and determine whether bile passages are open.
— To confirm a suspicion that anemia is due to the degradation of too many red blood cells (see p. 637).
— To decide whether a newborn needs a blood exchange.

Normal Range

0.1 to 1.4 mg/dl

Purpose and Reliability

If the values are above 1.4 mg/dl, it can be assumed that the liver and/or bile passages are not functioning perfectly. However, the reason for the disorder cannot be determined with this test. An enzyme test (see below) is better for an exact diagnosis of liver disease.

Causes of Error

Many medications can impede bile flow and thus increase the bilirubin content of the blood.

Blood Enzymes

Enzymes are catalysts for all the chemical reactions that make up the body's metabolism. They are found in all tissues and cells. Determination of blood-enzyme levels gives the physician an excellent indication of liver condition and permits confirmation of suspected heart attacks. Because of its function as the metabolic and detoxification "factory" of the body, the liver produces many enzymes in its cells. Some of these are released into the blood. If these enzymes are assayed, the physician can learn how well the liver is doing its job.

Other liver enzymes are normally present only inside liver cells (e.g., GOT ([see p. 643], or GPT [see below]). These enzymes can only enter the blood if the cells containing them become permeable or completely degraded. Thus, elevated levels of these indicate that cells are malfunctioning. The term "liver function tests" includes these enzymes.

Some of the enzymes present in the liver are also present in the heart and skeletal muscles, but the relative quantities are different for each organ, and this permits them to be differentiated.

The following enzymes are often determined in blood samples:
— *Glutamic pyruvic transaminase (GPT)*—its new name is Alanine aminotransferase (ALT).
— *Glutamic oxalacetic transaminase (GOT)*—its new name is Aspartate aminotransferase (AST).

Both of these together are designated by the term "transaminases."
— *Gamma glutamyl transpeptidase (GGTP).*
— *Lactate dehydrogenase (LDH).*
— *Creatine phosphokinase (CPK).*

Glutamic Pyruvic Transaminase (GPT)

Application

This is a test of liver function, usually in combination with other enzymes.

Normal Range

Adults: 7 to 35 U/l
Newborn: 6 to 62 U/l, decreasing to adult range in several months

Purpose and Reliability

Elevated levels of this enzyme are relatively specific for liver diseases.

Causes of Error

The following medications can elevate the GPT level: Oral contraceptives, medications that lower blood-fat levels, and certain sedatives. In a large proportion of the population, alcohol causes the GPT level to rise (see Alcohol, p. 756).

Glutamic Oxalacetic Transaminase (GOT)

Application
Evaluation of liver function.

Normal Range
Adults: 7 to 45 U/l
Newborns: 7 to 62 U/l, decreasing to adult values at 3 months

Purpose and Reliability
GOT levels are elevated in
— Acute liver diseases (20- to 30-fold)
— Liver damage caused by poisoning
— Chronic liver disease
— Heart or lung infarction
— Rapidly progressing muscular dystrophies
— Shock

The test for GOT is extremely sensitive, but not highly specific. The cells of many organs can release this enzyme, so elevated levels are significant only if other enzyme values are also altered, in a fashion typical for the disease under consideration. In case of heart attack, the GOT value is meaningful only when it is determined 24 to 48 hours after the attack. After three days, the body has already metabolized the enzyme. It is more useful to determine the CPK value (see below) if the symptoms or an EKG indicate that a heart attack has occurred.

Causes of Error
Alcohol and many medications damage the liver. The GOT level is highest 3 hours after alcohol consumption.

Gamma Glutamyl Transpeptidase (GGTP)

Application
Confirmation of suspected liver disease.

Purpose and Reliability
GGTP levels are elevated
— If alcohol is consumed regularly (see p. 756)
— In liver diseases and obstruction of bile ducts

A GGTP test by itself is hardly sufficient to confirm a liver disease, but if its value is normal, one can be reasonably sure that the liver is healthy. Obese people usually have somewhat elevated levels without being unhealthy.

Causes of Error
Alcohol consumed the day before the test, as well as many medications, elevate the GGTP level. In these cases liver damage is not indicated.

Normal Range
Women: 5 to 55 IU/L
Men: 15 to 85 IU/L

Lactic Dehydrogenase (LDH)
This enzyme is found in all tissues. Its concentrations are especially high in skeletal and cardiac muscle, and in the liver.

Application
This enzyme is assayed when a heart or lung infarction is suspected, or for some blood diseases.

Purpose and Reliability
LDH values can be elevated in many diseases. In order to diagnose a heart attack with confidence, LDH and several other enzymes should be tested (see creatine phosphokinase [CPK] values, below).

Normal Range
30 to 200 IU/l

Creatine Phoshokinase (CPK)
There are several subtypes of creatine phosphokinase that are present in different tissues in different relative quantities.

Application
Diagnosis of heart attack.

Purpose and Reliability
The total CPK value is always elevated when muscle cells are destroyed. The causes vary, so it is only appropriate to use this test when other indicators point to a certain disease. In the case of heart attack, for example, such indicators would be symptoms or an EKG.

Normal Range
Women: 20 to 210 U/L
Men: 35 to 230 U/L

Causes of Error
Sore muscles, or injection of a drug into a muscle a little while before the test, can elevate CPK values.

URINE TESTS

Applications
— Evaluation of kidney condition. The presence of kidney stones, for example, may be revealed by traces of blood in the urine.
— Testing of kidney function. If kidneys are functioning properly, some substances, e.g., creatinine, should be eliminated as completely as possible, while others, e.g., protein, should be retained as completely as possible in the body.
— Investigation of infections of the kidneys, bladder, or urinary tubes.

Purpose and Reliability
Because the patient collects the sample for a urine test, part of the responsibility for its accuracy lies with the patient.

Procedure
All methods for collecting urine are designed to keep it as free as possible of contamination by bacteria. If the doctor needs to be certain that any bacteria present in the urine come from the bladder, he or she may collect the urine through a catheter or a needle inserted directly into the bladder. If you as patient are collecting the sample, be sure to use a new container—either one given to you in the doctor's office or one you can buy at a pharmacy. If you use a washed-out jelly jar or soda bottle, traces of detergent and/or rinse water may give false results. Your doctor will tell you which type of urine to collect.

Morning urine is what you produce first thing in the morning, after at least six hours of sleep.

Spontaneous urine is what you can produce on demand in the doctor's office.

Initial urine is the first part of the urine released.

Mid-stream urine is collected after allowing the first portion to flow into the toilet.

Total urine is all the urine you produce over a period of 24 hours. The doctor will tell you what time period to use. Twenty-four-hour urine, for example, might be collected as follows: After rising in the morning, you empty your bladder into the toilet. Thereafter, all the urine you produce is collected, with the final collection being made the next morning after rising.

Bacteria

Application
To test for bladder or urinary-tract infections.

Purpose and Reliability
Test strips: Test strips have one field that shows whether protein is present in the urine, and another that reveals changes in the composition of the urine caused by bacterial action. These strips are useful for screening, but not for monitoring the success of treatment.

Causes of Error
False negative results with test strips can be caused by:
— Ingestion of large amounts of vitamin C
— Low consumption of vegetables the day before the test
— Urine that has been in the bladder for fewer than 4 hours

A false positive result can be caused by letting the urine stand for a long period before testing it.

Normal Range
Bladder urine is normally free of bacteria.

Up to 1,000 bacterial cells per milliliter can be tolerated. If more than 10,000/ml are present, the test should be repeated. If more than 100,000/ml are present, the patient should be treated for an infection.

Blood
Urine normally contains no blood, red blood cells, or hemoglobin. Therefore, detection of any of these components is significant.

Application
Routine in urine examinations.

Purpose and Reliability

Test strips can detect red blood cells and hemoglobin separately.

Red blood cells in the urine are symptoms of the following diseases:
— Kidney stones
— Inflammation of kidney tissues or the urinary tract
— Kidney tumors
— Severe circulatory disorders in the kidneys
— Kidney injuries

Hemoglobin in the urine is symptomatic of the following disorders:
— Anemia caused by degradation of red blood cells
— Severe poisoning, burns, or infectious disease
— Muscle injuries or severe muscle diseases

Causes of Error

— After unusually strenuous physical exertion or sports training, red blood cells may be found in the urine when no disease is present.
— Menstruation may interfere with this test.

Red coloration of the urine may be due to ingestion of laxatives containing phenolphthalein, or red beets, but will not interfere with this test.

Protein

Applications

This test is usually used to check kidney function. If a strip test shows protein is present in the urine, the next step is to measure the amount precisely. Subsequent tests may reveal the type of protein, which will indicate the region of the kidneys that has become permeable. People who are at high risk of developing kidney problems, such as diabetics, should have their urine tested for protein at regular intervals. Treatment while the condition is in its early stages can retard the otherwise inevitable progression toward kidney failure.

Purpose and Reliability

Impaired kidney function can be a side effect of diseases in other organs; if this is the case, kidney function will return to normal when the other disease is cured. Above-normal amounts of protein are found in morning urine in cases of
— Fever
— Inadequate heart function

Any disease of the kidneys can impair their function so that more protein than normal is found in the urine. Such conditions include
— Kidney infections (pyelonephritis) (see p. 421)
— Inflammation of the filter cells of the kidneys (glomerulonephritis) (see p. 422)
— Degenerative processes in kidney tissue
— Gout
— Heavy-metal poisoning
— Damage to kidney tissue caused by chronic use of painkillers (see p. 660) or diseases like diabetes (see p. 483) or high blood pressure (see p. 321)
— High blood pressure during pregnancy (see p. 571)
— Side effects of many medications

For protein testing, the amount of protein present in spontaneously collected urine is compared with that found in 24-hour urine. In addition, either total proteins or just one type, the albumins, may be assayed.

For patients with diabetes and similar causes of high risk of kidney damage, there are methods for detecting much smaller amounts of protein. Quantities between 30 and 300 mg/100 ml of albumin in 24-hour urine are called "microalbuminuria," and total protein between 50 and 500 mg/100 ml indicates "microproteinuria." If the amount of protein lost per day is 3.5 g or more, the diagnosis of kidney damage is certain.

Procedure

Morning urine gives the most reliable information about the filtration capacity of the kidneys.

Causes of Error

The following can considerably increase the amount of protein in the urine during the day:
— Physical stress or sports training
— Hypothermia or hyperthermia

Normal Range

Protein concentration in 24-hour urine: Up to 50 mg/100 ml

Albumin concentration in 24-hour urine: Up to 30 mg/100 ml

TRACINGS

When nerves and muscles are in operation, tiny amounts of electrical current are generated. These voltages can be measured and graphed to aid in diagnoses. These tests are used primarily to evaluate brain and heart function.

Electrocardiography (EKG)

The voltage in an excited heart-muscle fiber is different from that in a resting fiber. As the heart works, each part undergoes a cycle of voltage changes. The tissue surrounding the heart is also electrically conductive, so that the heart's electric field can be detected over the entire body. Changes in this field are measured by an electrocardiogram or EKG, which is taken by placing small metal electrodes on the arms, legs, and chest.

Purpose and Reliability

Experienced physicians can correctly diagnose coronary disease in most of their patients by taking an accurate medical history, with no need for an EKG. Nevertheless, anyone who enters a medical practice complaining of chest pain is soon hooked up to an EKG machine. The purpose of an EKG is usually to give information about the heart's current condition. The heart's capacity to handle a load requires a so-called stress EKG, in which the patient exercises for a fairly long period on a stationary bicycle or treadmill. Ten deep knee bends or a couple of trips up and downstairs won't do it. A stress EKG is taken for patients with coronary heart diseases, angina pectoris, cardiac arrhythmias, or high blood pressure; it is also used to check general regulation of the circulation. In an extended-period EKG, a heart with no noticeable symptoms is checked, over a period of 24 hours, for arrhythmias and adequate blood supply.

Electroencephalography (EEG)

The brain, like the heart and nerves, generates an electrical current as it works. Small metal electrodes placed on the skin can detect these currents, which are then amplified and recorded on a long strip of paper. The resulting zigzags and curves give the doctor information about brain function.

Applications

Monitoring head injuries: Bleeding in the region of the dura matter, the relatively inflexible "skin" of the brain, can cause pressure on the cerebral cortex and damage it. After an acute injury, such damage is detected by a computed tomography (CT) scan (see p. 649) or magnetic resonance imaging (MRI) (see p. 650).

Inflammation of the meninges and brain: This condition markedly changes the shape of the curves in the EKG. *Brain tumors:* Sometimes a tumor is detected by the fact that no current is flowing at that site, but usually it is noticed because of the pressure it places on the surrounding tissue.

Epilepsy: The EKG may reveal the increased susceptibility of the brain to seizures, allowing the physician to confirm the presence of the disease and to monitor treatment. EKGs are also used to locate brain abcesses, as a check after electroshock treatments, and to help confirm brain death. The technology is less useful in psychiatric illnesses or Alzheimer's disease.

IMAGING TESTS

Ever since it was discovered how to make invisible energies visible, X rays, tomograms, scintigrams, thermograms, MRI, nuclear studies, and ultrasound have made it possible to see what is going on in human bodies.

Many of these imaging technologies are used to monitor a disease's nature and the stage of its progression. Choosing the most suitable method for individual patients is becoming more and more difficult, however, as testing methods become ever more specialized. The general considerations applicable to any kind of test, given on page 635, also apply here; ideally, the primary-care physician would consult with colleagues specializing in these high-tech methods when deciding what is best for the patient.

X Rays

Technical Aspects

X rays are generated when electrons are separated from atoms, accelerated to extremely high speeds, and beamed from one end to the other of a vacuum tube. The electrons then crash into atoms at the other end of the tube, releasing their kinetic energy as X rays. When the rays exit the tube and hit a photographic film or specially coated glass, they leave a visible image.

Taking X Rays

The part of the body to be X-rayed is placed on the X ray platform or positioned in front of the photographic film, the apparatus is then adjusted precisely so that only the desired area is irradiated.

The Image

When X rays penetrate matter, they lose energy. Bones absorb more energy than any other tissue, so they appear white on the picture. Organs filled with air or gas, such as the lungs and stomach, absorb extremely little energy and appear black on the image. Other tissues differ very little in the amount of energy they absorb and are therefore hard to distinguish in an X ray. Contrast media are used in order to improve this situation and heighten the contrast (see p. 648).

All layers of body tissues penetrated by the rays are visible in the image, though they are usually indistinguishable.

Fluoroscopy

In fluoroscopy, an X ray image is projected onto a screen or television monitor, making it possible to see into the body for a continuous period of time, longer than is possible with an X ray. Photographic images can also be produced concurrently.

During surgery, an image amplifier lessens the danger of radiation exposure. This technique permits operations to be viewed on a television monitor by the entire surgical team.

Viewing the Image

X ray images include the letters "R" and "L" to indicate the right and left sides of the body; if the letters are legible (as opposed to reversed) they refer to the sides of the X-rayed patient as if he or she were facing toward the viewer.

When contrast media are used, the image might include a small clock face showing how much time elapsed between the administration of the contrast medium and the X ray exposure.

A lighted viewing screen is needed to view the details of an X ray.

Undesirable Effects

Human bodies have been exposed to radioactivity for thousands of years in air, water, and food. The difference today is that human beings are purposely exposing themselves to artificially generated radiation, most of which is delivered by medical procedures.

X rays cause tissue damage, which can lead to cancer. Any X ray exposure is harmful; unlike chemicals, there is no threshold below which X rays are considered harmless.

While the mutations caused by X rays may not damage the patient directly, they may cause birth defects, disease, or a high risk of cancer in the patient's future offspring. Such risks increase with each exposure of the gonads to radiation. Embryos are also especially sensitive to radiation. For this reason, pregnant women

Women

Relatively large amounts of radiation reach this organ	...when the following organs are X-rayed (in order of decreasing exposure):
Breast	Breast (mammogram), ribs (lungs), thoracic vertebrae, entire vertebral column
Thyroid gland	Cervical vertebrae, entire vertebral column, skull, ribs (lungs)
Lungs	Upper digestive tract, ribs (lungs), thoracic vertebrae, gallbladder, lumbar vertebrae, entire vertebral column
Bone marrow	Large intestine after intake of contrast medium, lumbar vertebrae, upper digestive tract

Men

Relatively large amounts of radiation reach this organ...	...when the following organs are X-rayed (in order of decreasing exposure)
Lungs	Upper digestive tract, ribs (lungs), thoracic vertebrae, gall bladder, entire vertebral column, lumbar vertebrae
Thyroid gland	Cervical vertebrae, entire vertebral column, skull, ribs (lungs)
Bone marrow	Large intestine after intake of contrast medium, lumbar vertebrae, upper digestive tract

Women

Relatively large amounts of radiation reach the ovaries when the following organs are X-rayed (in order of decreasing exposure):
Lumbar vertebrae
Pelvis, sacrum
Bladder and urinary tract
Hip joint and neck of the femur
Kidneys
Abdominal cavity
Large intestine, lower digestive tract
Gallbladder and bile ducts

Men

Relatively large amounts of radiation reach the testes when the following organs are X-rayed (in order of decreasing exposure):
Hip joint and neck of the femur
Bladder and urinary tract
Pelvis, sacrum
Large intestine, lower digestive tract
Lumbar vertebrae
Abdominal cavity

should only be X-rayed if their lives would otherwise be endangered.

The human body can repair the damage caused by radiation, but the success of these repairs may depend in part on the frequency and duration of the exposure. "Weaker" radiation usually causes less damage than "concentrated" radiation.

The risks posed by X rays may be subdivided into three categories: the general cancer risk to the whole body, the particular cancer risk for an individual organ, and the risk of damaging genetic material in egg or sperm cells. The information in the box above can help individuals estimate their own risk/benefit ratio for various medical uses of X rays.

Anyone desiring (more) children should be very wary of tests that deliver significant doses of radiation to the gonads. As a precaution, a lead apron or lead plate may be used to cover the ovaries or testes during the X ray. However, this is obviously feasible only if those are not the areas to be X-rayed.

There is a difference between having a single X ray and a series of X rays. A single image exposes the body to less radiation than, for example, a tomogram or a CT scan, which requires several exposures. Any organ-function examination, like a gastrointestinal-tract examination or a blood-vessel-permeability examination (angiography) requires several exposures.

Reducing Undesirable Effects

Ask your doctor to explain every X ray according to the criteria on page 647, and to justify the need for it. "One X ray can't hurt you" is not a valid answer. It has been observed that part-time radiologists—physicians who also do X rays—order X rays much more frequently than other physicians.

Protective measures used during X rays include

— Lead aprons to protect personnel standing close to the patient.
— Gonad protection, either by way of a small lead apron tied around the waist, or a lead plate placed over the ovaries or testes.
— A woman of childbearing age should have abdominal and pelvic X rays only during the first 10 days after onset of her menstrual period, unless her life is in danger or she is using oral contraceptives.
— X ray record. This is not required, but everyone should consider one. Physicians would ask for the patient's record before any X rays are done, and enter applicable data.
— It's best to keep your own X rays at home and bring any relevant ones when you visit a new doctor or check into a hospital. You can request copies of your X rays.
— Go to an experienced diagnostician. If an X ray needs to be repeated because it is unusable, the fault lies with the personnel 80 to 90 percent of the time. One out of every 10 X rays is discarded. However, since health insurance companies have begun monitoring, the quality of the X rays has improved.
— Patients with an abdomen 12 inches in diameter require 10 times the dose of radiation needed for someone whose abdomen is 8 inches in diameter. Very thin people need only a quarter of the normal dose.

Contrast Media

Contrast media create black and white contrasts in the X ray image where there would otherwise be only an undefined gray. Which contrast medium is used depends on the organ to be visualized.

Barium sulfate is insoluble in water. It is stirred into a slurry, sometimes flavoring is added, and it is swallowed in order to make the esophagus and gastrointestinal tract visible. The medium is then eliminated unchanged in the stool.

Iodine-containing contrast media are water-soluble and are injected into blood vessels to make them visible (angiography). Likewise, in order to make the kidneys, gallbladder or bile ducts visible, a contrast medium is chosen which is concentrated in the desired organ.

Undesirable Effects

The use of contrast media carries some risks, in part because of their iodine content and in part because they bring foreign substances into the bloodstream. Fatal complications were once relatively common and widely feared. In the meantime, the advent of "nonionic" contrast media has made these procedures much less risky. However, older "ionic" contrast media are still used by some doctors and in smaller hospitals, and may have the following side effects:

— Especially for blood vessel examinations: Pain and a sensation of heat in the vessel into which the medium was injected; complications with thromboses are possible.
— Allergic skin reactions, such as hives, affect 1 to 4 out of every hundred patients.
—The first indications of an allergy may be nausea and vomiting. This happens in about one patient in six who have kidney X rays, and up to one in five of those who have gallbladder X rays.
— The following are symptoms of a severe to life-threatening allergy: outbreaks of sweating, pale skin, dropping blood pressure, unconsciousness, cessation of breathing, and convulsions. Kidney X ray patients stand a 3 per thousand chance of this; gallbladder X ray patients, 5 per thousand.

The iodine content of contrast media is most hazardous for elderly people, who are given X rays more frequently than younger ones and are also more likely to undergo unnoticed thyroid changes as a result. The risk of initiating thyroid hyperfunction by iodine-containing contrast media is high.

How to Reduce Undesirable Effects

Before having an examination with contrast media, it is vitally important to tell your physician if
—You have ever overreacted to any substance.
—You have had unpleasant reactions to contrast media in the past.
— You are taking medication to lower your blood pressure or thin your blood.

During and after the injection of the contrast medium, you should remain under the physician's supervision for at least 10 minutes.

After the test, it is important to drink large amounts of liquid. The contrast medium changes the water content of your tissues and increases the excretion of uric acid. Large amounts of liquid are needed to counteract this process.

Reasonable Use

X rays with contrast media are only appropriate when necessary for diagnosis or therapy, if less stressful methods of testing will not yield enough information.

Comments on X Rays for Individual Organs

Chest X Rays

Routine chest X rays are not advisable, but they are still done. Analyses have shown that almost one third of these X rays reveal something unexpected, and some of these discoveries lead to further testing, but they still have no diagnostic value.

Mammograms

The density of breast tissue is highly variable. To obtain a clear image, a relatively high dose of radiation is required, and both breasts must be X-rayed in two dimensions. To decide when a mammogram makes sense, see p. 516.

Tomography

Tomography is an X ray examination of a particular layer of the body tissue. This technique permits layers that are not of interest to virtually disappear, while focusing on a single slice that may be no more than a millimeter thick.

Computed Tomography (CT) or CT Scan

The X rays are generated in a circular apparatus within which the patient lies, so as to irradiate the area of interest from all sides. The measured beam intensities are fed into a computer, which then generates an image of the body layer. The patient is irradiated for

3 to 5 seconds for each image.

Advantage: Computed tomography is the best available method for detecting tissue abnormalities such as cysts, hematomas, or tumors, including cancerous tumors.

Disadvantage: If the irradiated layers are close to each other, the radiation load may be greater than with a single X ray. The distribution of the radiation load over the various parts of the body in computed tomography is different from that in other types of X ray imaging.

Magnetic Resonance Imaging (MRI)

Technical Aspects
This method produces cross-sectional images without the use of X rays by subjecting body tissues to strong magnetic fields.

Procedure
The patient lies on a platform that is moved into a tube. The patient needs to lie still in the tube for about 30 minutes. The latest versions of these machines are more open, reducing the incidence of claustrophobia. The examination is painless.

Undesirable Effects
— This procedure is not appropriate for people who have metal pins or clips, or pacemakers in their bodies.
— Lying enclosed in a narrow tube may trigger anxiety.

Applications
Examination of the central nervous system, spinal column, joints, and the soft tissue around them, and blood vessels.

MRI gives better contrast than simple tomography, especially in the nervous system. If an MRI of the central nervous system shows nothing out of the ordinary, this is considered "proof" that everything is in order.

Metastatic cancers in the bones are more readily detected by MRI than by any other commonly used technology.

Scintigraphy (Radionuclide Imaging)

Technical Aspects
Atomic particles, including those generated by fission in a nuclear reactor, can be used to synthesize radioactive substances. Over time, these substances decay into nonradioactive substances, emitting radiation as they do so. A scintigraph registers radiation emitted from such substances and makes it visible. The procedure is similar to an X ray, but the radiation comes from within the body instead of an external source.

Procedure
The chemical and physical properties of radioactive substances are no different from those of corresponding nonradioactive substances. They may be swallowed, inhaled, or injected.

The Image
Radioactive substances are taken up by the body in the same way as their nonradioactive counterparts, and become diluted in the nonradioactive elements in the body. Certain substances accumulate in particular organs. The radiation makes it possible to observe where and how rapidly the radioactive substances are distributed and accumulated in the body as a whole, or in individual organs.

Undesirable Effects
The radiation involved with scintigraphy causes the same types of damage as X rays (see p. 646). Scintigraphy may lead to a higher dosage of radiation than an X ray, because once the radioactive substance is introduced into the body, it stays there until it has decayed. However, the radiation exposure may also end up being lower, if the information yielded by the scintigraphic image would otherwise have required repeated X rays. The radiation intensity in scintigraphy can also be calculated more precisely than is possible with X rays.

Applications
— Thyroid diseases
— Brain examinations
— Examination of bones, especially for detection of cancer metastases
— To determine whether a joint is inflamed, and if so, how severely
— Heart problems in which neither an EKG nor a stress EKG yield usable results
— Diagnosis of lung infarction
— Kidney diseases

Scintigraphy often results in useful information before X-ray images show anything significant.

Sonography, Ultrasound

Technical Aspects
The physical act of hearing consists of detecting sound waves in a particular range of frequency. Above and below this range, there are sound waves humans cannot hear, including ultrasound. Like light waves, these sound waves undergo reflection, refraction, and interference when they strike an object. When ultrasound passes from one medium into another, the boundary layer reflects part of it. If ultrasound waves enter the air after passing through tissues, for example, they are almost completely reflected. In this way, the air prevents the ultrasound from reaching tissue layers behind it. In an ultrasound examination, sound waves are sent into the body, where they are reflected to different degrees by the various tissues. These reflected waves are detected and electronically converted into an image.

Procedure
A contact gel is smeared onto the skin to improve its conductivity; the physician or technician passes a sound emitter over the region to be examined; the image appears on a monitor.

Undesirable Effects
Ultrasound is widely considered to have no undesirable effects, but some scientists disagree and recommend that the technique be used with the same caution as X rays (see Ultrasound in Pregnancy, p. 570).

Today, many physicians also order ultrasound examinations without having the necessary knowledge to fully evaluate the results.

Applications
— In cases where ultrasound will yield more information than other methods, such as in gallbladder or bile duct disease.
— In cases where ultrasound is likely to give as much information as an X ray, because ultrasound is less dangerous than X rays. For example, in the evaluation of malformed hips in infants, sonography is less dangerous than X rays.
— In cases where X rays cannot be used, e.g. because

the patient is allergic to contrast media, because iodine-containing contrast media are contraindicated, or during pregnancy.

During pregnancy, ultrasound should not be used routinely, but only when there is a justifiable medical need for information (see p. 570).

Ultrasound Breast Examination
With ultrasound it is possible to determine whether a breast lump is a cyst or another type of tissue change. Experienced diagnosticians using modern equipment can even distinguish between benign and malignant tumors. However, this type of equipment may be available in only a few clinics.

Ultrasound alone is not suitable as a method for early detection of breast cancer (see p. 516).

Thermography
All bodies radiate heat in the form of infrared (IR) rays, which can be made visible electronically. Thermography can detect very small temperature differences. However, processes occurring more than about 1 inch below the skin don't affect surface temperature enough to be detected, which limits thermography's range. This technique can supplement other methods of breast examination, but not replace them.
Advantages: Thermography is simple and noninvasive, and involves no radiation hazards.

A LOOK INSIDE
An endoscope is used to observe the interior of hollow organs. The endoscope is a thin tube, either rigid or flexible, and contains a light source. Optical fibers carry an image from its tip back to the other end.

It is inserted into the body through either a natural opening or an incision. The tips of flexible endoscopes, which can be pushed far into the body's interior, can sometimes be bent, allowing the physician to see in any desired direction. These instruments can often also flush an area and vacuum out the liquid, and can provide for simultaneous insertion of surgical instruments.

A big advantage of endoscopes is that biopsies can be collected on the spot when cancer is suspected. In some cases, patient and physician agree beforehand that, if needed, treatment will be carried out immediately on the basis of the endoscopic examination.

Endoscopy Tests

Organ:	Name of test:
Esophagus	esophagoscopy
Stomach	gastroscopy (see below)
Colon	proctoscopy (see below)
Rectum	rectoscopy
Colon	colonoscopy (see p. 653)
Abdominal cavity	laparoscopy (see p. 653)
Upper airways	bronchoscopy (see p. 654)
Bladder	cystoscopy (see p. 654)
Interior of joints	arthroscopy (see p. 655)

Complaints, Complications, Risks

The word "endoscopy" seems to conjure up images of sword-swallowing for many people. Anxiety may constrict their throats so tightly that a gastroscope is unable to slide down far enough; or they may experience colonoscopy as deeply shameful. Some people just grin and bear it; others are helped by relaxation techniques (p. 693); some need medication to relax.

Because endoscopy is only minimally invasive, some physicians who are not well trained in the method have been tempted to use it. In such cases, its undoubted value may not outweigh the risk.

There is always some risk associated with penetrating the interior of the body. Blood vessels or even organs may be injured. If a cancerous tumor is removed, some cancer cells may be spread through the incision. Inadequate sterilization of instruments can cause infections. This danger is distinctly greater in individual medical practices than in large clinics. Residues of disinfectant may cause damage to mucous membranes.

Gastroscopy

Gastroscopy is used to view the gastric mucosa, the valves leading in and out of the stomach, and the duodenum. The examination is used to determine whether an ulcer, cancer, or foreign body is present in the stomach.

Preparation

The patient must have fasted overnight and skipped breakfast. Usually the patient is given the following medications:

— A sedative against anxiety
— A local anesthetic in the throat, to reduce the vomit reflex
— A painkiller

Before the procedure, the patient should be examined to make sure there are no reasons not to proceed. The blood's clotting properties should also be determined in advance. A preliminary X ray is only rarely needed.

Procedure

Gastroscopy can be performed on an outpatient basis. The patient lies on his or her left side. The physician places the gastroscope, which is ⅝ inch in diameter and 4 feet long, at the upper end of the esophagus. The patient swallows to guide it into the esophagus. The rest is done by the physician, who can look through the instrument or follow its progress on a monitor.

The passage through the esophagus is usually painless, but most patients experience a choking sensation when the instrument reaches the entrance of the stomach. If the procedure involves filling the stomach with air or fluid, the patient will feel full and may have the urge to vomit. Biopsies can be taken from suspicious sites while the instrument is in place.

The procedure lasts from 3 to 15 minutes. The patient needs medical supervision for 1 to 2 hours afterward.

Complaints, Complications, Risks

There are problems in about 13 out of every 1,000 cases, usually caused by the medications used in preparation for the procedure.

Incompletely disinfected instruments can transmit the bacteria that cause duodenal ulcers (see p. 389). One out of every 14,000 patients dies during the procedure of heart or circulatory complications, or because of bleeding or puncture of an organ.

If you have been medicated, you are not in a condition to drive for the rest of the day.

Significance

Tissue changes are easier to recognize using gastroscopy than from an X ray.

Proctoscopy

Usually this procedure is used to determine the reason for inexplicable changes in the stool. It is used in people over 50 as a means of early detection of cancer (see p. 470).

Preparation

An enema is administered before the examination in order to remove fecal residue from the rectum.

Procedure

Usually the examination is done on a special table on which the patient rests on knees and elbows or knees and chest, with support in that position. Some physicians use a seat similar to a birthing stool. Fragile patients can be examined while they lie on their left sides.

The examination is made using a rigid instrument about 1 foot long. If the patient is able to breathe quietly or use relaxation techniques (see p. 693), the process is easier. It lasts at most 5 minutes. If a suspicious area is found, a biopsy is taken.

Complaints, Complications, Risks

If the anus is inflamed, or if areas of the intestine are fused, proctoscopy can be extremely painful.

There is some risk that the intestine will suffer an unnoticed injury. This occurs in 1 out of 10,000 to 50,000 patients, in cases where the physician attempts to overcome resistance with pressure, or make the intestine unfold with a strong stream of air.

Significance

More than half of all colon cancers and their precursors can be found by proctoscopy. Early detection offers the best chance of cure.

Colonoscopy

Colonoscopy examines the entire large intestine and the final segment of the small intestine. This procedure is used to discover the reason for intestinal illnesses which cannot otherwise be diagnosed or to monitor the intestine after a cancer has been surgically removed.

Preparation

The large intestine must be as clean as possible. This is accomplished by using a laxative; however, if an examination after use of a laxative alone is unsuccessful, it must be repeated after the patient has consumed nothing but liquids for 2 to 3 days and again used as a laxative. An enema is administered just before the exam.

If the patient is fairly relaxed, no medications are needed; otherwise, see Gastroscopy, p. 652.

Procedure

The examination begins with a proctoscopy (see p. 652). After this, a colonoscope is inserted through the anus and into the colon. This instrument is less than ½ inch in diameter and about 6½ feet long. During the examination, air is blown through the instrument into the intestine. The procedure takes between 15 minutes and an hour. If suspicious areas are seen, biopsies are taken. Small growths, like polyps, can be removed at once.

Complaints, Complications, Risks

The insertion of the instrument may cause abdominal pain and a sensation of pressure. The air blown into the intestine to expand it cannot all be removed immediately; it escapes over a period of several days and may cause severe abdominal pains during that time.

The technique of colonoscopy presents a considerable challenge to the experience and skill of the physician, and should therefore be undertaken only in a recognized hospital. In such institutions, complications such as bleeding and puncture of the intestinal wall occur only in about 3 out of every 1,000 examinations.

Significance

Changes in the intestinal tissues can be more easily recognized with colonoscopy than with X rays.

Laparoscopy

In laparoscopy, the instrument is inserted into the abdominal cavity through an incision. This technique is used to evaluate the condition of the liver and gall bladder, and suspected appendicitis can be checked. Gynecologists use laparoscopy to diagnose diseases of the reproductive organs, to tie the fallopian tubes, and to treat infertility.

Preparation

Before the examination, the patient must have skipped breakfast. Usually a sedative and/or analgesic are injected.

Procedure

The patient lies on a special table. The abdomen is uncovered and disinfected, and a local anesthetic is injected. A needle is inserted into the abdominal wall near the navel, and gas is blown through it into the abdominal cavity. This separates the abdominal organs somewhat; otherwise, they are too close together to permit clear views. A second incision near the navel is made and a collar is inserted, through which the laparoscope is threaded. After the examination, the incision is closed with staples. The patient must remain in the hospital, under medical supervision, for another day.

Complaints, Complications, Risks

There are complications in 5 of every 200 examinations. The most common of these is pain caused by the gas remaining in the abdomen; however, the gallbladder or intestine may be injured, and sometimes there is bleeding from injured blood vessels. Circulatory collapse may occur.

Significance

In general, ultrasound and computed tomography (CT) are preferable to the riskier laparoscopy for diagnostic purposes. However, the method has its place in gynecology.

Bronchoscopy

The throat and bronchial tubes can be observed down to the fifth or sixth branching by bronchoscopy. This method is used to search for an unexplained recurring bronchitis, for inhaled foreign bodies, or for cancerous changes.

Preparation

Before a bronchoscopy, the patient should be given a general examination to be sure there is no contraindication to the procedure. The patient must have fasted for at least 6 hours before the examination. A local anesthetic is first inhaled by the seated patient, then a local anesthetic is sprayed onto the gums and into the throat. Only then is the patient helped to lie down on the examination table. Sometimes general anesthesia is needed for the bronchoscopy.

Procedure

Before the examination, an X ray should already show in which lobe of the lung the suspected disorder is to be found. The physician inserts the apparatus into that lobe, while the patient breathes normally. Tissue biopsies can be withdrawn immediately from suspicious areas. After the examination, the patient must not eat or drink anything for at least 2 hours. The local anesthetic prevents the swallowing mechanism from working, and food or drink could easily go down the "wrong way." The examination lasts 3 to 15 minutes. Treatment using a bronchoscope can last longer.

Complaints, Complications, Risks

The bronchial tubes react fairly vigorously to this operation. They may cramp and bleed extremely easily. In up to 5 out of every 100 patients, an injured bronchial tube admits air into the chest cavity, which should be free of it. This complication must then be treated in a hospital.

Significance

If a cancerous tumor is located within reach of the bronchoscope, it can be recognized in more than 90 percent of the patients. Other lung diseases are less readily recognized by bronchoscopy. Only about 50 percent of cases are so recognized.

Cystoscopy

Preparation

The patient lies supine with legs spread out and bent, as on a gynecological examination table, so that the physician can work between the legs. The genital region is cleaned with a disinfectant, and the remaining parts of the body are covered with sterile cloths. A lubricant which also contains a local surface anesthetic is applied to the urethra.

For anxious and extremely sensitive people, and for young men, whose urethras are very narrow, general anesthesia is necessary.

Procedure

The instrument is ⅛ inch in diameter. It is inserted through the urethra into the bladder. At the same time, a pressurized stream of sterile water, at body temperature, is fed into the urethra, to make it unfold. After the examination, the patient should empty the bladder normally and, for the rest of the day, drink plenty of fluid.

Complaints, Complications, Risks

Cystoscopy is more painful for men than women, because of their longer urethras. After the examination, traces of blood are often found in the urine, and for a short time urination is more difficult than usual.

In spite of the best efforts to keep the area sterile, there is always some risk of introducing bacteria into the bladder and causing an inflammation.

The risk of injury to the ureter during the examination is fairly large. Nearly half of these injuries lead to scarring, which narrows the urethra and causes chronic problems.

Significance

The examination is justified when a tumor in the bladder is suspected.

Arthroscopy

A view of the interior of a joint allows the doctor to recognize damage to cartilage and meniscus which could otherwise not be detected, and which may be the cause of otherwise inexplicable pain.

Preparation

Depending on the patient's anxiety level, either general or local anesthesia may be used. For examination of the knees, a spinal block is used to numb the lower part of the body, instead of general anesthesia. The surface of the skin around the joint is disinfected and covered with sterile cloths.

Procedure

The instrument is inserted through an incision about ½ inch long into the interior of the joint. In order to improve visibility, the area is rinsed with liquid, which is vacuumed out as completely as possible afterward. The examination lasts 15 to 30 minutes, and the incision is sewed or stapled shut. Normally, the patient can then return home, but a few days of taking it easy are a good idea. Those whose jobs require heavy physical labor should take 2 days of sick leave.

Complaints, Complications, Risks

The fluid left behind in the joint may make a squishing noise for a few days.

Arthroscopy leads to complications in about one fourth of patients. The most common of these are damage to the cartilage and bleeding into the joint. However, ligaments may be torn, and broken tips of instruments have been left behind on occasion. Infections arise in about 1 case in 1,000, and, in addition,

there are the usual risks of general anesthesia.

Significance

A joint should only be examined by arthroscopy as a last resort. However, if it must be used, it gives the most information of any available method.

An advantage is that small surgical operations, such as the removal of torn-off pieces of cartilage or smoothing of an inflamed synovial membrane, can be accomplished at the same time.

Biopsy

Microscopic examination is needed to determine whether cells are normal or diseased. Some liver diseases can only be diagnosed securely by microscopic observation of the liver cells, and a microscope is required to distinguish between benign and malignant growths.

With the endoscopic techniques described above starting on p. 651, physicians gain access to the interior of the body during an examination, and can immediately remove samples where the tissue looks suspicious. Tissue samples are also often removed during an operation. In this case, the sample must be examined immediately so that the result can guide the remainder of the operation.

Complications and Risks

Removing tissue always amounts to injury to an organ. In order to keep damage to a minimum, a biopsy must be obtained with the same care as any other surgery. It can be problematic when the body's reaction is not noticed for several hours after the procedure, especially when serious bleeding has resulted.

There is also a risk that removing tissue will release microorganisms or cancer cells into the blood or lymph, where they can spread throughout the body. The modern method of fine-needle biopsy, however, has not been shown to influence the course of disease by spreading pathogens from an inflammation or malignant cells from a tumor, even though a certain number of cancer cells will always be present in the channel left by the needle.

Liver Biopsy

With a "blind" liver biopsy, a physician can recognize diseases that cause changes in all parts of the liver. If the path of the needle is guided by ultrasound, localized centers of disease can also be reached.

Preparation

Liver biopsies are always taken in a hospital. Blood tests must be made beforehand, and the chest should be X-rayed. The patient is not given any medications before the test.

Procedure

The patient lies supine, with a cushion raising the right side of the body slightly. The right arm lies under the head. The physician finds the site for insertion of the needle by tapping the skin, and injects a local anesthetic. The upper layers of skin are separated by an incision. Then, while the patient holds his or her breath, the physician inserts the needle extremely rapidly, takes the sample, and withdraws the needle equally quickly. The actual process of obtaining the sample must be completed in a fraction of a second.

Afterward, the patient lies on the right side for 2 hours, then spends 4 hours in bed. During this time, the patient's pulse and blood pressure are periodically checked to be sure everything is in order.

Complaints, Complications, Risks

After the procedure, 10 percent of patients have pain in their right shoulders and when they breathe. More dangerous complications include bleeding, peritonitis caused by leaking bile, and air introduced into the chest cavity.

Significance

Analysis of the biopsied tissue is extremely difficult, and not every physician succeeds at it. Liver biopsies should be taken only by experienced liver specialists.

MEDICATION SUMMARY

The purpose of medicines is the healing of disease and the easing of symptoms. Some medications are taken to prevent undesirable outcomes, such as a pregnancy or vitamin deficiency.

Some medicines are prescribed by physicians and paid for by health insurance. Some are over-the-counter remedies paid for by individuals. Self-medication is only helpful, however, when it is not a substitute for more effective treatment, and when it does more good than harm. The following tips should help keep this risk to a minimum:

— Do not attempt to self-medicate altered mental status, seizures, heart arrhythmias, or diffuse pains in the abdominal or chest region.
— If you have a fever that lasts longer than 3 days and for which you can't find a plausible reason, see your health-care provider.
— If your symptoms persist for more than 2 weeks, see your health-care provider.
— Be clear about what you expect from the medicine: If you simply want to get rid of uncomfortable symptoms and don't know their cause, you may lose valuable time that could be put to use seeking effective treatment.
— Never use a prescription medicine left over in your medicine cabinet without first consulting your health-care provider (see p. 626).
— Try to use as little as possible of any medication.
— Pay attention to label warnings, and don't use a medication if any of the contraindications is present. Also, be careful about interactions between this medicine and others; this information should also be printed on the label.

VARIETIES OF MEDICATIONS

Medications are available in many forms: tablets, lozenges, capsules, pills, powders, drops, syrups, suppositories, and injections. The variety of forms reflects the differences in solubility, ease of distribution and effectiveness of the medications' active ingredients. Medications should be chosen carefully and applied correctly in order to ensure optimum effectiveness.

Quick-Acting Medications

The sooner an active ingredient enters the bloodstream, the sooner it takes effect. For example, for fastest relief of a headache, drops or effervescent tablets are indicated; alternatively, tablets may be dissolved in half a glass of water and drunk at least a half hour before eating.

Time-Release Medications

Slow-acting or time-release preparations release their active ingredients into the bloodstream only gradually, as they move through the digestive system. These medications should not be taken in powder or dissolved form.

For Sensitive Stomachs

Medications dissolved in liquid are less stressful to a sensitive stomach than medication in solid form. If solid medicines are swallowed along with a meal, they take effect more slowly, and sometimes their effect is less than expected. Using suppositories will avoid any stress on the stomach; however, suppositories make it difficult to calculate exactly how much of the active ingredient enters the bloodstream.

MEDICATION USE

As a patient, you should be informed how to take prescription medications, and what to do in case of unpleasant side effects (see Outpatient Medicine, p. 626). In case of side effects from a nonprescription medication, stop taking it and consult your health-care provider or pharmacist.

Following are some guidelines for medication use:
— Take seriously all label warnings, such as "for short-term use only." Some medications can lead to addiction without your noticing it (see Medication Misuse, p. 658).
— Medication may affect your concentration level, which could be hazardous when driving or on the job. Some drugs cause drowsiness; others interfere with vision, alter the heartbeat, or cause itching, which can be distracting. Stimulants may cause you to overestimate your capacities; you should take this effect into account.
— The combination of medications and alcohol may be dangerous, especially when driving or operating machinery.

Medication Package Inserts

Large quantities of medications, duly prescribed by physicians and fully paid for by insurance plans, end up in the garbage every year. One reason for this is the informational inserts included with some medications, which list so many possible side effects that patients throw the product away rather than risk such a fate.

These comprehensive lists are required by Food and Drug Administration (FDA) regulations; they also reduce the pharmaceutical companies' liability. If the information on the insert does not correspond to "the state of medical knowledge," the manufacturer may be liable for damages.

Therefore, ask your doctor all questions about prescription drugs before you buy them (see Outpatient Medicine, p. 626), or if you're buying over-the-counter preparations, ask the pharmacist first. The package insert won't help you decide whether or not to buy the medication, because you won't see it until you open the package—at which point you can no longer return it.

Drugs and Driving

— If you are new to sedatives, antidepressants, or high-blood pressure medication, time your first dose so you can observe its effects at home. If you find that your capacities are impaired, don't drive. Driving is also out of the question if your doctor, or the medication label or insert, states that this medication causes drowsiness or affects reaction time.

— The same caution applies if you're increasing the dosage of a medicine you are already taking, especially if it's for epilepsy or diabetes.

— The above also applies when reducing the dosage of medications for blood pressure, diabetes, or epilepsy.

— Don't drive for several days after you have stopped taking sleeping pills or sedatives.

— Some medications can impair vision. For example, codeine, an ingredient in some analgesics and cough syrups, lessens the eyes' ability to adapt to changes in light and distance. Eye ointments may cloud your vision.

Medications for Children

Never give a child a medication meant for an adult without a pediatrician's permission. Some adult medications have no effect on children, some have a stronger effect on children, and some have the opposite effect on children from what they have on adults. In addition, adjusting the dosage is not a simple matter. About two thirds of all pharmaceutical products that might be given to children list no suggested children's dosages, since the manufacturers have not tested them on children and need to protect themselves from liability.

Medicines for the Elderly

People over 60 years of age experience about three times as many undesirable side effects from medications as younger people. The changes in our bodies as we become older (see Aging, page 606) change the uptake, distribution, and excretion patterns of medications.

Tell your doctor if you:

— Doubt that all the prescribed medicines are really necessary

— Experience impairments that lead you to suspect that the dose is too high

— Cannot keep straight the various instructions for several different medicines

— Have trouble opening packages or find tablets difficult to swallow

— Can barely distinguish the various medicines

A responsible and caring health-care provider will take your questions and fears seriously and make time to answer them.

Disposing of Medications

When disposing of a medication, recycle the paper and plastic packaging materials if possible. Wrap the pills or powder in moist newspaper and place them in your household garbage. Light and moisture hasten the decay of medications.

MEDICATION MISUSE

Even "everyday" medications can be abused or lead to addiction. The following can become habit-forming:

— Sedatives and sleeping medications
— Strong analgesics
— Analgesics containing caffeine (see Analgesics, p. 659).
— Appetite suppressants
— Laxatives
— Cold medications

These medications can easily fool users. If you stop taking them, after a while all the symptoms that originally led you to use them will come back worse than before. Although these are actually withdrawal symptoms, you may conclude that they're simply a recurrence of the original symptoms, and start taking the drug again. Package inserts often give insufficient information about this phenomenon.

Because users of most of these medications do not require increasing amounts to achieve the desired effect, they often can't tell that they're hooked.

Sedatives and Sleeping Medications

Both sedatives, which are intended to ease daytime restlessness and anxiety, and sleep inducers can cause addiction. Both contain a benzodiazepine (see Emotional Problems, p. 60), which is habit-forming.

Many people become dependent within 3 to 4 weeks when taking these products daily. If they discontinue use, anxiety, restlessness, and sleep disorders will return in intensified form for 10 to 14 days. The longer the patient has been on the medication, the more intense the withdrawal symptoms will be. If benzodiazepines have been used for a long time, the patient may require hospitalization during the withdrawal period.

Analgesics With More Than One Active Ingredient

Mild analgesics (see p. 660) almost never cause dependence if they contain only one active ingredient. When caffeine or codeine are added, however, these products become habit-forming (see Analgesics, page 660). Caffeine-containing analgesics can be obtained without a prescription. Those containing codeine require a prescription. For the results of analgesic misuse, see p. 660.

Appetite Suppressants

These stimulants are addictive: One must continuously increase the dose to keep the desired effect constant.

Laxatives

Laxatives cause the body to lose water and essential salts. This interference with the body's water-salt balance can lead to serious damage to nerves, circulation and kidneys, which in turn can impair digestive activity to the point that the patient is unable to eliminate without a laxative (see Constipation, page 406).

Cold Remedies

These products contract the blood vessels in the nasal mucous membranes. When their use is discontinued, the nasal mucosa swell. Often the patient will then take more of the product to counteract this effect, setting a vicious cycle in motion. Prolonged use of cold remedies makes the nasal mucosa unable to function (see Colds from Cold Medications, page 299).

Storing Your Medication

— The ideal place to store medications is cool, dry, and inaccessible by children. The bathroom "medicine cabinet" isn't ideal; neither is the kitchen drawer or night table. If possible, your home pharmacy should contain only the items listed on page 704, not the ancient remains of a dozen prescription medicines. If you can't bear to throw anything away, at least observe the following rules.
— Write on the medication container the purchase date, the name of the person for whom it was prescribed and the condition for which it was prescribed.
— Keep the package insert together with the medication.
— Never keep leftover eyedrops, eye ointments, antibiotics (see p. 661), or potentially habit-forming medications.
— Be aware that the active ingredient in a product will become more concentrated as any alcohol it contains evaporates.

Taking Your Medication

— Before taking a medication, check the expiration date on the label.
— Wash down all swallowed medications with half a glass of water.
— Don't swallow medications while lying down; keep the upper part of your body erect.
— If a pill or capsule won't go down easily, take a bite of banana, chew it and swallow it.

Signs of Medication Dependence

You have become dependent if you
— Are unable to stop taking analgesics, sleeping pills, or tranquilizers on your own
— Need to take a certain quantity of these medications in order to feel well or cope with stress
— Feel physically or psychologically unwell as soon as you stop taking the medication
— Worry when you can't get the medication easily
— Notice that a medication that used to calm you down has become a stimulant

— Make excuses to yourself about your medication use, or hide it from others
— Have a variety of ways to get your medication, such as buying it (or asking someone else to buy it) from different pharmacies within a short time, or asking different doctors to prescribe it.

For more on medication misuse, see p. 658.

Preventing Dependence
— Don't take sleep medication or sedatives for more than a week. If your doctor prescribes them for a longer period, ask why.
— Use analgesics containing only one active ingredient. (Exception: Analgesic plus codeine, if the analgesic alone isn't strong enough)
— Use laxatives only when absolutely necessary, and only for a short time.
— Don't take cold remedies for more than 3 days.

ANALGESICS

In the United States there are hundreds of analgesics on the market, and millions of packages are sold annually. They contained excessive amounts acetylsalicylic acid, acetaminophen, and ibuprofen. Doctors prescribe nearly 33 percent more analgesics for women between the ages of 40 and 55 than for men. Pain starts out as a warning signal from the body, but after time it can become a disease in its own right.

How To Use Analgesics
Medications cannot remove the cause of pain. For causes and treatment of headaches, see p. 193. For migraine headaches, see p. 225.

Undesirable Effects
See individual active ingredients under Simple Analgesics, starting below.

Analgesics containing caffeine tend to be habit-forming.

Consequences
Regular or long-term repeated use of most analgesics can lead to severe kidney damage, possibly including kidney failure. About 20 percent of dialysis patients have a history of chronic analgesic use over many years.

There are three common reasons for misuse of analgesics.

— Frequently recurring pain (see Migraines, p. 225) is often masked with analgesics instead of being diagnosed and treated, or instead of the patient's learning to cope with the pain. It is estimated that 2 out of 3 chronically ill patients are addicted to analgesics.
— Some analgesics relieve headaches but cause new ones as their effects wear off. To avoid pain, the patient keeps taking more tablets.
— To get through the day, a patient may become dependent on the stimulation provided by an analgesic. This is especially common with the many over-the-counter products that combine analgesics with caffeine.

Preventing Undesirable Effects
— Don't take analgesics for more than 1 week without consulting your health-care provider.
— If your doctor prescribes analgesics for longer than a week, ask why this is necessary, whether there is any risk of dependency, and whether there are alternatives.
— Use only analgesics with a single active ingredient.

The exception to this rule is that codeine-containing analgesics are indicated, for a short time only, when pain is too severe for a simple analgesic.

Use Products With a Single Active Ingredient
Aspirin: Ecotrin, Empirin, Bayer, acetylsalicylic acid (ASA)
Ibuprofen: Motrin, Advil, Nuprin, Rufen
Acetaminophen: Tylenol, Panadol, Tempra
These include acetylsalicylic acid (aspirin), ibuprofen or acetaminophen. Don't take aspirin or ibuprofen on an empty stomach. Dissolve the tablets in a little water, swallow them, then drink at least half a glass of water.

Simple Analgesics
This section deals with mild pain medications. Strong painkillers, such as those needed by cancer patients, are discussed on page 480. For rheumatism medications, see p. 449. Some simple analgesics are also prescribed for rheumatism.

Acetylsalicylic acid (aspirin)

Aspirin is an effective and relatively safe analgesic. It has been in use for more than a hundred years, so its side effects are well known. 500 to 1,000 milligrams (1 or 2 tablets) relieve pain effectively.

Undesirable Effects

The following side effects are relatively common, but disappear completely when the medication is discontinued:
— Stomach pain and nausea
— Signs of overdose: Ringing in the ears, faintness, confusion, vomiting
— Sncreased tendency to bleed

A very rare, but serious, side effect in children is Reye's syndrome. Its symptoms are severe vomiting, fever, convulsions and loss of consciousness. The risk of this side effect is particularly high when the child is ill with viral "flu" or chicken pox.

Caution: If you take more than 7,000 milligrams of aspirin a month for about 6 months, you may develop headaches caused by the drug.

Aspirin should not be taken
— If you have an inflammation or ulcers in the stomach or duodenum
— If you tend to bleed easily and profusely
— If you have asthma or are allergic to aspirin
— By children or adolescents with a viral "flu" or chicken pox.

Acetaminophen

This substance works as well and as quickly as aspirin, and is easier on the stomach. One or two tablets is sufficient to ease pain. It is not advisable to take more than 650 milligrams of acetaminophen at one time.

Undesirable Effects

The following side effects are relatively rare, but can have serious consequences:
— Interference with blood composition
— Liver damage caused by an overdose
— Kidney damage caused by chronic use.

Patients who take more than one tablet of acetaminophen per day, or consume a total of more than 1,000 tablets, double their risk of kidney failure necessitating dialysis.

Caution: If you take more than 5,000 milligrams of acetaminophen a month for half a year, you are at risk of developing headaches caused by the drug.

Acetaminophen should not be taken if the liver or kidneys are not functioning perfectly.

Ibuprofen

Ibuprofen has long been useful in inhibiting the inflammation caused by rheumatism. At a lower dose, it can be used as a general analgesic. However, it costs four times as much as aspirin per dose.

Undesirable Effects

The following side effects may be serious:
— Allergic skin reactions
— General allergic reactions, possibly including shock
— Bleeding in the gastrointestinal tract

Ibuprofen itself does not damage the kidneys, but, in combination with other analgesics, probably hastens the development of kidney damage.

Combination Products

There are only two exceptions to the general rule that no analgesic combination has an acceptable advantage over analgesics containing only one active ingredient. These are vitamin C–analgesic compounds in effervescent tablets, and combinations containing an ingredient that acts on the central nervous system, such as codeine, for use when a single analgesic (aspirin or acetaminophen) is insufficient for pain management.

Combining aspirin with acetaminophen significantly increases the risk of kidney damage; combining acetaminophen with caffeine increases it still further.

ANTIBIOTICS

Antibiotics can heal diseases and save lives. This fact, however, has led to their current undeserved reputation as cure-alls. Today, indiscriminate antibiotic use causes many problems. According to one estimate, 90 percent of the antibiotics prescribed are not medically justified.

Infectious diseases are caused mainly by bacteria and viruses. Antibiotics prevent bacterial reproduction or kill bacterial cells. In this way, they help the body to rid itself of the pathogens. However, antibiotics have no effect against viruses.

Antibiotics: Yes or No?

An otherwise healthy body will heal an uncomplicated infection on its own. The use of antibiotics is justified only when there is reason to think that a patient's body will not succeed in ridding itself of the infection, or when the infection may lead to other, serious secondary diseases.

About 60 percent of infections treated by physicians in private practice involve the upper respiratory passages—and these are almost always viral infections. Antibiotics are useless in these cases. Nevertheless, physicians almost always prescribe them for respiratory ailments.

Varieties of Antibiotics

Each individual antibiotic compound is effective against specific types of bacteria. Substances that are effective against many species of bacteria are called *broad-spectrum antibiotics.* They are especially popular because the chance is greater that they will succeed against an unidentified species. The disadvantage is that many different species and strains of bacteria have a chance to become resistant to the antibiotic.

Narrow-Spectrum Antibiotics

Penicillins and amoxicillin are relatively well tolerated and have been used for a long time. Cephalosporins work in similar fashion to penicillins, but should only be used when penicillin is incapable of stopping an infection, or when a patient is allergic to penicillin. Erythromycin is used when penicillins are not effective enough, or when a patient is allergic to penicillin. These are all well-tested substances which have been in use for a long time.

Broad-Spectrum Antibiotics

Tetracyclines are suitable only for adults. They are relatively well tolerated, have been well tested, and are frequently prescribed. They are especially suitable for acne.

Fluoroquinolones should only be prescribed when other antibiotics have failed; they can have significant side effects. However, sales figures indicate that physicians do not follow this guideline.

Sulfonamides

The combination cotrimoxazole is a sensible, solid broad-spectrum antibiotic combination that has been well tested.

Products Containing More than One Active Ingredient

It is sometimes necessary to treat especially severe infections with several antibiotics at once. This should generally be done, however, with several single preparations, rather than with ready-made mixtures.

How to Use Antibiotics

It is advisable to begin treatment of the following diseases with these antibiotics:
— Severe, chronic bronchitis: Amoxicillin
— Pneumonia: Amoxicillin, penicillin V, erythromycin
— Middle-ear infections: Amoxicillin, erythromycin
— Sinus infections: Amoxicillin
— Tonsillitis: Penicillin
— Pharyngitis and laryngitis: Amoxicillin, penicillin
— Dental infections: Penicillin
— Urinary-tract and bladder infections: Cotrimoxazole

Undesirable Effects

At the Population Level: Development of Drug-Resistant Strains

Bacteria are continually evolving new strategies to protect themselves against eradication. Many strains have already become immune to the antibiotics with which they used to be successfully treated. This type of resistance can only develop when the bacteria come into contact with the antibiotics relatively frequently, either in the form of medicines or as additives to animal feed. The result is that new antibiotics must constantly be developed in order to combat bacterial diseases. This situation is not yet terribly serious for everyday infections, but it has already become a grave problem in hospitals.

At the Individual Level

The mucous membranes of our bodies, e.g. those of the eyes, mouth, and intestines, are hosts to symbiotic bacteria that cause us no problems, and in fact protect us from infections by pathogenic bacteria or fungi. Antibiotics upset this equilibrium. The results are
— Diarrhea
— Increased fungal and viral infections

Penicillin Preparations
Penicillins—Natural (1ˢᵗ generation)
Benzathine penicillin
Benzylpenicilloyl polylysine
Penicillin G
Penicillin V
Procaine penicillin
Penicillins—Penicillinase-Resistant (2ⁿᵈ generation)
Cloxacillin
Dicloxacillin
Methicillin
Nafcillin
Oxacillin
Penicillins—Aminopenicillins (3ʳᵈ generation)
Amoxicillin
Amoxicillin clavulanate
Ampicillin
Ampicillin sulbactam (Unasyn)
Penicillins—Extended Spectrum (4ᵗʰ generation)
Carbenicillin
Mezlocillin
Piperacillin
Piperacillin tazobactam (Zosyn)
Ticarcillin
Ticarcillin clavulanate (Timentin)
Cephalosporin Preparations
Cephalosporins—1ˢᵗ generation
Cefadroxil
Cefazolin
Cephalexin
Cephalothin
Cephradine
Cephalosporins—2ⁿᵈ generation
Cefaclor
Cefamandole
Cefmetazole
Cefonicid
Cefotetan
Cefoxitin
Cefprozil
Cefuroxime
Loracarbef
Cephalosporins—3ʳᵈ generation
Cefdinir
Cefixime
Cefoperazone
Cefotaxime
Cefpodoxime

Ceftazidime
Ceftibuten
Ceftizoxime
Ceftriaxone
Cephalosporins—"4ᵗʰ generation"
Cefepime
Macrolides
Azithromycin
Clarithromycin
Dirithromycin
Erythromycin
Erythromycin base
Erythromycin estolate
Erythromycin ethylsuccinate
Erythromycin lactobionate
Erythromycin ethylsuccinate and Sulfisoxazole (Pediazole)
Tetracyclines
Demeclocycline
Doxycycline
Minocycline
Tetracycline
Fluoroquinolones
Ciprofloxacin
Enoxacin
Grepafloxacin
Levofloxacin
Lomefloxacin
Norfloxacin
Ofloxacin
Sparfloxacin
Trovafloxacin/Alatrofloxacin
Sulfonamides
Cotrimoxazole, Trimethoprim/Sulfamethoxazole
Erythromycin ethylsuccinate and Sulfisoxazole (Pediazole)
Sulfamethoxazole
Sulfisoxazole
Other Antimicrobials
Aztreonam
Chloramphenicol
Clindamycin
Fosfomycin
Furazolidone
Methenamine hippurate
Methenamine mandelate
Metronidazole
Nalidixic acid
Nitrofurantoin
Rifampin
Trimethoprim
Vancomycin

The diarrhea can possibly be avoided by eating large amounts of yogurt, which supplies new bacteria to settle in the intestines.

Additional Undesirable Effects: All Antibiotics

— Irritation of the digestive tract, leading to nausea and vomiting.

— Allergic reactions, more common for penicillin than for other antibiotics. There are 2 types of allergies

— The slow form develops over 12 to 48 hours after a dose of the antibiotic, and causes rashes and itching.

— The dramatic form develops within 2 hours after a dose, and causes anaphylactic shock: Cessation of breathing, loss of blood pressure and circulatory collapse.

Additional Undesirable Effects: Tetracyclines

— In growing children, discoloration of the teeth and increased susceptibility of the teeth to dental caries. For this reason, children under 9 must not be given tetracyclines.

— Increased sensitivity of the skin to sunlight. When taking tetracycline, you should avoid sunlight altogether.

Additional Undesirable Effects: Cotrimoxazole

— Impaired formation of blood.

— Severe allergic reactions.

Additional Undesirable Effects: Fluoroquinolones

— Headaches, restlessness, loss of equilibrium, confusion, convulsions, allergic reactions, shock. Fluoroquinolones should be used only in adults.

Interactions

If you are taking an antibiotic, be sure to tell any doctor or pharmacist that may recommend a new medication. Also tell any doctor that prescribes an antibiotic about any other medications you are taking.

Topical Application

The use of antibiotic medication on the skin makes sense for only a few diseases. These medications lead to especially rapid evolution of resistant pathogens, and allergies also develop more frequently.

Eyedrops: Bacterial inflammations of the eyes can be treated well with antibiotics; the same guidelines apply as for internal administration.

Eardrops: If antibiotics are needed to combat a middle-ear infection, they must be taken orally. Eardrop antibiotics are only helpful for an ear canal inflammation.

Internal Administration

— The antibiotic level in the body should not fall below a certain level; this is the reason antibiotics must be taken several times a day. "Three times a day" means every 8 hours.

— "Before a meal" means 1 hour before eating.

— "With a meal" means between a half-hour and immediately before the meal.

Drink at least half a glass of water when you swallow tablets or capsules, so they don't lodge in your throat (this is especially important with tetracyclines). If the tablets won't go down, you can take a bite of banana, chew it well, and then swallow the pill with it.

Injections

Antibiotics are injected when rapid action is needed, or when they are ineffective if swallowed.

Preventing Undesirable Effects

By managing antibiotic treatment correctly, physicians can prevent undesirable effects.

— First, the physician should be sure of the diagnosis of the disease.

— Normally, physicians base their choice of antibiotic on the knowledge that certain pathogens always attack the same organs, and almost always cause similar symptoms. In cases of doubt, or when the expected result is not obtained, the pathogen should be identified in the laboratory. If a patient has recurring urinary-tract infections, it is necessary to identify the pathogen.

— Antibiotics should be used when it can be foreseen that the body will not overcome the infection without help, and when other treatments are not sufficient.

— If the pathogen is known or its identity can be surmised with high probability, the antibiotic with the narrowest spectrum should be used.

— If the antibiotic does not work, or if it becomes apparent after a short time that it is not needed, you should stop taking it after consultation with your health-care provider.

— The dosage of any antibiotic should be set high enough from the beginning.

— Take the antibiotic as long as necessary and for as short a time as possible. If all indicators suggest the patient is cured, the physician should end the course of antibiotics. Usually they are needed for 7 to 10 days.

— If you are taking sulfonamides, drink plenty of fluids so the active ingredients will not crystallize out in your kidneys.

What You Should Know About Antibiotics

— Antibiotics combat bacteria. They are of no use against viruses, and usually have no effect on fungi.

— Before your doctor prescribes an antibiotic, ask whether it is really necessary.

— Physicians like to prescribe the newest antibiotic in order to increase the chance that the pathogen is not yet resistant to it. However, this simply perpetuates the problem. In addition, the patient will be taking a compound with which the profession is relatively unfamiliar, and whose side effects may not yet be well known.

— Even the smallest amounts of antibiotics, which may be present in foods (see Harmful Substances in Foods, p. 729), can promote the development of resistance.

— If you are taking antibiotics, provide yourself with functional intestinal flora by eating yogurt.

— Someone who has once had an allergic reaction to an antibiotic must never take that antibiotic again, nor any other that is chemically similar to it.

What Women Should Know About Antibiotics

If you are taking antibiotics, your intestinal flora will be irritated most severely during the first few days. This can impair the effectiveness of oral contraceptives, as can long-term use of the following antibiotics: Chloramphenicol, neomycin, sulfonamides, and tetracyclines.

CORTICOSTEROIDS (GLUCOCORTICOIDS, STEROIDS)

Corticosteroids are hormones produced by the adrenal cortex (see p. 502). Medical practitioners call them glucocorticoids. When they first became available in quantities sufficient for treatment, they were hailed as wonder drugs; but their indiscriminate application later had disastrous consequences. This caused the pendulum to swing in the opposite direction, and many people are still afraid to use corticosteroids. This fear is unfounded, if your physician weighs the benefits and risks for each individual patient. Corticosteroids are a blessing for those afflicted with certain diseases.

Applications

— Insufficiency of the adrenal cortex (see p. 502)
— Shock
— Following organ transplants
— Severe allergies (see p. 360)
— Asthma (see p. 307)
— Severe inflammations not caused by pathogens such as bacteria or viruses
— Autoimmune diseases, such as lupus erythrematosis or polymyalgia rheumatica
— Rheumatoid arthritis and acute phases of some rheumatic diseases (see p. 455)
— Acute phases of inflammatory intestinal diseases
— Acute phases of eczema

Corticosteroids should only be prescribed when other treatments fail or are contraindicated, and for as short a period as possible. In spite of this, some diseases make it necessary to take large doses of corticosteroids for a long time.

How Corticosteroids Work

Corticosteroids can ease symptoms, but they do not cure. They inhibit inflammatory processes and suppress the reactions of the immune system.

Undesirable Effects

The following side effects may appear with corticosteroid use, but will disappear when it is discontinued:

— Severe, frequent infections
— Psychological disorders
— Fat accumulation on the body and face—the "moon face" look; high blood pressure and edema
— Weakening of the arm and leg muscles
— Acne
— Menstrual disturbances; impotence
— Ulcers of the stomach or duodenum, with almost no symptoms; danger of a perforated ulcer
— Poor wound healing
— Interference with growth in children

The following side effects, which are irreversible, may appear after long courses of treatment.

— Osteoporosis
— Cataract or glaucoma
— Thinning of connective tissue; appearance of scar-like fissures like the stretch marks of pregnancy

— Development or worsening of diabetes

Interactions

Be sure to inform your doctor and pharmacist that you are using a corticosteroid before starting any new medications. Corticosteroids react seriously with numerous other medications.

Applications

The dosages of highly active medications like corticosteroids must be exactly calculated, and their effects closely monitored. Compound preparations are inadvisable.

External

Externally applied corticosteroids can have the same undesirable effects as those taken internally. The risk becomes greater as the length of use, strength of the preparation and area to which it is applied are increased. The face reacts most intensely to corticosteroids, and special caution is required with children.

Externally applied corticosteroids can be classified into four groups according to their strength. The following ground rules apply to externally applied corticosteroids:

— With the right diagnosis in place, the most suitable substance and preparation should be found.
— Strong preparations should be applied only to small areas, and if possible, for no longer than 2 days. It may be hazardous for an adult to exceed 15 grams per week of a strong corticosteroid preparation, 30 grams of a medium-strength preparation, or 50 grams of a milder preparation.
— It is best to apply the medication following a bath.
— It should be applied as thinly as possible, and then rubbed in.
— Do not apply more than twice a day.
— Protect the hand you are using to rub in the cream by wearing a rubber glove.
— End long-term treatment gradually (see p. 667).

Inhalation

In order to limit as far as possible the damage to the respiratory passages caused by asthma (see p. 307), the patient must regularly inhale a corticosteroid. The spray is inhaled in the morning and evening, but not used as an emergency treatment for an asthma attack. Corticosteroid inhalants include beclomethasone, budesonide, flunisolide, fluticason, and triamcinolone.

Undesirable Effects: Corticosteroid inhalants have less effect on the body than those taken orally and often promote fungal infections in the mouth. You can prevent this by rinsing your mouth out long and well after each inhalation of corticosteroid.

Oral

Patients who do not produce their own corticoids (see Addison's Disease, p. 504) take corticosteroids in a rhythm which mimics that of a healthy body: The largest dose in the morning, a smaller one at midday, the smallest in the evening. Patients who take corticosteroids for other reasons need to find a balance between the following two principles: The activity of the adrenal cortex is least disturbed when the dosage is timed to be as similar as possible to the natural rhythm of production, but the disease determines when the greatest amount of corticosteroid effect is needed. While the normal daily rhythm would be most closely matched by taking the entire daily dose before 8 a.m. (see Adrenal Cortex, p. 502), asthmatics must take the largest doses in the afternoon, to prevent attacks at night.

All forms of corticosteroid therapy suppress the formation of corticoids by the adrenal cortex. It can take weeks or months before the gland recovers its normal activity; during this time, the body cannot produce its "fight-or-flight" reflex (see Stress, p. 182). In order to stimulate the organ back to work, corticosteroid treatment must be tapered gradually. As a rule, the period over which the dosage is gradually reduced should be equal in length to the time of treatment.

For long-term therapy, doctors should prescribe preparations with prednisone, prednisolone, or methyl prednisolone, if possible. These have the least effect on the body's hormone control cycle.

Corticosteroid tablets should be taken for as short a time as possible, and in as low a dose as possible. The upper limit is considered to be 5 to 7.5 mg prednisone daily, except in life-threatening diseases, when it may be necessary to take large amounts of corticosteroids over extremely long time periods. These diseases include asthma, rheumatism, and autoimmune diseases.

Injection

In emergency medicine, high doses of corticosteroids

are injected in order to help the body overcome stress. Because of the short-term nature of this use, the usual side effects of corticosteroids need not be feared.

Specialists advise against the injection of time-release corticosteroid into the buttocks. This method of treatment is entirely contrary to the principle of adapting corticosteroid administration to the body's natural daily rhythm of hormone production. In addition, the skin or muscle tissue adjacent to the injection site often deteriorates.

There is also no acceptable reason for the use of combination corticosteroid preparations. Combining a corticosteroid with an analgesic or rheumatism medication has proven so dangerous that it is illegal in some countries.

Preventing Undesirable Effects

Any bodily changes caused by cortisone will only be recognized by a physician familiar with the patient. Before prescribing a corticosteroid, therefore, your physician should:
— Weigh you
— Take your blood pressure
— Test your blood
— Test your urine
— Have your eyes examined by an ophthalmologist
— Make sure you are free of viral and fungal diseases

Monitoring Long-Term Treatment

At every follow-up appointment, your doctor should ask about side effects you may be experiencing. In addition, he or she should
One month after beginning treatment: Weigh yourself, take your blood pressure.
Every 3 months: Test your blood, urine, and blood sugar; an ophthalmologist should measure the internal pressure of your eyes and check your lenses for cloudiness.

Immunizations (Vaccinations)

The body's immune system defends it against intruders. It possesses a kind of memory which permits it to recognize pathogens, even years after its first encounter with them, and to immobilize or detoxify them at once.

If You're on Corticosteroids
Watching your eating habits can alleviate some of the problems that may arise during long-term corticosteroid treatment.
— Keep your weight down.
— Eat plenty of protein.
— Avoid salt.
— Avoid sugar.
— Get plenty of potassium (see p. 744).
— Get plenty of calcium (see p. 745).
— Get plenty of vitamin C (see p. 743).

In this case we say we are immune to the pathogen. Full-blown cases of infectious diseases usually confer lifetime immunity on their survivors. The protection offered by vaccinations lasts for varying lengths of time, and weakens as time goes on.

Active Immunization

In so-called active immunization, germs that have been weakened or killed, or "detoxified" toxins, are injected into the body. The immune system forms antibodies against the intruders. This is what is taking place, for example, when a mild fever or feeling of malaise follows a vaccination. The protection against disease provided by such vaccinations lasts for varying lengths of time. This protection can be increased and lengthened by booster shots. Alternatively, if you have been immunized and happen to come into contact with the pathogen, the booster effect may occur unnoticed.

Passive Immunization

In passive immunization, antibodies formed by other human beings or animals against the pathogen are injected into the body. This option is chosen when someone is very likely to have been infected or is about to depart on a trip, and it is too late to build up immunity via active immunization. In the case of likely infection, the injected antibodies, immunoglobulins or gamma globulins, will lessen the severity of the disease. To be effective, immunoglobulins must be injected within 3 days of the presumed infection. The full effect only lasts 3 or 4 weeks.

When a foreign protein is injected into the body, there is always the danger of an allergic reaction, which, in the worst case, may lead to life-threatening shock. Injecting immunoglobulins is advisable only under certain circumstances; for a more detailed explanation, see the sections dealing with specific diseases.

TO VACCINATE OR NOT TO VACCINATE?

The question of whether or not to vaccinate usually doesn't come up with regard to diseases like tetanus, which is generally agreed to be a severe, often fatal, preventable disease. Such agreement is not present with "childhood" diseases like measles or whooping cough, however. In the years before vaccinations were available, most children went through all the childhood diseases before reaching puberty. Today, most parents in industrialized countries have their children vaccinated against these diseases. Vaccinations are required by public school systems in the United States and elsewhere.

As the number of immunized children has grown, "wild" pathogens have become rare, reducing the likelihood that unvaccinated children will contract the diseases while very young. Instead, they may be infected as older children or adults, when they are at greater risk for severe illness and consequences. In tropical countries, nearly all infants are infected with polio virus while they are still nursing, and thus protected by the antibodies in their mothers' milk. In these countries, paralysis caused by polio is almost unknown. However, as public hygiene improves, such early infection with the virus becomes less common, making vaccinations necessary as a means for conferring immunity to polio.

Not all vaccinations offer reliable protection. In some individuals the vaccine does not work, either because something is wrong with the vaccine or because the person didn't respond to it. A vaccine's effectiveness can only be determined by a blood test. If it is not effective, the patient is at risk for severe illness.

Vaccinations are voluntary measures except when they are required for entrance into public schools. If the choice is up to you, carefully weigh the risk of the disease against the risk associated with the vaccination itself. This cost-benefit calculation will not be the same for everyone, or for every disease (see below). If you are wondering whether or not to vaccinate, consider the following:

— Diseases are more easily contracted when the body is weakened or stressed. Vaccinations are given to healthy people so that their bodies can form antibodies at a time when they are strong.

— For a few diseases, immunoglobulins are injected into people who may have been infected but have not yet had the disease. The risk of undesirable side effects from this passive immunization is greater than risks associated with active immunization. (See sections on specific diseases for more information.)

Vaccination makes sense if

— The disease is common.
— The risk of severe consequences is great.
— There is no cure for the disease.
— The protection provided by the vaccination lasts a long time.
— The risk associated with the vaccination is less than that of the disease itself.

Vaccinate with caution if

— The patient is taking medications that weaken the immune system (e.g., corticosteroids for allergies or rheumatism; immunosuppressants for cancer, rheumatism, or organ transplants; other cancer medications).
— The patient has a disease of the central nervous system.
— The patient is allergic to certain proteins.
— The patient's immune system is compromised (e.g., in leukemia or lymphoma, AIDS).

Postpone vaccinations if

— The patient is not completely healthy.
— An allergy is especially severe at the moment.

Vaccination Tips for Parents

— Avoid routine vaccinations before your child has been thoroughly examined to be sure he or she is healthy.
— Ask your doctor to explain the risks of vaccination for your child.
— Ask about the first signs of damage caused by a vaccination, and what you should do if you suspect such damage.

ADVERSE SIDE-EFFECTS OF VACCINATION

No vaccination is risk-free. The most widely feared result is probably brain damage, in the form of convulsions or loss of intelligence, which leave a child with a severe, lifelong disability. In order to be officially classified as the result of a vaccination, brain-damage symptoms such as loss of consciousness, convulsions or paralysis must occur from 3 to 18 days following the vaccination, and all other possible causes of these symptoms must be positively ruled out. This is very difficult to do. Furthermore, these officially recognized symptoms are signs of adverse vaccination reaction in older children or adults. In small children the signs are much less distinct and harder to notice.

Not all vaccination complications cause permanent damage. Others include reddening of the skin, swelling and pain. The preservatives added to some vaccines can also cause allergies.

Most medical practitioners believe vaccinations are practically harmless. However, the number of claims submitted for compensation for adverse vaccination reactions indicate otherwise.

Observe Your Child After the Vaccination
— Is he or she unusually sleepy?
— Is he or she unusually apathetic?
— Does he or she cry for no discernible reason?
— Is he or she unusually restless?
— Is he or she unusually fearful?
— Is he or she unusually irritable?
— Is he or she vomiting?
— Does he or she have a fever?

WHEN TO VACCINATE FOR WHAT

Vaccination schedules are usually flexible according to individual patients' health requirements. They may also change as a result of new scientific or medical developments and/or the diseases present in a particular region. As a consumer, it's worth your while to stay abreast of new research on the benefits and risks of each type of vaccine. Your local health department can help.

VACCINATIONS BEFORE FOREIGN TRAVEL

Vaccinations are usually unnecessary for travel to Europe. Travel vaccinations serve two purposes: They protect the locals against imported diseases, and they protect travelers from local diseases which they're unlikely to encounter at home. Your local hospital or health department can give you up-to-date informa-

tion on what vaccinations are required for travel to which countries. This information changes frequently.

Travelers must comply with legally mandated vaccinations. However, some vaccinations are not required but merely recommended. Before getting these, consider the points listed on page 668, as well as the following:
— Your risk of contracting an infectious disease is low if you stay in the "westernized" districts of large cities or in areas frequented by many tourists. It rises once you travel into areas with poor sanitation.
— Cholera and typhus are transmitted through food and can be prevented by a few simple actions (see General Precautions When Traveling, page 718).
— If you are at all likely to have intimate bodily contact with local individuals, consider getting a hepatitis B vaccination.

YOUR IMMUNIZATION CERTIFICATE

All vaccinations should be entered into your vaccination certificate. Maintaining this record can help you avoid unnecessary repeat vaccinations as well as unpleasant or dangerous side effects (see Tetanus, p. 670). It also provides a reliable source of information for any physician treating you. Carry it with you at all times.

US Vaccination Schedule

Age	Vaccination
Birth	Hepatitis B
1 month	Hepatits B
2 months	Diptheria, Pertussis, Tetanus (DPT), Hemophilus b (Hib), Polio
4 months	DPT, Hib, Polio
6 months	DPT, Hib, Hepatitis B
12–15 months	Measles, Mumps, Rubella (MMR), Varicella vaccine, Hib
15–18 months	DPT, Polio
4–6 years	DPT, Polio, MMR
14–16 years	Diptheria, Tetanus (Td)

Recommended Booster Vaccinations

Every 10 years	Tetanus (Td)

Recommended Immunizations for Travelers to Developing Countries

Call Centers for Disease Control and Prevention (CDC) International Travelers Hotline, accessible 24 hours a day, 7 days a week at: (404) 332-4559.

INDIVIDUAL VACCINATIONS

Tuberculosis

How Common Is It?
Tuberculosis is relatively rare in North America, although the number of cases has climbed somewhat in recent years. The people most susceptible to tuberculosis include seniors, people living in crowded and unsanitary conditions, and people with weakened immune systems.

Many people come into contact with the tuberculosis bacterium without noticing it. Their bodies then form antibodies which prevent the illness from becoming life-threatening. However, the presence of these antibodies will cause the person to react positively to tuberculosis tests.

How Dangerous Is It?
The most widely feared reaction is tubercular meningitis, which occurs most frequently in small children.

Is Treatment Possible?
There are effective medications for tuberculosis, but the number of bacteria resistant to them is increasing. The main reason is that patients don't stay on the medication long enough to ensure that all bacteria have been killed.

Vaccination Procedure
Newborns can be vaccinated without a tuberculosis (TB) test. After the sixth week, the vaccine can only be administered after a tuberculosis test has been given.

Tolerance and Risks
A vaccination stresses an infant severely. A fever may develop as a result of the vaccination, even 3 or 4 weeks later. Four out of every thousand persons receiving the vaccination develop an ulcer at the site of the injection or in a nearby lymph node. Swollen glands are also an occasional result.

Reliability
The vaccination gives fairly reliable protection against a severe case of tuberculosis, but it only lasts about 5 years. It cannot prevent infection altogether, and immunized people can transmit the pathogens to others if they are infected.

Recommendation
You should consider having your baby immunized against tuberculosis if someone in your family or neighborhood has tuberculosis, or if you are planning to travel in countries where the disease is common. This immunization is not routinely done in the United States.

Tetanus

How Common Is It?
The bacteria that cause tetanus are found everywhere. It's easy to become infected by way of a deep, dirty wound, but even a small cut, which may go unnoticed, can get the bacteria into the body. Tetanus is not contagious. Survivors of one bout of tetanus are not immune to future bouts.

How Dangerous Is It?
About half the people who contract tetanus die of the disease. The first signs are muscle pains and cramps in the jaw and back muscles. After a long period of more and more intense muscle cramps in the entire body, the patient dies of respiratory or circulatory failure.

Is Treatment Possible?
Passive immunization, antibiotics, sedatives, and muscle relaxants can relieve the symptoms, but there is no antidote for the tetanus toxin.

Vaccination Procedure
Three injections of vaccine are needed for effective protection, and these should be administered at intervals of no less than 4 weeks and no more than 4 months apart. After this basic immunization, you should have a booster shot about every 10 years.

Many doctors give tetanus booster shots as a matter of course whenever they treat an injury. However, in cases of injury, the booster is only needed if the last one was given more than 5 years ago.

Tolerance and Risks
In rare cases, the skin becomes red and swells at the injection site. If a booster is given when blood antibody levels are still high from the last immunization (meaning the patient is still protected), the tissue around the injection site can become hard as a board, and the neighboring lymph nodes may swell. The reaction may

spread to the entire body. If your blood shows high levels of tetanus antibodies from a previous vaccination, it should be written in your vaccination certificate that you should not be given a booster in case of injury. Because the test for antibodies is relatively expensive, however, it is not routinely carried out, so many people aren't sure when their last tetanus shot was.

Reliability
People who are vaccinated for tetanus are protected for at least 10 years.

Recommendation
Adequate protection against tetanus should be part of any basic preventive health-care regimen.

Passive Immunization
An injured patient should only be given tetanus immunoglobulin if
— He or she has never been immunized against tetanus, or was only given the first shot.
— It is not known whether or when the patient was vaccinated.

Diphtheria

How Common Is It?
Diphtheria has become rare in North America. Most of those who develop the disease are adults below the age of 40. Most older people are immune because they were exposed to the pathogen at some point, without knowing it.

How Dangerous Is It?
About 22 percent of people who become infected with diphtheria suffer severe complications or die. Those who survive have lifelong immunity. However, survivors may still have pathogens in their bodies and excretions.

Is Treatment Possible?
There is no medication for diphtheria.

Vaccination Procedure
Infants are given three diphtheria immunizations in their first year, at intervals of 2 months. Booster shots are given in the second and fourth year. Diphtheria vaccine is usually administered in combination with whooping cough (pertussis) and tetanus vaccines (DPT). These three can be given in combination with polio, hemophilus b, and hepatitis B.

Tolerance and Risks
The injection site may become red or swell. If this reaction is extremely strong, the immunization series should be discontinued. Vaccinations are tolerated less well as people get older. Nerve paralysis or inflammations, and kidney inflammations, are more common in older people. In order to prevent these effects, a lower-dose vaccine is used in children of school age.

Reliability of Protection
The protection offered by the initial course of vaccine lasts for about 7 years, and the booster shots give at least another ten years of protection. The vaccine does not completely prevent infection, but the course of the disease will be mild if it occurs.

Recommendation
Diphtheria vaccination is advisable for children. Adults should also renew their protection every 10 years, if possible in conjunction with their tetanus booster.

Passive Immunization
Passive immunization is given only if an unvaccinated person is suspected of contracting the disease. The antibodies used for this come from horses, and contain foreign proteins that cause side effects fairly frequently, which may be severe.

Pertussis (Whooping Cough)

How Common Is It?
Whooping cough has become rare in children. However, the disease has become more common recently, and tends to occur in cycles.

How Dangerous Is It?
Babies are especially susceptible to this disease in the first six months of life, because they don't acquire passive immunization from their mothers. 90 percent of whooping cough fatalities are in babies; and 35 percent of all children who contract the disease are babies under 6 months of age.

Is Treatment Possible?

Whooping cough is rarely recognized as such at the stage at which antibiotics could make a difference. Later on, it no longer responds as well to medication (see Pertussis, p. 602).

Vaccination Procedure

To create adequate immunity, three vaccinations are administered at intervals of 2 months. Because of the side effects, a baby should not be given the first one before it is 2 months old. However, this means that even vaccinated children lack optimum protection for at least 6 months.

Tolerance and Risks

The injection site may hurt, the nearby lymph nodes may swell up, and fever may develop. In the older vaccine used before 1995, these reactions were relatively common and severe. In 1995, "acellular" pertussis vaccine became available. It is much better tolerated.

Reliability

The vaccine protects about 85 percent of the people who receive it. After the first three injections, children are protected for about 1½ years.

Recommendation

All infants should be vaccinated with the new acellular vaccine. The criticisms leveled at the pertussis vaccination were based on the side effects of the old vaccine, and are no longer valid.

Passive Immunization

Pertussis immunoglobulin is not a reliable means of protection and is of no use once the first signs of disease have appeared.

Polio

How Common Is It?

Since the oral polio vaccine was introduced, this disease is practically extinct in industrial countries. In developing countries, about one child in 10 under the age of 3 carries the virus without becoming ill.

How Dangerous Is It?

The resulting nerve damage can lead to paralysis.

Is Treatment Possible?

There is no medication for the polio virus.

Vaccination Procedure

Until recently, with very few exceptions, until recently polio vaccine was taken orally. Now it is mostly given by injection in the United States since no vaccine-associated paralysis occurs with this specific vaccine. It is usually given to children at the same time as their DPT vaccinations. At least 6 weeks should pass between doses of polio vaccine. Measles, mumps, and rubella (German measles) vaccines can be given at the same time as the polio vaccine. However, if this is not done, at least 4 weeks must pass between the polio and the other vaccinations, or the vaccine will not protect the child reliably. Boosters are needed by adults only under certain workplace conditions, or if travel plans include areas of endemic polio.

Tolerance and Risk

In rare cases, the stool may be thinner than usual after a polio vaccination. Paralysis is an extremely rare result with the oral form. A newly immunized person may be able to transmit the virus to others for at least 6 weeks. For this reason special attention should be given to the immune status of the person caring for the newly immunized child.

Reliability

The polio vaccine imparts immunity for at least 10 years, and probably for a lifetime.

Recommendation

Infants who contract polio nearly always recover with no ill effects. However, since the chances of becoming infected during infancy are very slight today, and since the disease frequently paralyzes older victims, this vaccination is advisable.

Measles

How Common Is It?

Fewer and fewer children get measles, which was once a typical disease of childhood.

How Dangerous Is It?

The older the patient, the greater the chance of severe

complications and permanent damage. For people over 6, the risk of central nervous system damage is about 1 in 800.

Is Treatment Possible?
The disease itself cannot be treated. Medications can help relieve complications.

Vaccination Procedure
It is now recommended that children be vaccinated twice, in order to protect any who did not react to the first dose.

Tolerance and Risk
Five to 15 percent of children vaccinated for measles run a fever about 1 week after the shot. Three to 5 percent develop a mild, measleslike rash about 10 days afterwards. Both symptoms disappear rapidly and don't require treatment. According to one British study, about 1 in 15,000 children will suffer severe complications.

Reliability
The more people are vaccinated, the less likely it becomes that a single vaccination will impart lifelong protection, because the booster effect of exposure to "wild" pathogens is no longer likely to occur.

Recommendation
Parents who do not wish to have a child vaccinated for measles can have the child's blood tested for measles antibodies when he or she is about 10. If the child is not already immune, he or she should be vaccinated at that time, since the risk of severe complications increases with age.

Passive Immunization
Passive immunization against measles is not advisable unless an infant has been exposed before it has had its first vaccination. In this case, the gamma globulin must be administered within 3 days after exposure.

Mumps

How Common Is It?
Fewer and fewer children get mumps.

How Dangerous Is It?
Mumps can cause a form of encephalitis in young chil-dren; however, this is usually mild. Older children some-times develop an inflammation of the gonads as a result of mumps. In adult men, testicular inflammation occurs in about one third of those infected, and the result is often sterility.

Is Treatment Possible?
There is no medication for mumps.

Vaccination Procedure
Mumps and measles vaccines are usually combined and administered after a child is 12 months old.

Tolerance and Risks
Complications are rare. In one test, 19 children vacci-nated for mumps developed diabetes, but it is unclear whether this was a result of the vaccination.

Reliability
Because getting the mumps does not confer lifelong immunity, it is assumed that the vaccine doesn't do so either. Studies in Switzerland have shown that the pro-tection offered by the vaccination is not as reliable as expected.

Recommendation
Grown men can be tested to determine whether they are immune to mumps, and vaccinated if they are not. If a man is in contact with many small children, he should seriously consider doing this.

Passive Immunization
Mumps immunoglobulin does not always prevent the disease, nor does it prevent inflammation of the ovaries or testes.

Rubella (German Measles)

How Dangerous Is It?
If a woman has rubella during the first weeks of preg-nancy, the embryo is at very high risk of birth defects. The vaccination is thus intended to protect unconceived children.

Is Treatment Possible?
Only an abortion can reliably prevent the birth of a child with birth defects, if a nonimmune woman is infected during the first trimester pregnancy.

Vaccination Procedure

The recommendation that both girls and boys be vaccinated against rubella in their second and fifth years of life is intended to reduce the number of cases of the disease to the point that the danger of infecting pregnant women is greatly reduced. The antibody titer in a girl's blood can be determined, and if she is not immune during puberty, a third dose should be given.

Tolerance and Risks

In 8 to 14 percent of women over the age of 25, the vaccination may produce temporary joint pains similar to rheumatism. If the pains last longer than 2 weeks and fever is present, a physician should check whether the rubella vaccine has led to a rheumatic illness. These complications are much less common in younger women and girls. Two to 5 percent of people who receive this vaccine develop a mild fever and skin rash.

Reliability

The actual disease gives better protection than the vaccination. Of those who have had rubella once, only 2 to 5 percent develop the disease again, but among those who have been vaccinated, half can contract the disease again. The (partial) protection offered by the vaccine lasts 15 years. If you are not certain that you are immune and are planning a pregnancy, you can ask a doctor for a blood test.

Recommendation

The disease itself is so mild that some recommend to expose healthy girls to a child who has it, so they can develop and maintain natural protection. The titer of blood antibodies should be checked in 10-year-old girls, and if it is deficient, they should be vaccinated.

Passive Immunization

Passive immunization should be considered only for a pregnant woman who is not immune to rubella, has been exposed to it, and will not consider an abortion. However, rubella immunoglobulins will not offer definite protection, either to the mother or child.

Hemophilus Influenza Type b (Hib)

How Common Is It?

The hemophilus vaccine gets its name from a pathogen that causes several childhood diseases, including one type of meningitis and inflammation of the epiglottis (see Epiglottitis, p. 597).

Before the Hib vaccination, Hib was the most common cause of bacterial meningitis in the United States. Since 1988, when Hib vaccination was introduced, the incidence of invasive disease has declined by 95 percent in infants and young children.

How Dangerous Is It?

It is estimated that every fifth child with Hib meningitis infection suffers mild, chronic mental, and physical disabilities. About one third are permanently disabled, with impaired equilibrium, hearing, vision or speech, or paralysis, or convulsions. Five percent of afflicted children die of this form of meningitis, in spite of early treatment.

Is Treatment Possible?

The earlier this type of meningitis is recognized and treated with antibiotics and corticosteroids, the better the chances of cure. A child with meningitis should be carefully treated in a hospital.

Vaccination Procedure

The recommended procedure includes four vaccinations, in the second, fourth, sixth, and fifteenth month. However, if the first dose is given after the child is 15 months old, a single dose is sufficient.

Tolerance and Risk

This vaccine is considered to be well tolerated. Side effects reported to date include reddening and swelling of the injection site, fever, skin rash, and intensified allergies.

Reliability

At least 85 percent of children who receive this vaccine are protected from invasive hemophilus infections.

Recommendation

Hib vaccination is advisable, but should not be considered a vaccination against meningitis, as it does not protect patients from meningitis caused by other pathogens.

Hepatitis B (Infectious Hepatitis)

How Common Is It?
About 5 to 8 percent of the U. S. population has been infected with hepatitis B. In Asia and Africa, much larger proportions of the population are infected.

How Dangerous Is It?
About two thirds of cases of hepatitis B infection go unnoticed. However, about 2 percent are rapidly fatal, and about 10 percent lead to chronic liver inflammation, which increases the chances of liver cancer. Cirrhosis of the liver can also develop as a result of this disease (see p. 396).

Hepatitis B is transmitted only by contact with infected blood and body fluids. Therefore, those at greatest risk are medical personnel, people who receive blood transfusions or blood products, addicts who inject drugs, people with risky sexual practices, and newborn infants of infected women.

Is Treatment Possible?
There is no reliable medication for hepatitis at this time.

Vaccination Procedure
The basic immunization consists of three vaccinations.

Tolerance and Risk
The injection site may be temporarily painful.

Reliability
Young, healthy people are well protected by the vaccination, but those over 50 are protected less well. The success of the vaccination can be monitored by checking the antibody titer.

Recommendation
The vaccination is highly recommended for those with a high risk of contracting hepatitis B. The recommendation that small children be vaccinated is based on the following considerations: The disease is fairly likely to become chronic in children, and they should be protected by the time they reach the age of sexual activity. The World Health Organization has stated its intention of reducing the number of carriers worldwide.

So long as there is no vaccine against HIV, however, all young people should be instructed in the use of condoms, which impart some protection against both hepatitis B and HIV.

Hepatitis A

How Common Is It?
About one fourth of all liver inflammations are caused by hepatitis A viruses. The infection is common in countries with poor sanitation, especially in Africa, Asia and South America. In these countries, the risk for "conventional" tourists is estimated at 3 to 6 cases per 1,000. However, for backpackers and the like, the risk is six times as high.

How Dangerous Is It?
In children under 5, hepatitis A infections usually go unnoticed. Adults usually develop jaundice. After a few weeks, or at most after 6 months, hepatitis A disappears without complications. It never becomes chronic (see Hepatitis, p. 395).

Is Treatment Possible?
There is no specific treatment for the disease.

Vaccination Procedure
For a basic immunization in preparation for a trip, the first shot is given 4 weeks before departure, and the second 2 weeks or less before departure. The vaccination should be repeated 6 months to 1 year later.

For those who tend to travel on the spur of the moment, quick immunizations are also available.

Tolerance and Risk
Fatigue, fever, and skin reactions are fairly common. More severe side effects are rare.

Reliability
After the first injection, about 70 percent of those receiving this vaccination are protected. After the second, nearly 100 percent are protected. After three injections, the level of protection is similar to that produced by the actual disease, and lasts about 10 years.

Recommendation
This immunization is recommended for people traveling in countries with poor hygiene if they plan to leave the major tourist areas, and for people working in those

countries. Someone who has spent extended periods in a foreign country can have a blood test to determine whether the antibody titers are sufficient.

Influenza

How Common Is It?
Most of the common illnesses of winter are colds. If there is a flu epidemic, only a laboratory test can distinguish between illnesses caused by influenza and cold viruses.

How Dangerous Is It?
True influenza can be quite serious in older people and chronically ill persons, and fatalities are possible.

Is Treatment Possible?
Only the symptoms can be treated (see Colds, p. 298).

Vaccination Procedure
One flu shot is usually given in October or November.

Tolerance and Risk
In about 10 percent of those vaccinated, the skin becomes red and swollen at the site of injection. A mild fever develops in 2 to 3 percent of cases.

Reliability
Influenza viruses are highly mutable, and for this reason, vaccines are adapted to the current versions each year. In spite of this, the vaccine has only about a 60 percent protection rate. The vaccination needs to be repeated on a yearly basis.

Recommendation
Flu shots are recommended only for people at especially high risk in case of a true influenza infection, e.g., seniors, chronically ill people, and those with asthma or other lung diseases and/or heart disease.

Cholera

How Common Is It?
The World Health Organization estimates that about one million people worldwide are infected with cholera. It has recently been discovered that cholera bacte-

ria can survive for long periods in water, so there is always a reservoir of the disease outside human beings.

How Dangerous Is It?
Even in centers of cholera epidemics, only about 15 people in 100 are affected by the disease. People in poor economic or social circumstances who lack adequate sanitation are at highest risk of contracting cholera.

Is Treatment Possible?
Death can be prevented by immediate replacement of the water and salts lost through diarrhea. There are effective antibiotics against the pathogen.

Vaccination Procedure
The basic immunization against cholera consists of two injections a week or two apart. If a booster is needed, it is given 6 months later. A better-tolerated oral vaccine has also been developed.

Tolerance and Risk
The injected cholera vaccine is not well tolerated. Nearly all injected patients develop headaches, fever, and pains. The injection site frequently swells considerably. The vaccination can cause damage to internal organs in persons with poor circulation, and inflammations latent in the body may flare up. Because of the strong side effects, this vaccination cannot be repeated at will.

Reliability
The cholera vaccine does not give complete protection against infection. The protection it does offer lasts 2 to 3 months.

Recommendation
The World Health Organization no longer recommends cholera vaccinations, but if you are traveling to a country that requires one, you must get one.

To prevent cholera infection, see General Precautions When Traveling, p. 718.

Yellow Fever

How Common Is It?
Yellow fever is a common disease in tropical regions of Africa and South America. It does not occur in Asia.

How Dangerous Is It?

The first signs of yellow fever are fever, pains and vomiting. Damage to the liver, kidneys, and blood vessels is fatal in about 10 percent of cases.

Is Treatment Possible?

Only the symptoms can be treated.

Vaccination Procedure

A vaccination for yellow fever can usually be obtained only at a specialized tropical medicine center, because the vaccine is more complicated to prepare and store than others, and the procedure requires special training for the physician.

Tolerance and Risk

The yellow fever vaccination is well tolerated.

Reliability

The vaccination gives protection for at least 10 years. International health regulations recommend a booster after 10 years.

Recommendation

The yellow fever vaccination is "the" tropical disease vaccination. See p. 717 for foreign travel vaccination information.

Typhus

How Common Is It?

Typhus and paratyphus have become rare in countries with good sanitation. The risk of contracting typhus is relatively high in North and Central Africa, and of paratyphus in Southeast Asia and the Far East.

How Dangerous Is It?

Inflammations of the intestines, heart muscle, lungs, meninges, and gallbladder may be caused by typhus.

Even where timely treatment is administered, about one percent of typhus patients die of the disease (see Gastroenteritis, p. 599).

Is Treatment Possible?

Antibiotics are effective against typhus.

Vaccination Procedure

Both oral and injectable typhus vaccines are available. The oral immunization consists of capsules taken three times a day on 3 days, spaced 1 day apart. The injected form of the vaccine needs to be administered only once.

Tolerance and Risk

The oral form of the vaccine is very well tolerated. The injected form causes side effects about 10 times more frequently, but they are mild.

Reliability

The oral vaccine protects the patient for 1 year; the injected form for 3 years. Both have only about a 60 percent reliability rate.

Recommendation

A typhus vaccination is needed only by travelers in countries with inadequate sanitation who are planning to venture beyond high-traffic tourist areas.

Rabies

How Common Is It?

Raccoons, skunks, foxes, bats, and other species are the main carriers of rabies. In some areas, these wild animals infect domestic dogs, cats, and ferrets. People who are in frequent contact with wild animals have the highest risk of catching rabies.

How Dangerous Is It?

Not all bites from an animal presumed to carry rabies will result in the disease in a human. The farther the bite is from the head, the less likely the chance of transmission of the pathogen. People bitten on the face, neck, or thumb have a 40 to 60 percent chance of contracting the disease.

Is Treatment Possible?

Rabies vaccination should be given to bite victims. Untreated, rabies is always fatal.

Vaccination Procedure

People who come in frequent contact with potentially infected animals should be vaccinated as a precautionary measure. The first vaccination is repeated after 1 week, and again after 3 weeks; a booster is administered after 1 year, and every 5 years thereafter.

Bite victims are given 6 injections: The first as soon as possible after the accident, and then 3, 7, 14, and 28 days later.

Tolerance and Risk

So-called human diploid cell (HDC) vaccines are well tolerated. However, in some countries other types of vaccines are still used. These carry a high risk of allergy or inflammation of the brain or spinal cord.

Recommendation

A preventive rabies shot is a good idea if you work with wild animals, and should be considered if you are planning to travel to remote regions of Asia.

NATURAL HEALING AND ALTERNATIVE MEDICINE

The human body has strong self-healing powers that can be stimulated and supplemented through natural healing. Natural remedies—including heat and cold therapy, movement, or massage, a wholesome diet (see p. 722) or specific relaxation techniques (see p. 693)—can restore the equilibrium of a system out of balance, or in which the organs are no longer functioning optimally.

When used regularly, these natural healing methods tone and strengthen the body, better enabling it to withstand stress and infections and overcome disease.

The central principle of natural healing is to go easy. A sick body needs rest, sleep, no stimulation or irritants, and a diet that won't place stress on the digestive system—just a complete focus on getting better, followed by initially gentle and increasingly rigorous exercises to restore inner balance. Rest, stimulation and strengthening are the basic principles of natural treatment. For example, Kneipp therapy consists of the following essential processes: Hydrotherapy (alternating hot and cold baths), exercise, diet, and relaxation.

Physical therapy developed from natural healing methodologies. Today its range of treatment has broadened to include electrical stimulation, ultrasound, and light therapy.

Many people prefer to treat their symptoms with natural methods if at all possible, using home remedies such as teas and compresses, building their resistance with alternating hot and cold baths or saunas, or changing their diet. Many also turn to alternative health practitioners to supplement conventional medical treatment (see p. 626), for a variety of reasons: To minimize side effects of medication, to support the body's ability to heal, and to enjoy a more holistic doctor-patient relationship, with more relaxed appointments and more attention to the patient's state of mind or overall well-being.

The faith people have in complementary and alternative medicine is the basis for its successes, and for its failures as well. Many patients drop or switch alternative methods if they don't get the results they're expecting.

The trust between patient and health-care provider is a significant factor in the success of any treatment, as is the mystique of the treatment plan itself: Arcane equipment, complicated instructions for taking medications, and behavioral guidelines focus the patient's attention and have a powerful suggestive impact, which explains why many patients report feeling better, at least initially.

However, there are those who point out that natural healing, alternative medicine, and complementary healing techniques are simply not supported by scientific evidence. And the old adage, "even if it doesn't work, at least it won't hurt you" is not necessarily applicable either. Some alternative methods can indeed be dangerous, particularly if the patient is blinded by hopes of miracle cures and doesn't seek conventional medical treatment in time.

APPLIED KINESIOLOGY (AK)

The premise of this unconventional diagnostic technique, used by some chiropractors and osteopaths (see p. 682) is that by muscle testing one can diagnose a diseased organ or a food sensitivity, detect developmental disorders or emotional problems, and even choose the most appropriate medication.

Techniques and Applications

In AK diagnosis, the patient extends an arm, and the practitioner exerts downward pressure on that arm while palpating the area of the body suspected of being diseased. Low resistance suggests disease; high resistance suggests the patient is healthy. In the same way, foods and/or medications can be held in the hand to test the patient's sensitivity.

Controls have shown this method to be open to subjective interpretation and, as such, unsound; nor are similar methods such as "Touch for Health" scientifically recognized.

None of these methods is recommended.

ACUPUNCTURE AND MOXIBUSTION

Acupuncture evolved in China from shamanic scarification rituals and from numerology: The number of acupuncture points corresponds to the days in a calendar year, and the number of connecting lines to the months. It was Westerners who first called these lines "meridians."

Acupuncture was used in China only as a secondary, or supplementary, treatment. It was further developed in the West, where many widely divergent variations arose. Some systems have only 20 acupuncture points, others more than a thousand. The number of meridians varies, as does the recommended depth of penetration by the needles. The goal of Chinese medicine is to keep the life energy, or "chi," unblocked and flowing.

Techniques

With the patient sitting or lying, needles ranging in length from half an inch to 4 inches are inserted into acupuncture points; the needles may be turned to intensify the effect. The point of insertion may become slightly irritated.

Treatments usually last 10 to 30 minutes, repeated 5 to 10 times over several days. Long-term needles with barbed hooks can be left in the body for several days.

Some acupuncturists inject acupuncture points with medicine to stimulate the immune system (see p. 351) or use additional aids such as pressure balls, glass rods, or clamps. Electro-acupuncture employs electrodes clamped to the needles to send mild electrical impulses to the whole area.

Laser acupuncture, in which a laser ray is used on the appropriate points, is a pain-free variation used primarily in children.

The premise of ear acupuncture is that the whole body can be treated via the ear (other variations hold that this can be done through the mouth or vagina as well). This paradigm, however, contradicts orthodox anatomical teachings.

Moxibustion is a traditional variation of acupuncture that involves placing burning cones of a dried and fermented herb, mugwort, on the acupuncture points as long as the skin can tolerate the heat.

Applications

The effectiveness of acupuncture in pain treatment has been proven. The use of needles can break the cycle of pain and improve nervous system disorders. It is especially effective in management of migraines, headaches, and back, joint, and nerve pain.

Acupuncture is used only rarely as an anesthetic, even in China. It has not proved effective in the treatment of addiction.

Laser acupuncture is classified as placebo treatment. It can be beneficial for children and adults with a fear of injections.

Recommendations

Before any acupuncture treatment, have a medical checkup. Needle-pricks, particularly in the ear and especially with long-term needles, can be painful. Acupuncture treatments can cause collapse and fainting. Electro-acupuncture can cause heart arrhythmia. Only single-use needles should be used. Incompletely sterilized needles can cause local infections and spread diseases such as hepatitis and AIDS.

There have been documented cases of acupuncturists injuring organs with needles so badly that their patients died.

Electro-acupuncture should not be performed on patients with pacemakers, or those suffering from arrhythmia, epilepsy or shock, or during pregnancy.

ACUPRESSURE AND SHIATSU

Acupressure has its origins in Chinese massage and was further developed by the Japanese as shiatsu. Like acupuncture (see p. 679), it involves applying pressure to specific body points to ensure optimal energy flow and organ function.

Techniques

Using fingers, knuckles, elbows, or feet, the practitioner applies pressure to acupressure points for 5 to 20 seconds.

Applications

Acupressure relaxes the muscles and improves circulation. It is helpful in treating nervousness and sleep disorders, easing headaches and pain, and strengthening the immune system.

Recommendations

Have a medical checkup prior to any acupressure treatment.

Treatment may cause or increase pain or nausea; both will clear up on their own.

Do not undergo acupressure treatment if you have

a systemic or infectious disease.

BREATHING THERAPY

One important technique of curative gymnastics (see p. 762) is breathing therapy, which is used for respiratory tract problems. In addition, breathing therapy is an integral part of relaxation techniques (see p. 693).

Techniques

The therapy may take the form of either a focus on conscious proper breathing, or a physical or vocal workout. This generally takes place in a group environment, with patients practicing together for an hour once a week for several weeks.

Applications

Breathing therapy can improve any restriction of the voice and airways, cardiovascular system, or digestion. It can improve posture, ease tension, reduce stress and help promote emotional balance.

Recommendations

Breathing therapy should be performed by educated, experienced psychotherapists. It is not recommended in case of serious psychological disorders.

ANTHROPOSOPHICAL MEDICINE

Anthroposophical medicine combines philosophical, mystical, religious, and scientific elements.

Health and illness is defined as a balance between the four elements of being, the "physical," the "spiritual," the "ethereal," and the "I." Imbalances between the four elements cause disease. In anthroposophical medicine, disease is viewed as a positive possibility for the body, soul, and spirit to overcome illness, and thereby achieve new strengths.

Techniques

Diagnostic and treatment modalities are based on conventional medicine, which are expanded by anthroposophical elements.

Specific anthroposophical diagnostic techniques include drawing a blood sample, specially handling it, placing a sample on paper, and analyzing the pattern to diagnose the illness.

Specific anthroposophical treatments and medicines are not scientifically proven.

In addition to medicines, anthroposophical treatment includes living with a healthy diet, eating foods that are "natural," and doing therapies using music, speech, painting, and sculpting. A specific type of therapy, curative eurythmy, is movement done to the sound of vowels and other sounds.

Applications

Since anthroposophical medicine is seen as something in addition to conventional medicine, it is more inclusive. The artistic therapies are very successful, specifically for rehabilitation.

Recommendations

The anthroposophical diagnostic techniques go beyond any scientific basis.

Some anthroposophical medicines contain heavy metals, and as such are toxic to the body, especially if used long-term. Exposure to these medicines is in addition to the toxins found in our environment (see The Most Common Pollutants, page 773).

Also problematic can be allergic reactions that can occur if ant- and bee-based medicines are injected.

AYURVEDA

Ayurveda is a 3,500-year-old Indian philosophy detailing a comprehensive approach to good health and living one's life. Ayurvedic medicine is practiced widely throughout the subcontinent and taught as a university subject.

Its basic concept is that the three "doshas"—vata, pitta, and kapha—correspond to the body's regulatory systems. When these are in balance, the individual is strong, vital, and healthy; imbalance leads to disease.

The type of ayurvedic medicine principally known in the West is the approach popularized by the guru Maharishi Mahesh Yogi.

Techniques

In addition to standard medical diagnoses, ayurveda uses pulse diagnosis to determine the patient's basic nature.

Treatment is with diet and herbal/botanical remedies (rasayanas) that are purported to regulate the doshas. Their effect has not been proven scientifically.

Yoga and meditation are also part of the treatment: They help reduce anxiety and tension.

Applications

The strength of ayurvedic medicine lies in its focus on maintaining health. It also promises relief and improvement of chronic diseases and functional disorders.

Although ayurvedic medicine claims success in treating a very broad range of diseases, the credibility of supporting evidence is dubious.

Recommendations

Ayurvedic medicine is not recommended for those suffering from a serious disease or psychological problems.

BACH FLOWER THERAPY

At the beginning of the twentieth century, the British physician Edward Bach expanded on the concept of flower therapy invented by the psychoanalyst Carl Jung. Bach held that diseases are caused by conflicts between one's personality and one's higher self, and he claimed to have isolated 38 negative emotional states that could be cured with specific plants. Healing was considered successful when a patient's character flaws were transformed into virtues.

To prepare the remedies, fresh flowers are distilled with water and alcohol. They must be diluted when taken internally. "Rescue Remedy," for example, is a Bach product that is used as a first-aid medication; it consists of the distilled essences of five different flowers.

Techniques

Flower therapists do not believe in conventional diagnosis; some claim to intuit a patient's condition. Bach flower therapy is predominantly a self-help modality.

Applications

Bach flower remedies are said to help in overcoming psychological crises and conflict. Diseases are said to be affected on a "higher energetic level."

"Rescue Remedy" is supposedly helpful in treating both physical and emotional crises.

There is no scientific evidence of the effectiveness of flower therapy.

Recommendations

Relying on "Rescue Remedy" in a medical crisis may mean putting yourself at great risk by not seeking ef-fective treatment in a timely manner. This applies equally to cases of psychological illness.

CHIROPRACTIC AND OSTEOPATHIC MEDICINE

These modalities of manipulative medicine (see p. 686) are recognized as a significant method of diagnosis and treatment for back and joint dysfunctions.

Techniques

Various methods serve to relax muscles and release blocked (not fused) joints and restore their function. The best-known of these is chiropractic manipulation, in which the affected joint, muscle, tendon or nerve ending is released through characteristic short, sharp tugs and the familiar pain-free "crack." In this method, special grips or holds keep the other joints in traction.

Osteopaths and chiropractors also use gentler techniques, such as applying fingertip pressure to release tensed muscle groups, or carefully flexing a stressed joint repeatedly until its full range of motion is restored.

Applications

This kind of treatment is appropriate only in cases where functional movement is restricted, and there is joint as well as back pain. It should not be employed once a joint is already compromised.

Recommendations

Chiropractic manipulation should be performed only by licensed professionals. Patients should have X rays prior to any treatment.

Chiropractic methods should never be employed following an accident or in the event of acute joint infections. In cases of extreme pain, four treatments should be the maximum.

Excessively frequent "cracking" can cause looseness of the joints; it can also have a deleterious effect if blood vessels in the neck have undergone damage. Patients over age 50 should not have neck manipulations.

STEAM BATHS OR SAUNAS

Techniques

Inside the average steam bath, temperatures run about 120°F and humidity 100 percent. You should stay in a steam bath only as long as you feel comfortable—

between 5 and 15 minutes.

Applications

Steam baths can enhance overall health and tone the system. The advantage of a steam bath over a sauna is that its high level of humidity relieves persistent congestion associated with chronic respiratory disease.

Recommendations

Some people tolerate steam baths less well than saunas because the high humidity restricts the evaporation of sweat, preventing the body from cooling itself down. As with saunas, cooling-off and rest periods should be strictly observed (see p. 690).

Avoid steam baths if you have an acute infectious disease, a cold, or cardiovascular disease.

RELAXATION

See p. 693.

ENZYME THERAPY

The idea behind enzyme therapy is that enzymes break down inflammatory substances and can therefore change the outer layer of cancer cells in such a way that the body can then render them harmless.

Techniques

Anti-inflammatory medication is applied topically or taken internally; cancer drugs are usually swallowed or injected.

Medication is given at high doses. When used for treating cancer, treatment usually lasts at least 2 years.

Applications

Enzyme therapy is used in cases of accidents and sport injuries, rheumatic infections, skin diseases, herpes, and burns. In the case of cancer, enzyme therapy is supposed to prevent metastasis, guard against relapse and improve the general health of terminally ill patients.

Enzyme therapy is controversial and not yet scientifically proven effective for treating injuries, infections, or cancer.

Recommendations

Enzyme injections present a relatively high risk of allergic reaction. Injections into body cavities can lead to fever and circulatory problems, and result in shock.

FASTING

Periodic fasting has a place in many religious practices. This is not to be confused with fasting as a crash-diet technique, however, which is not recommended. When practiced appropriately, fasting can be a means of cleansing the body and renewing the spirit.

Techniques

Going on a "fasting retreat" is an especially effective technique. Caloric intake should be reduced for 3 days prior to beginning the fast, usually accompanied by regular enemas, since empty intestines are supposed to result in fewer hunger pangs. Two to 3 liters of calorie-free liquid must be drunk daily. Exercise and bodywork such as massage are part of the treatment, which lasts about 3 weeks, after which a balanced diet consisting of wholesome foods is slowly reintroduced (see p. 723).

There are different types of fasts: Some involve drinking only vegetable broths to lower metabolic processes, others (such as a juice fast) allow fruit and vegetable juices.

A protein-modified fast involves daily intake of buttermilk or a special protein supplement: This prevents the otherwise significant protein loss and enables the body to metabolize more fat than protein.

Applications

During a fast, body tissue dehydrates, causing improved circulation, less stress to the heart, lower blood pressure and easier breathing. Fasting stimulates the immune system and can result in short-term improvement of rheumatoid arthritis. All diseases influenced by diet can be affected by fasting.

Recommendations

Fasting can lead to sleep and menstrual disorders. During the first 2 weeks of calorie-free fasts, the body loses significant amounts of protein. This puts at risk those people with serious organic diseases, especially heart disease. Gout can result.

People who should not fast include pregnant and nursing women, children under the age of 10, insulin-dependent diabetics, cancer patients, and anyone prone to bleeding, hyperthyroidism or circulatory disorders of the brain.

FOOT REFLEXOLOGY (HAND AND EAR REFLEXOLOGY)

Advocates of this method believe there are specific zones on the soles of the feet (as well as the hands or ears) that are connected to our internal organs (see diagram). Areas especially sensitive to pressure or pain indicate the presence of internal ailments that can be healed or lessened through intensive massage of these areas. Sensitive lumps on the feet suggest the buildup of toxins that can be eliminated through massage.

Techniques

Foot reflexology calls for intensive massage of the stressed areas, especially the heel. Special attention is given to painful areas. In hand and ear reflexology, certain areas are massaged intensively with the fingertips or little rods. Treatment can take up to an hour.

Applications

Foot reflexology has a relaxing effect. Applying pressure along the heel can ease pain in the lower back and help menstrual disorders, since these areas are connected via nerve pathways.

There is no evidence, however, that internal organs can be treated through any reflexology—hand, ear, or foot.

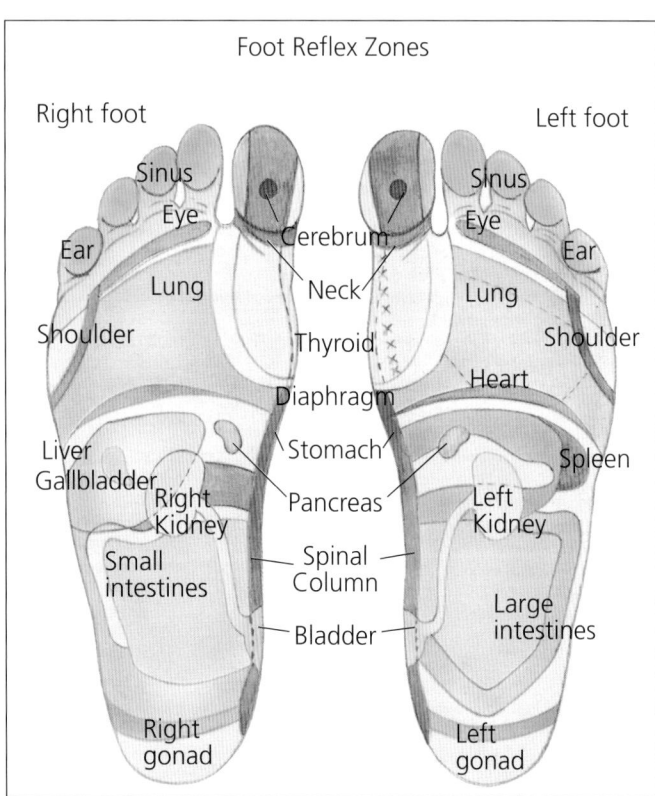

Foot Reflex Zones

Right foot — Left foot

Sinus, Eye, Ear, Lung, Shoulder, Cerebrum, Neck, Thyroid, Diaphragm, Stomach, Liver, Gallbladder, Right Kidney, Pancreas, Small intestines, Spinal Column, Bladder, Right gonad

Sinus, Eye, Ear, Lung, Shoulder, Heart, Spleen, Left Kidney, Large intestines, Left gonad

HOMEOPATHY

Homeopathy is widely divergent from conventional medicine, and was developed at the beginning of the nineteenth century by Samuel Hahnemann.

The homeopathic belief is that every person has a certain dynamic and functional "life force" that is brought out of balance by disease. The symptoms of illness can be cured by homeopathic remedies because they irritate the body into regulating it's unbalanced "life force." There are two main principals of homeopathic medicine. The first was based on evaluating remedies on healthy individuals. Here Hahnemann tested numerous plants and minerals, to see what there effects were on healthy individuals. His observations are the basis of his belief that administering minute doses of a remedy that would in healthy individuals produce symptoms similar to those of the disease, are curative for those individuals affected by those symptoms.

Homeopaths use extracts from plants and minerals, either very concentrated or extremely diluted. The healing effect of the remedy is not supposed to be affected by the decreasing concentration. Quite the opposite; some homeopaths believe that extremely diluted remedies are more efficacious than the more concentrated ones.

Homeopathic Medicines

Homeopathic medicines are produced according to the homeopathic medicine book, and diluted according to specific regulations. Homeopaths talk about "potentiating," because they believe that shaking the remedy increases its efficacy.

The dilutions are labeled with "D," "DH," or "X;" if they are diluted in a manner of 1:10. That is, 1 part of original substance is mixed and shaken with 10 parts of diluting material. If labeled with a "C," the dilution is 1:100; if labeled "LM," the dilution is 1:50,000.

Remedies labeled D6 or less are considered low potency, D12 middle, and anything above that is considered high potency. Homeopathic remedies are not FDA approved and many are available without a prescription.

Techniques

Before any homeopathic treatment is undertaken, it is suggested to have a conventional medicine evaluation to see whether or not homeopathic treatment is indicated.

To begin with, the homeopath evaluates the individual, both body and soul, to see what the problems are; and in conjunction with the specific symptoms, then determines what the best homeopathic remedy is for that individual.

Applications

Reports on the beneficial use of homeopathic medicine for disorders of well being, such as depression, chronic functional disorders, allergies, and poor immune defenses have been made. However, it has yet to be scientifically proven that the benefit was derived from the homeopathic medicine(s).

For numerous illnesses, homeopathy can be an adjunctive treatment.

Recommendations

Homeopathic medicines are not without risks and side effects.

If remedies containing arsenic, mercury, lead, or cadmium are used in concentrations less than D8 for longer periods of time, chronic toxicity is very possible.

Substances and plants that can damage the genes, or are potential carcinogens, are still used in the preparation of certain homeopathic remedies (such as arsenic compounds, and plants of the family Aristolochia).

Allergy-inducing plants, up to a D8 concentration, can be harmful to susceptible individuals. Particulary problematic are remedies containing bee or spider products, especially if injected.

Certain lower-potency remedies can acutely damage specific organs or organ systems (e.g., berberis can cause acute hepatitis).

COLD TREATMENTS

Cold has an immediate effect on acute inflammations and injuries. It constricts blood vessels, stops bleeding, reduces swelling, and eases pain. Ice packs (see p. 685), cold wet compresses (see p. 692), or cooling and anesthetic ethyl chloride spray can be used as first aid for sport injuries.

ICE PACKS

Techniques

Keep warm; the room should be warm as well.

Cover ice cubes in a towel; smash with a hammer.

Fill a plastic bag with ice chips, add an equal amount of water; then squeeze air out of the bag and seal it. Wrap the bag in a towel and place on the affected area. Dry ice or ready-made ice packs work just as well. Some contain a special gel that keeps them semiliquid even below freezing temperatures. Cold running water may also do the trick.

Applications

Ice packs are excellent first aid for sprains, contusions, strains, and acutely inflamed joints. Cold compresses on the wrists or temples help with circulatory problems and headaches.

Recommendations

Do not use cold packs in the event of reduced sensitivity to pain (e.g., in diabetics) or serious circulatory disorders (such as smoker's leg). Remove ice pack immediately if it causes pain or discomfort.

LIGHT THERAPY

Sunlight has healing properties involving various processes:
— Ultraviolet (UV) and infrared rays affect the skin.
— Exposure to light lifts one's spirits and improves productivity by stimulating the metabolism and hormone production.
— UV rays kill bacteria.

While sunlight produces all these effects simultaneously, each can also be produced individually by exposure to specific sources of artificial light.

Techniques

Start with daily sunbaths lasting 2 to 10 minutes. Increase the length of time every day, or every other day, until you are in the sun for a maximum of 1 hour a day.

Applications

Light therapy is used in treating mood disorders, vitamin D deficiency, skin disorders (acne, psoriasis), and depression.

Recommendations

Determine your skin's sensitivity before exposure (see Sunburn, p. 263).

Apply an appropriate sunscreen for your skin type. While sunbathing, wear glasses that absorb UV rays.

Long hours in the sun can be dangerous. Excessively strong UV rays increase the risk of skin cancer, as does every incidence of sunburn. This also applies to UV rays in solariums and tanning salons.

Excessive sun exposure causes irritability and fatigue and can lead to headaches, circulatory disorders, stomach problems, and heat stroke.

Ultraviolet light therapy should not be used in cases of acute internal/systemic and infectious diseases, shock, or allergic reactions.

MAGNETIC FIELD TREATMENT

In the 1960s it was discovered that bone fractures heal more quickly under the influence of low-level electrical currents, yielding the conclusion that magnetic fields have a general healing effect. To date, this has not been scientifically proven, but treatments with magnetic equipment and objects abound nonetheless.

Techniques

A magnetic field is set up around the affected area for a period of half an hour to several hours. Treatment is repeated several times over a period of weeks or months.

Applications

Magnetic field therapy is purported to help various problems, in particular wounds that are slow to heal, back problems, and bone fractures. However, there is still no definitive proof of its effectiveness. Any beneficial effect such as pain relief is probably because of the long rest periods the treatment requires.

This does not hold true for metal implants in complex bone fractures: In these cases, it is the electrical stimulus to the implant that has a beneficial effect.

MANIPULATIVE MEDICINE

Various techniques have evolved from the traditional bone-setting of folk medicine, where the emphasis is on restoring health through manipulation: these include chiropractic and osteopathy (see p. 682). Osteopathy also led to the unconventional methods of craniosacral therapy (see p. 691) and applied kinesiology (see p. 679).

MACROBIOTICS

The macrobiotic diet is part of a whole world view based on Zen buddhism in which foodstuffs are classified as having either yin or yang characteristics. A food is considered optimal when it has a ratio of five parts yin to one part yang; whole grains reflect this ratio and as such are considered the ideal food.

Techniques

Originally, a true macrobiotic diet meant one consisting exclusively of grains. Today's more moderate versions are more well rounded (see p. 722), but still deficient in certain food groups.

The drinking of excessive liquids is discouraged. The macrobiotic maxim is: drink only when you're thirsty.

Babies and small children are fed a macrobiotic mixture of ground grains, sesame seeds, and adzuki beans.

Applications

The macrobiotic diet promises health, longevity and the prevention and healing of all diseases including cancer, but there is no definitive proof of such claims.

Recommendations

A diet high in grains and low in fruits, vegetables and proteins leads to malnutrition. Similarly, an excessively low fluid intake poses the risk of kidney disorders. Feeding infants and small children exclusively on the diet mixture described above can be life-threatening.

MASSAGE

Touch is probably the most ancient form of healing. Every culture has developed some form of healing massage to facilitate the birthing process, as well as treating other specific conditions. The goal of massage is to regenerate the body and stimulate its self-healing powers. Massage can also release tension and anxiety, making it a holistic therapy which addresses the health of body and mind alike. The full benefit of massage is realized only after repeated treatments.

The various massage techniques are based on distinct philosophies. The Western tradition, based primarily on Swedish massage, is geared to address unhealthy changes in the skin, connective tissue, muscles, tendons, and joints. This tradition includes classical massage (see p. 687), lymph drainage, underwater pressure massage and reflexology (see p. 684).

Massage therapists, physical therapists, and sports injury specialists are required to be board-certified.

The Eastern tradition of massage is based on the belief that the cosmic energy circulating in the body gets blocked when muscles are tense: Massage releases this blockage, enabling the energy to flow freely again. Methods include acupressure and shiatsu (see p. 680). Many hybrid approaches have evolved, such as foot reflexology (see p. 684) and rolfing (see p. 690).

CLASSICAL MASSAGE

Massage involves stimulating the entire organism via nerve endings in the various skin layers and muscles. Sensations of warmth, contact, pressure, pulling, stroking, and pain are transmitted through the nerves; this boosts circulation and regulates the autonomic nervous system as well as muscle tension and organ function, stimulating lymph flow and hormone production.

Techniques

Before you have any massage that's designed as a healing treatment, get a medical checkup. Classical (or Swed-ish) massage involves various maneuvers (see below) that are always performed from the outer areas of the body toward the center. Gentle warm-up exercises are a good idea. Heat treatments are better following the massage than preceding it.

Applications

Massage helps relieve rheumatic pain, back and joint pain, tense muscles, sports injuries, respiratory problems, headaches, high blood pressure, and migraines. It is also effective as part of post-operative rehabilitation. Massage also helps in general relaxation and can improve one's psychological outlook.

Recommendations

Massages should not be given in cases of fever, acute inflammations, ulcers, skin disease, heart attack, atherosclerosis, or tumors, or if there is danger of thrombosis.

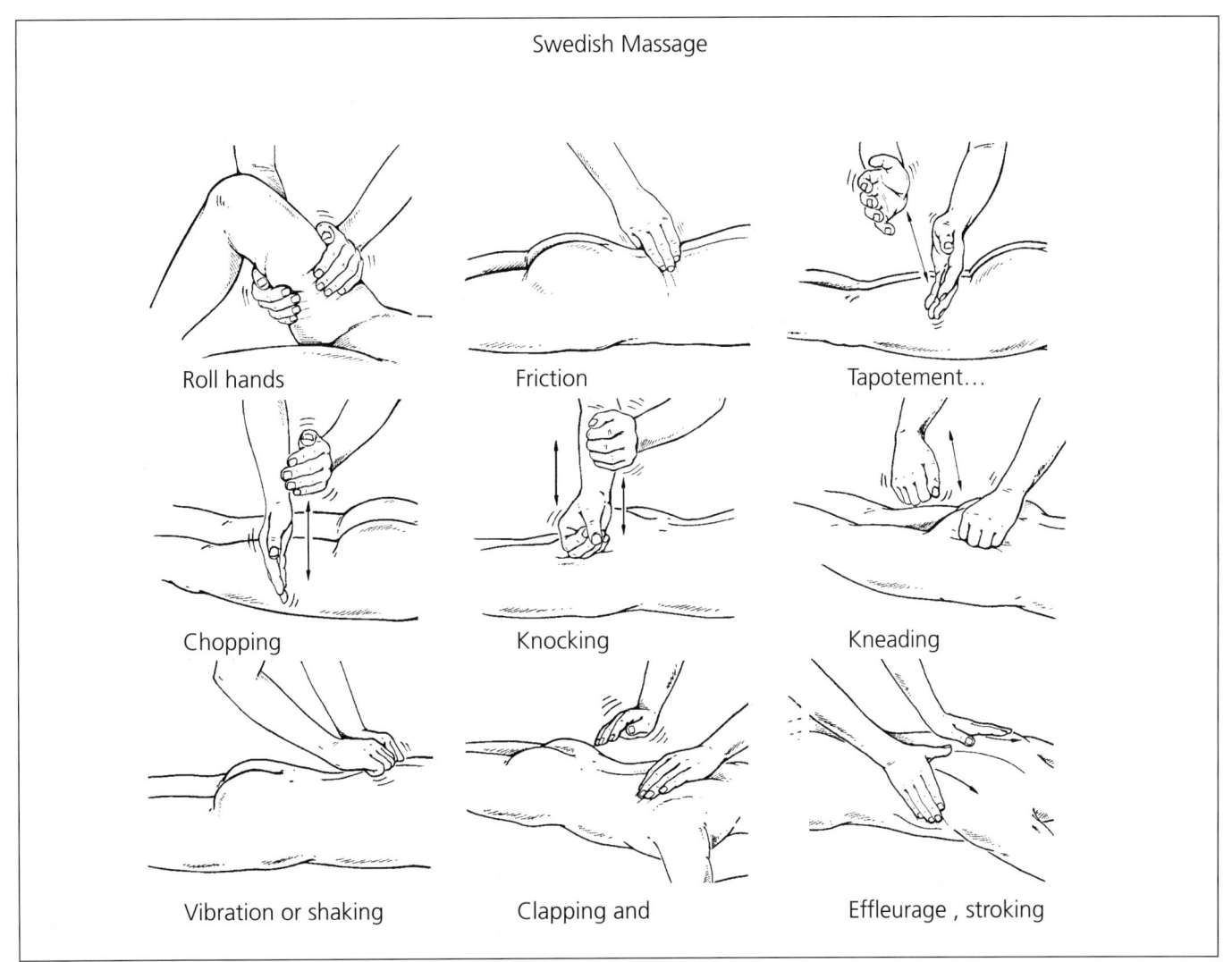

Swedish Massage

Roll hands   Friction   Tapotement...

Chopping   Knocking   Kneading

Vibration or shaking   Clapping and   Effleurage , stroking

Self-massage
Even rubbing your neck when it's tense is a form of self-massage. When consciously applied to your whole body, a massage can be refreshing and relaxing.

How to give yourself a massage
Before you begin, take a few deep breaths. Put a few drops of warm oil in your hands. Sit on the floor with your legs stretched out in front of you. Knead both feet, alternating frequently. Rub ankles, calves, knee joints, and inner and outer thighs. Always rub more firmly in the direction of your heart, less firmly away from the heart. Lie back with knees pulled up. Massage outward from the pubic bone around the hips to the tailbone. Turn on one side: Massage buttocks towards the sacrum, then around hip joint to the belly; repeat for other side. Lie on your back again and massage from the base of the stomach towards the collarbone. Massage the ribs, working out from the center. Knead the muscles of your shoulder in towards the neck. As far as possible, knead shoulder blades, side of throat and neck. Follow up by sitting up and, using both hands, massage from the hips up the sides of your back. Knead hands, forearms, upper arms, armpits and shoulder joints. Put a tennis ball, broomstick, or rolling pin under your back and roll up and down. Finish up with the head: Using both hands, stroke down from forehead to chin, always working from the middle of the face outward. Massage lower jaw and ears with upward strokes. End by gently stroking the scalp.

HEALING WITH HERBS
Plants are our most ancient medicines. Since the early 1900s, science has helped us identify and isolate the active ingredients in various types of plants. Pure herbal essences like digitalis or atropine are part of today's pharmaceutical arsenal. Although the active ingredients of many healing herbs are known, there are still many whose ingredients and effects are unknown or disputed. Sometimes the effect of a particular ingredient differs depending on whether it is isolated from the plant or not; often, the effectiveness of a whole plant is greater than that of its ingredients taken separately.

Herbal remedies are available either in dried form as teas or in ready-to-use commercial products. Approximately 400 different plants are used in the manufacture of these medications, known as phytochemicals (see p. 689).

Techniques
Herb teas are the most commonly used plant-based home remedy. Many people also use commercially prepared herbal products as their first choice of self-help remedies.

Teas
A tea is any water-based extract of dried plant matter—blossoms, leaves, herbs, bark, wood, roots, fruits, or seeds. The manner of preparation depends on which part (or parts) of the plant is used.

Infusions
Most herbal infusions are created by pouring boiling water over a container filled with a prescribed quantity of crushed or powdered plant matter. The solution is left to stand for 5 to 10 minutes before being stirred and strained.

Decoctions
Herbal preparations made with stem, root, or bark must be decocted. A prescribed quantity of the plant matter is put in cold water, brought to a boil and boiled while stirring for five to ten minutes. The decoction is then left to steep before being strained.

Chamomile Tea
— Pour 1 cup of boiling water over 1 tablespoon of dried chamomile flowers.
— Cover, let steep for 10 minutes, then strain.
Sage Tea
Preparation: As for chamomile tea.
Applications: For sore throat. Gargle with tea, every 2 hours, as warm as can be tolerated.
Individual tea recipes are listed under various complaints and illnesses.
Sedating: See Sleep Disorders, 588.
Cough: See Acute Bronchitis, 305.
Stomach: See Nervous Stomach, 386.
Gas: See Irritable Bowel Syndrome, 403.
Constipation: See Constipation, 406.
Bladder and kidney: See Bladder Infection, 418.

Cold infusion
This method works for mucilaginous plants like mallow or linseed. The plant is put in cold water and left to sit for several hours at room temperature before

being strained. This method does not kill bacteria or fungi; if it is necessary to do so, the liquid is boiled briefly before ingestion.

Prepared teas

A wide range of packaged teas is available in pharmacies and grocery stores.

Tea bags: A single tea bag contains a measured amount of plant material for one cup. The quality of such tea may be hard to determine.

Instant teas

Although these are quick to prepare, they can't compare with teas that require steeping. Nutrients and components are lost in the manufacturing process, and additives are mixed in to render the herb into a uniform powder. Granulated teas may contain large amounts (up to 97 percent) of sugar; some products also contain sugar substitutes.

Instant teas made of plant extracts are a better bet: The manufacturing process preserves essential ingredients more effectively, and the final product may contain up to 20 percent of the plant extract. Instant teas easily absorb moisture, resulting in clumping.

Alcohol-based tinctures

Many plants, such as valerian, are extracted using alcohol and then ingested as extracts or tinctures.

Preservation and Storage of Teas

— Shield from light, warmth, and humidity. Light can accelerate chemical processes, and thereby change the quality. The same holds true for warmth. With heat, some of the essential oils can evaporate. Molds and other microorganisms can easily accumulate and grow in a humid environment, decreasing the shelf-life substantially.

— Store teas in tightly sealed containers made of metal, wood, or darkly colored glass. Unstained glass allows too much exposure to light.

Phytochemicals

These are artificial products made with natural plant materials that are extracted, concentrated, dried or somehow processed. The same therapeutic claims cannot be made for them as those made for herbal teas, because the effectiveness of the ingredients may be compromised during production or processing. Before being marketed as medicines, phytochemicals must undergo clinical trials to prove their effectiveness as well as establishing any side effects.

General rules for using teas

Depending on how much you use and for how long, even harmless, beneficial herbs can cause side effects.

— Teas taken for medicinal purposes should not be used for long periods of time; excessive and long-term use can become toxic.

— When using tea for medicinal purposes, pay as much attention to dosage, instructions, and duration of treatment as you would with any other medicine.

— Teas with medicinal properties usually consist of one or two principal herbs (the "active ingredients") with an additional herb or two added to improve aroma and taste.

— Avoid mixtures containing 20 or more herbs. These are less effective.

— When experimenting, exercise caution. Keep in mind that herbs from unfamiliar cultures may lack sufficient documentation of effectiveness and side effects.

Applications

Herbal remedies are especially good for treating general malaise and minor, temporary illnesses. They supplement the treatment of chronic, psychosomatic, and functional disorders. They can cut back on medication use or minimize unavoidable side effects.

Recommendations

— Some plants should not be taken during pregnancy; others should be used only with great caution.

— Long-term regular use of herbal laxatives can contribute to cancer of the large intestine.

— Experiments using Indian and Mexican valerian caused genetic changes in laboratory animals; any similar effect on humans has not been determined.

— Plants can trigger allergies. Symptoms may consist of a skin rash that erupts and disappears quickly, or becomes chronic. After an initial reaction to pollen, be prepared for similar reactions, or cross-reactions. Just breathing the pollen of certain plants can trigger asthma attacks.

PHYSIOTHERAPY

Physiotherapy comes under the heading of "natural healing processes" along with other forms of treatment: Massage, regulated exercise, water, light, heat, and electricity. Physical treatments stimulate the body's metabolic processes and regulating systems, and possibly prevent disease. Most physical techniques work at skin level; electrotherapy penetrates more deeply. Notwithstanding, even the internal organs can be treated with physiotherapy (see Reflex Zone Therapies, below).

REFLEX ZONE MASSAGE

The best-known reflex zone massage is connective tissue massage. It focuses on sensitive areas in the subcutaneous tissue of the body to affect disorders of the internal organs.

Techniques

Therapists detect tense areas with their fingertips and work them over using specific techniques.

In muscle reflex zone massage, the muscles themselves are also massaged.

Periosteal massage follows the reflex connections between the organs and the fibrous membrane covering the skeletal system. Using the knuckles, the therapist applies pressure lasting several minutes.

Applications

Connective tissue massage can alleviate functional disorders of internal organs such as heart, stomach, and abdomen. It can also help gastritis, menstrual disorders, autonomic disorders, vein problems, and structural changes of the connective tissue. Periosteal massage eases pain caused by arthritis and back problems.

Recommendations

Only certified specialists should perform this sort of massage. It can be very painful, and often causes reactions such as sweating, heart arrhythmia, diarrhea, and induced menstruation.

Do not use in case of acute inflammations, osteoporosis, tumors, psychosis, pregnancy, or following a heart attack.

REFLEX ZONE THERAPIES

These treatments are based on the discovery that diseased organs cause pain and changes in very clearly delineated subcutaneous areas known as Head's zones. Treating or stimulating Head's zones can affect the internal organs via nerve pathways.

This can be achieved through heat and cold treatments, electrotherapy and, to some extent, neural therapy, acupuncture and similar methods.

Special reflex zone massages have been developed for specific problems; these include connective tissue massage, muscle reflexology, and periosteal massage.

ROLFING

This form of deep-tissue massage restores shortened or pulled tendons and muscles to their original shape, thus relieving pain.

Techniques

Using elbow or knuckles, intense pressure is placed on specific points of the connective tissue and on any tissue surrounding muscle. A standard course of treatment is 10 hour-long sessions that can be very painful and release strong emotions and memories.

Applications

Rolfing claims to improve both physical bearing and morale; however, there is no evidence of its efficacy.

Recommendations

Rolfing is very painful and should not be employed in the event of psychological disorders. This form of treatment is not scientifically recognized.

SAUNAS

Saunas are air-based heat treatments. In the dry, hot

(around 200°F) air, the body starts to sweat. When the humidity level inside the sauna is raised, the body sweats profusely. This is followed by a sudden immersion in cold water. If you're healthy, the dramatic change between hot and cold provides an excellent boost to the circulation.

Techniques

The length of sauna treatments depends on individual tolerance: In general, 8 to 10 minutes is enough. After about 5 minutes, pour water onto the stones or heat source (you can add essential plant oils, but avoid any that contain alcohol); using a towel, disperse the steam evenly. Follow up with a cold shower or quick swim, being sure to get your head wet. Then lie down and wrap yourself in a blanket.

After half an hour, the process can be repeated, up to two more times. The steam part of the process doesn't need to be repeated, however.

Applications

Regular saunas can build strength, improve resistance to colds, boost circulation and ease sciatica, rheumatic, and menstrual pain. Saunas are relaxing, as long as you devote enough time to doing them properly (2 to 3 hours, once or twice weekly).

Those in good physical condition—including small children, if they feel comfortable—can take several saunas a week without concern.

Recommendations

— Don't eat right before a sauna.
— Leave the sauna immediately if you don't feel well.
— Only if you are in top physical condition should you cool off by plunging into cold water.
— If you're a novice, break yourself in gradually.

Saunas do not promote weight loss. Replenish the water you lose through perspiration by drinking plenty of water or fruit juice after the sauna.

Saunas are off limits in case of acute inflammatory diseases, colds, and cardiovascular illnesses. When in doubt, ask your doctor.

CRANIOSACRAL THERAPY

This unconventional method, which flies in the face of medical opinion, holds that the seams of the skull are flexible rather than fixed, and that pulsing fluid from the brain connects the spine to the sacrum. A disorder in the head area can thus give rise to various diseases throughout the body.

Techniques

Treatment involves gently manipulating the plates of the skull, thus benefiting the entire spinal column and any posture-related problems.

Applications

Craniosacral therapy is purported to correct postural, hip, and spinal problems, as well as jaw misalignments and other diseases. However, there is as yet no proof of its effectiveness.

TRANSCUTANEOUS ELECTRIC NERVE STIMULATION (TENS)

Nerves are electrically stimulated through the skin to help alleviate chronic pain.

Techniques

Electrodes are placed over painful body areas. The device can be a portable one, that the patient can apply and control when pain is present. It should be used at least for a half an hour at a time.

Applications

TENS works best for various neuralgias, and for phantom pains experienced after a limb amputation.

Recommendations

Do not use if a pacemaker is present. Occasionally an allergic reaction can occur to the electrode gel.

HEAT BATHS

This treatment involves artificially inducing a fever to jump-start the metabolism and stimulate the immune and hormonal systems.

Techniques

The patient lies in body-temperature water; hot water is added, gradually raising the temperature to 109°F. *Warning:* Pulse and temperature must be checked every 5 minutes. Following the heat bath, a 1- to 2-hour rest period is mandatory.

Applications

This treatment is used against certain types of rheumatism, asthma, ulcerative colitis, and cancer.

Recommendations

This treatment is very taxing to the cardiovascular system, and should only be done under professional supervision.

HEAT TREATMENTS

Heat treatments include sunlight (see Light Therapy, p. 685), infrared rays, ultrasound, heat packs, saunas, steam baths, and heat baths.

FOOT BATHS, WARM AND WARM/COLD

Techniques

Warm foot bath: Stand in knee-deep water. Water temperature should be about 100°F; to enhance the effect, add hot water to raise temperature above 103°F. The bath should last no longer than 15 minutes.

Alternating warm and cold: Place legs into warm water for about 5 minutes; then plunge into cold water for 10 seconds. Repeat 5 to 10 times, finishing with cold water.

Applications

Warm foot baths stimulate circulation and help with bladder problems and colds. They can be done every night to ease backaches and cold feet. Be sure to keep water temperature moderate rather than hot.

Alternating warm and cold baths stimulates circulation and helps combat circulatory problems and low blood pressure.

HYDROTHERAPY

Because it transmits heat and cold directly through the skin, water is good for all sorts of stimulative therapy: Arm baths, foot or full baths, stepping water, cold infusions, or alternating baths. It helps build resistance to cold and helps regulate circulation and body temperature.

TREADING (STEPPING) IN WATER, COLD FOOT BATHS

Treading (stepping) water is essential to several forms of hydrotherapy and is easy to do in a bathtub, or even with two pails of water.

Techniques

Stand in cold (around 60°F) water to midcalf; walk like a stork, alternately raising each leg out of the water, for up to 3 minutes. Dry your legs gently; then jump, run or walk until feet are warm again.

Applications

This treatment is beneficial in treating headaches, low blood pressure, sluggish digestion, and sleep disorders. People who are tired, stressed, or grouchy on waking should incorporate a cold foot bath into their morning routine.

Recommendations

Have a cold foot bath only when your feet are warm: People with chronically cold feet should start off with alternating hot and cold foot baths (see above).

COMPRESSES

Compresses and wraps are tried-and-true home remedies for altering body temperature and improving circulation.

Techniques

Cold compresses: Place on the calves, feet, or torso to reduce fever, promote sleep and help with chronic digestive issues such as gallbladder and liver problems and bloating.

Warm compresses: These can ease the symptoms and pain of chronic diseases like arthritis, stomachaches, nervous stomach (see p. 386), irritable bowel (see p. 403), and kidney and bladder disease.

Recommendations

Use cold compresses only when the patient is feeling warm; remove immediately if shivering ensues.

Herbal essences may cause allergic reactions in some individuals.

Compresses

— Soak a linen cloth in water (40° to 50°F for cold compresses and 120° F for warm). Wring out and apply to affected body part.

— Cover the linen cloth with a flannel cloth and secure it (for the feet, use cotton socks instead of the two cloths).

— For a full-body compress, use a wet sheet, then wool blankets to wrap up the patient. Use a rubber pad to protect the bed.

— Cover patient well and protect from drafts.

— Cold compresses can be left on for about 2 hours before removing; they can also be left on the body until they dry.

— Warm compresses can be kept warm longer by applying hot-water bottles. Their effectiveness can be enhanced by adding herbal essences.

Relaxation

What's good for the body is good for the soul, and vice versa. For an active, well-balanced life, the rhythm between tension and relaxation is important. Nervous tension can cramp parts of the body, causing a physical imbalance which in turn affects the mood. If pressures persist or heighten, resulting health complaints may range from headaches, high blood pressure, heart ailments, skin problems, and backaches all the way to pain throughout the entire body (see Health and Well-Being, p. 182).

Sources of chronic stress may include relationships, personality issues, problems on the job, or simply the daily grind.

TAKE A BREAK

In stressful situations, taking a short break and breathing deeply several times are a simple way to protect yourself from overload. Small breaks throughout the day can be very enlivening. A brief chat totally unrelated to the situation at hand, or a few moments of physical activity, can help tune out stress.

Physical and psychological tension may pass if you can lie down with your feet up and listen to music for a little while, do some stretches (see Stretching, p. 765), or take a 15-minute nap. Find what works best for you. Your most effective form of relaxation might be taking a walk, or just hanging out and not filling every minute of the day with productive activity.

Active relaxation involves more than simply doing nothing, however. Initiating your own effective form of relaxation requires activity on your part.

THE IMPORTANCE OF BREATHING

When we are tense, our breathing is shallow. As a result, our circulation carries less oxygen to the brain, which can lead to headaches, difficulty concentrating, fatigue, nervousness, or sleep disturbances. Individual or group breathwork or breathing therapy can greatly improve breathing, as can biofeedback (p. 695); a few simple breathing and relaxation exercises can help as well.

Consciously take deep breaths, exhaling slowly while letting your jaw drop and making a sound. Take every opportunity to sing. If you can let out a scream, the relaxation effect will be even greater. Inside a closed car is an appropriate place for screaming, especially if you get angry while driving.

BREATHING EXERCISES

Sit comfortably in a chair, feet flat on the ground, placing backs of hands on knees.

Close your eyes. Breathe in deeply through the nose—first into the stomach, then into the chest, slowly arching the body. Count to four while doing this.

Hold your breath and continue counting, to six.

Continue counting to eight while slowly exhaling through your open mouth.

Release the air from the stomach first, then the chest. Let the lower jaw hang loosely.

Repeat five times and then relax the face: While exhaling, let head sink onto chest and let facial muscles hang loosely.

MUSIC AND DANCE

Sound and music have a powerful influence on the body and soul: They can alter pulse rates, breathing, and metabolism and secretion rates, which in turn can stimulate brain activity and trigger the release of feelings.

From marches to reggae, music with a strong rhythm is stimulating and enlivening; the effect is strengthened by dancing to the beat.

Tension and pain are alleviated by letting soft, flowing violin or piano music soothe the body while lying in a relaxed position.

Actively playing music or dancing in group or individual sessions can contribute to the healing of mental and psychological problems in conjunction with psychotherapy.

RELAXATION METHODS

If you find it hard to create relaxing situations or to keep to a daily exercise routine and you already suffer from tension, consider working with a trainer—alone or in a group—to learn a particular relaxation technique. It will then be easier to follow through on your own.

An easy way to relax is as follows: Sit with legs apart, feet splayed, elbows on thighs, and head hanging down. Lying stretched out on your back with arms at your sides is just as good. Gentle rhythmic music can be very helpful.

Be aware of the following:
— Relaxation methods are harder to learn when you are in a crisis, sick, or going through a stressful period.
— To learn any method, you must be committed to set aside time for simple daily exercises. Do this someplace you won't be disturbed.
— It can take anywhere from a few weeks to months to master a new technique; after that it's like riding a bike or playing tennis. Once you have learned a technique you will not forget it, although you might forget some individual exercises.
— Slow relaxation can even make some medications (such as those for high blood pressure) unnecessary. At some point while you're learning the technique, have your doctor check your physical symptoms.

Relaxation calls for stepping outside daily life for a time, not escaping from it. Quite the contrary: You'll gradually become more aware of yourself and your environment, your experience of reality will be enhanced, and your appreciation of being alive will intensify, resulting in a sense of well-being.

Learning Relaxation Methods Makes Sense in Cases of
— Psychological rigidity, possibly resulting in insomnia, poor appetite, autonomic nervous disorders, muscle tension, agitation, heart palpitations
— Psychosomatic illnesses such as stomach and duodenal ulcers, asthma, neurodermatitis, migraines,

Stay Fit and Relaxed All Day Long
The following sequence of exercises, performed daily, will keep you fit and relaxed—and they're fun. Note: They are designed for those in good physical condition.

Standing straight
Stand with feet slightly apart. Stretch tall with knees bent, back straight, neck long. Let your arms and jaw hang loose. Imagine you're suspended from a string attached to the top of your head.

Shaking out
Imagine the string is loosened a bit; shake your feet, legs, hips, waist, shoulders, arms and hands, neck and head one after the other. Straighten up again; repeat.

Stretching
Breathe in deeply, stand on tiptoes and stretch arms and fingers as far as possible—reach for the stars. Slowly let your arms drop. Repeat three times.

Bending
With bent knees, bend from the waist to wherever feels comfortable; let your head and arms hang loosely. Inhale through your mouth; slowly exhale—lowering your hands to your feet. Inhale and exhale three times. Don't sway back and forth.

Running in place
Run in place 200 steps, raising knees (and, alternately, heels) as high as possible. Increase over time to 400 steps. Finish up by shaking out your limbs.

Grounding
Lie relaxed on your back. Close your eyes for a while; then open them, consciously notice your surroundings, and finally stand up.
See also Physical Activity and Sports, p. 762.

polyarthritis, functional neurosis with cardiac symptoms, painful menstruation
— After injuries
— Relationship problems, work conflicts, separation anxiety

If psychotherapy is necessary, use relaxation methods only to supplement treatment.

Learning Relaxation Methods Doesn't Make Sense If
— You're not committed to changing. Relaxation only works when you are committed.

—You don't pay attention to pain and take it seriously, or don't recognize it as a sign of an emotional process. Full awareness is critically important during relaxation.

—You suffer from deep anxiety, profound depression, self-esteem problems, hypochondria, or suicidal tendencies.

—You are a habitual substance abuser and are not in an institutional setting.

How to choose the method that's right for you

Finding a method that's best for you calls for knowing yourself very well. The following list divides people by behavior, but most people don't fit into just one category. Trust your instincts when trying out a new technique. Don't hesitate to change instructors; and don't give up after the first time.

— Do you like rules and don't feel hampered by them? Try methods with fixed protocols such as tai chi and chi gong (see p. 696).

— Do you feel hampered by rules and prefer to do things your own way? Try biofeedback (see below).

— Do you dislike being active, and would you prefer to delegate control to the therapist? Try massage (see p. 686).

— Are you quietly rebellious, independent-minded, and fond of taking responsibility? Try meditation and yoga (see below).

Breathing exercises (see p. 693) are vital and form part of all other methods.

Risks of Relaxation Methods

— Relaxation can be used as a form of distraction and escapism; used in this way, it can paralyze individual initiative. If you find yourself using relaxation this way, try playing a sport with other partner(s).

— Relaxation can be used to mask the symptoms of an unhappy relationship, which is why it's important beforehand to be clear about what you're releasing.

Choosing a Method

Not every relaxation method is appropriate for every person. Use the list above to find the method that's right for you.

Choosing a Trainer

The relationship between trainer and trainee must be harmonious—both parties need to be able to work together. Serious therapists regularly work with a supervisor to monitor their work and resolve any issues before they become problems. Don't hesitate to ask your trainer whether he or she does this or not.

Don't give up if your first choice was a flop. Try again at least once. Ask for information and referrals from health maintenance organizations, mental health centers, counselors, adult education programs.

Costs

Costs are usually high and generally not covered by insurance; check first.

BIOFEEDBACK

This method teaches you to work with your body by using biological signals to monitor your progress and let you know how you're doing. Sensors attached to the skin monitor your breathing, blood pressure, brain waves, skin resistance, heart rate, muscle tension, and body temperature. The results appear as a graph on a screen or as audible beeps so you can observe any and all changes. For example, by making a fist, then relaxing the fingers and noting the variations on the screen or in the beeps, you get direct feedback on your actions and can quickly learn both to tense up and relax consciously. Body functions that are usually unconscious can be affected in the same way.

Biofeedback can help with nervousness, anxiety, sleep disorders, asthma, migraines, high blood pressure, cardiovascular disorders, tension and bruxism (teeth-grinding).

Training: Biofeedback is taught in a clinical setting.

YOGA

"Yoga is balance in all things," according to Hindu philosophy. One characteristic of this ancient tradition is that all exercises are done slowly, concertedly and in synchrony with the breath, improving breathing, calming the autonomic system and easing tension. It benefits psychosomatic disorders and asthma.

It is important to practice yoga regularly, fully and consciously stretching the different body parts while breathing deeply—the extreme acrobatics are less important. The goal of each position is to concentrate and center your mind, which leads to inner harmony and calm.

Training: Get a medical checkup before you start any

yoga program. Take instruction only from an experienced yoga practitioner.

Practice: Do yoga daily, on your own.

MEDITATION

Meditation has traditionally been practiced in a religious context, with specialized forms dating as far back as six thousand years in India. It also appeared later in such traditions as Judaism, Buddhism, Islam, and Christianity. In meditation, the breath becomes the medium between body and soul.

There are many different meditation techniques. The optimal technique involves sitting upright for about 15 minutes, in the lotus position: Legs crossed and hands either folded in front of the stomach or palms down on knees, thumb and index finger touching.

Concentrate on your breathing and repeat your mantra—a combination of sounds, a poem, or an image. The effect may be intensified with the sound of noninvasive music or flowing water, or the use of candlelight. Meditation can alleviate nervous tension, sleeplessness, and psychosomatic problems.

Training: Learn meditation from a teacher, either individually or in a group. Be aware that some schools of meditation, such as Transcendental Meditation, involve joining a religious sect.

Practice: On an individual basis.

CHI GONG AND TAI CHI

Chi gong is a form of Chinese meditation several thousand years old. Learned in stages, it is a fluid, tranquil sequence of about 16 postures, symbolizing various animals, which unfolds almost like a dance. The requisite concentration has a calming effect and increases flexibility. Underlying chi gong are the concepts of yin and yang balance and the flow of life energy through the body. Like chi gong, the 2,000-year-old practice of tai chi ("shadow-boxing") is based on the tension between yin and yang: The exercises represent the stylized battles of imaginary foes.

In modern China, tai chi is practiced regularly in factories to boost productivity.

Both techniques are good for reducing tension and preventing psychosomatic disorders.

Training: Both techniques are learned in a group setting.

Practice: On an individual basis, for about 20 minutes daily.

COUNSELING AND PSYCHOTHERAPY

A candid, meaningful conversation with your doctor may well contain the basic elements of psychotherapy: Attentive listening on the doctor's part, and honest sharing of problems and concerns on your part. On the other hand, you might feel more comfortable seeing a professional counselor or therapist to help you deal with issues and crises.

In addition to professional psychotherapists, self-proclaimed psychic healers abound, but all such claims should be carefully scrutinized. The dangers of dubious gurus, healers, and cult leaders are often underestimated: Dabbling in psychology with a poorly trained practitioner can result in profound emotional crises, extreme dependency, and ultimately the disintegration of daily life. The following overview of scientifically grounded therapies should help you separate the wheat from the chaff.

Objectives

Psychotherapists are generally attentive observers and listeners. They present you with opportunities to understand your problems, learn from them, and perceive yourself differently. Any psychotherapeutic methodology of worth will not dispense easy catch-all answers to life's questions; instead, it will endeavor to assist each client in finding his or her own path to health and emotional balance. Psychotherapy can help you overcome your problems, but only with your active participation.

Ideally, psychotherapy works as a mirror in which you identify and acknowledge your problems, discover how they evolved, and develop opportunities for change. A successful course of therapy depends on several critical factors.

— Before initiating therapy, establish how long the process will take and the number of hours involved; then adhere to that agreement.

— After about 10 sessions, you will hopefully have the feeling that this therapist and his or her approach are helping. If this is not the case, you should both decide whether it is time to consider another type of therapy.

— The therapy should focus not simply on your weaknesses, but also on recognizing and mobilizing all your resources and strengths to address your problems.

— The therapy should be appropriate for the issues it's addressing: Marital issues are best worked on in couples therapy, problems dealing with others in group therapy.

— In addition to helping you develop problem-solving strategies, the therapy should encourage you to apply them. The more active your role in changing your awareness and behaviors, the more supportive therapy can be.

— When shopping around for particular therapeutic approaches, don't agonize over which approach is the "right" one. The one that will work best for you is the one that appeals to you, makes sense, and sheds light on the issues you're dealing with.

COUNSELING

Churches, community mental-health organizations, social service institutions, and private counseling centers are equipped to offer compassionate care to people seeking help with problems involving family issues, marriage problems, conflict resolution, and crisis intervention.

Most counselors, including social workers, psychologists, doctors, therapists, and occasionally lawyers or theologians, have specialized training in psychotherapy.

A person is most likely to seek counseling when unable to cope alone:

— Following a separation, divorce, death of a partner, or loss of a child

— When making decisions that call for more input, such as a pregnancy, marriage crisis, or other family upheaval

— with learning and behavioral problems in children

— In times of isolation, loneliness, or upheaval

— In situations of acute emotional crisis, such as considering quitting a job, leaving school, running away from home, or after attempting to commit suicide

— In cases of performance anxiety before a test, or dealing with recurring patterns of failure or a recurring illness

Professional intervention can prevent crises from escalating or problems from becoming overwhelming to the point of breakdown. In a counseling session, you will first attempt to define your problem and the best way to deal with it. If therapy is advisable, the counselor can help you explore which type of therapy is appropriate. Planning this strategy may be a simple procedure that can be accomplished at one session or take up to ten sessions.

For extreme situations, crisis hotlines operate 24 hours a day.

Individual and Group Therapy

All psychotherapeutic procedures, with the exception of family therapy, can take place in either individual or group settings. In individual therapy, problems are analyzed, discussed and put in perspective with the therapist one-on-one.

Group therapy has the advantage that other participants can give voice to thoughts, feelings, opinions, desires, conflicts, or fantasies that might emerge only later, if at all, in individual therapy. This can be confrontational and challenging, but courage is contagious. In a group you can learn from others how to interact with others.

Many proven behavioral techniques are taught in groups, for example autogenic training for relaxation, quit-smoking programs, or pain management techniques.

Many psychoanalysts are trained in group as well as individual therapy; most counseling centers offer both.

Usually, a group therapy session involves 6 to 10 participants of both genders and lasts about 90 to 100 minutes.

Couples and Family Therapy

Couples therapy and family therapy are different from each other, and also differ from other approaches. Both incorporate various elements from the following techniques, discussed elsewhere in these pages:
— Conflict-centered Techniques, p. 699
— Practice-oriented Techniques, p. 700
— Experience-oriented Techniques, p. 701

Couples therapy and family therapy are both based on the notion that problems do not arise in isolation, but in the context of a complex interpersonal dynamic.

In relationships involving two or more people, distinct patterns of behavior emerge and tend to repeat endlessly until they are short-circuited. The same irritants always trigger disagreements, and certain issues consistently cause bickering, tears, shouting, or violence. One objective of marriage and family therapy is to establish the specific elements that trigger such disputes, and discover their underlying causes.

Marriage and family therapy is a good choice if you are dealing with
— School and behavioral problems in children. Parents and environment play a big role in nearly all learning and developmental problems, disorders such as bed-wetting, aggression, or social alienation. The child is acting out an imbalance in the family system.
— Problems in a marriage or relationship that always end up at the same seemingly unresolvable point, perhaps including sexual incompatibility or an impending separation.

Many counseling centers and individual therapists offer couples counseling or family therapy. The weekly sessions, averaging between 10 to 20, can provide relief and new solutions.

Women's Counseling and Therapy

Many communities have a women's health center, where professionals (psychologists, physicians, and social workers) focus specifically on women's role in the workplace and the home.

The focus of these centers, which tend to follow general, basic psychotherapeutic procedures, is on empowering women and helping them rediscover their own desires and needs. Women are supported in making their own decisions on how to live their lives.

Workshops and Training Groups

There is a huge market in so-called experience-oriented therapies, including rebirthing, and transactional analysis.

Workshops usually take place several weeks or months apart, with changing groups of participants spending several days together at a time. When considering participation in this sort of workshop, remember that the trainers or workshop leaders may have more training in marketing techniques than psychology.

One indication of the quality of a workshop is whether trainers meet with prospective participants beforehand. Serious practitioners are alert to the makeup of the group and are interested in ensuring that participants are psychologically stable.

People who are anxious, shy, sick, or in crisis should not be taken in by "one size fits all" approaches. Their emotional needs can easily get lost in a crowd, leading to emotional breakdowns or crises that are hard to resolve.

PSYCHOTHERAPY

The most important motivation for undergoing psychotherapy is the experience of psychological pain. This pain may be so strong that it manifests as a lack of desire or ability to go on living. This happens most often in people who have reached an impasse and are simply unable to cope any longer—perhaps because they repeatedly deal with difficult situations without support, or because they are trapped in the same agonizing daily patterns and relationships.

You Should Consider Psychotherapy if:

If something in your life is making you extremely unhappy and isn't serving your needs, that's a sound reason to seek therapy. Another good reason is a strong desire to change something or approach it differently. A fundamental motivation like this makes it more likely that you'll commit to the long, hard work psychotherapy often requires.

You should also consider therapy if someone in your family is obviously going through great psychological difficulties, even though this may seem to have nothing to do with you. A common example of such a situation is found in families with children with behavioral disorders. Often these children are acting out the psychological problems of their parents, who are either unaware or in denial.

You Need Psychotherapy if:

If you have a tic or a phobia, it may be serious enough to require treatment. On the other hand, countless people manage to live with anxieties, neuroses, and tics without resorting to professional help.

The need for psychotherapy can usually be established if any of the following conditions are present, either in your estimation or that of your family members:

— A particular behavior consistently disrupts your daily life. Examples include obsessive neatness, cleanliness, repetitiveness, or compulsive washing (see Neurotic Behavior, p. 195).

— Certain phobias make your daily life impossible. If you feel threatened in a crowded environment, you're unlikely to be able to carry out simple tasks like shopping or taking public transportation (see Phobias, p. 195).

— Certain behaviors on the job or in relationships consistently result in the same dead end, such as always getting the short end of the stick professionally or always being the one in a relationship to give in.

—You're trapped in the same behavior or relationship pattern, noting after the tenth relationship breakup that the same issues are always at the root of the problem.

— Psychosomatic problems manifest frequently, or a disease becomes chronic (see Health and Well-Being, p. 182).

The Psychotherapeutic Relationship

Your relationship with the therapist should be trusting and open. However, the therapist should always remain disinterested, neutral, and separated from the rest of your life and relationships. It is an ethical lapse for a psychotherapist to establish a familiar, intimate, or friendly rapport with a client. The most important reason for this is that only someone with no personal relationship to you can function completely independently of your expectations and demands.

There are other advantages as well:

— Regardless of how often you tell the therapist something, or in what detail, a professional will continue to give the matter full attention long after others would have stopped listening—because repetition means a problem is still unresolved.

— There is no danger that personal thoughts and feelings might get back to family and friends.

— It's often easier to share fantasies or fears with a therapist than with family or friends; therapy can be a refuge where you know you won't face embarrassment, ridicule, dirty looks, or other types of flak.

— Good therapists have no expectations of their clients—even after months or years—beyond getting paid for their professional services.

CONFLICT-CENTERED TECHNIQUES

Conflict-centered techniques evolved from psychoanalysis. They focus on unconscious conflicts, which are revisited and reexperienced in the course of therapy. The therapist tries to help by interpreting the unresolved conflicts.

Psychoanalytic Techniques

Psychoanalysis is based on the notion that each of us, because of character and experience, has basic idiosyncrasies and mechanisms that determine our relationships with others. Often inherent in these dynamics are unconscious conflicts.

An example of this is when a person consistently yet unconsciously provokes others to hurt them as they were hurt as children. Sooner or later, the client will try to recreate this pattern even in the psychoanalytic relationship. This mechanism—reliving childhood experiences, for example—is the centerpiece of analysis and its great promise.

Unconscious conflict can be brought to the level of consciousness through work with the analyst. For example, the therapist will reject any role the client tries to project or impose, such as that of the omnipotent father. Instead, the therapist tries to help the client recognize that by investing responsibility and power in others, he or she is establishing the patterns and relationships of dependency. Once the client recognizes and processes this, the conflict can be resolved.

Procedure and Timeframe

In classic psychoanalysis, the client reclines on a couch and the analyst sits to the side or behind, out of view. Sessions last 50 minutes and take place three to five times a week. Some health insurance plans cover a certain number of sessions.

In addition to the classic form, other versions of psychoanalysis have evolved in which analyst and client sit facing one another. They are known variously as
— Analytic psychotherapy
— Dynamic psychotherapy

These sessions usually take place once or twice a week and can conclude after 15 to 30 sessions or more. They are as effective as classic psychoanalysis.

Conversational Psychotherapy

This term is misleading, since nearly all therapy involves conversation. However, this method evolved independently and is highly effective.

In conversational psychotherapy, the focus is on the client's conscious, acknowledged problems. There is less emphasis on the past and more on the here and now. The therapist addresses the issues with honesty, compassion, perceptiveness, and warmth, attempting to comprehend the client's reality, worldview, sensibilities, and experiences. The following factors are especially important:
— Therapist and client work together to define the client's self-image and work out problems.
— The therapist observes and monitors not only what is said, but also body language and methods of verbal expression, and then uses these perceptions to mirror the client back to him or herself. With such compassionate and nonjudgmental guidance, the client is better able to comprehend, think through and change his or her subjective reality.

The objective of this therapy is expanded self-awareness and self-acceptance. In this sense, its goal is similar to that of psychoanalysis: What is most important is the transformation of individual reality and experience, and the recognition of conflicts rather than focusing on symptoms.

Procedure and Timeframe

Sessions are usually held once a week and last about 1 hour. The average length of therapy is about 20 hours, which can be prolonged if necessary.

PRACTICE-ORIENTED TECHNIQUES

Practice-oriented techniques like behavior therapy, cognitive therapy or confrontational therapy are premised on behaviorism. With special exercises, a disorder is affected through conscious behavioral modification.

In such approaches, early childhood and the unconscious play only a minor role; the focus is on concrete problems and overcoming them in actual life situations.

Behavior Therapy

Behavior therapy tries to analyze dysfunctional or aberrant behavior as closely as possible while also respecting the circumstances. The focus is primarily on the conditions and circumstances that give rise to a specific behavior and the mechanisms that perpetuate it.

A disorder, compulsion, or phobia (see p. 195) is not considered in isolation; self-perception, feelings and internal conflicts are taken into account. Rather than

concentrating on discovering the conflict, emphasis is placed on learning or unlearning behaviors
— The emphasis is on changing views, expectations and attitudes (e.g., breaking down anxieties).
— Current problems can often be solved quickly, or lost capacities regained through self-confidence training.
— Problem-solving can take the form of role-playing, learning techniques to enhance self-control or practicing taking charge of one's life.

Procedure and Timeframe
Behavior therapy always calls for high client involvement. Regardless of the issue—from quitting smoking to addressing eating disorders—the principle of self-control must be learned. This can be accomplished in a few sessions. More serious problems call for longer-term therapy.

SUGGESTIVE TECHNIQUES
While conflict-based therapies focus on bringing buried aspects of our personalities into the light of conscious scrutiny, the suggestive therapies seem to do just the opposite: They work beneath the surface and leave things buried in the subconscious. Many of these therapies purport to offer miracle cures, and should be examined very critically. They are often quite expensive, can wreak havoc, and are not very successful. Only hypnosis has been confirmed as effective when practiced by trained physicians, and is enjoying newfound respect.

Hypnosis
In hypnosis, the practitioner attempts to influence disorders or problems until they are resolved. The technique used in hypnosis is based on relaxation rather than active influence. In a relaxed state, the subject is more open to suggestions and new information that can lead to new behaviors and experiences.
— With a statement such as the hackneyed "You are getting very sleepy," the client is led into a trance-like state somewhere between sleep and conscious wakefulness.
— In this state the client can still hear and understand the therapist, who communicates instructions aimed at calming, stabilizing, or altering the client's behavior.

Hypnosis can actually rid some people of their symptoms completely: For example, it can resolve dental phobias. Frequently, however, the effect wears off after a short time. Not all people are good candidates for hypnosis.

Procedure and Time Frame
Nearly always, the client lies on a couch. At the beginning of treatment, about 6 hours are spent on learning how to achieve a trancelike state; which is spread out over several days. Usually it is only after this phase that the client can go into a trance deep enough to address problems or disorders.

Average length of treatment is between 10 and 40 hours.

EXPERIENCE-ORIENTED TECHNIQUES
Experience-oriented techniques are based on the idea that intense emotional experiences can have compelling curative effects.

These approaches include music therapy, poetry therapy, and gestalt therapy as well as various types of body therapy. They are well represented in institutional psychotherapy and in outpatient therapy in conjunction with other techniques. Exactly how they work is not yet clear.

Gestalt Therapy
This is the most widely employed experience-oriented technique. The focus is on the immediate experiencing of the here and now. All problems are seen in terms of currently experienced feelings or perceptions. Clients are encouraged to confront negative as well as positive impulses and live them out fully, making it possible to see their own behavior in a new light.

Gestalt therapy is not simply a therapeutic procedure; it's also a life philosophy. A basic tenet of gestalt therapy holds that change is possible only when you accept yourself as you are.
— Much attention is given to nonverbal behavior.
— Impressions, feelings, dreams, sensations, or experiences are acted out or staged using various techniques.
— The goal is to intensify the experience as much as possible so that previously rejected behaviors can now be accepted, marking the first step to change.

Procedure and Timeframe

Fantasy work, role-playing, and a specific type of dialogue all promote understanding and ownership of feelings and desires. There is no fixed duration of therapy. Therapy usually takes place in group, seminar, or workshop settings.

CHOOSING A THERAPY

Academics within the various disciplines of psychotherapy still debate which approach is best for which personality and disorder. An experienced specialist can usually gauge what approach would work best for someone based on a conversation with the individual in question.

If you are seeking professional help, ask yourself:

— Do I need immediate intervention, or can I wait a while? (See Counseling, p. 697)

— Do I need comprehensive therapy, or is my problem pretty narrowly defined?

— How much time do I want to spend on therapy? How many hours a week am I willing to spend working on my own issues?

— How much money do I want to spend on therapy?

— Do I need to be in a residential institutional setting, or can I get treatment on an outpatient basis?

Choosing a therapist

The choice of a therapist is often more important than the choice of therapy: Even the best procedure will probably be unsuccessful if the client/therapist relationship is not a trusting one.

— A lot will depend on your interpersonal interaction, so make sure you feel you can open up to the therapist.

— If you feel uncomfortable, alienated, or turned off during your first session, let the therapist know, and look for someone else.

— On the other hand, if you notice you're feeling this way at your first session with every therapist candidate, it is probably because of you and not the therapist.

— Don't feel disappointed or hurt if a therapist chooses not to work with you.

— The first session should not focus exclusively on your issues. Take this time to get your questions answered regarding procedures, time frame, cost, and the therapist's qualifications and continuing education commitments. Clear communication and basic agreements are a must for every form of therapy.

— Evasive answers or ambiguous statements are not a sign of professionalism; look for another therapist.

— Look for specialized training when assessing a therapist's qualifications. A basic degree and a professional practice aren't enough.

Self-Help

FIRST AID

In the United States, trauma is responsible for more deaths in the 5 to 34 year age group than all diseases combined. It is the leading cause of death up to age 44. The majority of trauma related deaths are due to motor vehicle crashes.

Many trauma related accidents happen inside the home. Working in the yard or garden, or around the home on stairs, landings, ladders, and scaffolds, can be more dangerous than is commonly assumed. First aid is very likely to be needed in the home, during leisure time.

SAFETY AT HOME
— When buying household goods or toys, make sure you check packaging for proof of compliance with safety standards.
— Before purchasing large appliances, have your electrical outlets checked by a professional to make sure they meet required safety standards.
— Cover smooth, slippery floors or stairs with secured carpeting or mats.
— Secure tall cupboards and shelving to the wall to prevent tipping if bumped accidentally.

EVERYDAY ACCIDENTS

Nosebleeds
Nosebleeds result when small arteries burst, usually in the tip of the nose (see Nose, p. 295).

What to Do
— Apply a cold neck compress.
— If bleeding from the tip of the nose, squeeze nose tightly closed for 10 minutes.
— If you have a nosebleed, DON'T lie down, sniff water, or stuff nose with cotton.

Choking

What to Do
— With the infant's head lower than his/her body, perform back blows and chest thrusts. For children older than 1 year, perform the Heimlich maneuver (abdominal thrusts). If this doesn't help, call emergency services immediately.

Home First Aid Kit
The best place to keep your home first aid kit is in a locked cabinet, inaccessible to children, in a cool, dry place—definitely not in the bathroom. It should contain:

Bandages and Instruments
Box of Band-Aids
Wound dressings—large dressings that consist of a gauze pad attached to a bandage
Antiseptic wipes
Packet of skin closures
Cotton
Gauze dressings
Open-weave (gauze) bandages
Surgical tape
Elastic bandages
Triangular bandages
Tweezers
Safety pins
Scissors
Thermometer
Disposable gloves
Personal-use mask for mouth-to-mask resuscitation

Medications
Simple analgesics (see p. 660), such as acetaminophen and/or ibuprofen
Medications for insect bites and stings (see p. 268)—such as calamine lotion
Antibiotic ointments for wounds
Syrup of ipecac to make your child vomit in case of poisoning with a noncorrosive substance.

Individualized Medications
Medications that are prescribed for you or someone in your family should also be in your locked first aid kit cabinet, and not on your bedside table or kitchen cabinet.

— If breathing stops, start mouth-to-mouth resuscitation immediately (see p. 715). It is almost always possible to get air past an object in the wind pipe.
— After removing the foreign body, always have the child see a doctor.

Choking in Children
If a child chokes on a piece of food or a small object, immediate action is necessary.

Heimlich Maneuver

Airway Obstruction
in Infants

Babies under one year: Hold infant face down, resting on forearm. Rest your forearm on your thigh to support infant. Support infant's head, which should be lower than the trunk. Forcefully deliver 5 back blows, with the heel of your hand, between infant's shoulder blades. Alternate with 5 chest thrusts until obstruction is retrieved.

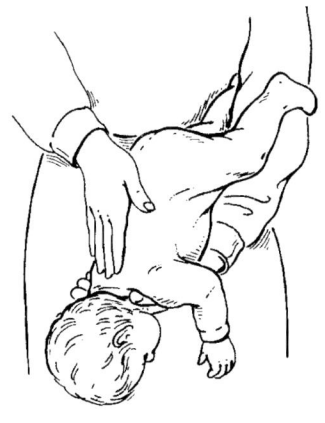
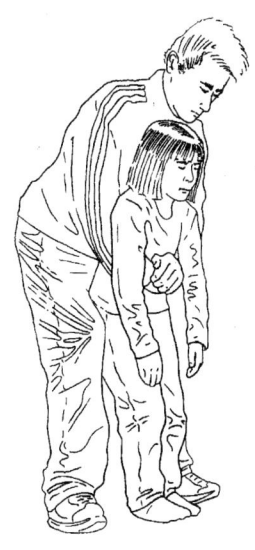

Airway Obstruction
in Children

Place the thumb side of one fist against the victim's abdomen slightly above the navel. With hands together, exert a series of quick upward thrusts. Each thrust should be a separate movement. Continue abdominal thrusts until the foreign body is expelled.

Foreign Bodies

In the mouth or pharynx: Kneel above victim's head. Open victim's mouth by pressing into cheeks with both your thumbs. Keeping mouth open with one thumb, reach into mouth and down throat as far as possible to remove foreign object.

In nose: Holding the unobstructed nostril shut, try to blow hard out of the blocked nostril.

In ear: Only a professional should remove foreign objects in the ear.

In eye: Pull lower eyelid down to remove small objects with tip of handkerchief or tissue. Or hold a matchstick or cotton swab across the upper eyelid, pull lid forward by lashes and fold lid upward over matchstick or swab; when victim rotates eyeball downward, the foreign object may become visible and may be removed with tip of handkerchief or tissue.

WOUND CARE

Heat, cold, chemicals, injuries, or surgery can damage the skin's protective function, allowing viruses, bacteria or fungi to penetrate the individual. If the body's immune system (see p. 351) is unable to fight off these intruders (for example, staphylococcus or salmonella in a wound), an infection will develop, which if not treated can cause blood infection (bacteremia) and potentially fatal septic-toxic shock.

Protection against tetanus (see p. 670) is provided by a three-phase tetanus vaccination. In most cases doctors automatically give tetanus shots in case of an injury, but this is really only necessary if more than five years have passed since the last shot.

When to Seek Medical Advice

— Small wounds can be cared for by oneself using bandages (see Bandages, p. 706).

— Larger wounds should be treated by a doctor within 6 hours.

— The warning signs of blood infection are fever, chills, pallor, tiredness, weakness, loss of appetite. See your health-care provider immediately.

Warnings When Treating a Wound

— Do not apply cotton or gauze bandages directly to a wound.

— You should not touch an open wound: Don't wash it (except for gently cleaning the outer edges with an antiseptic) and don't apply powders, salves or sprays. The only two exceptions to this rule are acid and base (alkali) burns, which should be washed out, and burns, which should be wetted and cooled with water.

— Larger objects inside a wound should only be removed by a professional.

Bandages

Bandages consist of a sterile surface and a means of attaching it to the patient's body. For minor wounds, a simple Band-Aid is all that's needed. For larger wounds, a full-size adhesive bandage is necessary: The sterile portion should be sufficiently large to cover the whole wound; the adhesive part should not touch the wound.

Triangular Bandage

A triangular bandage will hold dressings in place in various areas of the body. Make sure knots are not too tight and don't press on the wound.

Prepackaged Adhesive Bandage

When opening and applying a prepackaged adhesive bandage, make sure you avoid touching the sterile dressing area.

Gauze Bandage

Rolls of gauze bandage are used to hold wound dressings in place and should not be applied directly to the wound.

Minor Scrapes and Cuts

Minor injuries usually stop bleeding on their own within a few minutes.

What to Do

— The edges of the wound (not the wound itself) may be cleaned with an antiseptic solution.
— Either apply an adhesive bandage strip (Band-Aid), or let the wound air dry.
— Use an adhesive bandage to rejoin the edges of cut.
— Cuts longer than about a half inch should been seen by a doctor so they can be stitched if necessary, to minimize scarring.

Puncture Wounds

If a dirty object (e.g., rusty nail or piece of wire) has caused the puncture or stab wound, there is a higher risk of infection. Puncture wounds in joints or the body's hollows are especially dangerous, as they can develop internal infections.

What to Do

— Only a professional should remove foreign objects from a wound. If this is attempted by somebody untrained, surrounding tissues will probably be damaged.
— Cover the area immediately surrounding the foreign object with sterile pads, then arrange for the victim to be taken to a hospital. Foreign objects usually require surgical removal.

Scratches, Stings, and Bites

Although most animal bites and insect stings are not life-threatening, they should be seen by a doctor because of the risk of tetanus, gangrene, and/or rabies.

Some people are highly allergic to insect stings (see Anaphylactic Shock, p. 360). This requires emergency medical attention.

Mosquito Bites and Wasp Stings

Itching, swelling, and redness can be relieved by a cold water compress, or a topical itch reliever containing an antihistamine, or calamine.

Bee and Hornet Stings

If the stinger is still in the wound, it must be removed. To relieve symptoms, see Mosquito Bites and Wasp Stings, above.

Stings in or near the Mouth

Wasp, bee, or hornet stings can cause the tongue and oral mucous membranes to swell and interfere with breathing. Suck on ice cubes continuously until swelling subsides, and apply a cold compress to throat. If you experience difficulty breathing, call emergency medical services immediately.

Tick Bites

Engorged ticks can swell to the size of a pea. Do not try to remove a tick with tape or a nail—remove the tick using tweezers (Don't worry if the head stays behind; it will soon fall off.) Or:

— Touch the tick with a red-hot needle; it should release its hold.
— If, within a few days or weeks, the area of the bite turns bluish-red, or it is surrounded by a red bull's-eye rash, or fever develops, contact your health-care provider (see Lyme Disease, p. 223).
— To prevent tick bites, wear clothing that covers the entire body.

Burns and Scalds

Sunburn

Cool sunburned skin with moist compresses and apply cooling lotions or ointments to reddened areas (see Sunburn, p. 263).

Burn Wounds

In large burns (see Burns, p. 264) considerable amounts of tissue fluid, containing essential electrolytes, is lost. This can lead to shock (see p. 712).

What to Do

— Immediately pour clean, cold water over the burned area, or submerge area in cold water, until pain decreases.
— Never use household remedies such as flour, oil, powder, burn salves, or the like. They tend to worsen the damage.
— Do not pop any blisters that may form.
— Wrap the burn loosely in sterile towels.
— Do not cover a facial burn.
— If burn was caused by hot liquid, immediately remove any wet clothes covering the area.
— If clothes are stuck to the body, don't try to rip them off; place sterile cloths over them.
— Cover the burn victim immediately or wrap in blankets, avoiding the wounded areas, so no body warmth is lost.
— Give liquids to drink only if the burn victim is not in shock, unconscious, or nauseous, and has no facial burns or injuries to the stomach or intestines. Sipping uncarbonated mineral water is best to lessen fluid loss.
— Check pulse and breathing regularly.

HEAT DISORDERS AND COLD INJURIES

Heat Exhaustion

Symptoms of heat exhaustion include pronounced pallor, weakness, cold sweat, and chills, and a weak, rapid pulse accompanying a normal temperature.

What to Do

— Have patient lie down in the shade and cover him or her.
— Give mineral water to drink, with some salt added if possible, or give a sports drink such as Gatorade, to keep fluid levels up.

Heat Stroke

Heat stroke occurs when the body is overheated. Unlike a heat-exhaustion victim, a heat-stroke victim's face and head are red, the skin is hot and dry, the face is expressionless, the gait is unsteady and the temperature is very high. The patient may lose consciousness.

What to Do

— Move victim to a cool place in a raised position, and remove or loosen his or her clothing.
— Call emergency medical services. Heat stroke can be life-threatening.
— Apply cold compresses and fan the victim.

Sunstroke

Sunstroke is caused by strong, direct sun on an unprotected head. Symptoms are a very red, hot face and head, cool skin elsewhere, restlessness, headache, nausea, and possible vomiting and loss of consciousness. Small children are especially at risk: Their hair provides very little protection and their skulls are still thin. When exposed to long periods of sun, they may develop a high fever and turn pale.

What to Do

— Move victim into the shade.
— Raise victim's head and keep it cool with wet towels.
— If symptoms are severe, call emergency medical services.

Hypothermia

Hypothermia is caused by prolonged exposure to cold temperatures, e.g., in cold water or following a skiing accident or avalanche. At body temperatures between 93°F and 97°F, symptoms include shivering, pains in arms and legs and slightly raised pulse. If the body temperature drops below 93°F , the victim gradually loses consciousness, and shivering and pains disappear. At body temperatures of 81°F or lower, the victim is deeply unconscious.

What to Do

— For severe hypothermia, call emergency medical

services immediately.
— Move victim into a building or sheltered area, remove any wet clothing and cover victim with blankets.
— If victim is conscious, give hot, sweetened drinks, but never alcohol.
— Do not move hypothermia victims or massage their extremities. They should be allowed to rest while gradually warming up.
— If you cannot hear a heartbeat, practice cardiopulmonary resusitation (CPR).

Frostbite

Frostbite can occur at temperatures as high as 42°F in conditions of high humidity. Body parts at highest risk of frostbite are those with little protection from muscle or tissue, such as fingers, toes, nose, and ears, and those with excessively tight clothing or shoes (feet, for example).

What to Do
— Loosen tight clothing or footgear. The best way to bring warmth to the affected area is by covering or holding it with a warm hand.
— Encourage the victim to gently move limbs.
— In mild cases of frostbite, submerge affected areas in warm water.
— In severe cases, give warm water treatment and seek medical attention.

ELECTRICAL INJURIES

A severe electric shock can cause unconsciousness and stop breathing and circulation. Deep burns can result at the spot where the current entered the body.

What to Do
— Disconnect electrical current by pulling a plug, removing a fuse, or tripping a circuit breaker.
— If this is not possible, the victim must be separated from contact with the live wire or high-tension source.
— Warning: To avoid contact with high-voltage current, stand on a nonconducting substance such as dry wood, dry cloths, or a thick pile of newspapers.
— Don't touch anyone or anything while standing in this "insulated" position.

— Now either drag victim away from the current by pulling on his or her clothes, or lift and push the source off the victim using a nonconducting object like a dry stick or wooden broom.
— Let victim rest; check pulse and breathing (see Checking for Breathing, p. 713).
— If victim is unconscious, roll onto his or her side (see p. 714).
— If victim is not breathing, begin mouth-to-mouth resuscitation (see p. 715).
— If victim has no pulse, begin CPR (see p. 716).
— Minimize the risk of shock (see p. 712). Call emergency medical services immediately.

POISONING AND CAUSTIC SUBSTANCES

Poisoning and injuries from caustic substances are relatively frequent in the home, especially in small children. All solvents, cleaning products, and household chemicals should be kept locked and out of the reach of children, and instructions on product packaging should be closely followed.

Poisoning

General indicators of poisoning include nausea, vomiting, diarrhea, sudden abdominal cramps, headaches, dizziness, fading or loss of consciousness, difficulty or lack of breathing, symptoms of shock, rapid or slowed pulse, and agitation.

What to Do
— Maintain open airways by laying victim on his or her side (see p. 714).
— Maintain cardiovascular activity by laying victim flat and giving CPR if necessary (see p. 716).
— Call emergency medical services.
— Contact the nearest poison control center for information on what to do next.
When calling a poison control center, have the following information ready:
— Age of victim
— Type and concentration of poison or hazardous substance
— How much was ingested
— How long ago it was ingested
— What poisoning symptoms are present
— What has been done for the victim so far

When to Induce Vomiting

— If victim has been poisoned by medications, alcohol, mushrooms, or berries, vomiting may be induced immediately after the ingestion, but only if the victim is conscious.

— To induce vomiting, give ipecac syrup (2 tablespoons for adults, 1 tablespoon for children 1–12 years of age).

— Do not induce vomiting if victim has ingested gasoline, petroleum products, acid or lye.

Caustic Substances

If strong acids or alkalis (lye-type substances) are swallowed, internal injuries result. If they come in contact with skin, external injuries result. The most common sources of caustic burns are cleaning products (especially toilet cleansers and dishwasher detergents) and pesticides. Many products simultaneously cause caustic burns and poisoning.

Swallowing caustic substances can cause deep wounds in the esophagus, which may become infected and cause esophageal wall perforation.

What to Do

Seek medical help immediately.

External injury: Immediately and carefully remove all clothing from affected area and hold affected area under running water as long as possible. Take the container of poison along to the emergency room.

Internal injury: Give plenty of water to drink (not milk). Do not induce vomiting.

Injury to eye: Get medical help as soon as possible. In the meantime, rinse the eye continuously with water for at least 20 minutes. Tilt head back, hold eyelids apart, and carefully pour water into eye from about 4 inches away.

INJURIES OF BONES, JOINTS AND MUSCLES

Injured bones, joints, and muscles should be immobilized in a well-padded splint and a sling. Makeshift splints can be improvised out of newspapers or magazines, cardboard, wire mesh, and other pliable materials.

Strains, Sprains, Dislocations

Injuries to joints and associated muscles, tendons, and ligaments usually cause swelling, pain, and restricted movement.

What to Do

— Do not move or place pressure on injured joint; rest it, elevate it and/or place in a splint.

— Ice packs or cold compresses will ease acute pain and swelling.

— Have your health-care provider examine the injury (see Pulled or Torn Muscles, p. 437; Sprained or Strained Tendons and Ligaments, p. 441; Sprained or Strained Joints, p. 447; Dislocations, p. 448).

Bruises and Contusions

Torn layers of deep tissue or internal bleeding can cause effusions, bruising, swelling, and pain. Injuries to internal organs or fractured bones may not be externally visible, so these injuries should be handled like a sprain (see p. 441).

Closed Fractures

A broken bone may not be immediately obvious; often the injured part can still be moved. A fracture should be suspected if the patient favors the limb and complains of pain, and the affected body part appears swollen or mishapen.

What to Do

Rest the injured part; have the patient get into the least uncomfortable position. Take weight and pressure off the injured part.

— For a hip fracture, use a knee roll or support under the knee.

— For a broken leg or ankle, immobilize and support the injured part with rolled-up clothes, pillows and blankets, and anchor it in place with a heavy briefcase or similar object.

— For an upper-arm fracture, immobilize the arm with a triangular cloth sling.

Warning: Never move the victim with a suspected spinal injury.

Warning: Closed fractures may turn into open fractures if handled incorrectly (see Fractures, p. 429).

Open Fractures

In an open fracture, the bone penetrates the skin. This is considered a serious injury because of the high risk of infection.

What to Do

— Stop wound from bleeding and cover with a sterile dressing.

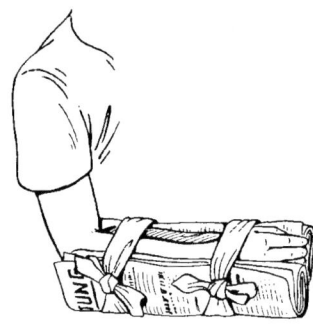

Improvised splint for lower arm or hand fracture

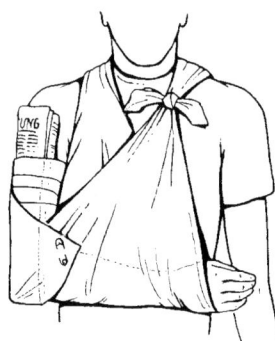

Temporary immobilization after upper arm fracture

— Prevent victim from going into shock (see Shock, p. 712).
— Take weight or pressure off injured part by moving victim into the least uncomfortable position (see Closed Fractures, p. 709).

Skull Fractures

Skull or brain injuries are often impossible to detect externally, especially if no injury is visible.

What to Do

— Make sure the victim's airway is unobstructed. If victim is not breathing, start mouth-to-mouth resuscitation (see p. 715).
— Elevate upper body slightly (about 30° above horizontal).
— Lay an unconscious victim on his or her side (see illustration, p. 714).
— Call emergency medical services.

Concussion

Symptoms of concussion include
— Short-term loss of consciousness
— Inability to remember events immediately preceding the accident or injury
— Nausea or dizziness; headaches

What to Do

— Lay victim horizontally in the least uncomfortable position, and have him or her remain there until a health-care professional states that he or she may get up.
— Monitor victim's breathing. If victim is unconscious, roll him or her onto side.
— Call emergency medical services.

Chest Injuries

Symptoms of injuries to the chest, including broken ribs, consist of
— Increasing difficulty breathing (the victim strains to get more air and tries to sit up in order to breathe better)
— Possible spitting up of bright, foamy blood
— Symptoms of shock (see p. 712)
— Possible whistling or blowing sound, if there's an open wound

What to Do

— Call emergency medical services. The victim should neither eat, drink, nor smoke.
— When the lungs can't expand completely, breathing gets harder and harder. Placing the victim in a sitting position with the back supported may make breathing easier.
— If blood is coughed up, suspect a lung injury and do not apply a support bandage.
— Loosen tight clothing; monitor victim's breathing. If victim stops breathing, begin mouth-to-mouth resuscitation (see p. 715).
— If there is an open wound, stop the bleeding. Apply a pressure bandage or clean cloth, or press steadily on the wound with a flat hand until medical help arrives. Watch out for symptoms of shock (see p. 712).

Spine Fractures

The symptoms of a spinal fracture are far from obvious.

Encourage the victim to move hands, arms, legs and feet. For example, ask victim to wiggle their toes, and squeeze your hand tightly.
— If victim is unable to move hands and arms, a cervical spine injury is likely.
— If victim is unable to move legs and toes, a lumbar vertebral injury is likely.

What to Do
— Call emergency medical services.
— Do not move victim or allow him or her to move. With a spinal cord injury, any movement may cause permanent paralysis.
— Keep victim warm, stay with him or her, and offer reassurance.
—Victim should be transported to the hospital only by trained professionals.

FIRST AID IN MOTOR VEHICLE CRASHES

In the United States, motor vehicle crashes account for the largest share of trauma deaths. Teenage drivers have the highest crash rate of all age groups. The elderly are also at increased risk of death and injury from motor vehicle crashes. Alcohol is implicated in about 40 percent of all motor vehicle crash deaths.

Volunteers trained in first aid, artificial respiration and CPR can play an important role in caring for accident victims until help arrives, since even with a well-functioning emergency medical system, an ambulance may take 10 minutes to get to the scene in a city, and 15 minutes or more in rural areas.

Most accidental injuries are minor and can be treated with simple methods, but it pays to be prepared for a serious accident. Timely action may even save a life; yet only a third of those who witness an accident will offer help. Even trained volunteers are often reluctant to speak up or step forward at the scene of an accident, due to a lack of self-confidence or the feeling of having forgotten too much of their training. It may spur you to take responsibility and action if you remember that your own life may one day depend on the help of a stranger.

Preventing the Risk of Acquired Immunodeficiency Syndrome (AIDS)

Two precautions can eliminate the risk of HIV infection when administering first aid to an accident victim:

— Avoid direct contact with the victim's blood; use disposable gloves (keep some in your vehicle first aid kit).
— Medical opinion is divided concerning the contagiousness of saliva. If the victim is bleeding from the mouth and you are performing mouth-to-mouth resuscitation (see p. 715), breathe through a cloth and/or through the nose (see p. 713). However, it is best to use the mouth-to-mask technique.

What to Do at the Scene of an Accident
Stay calm. Act swiftly, but without haste.
— First try to find out what happened, without endangering yourself.
— Protect victim(s) from further injury.
— If vehicle engines are still running, turn them off. Rescue victim(s) from vehicle(s). Douse any fires with an extinguisher, blankets, cloths, or sand. If possible, put up warning signs (reflective orange triangles) around accident.
— Call emergency medical services, or send somebody to get help.
— If necessary, get somebody to direct traffic, keeping one lane open for emergency vehicles.
Determine whether the situation is life-threatening:
— Is the victim conscious?
— Is he or she breathing?
— Does he or she have a pulse?
— Is there severe bleeding?
— Is the victim in shock?

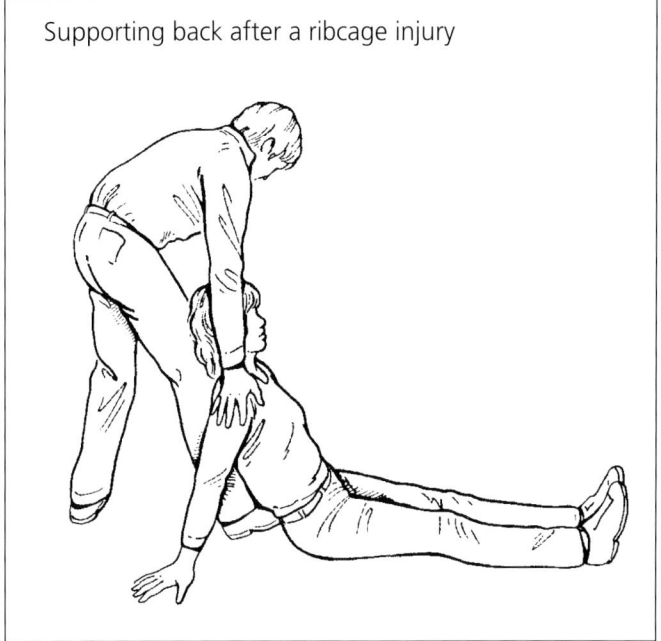

Supporting back after a ribcage injury

If victim is unconscious, roll him or her onto side (see p. 714).

— Stop severe bleeding as quickly as possible (see below).

— Apply cold pack to severe burns immediately (see p. 707).

— Monitor breathing and pulse. If breathing has stopped, begin mouth-to-mouth resuscitation immediately (see p. 715).

— If victim is in shock, stay with him or her and treat accordingly (see below).

— Try to organize how victim will be transported to an emergency room.

Warning: Transporting a Victim: Never transport an accident victim in your own vehicle if

— You suspect a spinal injury (victim cannot move hands, arms, legs, or feet)

— A stretcher is required (e.g. in case of a complicated fracture)

— You are alone with the victim, who is either in shock or unconscious

Calling Emergency Medical Services

When you make the call, be sure to have the following information on hand:

— What happened?

— Where did it happen?

— How many victims are there?

— What kinds of injuries do there seem to be?

— Name of the person reporting the accident.

How to Stop Bleeding

Very deep or extensive wounds can cause a victim to bleed to death. Severe bleeding may indicate damage to blood vessels or internal organs (e.g., a ruptured spleen following a motorcycle accident). In adults, losing a quart of blood may cause shock, and losing 2 quarts may be fatal, so bleeding should be stopped as soon as possible.

What to Do

— Victim should be lying down, with the injured part elevated.

— Apply a pressure bandage to the site of bleeding. Use gauze rolls or several handkerchiefs. The pressure should be strong enough to stop bleeding, but not to constrict the vessels underneath.

— If bandages are not available, press any clean, soft material onto the wound.

How to Stock Your Car First Aid Kit

Box of Band-Aids
Wound dressings—large dressings that consist of a gauze pad attached to a bandage
Antiseptic wipes
Packet of skin closures
Gauze dressings
Surgical tape
Elastic bandages—for supporting sprains and strains
Triangular bandage
Antibiotic ointment
Scissors
Safety pins
Disposable gloves
Personal-use mask for mouth-to-mask resuscitation
Booklet of first aid treatments
White chalk
Reflective traffic warning sign or flare

— If bleeding is not stopped by applying pressure, the blood supply to the wound may be cut off by tightly constricting the thigh or upper arm. This s h o u l d only be attempted in extreme emergencies.

— In an amputation injury, the severed limb should be wrapped, as is, in sterile bandages and kept cool. It may be possible for it to be sewn back on.

— Severe bleeding can lead to shock and death, so in addition to stopping bleeding it is important to try to prevent against shock.

Shock

Shock is a state of severely disturbed circulation that can deprive vital organs of oxygen and nutrients. Symptoms of shock include

— Rapid pulse, growing weaker and weaker until it is barely noticeable

— Pallor; cool skin; chills, sweat on the forehead

— Distinct uneasiness and restlessness, but usually no loss of consciousness

Shock has various causes, but always requires immediate medical attention.

What to Do

— Stop bleeding immediately.

— Raise victim's legs ("self-transfusion") and leave them slightly elevated ("shock position").

— Loosen tight clothing.

— Keep victim warm: Place him or her on a blanket and wrap it around him or her.
— Stay calm, talk quietly and soothingly to the victim, and never leave him or her alone.
— Do not give the victim food or drink.
— Check pulse and breathing regularly.

Checking the Pulse

An adult's pulse when at rest beats 60 to 80 times per minute. The pulse may be checked either on the neck or wrist, using three fingertips (not the thumb).

FAINTING AND LOSS OF CONSCIOUSNESS

Fainting is caused by a temporary lack of oxygen to the brain. This may occur, for example, if you have been standing for a long time, and your circulatory system is no longer able to keep a sufficient supply of oxygen flowing up to the brain. You become pale and unresponsive and suddenly collapse. This form of fainting usually passes quickly, because by bringing your whole body down to floor level, you have just stimulated better circulation to the brain.

However, fainting may also be caused by metabolic disorders, for example high or low blood sugar levels in diabetics (see p. 483).

If fainting lasts longer than a minute, it is referred to as unconsciousness. The same factors that trigger fainting may cause unconsciousness. Long-term unconsciousness is usually caused by an accident, a blow to the head, poisoning, or exposure to heat or cold.

Always call emergency medical services if someone is unconscious.

What to Do

— Immediately lay victim down and elevate the legs, thus supplying the brain with more oxygen.
— Monitor pulse and breathing (see above and below and p. 715).
— After regaining consciousness, have the victim lie still for a while; he or she should then breathe fresh air.

If victim is unconscious for more than a minute, but still breathing

— Roll victim onto side to keep airways open and enable any fluid in the mouth and throat to drain.

— Check constantly to make sure fluid is able to drain. The most frequent cause of death after an accident is choking on saliva, mucus, blood, or vomit.
— Monitor pulse and breathing (see above and below and p. 715).

Checking for Breathing

If an unconscious victim is not breathing:
— Clear the airway by removing dentures, retainers or chewing gum. Begin mouth-to-mouth resuscitation.
— Check pulse and breathing repeatedly.
— If victim has no pulse, begin CPR immediately.

If the Victim Is Not Breathing

Only immediate artificial respiration can save the life of someone who has stopped breathing. People with transient cessation of respiration or apnea have a bluish pale look (see Checking for Breathing, above).

What to Do

— Lay victim on back on a hard surface; gently stretch victim's neck out.
— If victim has been in an accident, do not move to avoid possible injury to the spinal column. Try to open victim's airway with both hands gently pulling forward on lower jaw ("jaw thrust maneuver").
— Begin mouth-to-mouth resuscitation (see Mouth-to-Mouth Resuscitation, p. 715).

Mouth-to-Mouth Resuscitation for Infants and Children

— Cover child's nose and mouth simultaneously with your open mouth.
— Breath less hard, but more quickly than for an adult— about 30–40 times per minute.

Mouth-to-Nose Breathing

If the victim has facial injuries, mouth-to-mouth resuscitation may be difficult or impossible. In this case, mouth-to-nose breathing may be performed.
— Close unconscious victim's mouth by holding his or her chin up.
— Blow forcefully into victim's nose ("breathes in").
— Now open victim's mouth so the air can escape (victim "breathes out").
— Repeat every 5 seconds, as with mouth-to-mouth resuscitation, stopping only once victim starts breathing spontaneously again.

Positioning the Unconscious Person

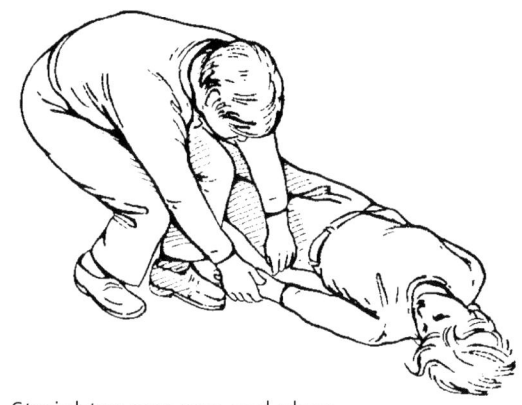

Straighten one arm and place under body as far as possible.

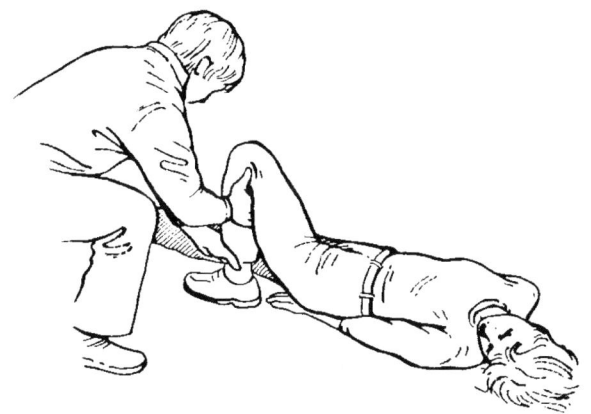

Bend leg of same side.

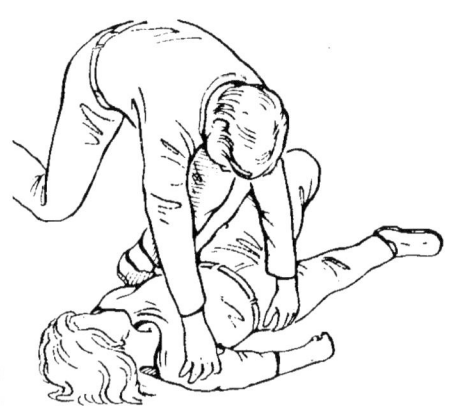

Holding opposite shoulder and hip, attempt turning person.

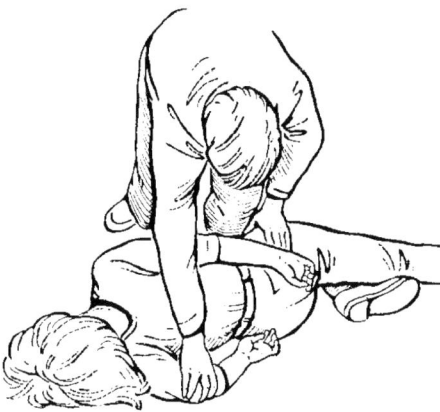

Carefully take out arm from underneath the body.

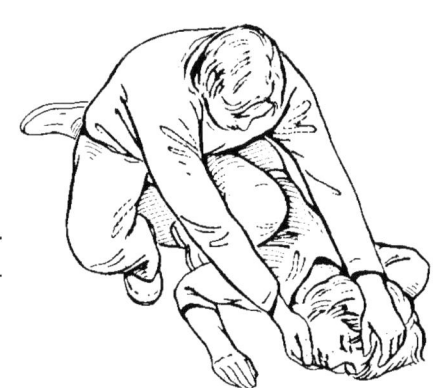

Mildly extend neck turning face towards ground.

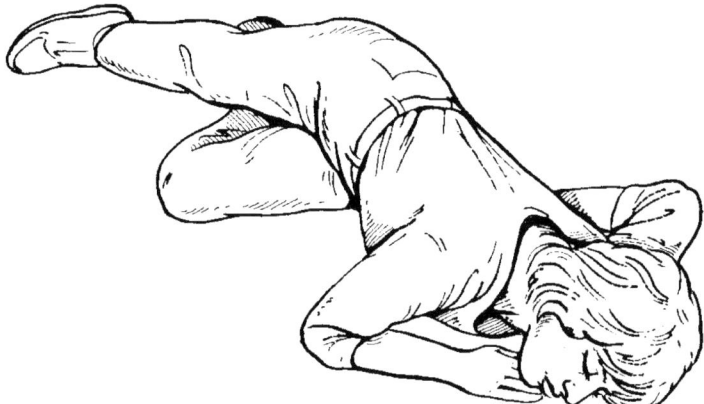

Place fingers under cheek.
Remove foreign objects from mouth.
Saliva should flow out from mouth.

Signs of Normal Breathing
— The skin's bluish tinge disappears and its normal rosy color returns.
— The pupils contract to their normal size; the chest visibly expands and contracts.

If the Victim has no Pulse
If the victim has no pulse, chest compressions of CPR can maintain circulation artificially to keep the internal organs oxygenated and nourished until the heart starts beating on its own again. The victim's ribs may be broken by the chest compressions, but if the choice is either the chance of broken ribs or the likelihood of death, CPR comes out ahead.

In chest compressions, the heart is squeezed between the breastbone and the spine, which press the blood out of the heart's chambers into circulation in the body and lungs. When pressure is released, the chest returns to its original position and the heart fills with blood again.

What to Do (for Adults)
— Place victim on back on a hard surface.
— Kneel at victim's side. Place the heels of both hands, one on top of the other, onto the lower half of the breastbone. Keeping your arms straight, push down hard in a vertical position at regular intervals. With each push, the breastbone should be compressed at least 1½ inches.
— Do 60 to 80 compressions per minute. Don't take breaks lasting longer than 5 seconds.
— Chest compressions won't supply the lungs with air. The other part of CPR involves mouth–to–mouth resuscitation, supplied if possible by another volunteer, in a ratio of 1 breath for every 5 chest compressions, or 12 breaths and 60 chest compressions per minute.
— If no other volunteer is available, give 2 breaths for every 15 chest compressions every 15 seconds (see illustration, right); this amounts to 8 breaths and 60 chest compressions per minute.

CPR for a Drowning Victim
If a victim is drowning, artificial respiration should begin while he or she is being rescued from the water. Don't waste precious time trying to get water out of the lungs and stomach—once it's in, it's in.

Mouth-to-Mouth Resuscitation

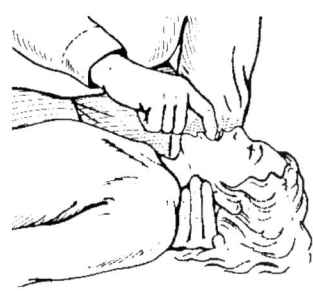

Remove foreign objects such as loose dentures and chewing gum from mouth.

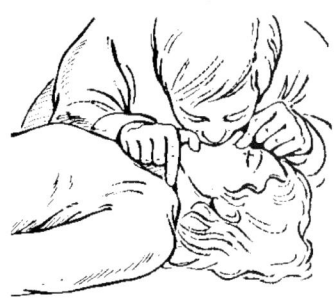

Close nose with thumb and index finger. Take a deep breath and tightly close your mouth over the victim's.

Give 12 to 15 breaths per minute.

After each minute, reassess if person is spontaneously breathing by looking to see if there is chest rise, or if you can hear or feel air coming out of victim's mouth.

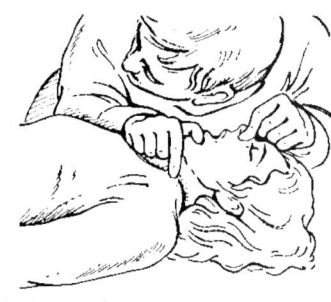

Continue rescue breathing until medical help arrives or until the victim breaths spontaneously on his/her own. Do not stop rescue breathing for longer than 5 seconds at a time.

What to Do

— Begin CPR within 3 to 5 minutes if possible.
— Start with two strong, slow breaths.
— Now begin chest compressions. Don't take breaks from the breathing or chest compressions for more than 5 seconds.

Resuscitation for cardiac arrest (chest compressions)

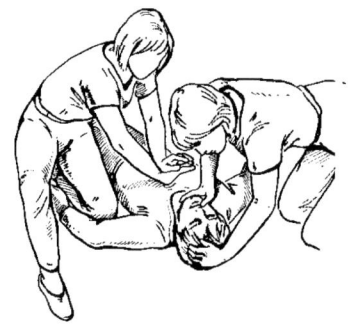

Push down strongly on lower half of sternum 80 times a minute.

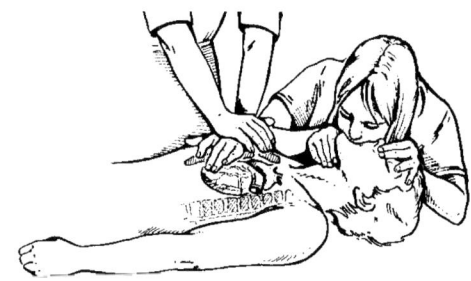

Continue chest compressions. A second person gives one breath for every 5 chest compressions.

TRAVEL

VACCINATIONS BEFORE FOREIGN TRAVEL

Some countries require specific vaccinations for foreign visitors, leaving them no choice in the matter. Sometimes, however, vaccinations are not required but simply recommended by the World Health Organization, or the Centers for Disease Control and Prevention (CDC). In such cases, the traveler should consider the following: Will the trip I've planned actually expose me to these diseases? Some vaccinations' side effects may be more harmful than contracting the disease itself (see Immunizations, p. 667).

General precautionary measures—e.g., avoiding suspect foods or insect stings (see p. 718)—are often more important for maintaining good health while traveling than the deceptive protection provided by vaccinations.

Malaria

The term malaria describes a group of infectious diseases in which red blood cells are invaded by the single-celled Plasmodium species. Malaria is spread by the bite of female Anopheles mosquitos. When the mosquito bites an infected person, it ingests the contaminated blood and the parasites further develop, and then collect in the mosquito's salivary glands.

When the mosquito bites the next person, it injects the parasites into that person's blood along with its saliva. The parasites end up in the patient's liver, where they multiply and finally invade the red blood cells, causing them to rupture and the patient to develop a sudden high fever. The fever then recurs at regular intervals. Depending on the type of parasite, 1 to 4 weeks may elapse between the mosquito bite and the onset of fever. The various types of malaria (e.g. quartan, tertian) are named according to the frequency of the outbreaks of fever. Malaria secondary to P falciparum is the most serious and life-threatening form.

Pieces of the ruptured red blood cells may get caught in the tiny blood vessels of the brain or essential organs; this can be fatal.

Preventive Measures

— The Anopheles mosquito bites only between dusk and dawn, so spend this time in a mosquito-free area indoors.
— In non-air-conditioned hotel rooms, your most important protection is a mosquito net, which is standard issue in many countries. To be on the safe side, bring one along on your trip, or buy one locally. Doors and windows should also be secured by mosquito netting or fine-mesh screens.
— Mosquitos cannot penetrate fabric thicker than 1 millimeter (0.04 inch). An insect repellent may be applied to exposed skin. It should be effective for 6 to 8 hours.
— Although insect-repellent sprays or fumigants are effective, they may also cause breathing difficulties, nausea, and headaches. Avoid high doses of vitamin B or so-called ultrasound insect repellents; neither has been proven effective.

Preventing Malaria with Medication

Medications can greatly reduce the risk of contracting malaria, while not preventing it totally. All malaria medications, however, have potentially significant side effects and may be contraindicated for certain individual patients.

Because medication-resistant malaria parasites are becoming more and more common, prevention is becoming increasingly problematic and recommendations are constantly changing. Consulting your doctor or the CDC for current recommendations about 6 weeks prior to traveling is probably your best bet.

Answering the following questions can help you decide whether to take preventive medication:
— Are you traveling to an area where malaria is prevalent?
— How high is the risk of contracting malaria there? The side effects of prophylactic malaria medications such as chloroquine hydrochloride or mefloquine can be so serious as to necessitate hospitalization in one ten-thousandth of the population; if your risk of contracting malaria is less than one in ten thousand, it probably makes more sense to avoid advance treatment and take medication along in case you need it (see Standby Therapy, p. 718).

Prophylactic medications are taken according to the following schedule:

— Start the medication 1 week before departure. This way, you will already have a certain degree of protection by the time you arrive at your destination, and you may be able to catch any side effects while you're still home.

— During your trip, follow the prescribed dosage.

— After returning home, continue the medication for another 4 weeks, to destroy any parasites remaining in the bloodstream.

If you are relying on "standby therapy," you should use the preventive medication usually recommended for your destination, but only as an emergency treatment under the following conditions:

— At least 6 days after arriving at your destination, you develop a fever and other malaria symptoms (headache, stomach ache, joint pain, outbreaks of sweating, diarrhea)

— Medical care is unavailable.

— "Standby" therapy might consist of three mefloquine tablets to begin with, followed by two tablets after 6 to 8 hours, followed by one tablet after another six to eight hours. Considerable side effects may accompany the medication: In almost 50 percent of such cases, vomiting and nausea occur, and almost all patients report a high level of discomfort. Psychotic events and seizures have been known to result as well.

Because malaria symptoms can be deceptive and "standby" medications at high dosages have undesirable side effects, a blood test to determine whether what you have is actually malaria is a good idea. A rapid screening test for malarial parasites, the quantitative buffy coat analysis, is available. But blood smears are more reliable. New diagnostic tests are in development, and may provide rapid and accurate diagnosis in the future.

SUGGESTED MEDICATIONS TO TAKE ALONG WHEN TRAVELING

When traveling, it is a good idea to take medications to treat minor ailments, as well as an appropriate supply of any medications you need to take regularly. Your travel kit might contain:

— Bandage rolls, adhesive strips, gauze and elastic bandages.

— Antiseptic solution or ointment.

— An analgesic such as aspirin or acetaminophen (Tylenol) that can also lower a fever (see Simple Analgesics, p. 660).

— Nasal decongestant.

— Salts to be mixed with water to maintain electrolyte levels and combat dehydration due to diarrhea (see Gastroenteritis, p. 599) or a premixed rehydration product.

— A diarrhea remedy such as Imodium, in case you don't have time to recover while traveling (do not take for more than 2 days unless under medical supervision, however) (see Gastroenteritis, p. 599).

— A mild laxative, if you tend to be constipated.

— Antifungal medication, if you tend to get fungal infections.

— Sunscreen with the right sun protection factor (SPF) number for your destination (see Sunburn, p. 263).

— Travel (motion) sickness remedies, if you are prone to this. For ship voyages, a special skin patch is available that releases motion sickness medication for 2 to 3 days.

— Insect repellent.

— Condoms to protect you against sexually transmitted diseases.

— Don't bring disinfectant tablets for drinking water; they have not been proven to be reliable.

GENERAL PRECAUTIONS WHEN TRAVELING

If you plan to stay in highly traveled tourist areas, fewer precautions are necessary than if you're planning a trip to less traveled areas of a foreign country.

A rule of thumb regarding food when traveling is: If it isn't peeled and cooked, don't eat it.

To lower your risk of diarrhea, typhus, cholera, and hepatitis A:

— Drink only bottled, canned, or just-boiled (not just warmed up) beverages.

— Eat only freshly prepared foods that have been cooked (steamed, broiled, fried, baked) at temperatures sufficient to kill potential germs.

— Avoid ice cubes, ice cream, and tap water.

— Avoid raw, unpeeled fruits and vegetables.

WHEN YOU ARRIVE AT YOUR DESTINATION

— After a long flight across several time zones, take a day off to rest and let your body catch up.

— When in Rome . . . try to connect with the local

daily rhythm. For example, in a hot climate, it makes sense to get up early, take it easy in the middle of the day, and increase your activity level in the evening.

—You will adjust more quickly to a new climate if you maintain a moderate level of physical activity. Neither strenuous labor nor complete inactivity are recommended.

— Drink plenty of liquids if you are in a hot, dry climate. It's easy to underestimate the amount you need. If your urine is pale yellow and not dark in color, you are getting enough fluids.

— Don't go barefoot in tropical countries because of the risk of hookworm infestation and bites from insects, poisonous reptiles, etc.

— Avoid swimming in African or South American rivers and lakes because of the risk of contracting schistosomiasis.

—Wear light, absorbent clothing in hot climates.

AIR TRAVEL

Should You Fly?

Just because you make it to the airport in one piece doesn't necessarily mean you should get on the plane. Air travel carries a variety of risks; the wise traveler will be forewarned.

The air pressure inside the cabin of a modern jetliner corresponds to an altitude of 8250 feet above sea level; this means there is less oxygen available to the body. In response, heart and breathing rates increase, raising the pressure in the lungs and placing stress on the right half of the heart.

Therefore, you should basically avoid flying if you have any of the following conditions:

— Blood pressure greater than 220/120 mmHg
— Coronary artery disease involving frequent angina pectoris attacks
—Weak heart
— Serious arrhythmias
— Heart attack within the past 6 months
— Collapsed lung (pneumothorax) (see p. 314)
— Insufficient breathing capacity, for example severe asthma
—Acute infectious diseases
— Pregnancy over 36 weeks

Even with one of these conditions, however, flying may be an option if you arrange in advance for adequate medical assistance with the cooperation of the airline.

Jet Lag

Long plane trips often involve crossing time zones. It's a simple matter to reset your watch, but the human body takes much longer to adjust to a new time zone (see Biorhythms, p. 183).

Symptoms experienced during this adjustment period are lumped together under the name "jet lag." Depending on the individual, jet lag may last a day or two or a week; in general, the older you are, the longer it will take your body to adjust. Build a few hours (at least) of rest and relaxation into your schedule following all long flights.

For reasons that are only partly known, the body seems to adjust more easily when flying westward rather than eastward. In general, however, jet lag remains unavoidable. To lessen jet lag, the following pointers may be useful:

— A few days before departure, start changing your eating and sleeping times. If you'll be traveling westward, eat, get up and go to bed 1 hour later every day; if traveling eastward, 1 hour earlier.

— If you start your flight well rested, jet lag will be lessened. Avoid eating a heavy meal or drinking alcohol before or during your flight.

— If you have trouble going to sleep once you've arrived at your destination, try exercising or taking a warm bath.

If You're On Medication

— Always carry a 10-day supply of medication with you.

— Crossing two or three time zones should cause no problems.

—With most medications, e.g., oral contraceptives, it is advisable to keep to your regular schedule according to the time it is at home, not the time at your temporary location. However, if you're taking birth control pills and are planning a long stay many time zones from home, gradually switch this way: On the day you arrive, take the pill in the afternoon. The following day, take it with dinner. From then on, take it at bedtime as usual.

— Patients with certain conditions, e.g., diabetes, may need to switch medications temporarily. Consult your health-care provider.

Risk of Thrombosis

Spending long hours seated in a plane may cause the formation of a blood clot, or thrombosis, especially in pregnant women or people with varicose or inflamed veins.

Any type of movement can help: stretching your legs, taking a little walk, doing some deep knee bends, wiggling your toes, flexing your feet. If you are at risk for thrombosis, wear support hose and consider getting a heparin injection as a precaution before the flight.

The low cabin humidity in some planes causes the body to lose additional fluids, which can increase the chance of thrombosis. Drink plenty of liquids, but avoid coffee and alcohol, which actually increase the body's elimination of fluids.

ALTITUDE SICKNESS

Many people are unaware of the risks of altitude sickness. "Flatlanders" traveling in mountainous regions often experience the first symptoms within a few hours of reaching altitudes of about 10,000 feet.

Complaints

The symptoms of mild altitude sickness include headaches, loss of appetite, nausea, tiredness, and restless sleep.

More serious symptoms include difficulty breathing, strong and rapid heartbeat, dizziness and vomiting, apathy, or euphoria.

Causes

Low oxygen levels in the air cause breathing and heartbeat to speed up; this leads to metabolic disorders and increased blood pressure in the lung blood vessels.

Because air contains less water as temperatures drop, the body loses more water during exhalation. This may cause the blood to thicken, making it more difficult to keep tissues supplied with oxygen.

Who's at Risk

Altitude sickness affects 50 percent of people at altitudes above 10,000 feet who have not undergone sufficient preparation. Children under age 6 are especially sensitive. Being in good physical condition alone will not protect you against altitude sickness.

Possible Aftereffects and Complications

In rare cases, altitude sickness can cause retinal hemorrhage, life-threatening pulmonary edema (characterized by whistling breath and blue lips), and cerebral edema. Cerebral edema should be suspected if painkillers are no longer effective against a headache.

Prevention

If you are climbing at high altitudes, take your time. Climb no more than 1,000 feet a day once you reach heights of 5,000 to 10,000 feet. If possible, sleep at levels slightly lower than those reached during the day: Your breathing rate and oxygen intake drop at night, increasing the risk of pulmonary edema.

While climbing, keep your fluid intake high. You should drink enough to eliminate between 1 and 2 quarts of urine a day.

Avoid alcohol; it slows breathing and dulls your early warning system.

Taking acetazolamide (Diamox) can reduce your adjustment period to the high altitude by 1 to 2 days and can reduce the incidence and severity of acute altitude sickness.

Start taking acetazolamide 2 days prior to starting your climb, and take it for up to 5 days at high altitudes. Potential side effects include tingling in the limbs, frequent urination, nausea, fatigue, and an intolerance for carbonated drinks, which taste unpleasant.

Acetazolamide should not be considered a substitute for adequate preparation and acclimatization, however.

Self-Help

Drink plenty of liquids. If you notice early symptoms of altitude sickness, stop your physical activity, including climbing. Aspirin (see Analgesics, p. 660) may ease the symptoms.

If your condition worsens, you should be transported 3,000 feet down as soon as possible.

Treatment

The most effective treatment for altitude sickness, and a life-saver in some cases, is an immediate descent to lower elevations. If pulmonary edema has developed, oxygen supplementation may be necessary. Nifedipine in chewable form may help relieve shortness of breath. Cerebral edema should be treated with injections of high doses of corticosteroids.

COMMON ILLNESSES WHILE TRAVELING

Seek medical care for any of the following combinations of symptoms:

— Constant headaches, especially if accompanied by confusion
— Kidney pain, especially if accompanied by fever and pain when urinating
— Chest pain when breathing in or out, especially if accompanied by fever or shortness of breath
— Acute abdominal pain accompanied by fever, nausea or vomiting
— Colds accompanied by severe headaches or yellow, puslike nasal discharge
— Painful throbbing in ear; sudden hearing loss; fluid draining from ear
— Sore throat with severe difficulty swallowing and swelling of the lymph nodes
— Severe diarrhea with bloody or mucous stool, accompanied by fever

Motion Sickness

A tendency toward motion sickness is quite pronounced in some individuals and totally absent in others. Some people get dizzy after a few minutes in a moving car; others don't get sick even after days aboard a ship in stormy seas.

A feeling of tiredness is usually the first symptom, together with loss of appetite, pallor and frequent yawning. Next come headaches, dizziness, nausea, vomiting and circulatory problems. Severe cases may cause apathy and anxiety attacks.

Prevention

— In a moving vehicle, choose a seat where motion is least perceptible: on a plane, between the wings; on a boat, in the middle; on a bus, up behind the front axle.
— Look out a window if possible, and focus on the horizon so your eyes and sense of balance can stay in synch with one another. This is very hard to do in an inside cabin on a ship, where your eyes tell you the cabin isn't moving, but your sense of balance tells you the opposite.
— Don't read in a moving car.
— An empty stomach won't prevent motion sickness; it helps to eat lightly before and during a trip.
— If you take motion-sickness medication, do so 1 to 2 hours before departure.

Self-Help

If possible, lie down flat with legs raised; breathe deeply and keep eyes closed. If swallowing medication makes you feel like vomiting, use suppositories instead.

Diarrhea

Diarrhea is the commonest illness of travelers, usually caused by bacteria in food or beverages (see Gastroenteritis, p. 599). It is sometimes accompanied by fever and/or vomiting and usually lasts no more than two to four days, even if untreated.

The general precautions recommended on p. 718 can greatly reduce the risk of diarrhea.

If you have diarrhea, the main thing to remember is to drink lots of liquids, with added salt and sugar (see Gastroenteritis, p. 599).

Diarrhea medications, such as Imodium, don't cure diarrhea, but they do limit the frequency of trips to the toilet. A rest of 2 or 3 days is preferable to taking medication; it will give your body the chance to combat the infection and stop the diarrhea at its source. Don't take diarrhea medication if you have a temperature or the stool contains blood or mucus; these symptoms usually indicate a serious infection, in which chemically slowing down the intestines can actually be dangerous (see Gastroenteritis, p. 599).

If diarrhea does not improve within 2 to 3 days, seek medical assistance.

Sunburn

Many travelers underestimate the power of the tropical sun. Make sure you have enough protection: a sun hat, appropriate clothing, and sunscreen (see Sunburn, p. 263).

BACK HOME

If you've spent more than 3 months in a tropical area, you should undergo blood, urine, and stool tests upon your return, even if you have no symptoms.

If you return from the tropics with unexplainable symptoms such as fever, diarrhea, nausea, vomiting, coughing, or a skin rash, consult your health-care provider and give him or her full details about your trip.

NUTRITION

Although hunger and thirst are signals of bodily needs, supplying the body with energy and fluids is only one of the many functions of food and drink. Eating and drinking satisfies various needs: social give-and-take when food is enjoyed with friends; stimulation and enrichment when we widen our horizons to try different dishes; evidence of status when we titillate our palates with luxurious delicacies. Eating and drinking can also help reduce stress or compensate for unmet needs in other areas of our lives. Thus, food and drink truly "hold body and soul together."

Results of Poor Diet

A high percentage of adults in Western society are overweight; most of us eat much more protein and fat than we need. Although bad dietary habits don't lead to ill health in all cases, some diseases are inexorably linked to diet.

An overly rich diet often raises cholesterol levels, potentially resulting in hardening of the arteries, heart disease, and heart attacks (see Arteriosclerosis, p. 318; Atherosclerosis, p. 318); excessive weight and a lack of exercise contribute to diabetes; too much animal protein stresses the kidneys and can lead to gout; too much sugar contributes to dental caries.

Although dietary deficiencies are less common in industrialized countries, people who eat insufficient seafood may risk iodine deficiency and develop a goiter (see p. 494), and insufficient intake of dairy products may lead to calcium deficiency and brittle bones. Poor nutritional habits can also lead to vitamin deficiencies. A balanced diet can prevent deficiencies of any type.

Diet as Prevention

It has been observed that French men eat relatively large amounts of animal fat and drink plenty of alcohol, yet are at lower risk for heart disease overall than some men who drink less. The clue lies in their blood low-density lipoproteins (LDL) levels (see p. 640). Small amounts of alcohol lower high blood LDL levels. (If LDL levels are already low, however, the risk of heart disease cannot be lowered further by consuming alcohol.) Before you rush off to the liquor store, be forewarned: No more than two glasses of red wine should be taken at a time, with meals. And if you want to lower your risk of coronary heart disease to an absolute minimum, eat as the Japanese do: lots of fish and vegetables, little fat, and little alcohol.

Often, however, eating and drinking can become a medical issue; overconsumption is a common phenomenon in our society.

Nutritional Habits

Already as children we lay the basis for our weight as adults (see Body Weight, p. 727), and up to about age 10 our sense of taste is established. The dietary habits of our families of origin determine whether we find only meat, pasta, and sweets appealing, or enjoy eating vegetables and grains. Nutritional studies have shown that children in our society eat too much in general, and consume excessive fat, salt, and sugar.

As children we also learn (or don't learn) the more subtle satisfactions of eating. Too often today, family meals are rushed, distracted affairs: We gulp our food and run, not bothering to present the meal attractively, chew each bite thoroughly, or even sit down together.

HEALTHY NUTRITION

Eating right always means eating a balanced diet. This doesn't mean each and every meal needs to be perfectly balanced; it means that over the course of time, your diet should meet or exceed certain standards. In addition to providing a wide range of nutrients, a balanced diet ensures that you won't be overdosing on one type of pesticide residue, or other undesirable (but often unavoidable) ingredient in food.

Nutritionists recommend that healthy adults eat a diet consisting of about 60 percent carbohydrates, 10 percent protein, and not more than 30 percent fat. Fiber should also be part of the picture (see Energy Suppliers, starting p. 725). For most of us, this means some changes are in order if we're going to start eating right (see p. 724).

Children and pregnant women require more than the recommended 10 percent of protein. It should be supplied by grains, legumes and dairy products to provide adequate calcium. Limit meat products to once or twice a week: This will supply essential iron and vitamin B12 without raising fat and cholesterol levels.

Changing Your Habits

Make dietary changes gradually, giving your body time to adjust. Refer to the chart on p. 724 for help. You may already be eating a fairly balanced diet, with only a few minor adjustments necessary, or you may be facing a major lifestyle shift. Make it as easy on yourself as possible. In any case, don't go on to the next stage until you've mastered the previous one and it has become second nature.

Breakfast is an especially effective place to start. Instead of grabbing a sugary doughnut or muffin, try muesli, granola or other whole-grain cereal with fruit and milk or yogurt, or whole-grain bread with cottage cheese or low-fat soft cheese and fruit. You'll find yourself feeling comfortably full for longer than after "empty calorie" breakfasts.

BALANCED NUTRITION

The foundations of a balanced diet are vegetables, fruits, whole-grain products, legumes (lentils, peas, beans), and dairy products. Keep meat, fish, and egg consumption to a maximum of twice a week; as much as possible, buy organically grown produce in season.

By eating this way you are both maximizing your chances of optimum health and minimizing misuse of the earth's resources. A concern for both these factors often leads people to avoid meat in their diet. Avoiding meat prevents excessive intake of the fat, cholesterol, purines, hormones, antibiotics, and other potentially harmful ingredients concentrated in meat, which sits at the top of the food chain. Avoiding meat is also an acknowledgment that the grain needed to fatten one steer for human consumption could feed a much larger number of human beings than those who will end up eating the steer.

Balanced nutrition also reflects a concern for agricultural and social conditions in many Third World countries that supply us with food, and for environmental problems caused by transporting food halfway around the world to the dinner tables of the more prosperous nations.

A balanced diet supplies twice the vitamin C and beta-carotene than a "conventional" diet, and almost a third more vitamin E.

ORGANIC PRODUCTS

Foods produced in accordance with organic farming standards may be labeled "organic." This implies that neither soil nor plants were sprayed or treated with

Guidelines for a Balanced Diet
— Eat plenty of fresh vegetables and fruits: at least one 7-ounce serving of vegetables daily, one 3-ounce serving of salad, and one to two pieces of fruit.
— Rediscover potatoes, legumes (lentils, peas, beans) and grain products such as bread, muesli, and oatmeal.
— Eat meat products no more than two or three times a week, preferably lean meat.
— Eat fish once or twice a week.
— Eat no more than three eggs a week (including those in baked goods, pasta, mayonnaise etc.).
— Eat no more than $3/4$ ounce of butter or margarine a day (including that used in cooking, frying and baking); eat $3/4$ ounce of unsaturated oil daily (see Fats, p. 725).
— Consume about a cup (8 ounces) of milk or milk products (yogurt, buttermilk, kefir) a day, plus two slices of cheese.
— Avoid cheese containing more than 45 percent fat.
— Use liquid oils (e.g., sunflower oil) instead of solid oils (lard, coconut oil).
— Eat as little sugar as possible.

synthetic fertilizers or pesticides. Compost, crop rotation, and ecologically friendly pest-reduction methods are used instead.

Farmers wishing to switch to organic farming methods must comply with strict regulations and undergo a transition period during which the soil purifies itself of poisons. Similar standards apply for animal-raising practices; as much as possible, animals are fed locally grown feed containing no hormones, antibiotics, or animal products (see BSE, p. 729).

Studies have shown that organic products contain significantly lower levels of nitrates and pesticide residues than conventionally grown products. They usually cost more, however.

VEGETARIAN DIETS

Being a vegetarian means avoiding animal products, but there are various interpretations of what that means. There are three types of vegetarian diets:

Lacto-ovo vegetarians eat no meat or fish, but do eat eggs and dairy products.

Lacto-vegetarians eat no meat, fish, or eggs, but do eat dairy products.

Vegans avoid all products originating from animals, including meat, fish, eggs, dairy products, and honey.

Simple Ways to Switch to a Balanced Diet (Work your way from left to right.)

Grab meals at a stand or fast-food restaurant.	Bring food from home.	Eat fresh fruits and vegetables for snacks.	When you go out to eat, choose whole-foods restaurants.
Eat mainly canned foods.	Eat mainly frozen foods.	Buy ready-made fresh foods and add your own freshly prepared foods.	Prepare your meals yourself using fresh ingredients.
Buy foods on impulse.	Buy fresh foods in season (see p. 732).	Buy conventionally grown fruits and vegetables.	Buy organically grown fruits and vegetables.
Eat meat, meat products, or eggs at every meal.	Have two meals a day containing no meat, meat products, fish, or eggs.	Twice a week, eat fish or poultry instead of red meat.	Eat meat or fish no more than four times a week.
Eat few fruits or vegetables.	Eat cooked fruit and vegetables.	Eat half your fruit and vegetables raw.	Eat organically grown fruits and vegetables.
Use sugar or sugar substitute as sweetener.	Use honey or fruit syrup as sweetener.	Use fewer and fewer sweeteners.	Use no sweeteners.
Eat white bread and rolls.	Eat whole-grain bread products.	Eat whole-grain breads, granola and/or muesli.	Eat organic whole-grain products, sprouted if possible.
Eat lard or similar animal fats.	Eat margarine and refined oils.	Eat butter, unhydrogenated margarine.	Eat cold-pressed, unrefined oils.

Vegetarians Live Longer . . .

Vegetarians have a 30 to 70 percent lower risk of coronary heart disease than meat-eaters. Their gastrointestinal tracts are less susceptible to disease; they get fewer cases of gout and kidney disorders; terminal cancers are 50 to 70 percent less common in vegetarians than in meat-eaters.

Risk factors known to contribute to disease are much less common in vegetarians, who tend to have
— Normal body weight
— Lower blood pressure
— Lower blood cholesterol levels

Nursing mothers who have been vegetarians for a long time have lower levels of harmful substances in their milk.

. . . But They Need to Pay Close Attention

Vegetarians need to be well informed about the nutritional values of the foods they eat so as not to risk any deficiencies. This is especially true in the case of vegans. If you are a vegetarian and eat eggs and/or milk products, you are probably getting adequate protein. If you are a vegan, make sure you are getting sufficient proteins in the right combinations. Legumes and soybeans are excellent sources of plant protein.

Pregnant women, nursing women, and babies should get some animal protein in their diets; similarly, growing children need lots of protein, and supplying sufficient amounts may be a problem if they eat no animal products. One serving of meat a week will supply enough iron to prevent deficiency.

The iron contained in plants is harder for the human body to absorb than the iron in animal products. If iron levels drop below a certain point, the body adjusts by increasing its demand for iron-rich foods. Vegetarian men tend not to be iron-deficient; vegetarian women have blood iron levels about 10 percent lower than nonvegetarian women, yet they still tend to get fewer diseases. For vegans, calcium may be more of an issue than iron.

Vegetarians usually obtain sufficient quantities of vitamin B^{12} from dairy products. Although vegans eat no dairy, they are usually not vitamin B^{12}-deficient, proving that they obtain enough vitamin B^{12} from fermented products such as sauerkraut.

ENERGY SUPPLIERS

Various foods and dietary supplements routinely make headlines as studies are published showing that they cause (or, alternatively, cure) this or that ailment. Time usually proves, however, that these "silver bullet" approaches don't tell the whole story. The human body is a uniquely complex organism.

Fats

Fats are present not only in animal products such as meat, fish, eggs, and milk, but also in fruits, nuts, and seeds. We consume fats "straight" when we spread butter on bread or eat marbled meat. We also consume large quantities of "hidden" fats in prepared foods, chocolate, mayonnaise, pastries, cheese, meat products, and fried or breaded foods.

Fats supply the body with energy. They are also basic building blocks for hormones and other substances produced by the body.

Fats can be either saturated or unsaturated. The body can produce saturated fats itself from other nutrients, but cannot produce most unsaturated fats. Unsaturated fats must be supplied externally, like vitamins. The following oils are rich in polyunsaturated fats: thistleseed oil (75 percent), flaxseed oil (72 percent), sunflower oil (60 percent), and corn oil (55 percent).

Cholesterol

Cholesterol is a fatty substance found only in animal products. The body manufactures sufficient cholesterol on its own and uses it in cell synthesis and production of bile, hormones and vitamin D. Blood cholesterol levels normally fluctuate greatly.

Cholesterol is a factor in the development of heart and vascular disease.

How much blood cholesterol is "normal" depends on the patient's age, but medical opinion is divided beyond this point. If levels are above 200, it is generally agreed that the patient should watch cholesterol intake (see Atherosclerosis, p. 318).

Three hundred mg of cholesterol is considered the upper limit for daily consumption, yet most people in our society consume at least twice that amount. You can lower your cholesterol intake by
— Avoiding cholesterol-rich foods like eggs and butter
— Eating fewer animal fats, which always contain cholesterol
— Eating a low-fat, high-fiber diet, which causes the body to eliminate more cholesterol
— Using vegetable fats

Butter/Margarine

If you eat too much fat, it doesn't matter whether you're eating butter or margarine. Although butter is high in cholesterol and contains 4 to 7 percent trans-fatty acids, eating between ¾ and 1 ounce a day will not have deleterious effects.

Margarine is often a mixture of animal and vegetable fats. During its manufacture, the unsaturated fats in the vegetable oil become partially saturated, destroying most of its natural vitamins, which are later added as artificial supplements.

Warning for people with nickel allergies: Nickel is used in margarine production, and traces of the metal remain in some brands of margarine.

The high levels of trans-fatty acids formed during margarine production may also cause problems. According to one study, 30,000 Americans die of heart attacks every year from eating margarine with high fatty-acid levels (30 percent).

Carbohydrates

Carbohydrates are found almost exclusively in plant products and milk. Sugars, starches, and fibers are carbohydrates; starches and fibers consist of giant molecules made from individual sugar (glucose and fructose) molecules. In the process of digestion, carbohydrates are broken down into their smallest components, the sugars, which are then transported by the blood to all the body's cells. The cells rely on these sugars for energy.

Sugar

Refined sugar, whether white or brown, supplies only "empty calories" and can be totally eliminated from the diet with no ill effects. The sugar required by the body's cells for nourishment is supplied by the carbohydrates in fruit, vegetables, and grains.

Sugar's negative effect on health is so apparent that it has rightly been called a toxin. Sugar encourages development of dental caries, and when overconsumed for a long time it is turned into fat deposits in the body.

Honey

Honey consists of 80 percent sugar, 20 percent water, small amounts of acetylcholine, enzymes, and minerals—especially potassium and phosphorus—and traces of vitamins. More than a hundred other substances are responsible for honey's distinctive aroma.

Although honey is more "natural" than refined sugar, it does not possess all the healthy properties attributed to it, and potentially causes more cavities than other sugars because it sticks to the teeth.

Fiber

Fiber consists of plant substances largely unusable by the body. Fiber is partly broken down by bacteria in the large intestines, or eliminated in stool. High-fiber foods include vegetables, fruits, and whole-grain products.

Eating fiber
— Keeps the stomach full longer, which prolongs the feeling of satiety after eating. In diabetics, a stomach full of fiber means carbohydrates are absorbed into the blood more slowly, keeping blood sugar levels balanced.
— Keeps the intestines filled. Fiber absorbs water and keeps the intestinal contents moving, which makes for more thorough digestion.
— Makes elimination of bile possible, since fiber absorbs bile. To compensate for this elimination, the body produces more bile using cholesterol, thus lowering cholesterol levels. Eliminating excess bile also prevents the formation of potential carcinogens.
— May cause bloating initially, as intestinal bacteria take longer to break down the fiber. Usually the body

Eat Less Sugar
— Instead of eating a sugary snack, have some fruit.
— Instead of jam or marmalade, spread cottage cheese, low-fat cheese, or fruit on bread.
— Use less sugar than recipes call for when baking.
— Check product packaging for sugars hiding behind pseudonyms: high-fructose corn syrup, fructose, glucose, invert sugar, maltodextrin, maltose, sucrose, dextrose.

adjusts within a short time and this undesirable side effect disappears.

Protein

Proteins are giant molecules built out of individual amino acids. The body breaks the proteins in food down into amino acids and then uses them to construct its own proteins, enzymes, and hormones. A few so-called essential amino acids are necessary for this process to take place: If even just one of them is missing, protein synthesis stops, even though plenty of other proteins may be available. A varied diet is desirable because it provides all the necessary amino acids. In any case, Americans tend to consume twice as much protein as needed. Ideally, no more than a third of the protein we eat should be from animal sources (milk, eggs, meat, fish). The following foods are highest in proteins: soybeans (37 percent), legumes (23 percent), lean meat (16 to 20 percent), eggs (13 percent), cheeses (10 to 35 percent), grains (7 to 12 percent).

Milk

Milk and milk products are an irreplaceable source of calcium. People who are unable to tolerate milk should consume other types of dairy products.

Milk that has undergone no processing is known as raw milk and may contain potentially harmful microorganisms. Historically, tuberculosis bacteria were transmitted in raw milk.

"Regular" milk is pasteurized, meaning all microorganisms have been destroyed. The pasteurization process changes some of the proteins, but leaves most of the milk's vitamins intact.

In homogenized milk most of the proteins have been changed, which accounts for its "boiled" taste. B vitamins and folic acid are considerably reduced, and homogenized milk may contain only a third as much vitamin C as regular milk. After it has been stored for a while, more vitamins are lost.

Eggs

Egg whites contain all the essential amino acids and no fat. Egg yolks, on the other hand, contain lots of fat and cholesterol.

Raw eggs should not be eaten because they contain a substance that neutralizes the vitamin biotin and another that inhibits a certain digestive enzyme. Cooking the egg renders both ingredients ineffective.

New eggs on the market include "cholesterol-neutral" and "omega-DHA" eggs—the former laid by hens who have been fed flaxseed or rapeseed oil, which slightly lower the eggs' cholesterol content, and the latter laid by hens who have been fed algae containing omega-3 fatty acids, which it is hoped will lower the risk of heart and vascular diseases, or at least not increase it. The jury is still out regarding the effectiveness of both.

Salt

The body needs sodium chloride, or table salt, to regulate its salt-water balance. Nutritionists advise against consuming more than 5 grams of salt per day, but the average person eats two to three times that amount, placing extra stress on the kidneys and heart. If you have high blood pressure or heart or kidney disease, limit your salt intake to 3 grams a day.

If your doctor advises you to lower your salt intake or your sodium intake, find out for sure which he or she means. A gram of table salt is not the same as a gram of sodium; it consists of only about two-fifths sodium.

Almost all foods contain at least trace amounts of salt. Although we're used to salting our food, spices often do the job just as well (see Low-Sodium Products, p. 736). Excessive salt is often used to add taste and zip to commercially prepared products. Especially high in salt content are sausages, cured and smoked meats, cheese, chips, mixes, soup, broth, sauces, TV dinners, and bread.

Body Weight

Some people can "pig out" several times a week and stay slim, while others seem to subsist on salad and water but can hardly keep their weight down. Almost all of us are familiar with the frustration of stepping onto the bathroom scale after going on a diet and watching the pointer inching back up.

Medicine has gradually discovered the factors responsible for body weight. They include genetic predisposition, patterns the body learns early in life, diet, and especially exercise.

Two developmental stages in every person's life apparently determine how much the person will weigh as an adult; after these stages are finished, the body will do everything in its power to maintain that weight, no matter what. The first stage occurs during pregnancy: if the mother is watching her calorie intake or her food supply is limited for other reasons, the baby's metabolism will get used to extracting as much nourishment as possible from available food. The second stage occurs at the end of puberty, when the body seems to establish another benchmark for future reference. Henceforth, the person's "normal" weight has been set; he or she who dares to question the body's decision embarks on an almost hopeless lifelong battle.

THE YO-YO EFFECT

Any reduction in food intake is interpreted by the body as life-threatening. In response, it drastically cuts its rate of energy consumption. That's why, after you've been dieting for a while, you reach the inevitable point at which you're only losing a few ounces a week. After you end the diet, your metabolism shifts into high gear to make sure it stores enough fat to survive the next "hunger emergency." After several diets, the body starts anticipating regular famines and extracting as much nourishment as possible from everything you eat, to store it as fat. The end result of a series of diets is that you usually weigh more than before you started.

The "Fat Gene"

Numerous people are significantly overweight due to a disturbance in their weight-maintaining mechanism. This mechanism is regulated by the so-called "fat gene," which has been isolated in humans and mice. If something is wrong with this gene, a hormone in the brain that tells the body to stop storing fat cannot develop sufficiently. As a result, the body keeps on storing fat.

Scientists have developed a synthetic hormone that mimics the effect of the naturally occurring hormone. So far, lab testing on mice has been successful; results in human subjects are not yet available.

"Ideal" Body Weight

There are various ways of calculating so-called "ideal" body weight and height for men and women. Some formulas take body build and other factors into consideration. In general, however, such formulas should be taken with a dose of common sense. If you feel good in your body, you don't need a scale. If the waistband of your pants leaves you room to breathe, if you can climb stairs with no problem, and if you have no health complaints during your regular medical checkups, your weight is probably right for you.

Obesity

Overweight people are generally at higher risk of disease than others. Their risk of dying of coronary heart disease is 60 percent higher than average; dying as the result of an accident, 30 percent higher; dying of liver disease or diabetes complications, two and a half times higher; dying as a result of surgery, two times higher. Diagnostic tests such as ultrasound or X rays are harder to perform and less reliable in obese people.

Forty-five percent of women who unexpectedly fail to menstruate for long periods at a time are significantly overweight. Obesity may occur more frequently in people with unmet or unresolved childhood needs.

Obesity is a risk factor in intestinal, endometrial, and breast cancer.

LOSING WEIGHT

Whether we consider ourselves fat or thin, our individual weight range has been established by our bodies, which will now defend the established weight against all odds. Changing it will require time, patience, and work.

If you want to lose weight, first of all you need to figure out what food means to you. For example, if eating is protecting you from anxiety, loneliness, boredom, or unfulfilled desires, you can't change your habits overnight without these emotions crashing down on you.

To discover which emotions are connected with eating for you, it may help to keep a food diary in which you record every single thing you eat and drink for a certain period of time. Or you may feel more comfortable joining a support group like Weight Watchers or Overeaters Anonymous. Sometimes a short course of psychotherapy can be very useful (see p. 699). Losing weight can have one significant drawback: Many toxins and hazardous substances (see p. 729) are stored in fat, and as fat deposits are metabolized, these substances are released into the blood, potentially resulting in problems such as difficulty concentrating, sleep disorders, headaches, and depression.

For this reason, nursing mothers should under no circumstances try to lose weight: Hazardous substances could enter their milk and cause damage to the baby.

High Activity, Low Fat Intake

Physical activity is the key to getting your body to establish a lower base weight. It has been proven over and over again that decreasing calorie intake while increasing physical activity is the quickest way to lose weight; in the long run, activity is more important than calorie intake.

The activity should be enough to make you sweat, and it should be done on a daily basis, continuously for half an hour.

The long-range goal of a change in diet is to alter your perception of what tastes good. In particular, a craving for fatty foods must absolutely be overcome. Fatty foods account for about 45 percent of conventional diets. Reducing fat intake produces the most impressive weight loss, because if the body is getting only proteins and carbohydrates, it immediately increases its metabolic rate. Fats, on the other hand, burn slowly. If you eat too much fat today, it will not be burned completely until all the body's fat deposits are gradually metabolized.

The path to a sensible reducing diet, therefore, leads away from fats whenever possible, and toward vegetables, fruits, potatoes, pasta, or bread. You won't need your calorie counter if you can stick to this basic rule.

Fad Diets

Every spring, fabulous new diets appear, promising instant weight loss. One look at the average person on the street, however, will tell you that all these fad diets can't possibly work—and will also show you why there's such a large market for them.

Be skeptical of any diet that claims you can eat "all you want" of certain foods, while avoiding others. By now, there seems to be a fad diet for every type of food.

Any diet that doesn't advocate eating small quantities of a variety of wholesome, balanced foods is bound to fail, at least over the long term (see The Yo-Yo Effect, p. 727).

Fasting

If you eat nothing at all, you will lose about a pound of weight a day under normal conditions. Before you consider fasting for a few days, however, consult your health-care provider to make sure this is advisable in your case. Fasting for periods as long as a week should only be attempted under close medical supervision.

When you fast, your metabolism changes completely. At first, it produces energy out of reserves of protein; only later does it begin to burn more fat than protein. Medical opinion is divided over the risks, especially to the heart, of significant protein loss. Fasting often causes sleep disorders; gout and kidney stones can result if you don't drink enough liquids. At least 3 quarts of liquid a day are absolutely necessary when fasting. The quick weight loss produced by fasting may provide the motivation needed for you to make lasting dietary changes; if not, however, fasting, like repeated dieting, will ultimately lead to weight gain.

Liquid Diets

Liquid or formula diets consist of powdered mixes containing nutritional ingredients and vitamins, minerals, trace elements, and fiber, not exceeding 100 calories per 3.5 ounces. The powder is mixed with water and drunk either cold or warm, taking the place of food. After a while, liquid diets get monotonous. A limited variety of flavors is available, and there's nothing to satisfy the need to chew. They are also relatively expensive. Long-term success is unlikely with this sort of diet, since it does nothing to alter your tastes or nutritional habits.

Energy Providers

Fats, carbohydrates and proteins provide the body with energy in the form of heat. The heat is measured in kilojoules or kilocalories; the common term for the unit is calories.

1 gram of fat provides about 9 calories.
1 gram of carbohydrate provides about 4 calories.
1 gram of protein provides about 4 calories.
1 gram of alcohol provides about 7 calories.

Hazardous Substances in Food

Not all toxins found in foods are necessarily foreign substances: The characteristic taste and smell of bitter almonds, for example, is produced by the hydrogen cyanide they contain, and green spots on potatoes and tomatoes are due to the toxin solanine and should not be eaten. Many contaminants do enter food from the outside, however; these include disease-causing bacteria such as salmonella or enterohemorrhagic *Echerichia coli* (EHEC), mold toxins such as aflatoxin, or carcinogens such as benzpyrene, which are produced during the preparation or processing of certain foods.

Other substances that compromise health to a greater or lesser degree are found in food as a result of environmental and production conditions.

BACTERIAL ILLNESSES

Bacteria are present in all raw or untreated foods; which bacteria, and how many, depends on production conditions. Salmonella enters poultry intestines primarily through feed containing infected animal parts. After slaughter, bacteria are spread from one infected animal carcass to others in the same tank.

Enterohemorrhagic *E. coli* (EHEC), a malignant form of the otherwise harmless intestinal bacterium *E. coli,* can cause serious illness, especially in children, through changes in the blood and kidney malfunction. The pathogens are transmitted most commonly but not exclusively by raw, untreated milk and beef.

Heat destroys most germs—how effectively depends on temperature and length of exposure. In this respect, cooking or heating foods in the microwave is less effective than the more conventional methods of boiling or broiling.

Bovine Spongiform Encephalopathy (BSE)

In early 1996 the news broke that over the previous 2 years, 55 people in England had died of Creutzfeldt-Jakob disease (CJD), which destroys the brain and causes death within a year. An official inquiry was able to establish that it was transmitted from cows to humans. In cattle, the disease caused by the same pathogen is known as bovine spongiform encephalopathy (BSE).

The route of transmission was probably a series of events starting in sheep, crossing to cattle, and ending up in humans.

Sheep, Cattle, Humans

The sheep disease known as scrapie destroys the brain, resulting in death. It is caused by a recently discovered infectious agent known as a prion. For years, the offal of infected sheep, insufficiently sterilized since 1979 as a cost-cutting measure, was ground into filler and sold as cheap cattle fodder.

Increasing numbers of cattle became infected with BSE caused by a malignant strain of scrapie. The disease soon appeared in other animals also fed with infected sheep remains. By March 1996, the epidemic had claimed 160,000 head of cattle in England.

The brains of these infected cattle were used in food for general human consumption until 1988 and in baby food until February 1989.

Only in 1994 did the European Community prohibit feeding this type of filler to herbivorous animals. Since 1996 there has been a prohibition on export of cattle, veal, and ground meat from Great Britain and Switzerland.

Although the connection between eating BSE-infected meat and contracting CJD has not been definitively proved, the indices definitely point to avoiding British beef and beef products. Beef consumption has since dropped.

The infectious agent in question is not affected by boiling, broiling, or the use of disinfectants. Its presence in humans or animals can be determined only after death.

Since it takes about twelve years for infected people to manifest signs of CJD, only time will tell whether the misguided use of animal protein to feed herbivores will cause another epidemic in humans.

Proper Food Handling

— Defrost frozen poultry in refrigerator. Discard thawed fluid.
— Thoroughly wash hands and work surfaces after handling uncooked poultry and raw eggs.
— For recipes using raw eggs (mayonnaise, tiramisu) use only fresh, refrigerated eggs.
— Cook meat and eggs thoroughly.
— Avoid unpasteurized milk and cheese; pasteurizing kills all germs but retains most vitamins.

THRESHOLD VALUES: "MAXIMUM PERMISSIBLE DOSES" AREN'T PROTECTIVE

Residues of hazardous substances in food are rated as harmless by the food-regulating industry if they don't exceed legally stipulated levels. However, these levels or threshold values are not absolute: They are entirely dependent on the current extent of scientific knowledge, and on varying interpretations of that knowledge. We still don't know the effects of various combinations of hazardous substances on the body. Moreover, the definition of the maximum permissible dose of a substance is always a compromise between the interests of all involved, including those for whom low limits mean financial gain.

Threshold values are calculated according to averages—the average dose an average person with average eating habits would receive in an average affected geographical area. Conditions for actual individuals, however, can vary widely from this theoretical norm.

Some prepared foods cannot be sold unless their content of certain substances is below limits set by the World Health Organization. However, if at the same meal you eat several different items, each containing quantities of hazardous substances just under the legal limit, your total consumption of toxins at that meal will exceed the daily limit. If you know which products are high in hazardous substances, you can keep your exposure to a minimum through eating a varied diet. Unfortunately, the legal guidelines are not always complied with by food producers (see Hormones, p. 732; Antibiotics, p. 661).

Lead

This heavy metal interferes with production of red blood cells and affects the nervous system.

Lead affects the developing fetus. Children born to women living in areas with heavy lead pollution tend to be developmentally disabled intellectually.

Sources: rust-proofing solvents; lead housing (as for pipes); lead-processing industries; garbage incinerators. In the home: lead pipes (see Drinks, p. 736), lead-glazed pottery.

Cadmium

Cadmium accumulates in the body. It takes about 30 years to expel half of the bioburden. Even small doses of cadmium affect fertility and immune function and cause nervous system disorders.

Sources: the metal-alloy industry; synthetic dyes; battery parts; incineration of these products. Cadmium is also used in fertilizers.

Mercury

Humans and animals metabolize this metal into a highly toxic compound that can cause brain damage and paralyze nerves. Even unborn children are in danger. Fertility may be affected in women who are exposed to mercury vapor from working in dental offices.

Sources: waste water from power plants and paper factories; incinerators; batteries.

Foods to avoid

— Kidneys (heavy metals, especially cadmium)
— Beef and pork liver (heavy metals, especially cadmium)
— Game such as rabbit, hare and deer (heavy metals, especially cadmium, mercury, radioactive cesium)
— Wild mushrooms (heavy metals, especially cadmium, mercury, radioactive cesium)
— Predatory fish such as salmon (halogenated hydrocarbons, dioxin)

Foods to eat infrequently

— Calf liver (heavy metals, especially cadmium; hormones)
— Fish from the North Sea or Mediterranean (heavy metals, especially mercury)
— Fish from inland waterways (heavy metals)

Foods containing significant amounts of hazardous substances (if conventionally grown)

Endive	(Nitrate)
Salad greens	(Nitrate)
Fennel	(Nitrate)
Cabbage	(Nitrate)
Potatoes	(Nitrate)
Kohlrabi	(Nitrate)
Boston lettuce	(Nitrate)
Watercress	(Nitrate)
Swiss chard	(Nitrate)
Mushrooms, wild	(Cadmium, mercury)
Radish	(Nitrate)
Daikon radish	(Nitrate)
Rhubarb	(Nitrate)
Beets	(Nitrate)
Celery	(Cadmium)
Spinach	(Nitrate, cadmium)
Savoy cabbage	(Nitrate)

Nitrates, Nitrites

Nitrates are converted to nitrites by bacteria in the mouth; nitrites are metabolized into nitrosamines when combined with protein components in the stomach. Because nitrosamines are toxic and carcinogenic, nitrates are considered a hazardous substance. High levels of nitrates increase the risk of goiter (see p. 494).

Sources: vegetables (spinach, Boston lettuce, beets, radishes) and drinking water. Extensive use of fertilizers and liquid manure increases the level of nitrates in the soil. Nitrites are used in cured or smoked meat and sausages.

Warning: Infants are especially sensitive to nitrites, which can change their blood composition and cause cyanosis. Never feed children nitrate-containing food (spinach, carrots) that has been reheated, thus causing nitrates to be transformed into harmful nitrites.

Pesticides

Almost all pesticides are believed to cause cancer through blood damage (see Leukemia, p. 349); they may affect fertility and can cause birth defects.

Sources: Because consumers demand unblemished, perfect-looking fruits and vegetables, toxins of various kinds are used to destroy anything and everything that could reduce their appeal.

The net result is that we eat the chemical residues in produce, as well as in the meat of animals fed with pesticide-sprayed plant matter. Meat is not inspected with this criterion in mind.

Antibiotics

Feeding animals antibiotics accelerates the development of pathogens resistant to common medications. These resistant germs pose an increased danger to humans as medications become less effective; the germs continue to develop resistance in humans who eat antibiotic-treated animal products.

People who are especially sensitive to antibiotics may react as if they themselves had taken the drug; even traces can trigger allergic reactions.

Sources: Antibiotics are given to animals to limit the risk of infection in overcrowded stalls, and to promote growth. Although a specified time must elapse between the animals' last antibiotic dose and their slaughter, inspections have shown that 1 percent of all meat tested contains antibiotics; in veal the figure exceeds 15 percent.

Hormones

To date, there is no evidence that the use of sex hormones, or anabolic steroids, in beef cattle production is harmful to humans. The hormones are used to accelerate growth rates. Although use of these hormones is legal in the United States and South America, it is banned in Europe.

Other Medications

Heart medication and sedatives are injected into pigs and cattle so they survive transportation to the slaughterhouse. Often they have not metabolized that medication before being killed. The part of the animal receiving the injection may still contain high levels of medication.

Medication residues in meat may have a long-term effect, possibly causing genetic mutations or cancer.

Radiation

The acute threat of radiation exposure following the 1986 Chernobyl nuclear reactor accident is past. However, more foods are radioactive today than before Chernobyl, particularly game and wild mushrooms. Levels of radioactivity in food depend on its place of origin.

For dangers of low-level radiation, see Radioactivity, p. 777.

REDUCING HAZARDOUS SUBSTANCES IN FOOD

Sensible buying and preparation of food can ensure a well-balanced diet. The exact meaning of "sensible" keeps changing; some guidelines that were valid only a few years ago already need modifying or strengthening.

Buying in Season

Consumers have come to expect the year-round availability of all kinds of fruits and vegetables. This has led to intensive use of fertilizers and a variety of toxins to make the forcing of greenhouse harvests economically viable.

Not all these toxins can be washed or peeled off, so we eat the chemicals along with the produce. Hothouse vegetables (e.g., lettuce, radishes, kohlrabi, and others) can contain nitrate levels twice as high as vegetables grown outdoors.

Imported products are sometimes grown under conditions potentially even more problematic than those in the United States. Legal standards of protection from high levels of toxins may not be enforced, or may not be a priority, in less industrialized countries.

In addition, produce must be harvested unripe so it can be transported without spoiling; because vitamins don't have time to develop, this always means less nutritious food. Often such produce also contains more chemical additives to survive transportation and ripen artificially at market.

Reducing Your Intake of Hazardous Substances

— Avoid imported products.
— Buy in season (see above).
— If possible, buy only products from growers whose practices you are familiar with.
— Do not combine high-risk foods in one meal.
— Do not eat more than 7 ounces of high-risk foods per week.
— Do not reheat or keep warm nitrate-containing foods: this process creates nitrites.
— Do not melt cheese over nitrate-containing vegetables or cured foods: carcinogenic nitrosamines may result.

Meat
— Veal that is light in color is anemic and comes from calves who have hardly ever seen daylight or green grass.
— Ninety percent of frankfurters, sausages, etc. are cured and contain nitrites (see Nitrates, p. 731).

Fish
— Non-predatory fish from the Atlantic and Pacific are relatively low in toxins. The leaner the fish, the fewer pesticides it has accumulated.

Fruit
— Wash thoroughly in hot water to reduce lead residue, nitrates, sprays.
— Rub thoroughly dry to remove lead; peel thickly.

Vegetables, including lettuce
— Discard outer leaves to reduce lead residue, nitrates, sprays.
— Discard tough centers and stems in lettuce, cabbage and similar vegetables to reduce nitrates.
— Blanch or boil vegetables; discard water to reduce nitrates, sprays.
— If you grow fruit and vegetables and live near a high-traffic road or in a polluted area, don't grow leafy vegetables that may contain high levels of lead.

Grains
— Only use organically grown whole grains. In conventionally grown products, toxins are concentrated in the outermost layer of the grain.

Food Additives

Hundreds of chemical substances function as food additives. They include preservatives, coloring agents, thickeners, sweeteners, taste enhancers, and more. Each one has its own code or number. Most prepared foods today contain additives and artificial flavors, of which there are over 2,000.

All additives are required by law to be listed, by name or number, as ingredients on food packaging.

Some additives are necessary for the production of prepared foods, but many are unnecessary, and the effectiveness of some is even in doubt. Coloring agents and some preservatives may trigger allergies; some may even promote carcinogenicity in other substances in food.

Food Colors/Dyes

Used in: Sweetened foods, desserts, fruit jams, jellies and conserves, seafood products, and liqueurs.
Required: No.
Disadvantages: Synthetic food colors often trigger allergies. Food colors are often used to enhance the appearance of food beyond its actual level of quality.

Preservatives

Used in: Salads, marinades, mustard, preserved fish, margarine, lemonade, jams and marmalades, marzipan, and sliced bread.
Required: Not if perishable food is bought fresh and used within a short time.
Advantages: Foods keep longer.
Disadvantages: Some may be hazardous to health.
Warning for people with allergies: Benzoic acid and its salts, benzoates, may trigger allergies. They may be used in mayonnaise, salads, marinades, and vegetable and fruit conserves.

Sulfur dioxide and its compounds (sulfites) may trigger nausea, headaches, and diarrhea in sensitive people. In asthmatics it may trigger choking attacks. Sulfur dioxide may also enhance the action of carcinogens. It is found in dried fruits and vegetables, potato products, jams and marmalades, wines and beers.

Natamycin is a fungicide added to hard cheese. It is also used as a medication and is known to be allergenic. People who are allergic to the medication may therefore have an allergic reaction to hard cheese.

Antioxidants

Usefulness: They keep foods from combining with atmospheric oxygen and spoiling quickly. For instance, fats with added antioxidants don't turn rancid as fast. Vitamin E is an antioxidant.
Required: No.
Disadvantages: None are known.

Emulsifiers

Required: In order for fats or oils to be mixed with water.
Disadvantages: None are known.

Taste-Enhancing Substances

Required: No.
Disadvantages: Sensitive people may react to taste enhancers such as monosodium glutamate (MSG) with symptoms like numbness in the neck area and below it, headaches, dizziness, weakness, heart palpitations, or a tight sensation in face and chest.

Sweeteners (Aspartame, Cyclamates, Saccharin, etc.)

Used in: Beverages, desserts, yogurt, "lite" products, and table sweeteners.
Advantages: Artificial sweeteners can be helpful for people who want to lose weight but can't do without sweets. In moderation, they are probably not harmful, but drinking more than 2 liters of artificially sweetened soda, perhaps in addition to an artificially sweetened snack, will easily put you out of the "moderate" range.
Disadvantages: Aspartame is still being tested for carcinogenicity. It has been suspected of causing a rare form of brain tumor. People on a phenylalanine-free diet should avoid aspartame. Saccharin may trigger carcinogenicity in other substances. Cyclamates were associated with bladder tumors in animals, and banned in the United States in 1969.

Sugar Substitutes

Used in: Candy, chewing gum that "doesn't promote tooth decay," beverages, diabetic products (see p. 735).
Required: No.
Usefulness: Helpful for people who can't do without candy and gum, but want to protect their teeth.

Advantages: Sugar substitutes can be advantageous for diabetics because they keep blood-sugar levels from rising too quickly.

Disadvantages: All are high in calories and may cause diarrhea.

Expiration Dates

All prepared, packaged, and canned foods must be dated. The date, however, neither guarantees the food's good quality beforehand nor its inedibility afterwards. "Expired" foods may still be sold. Make sure you not only check the date but also look for signs of spoilage when buying these products.

Returning Food Items

If you notice spoiled groceries when unpacking them at home, you should immediately return them to the store where they were purchased. It helps to have your receipt handy.

Food Preservation

Foods are susceptible to bacteria and fungi. Mold fungi produce the most poisonous and most carcinogenic substances known, which spread especially fast in products containing water. Always throw out moldy foods in their entirety (i.e., don't just remove the moldy part).

Foods that require long-term storage must therefore be preserved. Common methods of food preservation include cooking with sugar (jam), salting (cheese, fish, meat), pickling in vinegar (sweet pickles), or fermentation (sauerkraut, sour pickles). Heating, freezing and chemicals (see Preservatives, p. 733) also preserve food.

Canning

Whether you can foods at home or buy factory-canned foods, between 5 and 50 percent of vitamins are lost in the canning process. Storing cans for 1 to 2 years destroys another 20 percent of their vitamin content. Additives used in commercially canned products may be listed on labels (see Food Additives, p. 733). These usually include salt for vegetables and sugar for fruits.

Metal cans are better for canning than glass jars, which allow light through. The contents of an opened can should be used as quickly as possible; any leftovers should be stored in a nonmetal container.

Freezing

Vegetables are blanched (briefly immersed in boiling water) before being frozen. The heat destroys some of the vitamins, and minerals are drained off with the water, but the loss is much smaller than with canning. After 3 months in the freezer, vitamin C has been reduced by 2 to 28 percent; after six months, between 13 and 56 percent. Frozen produce may retain more vitamins than produce bought "fresh" at the supermarket, because it is frozen immediately after picking, while "fresh" produce has to stay "fresh" while traveling great distances to the market and then to your home before finally being eaten. Frozen foods also have the advantage of containing levels of nitrates and other hazardous substances certified to be at or below legal limits.

Frozen meat should be used as soon as it is thawed, and leftovers should neither be reheated nor refrozen. Freezing food consumes the most energy of all food storage methods.

Precooked Meals

These are preserved by cold (frozen) or heat (canned).

Due to the long storage capability of ready-made or prepared foods, vitamin loss is considerable.

Food scraps and leftovers are often ingredients in "gourmet" prepared foods: for example, ground fish with bones may be transformed by food additives into a presentable and appetizing dish. People who rely mostly on this type of food for their daily meals should make sure they get plenty of fresh fruits and vegetables; deficiencies are unavoidable otherwise.

Irradiation

Gamma radiation from cobalt-60 is now used to preserve easily spoiled foods such as fish, meat, fruits, vegetables, and herbs, and to keep potatoes and onions from sprouting. Neither the food nor the packaging becomes radioactive as a result. Irradiation destroys cells' genetic components and proteins. The higher the life form, the more harmful irradiation is. For this reason, insects and parasites are killed at lower dosages than those required to kill bacteria. Viruses are not affected by irradiation.

Irradiation destroys some amino and fatty acids, as well as vitamins, although these changes are invisible to the consumer. Smell, taste, color, and consistency may also change; this is corrected by additives where possible. The health effects of consuming large quantities of irradiated food are still not known.

Your eyes and nose normally tell you whether or not food is spoiled, but irradiated foods look and smell fine even when they're spoiled. The bacterial botulism spores, which cause food poisoning, are not killed by irradiation.

Today 80 to 90 percent of poultry is contaminated with microbes. If animals were fed, handled, and cared for with more attention to hygiene than to profits, irradiation would not be necessary to kill the microbes. Even a salmonella-infected chicken won't make you sick if you prepare and cook it properly and thoroughly (see Bacterial Illnesses, p. 729).

Dietetic Foods

Very few diseases still require specific diets, such as a low-protein diet for kidney-functioning deficiencies. Most restricted diets prescribed in the past are considered unnecessary by today's standards.

Instead, we have diet foods and "lite" products that encourage us to "indulge without guilt" and on which we spend huge amounts of money. We are led to believe that by eating and drinking these products we are somehow getting better nutrition, even though we're still eating too much—in fact, sometimes more than before—of the wrong kind of food.

"LITE," "LOW FAT" PRODUCTS

The terms "light," "lite" or "low-fat" are not trademarked; they can be used to describe just about anything. Only when "lite" is used to describe calorie content does it have a specific meaning, namely that the product in question contains at least 40 percent fewer calories than normal. A product calling itself "low calorie" may not contain more than 50 calories per 100 grams; low-calorie beverages may contain only 20 calories per 100 ml.

A reduction in calories is usually achieved by pumping a product full of air to increase its volume (e.g., foamy desserts), adding water (e.g., "low-fat" margarine), or substituting low-calorie chemicals for naturally occurring ingredients (e.g., "lite" sausage).

Many of these technologically fabricated meals fill the stomach, but are not really satisfying. The brain fails to register a sufficient amount of fat consumption to send the "stop eating" command, with the result that the consumer keeps eating, secure in the illusion that this food "won't make you fat." After a while, alas, the bathroom scale shows you actually weigh more than you used to, and you're no closer to effective, balanced nutritional habits (see p. 723).

The healthy alternatives to these products are nature's "low-fat" foods: fruits, vegetables, and grain products.

"Diet" Fats

"Diet" margarine contains at least 40 percent unsaturated fats. Products labeled "rich in unsaturated fats" contain at least 50 percent unsaturated fats. "Diet oils" contain at least 60 percent unsaturated fats. These all contain vitamin E.

Natural alternatives to these products can be found in thistle-seed oil or sunflower-seed oil, which are rich in unsaturated fats.

Fat Substitutes

The recently released Olestra fat substitute tastes and acts like actual fat. It is made out of vegetable oil but transformed into a molecule impermeable to digestive enzymes, which leaves the body without a trace. Once it is eliminated, normal septic systems cannot break it down. When Olestra is eliminated, fat-soluble vitamins such as vitamins A, D, E and K are eliminated as well, so they are artificially added to the product. Abdominal cramping and diarrhea have been reported as side effects.

DIABETIC FOODS

Diabetes doctors do not look fondly upon diabetic foods, since the most important treatment for diabetes consists of weight loss and exercise (see p. 486). So-called "lite" or "low fat" products will usually serve diabetics just as well as "diabetic" products. Diabetic chocolate contains just as much fat as regular chocolate, so it won't help you lose weight. The same goes for many other diabetic foods.

The one distinguishing factor of foods labeled "diabetic" is that the sugars they contain must not cause blood-sugar levels to rise too quickly. However, many foods containing sugar substitutes (see p. 733) contain just as many calories as regular foods.

LOW-SODIUM PRODUCTS

People who need to restrict their sodium intake would do best to avoid prepared foods entirely, due to their undeclared salt content. Salty products (see Salt, p. 727) should be shunned, and the salt shaker should disappear from the table.

Products are allowed to be called "reduced-salt" or "reduced-sodium" if they contain less than 1.25 grams of salt, or less than 0.5 gram of sodium, per 100 grams. They may be called "low-sodium" if they contain less than 0.12 gram of sodium, or less than 0.3 gram of salt, per 100 grams. They may be called "sodium-free" if they contain less than 0.04 gram of sodium, or less than 0.1 gram of salt, per 100 grams.

Salt Substitutes

Salt substitutes are usually about 40 percent potassium and may contain iodine as well. People who need to watch their potassium intake should avoid these products, as should people with kidney insufficiency. The taste of all salt substitutes leaves much to be desired.

IODIZED SALT

Using iodized salt helps prevent iodine deficiency. Some iodized salt also contains fluoride.

People who need to watch their iodine intake (see Goiter, p. 494) should read all labels carefully. With some products, it is hard to tell for sure whether iodized salt is an ingredient.

Eating consciously and including saltwater fish in your diet will cover daily iodine requirements without iodized salt (see Trace Elements, p. 747).

Feeding a Crowd

The way meals are prepared in modern institutions such as factories, schools, hospitals, prisons, and nursing homes can hardly be referred to as "cooking." Cafeterias often simply thaw, reheat and serve precooked, ready-to-serve meals shipped in by a food service.

The quality of these meals is less apparent to the eater than their taste. Surveying an institutional menu for a few weeks, however, will reveal the degree to which general dietary and nutritional recommendations are followed.

Institutional meals are usually planned according to the lowest common denominator theory: They need to taste good to the "average" person while costing as little as possible, with predictably poor results. Yet it doesn't have to be this way. Cafeteria food could be much better than it is today, without costing significantly more, if certain simple rules were followed.

If you work in an institution and would like to see its food service improved, working toward the ideal of more wholesome meals is a worthy goal. This doesn't mean throwing the baby out with the bathwater. Starting from wherever you are, gradual changes toward balanced, whole-foods nutrition can be amazingly effective.

FAST FOOD

There are many reasons for resisting the temptation to grab a bite at a fast food restaurant. From a nutritional point of view, burgers, fries, hot dogs, tacos, pizza, and so on provide too much fat, too much protein, and just plain too much to eat. If fast food is a staple for you, at least make sure your other meals help balance out your diet; otherwise, nutritional deficiencies are likely to result.

If you frequently eat at fast food chains, you can make more sensible food choices:

— Order a roast beef sandwich instead of a burger.
— If you're going for a burger, think small, not gigantic.
— Skip the mayonnaise.
— Have a salad on the side.
— Drink milk or seltzer instead of a soft drink or shake.
— Skip the fries and order a baked potato or roll instead.

Drinks

Drinking is an important part of the diet.

Children are very thirsty creatures. A 2-year-old drinks about as much as an adult: about a quart and a half of liquid a day. Six-year-olds need over 2 quarts a day; teens over age 14 need over 2.5 quarts.

Although older people often don't feel thirsty, they should still take care to drink at least 1.5 quarts of liquid a day. It may be helpful to keep a written log of liquid intake, to be sure you are drinking enough.

When we feel thirsty, it means the body is asking for water. Tap water and mineral water have no calories. Tea and coffee are, in effect, flavored and colored water; if we add sugar and/or milk, we're adding calories. Good thirst quenchers and sources of minerals are fruit juices diluted with water; all other drinks qualify as calorie-containing liquid foods.

Tap Water

Safety standards for tap water are calculated based on daily consumption over an entire lifetime. Regular testing of town and city water assures the purity of public drinking water supplies, but people who drink well water have the responsibility of getting their water tested regularly as well.

Nitrates and lead are common hazards; for information on these, see Hazardous Substances in Food, p. 729.

Some harmful substances get into drinking water not at the source, but during the trip into your home. Have your tap water tested if it

— Comes from your own well
— Passes through very old pipes
— Passes through lead pipes
— Is used to prepare infant formula or baby food

Very old water pipes or lead pipes should be replaced.

Tap Water and Infants

Nitrates are especially harmful for infants. Once in the body they develop into nitrites and combine with the blood's hemoglobin, potentially leading to nitrite poisoning (cyanosis). If your water comes from a public supply and contains over 50 mg/L of nitrates, you should use bottled water to prepare your baby's food and drinks. Acid water (with a pH below 6.7) can leach copper out of copper pipes and cause life-threatening liver damage in infants. In this case, too, stick to bottled water.

Water fed to infants and small children should have a lead content under 10 micrograms per liter (mg/L).

Water Hardness

Drinking water is an important source of calcium and magnesium. However, since home appliances often require soft (low-calcium) water, public water supplies are usually softened.

Using home water softeners is not advisable since they replace calcium and magnesium with sodium. Too much sodium may increase blood pressure. Infants are especially at risk.

Water filters for home use, e.g. Brita filters, will help remove sodium, calcium, and lead but will allow magnesium to pass. It is possible, however, that such filtered water may contain more bacteria than water straight from the tap.

Mineral Water

Mineral water comes out of the earth containing a variety of minerals; many different mineral levels and combinations exist, depending on the source of the water.

Mineral water may develop high levels of microorganisms if too much time elapses between bottling and consumption. People with compromised immune systems may be placed at risk. The probability of high microorganism levels is greater if the water is bottled in plastic rather than glass. Therefore, opened bottles of mineral water should be finished as quickly as possible and unused portions should be stored in the refrigerator.

Fruit Juices, Nectar, Lemonade, etc.

Beverages like these are actually liquid foods because of their high calorie content. Since they often contain additives and are highly processed, however, they aren't very nutritious foods.

If you want to drink "pure" fruit juice, your only option is making your own juice. Commercially produced juices usually contain varying amounts of sugar. You may purchase sugar-free juices at a health food store and some supermarkets.

"Lite" artificial lemonade contains little or no sugar.

Let the buyer beware: "Sugar free" products may contain sugar substitutes (see p. 733), which may be advantageous for diabetics but contain almost as many calories as sugared drinks. To qualify as "low-calorie," a beverage can contain no more than 200 calories per liter.

Colas

These brownish liquids are basically sugar water plus caffeine, phosphoric acid, and a host of chemical additives. The caffeine content of a liter of cola is equivalent to about one and a quarter cups of coffee. Although cola doesn't exactly qualify as harmful to health, it has no part in a sensible, balanced diet.

Bitters and Tonics

Despite its bitter taste, tonic water is basically sugared lemonade containing almost 4 ounces of sugar and up to 85 mg of quinine per liter. Europeans colonizing Africa invented bitters as a malaria preventative.

Baby Food

During the first six months of life, infants require nothing more than their mother's milk (see Nursing, p. 584) or, if that is not an option, infant formula. The later all other forms of nourishment are introduced, the better for the child.

The more closely infant formula resembles the mother's milk, the better the baby will digest it and the more nutrients he/she will derive from it. Formula is sold in different versions suitable for different ages. Some kinds contain corn or rice starch or maltodextrin, which may cause babies to gain weight too fast.

If you are mixing formula with water, make sure your water is suitable (see Tapwater and Infants, p. 73).

Solid Foods

Below a certain age, babies are unable to digest some foods. After a certain age, on the other hand, they should have some foods regularly in order to ensure complete nutrition.

If a baby food is labeled "From 6 months," it means a baby over 6 months can normally digest the food without problems, but it doesn't mean the baby needs this food in his or her diet. Babies do not require a varied menu. It is quite enough for toddlers simply to sample the family's meals at the dinner table.

It is common for solid foods to be introduced into a baby's diet much too soon, with the following potential risks:

— The baby's digestive system may become burdened by foods it can barely digest, causing cramping and bloating.
— Food allergies may develop. The risk of allergies is greater the earlier solids are introduced and the more varied the diet; exotic fruits and vegetables should be avoided.
— The baby may gain too much weight from being given too many carbohydrates.

In addition, if you are feeding a baby older than 6 months commercial baby food

— The baby may be getting used to very sweet foods, since most products are overly sweetened.
— The baby may be ingesting too many vitamins, since almost all products are artificially vitamin enriched.
— The baby may be ingesting too much salt, since baby food is salted to taste "right" to adults.

From Bottle or Breast to Table Foods

— In general, infants don't need solid foods before they are six months old.
— Single grains are usually introduced first, followed by one fruit or vegetable at a time to make any food allergies or sensitivities easier to spot.
— By age two, children can eat like adults, with food cut into bite-size pieces. Introduce tomatoes, legumes, and cabbage carefully—they may initially cause bloating.

Store-Bought vs. Homemade

Commercially prepared baby food is not only convenient, its ingredients are also subject to high standards. Fresh fruits and vegetables are processed immediately after harvesting and screened for nitrates and pesticide residues.

On the other hand, with homemade baby food you know exactly what's in it because you put it there. You can give your baby fruits or vegetables that aren't common in commercial products, e.g., potatoes. Make sure you buy high-quality organic produce whenever possible, to protect your baby against potentially harmful chemical residues. Carrots, the most important "baby vegetable," are unfortunately big nitrate collectors.

Children's Energy Requirements

Children need more high-energy foods than adults do. A child aged 5 to 7 needs as many daily calories as a grown woman doing light physical work. From age 10 until after puberty, the caloric requirement sometimes equals that of an adult doing hard labor.

Children's appetites tend to fluctuate more the younger they are. It's a safe bet, however, that three meals a day won't cover their energy requirements; morning and afternoon snacks are a must. Good snacks include whole-grain bread with nut butter or cheese, raw vegetables and fruit, dried fruits, nuts, milk, and yogurt.

Nutrition of the Elderly

When you're older everything tends to slow down a little, including digestion. Special diets are not necessary, however, as long as you're eating healthy, balanced meals. If you have trouble chewing, fruits, vegetables and nuts can be pureed, and whole grains can be consumed as flours. Eating several smaller meals a day instead of three big ones will keep the stomach from overloading.

Beware of the following claims, used to market products to senior citizens:
— "Seniors need more protein." Your protein requirements may indeed be slightly higher now, but since conventional diets are already too high in protein, this need not be a concern.
— "Seniors need more calcium." An adequate intake of dairy products and vegetables will meet this requirement.

Seniors also need to pay attention to the interaction between any medications they may be taking and the foods they eat. Discuss this with your doctor.

If you don't feel like cooking, either subscribe to an elderly-nutrition program such as Meals On Wheels or buy ready-to-eat meals, preferably frozen. This may be more expensive than eating bread and butter three times a day, but the nutritional advantages far outweigh the monetary cost.

Vitamins, Mineral Substances, and Trace Elements

Vitamins, minerals, and trace elements are essential to sustain life. Each must be available in sufficient quantity. To ensure this, the body has minimum requirements for each substance. If one is insufficient, oversupplying another won't make up for its lack. If the delicate balance of substances is disturbed by too much of one, the functional effect of other substances is affected.

A balanced diet will provide the body with all of these substances in sufficient quantity and proper ratio over the long term.

Product marketing is fond of attributing to vitamins all sorts of qualities they don't have. Vitamins

---

Deficiencies may occur
— If you eat enough food, but the wrong kind (see Balanced Nutrition, p. 723).
— In conjunction with certain diseases. The deficiency is likely to be cured during treatment for the illness.
— If you take certain medications. Read medication labels or inserts to see whether deficiencies may result from its use, or ask your doctor or pharmacist.
— If you need more vitamins and minerals than the recommended daily allowance (RDA). Reasons for this can include:
— Pregnancy
— Breastfeeding
— Alcoholism

---

cannot in fact make you more energetic or better able to handle stress, or make your kids smarter, or ward off colds or cancer, or bring happiness or prolong youth. The first signs of a vitamin deficiency are often fatigue, difficulty concentrating, and lowered resistance to infections. However, only rarely can it actually be established whether these symptoms are due to vitamin deficiency or other factors. There is no evidence of the curative effects of vitamins, minerals, and trace elements, even in situations of duress such as illness or stress. Megadoses of vitamins, on the other hand, can have negative side effects (see table of vitamins, p. 748).

How Much Is Enough?
The recommended daily allowances (RDA) apply to healthy adults and allow for individual variations, but not for the fact that some people's needs may be greater at certain times. For instance, smokers require more vitamin C than nonsmokers; at times of extreme stress, such as after surgery, the need for trace elements increases.

The recommended allowance need not be taken daily; it reflects optimal average daily intake over the long term.

If you suspect that you're not getting your RDA, consult your doctor.

If it is established that you do have a deficiency
— Increase your intake of those foods that provide the missing substances.
— If your doctor determines that you need to take a certain substance as a supplement, make sure you take it as a single supplement rather than in combination.

— Your doctor will monitor your treatment and take you off supplements when the desired results are achieved and your reserves are back to normal.

VITAMINS

Only vitamins D and K are produced by the body itself. All others must be provided through diet. The body stores vitamins so that it can make up for deficiencies in the short term. Because the average Western diet today is varied, serious vitamin deficiencies are rarely seen. Nevertheless, some people don't get enough of some vitamins simply because they don't eat a balanced diet.

Vitamins are either water- or fat-soluble. Water-soluble vitamins (B^1, B^2, B^6, B^{12}, folic acid, niacin, pantothenic acid, and C) are found primarily in foods high in carbohydrates. The body can rid itself of a surplus of these vitamins. However, an oversupply can still have negative side effects (e.g., vitamin B^6). Fat-soluble vitamins (A, D, E, and K) are found in fatty foods. Excess amounts are stored in the body rather than being excreted. This can result in poisoning.

Be careful not to simultaneously
— Eat a vitamin-rich diet and/or
— Consume vitamin-enriched foods and/or
—Take vitamin supplements or cod-liver oil.

Multivitamins

Multivitamins are combinations of various vitamins and sometimes other substances. Taking them for short periods can be beneficial in certain situations, such as
— Weight-loss programs
— An unavoidably unbalanced diet
— Serious gastrointestinal or liver diseases

Vitamin-Enriched Products

Eating vitamin-enriched foods may appear to be a ticket to good health, yet often products are enriched with vitamins because their natural nutritional value has been lost in processing. Added vitamins are unnecessary as long as you eat a balanced diet. Common vitamin-enriched products include
— Fruit juice, lemonade, soda
— Candy, granola bars, other sweets
— Jam, jelly, marmalade
—Yogurt, instant pudding, and similar prepared dairy foods

— Margarine, butter, and other spreads
—Vegetable oils

Vitamins and Cancer

By now we've all read the latest catch phrases in the headlines: "antioxidants" fight "free radicals." Free radicals develop constantly throughout the body, which uses them in part to protect itself against harmful metabolic products. However, aggressive radicals can also damage healthy cells or even transform them into cancer cells.

To combat such malignant effects, the body's protective mechanisms utilize vitamins C and E and beta carotene.

Several major studies have established, however, that supplemental doses of these substances have no preventive effect against cancer (see Preventing Cancer Through Diet, p. 472).

Secondary Trace Substances

This term *secondary trace substances,* refers to components in vegetables, fruits, or grains that are only present as trace amounts but are still essential for maintaining good health.
— The substances allyl in garlic and isothiocyanate in cabbage-family vegetables have antibacterial properties.
— Bioflavonoids, which occur in all vegetables, especiallyin broccoli and soybeans, can neutralize carcinogenic substances.
—The bioflavonoids in tea, onions, garlic, and red grapes can reduce the risk of heart attack.
— Substances found in kale, carrots, and tomatoes have the capacity to bind free radicals.
— Acids in strawberries, pineapple, and tomatoes neutralize carcinogenic nitrosamines.

Vitamin A (Retinol)

Needed for
— Development and repair of skin and mucous membrane
— Night vision.
RDA
— At least 2,500 IU for adults
— 5,000 IU for women in the last trimester of pregnancy and while breastfeeding

Sources
— Animal products. Vegetable products contain precursors of vitamin A, such as carotene, from which the body can produce vitamin A on its own. However, carotene is not easily assimilated from raw foods.
RDA found in each of the following:
— 1.4 ounces cooked carrots
— 4 ounces spinach
— 4.5 ounces butter
— 8 ounces Swiss cheese
— 0.1 ounce cod liver oil
Vitamin A deficiency can result from a diet totally lacking in
— Milk
— Dairy products
— Butter
— Enriched margarine
— Carrots
— Leafy vegetables
Signs of vitamin A deficiency
— Loss of appetite
— Dry skin
— Night blindness
— Growth disorders in children
Excessive vitamin A
Possible only if one takes megadoses of supplements (including cod liver oil) or vitamin-enriched foods.
Signs of excessive vitamin A
— Fatigue
— Loss of appetite
— Nausea
— Headaches
— Hair loss
— Dry skin
— Double vision
Warning: Women in the first months of pregnancy should not take more than the recommended dose of vitamin A. Birth defects have been found to result from daily doses in excess of 10,000 IU.

Vitamin B¹ (Thiamine)
Needed for
— Metabolizing carbohydrates and alcohol
RDA
— 1–2 mg
    Higher doses in the event of heavy physical exertion, fever, pregnancy, or hyperthyroidism.

RDA available in each of the following:
— An 8-ounce pork chop
— 8 ounces peanuts
— 16 ounces lentils
— 23 ounces whole-grain bread
    Vitamin B¹ deficiency can be caused by a diet including no pork products, grain or cereal products, or potatoes.
Signs of vitamin B¹ deficiency
— Headache
— Loss of appetite
— Stomachache
— Constipation
— Memory and concentration disorders
Excessive vitamin B¹
Possible only through overmedication.
Signs of excessive vitamin B¹
Nerves are hypersensitive to stimuli.

Vitamin B² (Riboflavin)
Needed for
— Metabolism of fat and protein
RDA
— 1-2 mg
— During pregnancy about 0.5 mg more
RDA available in each of the following:
— 8 ounces beef heart
— 1 ounce Parmesan cheese
    Vitamin B² deficiency can result from a diet lacking in meat, eggs, and dairy products.
Signs of vitamin B² deficiency
— Cracked lips and corners of mouth
— Dry, inflamed skin
— Burning, itching eyes; light sensitivity
    Excessive amounts of vitamin B² are not known to cause problems.

Vitamin B⁶ (Pyridoxine)
Needed for
— Protein metabolism
RDA
— About 2 mg
— Pregnant women need about 3 mg.
    Women taking birth control pills are occasionally deficient in vitamin B⁶; this doesn't mean all women on the pill need to take vitamin B⁶ supplements. If you suspect you are deficient in this vitamin, eat more whole-grain bread or bananas.

RDA available in each of the following
— 7 ounces salmon
— 11 ounces mackerel
— 17.5 ounces banana
— 17.5 ounces whole-grain bread
Vitamin B^6 deficiency is rarely caused by diet.
Signs of vitamin B^6 deficiency
— Loss of appetite
— Nausea
— Vomiting
— Inflammations of the oral mucosa
— Dry skin
Excessive vitamin B^6 can occur only through taking the vitamin as medication. It is purported to alleviate vomiting or premenstrual syndrome (PMS) (see Possible Premenstrual Symptoms, p. 506).
Signs of excessive amounts of vitamin B^6
— Tingling, "pins and needles" and burning pains in limbs
— Unsteady gait

Vitamin B^{12} (Cyanocobalamin)
Needed for
— Production of red blood cells
RDA
— About 0.003 mg
RDA available in each of the following
— 2 ounces beef or pork
— 1 ounce herring or mackerel
— 10.5 ounces yogurt made with whole milk
Sources
Vitamin B^{12} is found only in animal products and in vegetables fermented in lactic acid (sour pickles, sauerkraut).
Vitamin B^{12} deficiency is known to be nutritionally caused only when animal products are completely absent from the diet. Patients with severe intestinal diseases may not be able to absorb this vitamin. If the small intestine does not produce the substance needed to absorb vitamin B^{12}, the result is pernicious anemia (see p. 347).
Signs of vitamin B^{12} deficiency
— Antipathy towards meat
— Burning tongue
— All symptoms of anemia: fatigue, dizziness, weak heart
Excessive vitamin B^{12} is not known to cause health problems.

Folic Acid
Needed for
— Production of red blood cells (together with vitamin B^{12})
RDA
— About 0.2 mg
— Pregnant women need about twice that amount.
RDA available in each of the following
— 9 ounces spinach
— 7 ounces fennel
— 11.5 ounces kale
— 9 ounces asparagus
— 11.5 ounces whole-grain bread
Folic-acid deficiency does not occur in a well-balanced diet. Infants fed heated cow's milk (see Milk, p. 726) may not get enough folic acid; infant formula has folic acid added.
Patients with severe intestinal diseases may be unable to absorb this vitamin. Absorption may also be hindered by anticancer and arthritis medications.
Signs of folic-acid deficiency
— Same as signs of vitamin B^{12} deficiency
Women who show a folic-acid deficiency in the first months of pregnancy are at significantly higher risk of their child being born with birth defects (spina bifida, neural tube defects, hydrocephalus). A diet rich in folic acid and a supplement of 0.4 mg of folic acid should be taken for three months prior to a planned pregnancy and during the first trimester.
Excessive folic acid is not caused by diet.
Signs of excessive folic acid
— Gastrointestinal problems
Too much folic acid can be dangerous only in that it makes diagnosing pernicious anemia (see p. 347) difficult. In adults, excessive amounts of folic acid can mask a vitamin B-group deficiency.

Niacin (Nicotinamide, Nicotinic Acid)
Needed for
— Energy production in the cells
RDA
— Between 10 and 20 mg
RDA available in each of the following
— 8 ounces chicken
— 18 ounces herring
— 4.5 ounces peanuts
Niacin deficiency can be caused by a diet totally

deficient in meat or bread, or by severe stomach or intestinal diseases.

Signs of niacin deficiency
— Headaches
— Loss of appetite
— Stomach disorders
— Diarrhea
— Flushed skin
— Rough, red, flaky, inflamed skin

Excessive niacin can result from taking high doses of nicotinic acid–containing medications to treat circulatory disorders or high cholesterol levels.

Signs of excessive niacin
— Dry, red skin
— Hair loss
— Itching
— Diarrhea
— Vomiting
— Liver damage

Pantothenic Acid

Needed for
— All food metabolism

RDA
— About 5 mg

Neither deficiency nor excess are known to cause problems.

Vitamin C (Ascorbic Acid)

Needed for
— Formation of connective tissue

Vitamin C is vital for the body's absorption of folic acid and iron, themselves necessary for blood production.

RDA
— About 60 mg
— About 80 mg for pregnant women
— About 100 mg for nursing mothers and smokers

No research to date has established the efficacy of vitamin C in preventing colds or cancer.

RDA available in each of the following
— 0.7 ounce kiwi fruit
— 1 ounce black currants
— 1.5 ounces red pepper (capsicum)
— 2 ounces kale
— 3.5 ounces orange
— 14 ounces potatoes (unpeeled)

Vitamin C deficiency
— Possible in a diet low in fresh fruit, vegetables, and potatoes.

Signs of vitamin C deficiency
— Weakness
— Weight loss
— Bleeding, especially of the gums
— Wounds that are slow to heal
— Anemia

Excessive vitamin C can be caused by diet and taking it as medication.

Signs of excessive vitamin C
— Diarrhea
— Indigestion
— Kidney stones

Vitamin D (Calciferol, Cholecalciferol)

Needed for
— Metabolism of calcium and phosphate for bone development and dismantling.

RDA
— Infants: 100-200 IU
— Children, youths, pregnant and nursing mothers: 400 IU
— Other adults: 200 IU

Vitamin D's precursors are taken in through food, stored in the skin, and transformed into the actual vitamin with the help of ultraviolet rays in sunlight. Adults usually produce sufficient quantities.

Sources
— Fish, eggs, butter

Vitamin D deficiency can occur
— In nursing infants whose mothers have insufficient levels of vitamin D.
— In infants fed cows milk or homemade formula (commercially produced infant formula is enriched with vitamin D).
— In people who get no exposure to sunlight, or who live in heavily polluted areas where insufficient ultraviolet light filters through.
— In people with kidney or liver disorders, who are unable to produce vitamin D.

Signs of vitamin D deficiency in children
— Agitation, poor sleep habits, frequent sweating, slack muscles
— Rickets (see Osteomalacia, p. 433)

Signs of vitamin D deficiency in adults
— Thinning bone mass, bone deformities (see Osteomalacia, p. 433)

Excessive vitamin D can result only from medication (including cod-liver oil).

Signs of excessive vitamin D
— Excessive thirst and frequent urination
— Headaches
— Fatigue
— Loss of appetite
— Nausea
— Diarrhea
— Fever

In advanced stages, kidney stones, blockages of the arteries and changes to the bone mass can occur.

Vitamin E (Tocopherol)

Needed for
— Neutralizing substances toxic to cells.
RDA
— Estimated to be about 10 mg
RDA available in each of the following
— 0.25 ounce wheat germ oil
— 1 ounce sunflower oil

Vitamin E deficiency in animals can cause fertility disorders, among other symptoms; similar observations have not been made with regard to humans.

Serious gastrointestinal diseases in which fat absorption is disturbed can hinder the absorption of vitamin E.

Signs of vitamin E deficiency
— Changes to red blood cells
— Muscle weakness
— Changes in the retina

Excessive vitamin E obtained through diet is not known.

Biotin

Needed for
— Metabolism of all food
RDA
— Not established; produced by intestinal flora.
Sources
— Egg yolks, soybeans and peanuts

Signs of biotin deficiency or excess are rarely known to occur in humans.

Vitamin K

Needed for
— Blood clotting
RDA
— Not established, because it is produced by intestinal flora themselves.
Sources
— Green vegetables, especially of the cabbage family, and eggs

Vitamin K deficiency can occur as a result of serious gastrointestinal disease in which fat absorption is disrupted, or as a result of intestinal flora being killed off after long-term antibiotic use. In newborns, deficiency may occur in the first four to six weeks of life. It is possible that breastfed infants may develop different intestinal flora from bottle-fed infants.

Signs of vitamin K deficiency
— Hemorrhaging, visible as bruises; frequent nosebleeds

Excessive vitamin K is not known to cause problems.

MINERAL SUBSTANCES

Potassium

Needed for
— Electrolyte balance in the cells, to enable muscle and nerve function
RDA
— 3-4 gm daily, which a balanced diet provides
RDA available in each of the following
— 6 ounces dried apricots
— 23 ounces walnuts
— 25 ounces bananas
— 26 ounces whole-grain bread
Potassium deficiency can occur
— With regular use of laxatives
— When using diuretics (such as medication for high blood pressure or weak heart)
Signs of potassium deficiency
— Muscle weakness
— Fatigue
— Listlessness
— Flatulence
— Constipation

Excessive amounts of potassium can be caused by disease or medication causing the body to excrete too little potassium, or by medication containing potassium.

Signs of excessive potassium
— Fatigue
— Weakness
— Auditory problems
— Metallic taste in mouth

In advanced stages: irregular heartbeat, low blood pressure and confusion.

Prevention: If kidney function is impaired or you take diuretics, your blood potassium levels should be checked regularly.

Calcium

Needed for
— Bones and teeth
— Responsiveness of muscle and nerve cells
— Defense against infections and allergies
— Blood clotting

RDA
— About 800 mg
— 1200 mg for women in the last trimester of pregnancy and while breastfeeding, and for youths between ages 11 and 24

Vitamin D is necessary for the intestinal absorption of calcium.

RDA available in each of the following
— 3 ounces hard cheese
— 3.5 ounces sesame seeds
— 8.5 ounces sardines in oil
— 23 ounces whole milk

Calcium deficiency can be caused by a dairy-free diet, or drinking water treated with a water softener (see Water Hardness, p. 737).

Signs of calcium deficiency
— Pale, sweaty skin
— Agitation
— Vomiting
— Diarrhea
— Tingling ("pins and needles") in the extremities
— Painful cramps, especially in the arms

Excessive calcium in the blood can result from intake of excessive amounts of vitamin D.

Signs of excessive calcium
— Loss of appetite
— Weight loss
— Flatulence
— Constipation

— Heartbeat disturbances (arrhythmias)

There is an increased danger of kidney stones.

Phosphate

Needed for
— Bones
— Cell reproduction

Phosphate absorption and excretion are regulated like those of calcium. Vitamin D is necessary for its absorption in the intestine.

RDA
A diet with sufficient calcium and protein ensures proper phosphate intake.

Sources
— Animal and plant products contain phosphate

Excessive amounts of phosphate: Because phosphates are present in many prepared foods (cheese products, condensed milk, soft drinks, processed meats), most people ingest far too much phosphate in proportion to calcium; this may compromise bone strength.

Magnesium

Needed for
— Bones and cells (especially muscle cells)

RDA
— About 300 mg

RDA available in each of the following:
— 2.5 ounces sunflower seeds
— 8 ounces navy beans
— 17.5 ounces spinach

Magnesium deficiency can occur if
— You mainly eat produce grown in chemical fertilizer, which often contains less magnesium than organically grown produce.
— You eat a high-fat, high-protein diet.

Signs of magnesium deficiency
— Nervous disorders
— Heart problems
— Nausea
— Leg and stomach cramps

Fluoride

Needed for
— Development of bones and teeth

Teeth with high fluoride content are more resistant to cavities (see Cavities, p. 366).

RDA
— For infants, 0.2 mg
— For adults, 1 mg
Sources
— Drinking water
— Fish
— Sea salt
— Black tea

Three cups of tea supply the RDA of fluoride for adults. An average diet provides about 0.3 to 0.4 mg fluoride daily, the bulk of it from drinking water (see Tap Water, p. 737).

Fluoride deficiency is not known to result in disease.

Excessive amounts of fluoride: More than about 2 mg of fluoride daily can lead to fluoride toxicity; in children this manifests as bright white flecks on the teeth (fluorosis).

More than 8 grams of fluoride daily over the long term can cause fluorosis of the bones, which manifests as stiffening of the joints and spinal column.

Other signs of fluoride toxicity include
— Skin problems
— Hair and nail problems
— Constipation
— Tingling ("pins and needles") in hands and feet
— Thyroid disorders
— Kidney disorders

Warning: Toothpaste, mouthwash, and chewing gum often contain undisclosed amounts of fluoride for protection against cavities.

Iron

Needed for
— Hemoglobin in red blood cells
RDA
— 0.5 to 1 mg for men and nonmenstruating women
— 2 to 3 mg for youths
— 2 to 5 mg for pregnant women

Diet should provide about ten times the RDA, of which the body uses only about 5 to 10 percent.

Sources
A varied diet contains 10 to 20 mg iron, enough to cover the daily requirement. If more iron is needed, the body significantly increases its iron absorption.

RDA available in each of the following
— 3.5 ounces salt herring
— 7 ounces sesame seeds
— 7 ounces millet
— 7 ounces dried soybeans

Spinach is missing from this list—its reputation as an excellent source of iron endures, though the myth has long been debunked.

The body can assimilate iron better from meat than other sources.

Iron deficiency can occur
— If the diet does not provide as much iron as the body currently requires;
— If the body cannot assimilate sufficient iron, in the event of gastrointestinal diseases or insufficient stomach acid;
— Due to blood loss. This can be either unnoticed (bleeding in the gastrointestinal tract due to ulcers, hemorrhoids, pain medication such as nonsteroidal anti-inflammatory drugs [NSAIDs]), or evident (blood loss as a result of large wounds, surgery, or frequent, prolonged menstruation).
—As a result of long-lasting infection.
—As a result of rheumatism.

Signs of iron deficiency
— Fatigue
—Weakness
— Pallor
— Cold hands and feet
— Sleep disorders
— Brittle hair and nails
— Nausea, constipation
— Diarrhea
— Libido disorders, impotence

Treatment: A diagnosis of anemia should be made only after blood tests. Your health-care provider should also monitor the progress of any treatment he or she prescribes. Take iron supplements at least half an hour before breakfast with a large glass of water or juice containing vitamin C. Coffee, tea, milk, and vitamin E hinder the absorption of iron.

Excessive amounts of iron can be caused by diet or medication. The body stores excess iron in the internal organs, causing damage which can eventually result in cirrhosis of the liver (see p. 396) or other diseases.

TRACE ELEMENTS

Many elements that occur in the human body are found only in traces (barely measurable amounts). Some are essential to life:

Copper is involved in the production of hemoglobin.
Cobalt is important in blood production.
Zinc is a component of the hormone insulin.
Chromium is important in the functioning of insulin.
Manganese, molybdenum and selenium are components of enzymes.

All of these are present in sufficient amounts in a normal diet. There is no evidence that megadoses of trace elements prevent cancer. It has not yet been established whether the many other trace elements in the body have a function.

Iodine

The thyroid needs iodine to function (see Goiter, p. 494). Adults require 0.15 mg daily, children up to about age nine 0.1 mg, infants 0.05 mg. Women have iodine deficiency more frequently than men.

All sea products contain iodine (see iodine content of food, table on p. 748). Eating seafood once a week will not cover your daily requirement, however. A liter of milk per day can have noteworthy benefits, as can Japanese seaweeds found in health-food stores and used as spices. Other possibilities include iodine-containing mineral water or toothpaste. Iodized table salt can also supplement a balanced diet. Uniodized sea salt usually contains no more iodine than regular salt.

Following the nuclear reactor accident at Chernobyl, recommendations of iodine prophylaxis were issued to protect people in the event of another episode. Nuclear fission creates radioactive iodine as a by-product, which can be released as gas into the atmosphere during an accident. Thyroid glands low in iodine absorb 60 to 70 percent of the radioactive iodine breathed in, increasing the risk of cancer. To prevent this, the thyroid should be saturated with iodine so that it will absorb a maximum of 1 percent of the radioactive iodine. In practical terms this means that, prior to exposure to the radioactive gas, adults should take a one-time dose of 200 mg, followed every 8 hours by an additional 100 mg as long as the danger of inhaling radioactive iodine continues, not to exceed a total intake of 1,000 mg. Children should be given half that dose.

This procedure should not be self-administered, but should only be undertaken following orders of your local health authorities. It can seriously endanger the health of people with hyperthyroidism (see p. 496), many of whom don't even know they have this disorder.

Such preventive measures protect only the thyroid from radiation damage: The rest of the organs are not protected. It is a mistake to think that downing iodine pills will protect your whole body from the effects of radiation.

One hundred grams of the following foods contain:

Vitamin A
Carrots 6,600 IU
Spinach 2,300 IU
Butter 1,950 IU
Swiss cheese 1,065 IU
Egg 730 IU
Whole milk 100 IU

Vitamin B1
Peanuts 0.9 mg
Pork chop 0.8 mg
Bacon 0.8 mg
Lentils 0.4 mg
Hazelnuts 0.4 mg
Whole-grain bread
    0.3 mg

Vitamin B2
Beef heart 0.9 mg
Wheat germ 0.7 mg
Parmesan cheese
    0.6 mg
Mushrooms 0.4 mg
Egg 0.3 mg
Whole milk 0.2 mg

Vitamin B6
Salmon 1 mg
Sardines 0.9 mg
Hazelnuts 0.5 mg
Whole-grain bread
    0.4 mg
Bananas 0.4 mg

Vitamin B12
Oysters 0.015 mg
Herring, mackerel
    0.009 mg
Beef 0.005 mg
Pork 0.005 mg
Cheese 0.002 mg
Whole-milk yogurt
    0.001 mg

Folic acid
Fennel 0.1 mg
Asparagus 0.083 mg
Spinach 0.078 mg
Egg 0.0065 mg
Kale 0.06 mg
Whole-grain bread
    0.06 mg
Peanuts 0.053 mg

Niacin
Peanuts 15.3 mg
Chicken 8.8 mg
Herring 3.8 mg
Trout 3.41 mg
Whole-grain bread
    3.3 mg

Vitamin C
Kiwi fruit 250 mg
Black currants 180 mg
Red peppers 140 mg
Kale 105 mg
Brussels sprouts
    85 mg
Broccoli 60 mg
Lemon 53 mg
Orange 50 mg
Tomato 24 mg
Potatoes (unpeeled)
    14 mg

Vitamin D
Sardines 300 IU
Tuna 215 IU
Egg 71 IU
Butter 52 IU

Vitamin E
Wheat germ oil
    215 mg
Sunflower oil 56 mg
Margarine 16 mg
Butter 2 mg
Sweet corn 2 mg

Biotin
Egg 0.025 mg
Peanuts 0.035 mg

Vitamin K
Brussels sprouts
    0.57 mg
Spinach 0.35 mg
Cauliflower 0.3 mg
Broccoli 0.13 mg
Egg 0.045 mg

Iron
Salted herring 20 mg
Sesame seeds 10 mg
Millet 9 mg

Iodine
Shellfish 0.4 mg
Saltwater salmon
    0.26 mg
Shrimp 0.13 mg
Lemon 0.07 mg
Herring 0.05 mg
Spinach 0.02 mg
Egg 0.01 mg

Potassium
Apricots (dried)
    1,700 mg
Dates, dried figs,
    raisins 700 to
    800 mg
Peanuts 740 mg
Spinach 660 mg
Walnuts 450 mg
Apricots (fresh)
    440 mg
Bananas 420 mg
Mushrooms 400 to
    500 mg
Whole-grain bread
    400 mg
Peas 370 mg

GENETIC ENGINEERING

In nature, dogs and cats don't produce offspring together, and flounder and strawberries can never propagate. Genetic engineering (GE), however, makes possible what is impossible in the natural world: Organisms can be altered and recombined in ways nature did not foresee, pushing boundaries of traditional breeding practices. Biomedicine is redefining the nature of life.

Genetic Engineering is being touted as the technology of the future and research dollars are flowing into related projects. It is producing substances from living matter for use in industry, food production, and medicine: Currently these substances are used in diagnostic tools, and possibly one day in medical therapy.

Experts believe that in as few as 10 years, all food will be genetically modified in some way. But most consumers are not quite as enthusiastic: Surveys reveal negative public attitudes toward genetically modified foods.

To date, the GE industry has not turned a profit; and many of the investment dollars come from taxes.

GOALS

The arguments in favor of genetic engineering include ensuring high-quality food products worldwide, minimizing the suffering caused by disease, and ensuring productivity and economic success. Critics view such purported goals as hubris, with humans simply "playing God."

In any case, the huge amounts of money invested need to yield profit as soon as possible. One way to guarantee a return on investment is by patenting new life forms. Patents have been taken out not only on genetically engineered plants, but on diagnostic techniques and therapies as well. Treatments employing genetically modified organisms are likely to be significantly more expensive than conventional alternatives.
Farmers are already feeling the impact: Seeds from genetically engineered plants cost more. Unlike regular seed stock, genetically engineered seed must be purchased fresh every year and does not reproduce. Genetically engineered plants require a special herbicide: Because both seed and herbicide are manufactured by the same producer, this means twice the profit—for the manufacturer.

CONSEQUENCES

First among the consequences of GE are fundamental ethical considerations regarding the impact humanity should have on nature itself. Also, our knowledge of edible plants and animals is called into question: Once strawberries contain genetic material from fish (see Allergies, p. 360 and below), thousands of years of human experience are of no help and a brave new world has indeed arrived.

Moreover, where the use of genetically modified material poses separate risks, use and risk must be assessed individually: Different criteria must be applied to short-term use of medicine and to long-term daily consumption of food.

A panel of World Health Organization (WHO) experts has outlined the general risks as follows:
— As a result of GE, organisms may generate harmful substances.
— They may have unforeseen byproducts.
— The new substances may cause side effects, such as allergies.
— Genetic samples that develop a resistance to one antibiotic may be transferred to another microorganism, exacerbating the problem of antibiotic-resistant pathogens.
— Genetic modification of microorganisms can cause changes in the gastrointestinal tract.
— In food, nutritional ratios and values and the bio-availability of nutrients can be altered.

For specific risks, please refer to the sections dealing with individual products.

Allergies

If genetic material is transferred from an organism that is known to cause allergies, it is possible under certain circumstances to test whether the source of the allergy is the manipulated organism or its end product. However, if nothing is known about the allergenic potential of the transgene, testing cannot be done. Although allergies may not show up for years or even decades, we do know that the allergenic potential of transgenic plants is greater than that of plants raised under normal conditions—particularly if they have been designed to be resistant to illnesses and insects.

Two examples illustrate the risk of unexpected allergies: Strawberries have been implanted with a fish gene that makes them less sensitive to frost. Consumers who cannot tolerate fish protein need to avoid strawberries treated in this way—and can do so, as long as genetically engineered products are so labeled.

Another example: Soybean plants are altered with genetic material from brazil nuts to improve their value as feed. The genetically manipulated soybeans have very strong allergenic potential. Soy products are also used as milk substitute in the food industry.

Because it is impossible to distinguish between normal soybeans and those that have been genetically treated, they may be used as a milk substitute in baked goods, causing severe allergic reactions in those susceptible.

Unforeseen Risks

Fear of unforeseen risks goes hand in hand with genetic engineering. In the final analysis, researchers really only test and look for what they already know. New genes may destroy or "confuse" inherited genes so much that the organism starts to behave differently. It could be possible that the new gene may affect unknown metabolic functions and trigger reactions that are not tested for because they have never before been encountered.

One alarming case in point concerns the over-the-counter sleep aid L-tryptophan, which was used for 15 years with no hint of side effects until 1989, when a rare blood disorder (eosinophilic myalgia syndrome) began to be diagnosed as a side effect, with 1,500 cases of serious illness reported and 38 deaths worldwide. It's thought that possibly the source organism used to produce the drug by a particular manufacturer formed toxic by-products as a result of genetic modification. This has not been established definitively, since the manufacturer refused to allow the bacteria strand in question to be examined or tested.

In another instance, researchers in Japan found that genetically altered brewer's yeast resulted in toxic by-products 200 times more potent than the norm.

GENETIC ENGINEERING IN FOOD PRODUCTION

In the industrialized world, genetic engineering is used first and foremost to improve productivity, and secondarily to change food makeups to promote "guilt-free" consumption of prepared foods—e.g., by increasing fiber content, reducing saturated fats for the sake of "protecting the heart," and altering nutritional values to meet minimum dietary requirements.

In developing countries, there is greater emphasis on supplying necessary nutrients and additives—for example, compensating for prevalent Vitamin A deficiency by increasing its level in genetically modified rice. This raises the question of how poorer countries are to finance expensive genetic engineering: Where profit margins are low, the number of such projects is correspondingly low.

The issue of helping the poor is also called into question when one considers that most genetically engineered plants are being used to replace naturally reproducing raw-material crops (see Genetic Engineering in Industry, p. 751).

Transgenic Animals

Livestock and other animals useful to humans are subjected to genetic modification on the grounds of optimizing productivity and yield, and minimizing loss and waste. "Super-salmon" are implanted with the growth hormones of codfish so that they grow faster; livestock kept in high-density living conditions are implanted with a gene that makes them more disease-resistant; and cold-resistant genes help them endure harsh conditions.

Transgenic Plants

Edible plants—wheat, tomatoes, potatoes—also undergo genetic modification. Blocking the genes that cause decay and spoilage resulted in the "Flavor-Savor" tomato, which has been on the market since 1993 and is soon to be joined by similarly altered raspberries and peaches.

By implanting other kinds of genes, plants can be made resistant to

— Certain herbicides. When a field is sprayed with these products everything except the target crop is killed.
— Insects. The plant produces toxins that repel insects, making the plant itself a pesticide. Use of such plants is increasing.
— Fungi and viruses. This helps minimize loss of yield in rice and potato crops.

Deregulation

In the industrialized world, growers wishing to grow genetically engineered crops in the field rather than under laboratory conditions must obtain regulatory clearance. This used to be an arduous process, but it's becoming easier and more streamlined.

The number of such open-air producers has grown to several thousand worldwide. In China, huge tracts of land are used to cultivate genetically engineered tomatoes and tobacco. The developing countries are a favorite venue because they involve few restrictions—as a rule there are no laws governing genetic engineering—and there are significant advantages such as auspicious climatological conditions that permit two crops a year.

Europe, France, Belgium, and England are leaders in permitting genetically modified crops (primarily corn, rapeseed, and sugar beets).

Any field use of a genetically engineered crop is a potential time bomb: The extent of devastation can't be known until after the explosion.
Field use lays the groundwork for the following risks:
— Cross-pollination with transgenic plants can create aberrations and cause new traits to spread uncontrollably throughout the entire ecosystem.
— Due to its new traits, a genetically modified plant may be stronger than the original, forcing out other types of plants.
— The new genetic materials may be harmful to animals, plants, and microorganisms.
— If pathogens adapt to a plant that has been genetically modified to be theoretically more resistant, more aggressive life forms may develop as a result, making us all more vulnerable.

Aftereffects and Risks

If weed killers won't harm crops, herbicides will be applied liberally, without restraint. This means people consuming these crops will ingest larger amounts of herbicide residue, which will also affect soil and water supplies.

It is not known whether the toxins used to protect plants against insects are harmful if ingested by humans. The results of systematic testing to learn the effects of long-term use are not publicized.

In one case, a strain of corn was "immunized" against a particular insect; tests showed that after 17 generations—corresponding to only about 5 years in a warm climate—the insect had become resistant to the insecticide.

Transgenic Bacteria, Fungi, and Yeasts

Various living microorganisms—bacteria, fungi, and yeasts—are used in food production. Those that have been genetically modified are reportedly more effective at suppressing or destroying "unfriendly" germs. For example, yogurt bacteria can now produce their own preservatives.

Genetically modified microorganisms, or their by-products, are used in the production of yogurt, wine, cheese, beer, salami, sauerkraut, and bread.

Transgenic Microorganisms as Producers in the Food Industry

Genetically modified microorganisms are already producing many substances and additives used in the food industry: enzymes, aromas, vitamins, thickeners, sweeteners, fruit acids, amino acids, flavor enhancers, antioxidants, etc.

On average, the production of about 40 percent of our consumables involves enzymes and microorganisms, a large portion of which are genetically modified.

In the Netherlands, more than half the white bread is currently made with the help of a genetically produced enzyme. In the United States, molasses and fruit juices, among other products, are made with the help of genetically produced enzymes. In England, the first beer brewed with genetically modified yeast is on the market.

Aftereffects and Risks

It has not yet been determined whether we are affected by the genetically engineered traits in, say, the yogurt we eat. If the traits do have an effect, they might change the flora of the skin and mucous membranes of the mouth, intestines and stomach, and may manifest as recurrent infections.

Microorganisms used for enzyme production enter the environment through the wastewater stream. Manufacturers claim that the organisms are killed off in the fermenting process, but tests show that some survive and pass on their new characteristics to other microorganisms.

GENETIC ENGINEERING IN INDUSTRY

Nearly all common crops have undergone some kind of genetically engineered variation. In Europe, an industrially significant strain of potato—one with a very high starch content—has been developed. Soy, rapeseed, and sunflower seedlings have been genetically modified so that their amino acid profile matches industrial requirements as closely as possible.

Aftereffects and Risks

Genetic modification of oil-producing plants has a potentially huge impact on the global economy. It enables industrialized countries to produce—cheaply and in huge quantities—oils and fats that currently must be purchased as raw materials from less developed countries. Nations whose economies depend largely on the export of substances like cocoa butter, peanut oil or coconut oil are especially affected by this development. Dramatic drops in prices, high export tariffs and, in the worst case, balance-of-trade collapses are unfortunately inevitable parts of this scenario.

GENETIC ENGINEERING IN THE PHARMACEUTICALS INDUSTRY

Various by-products of healthy human or animal immune systems show promise in the treatment of cancer and immune system disorders—if they could be produced in the necessary volume and cost-effectively. Genetic engineering makes it possible for genetic data to be implanted into a fertilized animal embryo, causing the animal's mammary glands to produce the medical substance in abundance. Even something like growth hormone can be manufactured in this way.

Genetically modified microorganisms produce, among other things: insulin for diabetics, beta-interferon (a medication for multiple sclerosis), and erythropoietin for kidney dialysis patients. Various vaccinations are produced as well.

Cost-effectiveness is of paramount importance in the production of pharmaceuticals. Genetically engineered drugs are advertised widely; they are also more expensive, although not necessarily more effective. They can actually cause heretofore unknown problems; for example, genetically engineered insulin can cause dangerously low levels of blood sugar significantly more often. The medical press has even gone so far as to dub alpha-interferon "a drug looking for an indication."

Milk from super-cows

Cattle injected with the genetically engineered growth-hormone bovine somatotropin increase milk production by as much as 20 percent. The hormone does not affect humans: Its protein is destroyed during digestion.

However, products made from this milk are significantly higher in IGF-1, an insulinlike growth factor that increases the risk of breast cancer. Bovine somatotropin is used in the United States, although some dairy farmers have stopped using it because it increases the incidence of udder inflammations.

GENETIC ENGINEERING IN DIAGNOSTICS

Using the tools of GE, human chromosomes can be isolated and hereditary diseases identified. Both the genes that increase the risk of breast cancer by 85 percent in 5 percent of all women can already be identified, as can the gene that triggers cystic fibrosis (see p. 598).

Genetic testing identifies pathogens relatively quickly and cheaply. It is also useful in criminal ID checks and establishing paternity. Genetic testing is a major growth industry.

Aftereffects and Risks

Genetic testing currently gives us more data than we can use at this time. Even if a gene is discovered that signals a predisposition to a specific illness, we don't know for certain whether and when it will develop. Using the gene itself for "therapeutic" applications has not been successful to date.

Rennet fermented chymosin (rennin)

Nowadays, it is unlikely that any of us has escaped contact with genetically modified food products. In the United States, 40 percent of all commercially produced hard cheeses contain the genetically produced enzyme chymosin. Since genetically engineered foods are not required to be labeled, they are impossible to identify.

Chymosin is a natural enzyme in rennet fermentation and is manufactured from the rennet of calf stomachs; this is the first step in cheese production. Chymosin produced from genetically modified bacteria is now being used.

The market for genetically engineered chymosin is estimated at about $180 million worldwide.

Mice who have been fed cheese produced with this substance show slight changes to their internal organs; however, the manufacturer claims that these changes fall within the normal range of variation.

In some cases, women in whom genetic testing revealed an increased risk of breast cancer have had their breasts removed protectively.

The great interest in such tests evinced by insurance companies and employers has given rise to fears that such information will be used in selection processes, qualifying some individuals for work or insurance eligibility on the basis of their genetic appropriateness. This technology also makes it possible to gene-test an embryo before it becomes viable.

GENETIC ENGINEERING IN THE TREATMENT OF DISEASE

Congenital diseases caused by an absent or malfunctioning gene can be treated by adding or repairing the gene in question. This has been done in the case of a rare immunological disease and with cystic fibrosis—although without long-term success. Under laboratory conditions, insulin has been successfully produced in the livers of mice implanted with insulin-producing genes.

Cancer Therapy

Two thirds of all clinical genetic studies involve cancer patients.

There are various strategies in the fight against cancer: supplementing the body's own defense mechanisms, making tumor cells more vulnerable, or inducing them to self-destruct.

The results can be summed up simply: Genetic cancer therapy is still in the experimental stage. Some leading U.S. molecular biologists believe gene therapy to be fundamentally misguided.

Aftereffects and Risks

Gene replacement and repair in disease therapy have quickly led some researchers to thoughts of genetically engineered offspring. By modifying parents' sex cells, new characteristics could be passed on to the next generation, making the concept of "designer babies" a reality.

MOOD-ALTERING SUBSTANCES AND RECREATIONAL DRUGS

The term "drugs" usually refers to illegal substances such as heroin, cocaine, and LSD rather than recreational drugs like alcohol or tobacco, although they may have similar effects. Terming things "legal" or "illegal" makes a false distinction: The real issue is addiction. Most people with addictions are dependent on "legal" substances like alcohol and tobacco, but they are addicted nonetheless.

SMOKING (NICOTINE)

There are fewer smokers in the United States than there used to be. The prevalence is inversely related to education and to socioeconomic status.

People who are likely to smoke show this tendency early. The habit is easily picked up on the rocky road through puberty, if cigarettes hold out the promise of an easy way to deal with uncertainty and relax nerves. Experimenting with cigarettes can lead to lifelong, expensive dependency. If smoking doesn't start by age 20, it's likely that it never will.

A Daily Dose of Poison

Nicotine is a toxin that attacks the entire nervous and vascular systems. A dose of 50 mg can be lethal if taken in the bloodstream at one time. That's about the amount a heavy smoker gets daily, in small doses. Nicotine accelerates the heart rate and constricts blood vessels, impairing circulation and reducing the supply of oxygen and nutrients to tissues and organs. This especially affects the coronary arteries, brain and limbs.

Heavy smokers may experience menopause up to 6 years earlier than nonsmokers (see p. 510).

Warning signs
— Persistent, productive cough
— Shortness of breath during physical exertion
— Leg pain when walking
— Chest pain, stabbing heart feeling, following exertion

Even one of these symptoms signals serious damage and means that you should quit smoking immediately.

Smoking Causes Disease

Worldwide, about three million people die annually from smoking-related lung cancer, emphysema, chronic bronchitis or heart disease. Smoking significantly shortens life expectancy since in addition to the above diseases it hastens the onset of a variety of other ailments.

Smoker's Cough and Chronic Bronchitis

Normally, the cilia (tiny hairs) lining the airways and bronchi protect the lungs from foreign matter. Tar from cigarettes damages the cilia, impeding this function. Coughing is the body's attempt to rid itself of accumulated toxins that have lodged in the mucosa. Morning "smoker's cough" often leads over the long term to chronic bronchitis (see p. 306).

Shortness of Breath and Smoker's Leg

Carbon monoxide, a by-product of tobacco smoke, is responsible for the shortness of breath that accompanies physical exertion in smokers. This toxin passes from the alveoli in the lungs into the bloodstream, where it binds with red blood cells, affecting their ability to transport oxygen. This impairs the oxygen supply to the brain, resulting in fatigue, headaches, or nausea.

Carbon monoxide can also significantly raise blood cholesterol levels, resulting in circulatory disorders including the dreaded "smoker's leg" (see Circulatory Disorders, p. 326), which can necessitate amputation.

A toxic combination
In addition to tar, nicotine, and carbon monoxide, tobacco smoke contains more than a thousand other chemical compounds, including nitric oxide, formaldehyde, radioactive polonium, arsenic, hydrogen cyanide, and ammonia. Between 20 and 80 percent of these materials lodge deep in the lungs: The more deeply you inhale, the more you take in. Tar also damages the lungs and airways. People who smoke a pack a day breathe in the equivalent of one cup of tar a year.

Stomach Disorders and Cancer

Smokers run a higher risk of developing stomach disorders. In people who quit smoking, ulcers heal faster.

If you smoke up to 10 cigarettes a day, you are 5

times as likely as a nonsmoker to develop lung cancer; if you smoke over 35 cigarettes a day, you are 40 times as likely to do so. Cigar or pipe smokers are "only" 4 times as likely to develop lung cancer, but cigar smokers develop oral and esophageal cancer more often, and pipe smokers are more likely to develop cancer of the lips and tongue.

Smoking also increases the likelihood of malignancies on the larynx, bladder, kidneys, and pancreas.

Heart Attacks

The risk of a fatal heart attack is two to five times greater in smokers than in nonsmokers. The risk increases the more cigarettes that are smoked daily, and also in the presence of high blood pressure, elevated cholesterol levels, and oral contraceptive use.

Passive Smoking

Nonsmokers are often exposed to cigarette smoke against their will ("passive smoking"). Workers in bars and restaurants, and children whose parents smoke, are especially affected.

Long-term passive smoking compromises lung function and significantly increases the risk of heart disease and cancer. Asthma and allergies can be intensified by passive smoking, which can also trigger outbreaks. Breathing tobacco smoke can also influence the effectiveness of medications.

If you feel your health is compromised by exposure to passive smoke in the workplace, you should report this to the Occupational Safety and Health Administration (OSHA). Your employer is obliged to protect nonsmokers from the ravages of nicotine (see Cigarette Smoke, p. 789).

Effects on the Unborn

Pregnant women who smoke are exposing their babies to toxins that enter the child's circulatory system through the placenta, compromising oxygen supply.

Poorly oxygenated blood can result in malnourishment and defects. Babies born to women who smoke weigh an average of 6 to 14 ounces less at birth, and are 2 to 4 inches shorter, than babies of nonsmokers.

Quitting Smoking

If you quit smoking, you can count on an increased life expectancy. After 15 years of not smoking, your risk of

Let the driver beware
It takes very few cigarettes to raise the carbon monoxide level in a closed vehicle. Physical and mental capacity are quickly impaired when the oxygen supply is reduced; vision can be impaired after only three cigarettes.

lung cancer will be equivalent to that of nonsmokers; your risk of heart attack will return to normal levels after even fewer years. The annoying side effects of smoking, such as coughing, oily skin, and impaired taste or vision disappear after only a few days or weeks of not smoking.

What to Expect If You Quit

It takes a few weeks after your final cigarette for body functions to regulate and the metabolism to adjust. Most people experience classic withdrawal symptoms such as anxiety, nervousness and irritation, fatigue, poor tolerance, and exhaustion. Most also gain weight, even if they eat no more than before, because the metabolism slows down in the absence of nicotine. This weight gain is only temporary if counteracted by a balanced diet (see p. 723) and sufficient exercise (see Physical Activity and Sports, p. 762). All the uncomfortable symptoms of nicotine withdrawal are temporary.

Tips for Quitting "Cold Turkey"

If you decide to quit "cold turkey"—from one day to the next—the following may help during those first smoke-free weeks:
— Spend as little time as possible indoors; get lots of outdoor exercise.
— Make sure you get enough sleep and relaxation.
— Ask all the smokers you know not to offer you cigarettes.
— Satisfy your urge to smoke with sugar-free gum or candy, breath mints, etc.
— Substitute new behavior for your usual smoking breaks: Instead of an after-dinner cigarette, take a walk around the block; instead of puffing the evening away in front of the television, go to the movies.
— Don't allow yourself to get bored.
— Avoid places where people are smoking.
— Avoid coffee or alcohol, which may give rise to the urge for a cigarette.

— Reward yourself by spending the money you've saved on yourself.

Tips for Quitting Step by Step

If you want to quit more gradually, plan to reduce your daily cigarette intake progressively. Within 3 to 5 weeks you should be down to zero.

— Don't smoke your first cigarette of the day until an hour after breakfast; increase this waiting period every day.

— Designate smoke-free zones in your home, preferably those in which you spend the bulk of your time.

— Don't smoke while your hands are occupied, such as behind the wheel.

— Don't smoke while walking.

— If you want to smoke, force yourself to wait 5 minutes before you act on the impulse; keep extending this waiting period.

— Change your behavior during the usual cigarette breaks: For example, go for a walk after eating instead of lighting up.

If You Just Can't Quit

— Don't smoke if nonsmokers are present.

— Try to designate smoke-free times (e.g., mornings) or activities (e.g., taking a walk).

— Create smoke-free zones at home or work; seek them out if they already exist (e.g., nonsmoking areas in restaurants).

— Smoke only half of each cigarette.

— Draw on your cigarette less deeply, or gradually stop inhaling altogether.

— Avoid rolling your own cigarettes, even those with filters; they contain much higher levels of toxins than those produced commercially.

— Switch to a "light" cigarette, but be careful not to smoke more to compensate.

Behavioral Therapy

Behavioral therapy can help you kick the nicotine habit (see p. 700). Local clinics and hospitals may offer classes on smoking cessation.

Medication and Acupuncture

Of the wide range of quit-smoking devices to choose from, the following are recommended:

— Nicotine gum containing varying doses of nicotine, which is reduced over the treatment period.

— A nicotine patch which, like gum, can support nicotine withdrawal by slowly reducing the amount of nicotine delivered. This reduces the severity of withdrawal symptoms.

Acupuncture (see p. 679) can also help during the initial phases of withdrawal. Its efficacy varies according to the patient.

The most important component in breaking an addiction, however, is always your own will and commitment.

ALCOHOL

The consumption of wine, beer, and hard liquor is part of much of Western culture. This is one recreational drug we wouldn't dream of giving up. In spite of trends toward fitness and health, alcohol consumption continues to be very prevalent.

The Silent Poison

The capacity to drink moderately and enjoy it is something most alcoholics have lost or never learned in the first place. The transition from social drinking, for the purpose of releasing tensions and inhibitions, to addiction, in which the amount of alcohol required increases steadily, is swift; most alcoholics don't notice it when they cross that line.

In spite of this, alcohol abuse verging on alcoholism is often assessed as "normal" consumption. An equal misconception is the belief that so-called social drinkers who indulge only in the company of others are not really addicted (see Alcoholism, p. 205).

Alcohol Causes Disease

Consistent, long-term alcohol consumption is detrimental to

— The body's vitamin and potassium levels

— Organs involved in digestion and metabolism, especially the liver (see Cirrhosis of the Liver, p. 396), pancreas (see Pancreatitis, p. 400) and stomach

— The heart and cardiovascular system

— The mucous membranes, which alcohol irritates and inflames (gastritis)

— The skin (alcohol causes enlarged capillaries)

— Sex drive and potency

— Peripheral nerves and brain cells, resulting in

reduced perceptual capacity, disturbed capacity for critical thinking and judgment, mild irritability, and feelings of euphoria alternating with depression.

Alcohol use also increases the risk of oral, laryngeal, esophageal, and pancreatic cancer. And it leads to weight gain: 10 to 20 percent of excess calories consumed by adults come from alcohol.

Effects on the Unborn

Alcohol and its residuals are transferred to the fetus directly through the placenta. Effects include low birth weight, developmental disorders or delays (both physical and intellectual), and birth defects such as malformations of the face or internal organs. The longer and more heavily a woman has been drinking, the greater the possibility of damage to her child.

For this reason, a pregnant woman should categorically abstain from alcohol. In this she needs the support of the father-to-be. It will be a lot harder for her to abstain if he drinks.

How Alcohol Works

Much of the alcohol we drink is absorbed directly from the stomach into the bloodstream and transported to the brain. How fast it is consumed, and whether or not there is any food in the stomach, are important factors in determining how we are affected. A stomach full of food, in particular fatty food, or milk will significantly counteract alcohol intake. Low-proof alcohol, or alcohol thinned with water or ice, is absorbed more slowly than higher-proof alcohol, or alcohol containing sugar and carbonic acid, such as champagne.

How fast alcohol works also depends on an individual's body weight, blood vessels, and psychological condition.

Drinking and Driving

Half of all automobile-related deaths are probably due

Alcohol consumption

The following amounts of alcohol are considered to be medically insignificant: for men, about 40 grams daily; about half that for women. A glass of wine or a bottle of beer each contain about 20 grams of alcohol. Approximately 20 percent of men and 10 percent of women over 30 drink more than this amount daily.

What Happens When You Drink?

Although alcohol affects each individual differently, the following general guidelines apply:

— Beer contains about 5 percent alcohol; wine, about 12 percent; hard liquor, about 40 percent (80 proof). An average 155-pound adult will experience the following effects at various blood alcohol levels:

— 0.3 to 0.5 liter beer, 2 shots liquor, or 0.125 to .025 liter wine: 30 mg/dl. Behavior and reaction time are slightly impaired; first signs of unsteady walking and overestimation of own abilities.

— 0.4 to 0.8 liter beer, 4 shots liquor, or 0.2 to 0.35 liter wine: 50 mg/dl. Slowed behavior and reaction time; euphoria.

— 0.7 to 1.5 liter beer, 5 to 7 shots liquor, or 0.3 to 0.5 liter wine: 80 mg/dl. In most states, 100 mg/dl is the highest permissible blood-alcohol level for driving. Anything more constitutes driving while intoxicated (DWI). Reaction time is significantly slower; and you have impaired ability to make objective judgments or be self-critical.

— 1.4 to 2.8 liters beer, 8 to 15 shots liquor, or 0.5 to 1.0 liter wine: 100-200 mg/dl. Reactive capacities are sharply diminished, as is self-control; euphoria may be accompanied by aggression; the ability to deal with reality is almost entirely compromised.

— 3.6 to 10 liters beer, 20 shots liquor, or 1.5 to 3.5 liters wine: 300-500 mg/dl. The sense of balance is significantly impaired; consciousness is dimmed; sensory awareness is diminished. Four hundred-500 mg/dl in the blood may cause death from respiratory depression and circulatory collapse.

to driving under the influence of alcohol, despite the fact that many of those implicated have not exceeded legal blood alcohol limits of 100 mg/dl. Reaction time is impaired by blood alcohol levels as low as 30 mg/dl.

Blood Alcohol: It Lasts and Lasts

Blood alcohol breaks down very slowly: It takes between 60 and 90 minutes for the body to process a medium-sized glass of wine. This means that if you've had too much to drink the night before and get behind the wheel after a few hours' sleep, a cold shower, and a cup of coffee, you may feel fine but you're still under the influence of residual alcohol in your blood and in no condition to drive. Coffee won't make a difference; there's no way to speed up the body's processing of alcohol.

Danger in the Workplace

The rate of accidents in the workplace rises significantly if alcohol is present. The same is true of domestic mishaps. Alcohol causes a lack of alertness, a narrowed field of vision, and slower reaction times.

Interaction with Drugs

Alcohol intensifies the effects of sedatives, psychopharmaceuticals and strong painkillers; decreases the effectiveness of medications for epilepsy, diabetes, gout, and tuberculosis; and intensifies the side effects of tetracycline, circulatory drugs, beta-blockers, and medication for coronary heart disease. Conclusion: Avoid alcohol if you are taking medication. (See Medication Summary, p. 657).

What To Do For a Hangover

A hangover is caused by dehydration and a drop in blood sugar.

— Avoid having another drink the morning after: It will only cause your blood-alcohol level to rise.

— If you feel you need a painkiller to make it through the morning, choose only a product containing aspirin, acetaminophen, or ibuprofen (see Analgesics, p. 660).

— Drink lots of water and restore your blood sugar level by eating fruit or drinking a beverage containing sugar.

To help you drink in moderation:

— Don't drink alcohol to quench thirst.
— Never drink to help you cope with physical or psychological problems.
— Don't drink out of habit or boredom; consciously decide to have a drink, then savor it sip by sip.
— Don't drink habitually in the same situation: Choose anew each time.
— Don't drink on an empty stomach; dilute drinks with water or ice.
— Always drink less than you think you can handle, and drink it over the course of several hours.
— When entertaining, don't pressure guests to drink alcohol to keep you company; always offer juices and other alcohol-free drinks.
— If you don't want to drink, just say no!

CAFFEINE

Coffee, tea, cocoa, and colas all owe their basic effects to varying degrees of caffeine content. Tea is easier on the stomach than coffee because it contains no by-products of roasting; the tannins in tea also slows the body's absorption of caffeine, with the result that its stimulating effect is felt more slowly and for a longer period of time than that of coffee.

How Much Is Too Much?

— More than 0.5 grams of caffeine (equivalent to four or five cups of coffee) can lead to symptoms of caffeine intoxication, including agitation, restlessness, racing pulse, pounding heart, and premature cardiac contraction. Circulation and breathing are markedly affected.

— After more than 1 gram of caffeine (equivalent to 10 or more cups of strong coffee), symptoms may include muscle twitching or seizures, accompanied by dizziness, headaches, and possibly nausea, vomiting, and diarrhea. Ten grams of caffeine can be fatal.

— Chronic excessive coffee consumption can lead to addiction. If the customary stimulation from caffeine is skipped, mild withdrawal symptoms appear in the form of headaches and fatigue.

— Caffeine has a mild laxative effect due to some of its plant oil content.

— The opposite is true of tea: tannic acid can cause constipation.

— The by-products created when coffee beans are roasted act as irritants to the stomach and stomach acids. People with stomach and gall or bile problems should avoid coffee. In contrast, tea is usually well tolerated by those with biliary colic or painful gallstones.

— Children are especially susceptible to caffeine; the first signs of caffeine intoxication appear far more quickly than in adults.

— If you are pregnant, exercise caution when using caffeine: You are, in effect, feeding your baby caffeine, and he or she is much more sensitive to it than you are. There is evidence that daily intake of more than 600 mg of caffeine increases the risk of miscarriage and premature birth.

— If you suffer from sleep disorders, don't drink coffee, tea, or colas after early afternoon.

ILLICIT DRUGS

The term "drugs" usually refers to illegal substances like heroin, cocaine, synthetic (designer) drugs, and cannabis (marijuana/hashish). In spite of popular opinion, far fewer people are addicted to "hard" drugs than is widely assumed. Most narcotic crimes involve the "soft" drugs, such as cannabis, and fewer involve possession or dealing in the other drugs.

Use of cannabis, which is relatively harmless, seems to be holding steady. "Hard" drug use seems to be tending away from heroin and toward cocaine and "designer" drugs such as Ecstasy. "Downers" seem to be out, "uppers" appear to be in.

Cannabis (Marijuana/Hashish)

Cannabis, made from the female hemp plant, is, after alcohol, the most widely used drug. Use of cannabis in its various forms—marijuana (grass, pot, weed), hashish (hash) and hash oil—cuts across all age groups and strata of society.

Hashish is made from the resinous secretions of the hemp plant, marijuana is its dried leaves, stems, and blossoms. The "desired" effect comes from the chemical delta-9-tetrahydrocannabinol (THC), which constitutes 3 to 10 percent of hashish, depending on its provenance, age, and quality.

Possession in the United States is illegal.

Effects

Marijuana and hashish affect the autonomic nervous system relatively quickly; they have a calming effect while simultaneously increasing the heart rate. These drugs usually produce a feeling of relaxation; daily problems loom less large, and mild euphoria is combined with apathy. Sensory impressions are intensified, time seems to pass more slowly, and concentration and vigilance diminish. Higher doses can lead to apprehensiveness, hallucinations, and impaired awareness of reality.

Dependency

In contrast to alcohol, use of marijuana and hashish does not cause physical dependency. Intake does not have to be increased regularly in order to achieve the desired effect, and no withdrawal symptoms manifest if you quit suddenly.

It is possible, however, for a psychological dependency to develop. The desire for a pleasantly relaxed state, or for escape from the realities of everyday life, can lead to chronic use.

Complications

Marijuana and hashish are consistently implicated as stepping stones to harder drugs. If this is true, it is due less to the actual effects of cannabis than to the necessity of obtaining it illegally. Users are obliged to buy from drug dealers, who usually also sell harder drugs.

The biggest physiological danger posed by cannabis use is nicotine: the smoke of filterless, hand-rolled marijuana cigarettes or joints is inhaled more deeply and causes more damage to the lungs than cigarettes made from tobacco.

Driving Under the Influence

About 10 percent of drug-related traffic accidents involve the THC found in cannabis. Marijuana and hashish use affects spatial orientation, reaction time, muscle coordination and therefore the capacity to drive; these effects can linger 3 to 4 hours longer than the actual "high." In rare instances, users may experience flashbacks lasting several minutes, without recent use of cannabis.

Heroin (Opiates)

Raw opium is obtained by scoring the unripe seed pod of the poppy plant. Opium is the raw material for morphine and a range of partially synthetic morphine-like compounds, including heroin.

Effects

Heroin affects the part of the brain involved in registering desire and suppressing pain. Opiates quickly produce strong feelings of euphoria, peace, and freedom from cares and woes.

Dependency

Physiological dependency on heroin almost always starts at the first try. The body gets used to the drug almost immediately, regardless of whether it is snorted or injected. Thereafter, the ingested amount must constantly be increased to achieve the same effect, and ever-greater amounts can be tolerated. Going without a fix can result in extreme agitation, nervousness, sleeplessness, shivering, outbreaks of sweating, vomiting, seizures, and severe pain. To avoid these withdrawal symptoms, the addict is driven to seek regular fixes. Psychological dependency on heroin is just as pronounced as physiological dependency, and between the craving for the next high and the pain of withdrawal, the distinction between the two disappears.

Complications

The extent to which heroin addiction leads to physiological damage is still open to debate. A major risk of heroin use is that it is sold on the black market in highly contaminated form. To stretch or "cut" the drug, dealers usually add all kinds of substances from powdered milk to strychnine. A variety of physical disturbances and changes can result, which are impossible to quantify accurately.

Sharing unsterile needles fosters infections and increases the risk of ulcers and of jaundice and eventual liver damage. Shared needles also transmit diseases, the best known and one of the most fatal of which is AIDS.

Additional physiological damage is caused by overdoses, inconsistent drug concentrations, and the generally unhealthy lifestyle of a criminalized subculture.

Criminalization

The black market price of heroin varies relative to the frequency of police crackdowns and fluctuations in supply and demand. As the addict craves ever-increasing doses, a weekly paycheck soon fails to cover drug expenses; dealing, theft, burglary, and prostitution are often the next steps.

Addicts easily enter the criminal subculture when they buy or deal drugs or procure money to support their habits, for example through prostitution. Many experts believe that this downward spiral could be arrested if addicts were not dependent on the black market. In addition to methadone clinics, several countries are exploring the idea of drug therapy consisting of controlled distribution of heroin free to addicts in combination with long-term psychotherapy (see Addiction to Illegal Drugs, p. 208).

Cocaine

Cocaine is a natural substance derived from the leaves of the South American coca plant. Cocaine is traded on the black market as a white powder, usually containing a maximum of 25 percent pure cocaine. It may be cut with borax, lactose, fructose, or other stimulant or narcotic drugs. Cocaine is usually snorted and is absorbed through the mucous membranes into the bloodstream, traveling from there to the brain.

Effects

Cocaine produces clarity of thought, carefree elation, and intense physical well-being. Even small amounts increase breathing and heart rate and elevate body temperature; the pupils dilate and digestion slows. Larger doses cause pallor and a fast, weak pulse; trembling, vomiting, dizziness, breathing difficulties, and seizures are signs of toxicity that can lead to unconsciousness and respiratory failure.

Dependency

Cocaine addiction may take longer to develop than heroin addiction, but even recreational users require gradually increasing doses. Psychological dependency on cocaine can develop quickly.

Complications

Long-term snorting of cocaine affects the mucous membranes of the nose, which can become inflamed and ulcerated.

Regular cocaine consumption can cause concentration difficulties, agitation, and insomnia. The capacity to think clearly is lost. Users may experience panic attacks and hallucinations, leading to suicidal tendencies.

Cocaine suppresses hunger, which can result in malnourishment and consequent weakening of the body's defense system, leading to susceptibility to infections.

Where to get help
Many support groups and clinics can help. Check your local community for services.

Crack

Crack is made by combining leftovers from cocaine production with baking powder and water and heating the mixture. Crack comes as little white lumps and is smoked in special glass or tin pipes. Heat causes the lumps to crack—hence the name. Its use is far more prevalent in the United States than elsewhere.

Crack is extremely dangerous. Within 8 seconds of inhalation it reaches the brain, potentially negatively affecting the nerves for years to come. Crack use can lead to respiratory and circulatory disorders that can be fatal. Relative to other street drugs, crack carries the highest risk of death and is highly addictive.

Ecstasy

Ecstasy is a designer drug; originally developed as an appetite suppressant, it was never marketed because of its psychogenic side effects. Today, ecstasy is manufactured primarily in private laboratories. It comes in pill form.

Young people are its principal users. It is considered an aid for enhancing consciousness and performance. It has evolved as a party drug among dance-music fans who use it during all-night "rave" parties.

Researchers note a rapid increase in ecstasy use among young people but at the same time caution against excessive concern: The use of synthetic drugs tends to peak around age 25 and then drops off sharply.

Effects

Ecstasy kicks in within 20 minutes to an hour. For 3 to 4 hours, it produces feelings of emotional equilibrium, intellectual clarity, and intensified concentration, together with increased physical energy. Users feel euphoric; inhibited people find it easier to approach others while under the influence.

Dependency

While ecstasy in its pure form usually does not produce physical symptoms of addiction, psychological dependency can become considerable. Sedatives must often be taken to counteract the resulting feelings of agitation.

Psychological addiction can often lead to increased doses, which augment the side effects of the drug. The biggest danger, however, comes from mixing ecstasy with other substances such as LSD, which can also cause physical addiction.

Complications

Ecstasy is taken in extremely small doses, but even these can lead to undesirable side effects—high blood pressure, rapid pulse, elevated temperature, and jaw cramping, for example. If ecstasy is mixed with other drugs, the risk of unpredictable results, complications, and side effects rises sharply. Long-term use of ecstasy can cause nerve damage and lead to brain damage.

Ecstasy is an inhibition-busting drug taken to help the user feel well adjusted and accepted. Even moderate side effects can lead to serious difficulties; for example, dancing in overheated environments for hours on end can lead to dehydration, hyperthermia, and even heat stroke. The effects of the drug can mask warning signs of impending circulatory collapse, such as exhaustion, thirst, or pain.

The consequences of a weekend ecstasy-dance bash may be total exhaustion, depression, loss of appetite, and impaired capacity to work for the next few days.

If All Else Fails

Going to rave parties does not necessarily imply drug use; likewise, trying ecstasy once will not result in addiction. If you suspect your child is using ecstasy regularly, avoid overreacting. Instead, talk to your child about the drug's risks and suggest ways to reduce them, such as:

— Drinking lots of nonalcoholic, caffeine-free beverages to equalize the fluid loss caused by dancing for extended periods of time
— Taking periodic fresh-air breaks from dancing
— Taking only minimal doses of the drug

PHYSICAL ACTIVITY AND SPORTS

Without exercise, the body atrophies: It can stay in shape only with regular use and workouts. Very few people actually get enough exercise—those who do have made a conscious effort to incorporate exercise and sports into their daily lives.

Sports keep the heart and muscles strong and the tendons and ligaments flexible. Someone who is physically fit has better defenses against stress and heart attacks than someone who isn't. Walking, swimming or bicycling on a regular basis significantly improves the body's resources and capabilities.

PHYSICAL ACTIVITY

In today's society, machines do more and more of the work, and people do less and less. Much of our professional life and leisure time is spent in a sitting position. This sedentary lifestyle, coupled with repetitive motion, causes the body significant damage: The most common consequences are slack or painfully tense muscles, cardiovascular disease, metabolic disorders, poor posture and bone and ligament problems. These classic symptoms of insufficient exercise account for about 20 percent of total health-care costs.

The number of people who get regular or occasional exercise continues to drop. A good third of the population wants nothing to do with sports. Yet a healthy lifestyle doesn't have to mean feats of athletic prowess or the pursuit of trophies—just integrating the right amount of exercise and physical activity to fit one's personal lifestyle.

Moderate, regular exercise (climbing stairs, riding a bicycle to work, or going for a brisk 30-minute walk every day) has the same health benefits as nonstrenuous sports.

What to Train For

Every human action requires the cooperation of the skeletal muscles, bones and ligaments, nervous system and circulation. The body's ability to perform depends on the smooth interaction of these different components. Diffcrent activities build different strengths.

— Walking, running, aerobics, strenuous bicycling or swimming, rowing or skiing build endurance.
— Body building, wrestling, weight training or weight-lifting build strength.
— Riding, dancing, ice skating or skateboarding improve coordination.
— Gymnastics and stretching enhance flexibility.

Endurance

Endurance is essential to training. The term "endurance" itself is misleading: It doesn't mean marathon training sessions, but rather toning several large muscle groups through constant tensing and relaxing. Training for as little as two 30-minute sessions a week can improve circulatory capacity in someone just starting out.

The muscles are worked aerobically: They release energy by burning up carbohydrates with the help of oxygen. This accelerates circulation, improves the oxygen supply and increases breathing volume.

Activities that build aerobic endurance (as long as the heart rate is raised) include running, aerobics, hiking, walking, cross-country skiing, bicycling, rowing and swimming, as well as all ball games that involve running or jumping, such as soccer, basketball, tennis, or squash.

— They strengthen the autonomic nervous system and reduce stress hormones in the blood.
— They improve blood flow and cardiovascular fitness.
— They also have a positive effect on blood pressure: People who get exercise have only half as many heart attacks as those who don't (for nonsmokers, the risk is even lower).

Staying fit

Make sure you get enough daily exercise, particularly if you don't do sports.
— Avoid elevators and escalators. Get in the habit of going places on foot and taking the stairs.
— Park your car about 15 minutes' walk from work; walk the remaining distance at a good pace.
— Designate certain days of the week "car-free."
— If work confines you to your seat, put things just out of reach so you have to stretch or get up as much as possible; get up frequently and walk around the office.
— Try to organize your work space so that you have to keep getting up: Store important documents and records somewhere else; set up the printer and other machines at some distance from your desk.

Strength

When performed correctly, strength training benefits muscles, tendons, ligaments ,and posture. Strong muscles protect the joints and the spinal column. On its own, however, strength training has only a minor effect on the muscles' endurance capacity, and it does not increase oxygen intake. Bodybuilders who train exclusively with weights do not have a superior cardiovascular system unless they cross-train to build endurance as well as strength.

Cross-training for strength and endurance through repetitive lifting of relatively light weights strengthens the whole musculature. By following strength and endurance training programs offered by many health clubs, seniors can prevent muscle deterioration and bone loss (Osteoporosis, p. 430).

In strength training, it is essential to avoid overstraining joints, tendons, and ligaments, as well as overdeveloping certain muscle groups. An imbalance in the musculature can affect overall posture and result in the stereotype Charles Atlas type who is so well muscled he or she can't budge (see Fitness, p. 765).

How Much To Train

For maximum benefit, exercise must be regular. Running once every blue moon won't do it.

Individual capacities vary greatly. You should be challenged to at least 50 percent of your capability; 70 percent is even better. The more regular the exercise, the better; aim for a minimum of 30 minutes, two to three times a week.

Pulse rate is a good indicator of when you've reached peak cardiovascular output. As a general rule, when building endurance, your pulse should increase to a number equivalent to about 170 beats per minute, minus your age in years. If you're younger and/or in good physical condition, the rate should be 180, minus your age. For older people, peak pulse rate should be lower.

You know you've reached optimal training intensity when your pulse accelerates as you start exercising and then remains constant throughout your training session.

— Measure your pulse 5 minutes after you start training and then again when you finish (each time for 60 seconds).
— If the number is the same both times, you know

you've trained at your optimal level.
— The simplest way to take your pulse is at the artery on the side of your throat, or the inside of your wrist, using a stopwatch or a wristwatch with a second hand.
— Always see your doctor before launching or returning to an exercise regimen, particularly if you have doubts about your cardiovascular fitness.

The longer and more frequent the training sessions, the better the benefits to heart, muscles and the whole body. But you can't rest on your laurels: To maintain physical fitness, you need to exercise on a regular basis.

Choosing a Sport

It's easier to start exercise programs than to stick with them: Many people quit before they've really begun. Try not to view exercise as all drill and discipline: Do it just for fun, as a social activity with a partner, or as a way of relaxing.

— Most important: Choose a sport you like, be it dancing to world music, volleyball, bicycling, whatever. What's essential is that you enjoy doing it regularly.
— Decide whether you prefer individual or team sports.

If you decide to swim or run on your own, it's up to you to incorporate the time into your schedule. If you prefer to train with a partner or play on a team, ball sports are a good choice. Many communities have teams sponsored by local businesses.

— Choose something you can do close to home or work. It's easier to keep exercising if it's convenient.
— Variety keeps you motivated: If you don't want to jog in the park three times a week, alternate with dancing, a game of handball and an early morning solo swim.
— Your age and condition will help determine what sort of exercise you choose.

Aging

Contrary to popular belief, the best place for an old body is not necessarily in a rocking chair on the porch. "Use it or lose it" holds just as true in the senior years as beforehand: An inactive body will start to deteriorate. A physically fit 60-year-old will be in better shape than a 40-year-old couch potato.

Exercise helps slow down, prolong and even stop the processes of physical degeneration. Even if

Before and after your workout

— Don't overload your body with a big meal before a workout; if you need to eat something, have something light, and even then eat only a little.
— Always warm up with stretching and loosening-up exercises (see Stretching, p. 765). They're also useful for "warming down" afterwards, particularly if your workout involves only certain muscle groups.
— Step up the intensity of your workouts gradually; pay attention to your body and don't push yourself to the point of exhaustion.
— After a brisk run, cool down with a walk.
— Stay alert to your body's signals: Discomfort, dizziness, nausea or pain during or after sports is a sign of overexertion, or an indication that your technique isn't right yet or that this activity simply isn't for you.
— Drink plenty of liquids following a workout—or even during, if it's for long periods. As an alternative to "sports drinks," a mixture of one part fruit juice to two parts mineral water is cheaper and just as effective.
— A hot bath, shower, or sauna relaxes the muscles.
— Don't work out in the evening or just before going to bed: This may disrupt sleep patterns (see Sleep Disorders, p. 190).

age-induced changes limit your capabilities, benefits can be derived from just about any activity that's painless and enjoyable.

Exercise that builds endurance and has a low accident ratio is particularly beneficial, including

— Swimming, vigorous long walks, hiking, running, bicycling, cross-country skiing, or rowing.
— Competitive sports such as tennis, table tennis, or soccer.
— Don't take up any sport without proper preparation.
— Train under professional supervision—join a health club or take a class. This way, you learn proper technique and find your own pace. If you're older, see a sports doctor and have them gauge your physical condition before starting out.
— Watch for signs of exertion, such as exhaustion, dizziness, headaches, or chest pain.
— Always take breaks and never exceed your limits. Learn to recognize your individual tempo, and pace yourself.

Children

Lots of exercise is essential for healthy development. Regardless of age, every child has a natural need to play and be active: Providing plenty of freedom and space to do so is the best thing you can do for the development of a strong, healthy body. Special physical training or gymnastics programs are then not necessary; they may even hinder a child's natural development.

As early as kindergarten, and certainly by the time they enter grade school, children start to adopt the sedentary habits of adults and their natural need to be active is thwarted. Apartments and city living aren't conducive to freewheeling movements; television screens or computer monitors monopolize children's attention, keeping them in a rigid position with poor posture, often for hours.

Physical stimulation improves the tone of the whole body—musculoskeletal system—bones, joints, cartilage, ligaments and tendons.

— Even if your child "hates sports," he or she doesn't by nature hate all physical activity. Try to involve her in a sport that's right for her.
— If the "play" aspect of sports is emphasized, children can become enthusiastic about any kind of activity—bicycling, playing ball, swimming, sledding, skiing, or skating. The emphasis needs to be on playing the game, not winning or losing. All too often, parents get way too emotionally involved in their children's sports.
— Exercise that builds endurance and strengthens the cardiovascular system is best—jogging, swimming, bicycling, gymnastics, playing ball, skiing, and skating. Children have a natural safeguard against overexertion: they simply get tired and stop before they exceed their limits.

Sports also teach children important life skills and behavior.

— Team sports can improve social skills; they teach team spirit and increase awareness of one's own strengths and weaknesses as well as those of team members.
— Strenuous sports such as tennis or squash help release aggression.
— Endurance sports encourage perseverance and self-motivation.
— Lifting weights is harmful for children under age 15; neither their muscles nor their bones are ready for strength training or sprinting.

— Intensive high-performance sports are almost always harmful; the child's body is rendered too flexible while it's still developing, which can have lasting negative impact on body alignment.

Exercising during pregnancy

If you are pregnant, you can maintain your usual exercise routine unless it involves high-performance sports or training.

Women in high-risk pregnancies should always seek medical advice about how much and how hard to exercise.

Sports that build endurance are recommended during pregnancy, because they
— Help prevent thrombosis, varicose veins, and hemorrhoids
— Improve oxygen supply to mother and child alike
— Reduce psychological stress and enhance physical capacity

About a month after childbirth, sports-minded women can gradually start exercising again. However, a 3-month break is recommended before taking up t sports that stress ligaments, tendons, and muscles.

Stretching

Everybody needs to stretch after long periods of inactivity. Start by stretching thoroughly in the morning while you're still in bed. Stretching exercises emulate this movement and are a gentle form of physical training appropriate for all ages and conditions. While stretching doesn't build muscle strength, it reduces tension and improves the elasticity of muscles, tendons ,and ligaments.

The more frequently you do the exercises, the better; daily is best, but you'll see definite improvement even if you stretch only two or three times a week.
— Improved mobility is noticeable very quickly.
— Regular stretching can help prevent injuries and accidents; daily activities are easier to accomplish.
— Stretching exercises are ideal for warming up.

Stretching isn't strenuous and you can do it anywhere. In as little as 20 minutes, you can give all the large muscle groups a workout; adapt your routine to your individual capacity.

The basic pattern for all stretching exercises is the same:
— Get into position; gently stretch the target muscle(s).

— Hold the position until you feel a release of tension (usually after about 20 seconds). Breathe normally throughout the whole exercise.
— Never stretch to the limit of pain, and ease back if you don't feel the muscle tension releasing.
— Always stretch both sides of the body equally to maintain symmetry.
— Stretching should always be slow and steady. Avoid quick or jerky motions.
— Consciously experience the stretch as well as the ensuing release; take all the time you need.
— Stretch whenever you feel like it: after getting up, during breaks, after work, or before and after training. The program of Basic Stretching Exercises on p. 767 alternates between easy and more strenuous exercises.

Isometric Training

A movement that overcomes resistance—such as jumping, or throwing a ball—is known as a *dynamic* or *isotonic force.* When a muscle presses against or is equal to a resistive force, this is known as *static* or *isometric force.* Muscle tone is strengthened without shortening the muscle.

Isometric exercises that build static strength can be performed anywhere, at any time and throughout life. Build up to major exertion gradually, otherwise the cardiovascular system can suffer significant damage.

The following isometric exercise can easily be done at the office, while talking on the phone: While standing with the receiver in one hand, press against the wall in front of you with the other hand. Alternate every 4 seconds.

FITNESS

Terms such as aerobics, bodywork, or bodystyling are still relatively new but already well known to the younger generation. They are contemporary ways of staying fit and offer many health benefits. Cardiovascular exercise can improve circulation and oxygen supply; it also regulates blood pressure and stimulates breakdown of body fat. These sorts of exercises principally increase endurance and build up various muscle groups (stomach, buttocks, shoulders, and back, depending on the exercise).

Most health club programs are also geared to help strengthen and build up certain muscles. Training for

Rating your health club

— Sign up for a trial membership (the fee may be applicable toward membership, should you decide to join). During the introductory session the trainer should devote full attention to you, explaining how each machine works and which body parts it trains.

— A complete fitness facility should include equipment for endurance training such as a treadmill, rowing machine or exercise bike.

— In addition to strength and endurance, you also need to train for flexibility. Check to see what the club offers in terms of gymnastics, stretching and/or relaxation classes. You should also be able to participate in group programs like aerobics, modern dance and/or gymnastics.

— The use of additional equipment such as a sauna or swimming pool should be included in membership.

— Ask about the professional qualifications of the staff.

— Find out about the scope and type of tests that constitute your personal evaluation, which should be performed the day you sign up. At a minimum, these should test your endurance, strength and flexibility. The test should take about an hour—at the very least, 20 minutes. Usually, the more comprehensive the test, the better your individual training program will be.

— After your evaluation, get your personalized training program in writing. Request a reevaluation and modification to your program after three to four months.

— Do not sign a contract for longer than a 6-month period. You should be able to renew the contract with quarterly cancellation options. The contract should have provisions for automatic, penalty-free cancellations in the event of pregnancy, military call-up or transfer; it should lapse without penalty in the event of long-term illness or serious accident. In addition to long-term contracts, membership options should include monthly subscriptions and passes.

strength can help alleviate back problems or painful shoulder/neck problems. However, the prerequisites of a worthwhile program are good instruction and access to the right equipment; unfortunately, health-club instructors are often not very well trained.

TYPES OF SPORTS

Walking, Running, and Hiking

Walking and running are among the healthiest, simplest, and most environmentally friendly modes of human activity: They call for dynamic use of the muscles, are easy, and can be done anywhere, at any time without expensive equipment.

— Speedwalking (in which one foot is always on the ground) and running are good for the cardiovascular system and overall conditioning.

— Hiking is a good hobby for people who don't have excellent endurance and are not especially active but still want to maintain cardiovascular fitness. Energy output increases with pace, body weight (including clothing and backpack), and the incline of the terrain.

— Running and jogging involve the major muscle groups, don't require much strength and make for excellent endurance training; blood pressure stays about constant and speed can be easily adjusted.

It's important to check your pulse regularly: Don't overdo. Many runners run far too quickly, not realizing that they simply end up being exhausted sooner.

— Set your workout by the length of the course, rather than an allotted period of time.

— Stop if you feel tired: your physical condition varies from day to day.

Risk of Injury

Running seldom causes injury. Avoid pulled muscles and tendons by doing warm-up exercises for 5 to 10 minutes and starting off slowly. At the first signs of wear in hip and leg joints, switch to other forms of endurance training such as swimming or bicycling. Make sure you run on the right surface: A springy, yielding path in the woods or fields is best. Running on asphalt or other hard surfaces can cause considerable damage. The severity of impact is determined by road surface and the quality of your shoes.

Good shoes protect the spinal column, feet, knee, and hip joints. It is important to have good tread and flexible soles as well as a stable heel to hold the foot securely in place.

Bicycling

Cycling doesn't require a major financial investment, and is also an ecologically sound form of transportation.

Although bicycling gives the buttock muscles less of a workout than running, it is much easier on the hip and knee joints. With proper posture and technique,

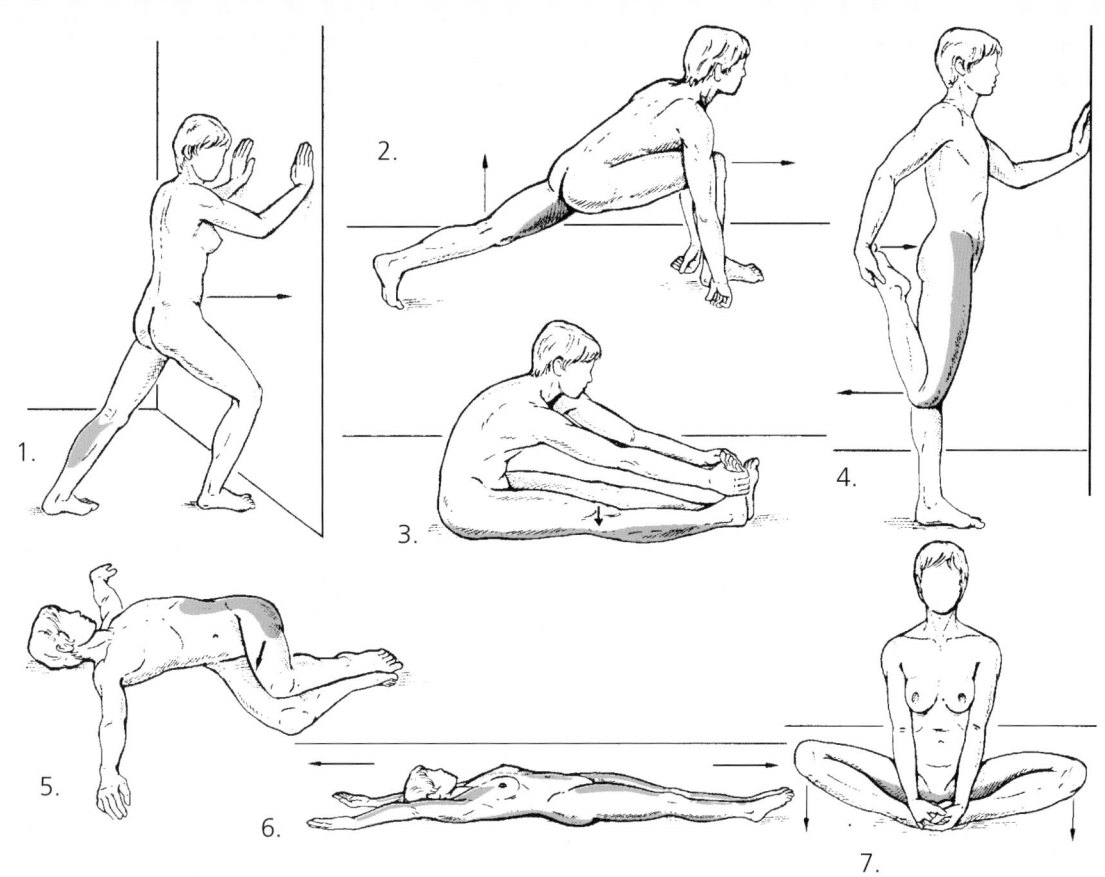

Basic Stretching Exercises

1. Stand with your feet flat on the floor; lean against the wall with both hands; flex one knee; regulate tension by moving your pelvis (this stretches the calf muscles).
2. Crouch in the starter's position; facing forward, stretch your back knee (thigh muscles).
3. Sit on the floor with your legs extended in front of you; with knees flexed, grasp feet with both hands and simultaneously bend your hips outward; avoid tensing your quadriceps (thigh and calf muscles).
4. Standing straight and relaxed, place one hand on the wall in front of you; press heel to buttock and move knee backward without stressing the lower back (thigh muscles; hip).

5. Lie on your back and extend arms to either side; pull knees up to your belly and then to one side (the more extended the hip, the better the stretch); alternate (buttocks and abdominal muscles).
6. Lie flat on your back and stretch; point toes and fingers and try to extend yourself as much as possible until you can feel the stretch all through your body (full-body stretch).
7. Sitting on the floor, bend your legs and grasp both heels, bringing them as close to your body as possible; relax your knees and let them fall to either side; maximize the stretch by tipping your pelvis forward and bending your upper body (adductor muscles).

cycling barely stresses the spinal column at all. The bicycle should be adjusted so that the upper body (with the back straight) leans forward at a 45 degree angle.

Because they enforce unnatural posture and put too much stress on neck and shoulder muscles, racing handlebars aren't advisable for people with back problems.

In comparison to running, the intensity of cycling is a little more difficult to control because the rider is more susceptible to conditions like elevation and wind. After long rides, make up for the relatively unnatural position with loosening-up exercises to straighten and relax your back.

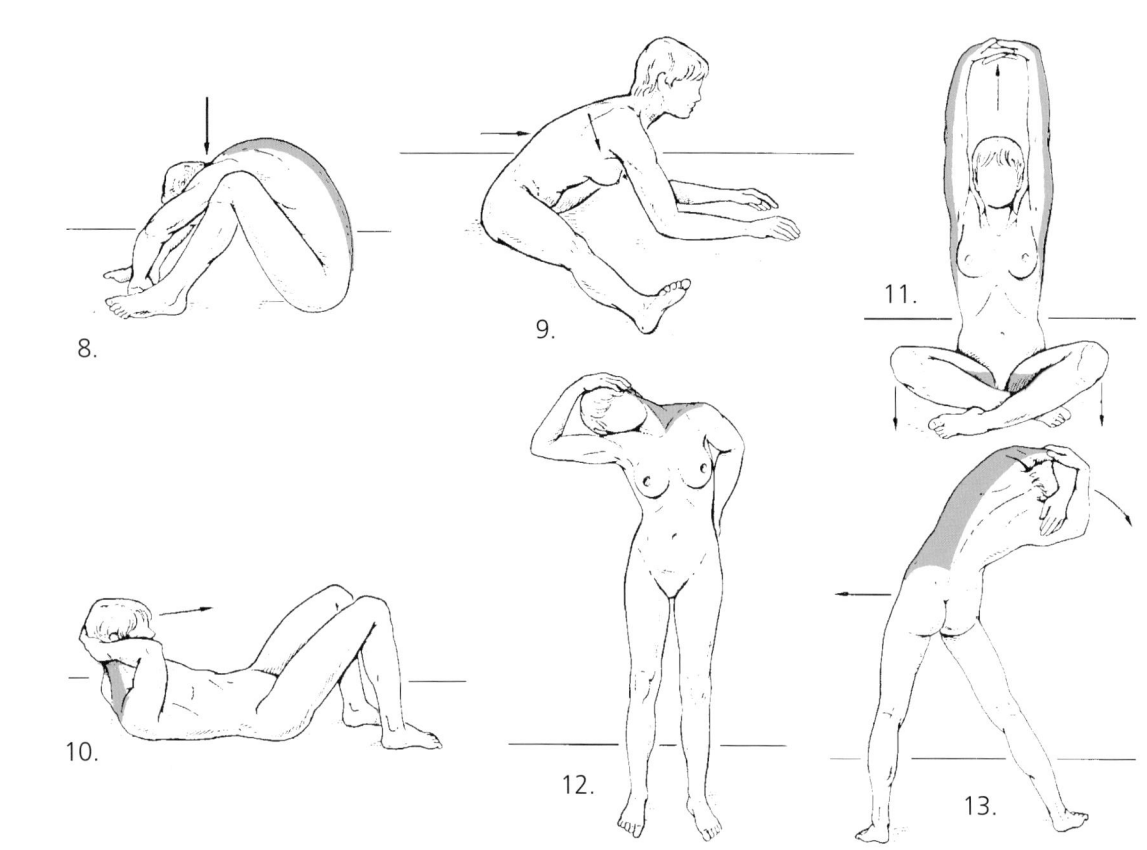

8. Sit on the floor; placing your feet in line with your hips, let your knees fall to either side; tuck your head down and arch your back (back and adductor muscles).
9. Sit on the floor with legs spread wide; bracing hands against floor, tip pelvis forward and extend the whole upper body (adductor muscles).
10. Lie on your back with knees bent and feet on the floor; folding hands behind neck, raise head up and forward until you can feel the stretch (neck muscles).
11. Sit cross-legged; pull feet close to your body; with back straight and fingers interlaced palm side out, stretch arms over head and extend your whole torso upward (adductors, the lateral back muscles, arm muscles).

12. Stand with legs slightly apart; place one hand on hip; place the other arm over your head and stretch (muscles on the side of the neck).
13. Stand with legs wide apart; bend one arm behind head and bend the whole torso to one side as far as you can; intensify the stretch by extending your hip (abdominal muscles, lower back, lateral back muscles, upper arm, and adductor muscles).

Risk of Injury

Most injuries incurred while cycling are due to traffic accidents. Cyclists should follow traffic rules and regulations, just as they expect drivers to observe them.
— Wear a helmet: Evidence shows that they can protect against head trauma in accidents.

Swimming

For many, swimming is more than just a leisure activity. Indoor swimming pools make it a year-round activity open to all ages and nearly all physical conditions. Swimming strengthens the lungs, cardiovascular system, and the entire musculature. The constant water resistance builds limb strength.

The prerequisite for serious training is that you actually work at it and not just take a dip. To strengthen your endurance, swim laps and get your heart rate up. Almost everyone finds water both relaxing and refreshing. Many people experience a feeling of euphoria and inner peace after swimming, which can last several hours.

People with asthma usually have fewer attacks when swimming than running or cycling, because the moist air traps dust and allergens.

While swimming is one of the most comfortable sports for people who are overweight, doctors often recommend forms of exercise that involve being on their feet, to enhance awareness of body, weight, and self.

Risk of Injury

Chlorine or other additives can irritate the eyes. Bacterial or fungal genital infections are easily transmitted in water.

— Don't leave on a wet bathing suit: This can cause bladder irritations.
— For those with knee problems, the crawl is preferable to the breaststroke.
— Swimming fast in relatively hot water (92°–94°F) can lead to overheating and profuse sweating.
— People who have had a heart attack must be careful when swimming because the filling pressure in the heart increases.

Track and Field

Running, jumping, and throwing a javelin or discus are among the oldest forms of sports. Today, many people participate in modern track and field events incorporating a range of different disciplines.

Track and field strengthens and refines a range of functions, from circulation and nervous system to the basic physical characteristics of strength, speed, endurance, flexibility, and grace.

Track and field is ideal for the single competitor and less suited as a family sport. Training isn't limited to the gym, field, or stadium: You can also train in fields and forest.

Risk of Injury

The biggest risk is posed by sprinting, which places excessive strain on the joints. The danger of injury increases proportionally with fatigue.

Rowing and Crew

Rowing strengthens the whole body. This endurance sport is suitable for older people as well as children. It calls on nearly all the muscles, particularly those of the arms, shoulders, and (because of the roller seat) legs. It stimulates the autonomic nervous system as well as circulation, prevents postural damage and maintains flexibility.

Despite this sport's many benefits, relatively few people row. Many of those who do have made it into a competition sport. Most rowing clubs participate in regattas.

Risk of Injury

The risk of injury is very small. The most common injuries are relatively harmless scrapes, bruises (especially of the thumb), blisters and calluses.

Horseback Riding

Riding is fun for people of all levels of training and experience, and encourages a rapport with the great outdoors. It is a good activity for groups—even those with varying skill levels—and can be enjoyed well into old age.

Riding teaches coordination and skill through close interaction with the horse, which requires intense concentration on the rider's part. At the same time, all the muscles of the buttocks, arms, and legs get a thorough workout. The constant muscle work involved stimulates circulation. The proper posture required for riding—erect with bent legs—has a beneficial effect on the spinal column, and the constant need to stay balanced promotes overall good posture.

Risk of Injury

Although falls from a horse occur relatively rarely, they can cause serious injuries and fractures; a helmet or riding hat is essential gear. Knee and leg injuries can be caused by slipping off or getting tangled in the stirrups.

Cross-Country Skiing

Cross-country skiing is considered the healthiest winter sport and the best for building endurance in all age groups. It calls for rhythmic coordination of nearly all the muscle groups—particularly leg, arm, and shoulder muscles. Forward motion through coordinated arm/leg movement coupled with the straight (albeit slightly inclined) spine makes this sport especially easy on the back.

Because the feet glide rather than being planted, the spinal column is not jolted.

Those who don't want their skiing limited to the winter months can invest in indoor roller-ski equipment.

Risk of Injury

The danger of injury while cross-country skiing is relatively low. As with all other sports, however, take some classes before you set out. The important trick of taking a fall gently (roll with it) must be mastered beforehand. If you feel unsure, or the trail is dangerous, take off your skis. Always keep to marked trails.

Downhill Skiing

Since downhill skiing can normally be done only a few days or weeks of the year, it is not particularly beneficial to the cardiovascular system. Its main benefits are leg-muscle strength and coordination. The attraction of the sport lies in the mastery of difficult techniques, its dynamism and speed, plus the intense rush of energy in pure mountain air and the dazzlingly beautiful winter landscape. However, there is a price to be paid for the lure of white mountainsides: The requisite huge tracts of land and long roads to ski destinations have turned downhill skiing into an environmentally harmful industry. Miles of trails, buildings and ski lifts can cause massive erosion and disruptions in the water table.

Risk of Injury

The risk of fractures and soft-tissue injuries is high. Forty percent of ski accidents stem from undisciplined skiing, exceeding one's capacities, or technical, or physical problems.

To prevent accidents

— Well before going skiing, start doing ski exercises.
— Take lessons. A good instructor can teach you the essential skill of gauging your own skill level correctly.
— Observe rules on the slopes; stay on trails. Don't ski after consuming alcohol.
— When you notice signs of wear and tear in the knees, hips, and spinal column, switch to cross-country skiing.

Ice Skating

Ice skating strengthens the lungs and cardiovascular system and teaches coordination and balance. It mainly uses the leg muscles. (You remember just how demanding on the legs this sport can be as soon as you get back on the ice after the summer off: You're virtually guaranteed a charley horse.)

Risk of Injury

If skating is a pastime rather than a profession, the risk of injury is relatively low. While falls are frequent, they normally incur nothing worse than small bruises or sprains of ankles and wrists. However, severe falls can cause broken arms and concussions. There is also a danger of lacerations from the skate blades. Ice skating should be discouraged if you have joint problems, and is out of the question if you have osteoporosis. Elbow and knee protection is advisable. Ice skates should fit snugly so that even the slightest movement is transferred directly to the blade.

In-Line Skating, Roller Skating

Like ice skating, in-line and roller skating are good for the lungs, cardiovascular system and leg muscles in addition to teaching coordination.

This new sport is fun not only for children: Many adults use skates as an alternative means of transportation in the asphalt jungle. A smooth surface is essential. As a means of experiencing nature in its purest form, skating has inherent limitations: It's a city sport.

Risk of Injury

Falls can result in scrapes, bruises, and fractures. Collisions with other skaters, pedestrians or cyclists can be dangerous. Speeds of up to 30 mph are possible, but speed enthusiasts should wear helmets. Elbows, knees, wrists, and palms should also be protected.

Dance

Jazzercise, African dance, modern dance, rock-and-roll, swing dancing, dance improvisation, tango, salsa, flamenco or belly dancing can all have significant and positive effects on physical and emotional well-being. Dancing teaches coordination and grace. The physiological benefits depend on the type and intensity of the dance: Competitive ballroom dancing is usually classified as a sport; aerobics and jazz dance as gymnastics.

You don't need a class or a studio—dancing at home to relax or cross-train can be just as fun and beneficial. Free-form dancing is a great way to express feelings and emotions.

Risk of Injury

Risks of injury are low. In show or acrobatic dancing, involving lifting and swinging partners around, accidents or overexertion can result. As with all types of physical activity, exercise in moderation.

TEAM SPORTS

Competitive games such as tennis, table tennis, soccer, volleyball or other team sports are exciting and have a social element. However, by their nature they make it harder to pay attention to stress on the cardiovascular system.

Overzealous play places excessive strain on the body. If you have heart problems, always seek medical advice before starting a sport of this type. For people with a history of cardiac trouble, a sports program endorsed by the hospital is recommended.

The following applies to all sports:

— Take plenty of time to warm up, and start at a moderate pace.
— Always build up your playing style gradually. Choosing the right partner and agreeing beforehand to the duration and pace of a match or game can prevent overdoing it.

Soccer

Soccer is one of the most popular team sports world wide. Once primarily a man's sport, it now attracts more and more women. It builds speed, endurance, flexibility, and strength. Some of soccer's health benefits come from running up to 7 miles per game.

Risk of Injury

The lower extremities are especially at risk. Torn ligaments, damaged cartilage, muscle strains, and torn leg muscles are common injuries.

Tennis

The distinctive movements required in tennis—stretch-ing and bending, running and turning—make use of various muscle groups, particularly those in the legs, shoulders, abdomen, and back. They make tennis a versatile sport that's good for cross-training. However, it should not be taken up without professional instruction, to avoid injury to the dominant arm and the spine. Tennis can be enjoyed from youth into old age, but if you are coming to the sport late, or taking it up again after some time, be careful. Because of its intensity, competitive tennis is not appropriate for people with cardiac problems.

Tennis is also not ideal for people with back problems: Especially when serving, the spine can be twisted and hyperextended.

Leaping, sprinting, lunging, and stopping on a dime all put great stress on the back.

Risk of Injury

Most tennis injuries occur in the arms and legs, the most common being "tennis elbow" (see p. 462), which is usually caused by poor serving technique or using the wrong racquet.

Squash

Squash can be learned much more quickly than tennis. It requires and builds good reaction time, coordination and speed. The ball can reach speeds of up to 120 mph. During a fast-paced game, cardiovascular strain can be very high. The duration and pace of a match should be determined by the skill levels of the players.

Risk of Injury

Because of the abrupt starts and stops and the lunging inherent in the sport, the cardiovascular system, spine and ankles come under particular strain. This may cause sprained ankles, torn calf muscles, and even torn Achilles tendon (see Tendons and Ligaments, p. 441).

Table Tennis

Like tennis, table tennis (or ping-pong) calls for a variety of movements, but unlike tennis it involves little or no running. It requires concentration, good reaction time, technique, and coordination rather than overall endurance. The risk of injury is slight.

HEALTHY LIVING

Although we usually think of "environmental issues" as having to do with the outdoors, concentrations of hazardous substances are often much higher indoors, where many of us spend most of our time. Among those substances that are particularly dangerous are certain types of particle board, wood preservatives, varnishes, floor coverings, carpeting, wallpaper, paint, adhesives, furniture, sealants, and other building materials. Personal-care products, household chemicals and textiles are another source of harmful substances and potential health risks.

Pollution in the Home

The presence of harmful substances in the home barely impinges on our consciousness. If there were laws regulating home air quality as there are for automobile and industrial pollution, millions of us wouldn't be allowed to live where we do.

Odorless, Colorless, and Lethal

Many people live in a toxic environment for years without knowing it. Appliances often emit fumes at very low levels; years of exposure can lead to health problems. Those who spend a lot of time—sleeping, reading, watching television—near a source of toxic fumes are especially at risk.

The human sense of smell quickly becomes inured to a familiar odor so it is no longer noticeable. Many harmful substances, of course, are completely odorless.

Unidentified Causes of Disease

Toxins in the home often go unrecognized as the cause of many diseases. The average person, but also many doctors, aren't sufficiently informed about the consequences of living in a toxin-laced environment.

Diagnosis can be difficult, since a combination of different factors is often at work: Usually there is no single cause of illness. The easiest culprits to identify are wood preservatives (see p. 781) or products containing formaldehyde (see p. 773). Gases are released during the large-scale application of paint or adhesives. If air circulation is poor, the fumes can become so concentrated that they cause acute health problems such as dizziness, inability to concentrate, headaches, and nausea.

Much more common is a complex of health problems known as "sick building syndrome," which manifest as irritations of the airways and conjunctiva. Those affected by the large number of environmental toxins suffer from headaches, general malaise, sleep, and concentration disorders. Smoking and badly installed air conditioners, particularly in offices (see p. 789), only make it worse. One analysis suggests that 10 to 20 percent of the population suffers from this syndrome.

General tips

If you suffer from general symptoms, try to determine whether some might be related to toxins in your home.

If you see a doctor about your symptoms, don't forget to discuss your living environment. Have you moved recently? Have you been working with paints and sealants? Is there a noticeable smell in your kitchen or bedroom?

Healthy Living is Possible

Clean air in your living space is possible, but you'll most likely have to take responsibility for it yourself. The fact is, nontoxic alternatives exist for all building materials, furnishings, household chemicals, and textiles. Usually these products are relatively expensive. If you can't afford new furniture made from solid wood, buy it second-hand.

Your first attempt at using all-natural products may be discouraging: Nontoxic paint doesn't cover as well, or the final effect isn't as nice. Make sure the product is the right one for the job. Conventional stores or building-supply outlets often do not have knowledgeable personnel to help you, but businesses specializing in environmentally sound products often do. The best time to create a healthy living space is when you are building, renovating or remodeling. Before renting a home or apartment, it's a good idea to reach an agreement with your landlord about whether and how you can renovate.

Once you determine that your health is being affected by your living space, you may want to start making changes in the bedroom, since this is where most people spend most of their home time.

A harmless, cost-efficient and beautiful way of

improving indoor air quality is plants (see p. 789): A single plant is all it takes to purify 10 cubic meters of air.

Your Contribution to Caring for the Environment

By using environmentally friendly and organic building materials, the whole cycle of production-consumption-waste becomes nontoxic. Careful selection of materials for both home and office use makes a big difference; in addition to benefitting your family's health, you are also do your part to protect the environment.

THE MOST COMMON POLLUTANTS

FORMALDEHYDE

Formaldehyde is the most ubiquitous and commonly produced chemical in the world. It can be found in the following products, among others:

Products that contain formaldehyde	
Medications	Leather
Car-care products	Glue
Bath oils	Metals
Deodorants	Mouthwashes
Disinfectants	Nail hardeners
Paints	Paper
Felt-tip pens	Photographic paper
Floor sealants	Shoe polish
Dishwasher	Soap
detergents	Softeners
Rubber	Shampoo
Household cleaners	Fillers
Wood preservatives	Particle boards
Foam insulation	Textiles (especially easy-care)
Tape/Adhesives	Cosmetics
Lighter Fluid	Laundry detergent
Varnishes	Toothpaste
Synthetics	Food (trace amounts)

Formaldehyde is also formed in the combustion process, such as when cooking or heating with gas, and in cigarette smoke and car exhaust.

The principal cause of long-term formaldehyde contamination indoors remains particle boards used for furniture, walls and ceilings. High levels of formaldehyde have been detected in homes built with particle board as much as 15 years later.

Formaldehyde is often present in the polyurethane sprays frequently used as cold barriers in old buildings around windows, doors, walls and in attics. Formaldehyde is released into the surrounding space at various rates, and the threshold of irritation varies from person to person. In higher concentrations, formaldehyde has a sharp, stinging smell; in concentrations greater than 4 to 5 parts per million it causes the eyes to tear.

Possible Health Effects

The effects of formaldehyde include breathing difficulties, irritating cough, red eyes, stinging in nose, chronic cold, asthma, skin allergy (contact dermatitis), hair loss, sore throat, headaches, nausea, vomiting, conjunctivitis, sleep disorders, difficulties concentrating, dizziness, and stomach and heart problems. Formaldehyde is also suspected of causing cancer and genetic damage.

If you are experiencing any of the above symptoms, ask yourself:

— Are your symptoms worse at the beginning and end of the heating season, as well as in warm and humid weather?

— Does your condition improve when you leave home? If the answer to either question is "yes," suspect formaldehyde. If you are uncertain and cannot find out for sure or remove the source yourself, have formaldehyde levels measured).

Recommendations

Formaldehyde levels should ideally be as low as possible. Note that foam insulation containing formaldehyde may not be removable without considerable expense.

— Use real, native wood wherever possible.

— If using particle board is unavoidable, use those which do not contain formaldehyde.

— Be especially alert when buying inexpensive children's furniture: Children are particularly sensitive to formaldehyde.

— In case of future claims, make sure that any particle board you are buying is safe for interior use.

— Air out the house as often as possible, first raising temperature and humidity levels (this increases release of gas, so do it while the place is empty).

— Remove old particle boards where possible.

THE OZONE KILLERS: HALOGENATED HYDROCARBONS

This group of harmful substances consists mostly of chlorofluorocarbons and fluorocarbons (the Freons). These gases are some of the most versatile and lucrative products the chemical industry has to offer, used in aerosol sprays, Styrofoam production and insulating materials.

They have also been used in fire extinguishers and as cooling agents in freezers, refrigerators and air conditioners. These gases are relatively nonpoisonous and nonflammable; however, they destroy the ozone layer and actively exacerbate the greenhouse effect.

Possible Health Effects

The Freons contribute to the holes in the ozone layer, which filters the dangerous ultraviolet rays. Because these gases rise slowly, even if a worldwide production ban were implemented today they would continue to cause damage for at least 20 years. This is why we can count on an increase in skin cancer and eye problems in the future.

Recommendations

The Freons can almost always be replaced by less harmful substances.
— Don't use spray cans.
— When buying a refrigerator, freezer or air conditioner, choose one that uses a nonchlorinated fluorocarbon coolant. Those using helium are more effective and energy-saving; propane-butane mixtures are also effective agents.
— Hard foam used as insulation loses some of its heat value when produced without chlorofluorocarbons. Try choosing other insulating materials such as fiberglass, and increase the amount you use.

CHLORINATED HYDROCARBONS

Chlorinated hydrocarbons are ubiquitous. They break down very slowly, which is why they are everywhere—in drinking water, food, and air. Household uses include cleaning products, paint removers, and solvents.

Possible Health Effects

Chlorinated hydrocarbons can penetrate the skin and attack the central nervous system. Inhaled as fumes, they cause irritated mucous membranes and lung infections.

They accumulate in the brain, liver, kidneys, heart and gonads. Long-term exposure can lead to chronic damage.

Many solvents containing chlorinated hydrocarbons are suspected of being carcinogenic. Chloroform has been shown to be carcinogenic in animals.

Recommendations

— Use only products free of solvents, or those with solvents in very low concentration.
— Chlorinated solvents can be replaced by terpenes made from citrus peels or conifers, among other things, which break down organically.
— Solvents such as alcohol, ester, and ketone are considered much less harmful.

POLYCHLORINATED BIPHENYLS (PCB)

For years, polychlorinated biphenyls were used to strengthen paints and varnishes as well as make them fire-resistant. They were also used as softeners in synthetics. Despite stricter controls today, they are still generally present in fat-containing foodstuffs, mother's milk, and human fatty tissue. They are also released by various garbage disposal techniques.

Possible Health Effects

If large amounts of PCBs enter the body through the food chain, acute toxicity may result, causing damage to liver, spleen, and kidneys. A chronic low dose causes reproductive disorders and compromises the immune system, concentration, and memory.

PENTACHLOROPHENOL (PCP)

In the 1970s, thousands of people painted their wood-paneled ceilings and walls with wood preservatives containing pentachlorophenol, a substance that kills bacteria and fungi. Over the years the treated wood released toxic vapors, making many houses and apartments uninhabitable.

Possible Health Effects

Acute toxicity: hyperventilation, nausea, headaches, seizures, loss of consciousness. Long-term exposure causes liver and kidney damage. The patient is continuously tired and loses weight.

Harmful substances in the home

Harmful substance	Source	Health effects	Concentration (in closed rooms)
Solvents, such as benzene dichloroethane, toluene	Paints, varnishes, resins, polishes, cleaners	Headaches, irritations of mucous membranes, nervous system disorders, liver and kidney damage, possible cancer with benzene and dichloroethane	Critical
Formaldehyde	Glues, varnishes, foams, particle boards	Irritations of the mucous membranes, inflammation of airways and conjunctiva, headaches, lung damage	Critical
Carbon dioxide (CO_2)	Heating, gas stoves, exhaled air, outdoor air	Headaches, dizziness, elevated blood pressure	Critical
Carbon monoxide (CO)	Car exhaust, heating, fires/fireplaces/woodstoves	Blockage of oxygen supply, circulatory disorders	Usually not critical
Nitric oxide (NO)	Heating, gas stoves, tobacco smoke, outdoor air	Cough, salivation, cold, breathing disorders, lung damage	Critical
Sulfur dioxide (SO_2)	Heating, gas stoves, human metabolism, tobacco smoke, outdoor air	Irritations of the mucous membranes, inflammation of airways and conjunctiva, bronchitis, breathing difficulties	Usually not critical
Polychlorinated biphenyls, phenol, styrene, etc.	Softeners in synthetics	Liver, spleen and kidney damage, headaches, dizziness, tiredness, reproductive disorders, weakened immune system, reduced concentration and awareness, possible cancer with phenol and styrene	Critical
Radon	Tiles, natural stones, natural gas	Nausea, stomach and intestinal disorders, weakness, all other signs of radiation poisoning	Critical

Recommendations

— Avoid using wood preservatives containing PCP.

— When buying wood products and furniture, ask for a written statement that it has not been treated with PCP or other wood preservatives.

Warning: Imported wood may still contain PCP.

POLYVINYLCHLORIDES (PVC)

PVCs are some of the best-known synthetics: they are used in various household items such as plumbing pipes, window shades, tablecloths, curtains, packaging, and toys. Because of the extremely toxic gases (dioxins, hydrogen chloride) given off when PVC is burned, it is no longer in use.

Possible Health Effects

When PVC-containing products burn, hydrogen chloride gas is released, irritating the airways; long-term exposure causes bronchial problems. Fires in houses with PVC floors are especially dangerous—they can cause additional fire damage and poisoning.

Vinylchloride monomers are carcinogenic and released only in very small quantities from modern PVC products.

Various synthetic materials are suspected of having estrogenic effects, thereby impairing reproductive capacity.

SOFTENERS

Softeners are often used in synthetics, textiles, and tobacco products; phthalic acid esters are used most often. They are present in large quantities in the environment and do not break down easily. If food is wrapped in foil or coated paper that contain these substances, they are transferred to—and consumed along with—the food.

Possible Health Effects

Little research has been done; possible risk of cancer.

DIOXIN

What is generally called "dioxin" should really be referred to scientifically as 2,3,7,8-tetrachlorodibenzo-para-dioxin (2,3,7,8 TCDD). Besides this, there are about a dozen other dioxins and dibenzofuranes, which are among the most dangerous substances known in organic chemistry. The chemical accident in Seveso, Italy in 1976 made it clear that dioxin is a chemical poison and that even the smallest amounts can be harmful.

It is known mainly as an environmental toxin; however, it can also occur indoors if solvents containing chlorinated hydrocarbons (see p. 774) or PCP-treated wood (see p. 781) are burned.

Possible Health Effects

The primary source (over 90 percent) is food: Dioxin becomes concentrated through the food chain. It is a carcinogen; high doses cause birth defects. Chronic low doses may affect metabolism and thyroid function. Amounts about 10 times greater than "normal" exposure can affect the reproductive, immune and central nervous systems. Amounts about a hundred times greater than "normal" exposure result in chloracne (a skin condition) and liver damage.

ASBESTOS

For many years, asbestos was considered an all-purpose material for insulating, soundproofing, and fireproofing. This versatile substance was installed not only in countless apartments, but also in auditoriums, schools, swimming pools, offices and exterior walls of buildings. It was also used freely in household objects like hairdryers, and heat sources. Although the danger of asbestos has long been well-known, it continues to be mined and used in flooring and other construction materials.

Possible Health Effects

Abrading asbestos creates a very fine dust that invades the lungs. No amount is tolerable: Even the tiniest particle can trigger lung cancer. In the industrialized countries, airborne asbestos fibers cause thousands of deaths.

Recommendations

— Check your home for asbestos-containing objects such as hairdryers or window boxes made in the 60s and 70s; discard.

Warning: Products containing asbestos are hazardous waste and must not go into the regular trash.

— If you need to dispose of large surfaces containing asbestos (e.g., floors), make sure to employ qualified professionals using the appropriate suction equipment. Well-equipped companies also provide protective clothing and masks when removing asbestos boards so that all harmful dust particles are removed. Similar precautions should be followed when electric space heaters are broken or dismantled. Pressing, tearing or sanding asbestos material is especially dangerous.

Over the past few years, asbestos removal has become a thriving industry. Beware of contractors who propose painting over the walls and cracks with synthetics: These often crack off again, exposing the underlying asbestos.

RADIOACTIVITY

Radioactivity released by nuclear power plants is far more devastating than the "background" levels of radioactivity found in nature.

Radioactive Building Materials

Natural radiation levels will vary depending on where you live. They may increase in buildings incorporating materials with high levels of radioactivity. Certain minerals, chemicals, and natural rock increase radioactivity; wood reduces it somewhat.

Possible Health Effects

The health effects of natural radiation are highly controversial. Most likely, there is no such thing as a "harmless" dose of radiation, although state or industry regulations may create that impression. On the other hand, no damage can be definitively attributed to natural radiation.

Radon

One of the so-called noble gases, radon is released from rocks and construction materials into the air we breathe. Relatively high levels are found in slag (rock waste), industrial gypsum, power-plant waste and blast furnace cement, as well as in naturally occurring rock such as granite and pumice. These materials often increase radon concentrations inside buildings to levels many times higher than those in the surrounding atmosphere.

HOUSEHOLD CHEMICALS

Product
Laundry detergent

Ingredients
Surfactants, bleach, fillers, phosphates

Possible health hazards
Skin irritations from frequent contact; potentially fatal poisoning in children, particularly from swallowing concentrated liquid detergent

Recommendations
Use less; adjust amount for hard water; avoid contact with skin; keep away from children

Product
Dishwasher detergent

Ingredients
Phosphates

Possible health hazards
Risk of poisoning (highly caustic)

Recommendations
Use correct amount; rinse dirty dishes beforehand; don't use finishing rinse agents (for extra shine, add vinegar to rinse water)

Product
All-purpose cleansers, abrasives

Ingredients
Surfactants

Possible health hazards
None, if used properly

Recommendations
Avoid cleaners that contain formaldehyde or organic chlorine; general-purpose cleaners are preferable to special-purpose products

Product
Toilet cleansers

Ingredients
Primarily chlorine

Possible health hazards
When used in conjunction with acid-based cleansers can release chlorine gas, which can cause lung damage and death

Recommendations
Avoid chlorinated toilet cleansers and drop-in-type products; use white vinegar and a toilet brush instead (but never together with chlorinated cleansers)

Product
Air freshener

Ingredients
Acetaldehyde, paraldehyde

Possible health effects
Liver damage, after long-term exposure

Recommendations
As an alternative, put a few drops of eau de cologne on a light bulb, or essential plant oils in a humidifier

Product
Drain openers/cleansers

Ingredients
Sodium hydroxide (caustic)

Possible health effects
Burns to skin; eye injuries from spray

Recommendations
Wear eye protection; avoid spray-type products; give the product enough time to work and don't try to unblock the drain manually at the same time

Product
Floor-care products

Ingredients
Solvents (e.g., chlorinated hydrocarbons)

Possible health effects
Long-term inhalation may cause nerve, liver, and kidney damage

Recommendations
Substitute all-purpose cleansers and waxes

Product
Rug cleaners (spray and shampoo)

Ingredients
Surfactants, solvents

Possible health effects
Possibly associated with fevers and febrile conditions in children

Recommendations
Deep-clean rugs as seldom as possible; treat individual spots with soap; keep children away; avoid open flame in vicinity

Product
Decalcifier (to remove scale or lime buildup on faucets or in coffee machines)

Ingredients
Various; formic acid

Possible health effects
Acid burns, vomiting, cough, circulatory collapse following accidental ingestion, damage to kidneys and bone marrow

Recommendations
Substitute diluted vinegar or a pinch of cream of tartar dissolved in water; for coffee machines, run as usual, then flush several times with water

Product
Spray-on oven cleaner

Ingredients
Sodium hydroxide, surfactants, solvents (among others)

Possible health effects
Skin and mucous membrane irritation from contact (through hands and eyes) with spray mist; solvent

residues turn up in food prepared in oven

Recommendations
Clean oven after each use; loosen baked-on food with water and remove with abrasive

Product
Spot remover

Ingredients
Chlorinated solvents

Possible health effects
Long-term exposure causes liver damage; suspected carcinogen

Recommendations
First try ordinary household products (soap, detergent, or isopropyl alcohol), then try dry cleaning

Product
Waterproofing spray for leather

Ingredients
Solvents

Possible health effects
Lung damage, fever, chills, headache, breathing difficulties, general collapse

Recommendations
Have leather items waterproofed at your dry cleaners; use sprays only on suede items

Product
Insecticides

Ingredients
Lindane, pyrethrins, permethrin

Possible health effects
Breathing difficulties, malaise, nausea, headaches if not used according to directions

Recommendations
Avoid wherever possible: insecticides kill off useful insects as well and are toxic to house pets, especially fish

Product
Insect repellent

Ingredients
Pyrethrins

Possible health effects
Bronchial asthma

Recommendations
Ultrasonic mosquito repellents are harmless, but they're also ineffective.

Keep your home sparkling with a minimum of chemicals
— A mild all-purpose cleanser, or even liquid soap or dish detergent containing surfactants, can be used in the kitchen, bathroom and toilet, on tiles and for spots on rugs. Check the product's pH factor: the more it deviates from 7, the more caustic the product—and the more environmentally hazardous.
— Nonchlorinated whiteners can be used to bleach sinks, bathtubs, irons, and stove tops.
— Use a mild abrasive if scrubbing with a sponge doesn't do the trick.
— Distilled white vinegar—a natural, environmentally safe product—will clean brass, remove scale and buildup, and clean toilets.
— Expensive window cleaners are unnecessary. Use rubbing alcohol to clean windows, mirrors and stubborn spots. Windows can also be cleaned using a little dish detergent or ammonia in water.

RADON
Radon causes lung cancer. Levels of radon vary by geographical region. Indoor radon concentrations can reach dangerous levels without adequate ventilation.

Recommendation
— Make sure your home has adequate ventilation. Air it out regularly (see p. 782).
— Have your home checked for radon levels (see p. 777).
— Select building materials with care.

CIGARETTE SMOKE
Cigarette smoke consists of about 2,000 chemical compounds, including carbon monoxide and nicotine,

irritants such as formaldehyde and acrolein, and carcinogenic hydrocarbons and nitrosamines. Cigarette smoke is by far the major source of indoor environmental toxins, and nonsmokers as well as smokers are at risk (see Smoking, p. 754).

PARTICLE BOARD

Plywood and particle board, which consists of wood fibers and binding agents, is extremely popular because it is easier to work with and considerably less expensive than solid wood.

Particle board is used to make lightweight and easily removable partitions, to cover old walls, floors, and ceilings, and in furniture construction (more than half of all particle board produced). Often it is covered with a wood veneer.

Harmful Binders

Artificial resins are the principal binders used in plywoods and particle boards. Most used to contain formaldehyde. The vapors these compounds emit into home and building interiors can cause a range of health problems.

Numerous particle board producers now use isocyanates as binders. Even low concentrations can cause serious health problems, irritating mucous membranes of the nose, throat and lungs and leading to shortness of breath and chest pains. Long-term exposure can cause coughing paroxysms, bronchitis and allergic reactions such as asthma.

Recommendation

See formaldehyde, p. 773.

Alternative solutions

Often, walls and furniture that are outgassing formaldehyde can't be removed easily—for instance, expensive, new built-in cabinets.

Here are some alternatives:
— Cover the offending area with coated wallpaper, plastic paneling or laminated wood. Uncoated wallcoverings or wood veneers won't do the trick.
— Refacing built-in structures is somewhat less effective: Any damage to the surface will reduce its effect. Paints and varnishes may contain solvents. PVC laminates bring their own problems (see p. 776).

— Airing rooms frequently is a short-term solution, but ineffective over the long term.

LACQUERS AND PAINTS

Lacquers and paints consist of pigments, solvents, binders, and other ingredients. Lacquers, which can contain up to 70 percent solvent, are especially noted for their covering properties.

Many paints, particularly those in the yellow, red and orange color range, also contain heavy metals such as cadmium, chromate, and lead.

Possible Health Effects

Solvents vary widely in their impacts on health. Not only can they cause serious work-related illnesses (see Health in the Workplace, p. 789), but they can also compromise the home environment by releasing fumes for weeks following application.

Recommendation

— Use lacquers or paints that are either solvent-free or contain only minimal solvents. Provide adequate ventilation when applying.
— Product designations for either "interior" or "exterior" use simply refer to the fact that some are more weather-resistant than others, and have little to do with the toxicity of the product.

Environmentally safe particle board

Use particle board containing magnesite, potassium silicate, calcium, gypsum or cement instead of artificial resins.

Products containing magnesite are not waterproof and should not be used in kitchens or bathrooms.

When using products containing cement binders, make sure it's natural or Portland cement: Other types may pose a health risk due to their higher radioactivity. Don't be daunted if the store clerk draws a blank when you ask for "cement-bound particle board": sometimes these products are identifiable only by brand name.

Disadvantage: Environmentally safe products are often more expensive.

Environmentally Friendly Lacquers and Paints

Water-based lacquers and paints can be used for almost all interior purposes. They have several advantages over oil-based paints:

— They dry faster (a second coat can be applied after only 3 hours).
— They are more weather-resistant.
— They are more colorfast and less subject to yellowing.
— The fumes are not health hazards.
— They don't pollute the air or water.
— They are diluted with water.
— Brushes can be cleaned with water.
— They create fewer disposal problems.

Disadvantages: Water-based paints are expensive and have a less glossy finish than oil-based products.

Warning: "Natural" alternatives aren't necessarily impact-free. Turpentine oil, titanium dioxide, mineral oil and citrus oil can irritate the skin and kidneys and cause nerve disorders and cancer. Before beginning a big paint job, read product directions thoroughly, inform yourself about possible health effects, and take all necessary precautions.

Tips for Paint Use

— Use water-soluble paints whenever possible.
— When using oil-based paints or lacquers indoors, make sure ventilation is adequate. Continue to ventilate the area even after the product has been applied: It will continue to release small amounts of fumes.
— Avoid open flames and don't smoke while using solvent-containing products: The fumes are highly flammable and explosive and may form poisonous gases when burned.
— Avoid skin contact with paints and solvents. Wear gloves.
— Do not pour a leftover solvent (such as after cleaning brushes) down the drain. They contaminate the water supply and are nonbiodegradable; their toxic fumes are also an explosion hazard in the sewage system.

WOOD PRESERVATIVES

The health hazards of wood preservatives have recently been brought to public attention by the pentachlorophenol (PCP) scandal (see p. 774). Many other substances used in interiors also pose health risks but are still in widespread use.

Dry Interior Environments

Avoid using pressure-treated lumber and other fungicide-impregnated woods for interiors, if possible. In the average household interior, wood will usually not get damp enough to sustain fungus growth. Use only wood-care products containing no fungicide or insecticide.

As a paint alternative, water-based wood stains are practical and inexpensive.

Damp Interior Environments

Rooms that get damp (bathrooms, kitchens, basements) need protection against mildew, but products containing fungicides and pesticides increase your health risk needlessly. Stick to products that protect only against mildew; while they aren't impact-free, they are less hazardous than combination products. Use an inert glaze for a sealant over the mildew-proofing coat.

Solvent	Health Risks
Benzene Toluene Inhalation	Carcinogen that can cause fatigue, nausea, delayed reaction time, manic behavior, or excitability. Prolonged exposure: nerve and liver damage, skin disorders.
Xylene	Prolonged inhalation can cause concentration problems and headaches, affect eyesight and equilibrium, affect blood makeup. Suspected carcinogen.
Methylisobutyl ketone	Eye and nasal irritant
Butyl acetate	Mucous membrane irritant
Butanol	Mucous membrane irritant; headaches

Chlorinated hydrocarbons such as carbon tetrachloride and chloroform can penetrate skin and attack the central nervous system. Prolonged exposure can cause nerve and brain damage. Carbon tetrachloride is toxic to the liver. Tests on laboratory animals suggest chloroform is carcinogenic.

Toxic ingredients in wood preservatives

— Lindane, added to wood preservatives to kill insects, is considered an environmental toxin. It can also cause nerve damage and affect the blood and immune system. The active ingredients give off toxic fumes.

— Silicone fluorides are especially problematic because they release considerable amounts of hydrofluoric gases into the environment.

— Arsenic can crystallize on treated surfaces, posing a health threat to children or animals who might ingest it by licking the surfaces.

— Tributyl zinc oxide is as toxic as lindane and is absorbed through the skin and airways. Skin irritations may erupt several days after exposure. Avoid breathing fumes; wear a protective mask during use.

Saunas

Wood fungi or parasites cannot survive in a sauna: Air temperatures are too high and humidity too low. Due to the high evaporation rate from wood in a sauna, use of wood preservatives is extremely dangerous.

Attic Areas

In attic spaces that aren't likely to become damp, use products containing boric acid.

Environmentally Friendly Products?

Beware of products labeled "environmentally friendly": this may refer to only one ingredient, rather than the entire product. There are few laws restricting the use of this term in marketing.

FOAM INSULATION

Ideally, the hollow spaces underneath bathtubs and those lining window or door frames, walls and crawl spaces should be stuffed with an insulating material. Spraying foam insulation into such crevices is actually a poor substitute.

Possible Health Effects

Foam insulation releases various toxic ingredients during application. If it is applied incorrectly—for example, if the temperature is too low during application—toxins will continue to be released into the environment even after application.

Products with a polyurethane base usually include halogenated hydrocarbons as propellants (see p. 774),

known to cause damage to the ozone layer.

Foam insulation may also contain

— Foaming agents that can dry out the skin, irritate mucous membranes and cause narcotic effects in high concentrations

— Active ingredients with an unpleasant, fishy smell that can irritate mucous membranes, cause stomachaches and headaches, and potentially lead to allergic reactions.

Many polyurethane foams contain isocyanates, which mainly irritate the skin and mucous membranes. Their inhalation irritates the airways and may cause bronchitis or asthmalike symptoms as well as allergies. Individuals highly sensitive to isocyanates will react even to very low quantities of fumes, dust or airborne droplets.

Formaldehyde-based products contain formaldehyde (see p. 773).

Recommendation

— Avoid using foams. If you can't avoid them, wear protective clothing and a face mask.

— Consider using chemically inert alternatives like cellulose and fiberglass. The most commonly used fiberglass insulation, however, usually contains formaldehyde as a binding agent (see p. 773).

ADEQUATE VENTILATION

The danger of toxins accumulating to dangerous levels indoors increases dramatically the more tightly sealed the windows are. Thirty to 60 percent of the air in a room should be exchanged hourly, so that critical levels of toxins don't build up. This will not significantly increase heat loss. Air exchange rates of over 60 percent will affect the heating bill.

The drafts that come through normal, loose-fitting window seals account for 80 percent of the requisite air exchange; opening the windows accounts for only 20 percent.

Supertight Windows May Be Hazardous to Your Health

For years, snugly sealed windows were touted for their energy-efficient and noise-reducing qualities. But most tight-fitting plastic and aluminum windows cause hourly air exchange rates to drop to 10 to 15 percent, resulting in high levels of humidity, mildew and accumulation of toxic fumes.

To achieve adequate air exchange rates, supertight windows would need to be opened completely for 15 minutes out of every hour; the alternative of leaving them slightly ajar (at a 10 degree angle) all day would result in about 200 cubic meters of fresh air flowing through the room every hour—much too much on a cold day. The ideal air exchange rate—sufficient to change the air yet still retain warmth—is about 20 cubic meters per person. This can be attained by leaving the windows "cracked" open a few inches.

Tips on Window Seals
— Windows are too tight if the panes fog up on cold days, or when ambient humidity exceeds 60 percent.
— Most windows can be adjusted to regulate air exchange.
— When installing new windows, choose adjustable ones, with wood or aluminum rather than plastic frames.

Air Pollution

Innumerable toxins are present in the air we breathe—not only in our cities, but in rural environments as well. The possible connection between long-term exposure to air pollution and persistent, chronic health problems is often underestimated, in spite of the efforts of many environmental groups. Pollution from automotive exhaust fumes has become a major environmental problem. If you drive to work on a daily basis, you generate five times as much pollution as you would if you took the train—even if your car has a catalytic converter.

The average non-catalytic-converter car expels an average of 2.2 grams of nitrogen and 9 grams carbon monoxide per kilometer into the atmosphere, in effect polluting 27,000 cubic meters of clean air. In addition, leaded gasoline is a source of heavy metal (see p. 786).

Despite advances such as the use of catalytic converters, the widespread use of unleaded gas and stricter emission-control laws, pollution is on the rise due to the ever greater number of cars on the road.

Automobiles contribute not only to traffic-related problems—accidents, traffic jams, noise and pollution—but also to the impending climatological crisis. Even cars with catalytic converters contribute to the greenhouse effect. If there is not a drastic cutback in the production of carbon dioxide production, global warming is an inevitability with unforeseeable ramifications for humankind.

CARBON DIOXIDE (CO_2)

All fuels that burn—coal, oil, gas or gasoline—release carbon dioxide (CO_2). This gas is also the byproduct of the metabolism, or breakdown of carbohydrates, which simultaneously uses up oxygen. Exhaled air contains about 4.5 percent CO_2 by volume.

Without the impact of human society, a perfect equilibrium would exist in nature, with exactly as much CO_2 produced as that used by plant life for photosynthesis. As it is, carbon dioxide is our most abundant pollutant today: Its levels in the air have increased by about 15 percent over the last hundred years.

Possible Health Effects

In concentrations of greater than 3 to 4 percent by volume, this colorless, heavy, noncombustible gas can cause headaches, ringing in the ears, high blood pressure, shortness of breath and loss of consciousness. Concentrations at 20 to 50 percent can be lethal.

CARBON MONOXIDE (CO)

This colorless, odorless gas is created when fossil fuels (coal, oil, gas, gasoline) burn incompletely. Once released into the air, it is transformed chemically into carbon dioxide.

The internal combustion engine accounts for about 70 percent of the carbon monoxide in the atmosphere. Catalytic converters neutralize up to 90 percent of that.

Possible Health Effects

When inhaled, carbon monoxide prevents oxygen absorption in the blood, resulting in headaches and dizziness. High concentrations can lead to death from suffocation or oxygen deprivation. In extremely high-smog traffic conditions (see Smog, p. 787), it threatens heart function and circulation. If concentrations exceed 14 milligrams of carbon monoxide per cubic meter of fresh air, the incidence of fatal heart attacks rises.

HYDROCARBONS

If fuel combustion is incomplete due to insufficient oxygen levels or low combustion temperatures, unburned hydrocarbons accumulate. They are also released as vapor when gasoline tanks are filled at service stations. These substances are highly flammable and can form explosive mixtures when combined with air.

Hydrocarbons include substances like formaldehyde (see p. 773), the carcinogen benzene, and benzopyrene.

Motor vehicles account for about 40 percent of total air pollution from hydrocarbons. Catalytic converters neutralize about 90 percent.

Possible Health Effects

Hydrocarbons contribute to the development of smog and ozone (see p. 787) and affect vegetation. Some hydrocarbons, such as the benzene in gasoline, are carcinogenic.

NITROUS OXIDE (NO$_x$)

All combustion creates nitrous monoxide (NO) as a by-product, which recombines in the atmosphere as the toxic nitrous dioxide (NO$_2$).

In order to increase fuel efficiency, car manufacturers are raising combustion temperatures and improving engine compression. However, this contributes to nitrous oxide formation.

Possible Health Effects

Nitrous oxides are irritants, responsible in part for forest destruction in acid rain and, in combination with sunlight, for the breakdown of the ozone layer (see Ozone, p. 787).

Nitrous oxide levels in excess of 150 micrograms per cubic meter of fresh air contribute to acute respiratory illness. Symptoms include coughing, excessive salivation, colds, breathing disorders, and even lung damage.

Signs of chronic nitrous oxide poisoning include headaches, sleeplessness and/or ulcers of the mucous membrane.

Tests in children under age seven have shown that they suffer more frequently from respiratory illnesses in areas where nitrous oxide levels exceed 30 micrograms per cubic meter.

SOOT

Soot consists of very fine solid particles (or particulates) in the air. Diesel, and some gasoline, engines emit soot particles. The amounts they emit depends on the age and type of the engine and its fuel-injection system. Use of ceramic filters can reduce soot emission. This has been standard practice in the United States for quite some time.

If diesel fuel contains sulfur, another byproduct of its combustion is sulfur dioxide (SO$_2$). Diesel vehicles account for about 3 percent of total atmospheric sulfur dioxide emissions.

Possible Health Effects

Soot particles may attach to other harmful substances, primarily carcinogens such as polycyclic hydrocarbons.

In a recent marketing move, oil companies have developed a better-smelling type of diesel fuel which, though well received by the public, poses no less of a health risk than the old kind.

For more information on the dangers of sulfur dioxide, see p. 785.

ASBESTOS

Airborne asbestos particles from brake and clutch linings are among the major causes of cancer. Friction caused by frequent brake and clutch use, such as when inching along in heavy traffic, causes very fine asbestos fibers to be released into the air by the pound.

Possible Health Effects

Even a tiny particle of asbestos can trigger lung cancer (see Asbestos, p. 776).

People who work on automobile brakes are at high risk since, in addition to the asbestos hazard, brake fluids often contain trichloroethane or tetrachloroethane. It takes very little heat—a cigarette or a hot metal surface are enough—for these substances to form phosgene, the highly poisonous compound used as a chemical weapon in World War I.

Pollutants in the Car

VENTILATION

Vehicles pose a threat not only to the environment, but to their occupants as well. In addition to running the risk of traffic-related accidents during daily commutes or heavy holiday traffic, passengers and drivers are exposed to smog (see p. 787) and over 800 types of fumes, including nerve-damaging substances like toluene and carcinogens such as benzene and benzopyrene. Some pollutants may be left over from the automobile manufacturing process if outgassing hasn't been complete.

Many pollutants enter the interior when the car's air vents are open and the fan is on. One test showed peak levels of CO_2 at 265 parts per million (ppm). The maximum allowable levels of carbon monoxide in the workplace stand at 30 ppm.

Over the long term, exposure to nitrous oxide is even more dangerous. If you commute on the highway, you exceed the maximum allowable workplace limit for NO_2 within the first half of your commute. If you commute in city traffic, you exceed it within the first 15 minutes.

Recommendation

Ventilate your car as little as possible. An air filter can protect against particulates—asbestos fibers from brakes, soot from diesel engines, bacteria or pollen—so as to prevent eye inflammations, hayfever and asthma attacks.

Filtering gaseous pollutants requires a complicated filter system involving activated charcoal, sodium-calcium layers or other catalysts.

In contrast to the people inside the cars, cyclists breathe in only about one-third as many airborne pollutants, even in extreme traffic conditions. Moreover, bicycles as a means of transportation do not tax the environment.

CAR MAINTENANCE

Car-care products often contain hazardous ingredients, including chlorinated hydrocarbons (see Chlorinated Hydrocarbons, p. 774).

Windshield de-icers and antifreeze-containing washer fluid are among the most hazardous. Many contain toxic methanol or ethylene glycol. Every year, accidental ingestion of these substances causes numerous poisonings. Yet adding a squirt of distilled alcohol to regular water to make washer fluid would work as well.

Industrial Fumes

Industry is the biggest source of particulates and sulfur dioxide emissions, and a major contributor to atmospheric levels of nitrous oxide (see p. 784), carbon monoxide (p. 783) and hydrocarbons (p. 784). In addition to these, hundreds of other pollutants are released into the atmosphere daily, mainly from chemical plants.

DUST

Dust consists of tiny solid particles (or particulates) suspended in air. Only about 30 percent of dust comes from organic sources like plants. The majority is from crushed rock, sand, soot and ashes. Changes in production techniques and wider use of filters has significantly reduced pollution from coarser-grained particulates.

Possible Health Effects

Very fine dust (particles smaller than 5 micrometers across) is especially dangerous: It can enter the lungs, lodge in the alveoli and cause health problems. These particles can also easily combine with heavy metals such as lead and cadmium. Dust-filled air is a breeding ground for respiratory illnesses. There are correspondingly higher mortality rates in areas where high levels of dust and sulfur dioxide are found together.

SULFUR DIOXIDE (SO$_2$)

One by-product of fossil fuel combustion is the release of sulfur dioxide into the atmosphere. Sulfur dioxide is a colorless, sharp-smelling gas. Overall emission levels can be reduced by installing filters and using low-sulfur fuels.

Possible Health Effects

Sulfur dioxide irritates and can damage the mucous membranes, causing a cough or respiratory illness. This is especially true in winter, when prevailing weather patterns can cause levels to remain high for several days in a row. Acute reactions in asthmatics and others have been documented. People exposed to high levels of sulfur dioxide for prolonged periods initially may lose their sense of taste and develop breathing difficulties; later, lung inflammations appear, followed by pulmonary edema and, ultimately, cardiovascular failure and death.

Sulfur dioxide combines with water and oxygen in the atmosphere to form sulfuric acid, a component of acid rain.

HEAVY METALS

Heavy metals such as lead, cadmium, and mercury can enter the environment via processes used to refine them. Mainly, however, they enter the food chain through waste water and contaminated soil (see Hazardous Substances in Food, p. 729).

Possible Health Effects

Lead

In the past, 75 percent of the lead in the atmosphere was the result of automobile emissions. This number fell dramatically following the introduction of unleaded gasoline. Steel and iron production and incinerators are major contributors to lead pollution. Lead particles suspended in the atmosphere end up in soil, water, and plants.

Humans absorb lead from food (see p. 730), where it is distributed throughout the body and then incorporated into the bones. Even very low blood levels of lead can affect fetal brain development.

Children having a blood lead count greater than 10 mcg/dl at birth have been observed to be hyperactive and unable to concentrate or perform well academically. For this reason, maximum tolerable lead levels have been lowered from 30 to 10 micrograms in recent years.

Lead levels exceeding 50 micrograms can also affect brain function and fertility in adults. However, levels this high are usually found only at worksites involving direct contact with lead. Thanks to widespread protective measures, acute lead poisoning occurs only rarely.

Symptoms of lead poisoning include excessive salivation, discolored gums, vomiting, intestinal colic, constipation, nerve paralysis and acute kidney failure.

Cadmium

Inhaling cadmium-laden air over many years leads to lung and kidney damage. Cadmium and its chemical compounds are suspected carcinogens.

Mercury

Mercury vapors are extremely dangerous: If inhaled from a source such as vacuuming a broken thermometer, about 80 percent is absorbed and retained by the body.

Symptoms of mercury poisoning include a metallic taste in the mouth, nausea, vomiting, abdominal pain, bloody diarrhea, loosening of the teeth, and a characteristic black line on the gums.

Smaller amounts of mercury can lead to chronic mercury toxicity which, while not as dramatic, can nonetheless cause significant symptoms.

Electric Power Stations and Home Heating

In addition to motor vehicles and industry, power stations and home heating constitute major contributors to air pollution. Emissions depend on the quality of fuel (ideally, low-sulfur coal or fuel oil), plant design, and built-in smoke detectors or scrubbing devices.

For more information on individual pollutants and their health effects, see Carbon Dioxide, p. 783; Hydrocarbons, p. 784; Nitrous Oxide, p. 784; Dust, p. 785; Sulfur Dioxide, p. 785.

Clean Air

For the most part, we have the technology to reduce air pollution from almost all power and industrial plants; the only stumbling block is the question of who pays for it.

State-of-the-art technology with the help of smoke-stack scrubbers can reduce
—Dust by 99 percent (electric filters)
— Sulfur dioxide by 95 percent (absorption)
—Nitrous oxide by 90 percent (modern burning techniques)
— Hydrocarbons by 90 to 99 percent (absorption, afterburning)

By contrast, there are fewer options for reducing home-heating pollution. In the 1950s, the city of London was in danger of suffocating in smog; fuel oil and coal were replaced with electric and gas heating, with the result that air quality has improved.

Smog

Despite all efforts to curb pollution, smog is on the rise in many areas. Even minor gains are quickly offset by increases in traffic and industrialization. If no far-reaching political and environmental changes are made, we will be living with the health risks associated with increased air pollution.

Smog is created by weather patterns known as inversions, in which warmer air settles over cold air, trapping it and preventing air flow, thus impeding the dispersal of hazardous substances.

OZONE

In recent years, ozone, which is only one component of smog, has come into the spotlight. It is important to differentiate between the "ozone hole" (a thinning of the ozone layer in the atmosphere), and the levels of ozone in the lower atmospheric layers. The "good ozone" layer lies about 20 to 45 kilometers above the earth's surface, shielding the environment from dangerous ultraviolet rays. When ozone occurs in the lower atmosphere, it is toxic. Higher concentrations can lead to eye irritations, breathing difficulties, throat and pharyngeal problems. Prolonged breathing of ozone can cause infections of the alveoli. Ozone reduces lung function and overall endurance; it can cause headaches, nausea, excessive fatigue and a weakening of the immune system. In some sources, it is listed as a carcinogen. Exposure to lower levels over prolonged periods has the same effect as short-term higher levels of exposure.

During high-ozone or smog alert days, when the ozone level exceeds 150 micrograms per cubic meter of air, the elderly, infirm, and children should avoid outdoor activities between 1:00 and 7:00 P.M.

Ozone is toxic to trees and plants at the cellular level and, along with sulfur dioxide and nitrous oxide, is one of the main causes of forest destruction.

The prime source of lower-atmosphere ozone is vehicular traffic, followed by combustion processes of all types, power stations, the use and production of products containing solvents, and fuels like butane and propane. Landfills and even cattle are also sources of methane, that contribute to higher ozone levels.

Smog

Effectively cutting back on ozone production is possible only by drastically reducing traffic over the long term and improving public transportation.

Winter smog: In winter months, sulfur dioxide, suspended dust and carbon monoxide in the air can quickly reach dangerous levels, affecting breathing, irritating mucous membranes and causing circulatory disorders. Death rates are higher during this time. Especially at risk are the elderly, infirm, and small children.

Summer smog: Summertime smog is an unpleasant fact of life in most major cities. Its principal cause is automobile traffic, but climatological changes, believed by some scientists to be the first signs of global warming, are also factors.

Lower-atmosphere ozone is generated when the sun's rays interact with nitrous oxide and hydrocarbons.

Garbage Incinerators

The processing of incinerator exhaust still needs improving. In addition to carbon monoxide, hydrocarbons, nitrous oxides, and sulfur dioxide, the emission of heavy metals and dioxin is of serious concern.

Dry Cleaning

The dry cleaning industry is fully aware of the harmful health effects of solvents (particularly tetrachloroethylene) used in the dry cleaning process.

Legislative changes and new guidelines as well as environmentally friendly products have gone some way toward mitigating this process.

Possible Health Effects

Tetrachloroethylene is suspected of causing cancer. It causes headaches, irritations of the eyes and mucous membranes, and stomach and circulatory problems. Prolonged exposure damages the liver, kidney, and nervous system.

Recommendation

— Make sure your dry cleaner conforms to government guidelines (including those for cleaning leather).

Nuclear Power Plants

Even when functioning normally, nuclear power plants continuously emit radioactive substances into the air and water. We have no idea what effect this will have thousands of years from now.

Possible Health Effects

An increased incidence of cancer and a higher mortality rate among children has been documented in areas surrounding nuclear power plants, even those with good operating records.

In the event of accidents, the type of health damage depends on the relative amounts of different radioactive substances.

Following the nuclear accident in Chernobyl in 1986, more than 40 people died within a few days. In the intervening years, the incidence of leukemia and thyroid cancer, especially in children, has increased dramatically. Hundreds of thousands of residents live with significantly higher risks of cancer, leukemia, miscarriage, and birth defects, and can expect to do so for years to come.

HEALTH IN THE WORKPLACE

Long before environmental toxins polluted large tracts of land and infiltrated homes and buildings, they existed in the workplace. Today, the majority of offices and factories are still sources of exposure to chemicals.

Almost half of today's workforce is employed in offices. Although modern offices bear little resemblance to the noisy, filthy workplace of the past, the average employee spends about 70,000 hours in a lifetime—more time than is spent at home—in environments where basic human needs are simply disregarded. For example, the levels of airborne toxins often exceed external air pollution limits. Badly designed furniture contributes to poor posture and lack of muscle tone. High noise levels are stress-inducing; colors induce fatigue. Even laboratory animals are exposed to better lighting.

More than half of all office workers suffer from health problems directly attributable to the workplace. Studies have found that fully a quarter of the workforce is no longer employable after age 54. Assembly-line workers last only about a year longer. Despite such findings, however, most working people seem basically resigned to the fact that job-related health risks are an unavoidable fact of life.

Sick-building syndrome

Headaches, difficulty breathing, depressed mood, allergic skin reactions, fatigue, and general malaise, are the most common symptoms of sick-building-syndrome (SBS). Almost a third of the people working in new or newly renovated office buildings suffer from SBS. The adhesives used when applying new floor or wall coverings, various hazardous furniture fumes, and toxic substances released from office equipment, such as ozone, are the most common causes of SBS. Also contributing to these are pollen, mold spores and airborne germs from outside air, as well as from poorly filtered air, and poorly functioning air conditioners. The ever increasing number of people with allergies are those affected most by SBS.

THE OFFICE ENVIRONMENT

The office environment is a source of innumerable chemical pollutants: fumes from paint, carpeting, and furniture, toxins in toner dust, ozone from laser printers and copiers. Some toxins can be avoided completely through user-friendly construction; others can be greatly reduced by choosing the right equipment and furnishings.

The air in offices is used up rapidly and must be replenished regularly. Although satisfactory air replenishing and temperature regulation could actually be achieved simply by adjusting windows and blinds, most offices are in urban environments where opening a window will admit large quantities of dust, exhaust and noise instead of fresh air. This calls for the creation of an artificial, air-conditioned microclimate.

PLANTS AS CLIMATE REGULATORS

For the past twenty years, National Aeronautics and Space Administration (NASA) scientists have been researching the use of plants as regulators of climate conditions. Their findings should be of interest to all office employees suffering from work-related ailments. Plants elevate ambient humidity levels, reducing the need for humidifiers. They also filter pollutants, carbon monoxide and cigarette smoke out of the air while simultaneously producing oxygen. This filtering action is optimized by plants whose roots contain a specialized aeration system.

The plants best adapted for filtering specific toxins are
— For benzene: ivy, spathiphyllum, dracaena, and gerbera
— For formaldehyde: aloe, banana, philodendron, and dracaena
— For trichlorethylene: chrysanthemum, gerbera, dracaena, and spathiphyllum

CIGARETTE SMOKE

Cigarette smoke contains about 2,000 chemical compounds, including nitrous oxide, carbon monoxide and nicotine. Irritants such as formaldehyde and acrolein; carcinogenic hydrocarbons and nitrosamines. More than any other toxin, cigarette smoke is often the major source of workplace pollution.

Nonsmokers are severely affected by second-hand smoke (see Smoking, p. 754) and should insist on a smoke-free work place, or at the minimum a ban on smoking except during designated breaks, or in designated areas.

Fortunately, smoke-free areas in offices and public places have become increasingly common.

LIGHTING

Many office workers get appreciable amounts of daylight only on weekends and vacations. The average eight-hour office day is spent under artificial light.

For people sensitive to such things, light deprivation can lead to psychological symptoms including depression (see p. 197). Workplace lighting is important not only in terms of employee health and productivity, it's an environmental issue as well. The right kind of lighting can also mean energy cost savings of 80 to 90 percent.

Studies have shown that people who work near windows suffer less work-related stress. Workers whose desks are not near a window should have optimal artificial lighting for their work spaces. Ideally, this is a combination of indirect overhead lighting and individually adjustable work lamps.

The closer indoor lights come to replicating full-spectrum daylight, the better will be the workers' sense of well-being—and their productivity. Full-spectrum bulbs mounted in reflecting fixtures give the best results. Full-spectrum fluorescent lights are also obtainable.

Energy-efficient bulbs and fluorescent lights provide more full-spectrum light than regular incandescent bulbs, which use lots of energy, are short-lived and don't give particularly "natural" light. The significant disadvantage of fluorescent light, however, is its stroboscopic effect (rapid flickering) which, though just below the threshold of perception, can be annoying. Electronic regulators can be installed to reduce flickering.

Until 1983, all fluorescent tubes contained (polychlorinated biphenyls) PCB (see p. 774). To avoid the inadvertent release of PCB, all old fluorescent lights should be professionally replaced. Care should also be taken when handling the newer tubes, which contain mercury vapor.

Halogen lamps are rarely installed in offices because of their price. Also, their narrow light spectrum and relatively high UV-ray component makes them poorly suited for office lighting or as table lamps.

Recommendation

Check all fluorescent lights for age and defects, especially in children's rooms. Defective tubes can contaminate dust with PCB.

NOISE IN THE WORKPLACE

Noise pollution tops the list of work-related health problems. Extremely loud noise can impair hearing, but lower levels, too, cause health problems. The autonomic nervous system registers stress when exposed to noise levels as low as 55 decibels (see Hearing Loss, p. 250). Elevated blood pressure, muscle tension, and impaired digestion are direct effects of noise that may lead to chronic and acute stress disorders.

In offices, noise pollution is caused primarily by equipment such as printers, copiers and telephones. To reduce office noise levels

— Install acoustic tiles, noise-absorbing curtains, rugs and plants.
— Invest in the quietest equipment available.
— Move printers and copiers behind partitions. Sound baffles near noise sources are effective.
— Install felt pads under furniture to muffle sound.
— Store computer CPUs under desks or out of the way to minimize noise.
— Whenever possible, replace audio signals with visual ones.
— Low-level ambient music can reduce stress by lessening the impact of individual noises such as telephones.

COMPUTERS

Most offices now contain computer equipment. The widespread use of computers increases society's demand for electricity, as well as contributing to environmental pollution from substances involved in the manufacture of computers and chips, including heavy metals such as barium, lead, cadmium, copper, nickel, mercury, strontium, thalium, tin, and zinc. Hazardous substances cause health problems in over 6 percent of Silicon Valley employees involved in chip production, and their rate of miscarriages is higher than anywhere else in the United States.

Air pollution from computer production is caused by accumulations of carbon dioxide, nitrous oxides, sulfur dioxide, carbon monoxide, dust, and hydrocarbons.

The plastic parts of computers contain substances as flame retardant. In older computers, some of these substances can cause carcinogens to be emitted as fumes just through normal use, and in newer computers, in the event of a fire. Newer models no longer contain these substances, but it may be hard to tell with imported ones.

The unnatural posture and eyestrain brought on by sitting at the PC has an adverse effect on overall health.

VIDEO SCREENS

Standard computer screens emit various kinds of rays:
— Microwaves and radio waves, presumably in amounts too low to be detected
— X rays (at voltages higher than 24 kV)
— Electromagnetic radiation. So far research has not proved whether or not electromagnetic fields are harmful to health, but suggests that pregnant women should spend as little time as possible in front of the screen. Monitors emit most of their radiation through the sides and back, so seats in these positions should be avoided. The greater the distance from the monitor, the better.

In any case, look for "low radiation" labels on monitors.

Due to high voltage in the monitor's cathode-ray tube, static electricity is created on the surface of the screen. This can cause skin disorders such as acne or eczema in sensitive people. While the monitor is being switched off, the screen surface repels dust particles, which can lead to eye and skin disorders.

The following can reduce static electricity:
— Proper grounding of computer equipment
— A screen filter (but this adds to eyestrain by reducing brightness and contrast)
— Plenty of humidity in the air
— Antistatic office equipment
— Natural-fiber clothing and shoes with leather or natural rubber soles

PRINTERS

The much-heralded "paperless office" has not become a reality. Today, printers are standard office equipment and often in constant use.

Impact printers (daisy wheel, dot matrix) are still widely used and as loud as ever. Laser printers, like copiers, are sources of ozone and toner dust, which pose health risks.

Laser printers can raise ozone levels beyond acceptable limits, especially when several printers or copiers are being used simultaneously. Ozone (see p. 787) affects airways, eyes, and mucous membranes, causing headaches, eye problems, and higher incidences of colds. Proper temperature range and adequate ventilation can lower the risk of high ozone concentrations, as can activated carbon filters, if changed regularly.

Toner dust, released into the air during the printing process, contains a suspected carcinogen nitropyrene. Other suspected carcinogens, polycyclic hydrocarbons, may also be released. Dust emissions from toner can cause respiratory problems in sensitive people. Breathing or skin contact with toner should be avoided, particularly when changing the cartridge.

The ergonomically correct workstation
— Eyes should be level with upper edge of monitor screen; monitor should be 20 to 30 inches away.
— Office chairs should have adjustable height and back support.
— Document holders should be placed at the same height as the screen.
— Use an ergonomic keyboard or one with a palm rest; the middle row of keys should be no more than 1 inch above the desk surface.
— Screen diameter should be at least 14 inches; video frequency should be at least 70 hertz; screen surface should be nonglare and display dark characters on a light background.
— Lighting should be indirect, with an additional adjustable table lamp.
— Desk height should be adjustable; desk should be at least 32 inches deep.
— Leg room should be at least 26 inches high, 28 deep and 32 wide.
— Use a foot support with adjustable angle.

PHOTOCOPY MACHINES

The toner in photocopy machines consists of carbon, artificial resins and iron oxide, and is suspected of causing cancer. Its fine particles can harm the lungs, which is why contact with toner should be avoided as much as possible. Two-component toners are more harmful than single-component toners: Their particles are much smaller and can enter the lungs more easily. Also, single-component toners usually don't overflow, releasing dust. In equipment with a closed toner cartridge system, toner dust cannot reach the air.

Medically significant levels of ozone (see p. 787) are created during the copying process. In sensitive people this irritating gas affects the mucous membranes and eyes, possibly leading to headaches, burning eyes, and increased susceptibility to colds. Modern equipment contains activated carbon filters that can reduce ozone output when used according to directions.

Recommendation
— Buy equipment that meets EPA requirements.
— Use only toner without polycyclic aromatic hydro-carbons or nitropyrene. If in doubt, ask your supplier for documentation.
— Older copiers use a lot more chemicals and should be replaced with newer "dry copiers."
— Use closed toner systems when possible: They burden the lungs and the environment a lot less than open ones. In open systems, avoid spilling dust when changing toner.
— Equipment containing activated carbon filters will emit considerably less ozone, as long as product directions are followed carefully.
— Do not eat or smoke while photocopying or changing toner cartridges.
— Wash hands carefully after replacing toner and, as a precaution, after handling a large number of copies.
— Copiers should be set up outside the common work area and only in areas with more than 80 cubic feet of air.
— If you smell ozone, ventilate the area.
— Avoid unnecessary photocopying.

PAPER
There are hundreds of kinds of paper and cardboard on the market; some 2,000 chemicals are used in manu-facturing these products. There is now some evidence of possible health effects associated with the use of chemically treated papers.

Glues in self-adhesive paper often contain organic solvents; formaldehyde (see p. 773) and polychlorinated biphenyls (see p. 774) are among the substances found in the "carbonless" paper used in receipts and other applications.

FELT-TIP PENS, CORRECTION FLUID
Many markers and pens contain solvents, easily identi-fiable by their acrid smell.

Ordinary correction fluids often contain chlorinated hydrocarbons as solvents, as do fluid thinners.

Possible Health Effects
The different solvents vary in their effects. Chlorinated hydrocarbons such as trichloroethane are suspected of causing cancer and genetic changes. They can also cause dizziness and intoxication, making them a classic "sniff-ing" drug and potential introduction to drug experi-mentation in children.

Recommendation
If you must use solvent-containing pens, for use with overhead projectors for example:
— Make sure the room is well ventilated.
— Use water-soluble felt-tip pens where possible. Avoid inexpensive pens, especially imported ones: Most still contain formaldehyde (see p. 773).
— Use water-soluble correction fluid even though it dries more slowly.

ADHESIVES
All-purpose glues, contact adhesives and special-use glues often consist of up to 70 percent solvent. These can be detected by their strong (not necessarily unpleasant) odor, or the presence of the word "flammable" on the label.

Possible Health Effects
Depending on individual sensitivity and the levels of solvent in the air, solvents can cause watery eyes and a scratchy throat. They can also cause dizziness and intoxication—solvents are a classic "sniffing" drug and potential introduction to drug experimentation in children.

Two-part epoxies, used for gluing stone, porcelain or metal, can cause skin irritation or contact dermatitis (see p. 271) after even a tiny amount of skin contact. The second component often releases fumes consid-ered carcinogenic.

Recommendation

Regular white glue is adequate for most office use. It is water-based and comes in liquid, paste or stick form. Note that some imported products may still contain formaldehyde (see p. 773).

Chemicals in the Workplace

Workplace pollutants cause disease. Vectors include gases and fumes, dust, dirt, drafts, and excessive heat and cold. Pollutants can be inhaled (e.g. asbestos dust), ingested from contaminated hands, or absorbed through skin contact with liquids.

ALLERGIES IN THE WORKPLACE

For many people, allergies have become a serious health problem (see p. 360). Typical industry-specific allergens include

Metal industry: cleaning agents and solvents, hydrazine hydrobromide (used in soldering), chrome, nickel, cobalt, cadmium, beryllium, uranium

Electronics industry: chlorparaffin, epoxy resins, triethylene tetramine hardener, formaldehyde

Pharmaceuticals/chemicals: isocyanate, aldehyde, aromatic nitro combinations, P-amine, hydrazine, peptides, proteases, heavy metals, turpentine, benzene, toluene, synthetics, metals

Plastics: phenol, formalin, epoxy resins, all synthetics.

Printing: turpentine, xylol, aniline derivatives, chrome, cobalt, nickel in black ink, rubber

Photography: developer, fixatives, toning agent, enhancers, solvents

Rubber: accelerators, azo substances, rubber

Textiles: aniline dyes, antiseptics, mothproofing substances, cobalt, finishes, chrome, nickel, mercury, formaldehyde, organic dusts

Woodworking: formalin, pyridine, phenol, chrome

Construction/painting: phenol, solvents, lacquers, formalin, turpentine, metals, pigments, glues, concrete materials

Medical: disinfectants, medications such as antibiotics or analgesics

Hair care: dyes, bleach, shampoos, holding sprays/gels, cosmetics, preservatives, mercury

Household: cleaning materials, disinfectants, waxes, bleaches, rubber gloves

Agriculture: organic dust, pesticides, fertilizer, saltpeter, cobalt (in mineral-enriched feed), antibiotics, preservatives

If you can't avoid contact with these substances

— Follow safety regulations carefully.

— Seek medical attention immediately if unusual symptoms (skin changes, breathing difficulties, eye problems) appear, and report problems of working conditions to the relevant authority.

Lowering Your Risk of Job-Related Cancers

— Find out the legally acceptable maximum levels for your industry if you have to work with chemicals, inhaling their dust and fumes. Find out whether you are working with substances known to trigger cancer.

— Ask your employer to conform to the maximum acceptable levels.

— Ask your employer to follow safety guidelines (e.g., installation of vents for fresh air exchange).

— Follow safety regulations to the letter. Wear protective masks, eye wear, gloves, and uniforms even if they are a nuisance. Work in properly vented areas as directed.

— Participate in regular safety drills. Seek medical attention immediately at the first sign of unusual symptoms.

CANCER IN THE WORKPLACE

Work-related cancers have been identified for 200 years. To date, of the 600,000 common chemical compounds, scientists have established that 1,000 of these are known to cause cancer. Every year, 1,000 new substances are developed but only approximately 77 of them are tested for possible carcinogenic properties. The effects of these substances in combination with others are also not known.

Some carcinogens encountered in industry have definite exposure limits that must not be exceeded; others are less restricted.

Carcinogens should be avoided wherever possible. If they cannot be avoided, the following safety precautions should be followed:

— Regularly monitor air quality in the workplace.

— Establish time limitations on exposure to hazardous substances.

— Each employee should have his or her own protective masks and clothing.

— Make sure intensive medical monitoring is in place.

Keep in mind that in cases of work-related exposure leading to cancer, 20 years usually elapse between the initial contact with the carcinogens and the diagnosis of cancer. Aggressive precautions have recently lowered the incidence of work-related cancers.

Cancer-causing substances

Seventeen substances are known to cause cancer in humans, including:

— 4-aminodiphenyl, arsenic acids and salts, asbestos, benzidine, benzene, dichloromethyl ether, coal tar, beech and oak wood dust, 4-chlorotoluidine, dichlorethylsulfide, N-methyl-bis-monochlordimethylether, ß-naphthylamine, nickel, pitch and oils, vinylchloride, zinc chromate.

Seventy-five substances cause cancer in laboratory animals (and probably in humans as well). These include:

— beryllium compounds, cadmium chloride, chrome II and IV compounds, cobalt, emissions from diesel engines, hydrazine, nitroso-compounds.

Fifty-nine substances are classified as suspected carcinogens.

KNOWN CARCINOGENS IN THE WORKPLACE

Bis(Chlormethyl) ether (BCME)

People who work with BCME are six to nine times more likely to get lung cancer than others; smoking increases this risk still further. BCME is used in numerous biological and chemical manufacturing processes and insect breeding labs as well as in the production of paper and particle board.

Coke furnaces

People who work around coke ovens in the steel industry for longer than 5 years are 11 times more likely to get lung cancer than others.

Benzene

Benzene, a petroleum derivative, can cause leukemia.

Benzopyrene

Benzopyrene is a volatile hydrocarbon created by in-complete combustion. It is found throughout our environment, polluting air, water and soil—and therefore the food chain—through industrial smokestack emissions and automobile exhaust. Workers in the following areas are especially prone to exposure: roofing, insulation, steel refineries, blast furnaces, and road resurfacing. All are at higher risk of developing cancers of the lungs, mouth, lips, throat, larynx, and esophagus.

Metals

Nickel, arsenic and chromates are powerful carcinogens, causing primarily lung cancer in humans. Cadmium (used in galvanizing metals, the rubber industry, and the manufacture of batteries and plastics) may encourage lung and prostate cancer. Beryllium, cobalt, zinc, and titanium are also likely carcinogens.

Increased risks of bladder and tongue cancer is noted among plumbers, metal workers, and welders.

Cancer of the pancreas occurs more frequently in aluminum and sheet metal workers. Aluminum workers are also at an increased risk of developing tumors of the lymph system.

Asbestos

Asbestos is widespread in the environment (see p. 776). Lung cancer is the cause of death in one out of five people subjected to long-term asbestos exposure.

Radioactive dust

Radioactive particles can get into the lungs through dust; mine workers are particularly at risk. Radon gas is found in deposits of iron, feldspar, tungsten, copper, and zinc as well as in clay pits. In uranium mines, the radioactive emissions are 20 times those of directly inhaled radon.

Sawdust

Workers in the wood industry have a higher than normal risk of cancer. Carpenters, lumberjacks, forestry workers, paper mill workers, and those involved in plywood production are more prone to cancer of the stomach, lymph system and organs involved in blood production. Furniture and cabinet makers often suffer from nasal and paranasal cancer. To date, it is unclear whether the carcinogen is the sawdust itself, another substance used in wood processing, or some unidentified end-product or by-product.

OCCUPATIONAL DISEASES

Statistics don't reveal the whole picture of occupational diseases: Many diseases are not recognized as work-related, or are attributed to other causes. The causes are only incontrovertible in extreme cases like dioxin or lead poisoning. However, many chemicals show their effects only after a few years, or more than a few in the case of carcinogenic or genetically harmful substances. Sometimes, a single contact with a carcinogen is enough to trigger cancer.

Getting Your Voice Heard

Obtaining compensation for an occupational disease can be a long and arduous process. Your doctor must be able to establish a causal relationship between your occupation and the ailment. If this is deemed inconclusive, you may be left to the mercies of the legal system, and the courts, which can take years to conclude a case.

As always, an ounce of prevention is worth a pound of cure. As a worker, you are in the best position to find out for yourself whether or not you are running needless risks on the job. Take all necessary precautions to protect yourself and ensure that accidents don't happen, and be proactive: Speak up to ensure the best possible working conditions for all.

Index

About the Authors

Verena Corazza

Verena Corazza studied at the Pedagogical Academy in Vienna. She contributed to several issues of *Bittere Pillen* and several volumes of *Bittere Pillen-Patientenreihe*, and is a coauthor of *In der Regel, Wenn die Menstruation Probleme macht* (1987). She has taught in Vienna since 1990.

Renate Daimler

Renate Daimler is an author and journalist, and lives with her two children in Vienna. She is the author of *Altern ist keine Krankheit* (1988) and coauthor of *Alles rund ums Kinderkriegen* (1996). Her more recent publications include *Verschwiegene Lust: Frauen über 60 erzählen von Liebe und Sexualität; Wie's den Männern mit den Frauen geht;* and *Die unsichtbaren Mitspieler: Warum wir streiten, wenn wir lieben.*

Andrea Ernst

Andrea Ernst studied social sciences in Vienna. She is the author and publisher of numerous nonfiction books. She has been a scientific journalist since 1985, with an emphasis on medicine, health and social issues. Since 1997, she has worked as an editor at WDR-Television (*Frau-TV*). Publications include (some as coauthor): *Gift Grün: Chemie in der Landwirtschaft* (1986), *In der Regel: Wenn die Menstruation Probleme macht* (1987), *Sozialstaat Österreich: Bei Bedarf geschlossen* (1987), *Schlucken und schweigen: Wie Arzneimittel Frauen zerstören können* (1988), *Kinder-Report: Wie Kinder in Deutschland leben* (1991), *Kursbuch Kinder* (1993), *Gesunder Rücken* (1996), *Kursbuch Frauen* (1997).

Krista Federspiel, PhD

Krista Federspiel, PhD, is an independent journalist in Vienna covering social and women's politics and medicine. Her work has appeared in *Arbeiterzeitung, Die Frau, Profil, Stern, Gesundheits-magazine, ORP,* and *Club 2-Moderation..* Her publications include (some as coauthor): *Zahn um Zahn* (1986 in *Bittere-Pillen-Patientenreihe*), *Mit anderen Augen* (1987), *Der Krampf mit dem Magen* (1987), *Frauen der ersten Stunde 1945-1955, Wer? Ein Anti-Who's Who von Österreich* (1987), *Sozialstaat Österreich: Bei Bedarf geschlossen* (1987), *Öko-Bilanz-Österreich* (1988), *Lückenlos* (1988), *Arbeit* (1990), *Handbuch die andere Medizin* (1996), *Kursbuch Seele* (1996).

Vera Herbst

Vera Herbst studied pharmacology in Braunschweig and has worked for many years as a pharmacist. She has been an independent journalist and nonfiction author since 1986. Her areas of emphasis include pharmacology, medicine and health. Her publications include (some as coauthor) *Botanik und Drogenkunde* (1987), *Mit anderen Augen* (appeared in *Bittere-Pillen-Patientenreihe,* 1987), *Unsern Kindern helfen* (1988), *Beweglich bleiben* (1989), *Zuckerkrank* (1989), *Kursbuch Kinder* (1993), *Handbuch die andere Medizin* (1996), *Kursbuch Frauen* (1997).

Kurt Langbein

Kurt Langbein studied sociology in Vienna. From 1979 to 1989 he worked on documentary films and was a magazine journalist for Österreichischen Rundfunk ORF, and from 1989 to 1992 he was head of the domestic government department for the Austrian news magazine *Profil*. Since 1992, he has worked at *Die Woche, Focus* and *Profil*, and filmed documentaries for RTL, TV Asahi, Pro 7 and ORF, among others. He is manager of the editorial staff of Langbein & Skalnik in Vienna, and publisher and author of numerous nonfiction books. Publications include (some as coauthor) *Gesunde Geschäfte: Die Praktiken der Pharmaindustrie* (1981), *Bittere Pillen: Nutzen und Risiken der Arzneimittel* (1983), *Sozialstaat Österreich: Bie Bedarf geschlossen* (1987), *Kursbuch Kinder* (1993), *Kursbuch Lebensqualität* (1995), *Kursbuch Küche* (1995), *Bittere Naturmedizin* (1995), *Leben verlängern — um welchen Preis* (1996), *Einfach genial — die sieben Wurzeln der Intelligenz* (1997).

Hans-Peter Martin, J.D.

Hans-Peter Martin, J.D., received a scholarship to study in California, then continued his studies in Vienna. Since 1986 he has been an editor at *Der Spiegel*, where he has worked as a correspondent in South America, and currently as office manager in Vienna and Prague. In 1980 he was awarded the Dr. Karl-Renner-Preis für Publizistik, and in 1997 the Bruno-Kreisky-Preis für das politische Buch. He is a member of the Club of Rome. His publications include (some as coauthor): *Nachtschicht: Eine Betriebsreportage* (1979), *Gesunde Geschäfte: Die Praktiken der Pharmaindustrie* (1981), *Bittere Pillen: Nutzen und Risiken der Arzneimittel* (1983), *Die Globalisierungsfalle: Der Angriff auf Demokratie und Wohlstand* (1996).

Hans Weiss

Hans Weiss studied psychology in Innsbruck, followed by postgraduate studies in medical sociology at the "Institut für Höhere Studien" in Vienna. He received a research scholarship from the Italian Foreign Ministry Office to study psychiatric care in Italy. He also received a research scholarship from the British Council at the Fulbourne Hospital in Cambridge, and at Bedford College in London. He is a pharmalogical consultant for the companies of Sandoz and Bayer. He has also worked as an independent journalist since *1981* for Austrian television and the magazines *Profil, Der Spiegel, Die Zeit* and *Stern,* among others. In 1982, he won an Austrian Public Education prize for the documentary *Irre Welt-Psychiatrie* 1981. Publications include (some as coauthor) *Gesunde Geschäfte: Die Praktiken der Pharmaindustrie* (1981), *Bittere Pillen: Nutzen und Risiken der Arzneimittel* (1983), *Mit Hochdruck leben* (1986), *Gift-Grün: Chemie in der Landwirtschaft* (1986), *Die Leute von Langenegg* (1988), *Kriminelle Geschichten: Ermittlungen über die Justiz* (1987), *Öko-Bilanz-Österreich* (1988), *Wer? Ein Anti-Who's Who von Österreich* (1988), *Arbeit, Fünfzig deutsche Karrieren* (1990), *Rheuma* (1992).